M000288734

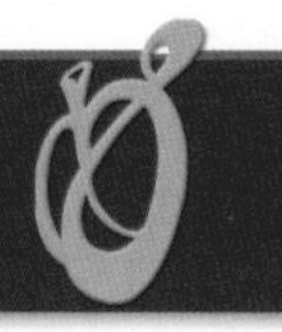

Clinical Arrhythmology and Electrophysiology

A Companion to Braunwald's Heart Disease

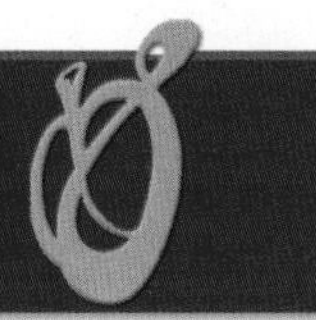

Clinical Arrhythmology and Electrophysiology

A Companion to Braunwald's Heart Disease

Ziad F. Issa, MD
Clinical Assistant Professor
Internal Medicine
Southern Illinois University School of Medicine
Cardiac Electrophysiology
Prairie Cardiovascular Consultants
Memorial Medical Center
Prairie Heart Institute, St. Johns Hospital
Springfield, Illinois

John M. Miller, MD
Professor
Division of Cardiology
Department of Medicine
Krannert Institute of Cardiology
Indiana University School of Medicine
Director
Clinical Cardiac Electrophysiology and Training Program
Clarian Health Partners
Indianapolis, Indiana

Douglas P. Zipes, MD
Distinguished Professor
Professor Emeritus of Medicine, Pharmacology, and Toxicology
Department of Medicine
Indiana University School of Medicine
Director Emeritus
Division of Cardiology and the Krannert Institute of Cardiology
Indiana University School of Medicine
Indianapolis, Indiana

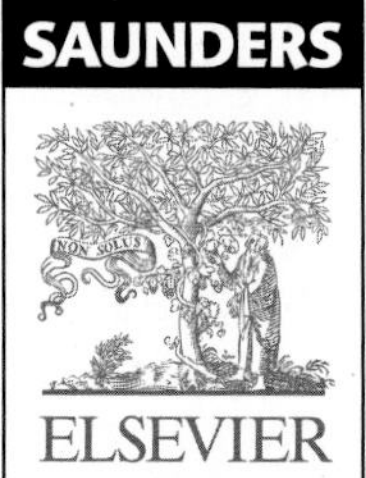

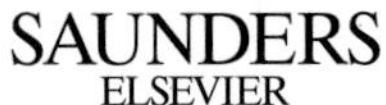

1600 John F. Kennedy Blvd.
Suite 1800
Philadelphia, PA 19103-2899

CLINICAL ARRHYTHMOLOGY AND ELECTROPHYSIOLOGY:
A COMPANION TO BRAUNWALD'S HEART DISEASE ISBN: 978-1-4160-5998-1

Notice

Knowledge and best practice in this field are constantly changing. As new research and experience broaden our knowledge, changes in practice, treatment and drug therapy may become necessary or appropriate. Readers are advised to check the most current information provided (i) on procedures featured or (ii) by the manufacturer of each product to be administered, to verify the recommended dose or formula, the method and duration of administration, and contraindications. It is the responsibility of the practitioner, relying on their own experience and knowledge of the patient, to make diagnoses, to determine dosages and the best treatment for each individual patient, and to take all appropriate safety precautions. To the fullest extent of the law, neither the Publisher nor the Authors assumes any liability for any injury and/or damage to persons or property arising out of or related to any use of the material contained in this book.

The Publisher

Library of Congress Cataloging-in-Publication Data

Issa, Ziad.
Clinical arrhythmology and electrophysiology : a companion to Braunwald's heart disease / Ziad Issa, John M. Miller, Douglas P. Zipes.—1st ed.
p. ; cm.
Includes bibliographical references and index.
ISBN 978-1-4160-5998-1
1. Arrhythmia. 2. Heart–Electric properties. I. Miller, John M. (John Michael). II. Zipes, Douglas P. III. Braunwald's heart disease. IV. Title.
[DNLM: 1. Arrhythmias, Cardiac—diagnosis. 2. Arrhythmias, Cardiac—physiopathology. 3. Electrophysiologic Techniques, Cardiac. WG 330 I86c 2009]
RC685.A65I87 2009
616.1′28–dc22 2008027014

Acquisitions Editor: Natasha Andjelkovic
Developmental Editor: Robin Bonner
Publishing Services Manager: Frank Polizzano
Senior Project Manager: Robin Hayward
Design Direction: Steven Stave

Printed in China.

Last digit is the print number: 9 8 7 6 5 4 3 2 1

We would like to thank our families for their support during the writing of this book, since it meant time away from them.

My wife Dana and my sons Tariq and Amr
Ziad F. Issa

My wife Jeanne and my children Rebekah, Jordan, and Jacob
John M. Miller

My wife Joan and my children Debbie, Jeff, and David
Douglas P. Zipes

We would also like to thank Julie Reed, Donna Hillyer, Leslie Ardebili, Alice Towers, and Ralph Chambers for their help in preparing this manuscript.

Foreword

Disturbances in cardiac rhythm occur in a large proportion of the population. Arrhythmias can have sequelae that range from inconsequential to life-shortening. Sudden cardiac deaths and chronic disability are among the most frequent serious complications resulting from arrhythmias.

Braunwald's Heart Disease: A Textbook of Cardiovascular Medicine includes an excellent section on rhythm disturbances edited and largely written by Douglas Zipes, the most accomplished and respected investigator and clinician in this field. However, there are many subjects that simply cannot be discussed in sufficient detail, even in a 2000-page densely packed book. For this reason, the current editors and I decided to commission a series of companions to the parent title. We were extremely fortunate to enlist Dr. Zipes' help in editing and writing *Clinical Arrhythmology and Electrophysiology*. Dr. Zipes, in turn, enlisted two talented collaborators, Drs. Ziad F. Issa and John M. Miller, to work with him to produce this excellent volume.

This book is unique in several respects. First and foremost is the very high quality of the content, which is accurate, authoritative, and clear; second, it is as up-to-date as last month's journals; third, the writing style and illustrations are consistent throughout with little, if any, duplication. The first four chapters on Electrophysiological Mechanisms of Cardiac Arrhythmias, Electrophysiological Testing, Mapping and Navigation Modalities, and Ablation Energy Sources provide a superb introduction to the field. This is followed by eighteen chapters on individual arrhythmias, each following a similar outline. Here, the authors lead us from a basic understanding of the arrhythmia to its clinical recognition, natural history, and management. The latter is moving rapidly from being largely drug-based to device-based, although many patients receive combination device-drug therapy. These options, as well as ablation therapy, are clearly spelled out as they apply to each arrhythmia.

We are proud to include *Clinical Arrhythmology and Electrophysiology* as a Companion to *Braunwald's Heart Disease,* and we are fully confident that it will prove to be valuable to cardiologists, internists, investigators, and trainees.

EUGENE BRAUNWALD, MD

PETER LIBBY, MD

ROBERT O. BONOW, MD

DOUGLAS L. MANN, MD

Preface

Many books have been written about cardiac arrhythmias and cardiac electrophysiology, and many chapters in general cardiology textbooks discuss the same subjects. However, they often focus on individual topics, such as a specific arrhythmia, rather than integrate, as they should, the electrophysiologic processes that underlie the clinical events.

In the chapters published in the parent title to this book, *Braunwald's Heart Disease: A Textbook of Cardiovascular Medicine,* 8th Edition, we presented a synthesis of clinical arrhythmias with underlying electrophysiology. Size limitations, however, prevented us from discussing these topics in great detail. Thus, we present this companion volume not only to provide more depth to these topics but also to present them in a format suitable for trainees, internists, and general cardiologists who specialize or are interested in arrhythmias and electrophysiology, as well as for electrophysiologists who need an up-to-date resource.

Unlike many other clinical texts that feature chapters contributed by dozens of respected authors in the field, this text was written by the three of us. By using this approach we could explain, integrate, coordinate, and educate in a comprehensive, cohesive fashion while avoiding redundancies and contradictions. We were able to choose our illustrations in a way that is certain to be understandable and explanatory. In addition, our practical experience allowed us to detail the actual application of the diagnostic and therapeutic concepts, from interpreting the scalar ECG to understanding intracavitary electrograms, from drug choices to implantable devices or placement of a catheter to shock, record, or ablate. In all chapters the readers can decide how much detail they want, from straightforward electrocardiography to practical electrophysiology to reading about mechanisms of arrhythmias. Other books in this field give abundant information on mechanisms but are of limited practical use, while others have a very pragmatic focus without much emphasis on the mechanistic underpinnings of therapy. We believe that this book provides a balanced, comprehensive perspective on the expanding field of diagnosis and treatment of clinical arrhythmias by featuring consistently organized chapters and juxtaposing theory and practical aspects of arrhythmia management, all enhanced by detailed full-color figures and useful references. We think that this book will find its place in the libraries of physicians and trainees and we hope readers will enjoy and learn from it.

ZIAD F. ISSA

JOHN M. MILLER

DOUGLAS P. ZIPES

Abbreviations

A	Atrial
AES	Atrial extrastimulation, extrastimulus
AF	Atrial fibrillation
AFL	Atrial flutter
AH	Atrial-His bundle interval
AT	Atrial tachycardia
AV	Atrioventricular
AVN	Atrioventricular node
AVNRT	Atrioventricular nodal reentrant tachycardia
AVRT	Atrioventricular reentrant tachycardia
BBB	Bundle branch block
BBR	Bundle branch reentry
BT	Bypass tract
CL	Cycle length
CS	Coronary sinus
CS os	Coronary sinus ostium
EP	Electrophysiology
H	His bundle potential
HA	His bundle-atrial interval
HB	His bundle
HPS	His-Purkinje system
HV	His bundle-ventricular interval
IVC	Inferior vena cava
LA	Left atrium
LAO	Left anterior oblique
LB	Left bundle branch
LBBB	Left bundle branch block
LV	Left ventricle
LVOT	Left ventricular outflow tract
MI	Myocardial infarction
NSR	Normal sinus rhythm
PAC	Premature atrial complex
PPI	Post-pacing interval
PV	Pulmonary vein
PVC	Premature ventricular complex
RA	Right atrium
RAO	Right anterior oblique
RB	Right bundle branch
RBBB	Right bundle branch block
RV	Right ventricle
RVOT	Right ventricular outflow tract
S-A	Stimulus-atrial interval
S-H	Stimulus-His bundle interval
SMVT	Sustained monomorphic ventricular tachycardia
SVC	Superior vena cava
SVT	Supraventricular tachycardia
V	Ventricle, ventricular
VA	Ventricular-atrial interval
VES	Ventricular extrastimulation, extrastimulus
VF	Ventricular fibrillation
VT	Ventricular tachycardia
WPW	Wolff-Parkinson-White
3-D	Three-dimensional

Contents

BRAUNWALD'S HEART DISEASE COMPANIONS

Upcoming Titles

2009

Theroux: Acute Coronary Syndromes, 2nd Ed.
Otto & Bonow: Valvular Heart Disease, 3rd Ed.
Mann: Heart Failure, 2nd Ed.
Taylor: Atlas of Cardiac CT (Imaging Companion with DVD)
Kramer & Hundley: Atlas of Cardiovascular MR (Imaging Companion with DVD)
Cerqueira: Atlas of Nuclear Cardiology (Imaging Companion with DVD)
Thomas: Atlas of Echocardiography (Imaging Companion with DVD)

2010

Kormos: Mechanical Circulatory Support and Artificial Hearts
Blumenthal: Prevention of Cardiovascular Disease

Published Titles

Ballantyne: Clinical Lipidology (2008, ISBN 9781416054696)
Antman: Cardiovascular Therapeutics, 3rd Ed. (2007, ISBN 9781416033585)
Black & Elliott: Hypertension (2007, ISBN 9781416030539)
Creager, Dzau & Loscalzo: Vascular Medicine (2006, ISBN 9780721602844)
Chien: Molecular Basis of Cardiovascular Disease, 2nd Ed. (2004, ISBN 9780721694283)
Manson: Clinical Trials in Heart Disease, 2nd Ed. (2004, ISBN 9780721604084)
St. John-Sutton & Rutherford: Clinical Cardiovascular Imaging (2004, ISBN 9780721690681)

CHAPTER 1

Electrophysiological Mechanisms of Cardiac Arrhythmias

The mechanisms responsible for cardiac arrhythmias are generally divided into categories of disorders of impulse formation (automaticity and triggered activity), disorders of impulse conduction (reentry), or combinations of both. The term *impulse initiation* is used to indicate that an electrical impulse can arise in a single cell or a group of closely coupled cells through depolarization of the cell membrane and, once initiated, can spread through the rest of the heart. There are two major causes for the impulse initiation that can result in arrhythmias, automaticity and triggered activity. Each has its own unique cellular mechanism that results in membrane depolarization. Reentry is the likely mechanism of most recurrent clinical arrhythmias.

Diagnosis of the underlying mechanism of an arrhythmia can be of great importance in guiding appropriate treatment strategies. Spontaneous behavior of the arrhythmia, mode of initiation and termination, and response to premature stimulation and overdrive pacing are the most commonly used tools to distinguish among the different mechanisms responsible for cardiac arrhythmias. Our present diagnostic tools, however, do not always permit unequivocal determination of the electrophysiological mechanisms responsible for many clinical arrhythmias or their ionic bases. In particular, it can be difficult to distinguish among several mechanisms that appear to have a focal origin with centrifugal spread of activation (automaticity, triggered activity, reentry). This is further complicated by the fact that some arrhythmias can be started by one mechanism and perpetuated by another.

AUTOMATICITY

Automaticity, or spontaneous impulse initiation, is the property of cardiac cells to undergo spontaneous diastolic depolarization (phase 4 depolarization) and initiate an electrical impulse in the absence of external electrical stimulation. Altered automaticity can be caused by enhanced normal automaticity or abnormal automaticity.[1]

Enhanced normal automaticity refers to the accelerated generation of an action potential by normal pacemaker tissue and is found in the primary pacemaker of the heart, the sinus node, as well as in certain subsidiary or latent pacemakers that can become the functional pacemaker under certain conditions. Impulse initiation is a normal property of these latent pacemakers.

Abnormal automaticity occurs in cardiac cells only when there are major abnormalities in their transmembrane potentials, in particular in steady-state depolarization of the membrane potential. This property of abnormal automaticity is not confined to any specific latent pacemaker cell type but can occur almost anywhere in the heart.

The discharge rate of normal or abnormal pacemakers can be accelerated by drugs, various forms of cardiac disease, reduction in extracellular potassium, or alterations of autonomic nervous system tone.

Enhanced Normal Automaticity

Pacemaker Mechanisms

Normal automaticity involves a spontaneous, slow, progressive decline in the transmembrane potential during diastole (spontaneous diastolic depolarization or phase 4 depolarization). Once this spontaneous depolarization reaches threshold (about −40 mV), a new action potential is generated.[2]

The ionic mechanisms responsible for normal pacemaker activity in the sinus node are still controversial. The fall in membrane potential during phase 4 seems to arise from a changing balance between positive inward currents, which favor depolarization, and positive outward currents, with a net gain in intracellular positive charges during diastole (i.e., inward depolarizing current; Fig. 1-1).[1,3-7]

There is evidence that diastolic depolarization results from activation of an inward current, called the pacemaker current, I_f, which is carried largely by Na^+ but is relatively nonselective for monovalent cations. The I_f channels are deactivated during the action potential upstroke and the initial plateau phase of repolarization but begin to activate as repolarization brings the membrane potential to levels

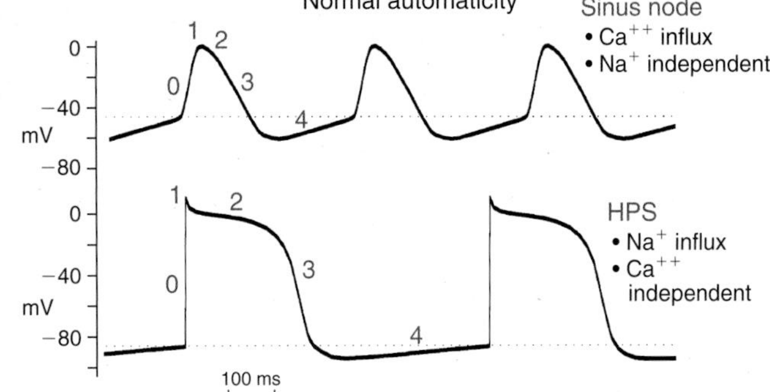

FIGURE 1–1 Normal cardiac automaticity. Action potentials from typical sinus nodal and His-Purkine cells are shown with the voltage scale on the vertical axes; dashed lines are threshold potential and numbers on figure refer to phases of the action potential. Note the qualitative differences between the two types of cells, as well as different rates of spontaneous depolarization.

more negative than about −60 mV; however, because the maximum diastolic potential is about −60 mV, the role of I_f current in normal pacemaker activity has been challenged.[6-9]

Important roles for other membrane currents, including the K^+ current, I_K, and the T- and L-type Ca^{2+} currents in causing spontaneous diastolic depolarization, also have been proposed. One hypothesis is that the first third of diastolic depolarization results from an inward leak of Na^+ coupled with a time-dependent decay in the outward K^+ current that is activated during the action potential. During the latter two thirds of diastolic depolarization, a slow inward movement of Ca^{2+} occurs (T-type Ca^{2+} channels). This process moves the membrane potential to the threshold potential, at which time there is a more rapid inward Ca^{2+} current (L-type Ca^{2+} channels), generating a slow action potential.[2,10] Therefore, there can be no single pacemaker current in the sinus node; rather, a number of currents can contribute to the occurrence of automaticity.[4-6]

Automaticity in subsidiary pacemakers appears to arise via a mechanism similar to that occuring in the sinus node. Diastolic depolarization is likely the result of an increase in an inward current, I_f, and a decrease in outward currents (I_{K1} and I_K).[1,11]

Hierarchy of Pacemaker Function

Automaticity is an intrinsic property of all myocardial cells. In addition to the sinus node, cells with pacemaking capability in the normal heart are located in some parts of the atria and ventricles. However, the occurrence of spontaneous activity is prevented by the natural hierarchy of pacemaker function, causing these sites to be latent or subsidiary pacemakers.[1,3] The spontaneous discharge rate of the sinus node normally exceeds that of all other subsidiary pacemakers (see Fig. 1-1). Therefore, the impulse initiated by the sinus node depolarizes and keeps the activity of subsidiary pacemaker sites depressed before they can spontaneously reach threshold. However, slowly depolarizing and previously suppressed pacemakers in the atrium, atrioventricular node (AVN), or ventricle can become active and assume pacemaker control of the cardiac rhythm if the sinus node pacemaker becomes slow or unable to generate an impulse (e.g., secondary to depressed sinus node automaticity) or if impulses generated by the sinus node are unable to activate the subsidiary pacemaker sites (e.g., sinoatrial exit block, or AV block). The emergence of subsidiary or latent pacemakers under such circumstances is an appropriate fail-safe mechanism, which ensures that ventricular activation is maintained. Because spontaneous diastolic depolarization is a normal property, the automaticity generated by these cells is classified as normal.

There is also a natural hierarchy of intrinsic rates of subsidiary pacemakers that have normal automaticity, with atrial pacemakers having faster intrinsic rates than AV junctional pacemakers, and AV junctional pacemakers having faster rates than ventricular pacemakers.

Subsidiary Pacemakers

Subsidiary Atrial Pacemakers. Subsidiary atrial pacemakers have been identified in the atrial myocardium, especially in the crista terminalis, at the junction of the inferior right atrium (RA) and inferior vena cava (IVC), near or on the eustachian ridge, near the coronary sinus ostium (CS os), in the atrial muscle that extends into the tricuspid and mitral valves, and in the muscle sleeves that extend into the cardiac veins (venae cavae and pulmonary veins).[12]

Latent atrial pacemakers can be expected to contribute to impulse initiation in the atrium if the discharge rate of the sinus node is reduced temporarily or permanently. In contrast to the normal sinus node, these latent or ectopic pacemakers usually generate a fast action potential (referring to the rate of upstroke of the action potential, dV/dT) mediated by sodium ion fluxes. However, when severely damaged, the atrial tissue may not be able to generate a fast action potential (which is energy-dependent) but rather generates a slow, calcium ion–mediated action potential (which is energy-independent). Automaticity of subsidiary atrial pacemakers can also be enhanced by coronary disease and ischemia, chronic pulmonary disease, or drugs such as digitalis and alcohol, possibly overriding normal sinus activity.[13,14]

Subsidiary Atrioventricular Junctional Pacemakers. Some data suggest that the AVN itself has pacemaker cells, but that is controversial. However, it is clear that the AV junction, which is an area that includes atrial tissue, the AVN, and His-Purkinje tissue, does have pacemaker cells and is capable of exhibiting automaticity.

Subsidiary Ventricular Pacemakers. In the ventricles, latent pacemakers are found in the His-Purkinje system (HPS), where Purkinje fibers have the property of spontaneous diastolic depolarization. Isolated cells of the HPS discharge spontaneously at rates of 15 to 60 beats/min, whereas ventricular myocardial cells usually do not normally exhibit spontaneous diastolic depolarization or automaticity. The relatively slow spontaneous discharge rate of the HPS pacemakers, which further decreases from the His bundle (HB) to the distal Purkinje branches, ensures that pacemaker activity in the HPS will be suppressed on a beat-to-beat basis by the more rapid discharge rate of the sinus node and atrial and AV junctional pacemakers. However, enhanced Purkinje fiber automaticity can be induced by certain situations, such as myocardial infarction (MI). In this setting, some Purkinje fibers that survive the infarction develop moderately reduced maximum diastolic membrane potentials and therefore accelerated spontaneous discharge rates.

Autonomic and Other Influences

The intrinsic rate at which the sinus node pacemaker cells generate impulses is determined by the interplay of three factors—the maximum diastolic potential, the threshold potential at which the action potential is initiated, and the rate or slope of phase 4 depolarization (Fig. 1-2). A change in any one of these factors will alter the time required for phase 4 depolarization to carry the membrane potential from its maximum diastolic level to threshold and thus alter the rate of impulse initiation.[1,7,15]

The sinus node is innervated by the parasympathetic and sympathetic nervous systems, and the balance between

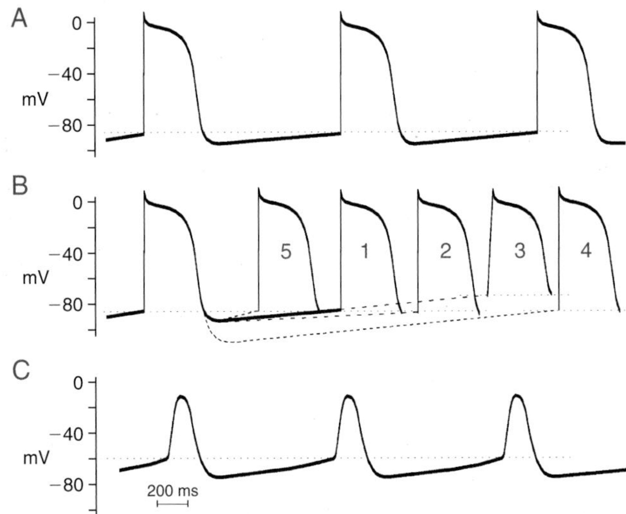

FIGURE 1–2 Abnormalities of automaticity. **A,** Normal His-Purkinje action potential. **B,** Modulation of rate of depolarization from baseline (1) by slowing rate of phase 4 depolarization (2), increasing threshold potential (3), starting from a more negative resting membrane potential (4), all of which slow discharge rate, or by increasing rate of phase 4 depolarization (5), yielding a faster discharge rate. **C,** Abnormal automaticity with change in action potential contour (resembling sinus nodal cell) when resting membrane potential is less negative, inactivating most sodium channels.

these systems importantly controls the pacemaker rate. The classic concept has been that of a reciprocal relationship between sympathetic and parasympathetic inputs. More recent investigations, however, stress dynamic, demand-oriented interactions, and the anatomical distribution of fibers that allows both autonomic systems to act quite selectively. Muscarinic cholinergic and beta$_1$-adrenergic receptors are nonuniformly distributed in the sinus node and they modulate both the rate of depolarization and impulse propagation.[1,16]

Parasympathetic Activity. Parasympathetic tone reduces the spontaneous discharge rate of the sinus node, whereas its withdrawal accelerates sinus node automaticity. Acetylcholine, the principal neurotransmitter of the parasympathetic nervous system, inhibits spontaneous impulse generation in the sinus node by increasing K^+ conductance. Acetylcholine acts through M_2 muscarinic receptors to activate the G_i protein, which subsequently results in activation of $I_{K/Ach}$ (an acetylcholine-activated subtype of inward rectifying current) in tissues of the sinus node and AVN as well as of the atria, Purkinje fibers, and ventricles. The increased outward repolarizing K^+ current leads to membrane hyperpolarization (i.e., the resting potential and the maximum diastolic potential become more negative). The resulting hyperpolarization of the membrane potential lengthens the time required for the membrane potential to depolarize to threshold, thereby decreasing the automaticity of the sinus node (see Fig. 1-2). In addition, activation of G_i protein results in inhibition of beta receptor–stimulated adenylate cyclase activity, reducing cyclic adenosine monophosphate (cAMP) and inhibiting protein kinase A, with subsequent inhibition of the inward Ca^{2+} current, I_{Ca}. This results in reduction of the rate of diastolic depolarization because of less calcium entry and subsequent slowing of the pacemaker activity. Inhibition of beta receptor–stimulated adenylate cyclase activity can also inhibit the inward I_f current.[15,16]

Sympathetic Activity. Increased sympathetic nerve traffic as well as the adrenomedullary release of catecholamines increases the sinus rate. Stimulation of beta$_1$ receptors by catecholamines enhances the L-type of inward Ca^{2+} current by increasing cAMP and activating the protein kinase A system; the increment in inward Ca^{2+} current increases the slope of diastolic depolarization and enhances pacemaker activity (see Fig. 1-2). The redistribution of Ca^{2+} can also increase the completeness and the rate of I_K deactivation; the ensuing decline in the opposing outward current can result in a further net increase in inward current. Catecholamines can also enhance the inward I_f current by shifting the voltage dependence of I_f to more positive potentials, thus augmenting the slope of phase 4 and increasing the rate of sinus node firing.

Sympathetic stimulation explains the normal response of the sinus node to stress such as exercise, fever, and hyperthyroidism. In addition to altering ionic conductance, changes in autonomic tone can produce changes in the rate of the sinus node by shifting the primary pacemaker region within the pacemaker complex. Mapping of activation indicates that at faster rates, the sinus node impulse originates in the superior portion of the sinus node, whereas at slower rates it arises from a more inferior portion of the sinus node. The sinus node can be insulated from the surrounding atrial myocytes, except at a limited number of preferential exit sites. Shifting pacemaker sites can select different exit pathways to the atria. As a result, autonomically mediated shifts of pacemaker regions can be accompanied by changes in the sinus rate. Vagal fibers are denser in the cranial portion of the sinus node and stimulation of the parasympathetic nervous system shifts the pacemaker center to a more caudal region of the sinus node complex, resulting in slowing of the heart rate, whereas stimulation of the sympathetic nervous system or withdrawal of vagal stimulation shifts the pacemaker center cranially, resulting in an increase in heart rate.[16]

Atrial, AV junctional, and HPS subsidiary pacemakers are also under similar autonomic control, with the sympathetics enhancing pacemaker activity through beta$_1$-adrenergic stimulation and the parasympathetics inhibiting pacemaker activity through muscarinic receptor stimulation.[1]

Adenosine (Ado) binds to A_1 receptors, activating $I_{K/Ado}$, a subtype of I_K identical to $I_{K/Ach}$, increasing outward K^+ current in a manner similar to that of marked parasympathetic stimulus. It also has similar effects on I_f channels.[7,15]

Digitalis exerts two effects on the sinus rate. It has a direct positive chronotropic effect on the sinus node, resulting from depolarization of the membrane potential caused by inhibition of the Na^+-K^+ exchange pump. The reduction in the maximum diastolic membrane potential decreases the time required for the membrane to depolarize to threshold, thereby accelerating the spontaneous discharge rate.[14] However, it also enhances vagal tone, which decreases spontaneous sinus discharge. The latter effect can dominate when sympathetic activity has been enhanced, such as during heart failure.[5]

Enhanced subsidiary pacemaker activity may not require sympathetic stimulation. Normal automaticity can be affected by a number of other factors associated with heart disease.[8] Inhibition of the electrogenic Na^+-K^+ exchange pump results in a net increase in inward current during diastole because of the decrease in outward current normally generated by the pump, and therefore can increase automaticity in subsidiary pacemakers sufficiently to cause arrhythmias. This can occur when adenosine triphosphate (ATP) is depleted during prolonged hypoxia or ischemia, or in the presence of toxic amounts of digitalis. Hypokalemia can reduce the activity of the Na^+-K^+ exchange pump, thereby reducing the background repolarizing current and enhancing phase 4 diastolic depolarization. The end result would be an increase in the discharge rate of pacemaking cells. Additionally, the flow of current between partially depolarized myocardium and normally polarized latent pacemaker cells can enhance automaticity. This mechanism has been proposed to be a cause of some of the ectopic complexes that arise at the borders of ischemic areas in the ventricle. Slightly increased extracellular K^+ can render the maximum diastolic potential more positive (i.e., reduced or less negative), thereby also increasing the discharge rate of pacemaking cells. A greater increase in extracellular K^+, however, renders the heart inexcitable by depolarizing the membrane potential and inactivating the Na^+ current.[15]

Evidence indicates that active and passive changes in the mechanical environment of the heart provide feedback to modify cardiac rate and rhythm, and are capable of influencing both the initiation and spread of cardiac excitation. This direction of the crosstalk between cardiac electrical and mechanical activity is referred to as mechanoelectric feedback, and is thought to be involved in the adjustment of heart rate to changes in mechanical load, which would help explain the precise beat-to-beat regulation of cardiac performance. Acute mechanical stretch enhances automaticity, reversibly depolarizes the cell membrane, and shortens the action potential duration. Feedback from cardiac mechanics to electrical activity involves mechanosensitive ion channels, among them K^+-selective, chloride-selective, nonselective, and ATP-sensitive K^+ channels. In addition, Na^+ and Ca^{2+} entering the cells via nonselective ion channels are thought to contribute to the genesis of stretch-induced arrhythmia.[15,17-19]

Abnormal Automaticity

In the normal heart, automaticity is confined to the sinus node and other specialized conducting tissues. Working atrial and ventricular myocardial cells do not normally have spontaneous diastolic depolarization and do not initiate spontaneous impulses, even when they are not excited for long periods of time by propagating impulses.[8] Although these cells do have a pacemaker current, I_f, the range of activation of this current in these cells is much more negative (−120 to −170 mV) than in Purkinje fibers or in the sinus node. As a result, during physiological resting membrane potentials (−85 to −95 mV), the pacemaker current is not activated and ventricular cells do not depolarize spontaneously.[1] When the resting potentials of these cells are depolarized sufficiently, to about −70 to −30 mV, however, spontaneous diastolic depolarization can occur and cause repetitive impulse initiation, a phenomenon called depolarization-induced automaticity or abnormal automaticity (see Fig. 1-2). Similarly, cells in the Purkinje system, which are normally automatic at high levels of membrane potential, show abnormal automaticity when the membrane potential is reduced to around −60 mV or less, which can occur in ischemic regions of the heart. When the steady-state membrane potential of Purkinje fibers is reduced to around −60 mV or less, the I_f channels that participate in normal pacemaker activity in Purkinje fibers are closed and nonfunctional and automaticity is, therefore, not caused by the normal pacemaker mechanism. It can, however, be caused by an "abnormal" mechanism. In contrast, enhanced automaticity of the sinus node, subsidiary atrial pacemakers, or the AVN caused by a mechanism other than acceleration of normal automaticity has not been demonstrated clinically.[5]

A low level of membrane potential is not the only criterion for defining abnormal automaticity. If this were so, the automaticity of the sinus node would have to be considered abnormal. Therefore, an important distinction between abnormal and normal automaticity is that the membrane potentials of fibers showing the abnormal type of activity are reduced from their own normal level. For this reason, automaticity in the AVN—for example, where the membrane potential is normally low—is not classified as abnormal automaticity.

Several different mechanisms probably cause abnormal pacemaker activity at low membrane potentials, including activation and deactivation of delayed rectifier K^+ currents, intracellular Ca^{2+} release from the sarcoplasmic reticulum, causing activation of inward Ca^{2+} currents and inward Na^+ current (through Na^+-Ca^{2+} exchange), and potential contribution by the pacemaker current I_f.[5,20] It has not been determined which of these mechanisms are operative in the different pathological conditions in which abnormal automaticity can occur.[1]

The upstroke of the spontaneously occurring action potentials generated by abnormal automaticity can be caused by Na^+ or Ca^{2+} inward currents or possibly a combination of the two.[1] In the range of diastolic potentials between approximately −70 and −50 mV, repetitive activity is dependent on extracellular Na^+ concentration and can be decreased or abolished by Na^+ channel blockers. In a diastolic potential range of approximately −50 to −30 mV, Na^+ channels are predominantly inactivated; repetitive activity depends on extracellular Ca^{2+} concentration and is reduced by L-type Ca^{2+} channel blockers.

The intrinsic rate of a focus with abnormal automaticity is a function of the membrane potential. The more positive the membrane potential, the faster the automatic rate (see Fig. 1-2). Abnormal automaticity is less vulnerable to suppression by overdrive pacing (see later). Therefore, even occasional slowing of the sinus node rate can allow an ectopic focus with abnormal automaticity to fire without a preceding long period of quiescence.[5]

The decrease in the membrane potential of cardiac cells required for abnormal automaticity to occur can be induced by a variety of factors related to cardiac disease, such as ischemia and infarction. The circumstance under which membrane depolarization occurs, however, can influence the development of abnormal automaticity. For example, an increase in extracellular K^+ concentration, as occurs in acutely ischemic myocardium, can reduce membrane potential; however, normal or abnormal automaticity in working atrial, ventricular, and Purkinje fibers usually does not occur because of the increase in K^+ conductance (and hence net outward current) that results from an increase in extracellular K^+ concentration.[8] Catecholamines also increase the rate of discharge caused by abnormal automaticity and therefore can contribute to a shift in the pacemaker site, from the sinus node to a region with abnormal automaticity.

Overdrive Suppression of Automatic Rhythms

Suppression of Normal and Abnormal Automatic Subsidiary Pacemakers

The sinus node likely maintains its dominance over subsidiary pacemakers in the AVN and the Purkinje fibers by several mechanisms. During sinus rhythm in a normal heart, the intrinsic automatic rate of the sinus node is faster than that of the other potentially automatic cells. Consequently, the latent pacemakers are excited by propagated impulses from the sinus node before they have a chance to depolarize spontaneously to threshold potential. The higher frequency of sinus node discharge also suppresses the automaticity of other pacemaker sites by a mechanism called overdrive suppression. The diastolic (phase 4) depolarization of the latent pacemaker cells with the property of normal automaticity is actually inhibited because they are repeatedly depolarized by the impulses from the sinus

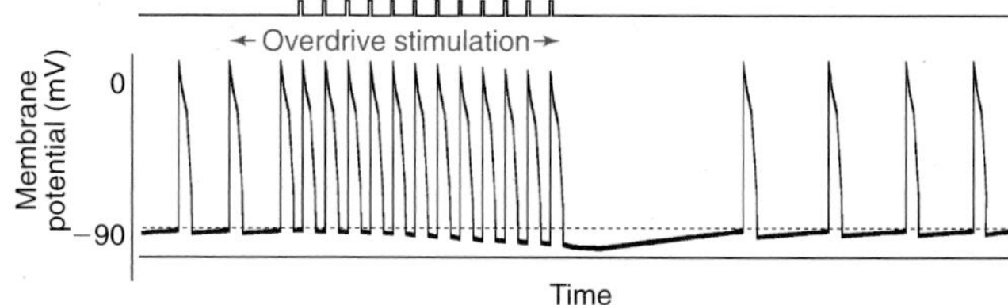

FIGURE 1–3 Overdrive suppression of automaticity. A spontaneously firing cell is paced more rapidly, resulting in depression of resting membrane potential; after pacing is stopped, spontaneous depolarization takes longer than usual and gradually resumes baseline rate. Dashed line = threshold potential.

node.[1] Electrotonic interaction between the pacemaker cells and nonpacemaker cells in the surrounding myocardium via intercalated discs can also hyperpolarize the latent pacemakers and contribute to their suppression (Fig. 1-3).

Mechanism of Overdrive Suppression

The mechanism of overdrive suppression is mediated mostly by enhanced activity of the Na^+-K^+ exchange pump that results from driving a pacemaker cell faster than its intrinsic spontaneous rate. During normal sinus rhythm (NSR), latent pacemakers are depolarized at a higher frequency than their intrinsic rate of automaticity. The increased frequency of depolarizations leads to an increase in intracellular Na^+, which enters the cell with every action potential, because more Na^+ enters the cell per unit time.[1,8] The increased intracellular Na^+ stimulates the Na^+-K^+ exchange pump. Because the Na^+-K^+ exchange pump is electrogenic—moves more Na^+ outward than K^+ inward—it generates a net outward (hyperpolarizing) current across the cell membrane. This drives the membrane potential more negative, thereby offsetting the depolarizing pacemaker currents (I_f) being carried into the cell and slowing the rate of phase 4 diastolic depolarization. This effectively prevents the pacemaker currents from depolarizing the cell to its threshold potential, and thereby suppresses spontaneous impulse initiation in these cells.

When the dominant (overdrive) pacemaker is stopped, suppression of subsidiary pacemakers continues because the Na^+-K^+ exchange pump continues to generate the outward current as it reduces the intracellular Na^+ levels toward normal. This continued Na^+-K^+ exchange pump–generated outward current is responsible for the period of quiescence, which lasts until the intracellular Na^+ concentration, and hence the pump current, becomes low enough to allow subsidiary pacemaker cells to depolarize spontaneously to threshold. Intracellular Na^+ concentration decreases during the quiescent period because Na^+ is constantly being pumped out of the cell and little is entering. Additionally, the spontaneous rate of the suppressed cell will remain lower than it might be otherwise until the intracellular Na^+ concentration has a chance to decrease. Intracellular Na^+ concentration and pump current continue to decline even after spontaneous discharge begins because of the slow firing rate, causing a gradual increase in the discharge rate of the subsidiary pacemaker. At slower rates and shorter overdrive periods, the Na^+ load is decreased, as is the activity of the Na^+-K^+ pump, resulting in a progressively rapid diastolic depolarization and warm-up.[11] The higher the overdrive rate or the longer the duration of overdrive, the greater the enhancement of pump activity, so that the period of quiescence after the cessation of overdrive is directly related to the rate and duration of overdrive.[11]

The sinus node itself also is vulnerable to overdrive suppression.[8] When overdrive suppression of the normal sinus node occurs, however, it is generally of lesser magnitude than that of subsidiary pacemakers overdriven at comparable rates. The sinus node action potential upstroke is largely dependent on slow inward current carried by Ca^{2+} through the L-type Ca^{2+} channels, and far less Na^+ enters the fiber during the upstroke than occurs in latent pacemaker cells such as the Purkinje fibers. As a result, the accumulation of intracellular Na^+ and enhancement of Na^+-K^+ exchange pump activity occurs to a lesser degree in sinus node cells after a period of overdrive; therefore, there is less overdrive suppression caused by enhanced Na^+-K^+ exchange pump current. The relative resistance of the normal sinus node to overdrive suppression can be important in enabling it to remain the dominant pacemaker, even when its rhythm is perturbed transiently by external influences such as transient shifts of the pacemaker to an ectopic site. The diseased sinus node, however, can be much more easily overdrive-suppressed, such as in so-called tachycardia-bradycardia syndrome.[11]

Abnormally automatic cells and tissues at reduced levels of membrane potential are less sensitive to overdrive suppression than cells and tissues that are fully polarized, with enhanced normal automaticity.[8] The amount of overdrive suppression of spontaneous diastolic depolarization that causes abnormal automaticity is directly related to the level of membrane potential at which the automatic rhythm occurs. At low levels of membrane potential, Na^+ channels are inactivated, decreasing the fast inward Na^+ current; therefore, there is a reduction in the amount of Na^+ entering the cells during overdrive and the degree of stimulation of the Na^+-K^+ exchange pump. The more polarized the membrane during phase 4, the larger amount of Na^+ enters the cell with each action potential, and the more overdrive suppression. As a result of the lack of overdrive suppression of abnormally automatic cells, even transient sinus pauses can permit an ectopic focus with a slower rate than the sinus node to capture the heart for one or more beats. However, even in situations in which cells can be sufficiently depolarized to inactivate the Na^+ current and limit intracellular Na^+ load, overdrive suppression can still be observed because of increased intracellular Ca^{2+} loading. Such Ca^{2+} loading can activate Ca^{2+}-dependent K^+ conductance (favoring repolarization) and promote Ca^{2+} extrusion through the Na^+-Ca^{2+} exchanger and Ca^{2+} channel phosphorylation, increasing Na^+ load and thus Na^+-K^+ exchange pump activity. The increase in intracellular Ca^{2+} load can also reduce depolarizing L-type Ca^{2+} current by promoting Ca^{2+}-induced inactivation of the Ca^{2+} current.

In addition to overdrive suppression being of paramount importance for maintenance of NSR, the characteristic response of automatic pacemakers to overdrive is often useful to distinguish automaticity from triggered activity and reentry.

Arrhythmias Caused by Automaticity

Inappropriate Sinus Node Discharge. Such arrhythmias result simply from an alteration in the rate of impulse initiation by the normal sinus node pacemaker, without a shift of impulse origin to a subsidiary pacemaker at an ectopic site, although there can be shifts of the pacemaker site within the sinus node itself during alterations in sinus rate. These arrhythmias are often a result of the actions of the autonomic nervous system on the sinus node. Examples of these arrhythmias include sinus bradycardia, sinus arrest, inappropriate sinus tachycardia, and respiratory sinus arrhythmia. The latter is primarily caused by withdrawal of vagal tone during inhalation and reinstitution of vagal tone during exhalation.[14,21]

Escape Ectopic Automatic Rhythms. Impairment of the sinus node can allow a latent pacemaker to initiate impulse formation. This would be expected to happen when the rate at which the sinus node overdrives subsidiary pacemakers falls considerably below the intrinsic rate of the latent pacemakers or when the inhibitory electrotonic influences between nonpacemaker cells and pacemaker cells are interrupted.

The rate at which the sinus node activates subsidiary pacemakers can be decreased in a number of situations, including sinus node dysfunction, with depressed sinus automaticity (secondary to increased vagal tone, drugs, or intrinsic sinus node disease), sinoatrial exit block, AV block, and parasystolic focus. The sinus node and AVN are most sensitive to vagal influence, followed by atrial tissue, with the ventricular conducting system being least sensitive. Moderate vagal stimulation allows the pacemaker to shift to another atrial site but severe vagal stimulation suppresses sinus node and blocks conduction at the AVN, and therefore can allow a ventricular escape pacemaker to become manifest.[11]

Interruption of the inhibitory electrotonic influences between nonpacemaker cells and pacemaker cells allows those latent pacemakers to fire at their intrinsic rate. Uncoupling can be caused by fibrosis or damage (e.g., infarction) of the tissues surrounding the subsidiary pacemaker cells, or by reduction in gap junction conductance secondary to increased intracellular Ca^{2+}, which can be caused by digitalis. Some inhibition of the sinus node is still necessary for the site of impulse initiation to shift to an ectopic site that is no longer inhibited because of uncoupling from surrounding cells, because the intrinsic firing rate of subsidiary pacemakers is still slower than that of the sinus node.[11]

Accelerated Ectopic Automatic Rhythms. These rhythms are caused by enhanced normal automaticity of subsidiary pacemakers. The rate of discharge of these latent pacemakers will then be faster than the expected intrinsic automatic rate. Once the enhanced rate exceeds that of the sinus node, the enhanced ectopic pacemaker will prevail and overdrive the sinus node and other subsidiary pacemakers. A premature impulse caused by enhanced automaticity of latent pacemakers comes early in the normal rhythm, whereas an escape beat secondary to relief of overdrive suppression occurs late in normal rhythm.

Enhanced automaticity is usually caused by increased sympathetic tone, which steepens the slope of diastolic depolarization of latent pacemaker cells and diminishes the inhibitory effects of overdrive. Such sympathetic effects can be localized to subsidiary pacemakers in the absence of sinus node stimulation. Other causes of enhanced normal automaticity include periods of hypoxemia, ischemia, electrolyte disturbances, and certain drug toxicities. There is evidence that in the subacute phase of myocardial ischemia, increased activity of the sympathetic nervous system can enhance automaticity of Purkinje fibers, enabling them to escape from sinus node domination.[11]

Parasystole. Parasystole is a result of interaction between two fixed rate pacemakers having different discharge rates. The latent pacemaker is protected from being overdriven by the dominant rhythm (usually NSR) by intermittent or constant entrance block (i.e., impulses of sinus origin fail to depolarize the latent pacemaker secondary to block in the tissue surrounding the latent pacemaker focus). Such block, however, must be unidirectional, so that activity from the ectopic pacemaker can exit and produce depolarization whenever the surrounding myocardium is excitable. The protected pacemaker is said to be a parasystolic focus. In general, under these conditions, a protected focus of automaticity of this type can fire at its own intrinsic frequency and the intervals between discharges of each pacemaker are multiples of its intrinsic discharge rate. It is also possible that the depolarized level of membrane potential at which abnormal automaticity occurs can cause entrance block, leading to parasystole. This would be an example of an arrhythmia caused by a combination of an abnormality of impulse conduction and initiation.

Occasionally, the parasystolic focus can exhibit exit block, during which it can fail to depolarize excitable myocardium. Importantly, the parasystolic focus may not be at a truly fixed discharge rate because electrotonic current flow from surrounding regions can modulate the cycle length of a protected focus, either prolonging or abbreviating it, depending on whether the surrounding electrotonic activity occurs during the early or late stage of diastolic depolarization.[8] All these features of abnormal automaticity can be found in the Purkinje fibers that survive in regions of transmural MI and cause ventricular arrhythmias during the subacute phase.

Arrhythmias Caused by Abnormal Automaticity. There appears to be an association between abnormal Purkinje fiber automaticity and the arrhythmias that occur during the acute phase of myocardial infarction—for example, an accelerated idioventricular rhythm. However, the role of abnormal automaticity in the development of ventricular arrhythmias associated with chronic ischemic heart disease is less certain.[8] Additionally, isolated myocytes obtained from hypertrophied and failing hearts have been shown to manifest spontaneous diastolic depolarization and enhanced pacemaker currents, suggesting that abnormal automaticity can contribute to the occurrence of some arrhythmias in heart failure and left ventricular hypertrophy.[22,23]

Abnormal automaticity can underlie atrial tachycardia (AT), accelerated idioventricular rhythms, and ventricular tachycardia (VT), particularly that associated with ischemia and reperfusion. It has also been suggested that injury currents at the borders of ischemic zones can depolarize adjacent nonischemic tissue, predisposing to automatic VT.

Although automaticity is not responsible for most clinical tachyarrhythmias, which are usually caused by reentry, normal or abnormal automaticity can lead to arrhythmias caused by nonautomatic mechanisms. Premature beats, caused by automaticity, can initiate reentry. Rapid automatic activity in sites such as the cardiac veins can cause fibrillatory conduction, reentry, and atrial fibrillation (AF).[24,25]

TRIGGERED ACTIVITY

Triggered activity is impulse initiation in cardiac fibers caused by afterdepolarizations that occur consequent to a preceding impulse or series of impulses.[1,3] Afterdepolarizations are depolarizing oscillations in membrane potential that follow the upstroke of a preceding action potential.[3] Afterdepolarizations can occur early during the repolarization phase of the action potential (early afterdepolarization, EAD) or late, after completion of the repolarization phase (delayed afterdepolarization, DAD; Fig. 1-4). When either

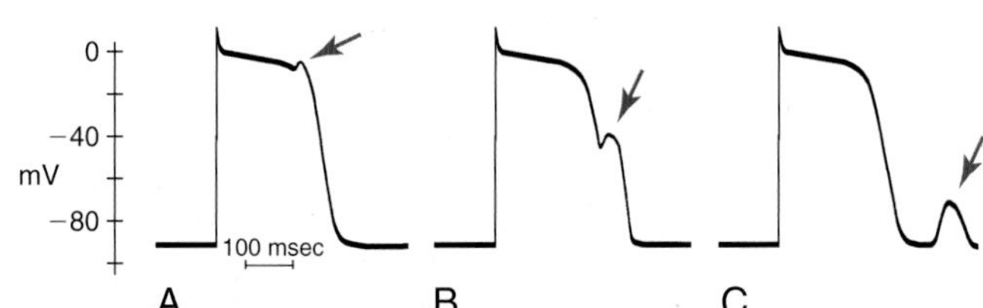

FIGURE 1–4 Types of afterdepolarizations. Afterdepolarizations are indicated by arrows. Purkinje cell action potentials are shown with phase 2 early afterdepolarizations (EADs) **(A)** and phase 3 EADs **(B)**, as well as delayed afterdepolarizations DADs **(C)**, which occur after full repolarization.

type of afterdepolarization is large enough to reach the threshold potential for activation of a regenerative inward current, a new action potential is generated, which is referred to as *triggered*.

Unlike automaticity, triggered activity is not a self-generating rhythm. Instead, triggered activity occurs as a response to a preceding impulse (the trigger). Automatic rhythms, on the other hand, can arise de novo in the absence of any prior electrical activity.

Delayed Afterdepolarizations and Triggered Activity

DADs are oscillations in membrane voltage that occur after completion of repolarization of the action potential (i.e., during phase 4). The transient nature of the DAD distinguishes it from normal spontaneous diastolic (pacemaker) depolarization, during which the membrane potential declines almost monotonically until the next action potential occurs. DADs may or may not reach threshold. Subthreshold DADs do not initiate action potentials or trigger arrhythmias. When a DAD does reach threshold, only one triggered action potential occurs (Fig. 1-5). The triggered action potential can also be followed by a DAD that, again, may or may not reach threshold and may or may not trigger another action potential. The first triggered action potential is often followed by a short or long train of additional triggered action potentials, each arising from the DAD caused by the previous action potential.

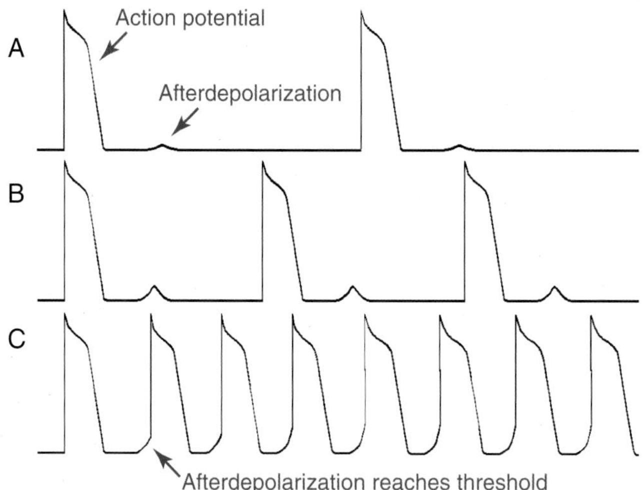

FIGURE 1–5 Behavior of delayed afterdepolarizations (DADs). **A,** The DAD is seen following the action potential at slow rates. **B,** At faster rates, the DAD occurs slightly earlier and increases in amplitude. **C,** At still more rapid rates, the DAD occurs even earlier and eventually reaches threshold, resulting in sustained firing.

Ionic Basis of Delayed Afterdepolarizations

DADs usually occur under a variety of conditions in which Ca^{2+} overload develops in the myoplasm and sarcoplasmic reticulum. During the normal action potential, Ca^{2+} flows through the L-type Ca^{2+} channels, causing a rapid rise in the concentration of intracellular Ca^{2+}, which in turn triggers Ca^{2+} release from the sarcoplasmic reticulum (so-called calcium-induced calcium release), causing a further rise in intracellular Ca^{2+} and initiating contraction (electromechanical coupling).[1,8,26-28] Ca^{2+} uptake by the sarcoplasmic reticulum then occurs during repolarization, and this process is enhanced by very high intracellular Ca^{2+}, catecholamine, or cAMP concentration (Fig. 1-6). Under such conditions, the Ca^{2+} in the sarcoplasmic reticulum can rise to a critical level during repolarization, at which time a secondary spontaneous release of Ca^{2+} from the sarcoplasmic reticulum occurs after the action potential. This secondary release of Ca^{2+} generates an aftercontraction as well as the transient inward (TI) current (an oscillatory membrane current of unclear ionic basis), either by increasing membrane permeability to inward Na^+ current or through electrogenic exchange of Ca^{2+} for Na^+. After one or several DADs, myoplasmic Ca^{2+} can decrease because the Na^+-Ca^{2+} exchanger extrudes Ca^{2+} from the cell, and the membrane potential stops oscillating.[20]

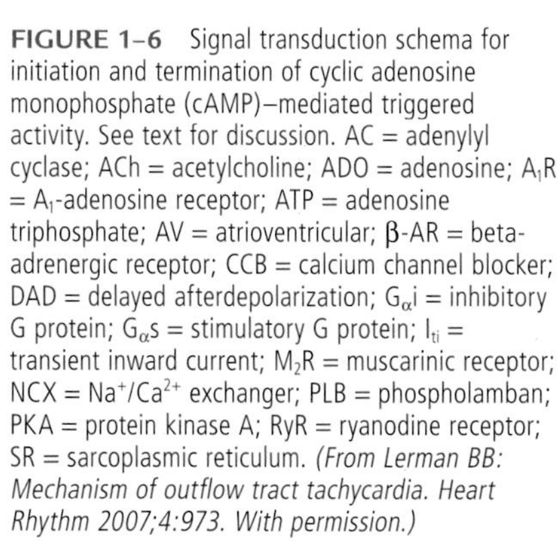

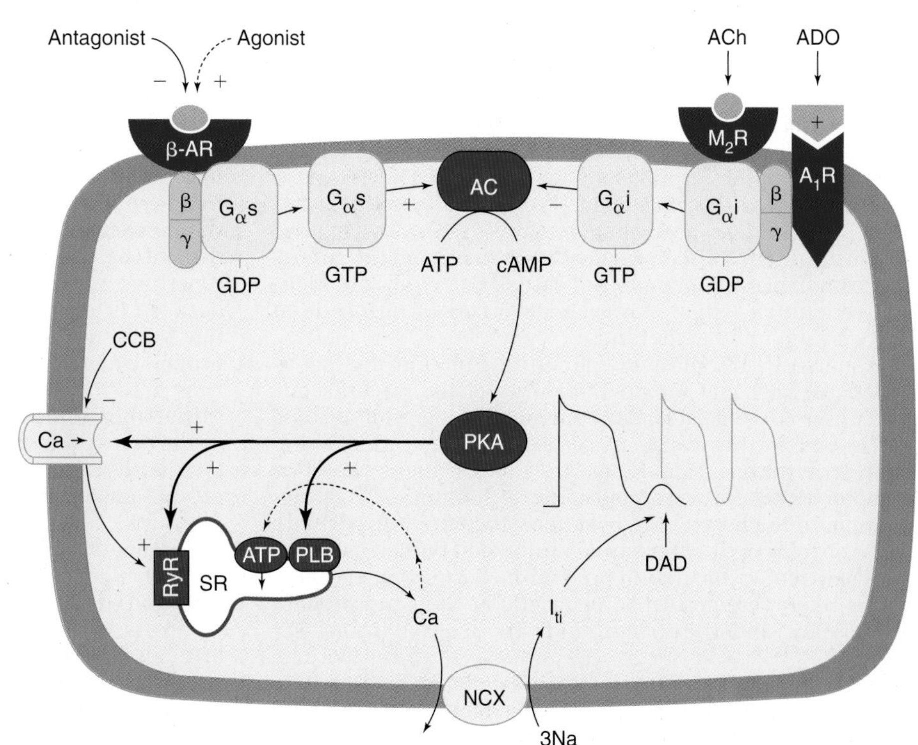

FIGURE 1–6 Signal transduction schema for initiation and termination of cyclic adenosine monophosphate (cAMP)–mediated triggered activity. See text for discussion. AC = adenylyl cyclase; ACh = acetylcholine; ADO = adenosine; A_1R = A_1-adenosine receptor; ATP = adenosine triphosphate; AV = atrioventricular; β-AR = beta-adrenergic receptor; CCB = calcium channel blocker; DAD = delayed afterdepolarization; $G_\alpha i$ = inhibitory G protein; $G_\alpha s$ = stimulatory G protein; I_{ti} = transient inward current; M_2R = muscarinic receptor; NCX = Na^+/Ca^{2+} exchanger; PLB = phospholamban; PKA = protein kinase A; RyR = ryanodine receptor; SR = sarcoplasmic reticulum. *(From Lerman BB: Mechanism of outflow tract tachycardia. Heart Rhythm 2007;4:973. With permission.)*

When the DADs are of low amplitude, they usually are not apparent or clinically significant. However, during pathological conditions (e.g., myocardial ischemia, acidosis, hypomagnesemia, digitalis toxicity, and increased catecholamines), the amplitude of the Ca^{2+}-mediated oscillations is increased and can reach the stimulation threshold, and a

spontaneous action potential is triggered. If this process continues, sustained tachycardia will develop.[8] Probably the most important influence that causes subthreshold DADs to reach threshold is a decrease in the initiating cycle length (CL), because that increases both the amplitude and rate of the DADs. Therefore, arrhythmias triggered by DADs can be expected to be initiated by a spontaneous or pacing-induced increase in the heart rate.

Digitalis causes DAD-dependent triggered arrhythmias by inhibiting the Na^+-K^+ exchange pump. In toxic amounts, this effect results in a measurable increase in intracellular Na^+, and diminishes Ca^{2+} extrusion from the cell by Na^+-Ca^{2+} exchange (secondary to reduction in the concentration-dependent driving force for Na^+ across the sarcolemma). Consequently, there is a net inward Ca^{2+} movement and intracellular Ca^{2+} overload.[8,20,29-31] Spontaneously occurring accelerated ventricular arrhythmias that occur during digitalis toxicity are likely to be caused by DADs. Triggered ventricular arrhythmias caused by digitalis also can be initiated by pacing at rapid rates. As toxicity progresses, the duration of the trains of repetitive responses induced by pacing increases.[31]

Catecholamines can cause DADs by increasing intracellular Ca^{2+} overload secondary to different potential mechanisms.[32-35] Catecholamines increase the slow, inward, L-type Ca^{2+} current through stimulation of beta-adrenergic receptors and increasing cAMP, which results in an increase in transsarcolemmal Ca^{2+} influx and intracellular Ca^{2+} overload (see Fig. 1-6). Catecholamines can also enhance the activity of the Na^+-Ca^{2+} exchanger, thus increasing the likelihood of DAD-mediated triggered activity. Additionally, catecholamines enhance the uptake of Ca^{2+} by the sarcoplasmic reticulum, leading to increased Ca^{2+} stored in the sarcoplasmic reticulum and the subsequent release of an increased amount of Ca^{2+} from the sarcoplasmic reticulum during contraction.[20] Sympathetic stimulation can potentially cause triggered atrial and ventricular arrhythmias, possibly some of the ventricular arrhythmias that accompany exercise and those occurring during ischemia and infarction.[11]

Elevations in intracellular Ca^{2+} in ischemic myocardium are also associated with DADs and triggered arrhythmias. Accumulation of lysophosphoglycerides in the ischemic myocardium, with consequent Na^+ and Ca^{2+} overload, has been suggested as a mechanism for DADs and triggered activity. Cells from damaged areas or surviving the infarction can display spontaneous release of Ca^{2+} from sarcoplasmic reticulum, which can generate waves of intracellular Ca^{2+} elevation and arrhythmias.

Abnormal sarcoplasmic reticulum function caused by genetic defects that impair the ability of the sarcoplasmic reticulum to sequester Ca^{2+} during diastole can lead to DADs and be the cause of certain inherited ventricular tachyarrhythmias. Mutations in the cardiac ryanodine receptor (RYR2), the sarcoplasmic reticulum Ca^{2+} release channel in the heart, have been identified in kindreds with the syndrome of catecholamine-stimulated polymorphic VT and ventricular fibrillation (VF) with short-QT intervals. It seems likely that perturbed intracellular Ca^{2+}, and perhaps also DADs, underlie arrhythmias in this syndrome (see Fig. 1-6).[36-40]

Several drugs can inhibit DAD-related triggered activity via different mechanisms, including reduction of the inward Ca^{2+} current and intracellular Ca^{2+} overload (Ca^{2+} channel blockers, beta-adrenergic blockers; see Fig. 1-6), reduction of Ca^{2+} release from the sarcoplasmic reticulum (caffeine, ryanodine, thapsigargin, cyclopiazonic acid), and reduction of the inward Na^+ current (terodotoxin, lidocaine, diphenylhydantoin).

DAD-related triggered activity is thought to be a mechanism for tachyarrhythmia associated with MI, reperfusion injury, right ventricular outflow tract (RVOT) VT and some atrial tachyarrhythmias. DADs are more likely to occur with fast spontaneous or paced rates, or with increased premature beats.

Properties of Delayed Afterdepolarizations

The TI current that causes DADs is dependent on the membrane potential (maximal at around −60 mV); therefore, the amplitude of DADs and the possibility of triggered activity are influenced by the level of membrane potential at which the action potentials occur.[41,42]

The duration of the action potential is a critical determinant of the presence of DADs. Longer action potentials, which are associated with more transsarcolemmal Ca^{2+} influx, are more likely to be associated with DADs. Drugs that prolong action potential duration (e.g., class IA antiarrhythmic agents) can increase DAD amplitude, whereas drugs that shorten action potential duration (e.g., class IB antiarrhythmic agents) can decrease DAD amplitude.[43]

The number of the action potentials preceding the DAD affects the amplitude of the DAD; that is, after a period of quiescence, the initiation of a single action potential can be followed by either no DAD or only a small one. With continued stimulation, the DADs increase in amplitude and triggered activity can eventually occur.

The amplitude of DADs and the coupling interval between the first triggered impulse and the last stimulated impulse that induced them are directly related to the drive CL at which triggered impulses are initiated.[8,30] A decrease in the basic drive CL (even a single drive cycle—i.e., premature impulse), in addition to increasing the DAD amplitude, results in a decrease in the coupling interval between the last drive cycle and the first DAD-triggered impulse, with respect to the last driven action potential, and an increase of the rate of DADs. Triggered activity tends to be induced by a critical decrease in the drive CL, either spontaneous, such as in sinus tachycardia, or pacing-induced. The increased time during which the membrane is in the depolarized state at shorter stimulation CLs or after premature impulses increases Ca^{2+} in the myoplasm and the sarcoplasmic reticulum, thus increasing the TI current responsible for the increased afterdepolarization amplitude and causing the current to reach its maximum amplitude more rapidly, decreasing the coupling interval of triggered impulses. The repetitive depolarizations can increase intracellular Ca^{2+} because of repeated activation of the inward Ca^{2+} current that flows through L-type Ca^{2+} channels. This characteristic property can help distinguish triggered activity from reentrant activity, because the relationship for reentry impulses initiated by rapid stimulation is often the opposite; that is, as the drive CL is reduced, the first reentrant impulse occurs later with respect to the last driven action potential because of rate-dependent conduction slowing in the reentrant pathway.

In general, triggered activity is influenced markedly by overdrive pacing. These effects are dependent on both the rate and duration of overdrive pacing. When overdrive pacing is performed for a critical duration of time and at a critical rate during a catecholamine-dependent triggered rhythm, the rate of triggered activity slows until the triggered rhythm stops, because of enhanced activity of the electrogenic Na^+-K^+ exchange pump induced by the increase in intracellular Na^+ caused by the increased number of action potentials. When overdrive pacing is not rapid enough to terminate the triggered rhythm, it can cause overdrive *acceleration*, in contrast to overdrive suppression observed with automatic rhythms. Single premature stimuli also can terminate triggered rhythms, although termination is much less common than it is by overdrive pacing.

Early Afterdepolarizations and Triggered Activity

EADs are oscillations in membrane potential that occur during the action potential and interrupt the orderly repolarization of the myocyte, manifesting as a sudden change in the time course of repolarization of an action potential such that the membrane voltage suddenly shifts in a depolarizing direction.[3]

Ionic Basis of Early Afterdepolarizations

The plateau of the action potential is a time of high membrane resistance, when there is little current flow. Consequently, small changes in repolarizing or depolarizing currents can have profound effects on the action potential duration and profile. Normally, during phases 2 and 3, the net membrane current is outward. Any factor that transiently shifts the net current in the inward direction can lead to EAD. Such a shift can arise from blockage of the outward current, carried by Na^+ or Ca^{2+} at that time, or enhancement of the inward current, mostly carried by K^+ at that time.[1]

EADs have been classified as phase 2 (occurring at the plateau level of membrane potential) and phase 3 (occurring during phase 3 of repolarization; see Fig. 1-4). The ionic mechanisms of phase 2 and 3 EADs and the upstrokes of the action potentials they elicit can differ.[1,8,28] At the depolarized membrane voltages of phase 2, the Na^+ current is inactivated and EADs can result from reactivation of the L-type Ca^{2+} current. EADs occurring late in repolarization occur at membrane potentials more negative than −60 mV in atrial, ventricular, or Purkinje cells that have normal resting potentials. Normally, a net outward membrane current shifts the membrane potential progressively in a negative direction during phase 3 repolarization of the action potential. Despite less data, it has been suggested that current through the Na^+-Ca^{2+} exchanger and possibly the Na^+ current can participate in the activation of phase 3 EADs.

The upstrokes of the action potentials elicited by phase 2 and phase 3 EADs also differ.[1] Phase 2 EAD-triggered action potential upstrokes are exclusively mediated by Ca^{2+} currents. Even if these triggered action potential do not propagate, they can substantially exaggerate heterogeneity of the time course of repolarization of the action potential (a key substrate for reentry), because EADs occur more readily in some regions (e.g., Purkinje, mid-LV myocardium, RVOT epicardium) than others (e.g., LV epicardium, endocardium). Action potentials triggered by phase 3 EADs arise from more negative membrane voltages. Therefore, the upstrokes can be caused by Na^+ and Ca^{2+} currents and are more likely to propagate.[3]

Under certain conditions, when an EAD is large enough, the decrease in membrane potential leads to an increase in net inward (depolarizing) current, and a second upstroke or an action potential is *triggered* before complete repolarization of the first. The triggered action potential also can be followed by other action potentials, all occurring at the low level of membrane potential characteristic of the plateau or at the higher level of membrane potential of later phase 3. The sustained rhythmic activity can continue for a variable number of impulses and terminates when repolarization of the initiating action potential returns membrane potential to a high level. As repolarization occurs, the rate of the triggered rhythm slows because the rate is dependent on the level of membrane potential. Sometimes repolarization to the high level of membrane potential may not occur, and membrane potential can remain at the plateau level or at a level intermediate between the plateau level and the resting potential. The sustained rhythmic activity then can continue at the reduced level of membrane potential and assumes the characteristics of abnormal automaticity. However, in contrast to automatic rhythms, without the initiating action potential, there could be no triggered action potentials.[8]

The ability of the triggered action potentials to propagate is related to the level of membrane potential at which the triggered action potentials occur.[8,44,45] The more negative the membrane potential, the more fast Na^+ channels are available for activation, the greater the influx of Na^+ into the cell during phase 0, and the higher the conduction velocity. At more positive membrane potentials of the plateau (phase 2) and early during phase 3, most fast Na^+ channels are still inactivated, and the triggered action potentials most likely have upstrokes caused by the inward L-type Ca^{2+} current. Therefore, those triggered action potentials have slow upstrokes and are less able to propagate.[3]

A fundamental condition that underlies the development of EADs is action potential prolongation, which is manifest on the surface electrocardiogram (ECG) by QT prolongation. Hypokalemia, hypomagnesemia, bradycardia, and drugs can predispose to the formation of EADs, invariably in the context of prolonging the action potential duration; drugs are the most common cause.[8] Class IA and III antiarrhythmic agents prolong the action potential duration and the QT interval, effects intended to be therapeutic but frequently causing proarrhythmia. Noncardiac drugs such as some phenothiazines, some nonsedating antihistamines, and some antibiotics can also prolong the action potential duration and predispose to EAD-mediated triggered arrhythmias, particularly when there is associated hypokalemia, bradycardia, or both.[46] Decreased extracellular K^+ concentration paradoxically decreases some membrane K^+ currents (particularly the delayed rectifier K^+ current, I_{Kr}) in the ventricular myocyte, explaining why hypokalemia causes action potential prolongation and EADs. EAD-mediated triggered activity likely underlies initiation of the characteristic polymorphic VT, torsades de pointes, seen in patients with congenital and acquired forms of long-QT syndrome. Although the genesis of ventricular arrhythmias in these patients is still unclear, marked transmural dispersion of repolarization can create a vulnerable window for development of reentry. EADs arising from these regions can underlie the premature complexes that initiate or perpetuate the tachycardia.[1,3,47] Structural heart disease such as cardiac hypertrophy and failure can also delay ventricular repolarization—so-called electrical remodeling—and predispose arrhythmias related to abnormalities of repolarization.[48] The abnormalities of repolarization in hypertrophy and failure are often magnified by concomitant drug therapy or electrolyte disturbances.

EADs are opposed by activators of ATP-dependent K^+ channels (pinacidil, chromakalim), magnesium, alpha-adrenergic blockade, tetrodotoxin, nitrendipine, and antiarrhythmic drugs that shorten action potential (e.g., lidocaine and mexilitine).[49,50] Alpha-adrenergic stimulation can exacerbate EADs.[51]

It has been traditionally thought that unlike DADs, EADs do not depend on a rise in intracellular Ca^{2+}; instead, action potential prolongation and reactivation of depolarizing currents are fundamental to their production. More recent experimental evidence has suggested a previously unappreciated interrelationship between intracellular Ca^{2+}

loading and EADs. Cytosolic Ca^{2+} levels can increase when action potentials are prolonged, which in turn appears to enhance L-type Ca^{2+} current (possibly via calcium-calmodulin kinase activation), further prolonging the action potential duration as well as providing the inward current driving EADs. Intracellular Ca^{2+} loading by action potential prolon-

gation can also enhance the likelihood of DADs. The interrelationship among intracellular Ca^{2+}, DADs, and EADs can be one explanation for the susceptibility of hearts that are Ca^{2+}-loaded (e.g., in ischemia or congestive heart failure) to develop arrhythmias, particularly on exposure to action potential–prolonging drugs.

Properties of Early Afterdepolarizations

EAD-triggered arrhythmias exhibit rate dependence. In general, the amplitude of an EAD is augmented at slow rates when action potentials are longer in duration.[8,52] Pacing-induced increases in rate shorten the action potential duration and reduce EAD amplitude. Action potential shortening and suppression of EADs with increased stimulation rate are likely the result of augmentation of delayed rectifier K^+ currents and perhaps hastening of Ca^{2+}-induced inactivation of L-type Ca^{2+} currents. Once EADs have achieved a steady-state magnitude at a constant drive CL, any event that shortens the drive CL tends to reduce their amplitude. Hence, the initiation of a single premature depolarization, which is associated with an acceleration of repolarization, will reduce the magnitude of the EADs that accompany the premature action potential; as a result, triggered activity is not expected to follow premature stimulation. The exception is when a long compensatory pause follows a premature ventricular contraction (PVC), which can predispose to the development of an EAD and can be the mechanism of torsades de pointes in some patients with the long-QT syndrome. Thus, EADs are more likely to trigger rhythmic activity when the spontaneous heart rate is slow, because bradycardia is associated with prolongation of the QT interval and action potential duration (e.g., bradycardia or pause-induced torsades de pointes). Similarly, catecholamines increase heart rate and decrease action potential duration and EAD amplitude, despite the effect of beta-adrenergic stimulation to increase L-type Ca^{2+} current.

REENTRY

Basic Principles of Reentry

During each normal cardiac cycle, at the completion of normal cardiac excitation, the electrical impulse originating from the sinus node becomes extinct and the subsequent excitation cycles originate from new pacemaker impulses.[1,3] Physiological excitation waves vanish spontaneously after the entire heart has been activated because of the long duration of refractoriness in the cardiac tissue compared with the duration of the excitation period; therefore, after its first pass, the impulse, having no place to go, expires. Reentry occurs when a propagating impulse fails to die out after normal activation of the heart and persists to reexcite the heart after expiration of the refractory period. In pathological settings, excitation waves can be blocked in circumscribed areas, rotate around these zones, and reenter the site of original excitation in repetitive cycles. The wavefront does not extinguish but rather propagates continuously, and thus continues to excite the heart because it always encounters excitable tissue.

Reentrant tachycardia, also called reentrant excitation, reciprocating tachycardia, circus movement, or reciprocal or echo beats, is a continuous repetitive propagation of the activation wave in a circular path, returning to its site of

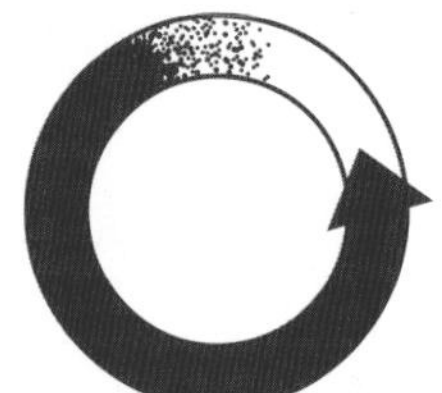

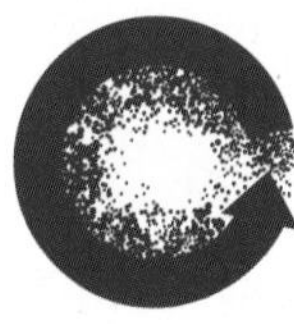

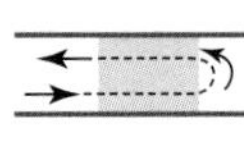

FIGURE 1–7 Models of reentry; solid area is completely refractory tissue, mottled area is partially refractory. In anatomical reentry, the circuit is determined by structures or scar in the heart and a portion of the circuit that has fully recovered excitability can be stimulated while it awaits the next cycle. In functional reentry, however, the rate is as rapid as it can be and still allow all portions of the circuit to recover.

TABLE 1–1	Criteria for Diagnosis of Reentrant Tachycardia

- Mapping activation in one direction around the continuous loop
- Correlation of continuous electrical activity with occurrence of tachycardia
- Correlation of unidirectional block with initiation of reentry
- Initiation and termination by premature stimulation
- Dependence of initiation of the arrhythmia on the site of pacing
- Inverse relationship between the coupling interval of the initiating premature stimulus and the interval to the first tachycardia beat
- Resetting of the tachycardia by a premature beat, with an inverse relationship between the coupling interval of the premature beat and the cycle length of the first or return beat of the tachycardia
- Fusion between a premature beat and the tachycardia beat followed by resetting
- Transient entrainment (with external overdrive pacing, the ability to enter the reentrant circuit and capture the circuit, resulting in a tachycardia at the pacing rate with fused complexes)
- Abrupt termination by premature stimulation
- Dependence of initiation on a critical slowing of conduction in the circuit
- Similarity with experimental models in which reentry is proven and is the only mechanism of tachycardia

origin to reactivate that site.[1,3,53,54] Traditionally, reentry has been divided into two types: (1) anatomical reentry, when there is a distinct relationship of the reentry pathway to the underlying tissue structure; and (2) functional reentry, when reentrant circuits occur at random locations without clearly defined anatomical boundaries (Fig. 1-7). Although this distinction has a historical background and is useful for didactic purposes, both the anatomical and functional forms can coexist in a given pathological setting and share many common basic biophysical mechanisms.

The original three criteria for reentry proposed by Mines[53,54] still hold true: (1) unidirectional block is necessary for initiation; (2) the wave of excitation should travel in a single direction around the pathway, returning to its point of origin and then restarting along the same path; and (3) the tachycardia should terminate when one limb of the pathway is cut or temporarily blocked. The twelve conditions that were proposed to prove or identify the existence of a reentrant tachycardia in the electrophysiology (EP) laboratory are listed in Table 1-1.

Requisites of Reentry

Substrate. The initiation and maintenance of a reentrant arrhythmia require the presence of myocardial tissue with adjacent tissue or pathways having different electrophysiological properties, conduction and refractoriness, and be joined proximally and distally, forming a circuit. These

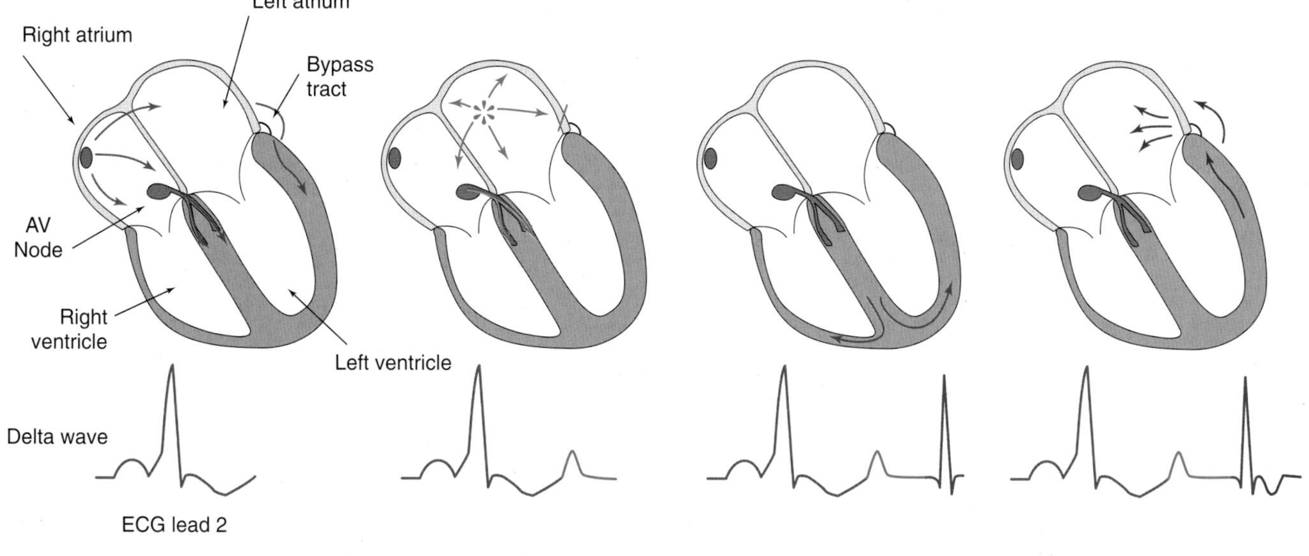

FIGURE 1–8 Reentry in the Wolff-Parkinson-White syndrome.

circuits can be stationary or can move within the myocardial substrate.

The reentrant circuit can be an anatomical structure, such as a loop of fiber bundles in the Purkinje system or accessory pathways, or a functionally defined pathway, with its existence, size, and shape determined by the electrophysiological properties of cardiac tissues in which the reentrant wavefront circulates, or it can be an anatomical-functional combination.[55] The cardiac tissue that constitutes the substrate for reentrant excitation can be located almost anywhere in the heart.[1,3] The reentrant circuit can be a variety of sizes and shapes and can include a number of different types of myocardial cells (e.g., atrial, ventricular, nodal, Purkinje; Fig. 1-8).

Central Area of Block. A core of inexcitable tissue around which the wavefront circulates is required to sustain reentry. Without this central area of block, the excitation wavefront will not necessarily be conducted around the core of excitable tissue; rather, it could take a shortcut, permitting the circulating excitation wavefront to arrive early at the site where it originated. If it arrives sufficiently early, the latter tissue will still be refractory, and reentrant excitation will not be possible.

As mentioned earlier, the area of block can be anatomical, functional, or a combination of the two.[8,56] Anatomical block is the result of a nonconductive medium in the center of the circuit, such as the tricuspid annulus in typical atrial flutter (AFL). Functional block at the center of a circuit occurs when there is block of impulses in otherwise excitable cardiac muscle. The central area of functional block develops during the initiation of the reentrant circuit by the formation of a line of block that most likely is due to refractoriness. When the reentrant circuit forms, the line of block then is sustained by centripetal activation from the circulating wavefront that, by repeatedly bombarding the central area of block, maintains the state of refractoriness of this region. A combination of an anatomical and a functional central area of block in the reentrant circuit has been described in some models of AFL such as the orifice of one or both venae cavae and an area of functional block continuous with or adjacent to either or both caval orifice(s). Additionally, it has now been shown that a functional extension of an anatomical line of block can occur such that it plays a role in creating the necessary or critical substrate for reentry. Thus, a surgical incision in the right atrium (RA) made to repair a congenital heart lesion can, under certain circumstances, develop a functional extension to one or both of the venae cavae, such that the substrate to develop and sustain AFL develops.

Unidirectional Conduction Block. Transient or permanent unidirectional block is usually a result of heterogeneity of electrophysiological properties of the myocardium, and is essential for the initiation of reentry. The excitation wavefront propagating in the substrate must encounter unidirectional block; otherwise, the excitation wavefronts traveling down both limbs of the reentrant circuit will collide and extinguish each other.[56]

Area of Slow Conduction. In a successful reentrant circuit, the wavefront of excitation must encounter excitable cells or the tachycardia will terminate. Therefore, a condition necessary for reentry is the maintenance of excitable tissue ahead of the propagating wavefront. In other words, the tissue initially activated by the excitation wavefront should have sufficient time to recover its excitability by the time the reentrant wavefront returns. Thus, conduction of the circulating wavefront must be sufficiently delayed in an alternate pathway to allow for expiration of the refractory period in the tissue proximal to the site of unidirectional block, and there must always be a gap of excitable tissue (fully or partially excitable) ahead of the circulating wavefront (i.e., the length of the reentrant pathway must equal or exceed the reentrant wavelength). This is facilitated by a sufficiently long reentrant pathway, which is especially important when conduction is normal along the reentrant path, sufficiently slow conduction in all or part of the alternative pathway, because sufficiently long pathways are usually not present in the heart, sufficient shortening of the refractory period, or a combination of these factors.[1,3]

The wavelength of the electrical impulse is defined as the product of the conduction velocity and the refractory period of the tissue involved in the circuit, which defines the anatomical size of the circuit. Note that this formula can be misleading in situations in which either value changes along the length of the circuit. In a macroreentrant circuit, such as atrioventricular reentrant tachycardia (AVRT; see Fig. 1-8), the anatomical circuit is clearly longer than the wavelength of the tachycardia. However, most forms of intramyocardial reentry require a substantial decrease in conduction velocity to enable sustained reentry. The wavelength formula makes it clear that a decrease in conduction velocity or shortened refractory period results in a decrease in the wavelength or lessening of the amount of tissue needed to sustain reentry. This situation favors initiation and maintenance of reentry. In contrast, an increase in conduction velocity or prolongation of refractoriness will prolong the wavelength of excitation and, in this situation, a larger anatomical circuit will be necessary to sustain reentry. If a larger circuit is not possible, initiation or maintenance of tachycardia cannot occur.

Critical Tissue Mass. An additional requisite for random reentry is the necessity of a critical mass of tissue to sustain the one or usually more simultaneously circulating reentrant wavefronts. Thus, it is essentially impossible to achieve sustained fibrillation of ventricles of very small, normal, mammalian hearts and equally difficult to achieve sustained fibrillation of the completely normal atria of humans or smaller mammals.

Initiating Trigger. Another prerequisite for reentrant excitation to occur is often, but not always, the presence of an initiating trigger, which invokes the necessary electrophysiological milieu for initiation of reentry.[1,3] Susceptible patients with appropriate underlying substrates usually do not suffer from incessant tachycardia because the different electrophysiological mechanisms required for the initiation and maintenance of a reentrant tachycardia are infrequently present at exactly the same time. However, changes in heart rate or autonomic tone, ischemia, electrolyte or pH abnormalities, or the occurrence of a premature depolarization can be sufficient to initiate a reentrant tachycardia.

The trigger frequently is required because it elicits or brings to a critical state one or more of the conditions necessary to achieve reentrant excitation. In fact, premature depolarizations frequently initiate these tachyarrhythmias because they can cause slow conduction and unidirectional block. Thus, a premature impulse initiating reentry can arrive at one site in the potential reentrant circuit sufficiently early that it encounters unidirectional block, because that tissue has had insufficient time to recover excitability after excitation by the prior impulse. Furthermore, in the other limb of the potential reentrant circuit, the premature arrival of the excitation wavefront causes slow conduction or results in further slowing of conduction of the excitation wavefront through an area of already slow conduction. The resulting increase in conduction time around this limb of the potential reentrant circuit allows the region of unidirectional block in the tissue in the other limb activated initially by the premature beat to recover excitability. It should be noted that the mechanism causing the premature impulse can be different from the reentrant mechanism causing the tachycardia. Thus, the premature impulse can be caused by automaticity or triggered activity.

Types of Reentrant Circuits

Anatomical Reentry

In anatomically determined circuits, a discrete inexcitable anatomical obstacle creates a surrounding circular pathway, resulting in a fixed length and location of the reentrant circuit. The length and location of the reentrant pathway are relatively fixed and the characteristics of the reentrant circuit are determined by the characteristics of the anatomical components of that circuit.

A reentrant tachycardia is initiated when an excitation wavefront splits into two limbs after going around the anatomical obstacle and travels down one pathway and not the other, creating a circus movement. Tachycardia rates are determined by the wavelength and length of the reentrant pathway (the path length). The initiation and maintenance of anatomical reentry is dependent on conduction velocity and refractory period. Thus, as long as the extension of the refractory zone behind the excitation wave, the so-called wavelength of excitation (wavelength = conduction velocity × refractory period), is smaller than the entire length of the anatomically defined reentrant pathway, a zone of excitable tissue, the so-called excitable gap, exists between the tail of the preceding wave and the head of the following wave.[56] In essence, circus movements containing an excitable gap are stable with respect to their frequency of rotation and can persist at a constant rate for hours. In the case in which the wavelength of excitation exceeds the path length, the excitation wavefront becomes extinct when it encounters the not yet recovered inexcitable tissue. A special case is present in the intermediate situation, when the head of the following wavefront meets the partially refractory tail of the preceding wavefront (i.e., the wavelength approximates the path length). This situation is characterized by unstable reentrant cycle lenghts and complex dynamics of the reentrant wavefront. There is often a long excitable gap associated with anatomical reentry.

Anatomical circuits therefore are associated with ordered reentry. Examples of this type of reentry are AVRT associated with an AV bypass tract (BT), AV nodal reentry tachycardia (AVNRT), AFL, VT originating within the HPS (bundle branch reentry [BBR] VT), and post-MI VT.

Functional Reentry

In functionally determined circuits, the reentrant pathway depends on the intrinsic heterogeneity of the electrophysiological properties of the myocardium, not by a predetermined anatomical circuit (i.e., without involvement of an anatomical obstacle or anatomically defined conducting pathway). Such heterogeneity involves dispersion of excitability or refractoriness and conduction velocity, as well as anisotropic conduction properties of the myocardium.[57-59]

Functional circuits typically tend to be small and unstable; the reentrant excitation wavefront can fragment, generating other areas of reentry. The location and size of these tachycardias can vary. The circumference of the leading circle around a functional obstacle can be as small as 6 to 8 mm and represents a pathway in which the efficacy of stimulation of the circulating wavefront is just sufficient to excite the tissue ahead, which is still in its relative refractory phase. Therefore, conduction through the functional reentrant circuit is slowed because impulses are propagating in partially refractory tissue. Consequently, this form of functional reentry has a partially excitable gap. The reentry cycle lengths are, therefore, significantly dependent on the refractory period of the involved tissue.[58]

The mechanisms for functionally determined reentrant circuits include the leading circle type of reentry, anisotropic reentry, and spiral wave reentry. Functional circuits can be associated with ordered reentry (the reentrant circuit remains in the same place) or random reentry (the reentrant circuit changes size and location). Random reentry can occur when leading circle reentry causes fibrillation.

Leading Circle Concept. To explain the properties of a single functional reentrant circuit, Allessie and colleagues have formulated the leading circle concept (see Fig. 1-7).[58] It was postulated that during wavefront rotation in tissue without anatomical inexcitable obstacles, the wavefront impinges on its refractory tail and travels through partially refractory tissue. The interaction between the wavefront and the refractory tail determines the properties of functional reentry. In this model, functional reentry involves the propagation of an impulse around a functionally determined region of inexcitable tissue or a refractory core and among neighboring fibers with different electrophysiological properties. The tissue within this core is maintained in a state of refractoriness by constant centripetal bombardment from the circulating wavefront. The premature impulse that initiates reentry blocks in fibers with long refractory periods and conducts in fibers with shorter refractory periods eventually returns to the initial region of block after excitability has recovered there. The impulse then continues to circulate around a central area that is kept refractory because it is bombarded constantly by wavelets propagating toward it from the circulating wavefront. This central area provides a functional obstacle that prevents excitation from propagating across the fulcrum of the circuit.

The leading circle was defined as "the smallest possible pathway in which the impulse can continue to circulate" and "in which the stimulating efficacy of the wavefront is just enough to excite the tissue ahead which is still in its relative refractory phase."[58] Thus, the "head of the circulating wavefront is continuously biting its tail of refractoriness" and the length of the reentrant pathway equals the wavelength of the impulse; as a result, there is usually no fully excitable gap.[58] Because the wavefront propagates through partially refractory tissue, the conduction velocity is reduced.

The velocity value and the length of the circuit depend on the excitability of the partially refractory tissue and on the stimulating efficacy of the wavefront, which is determined by the amplitude and the upstroke velocity of the action potential and by the passive electric properties of the tissue (e.g., gap junctional conductance). The partially refractory tissue determines the revolution time period. Because of the absence of a fully excitable gap, this form of reentry is less susceptible to resetting, entrainment, and termination by premature stimuli and pacing maneuvers. Leading circle reentry is thought to be the underlying mechanism of AF and VF and of at least some of the ventricular arrhythmias associated with acute ischemia.

Anisotropic Reentry. Isotropic conduction is uniform in all directions; anisotropic conduction is not. Anisotropy is the normal feature of heart muscle and is related to the differences in longitudinal and transverse conduction velocities, which are determined by the orientation of myocardial fibers and the manner in which these fibers and muscle bundles are connected to each other (Fig. 1-9). Anisotropic conduction occurs in myocardium composed of tissue with structural features different from those of adjacent tissue, resulting in heterogeneity in conduction velocities and repolarization properties, which can result in blocked impulses and slowed conduction, thereby setting the stage for reentry. Anisotropy can cause conduction slow enough to result in reentry in small anatomical circuits.[60]

Unlike the functional characteristic that leads to the leading circle type of reentry—local differences in membrane properties cause a difference in refractoriness in adjacent areas—in functional reentry caused by anisotropy, the

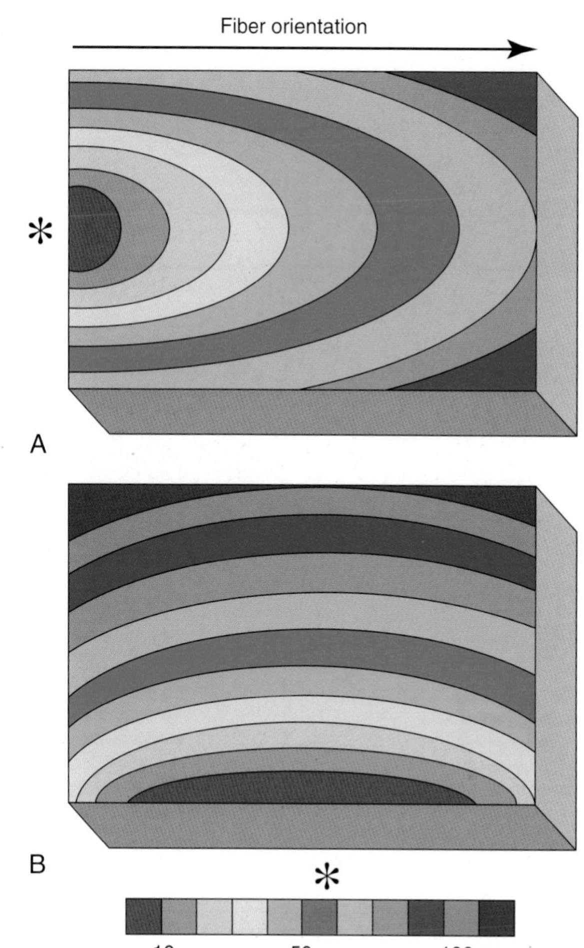

FIGURE 1–9 Anisotropic conduction. Progression of activation wavefronts in blocks of ventricular myocardium with longitudinal fiber orientation are shown. A wavefront stimulated (*) at the left edge progresses more rapidly (wider isochrone spacing, **A**) than one starting perpendicularly (**B**) because of more favorable conduction parameters in the former direction.

functional characteristic that is important is the difference in effective axial resistance to impulse propagation dependent on fiber direction. In its pure form, the unidirectional conduction block and slow conduction in the reentrant circuit result from anisotropic, discontinuous propagation, and there is no need for variations in membrane properties, such as regional differences in refractoriness or depression of the resting and action potentials.[60]

Anisotropic circuits are elliptical or rectangular because of the directional differences in conduction velocities, with the long axis of the ellipse in the fast longitudinal direction and a central line of functional block parallel to the long axis of fibers. Circuits with this shape can have a smaller dimension than circular circuits, such as the leading circle. Reentrant circuits caused by anisotropy also can occur without well-defined anatomical pathways and may be classified as functional.[60]

Anisotropic reentrant circuits usually remain in a fixed position and cause ordered reentry. The degree of anisotropy, the ratio of longitudinal to transverse conduction velocity, varies in different regions of the heart, and the circuit can reside only in a region in which the conduction transverse to the longitudinal axis is sufficiently slow to allow reentry. Stability of anisotropic reentrant circuits is also assisted by the presence of an excitable gap, which does not occur in the leading circle functional circuit. The excitable gap is caused by the sudden slowing of conduction velocity and a decrease in the wavelength of excitation as

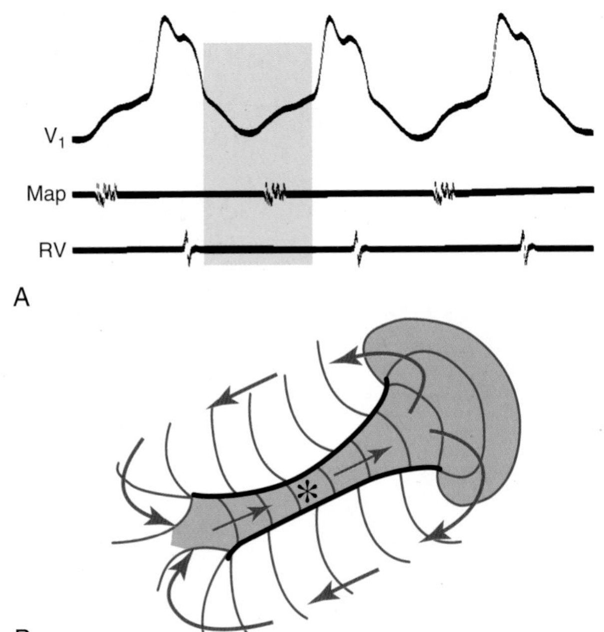

FIGURE 1–10 Figure-of-8 reentry. **A,** An ECG and intracardiac recordings from a left ventricular mapping catheter (Map) and the right ventricle (RV) are shown during scar-based ventricular tachycardia. **B,** A stylized tachycardia circuit is shown in which propagation proceeds through a central common pathway (small arrows) constrained by scar or other barriers and then around the outside of these same barriers. Activation in the circuit during electrical diastole is shaded (also in **A**).

the reentrant impulse turns the corner from the fast longitudinal direction to the slow transverse direction and from the slow transverse direction to the fast longitudinal direction.[61] Anisotropic reentry is typically initiated by a premature stimulus that blocks in the direction of propagation parallel to the long axis of the cells, and then propagates slowly in the transverse direction of fiber orientation because of high axial resistance (see later).

Anisotropic reentry can be responsible for sustained VT that occurs in the epicardial border zone region of healed infarcts, where viable normal myocytes are intermingled with islands of fibrous connective tissue, separating muscle-fiber bundles preferentially in the longitudinal direction and decreasing the density of side-to-side junctional connections, therefore creating nonuniform anisotropy.

Figure-of-8 Reentry. The model of figure-of-8 or double-loop reentry involves two concomitant excitation wavefronts circulating in opposite directions, clockwise and counterclockwise, around a long line of functional conduction block rejoining on the distal side of the block. The wavefront then breaks through the arc of block to reexcite the tissue proximal to the block. The single arc of block is thus divided into two and reentrant activation continues as two circulating wavefronts that travel clockwise and counterclockwise around the two arcs in a pretzel-like configuration.[62] This form of reentry has been shown in atrial and ventricular myocardia (Fig. 1-10).

Reflection. Reflection is a special subclass of reentry in which the excitation wavefront does not require a circuit but appears to travel along the *same* pathway in both directions. As in reentry, an area of conduction delay is required, and the total time for the excitation wavefront to leave and return to its site of origin must exceed the refractory period of the proximal segment (see Fig. 1-7).

Spiral Wave (Rotor) Activity. The leading circle concept was based on properties of impulse propagation in a one-dimensional tissue that forms a closed pathway (e.g., a ring). The concept was a major breakthrough in the understanding of the mechanisms of reentrant excitation. However, it became evident that these considerations alone do not fully describe wave rotation in two- and three-dimensional cardiac tissue.

Spiral waves typically describe reentry in two dimensions. The term *rotor* initially described the rotating source, and the spiral wave defined the shape of the wave emerging from the rotating source. In many publications, this difference has been blurred, and terms used in the literature include *rotors, vortices,* and *reverberators.*[56,63] The center of the spiral wave is called the core and the distribution of the core in three dimensions is referred to as the filament. The three-dimensional form of the spiral wave is called a *scroll wave.*[62]

Under appropriate circumstances, a pulse in two-dimensional, homogeneous, excitable media can be made to circulate as a rotor. When heterogeneities in recovery exist, the application of a second stimulus over a large geometric area to initiate a second excitation wave only excites a region in which there has been sufficient time for recovery from the previous excitation, not regions that have not yet recovered. An excitation wave is elicited at the excitable site in the form of a rotor because the wave cannot move in the direction of the wake of the previous wave but only in the opposite direction, moving into adjacent regions as they in turn recover. The inner tip of the wavefront circulates around an organizing center or core, which includes cells with transmembrane potentials that have a reduced amplitude, duration, and rate of depolarization (i.e., slow upstroke velocity of phase 0); these cells are potentially excitable, but remain unexcited, instead of a region of conduction block. In the center of the rotating wave, the tip of the wave moves along a complex trajectory and radiates waves into the surrounding medium. In addition, the spiral waves can give rise to daughter spirals that can result in disorganized electrical activity.

The curvature of the spiral wave is the key to the formation of the core and the functional region of block.[56,62] Propagation of two- and three-dimensional waves also depends on wavefront curvature, a property that is not present in one-dimensional preparations.[56] Because the maximal velocity of a convex rotating wavefront can never exceed the velocity of a flat front and the period of rotation remains constant in a stable rotating wave, the velocity has to decrease from the periphery (where the highest value corresponds to linear velocity) to the center of a rotating wave. As a consequence, any freely rotating wave in an excitation-diffusion system has to assume a spiral shape. A prominent curvature of the spiral wave is generally encountered following a wave break, a situation in which a planar wave encounters an obstacle and breaks up into two or more daughter waves. Because it has the greatest curvature, the broken end of the wave moves most slowly. As curvature decreases along the more distal parts of the spiral, propagation speed increases.[62] The rotor, by definition, has a marked curvature, and this curvature slows down its propagation. Slow conduction results from an increased electrical load; that is, not only must a curved wavefront depolarize cells ahead of it in the direction of propagation, but current also flows to cells on its sides.

Because the slow activation by a rotor is not dependent on conduction in relatively refractory myocardium, an excitable gap exists, despite the functional nature of reentry. This type of functional reentrant excitation does not require any inhomogeneities of refractory periods as in leading circle reentry, inhomogeneities in conduction properties as in anisotropic reentry, or a central obstacle, whether functional or anatomical. The heterogeneity that allows initiation can result from a previous excitation wave and the pattern of recovery from that wave. Even though nonuniform dispersions of refractoriness or anisotropy are not necessary for the initiation of reentrant excitation caused by rotors in excitable media, the myocardium, even when normal, is never homogeneous, and anisotropy and anatomical obstacles can modify the characteristics and spatiotemporal behavior of the spiral.

The location of the rotor can occur wherever the second stimulated excitation encounters the wake of the first excitation with the appropriate characteristics. Spirals can be *stationary*, continuously drift or migrate away from their origin, or be *anchored*, initially drifting and then becoming stationary by anchoring to a small obstacle.

In the heart, spiral waves have been implicated in the generation of cardiac arrhythmias for a long time. Both two-dimensional spiral waves and three-dimensional scroll waves have been implicated in the mechanisms of reentry in atrial and ventricular tachycardia and fibrillation.[56,64] Monomorphic VT results when the spiral wave is anchored and cannot drift within the ventricular myocardium away from its origin. In contrast, a polymorphic VT, such as the torsade de pointes encountered with long-QT syndromes, is thought to be caused by a meandering or drifting spiral wave. VF seems to be the most complex representation of rotating spiral waves in the heart. VF develops when the single spiral wave responsible for VT breaks up, leading to the development of multiple spirals that are continuously extinguished and recreated.[62]

Excitable Gaps in Reentrant Circuits

Wavelength Concept

The wavelength is the product of the conduction velocity of the circulating excitation wavefront and the effective refractory period of the tissue in which the excitation wavefront is propagating.[8] The wavelength quantifies how far the impulse travels relative to the duration of the refractory period. The wavelength of the reentrant excitation wavefront must be shorter than the length of the pathway of the potential reentrant circuit for reentrant excitation to occur; that is, the impulse must travel a distance during the refractory period that is less than the complete reentrant path length to give myocardium ahead of it sufficient time to recover excitability. Slowing of impulse conduction or shortening of refractoriness shortens the wavelength and increases the excitable gap.

For almost all clinically important reentrant arrhythmias resulting from ordered reentry and in the presence of uniform, normal conduction velocity along the potential reentrant pathway, the wavelength would be too long to permit reentrant excitation. Thus, almost all these arrhythmias must have, and do have, one or more areas of slow conduction as a part of the reentrant circuit. The associated changes in conduction velocity, as well as associated changes in refractory periods, actually cause the wavelength to change in different parts of the circuit. However, the presence of one or more areas of slow conduction permits the average wavelength of reentrant activation to be shorter than the path length.

The wavelength concept is a good predictive parameter of arrhythmia inducibility. A short wavelength indicates that initiation of reentry would require a small area of functional conduction block and, therefore, a little dispersion of refractoriness could easily lead to reentry.

Excitable Gaps

The excitable gap in a reentrant circuit is the region of excitable myocardium that exists between the head of the reentrant wavefront and the tail of the preceding wavefront and, at any given time, is no longer refractory (i.e., is capable of being excited) if the excitation wavelength is shorter than the length of the reentrant circuit (Fig. 1-11).

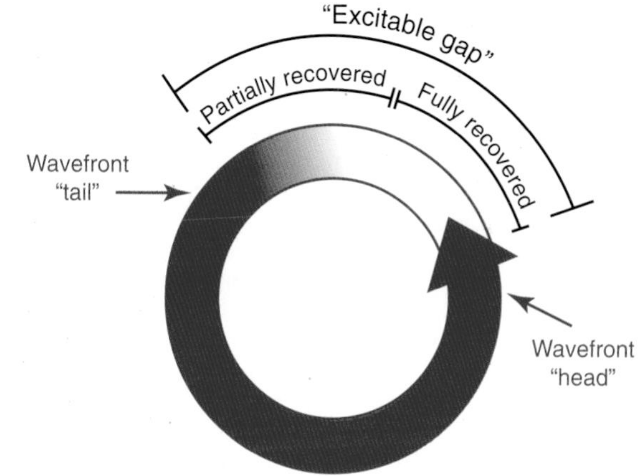

FIGURE 1–11 Excitable gap of recovered tissue in anatomically determined reentry.

The occurrence of an excitable gap is dependent on the recovery of excitability of the myocardium from its previous excitation by the reentrant wavefront. A fully excitable gap is defined as the segment of the reentrant circuit in which the tail of the preceding wavefront does not affect the head and velocity of the following wavefront (absence of head-tail interaction). A partially excitable gap is defined as the zone where the rotating wave can be captured by local stimulation in the presence of head-tail interaction. Whereas the excitable gap denotes a length of a segment within the reentrant circuit, the fully or partially excitable period denotes the time period during which a segment within the reentrant circuit is fully or partially excitable, respectively (see Fig. 1-11).

There are two different measurements of the excitable gap. The spatial excitable gap is the distance (in millimeters) of excitability occupied at any moment of time in the circuit ahead of the reentrant wavefront. On the other hand, the temporal excitable gap is the time interval (in milliseconds) of excitability between the head of activation of one impulse and the tail of refractoriness of the prior impulse. Both the spatial and temporal gaps can be composed of partially excitable or fully excitable myocardium, depending on the time interval between successive excitations of the circuit. The size of the spatial gap and the duration of the temporal gap vary in different parts of the circuit as the wavelength of the reentrant impulse changes because of changes in conduction velocity, refractory periods, or both.

The characteristics of the excitable gap can be different in different types of reentrant circuits. Many anatomically determined reentrant circuits have large excitable gaps with a fully excitable component although, even in anatomically determined circuits, the gap can sometimes be only partially excitable. On the other hand, functional reentrant circuits caused by the leading circle mechanism have very small gaps that are only partially excitable, although parts of some functionally determined reentrant circuits (anisotropic reentrant circuits) can have fully excitable gaps. An excitable gap has been shown to occur during AF, VF, and AFL; these are examples of arrhythmias caused by functional reentrant mechanisms, possibly including spiral waves.[65,66] The relationship between the excitable gap and the excitable period can be complex if the velocity of propagation changes within the reentry circuit.[56]

The existence and the extent of an excitable gap in a reentrant circuit have important implications.[56] The presence of an excitable gap enables modulation of the frequency of a reentrant tachycardia by a locally applied stimulus or by field stimulation; the longer the excitable gap, the more likely it is for an extrastimulus to be able to enter the reentrant circuit and initiate or terminate a reentrant arrhythmia. In addition, resetting and entrainment are more likely

to occur when the excitable gap is longer. The excitable gap can be exploited to terminate a reentrant tachycardia. The presence of a significant temporal and spatial excitable gap in some reentrant circuits enables reentry to be terminated by a single premature stimulus or by overdrive stimulation. Termination of arrhythmias by stimulation would be expected to be much more difficult when the reentrant circuit has only a small partially excitable gap. Additionally, the excitable gap can influence the effects of drugs on the reentrant circuit, so that reentry with a partially excitable gap and mainly functional components may respond more readily to drugs that prolong repolarization, without slowing conduction, whereas fixed anatomical reentry with a large excitable gap will respond to drugs that decrease conduction velocity, preferentially at pivot points.

The properties of the excitable gap influence the characteristics of arrhythmias caused by reentry. Arrhythmias caused by leading circle reentry, in which the wavefront propagates in the just-recovered myocardium of the refractory tail and in which there is only a small partially excitable gap, are inherently unstable and often terminate after a short period or go on to fibrillation. On the other hand, the reentrant wavefront in anatomical and nonuniform anisotropic reentrant circuits, in general, is not propagating in myocardium that has just recovered excitability and the excitable gap can be large. This property can contribute to the stability of these reentrant circuits.[56]

The shape of the anatomical obstacle determines the path of a reentrant wave in fixed anatomical reentry. Therefore, instability of anatomical reentry is confined to variations of the rotating interval and wavelength of excitation. This instability is characterized by the wavefront invading the repolarizing phase of the preceding wave, resulting in oscillations of the rotation period.[56]

Resetting Reentrant Tachycardias

Definition

Resetting is the advancement, made to occur earlier, of a tachycardia impulse by timed premature electrical stimuli. The extrastimulus is followed by a pause that is less than fully compensatory before resumption of the original rhythm. The tachycardia complexes that return first should have the same morphology and CL as the tachycardia before the extrastimulus, regardless of whether single or multiple extrastimuli are used.[67-69]

The introduction of a single extrastimulus (S_2) during a tachycardia yields a return cycle (S_2X_3) if the tachycardia is not terminated (Fig. 1-12). If S_2 does not affect the arrhythmogenic focus, the coupling interval (X_1S_2) plus the return cycle (S_2X_3) will be equal to twice the tachycardia cycle ($2 \times [X_1X_1]$); that is, a fully compensatory pause will occur. Resetting of the tachycardia occurs when a less than fully compensatory pause occurs. In this situation, $X_1S_2 + S_2X_3$ will be less than $2 \times (X_1X_1)$, as measured from the surface ECG. Tachycardia CL stability should be taken into account when the return cycle is measused. To account for any tachycardia CL instability, at least a 20-millisecond shortening of the return cycle is required to demonstrate resetting.[70]

When more than a single extrastimulus is used, the relative prematurity should be corrected by subtracting the coupling interval(s) from the spontaneous tachycardia cycles when the extrastimuli are delivered.

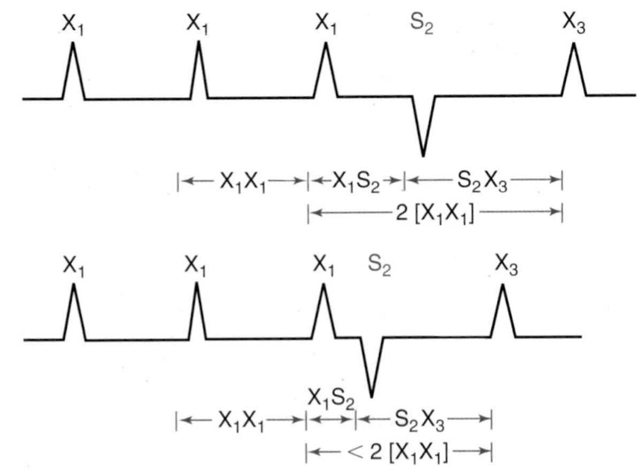

FIGURE 1–12 Response of tachycardia to a single extrastimulus (S_2). The tachycardia cycle length (CL) is [X_1X_1]. The coupling interval of the extrastimulus is [X_1S_2]. The return CL of the first complex of tachycardia after the extrastimulus is [S_2X_3]. In the top portion of the figure, the extrastimulus does not affect the tachycardia circuit and a compensatory pause occurs. Resetting (i.e., advancement) of the tachycardia is shown at the bottom of the figure. *(Reproduced with permission from Frazier DW, Stanton MS: Resetting and transient entrainment of ventricular tachycardia. Pacing Clin Electrophysiol 1995;18:1919.)*

Reentrant Tachycardia Resetting

To reset a reentrant tachycardia, the stimulated wavefront must reach the reentrant circuit, encounter excitable tissue within the circuit (i.e., enter the excitable gap of the reentrant circuit), collide in the antidromic (retrograde) direction with the previous tachycardia impulse, and continue in the orthodromic (anterograde) direction to exit at an earlier than expected time and perpetuate the tachycardia (Fig. 1-13).[67-69,71] If the extrastimulus encounters a fully excitable tissue, which commonly occurs in reentrant tachycardias with large excitable gaps, the tachycardia is advanced by the extent that the stimulated wavefront arrives at the entrance site prematurely. If the tissue is partially excitable, which can occur in reentrant tachycardias with small or partially excitable gaps or even in circuits with large excitable gaps when the extrastimulus is very premature, the stimulated wavefront will encounter some conduction delay in the orthodromic direction within the circuit (see Fig. 1-13). Therefore, the degree of advancement of the next tachycardia beat will depend on both the degree of prematurity of the extrastimulus and the degree of slowing of its conduction within the circuit. The reset tachycardia beat consequently can be early, on time, or delayed.

Termination of the tachycardia occurs when the extrastimulus collides with the preceding tachycardia impulse antidromically and blocks in the reentrant circuit orthodromically (see Fig. 1-13). This occurs when the premature impulse enters the reentrant circuit early in the relative refractory period; it fails to propagate in the anterograde direction because it encounters absolutely refractory tissue. In the retrograde direction, it encounters increasingly recovered tissue and can propagate until it encroaches on the circulating wavefront and terminates the arrhythmia.[70]

Resetting does not require that the pacing site be located in the reentrant circuit. The closer the pacing site to the circuit, however, the less premature a single stimulus can be and reach the circuit without being extinguished by collision with a wave emerging from the circuit. The longest coupling interval for an extrastimulus to be able to reset a reentrant tachycardia will depend on the tachycardia CL, duration of the excitable gap of the tachycardia, refractoriness at the pacing site, and conduction time from the pacing site to the reentrant circuit.[70]

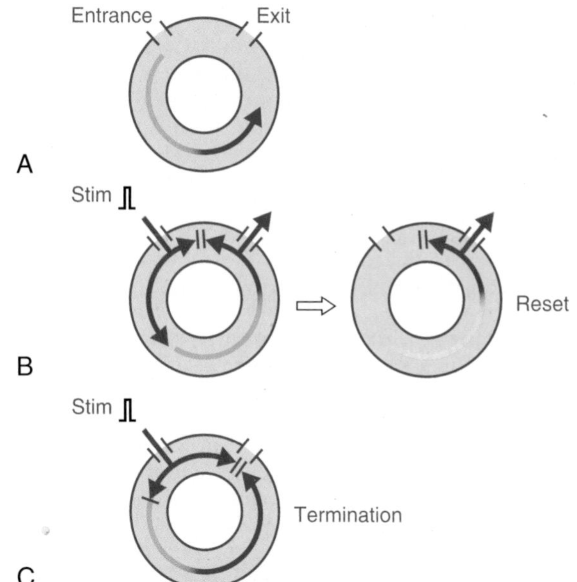

FIGURE 1–13 **A,** Schematic representation of the reentrant circuit is illustrated with separate entrance and exit sites. During tachycardia, a wavefront is shown propagating through the tissue of the reentrant circuit (arrow). The dark portion of the arrow represents fully refractory tissue and the fading portion represents partially refractory tissue. **B,** A premature stimulus (Stim) introduced during the tachycardia results in a wavefront of depolarization (red arrow), which enters the reentrant circuit and conducts antegradely over fully excitable tissue while it collides retrogradely with the already propagating wavefront (blue arrow). The premature wavefront (red arrow) then propagates around the circuit to the exit site, leading to the less than compensatory pause and resetting of the tachycardia. **C,** A more premature extrastimulus (Stim) results in a wavefront of depolarization (red arrow), which enters the circuit at a time when it collides retrogradely with the previously propagating wavefront (blue arrow) and encounters antegrade tissue incapable of sustaining further propagation. As a result, circus movement in the circuit is extinguished and tachycardia terminates. *(Reproduced with permission from Rosenthal ME, Stamato NJ, Almendral JM, et al: Coupling intervals of ventricular extrastimuli causing resetting of sustained ventricular tachycardia secondary to coronary artery disease: Relation to subsequent termination. Am J Cardiol 1988;61:770.)*

Resetting Zone and Excitable Gap. For an extrastimulus to be able to reset the reentrant circuit, it has to penetrate the circuit during its excitable gap. The difference between the longest and shortest coupling intervals resulting in resetting is defined as the resetting interval or resetting zone.[68,70] Thus, the coupling intervals over which resetting occurs, the resetting zone, can be considered a measure of the duration of the temporal excitable gap existing in the reentrant circuit. Therefore, the entire extent of the fully excitable gap would be the zone of coupling intervals from the onset of tachycardia resetting until tachycardia termination. The excitable gap, however, can be underestimated by using only a single extrastimulus or by using single or double extrastimuli in the absence of tachycardia termination by the extrastimuli.

All tachycardias reset by a single extrastimulus can be reset by double extrastimuli, unless tachycardia termination occurs. Double extrastimuli produce resetting over a longer range of coupling intervals and should therefore be used to characterize the excitable gap of the reentrant circuit more fully. During EP testing, only the temporal excitable gap of the entire circuit can be evaluated. It is impossible to assess the conduction velocity and refractoriness at any point in the circuit, which certainly must vary, with available technology.

Return Cycle. The return cycle is the time interval from the resetting stimulus to the next excitation of the pacing site by the new orthodromic wavefront. This corresponds to the time required for the stimulated impulse to reach the reentrant circuit, conduct through the circuit, exit the circuit, and travel back to the pacing site.[68,70] The noncompensatory pause following the extrastimulus and the return cycle are typically measured at the pacing site; however, they may also be measured to the onset of the tachycardia complex on the surface ECG.

When the return cycle is measured from the extrastimulus producing resetting to the onset of the first return tachycardia complex on the surface ECG, conduction time into the tachycardia circuit is incorporated into that measurement. Conduction time between the pacing site and the tachycardia circuit may or may not be equal to that from the circuit to the pacing site. Differences in location of the site of stimulation, as well as the tachycardia circuit entrance and exit, can result in differences in conduction time to and from the pacing site.

Orthodromic and Antidromic Resetting. Antidromic resetting occurs when intracardiac sites are directly captured by the premature stimulus without traversing the reentrant circuit and the zone of slow conduction.[68] Therefore, antidromic resetting of intracardiac sites occurs with a conduction interval from the pacing stimulus to the captured electrogram that is less than the tachycardia CL and with differing morphology of the captured as compared with the spontaneous electrogram. Although demonstration of an antidromic resetting response can indicate a tachycardia mechanism other than reentry, an antidromic resetting pattern can also be observed during reentry with an excitable gap if the pacing site is located distal to a region of slow conduction in the reentry circuit. Conversely, if the recording sites are located in regions activated proximally to a region of slow conduction, an antidromic resetting response will be observed.

Orthodromic resetting occurs when the premature stimulus traverses the reentrant circuit, including the zone of slow conduction, in the same direction as the spontaneous tachycardia impulse and with an identical exit site.[68] Intracardiac areas that are orthodromically reset are advanced by the premature extrastimulus but retain the same morphology because they are activated from the impulse emerging from the same reentrant circuit exit site. The conduction interval from the pacing stimulus to the orthodromically captured electrogram exceeds the tachycardia CL by the time required for the extrastimulus to travel from the pacing site to the reentrant circuit. Thus, an orthodromic resetting response implies that the pacing site is located proximal to a region of slow conduction in the reentry circuit and that the recording site is located distal to this region. The ability to demonstrate orthodromic resetting is critically dependent on the location of pacing and recording electrodes relative to the region of slow conduction in the circuit. Therefore, failure to demonstrate an orthodromic resetting response does not exclude reentry with an excitable gap as a possible tachycardia mechanism.

Resetting Response Curves

Response patterns during resetting are characterized by plotting the coupling interval of the extrastimulus producing resetting versus the return cycle measured at the pacing site. Alternatively, the return cycle is measured to the onset of the first tachycardia complex following stimulation on the surface ECG; then, qualitatively similar but quantitatively different response curves are obtained.[70] Demonstration of a noncompensatory pause following the extrastimulus is required, and the interval encompassing the extrastimulus should be 20 or more milliseconds earlier than the expected compensatory pause following a single extrastim-

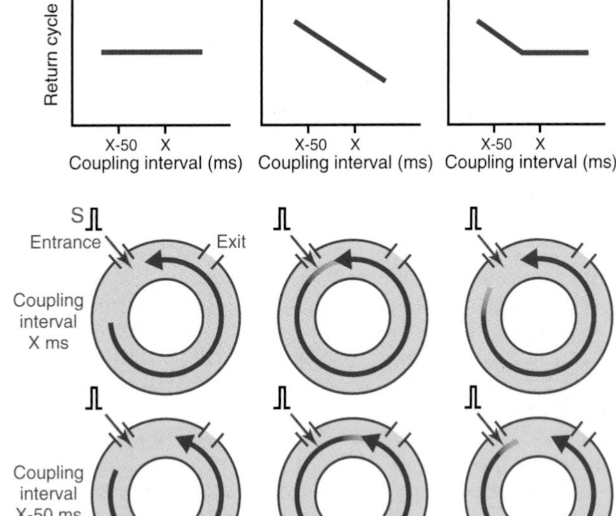

FIGURE 1–14 Mechanisms of various resetting response patterns. **Upper panel,** Schemas of three types of resetting response curves. **Lower panels,** A theoretical mechanism of resetting patterns in response to extrastimuli at coupling intervals of X and X-50 ms. The reentrant circuit is depicted as having a separate entrance and exit in each pattern. Each tachycardia wavefront is followed by a period of absolute refractroriness (blue arrow), which is then followed by a period of relative refractoriness (fading tail of the arrow) of variable duration. On the left side, a flat curve results when the stimulated wavefront reaches the tachycardia circuit and finds a fully excitable gap between the head and tail of the tachycardia wavefront. The gap is still fully excitable at a coupling interval of X-50. Therefore, the conduction time from the entrance to exit is the same. An increasing curve is shown in the middle; this results when the initial stimulated wavefront enters the reentrant circuit when the excitable gap is partially refractory. The curve continues to increase at a coupling interval of X-50 because the tissue is still in a relative refractory state. A mixed curve (right side) results when the less premature extrastimuli find the reentrant circuit fully excitable, whereas the more premature one (at coupling intervals of X-50) finds it in the relative refractory period. *(Reproduced with permission from Josephson ME: Recurrent ventricular tachycardia. In Josephson ME [ed]: Clinical Cardiac Electrophysiology, 3rd ed. Philadelphia, Lippincott, Williams, & Wilkins, 2004, pp 425-610.)*

ulus and 20 or more milliseconds less than three tachycardia CLs when double extrastimuli are used.[70] As always, it is important to establish the stability of tachycardia CL before assessing any perturbation in tachycardia presumed to be caused by resetting.

Four resetting response patterns are possible (Fig. 1-14)[70,71]:

1. During the flat response pattern, the return cycle is constant (less than 10 milliseconds difference) over a 30-millisecond range of coupling intervals.
2. With the increasing response pattern, the return cycle increases as the coupling interval increases.
3. With a decreasing response pattern, the return cycle decreases as the coupling interval increases.
4. A mixed response pattern meets the criteria for a flat response at long coupling intervals and for an increasing response at shorter coupling intervals.

Occasionally, a response pattern to a single extrastimulus cannot be characterized because resetting occurs over too narrow a range of coupling intervals as a result of significant variability of the baseline tachycardia CL or of variability in the return cycle. Triggered rhythms secondary to DADs usually have a flat or decreasing response. A flat response can be observed in automatic, triggered, or reentrant rhythms.

In all cases in which a single extrastimulus resets the tachycardia, double extrastimuli from the same pacing site produce an identical or expected resetting curve. Thus, if a single extrastimulus produces a flat curve, double extrastimuli produce a flat or mixed curve. If a single extrastimulus produces an increasing or mixed curve, double extrastimuli will produce the same curve.

The type of resetting curves can vary depending on the site of stimulation. Extrastimuli from different pacing sites likely engage different sites in the reentrant circuit that are in different states of excitability or refractoriness and, therefore, result in different conduction velocities and resetting patterns.[70]

Flat Response Curves in Reentrant Rhythms. A flat resetting curve implies the presence of a fully excitable gap within the reentrant circuit over a range of coupling intervals. The total duration of the excitable gap should exceed the range of coupling intervals that produce resetting with a flat response. Large excitable gaps are more likely to result in flat response curves, because the increasingly premature extrastimuli are less likely to encroach on the trailing edge of refractoriness and encounter decremental conduction (see Fig. 1-14). The flat return cycle also suggests the presence of fixed sites of entrance and exit from the circuit and fixed conduction time from the stimulation site through the reentrant circuit over a wide range of coupling intervals.

If a single extrastimulus produced resetting with a flat response, the response to double extrastimuli would also be flat. However, because the use of double extrastimuli allows engagement of the reentrant circuit at relatively long coupling intervals with greater prematurity, resetting will begin at longer coupling intervals and will continue over a greater range of coupling intervals than that observed with a single extrastimulus. Therefore, double extrastimuli can produce a flat and then increasing response curve.

Increasing Response Curves in Reentrant Rhythms. Increasing resetting curves result from progressively longer return cycles in response to increasingly premature extrastimuli and indicate a zone of decremental slow conduction, usually located within the reentrant circuit. The most probable mechanism underlying the decremental conduction is encroachment of the advancing wavefront from the premature extrastimuli on an increasingly more refractory tissue within the reentrant circuit, most likely within the zone of slow conduction (see Fig. 1-14).[70] This response pattern is possible only for reentrant arrhythmias and is not observed in triggered or automatic rhythms.

Mixed Response Curves in Reentrant Rhythms. In a mixed response curve, the initial coupling intervals demonstrate a flat portion of the curve of variable duration (but >30 milliseconds), followed by a zone during which the return cycle increases (see Fig. 1-14). Occasionally, a flat curve is seen with a single extrastimulus; it is only by using double extrastimuli that an increasing response can be observed.

Decreasing Response Curves in Reentrant Rhythms. Decreasing reset curves are not observed in reentry but can be seen in triggered rhythms, although flat responses are the most common response for triggered activity. The return cycle in triggered activity is typically 100% to 110% of the tachycardia CL.

Resetting with Fusion

Fusion of the stimulated impulse can be observed on surface ECG or intracardiac recordings if the stimulated impulse is intermediate in morphology between a fully paced complex and the tachycardia complex. The ability to recognize ECG fusion requires a significant mass of myocardium to be depolarized by both the extrastimulus and the tachycardia.[68,70-72] With early extrastimuli, the paced antidromic

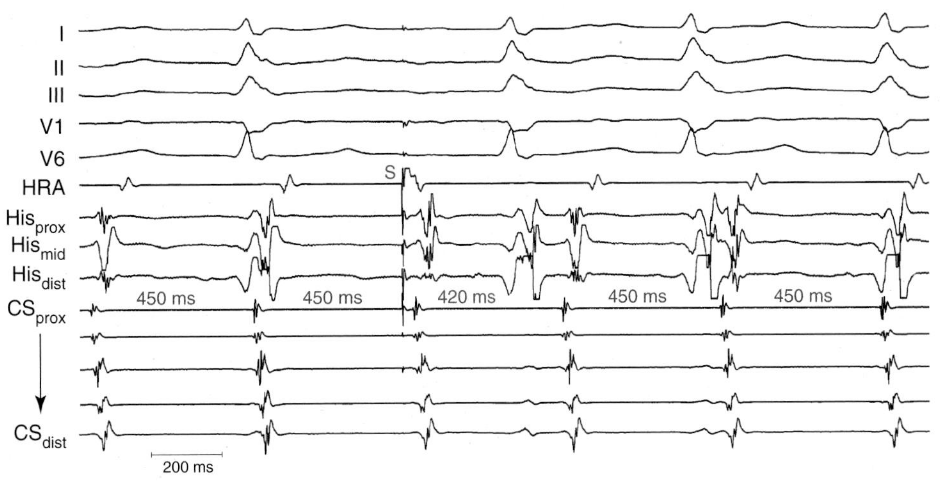

FIGURE 1–15 Resetting with fusion. An atrial tachycardia is shown with a stable cycle length (450 msec). A single extrastimulus (S) is delivered from the high right atrium (HRA) that resets, or advances the timing of the next cycle (420 msec); however, the coronary sinus (CS) electrogram occurs on time when the extrastimulus is given. Thus, intracardiac fusion is evident when resetting occurs, signifying macroreentry.

wavefront captures all or most of the myocardium prior to the orthodromic wavefront of the tachycardia impulse exiting from the reentrant circuit. Thus, no ECG fusion will be present, although resetting can occur. With later coupled extrastimuli, the orthodromic wavefront exits from the reentrant circuit, capturing a certain portion of myocardium before colliding with the paced antidromic wavefront. In this situation, ECG fusion will occur. Resetting with ECG fusion requires wide separation of the entrance and exit of the reentrant circuit, with the stimulus wavefront preferentially engaging the entrance.

If presystolic activity in the reentrant circuit is recorded before delivery of the extrastimulus that resets the tachycardia, one must consider this to represent local fusion (Fig. 1-15).[70] Thus, an extrastimulus that is delivered after the onset of the tachycardia complex and enters and resets the circuit will always demonstrate local fusion. Resetting with local fusion and a totally paced complex morphology provides evidence that the reentrant circuit is electrocardiographically small.

The farther the pacing site from the reentrant circuit, the less likely resetting with ECG fusion will occur, because the extrastimulus should be delivered at a shorter coupling interval to reach the circuit with adequate prematurity. Consequently, the stimulated impulse is more likely to capture both the exit and entrance sites and, therefore, have a purely paced ECG complex morphology without fusion.

Reentrant circuits reset with fusion have a higher incidence of flat resetting curves, longer resetting zones, and significantly shorter return cycles measured from the stimulus to the onset of the tachycardia complex. Resetting with fusion is a potential indication that the pacing site is located proximal to the zone of slow conduction (i.e., prior to the entrance site) within the reentrant circuit, whereas resetting without fusion potentially suggests pacing distal to the zone of slow conduction, because pacing closer to the exit is more likely to capture both the exit and entrance sites and produce resetting without fusion.

Resetting of Tachycardias with Diverse Mechanisms

Resetting can be demonstrated for tachycardias based on different mechanisms, including reentry, normal or abnormal automaticity, and triggered activity. Although the ability to reset an arrhythmia is not helpful in distinguishing the underlying mechanism, certain features of the resetting response can be useful for the differential diagnosis.[70]

Site Specificity of Resetting. Triggered activity and automaticity do not demonstrate site specificity for resetting, whereas reentry can. Site specificity for resetting is decreased with the use of multiple extrastimuli.

Resetting Response Curves. Triggered rhythms secondary to DADs usually have a flat or decreasing resetting curve. A flat resetting curve can be seen in automatic, triggered, or reentrant rhythms. Reentrant rhythms never demonstrate a decreasing resetting curve to single or double extrastimuli.

Resetting with Fusion. The ability to reset a tachycardia after it has begun activating the myocardium (i.e., resetting with fusion) is diagnostic of reentry and excludes automatic and triggered mechanisms.[68,70-72]

In automaticity or triggered activity, resetting of the arrhythmia by an extrastimulus requires depolarization of the site of origin by the paced wavefront. Because the entrance and exit sites of focal rhythms (automatic or triggered) are not separate, a tachycardia wavefront cannot exit the focus once the exit or entrance site has already been depolarized and rendered refractory by the paced wavefront.

During automatic or triggered tachycardias, when an extrastimulus is delivered late in the tachycardia cycle, it can collide with the tachycardia impulse exiting the tachycardia focus and produce fusion of a single beat on the surface ECG or intracardiac recordings. In this case, however, resetting cannot occur because the surrounding myocardium will be refractory to the advancing extrastimulus; that is, entrance block will occur. This would produce a fully compensatory pause.

Entrainment of Reentrant Tachycardias

Basic Principles of Entrainment

Entrainment of reentrant tachycardias by external stimuli was originally defined in the clinical setting as "an increase in the rate of a tachycardia to a faster pacing rate, with resumption of the intrinsic rate of the tachycardia upon either abrupt cessation of pacing or slowing of pacing beyond the intrinsic rate of the tachycardia" and taken to indicate an underlying reentrant mechanism. The ability to entrain a tachycardia also establishes that the reentrant circuit contains an excitable gap.[56,70,73]

Orthodromic resetting and transient entrainment are manifestations of the same phenomenon—that is, premature penetration of a tachycardia circuit by a paced wavefront—and the ability to demonstrate resetting is a strong indication that entrainment can occur from that specific pacing site. Entrainment is the continuous resetting of a reentrant circuit by a train of capturing stimuli. However, following the first stimulus of the pacing train that penetrates and resets the reentrant circuit, the subsequent stimuli interact with the reset circuit, which has an abbreviated excitable gap.[56,73]

During entrainment, each pacing stimulus creates two activation wavefronts, one in the orthodromic and the other in the antidromic direction. The wavefront in the antidromic direction collides with the existing tachycardia wavefront. The wavefront that enters the reentrant circuit in the orthodromic direction (i.e., the same direction as the spontaneous tachycardia wavefront), conducts through the reentrant pathway, resets the tachycardia, and emerges through the exit site to activate the myocardium and collide with the antidromically paced wavefront from the next paced stimulus. This sequence continues until cessation of pacing or block somewhere within the reentrant circuit develops.[68] The first entrained stimulus results in retrograde collision between the stimulated and tachycardia wavefronts, whereas for all subsequent stimuli, the collision occurs between the presently stimulated wavefront and the one stimulated previously. Depending on the degree that the excitable gap is preexcited (and abbreviated) by the first resetting stimulus, subsequent stimuli fall on fully or partially excitable tissue. Entrainment is said to be present when two consecutive extrastimuli conduct orthodromically through the circuit with the same conduction time, while colliding antidromically with the preceding paced wavefront. Because all pacing impulses enter the tachycardia circuit during the excitable gap, each paced wavefront advances and resets the tachycardia. Thus, when pacing is terminated, the last paced impulse will continue to activate the entire tachycardia reentrant circuit orthodromically at the pacing CL, and also will activate the entire myocardium orthodromically on exiting the reentrant circuit.

Overdrive pacing at long CLs (approximately 10 to 20 milliseconds shorter than the tachycardia CL) can almost always entrain reentrant circuits with large flat resetting curves and a post-pacing interval (PPI) equal to the return cycle observed during the flat part of the resetting curve.[70] During overdrive pacing, once the nth pacing stimulus resets the circuit, the following pacing stimulus $(n + 1)^{th}$ will reach the circuit more prematurely. Depending on how premature it is, this $(n + 1)^{th}$ extrastimulus may produce no change in the return cycle (compared with that in response to the nth extrastimulus), encounter progressive conduction delay (until a fixed, longer return cycle is reached), or terminate the tachycardia. The larger the flat curve observed during resetting and/or the longer the pacing CL, the more likely the return cycle of the nth and $(n + 1)^{th}$ extrastimuli will be the same. In this case, no matter how many subsequent extrastimuli are delivered, the return cycle will be the same and equal to that observed during the flat portion of the resetting curve. However, if the flat portion of the resetting curve is small, the pacing CL is short, or both, the $(n + 1)^{th}$ extrastimulus will fall on partially refractory tissue and the return cycle will increase. Continued pacing at the same CL will result in a stable but longer return cycle than the nth extrastimulus or termination of the tachycardia. Consequently, circuits with large fully excitable gaps (i.e., large flat resetting curves) can demonstrate prolonged return cycles or even termination at pacing CLs equal to coupling intervals of a single extrastimulus demonstrating a fully excitable gap.

Entrainment Response Curves

During entrainment, the orthodromic wavefront of the last extrastimulus propagates around the circuit to become the first complex of the resumed tachycardia. The conduction time of this impulse to the exit site of the circuit is termed the *last entrained interval*, and it characterizes the properties of the reset circuit during entrainment.[68,70] Measurement of the interval between the last paced extrastimulus to the first nonpaced tachycardia complex (on the surface ECG or presystolic electrogram) during entrainment at progressively shorter pacing CLs characterizes an entrainment response curve, analogous but not identical to resetting response curves with single extrastimuli. In this case, the return cycle depends critically on the number of extrastimuli delivered that reset the circuit before the return cycle is measured, because following the first extrastimulus producing resetting (the nth extrastimulus), subsequent extrastimuli are relatively more premature and can lead to a different return cycle.

During entrainment, the return cycle measured at an orthodromically captured presystolic electrogram should equal the pacing CL regardless of the site of pacing, as long as the presystolic electrogram is orthodromically activated at a fixed stimulus-to-electrogram interval (i.e., fixed orthodromic conduction time). This would not be observed if the electrogram were captured antidromically. If the time from the orthodromically activated electrogram to the onset of the return cycle on the surface ECG remains constant, which is a requirement to prove that the electrogram is within or attached to the reentrant circuit proximal to the exit site, then the interval from the stimulus to the surface ECG complex will remain constant. The same is true for the electrogram measured at the stimulation site. In the absence of recording of a presystolic electrogram, other measurements may be used to characterize the last entrained interval at any pacing CL. Therefore, during entrainment, curves relating the pacing CL to the last entrained interval can be measured from the stimulus to the orthodromic presystolic electrogram, to the onset of the surface ECG of the first tachycardia (nonpaced) complex, or to the local activation time at the pacing site of the first tachycardia (nonpaced) complex. These measurements will be qualitatively identical but have different absolute values. As always, it is important to establish the stability of tachycardia CL and document the presence of entrainment before assessing the return cycle and PPI.

Termination is the usual response to overdrive pacing of circuits that demonstrate an increasing curve in response to resetting by a single extrastimulus. However, if the number of extrastimuli following the nth extrastimulus is limited to one or two (especially at long pacing CLs), termination may not occur, although the return cycle will be progressively longer following each extrastimulus. Entrainment is not present until two consecutive PPIs are identical. In such cases, when termination does not occur, the return cycle will be longer than that observed if pacing were discontinued following the nth extrastimulus at that pacing CL.[68,70] Thus, if only the return cycle following entrainment is used to analyze the excitable gap, an increasing curve suggesting decremental conduction can result, even though a flat curve is observed with single or double extrastimuli, or both. Therefore, only resetting phenomena describe the characteristics of the reentrant circuit. Entrainment analyzes a reset circuit that has a shorter excitable gap. Flat, mixed (flat and increasing), and increasing curves can be seen during entrainment of macroreentrant circuits. Increasing curves are almost always observed during entrainment of small or microreentrant circuits.

Relationship of Pacing Site and Cycle Length to Entrainment

As with resetting, entrainment does not require the pacing site be located in the reentrant circuit. The closer the pacing site to the circuit, however, the less premature a single stimulus can be and reach the circuit and, with pacing trains, the fewer the number of stimuli required before a stimulated wavefront reaches the reentrant circuit without being extinguished by collision with a wave emerging from the circuit.

Overdrive pacing at long CLs (approximately 10 to 20 milliseconds shorter than the tachycardia CL) can almost always entrain reentrant tachycardias. However, the number of pacing stimuli required to entrain the reentrant circuit depends on the tachycardia CL, duration of the excitable gap of the tachycardia, refractoriness at the pacing site, and conduction time from the stimulation site to the reentrant circuit.[70]

Diagnostic Criteria of Entrainment

Entrainment is the continuous resetting of a tachycardia circuit. Therefore, during constant rate pacing, entrainment of tachycardia will result in the activation of all myocardial tissue responsible for maintaining the tachycardia at the pacing CL, with the resumption of the intrinsic tachycardia morphology and rate after cessation of pacing. Unfortunately, it is almost impossible to document the acceleration of all tissues responsible for maintaining the reentrant circuit to the pacing CL. Therefore, a number of surface ECG criteria have been proposed for establishing the presence of entrainment: (1) fixed fusion of the paced complexes at a constant pacing rate; (2) progressive fusion or different degrees of fusion at different pacing rates (i.e., the surface ECG and intracardiac morphology progressively look more like the purely paced configuration and less like the pure tachycardia complex in the course of pacing at progressively shorter pacing CLs); and (3) resumption of the same tachycardia morphology following cessation of pacing, with the first post-pacing complex displaying no fusion but occurring at a return cycle equal to the pacing CL.[74] These criteria are discussed in more detail in Chapter 3.

Mechanism of Slow Conduction in the Reentrant Circuit

As mentioned earlier, a condition necessary for reentry is that the impulse be delayed sufficiently in the alternative pathway(s) to allow tissues proximal to the site of unidirectional block to recover excitability.[56] Conduction of the cardiac impulse is dependent on both the active membrane properties of cardiac cells (generating the action potential) and the passive properties determined by architectural features of the myocardium. All types of reentrant arrhythmias have a basic feature in common—the wavefront must encounter a zone of tissue where local electrical inhomogeneity is present. This inhomogeneity can be related to: (1) electrical properties of the individual cardiac myocyte that generates the action potential (inhomogeneity in electrical excitability and/or refractoriness); (2) passive properties governing the flow of current between cardiac cells (cell-to-cell coupling and tissue geometry); or (3) combinations of those conditions.[75] Such changes can be permanent (e.g., in remodeling after ventricular hypertrophy) or they can be purely functional (e.g., inhomogeneity of refractoriness in acutely ischemic tissue). Additionally, some of those changes are only needed to set the initial condition for the deviation of the impulse, the so-called unidirectional conduction block. Once the disturbance is initiated, an arrhythmia can develop in a perfectly homogenous electrical medium.[75]

Slow conduction within the reentrant circuit is also an important determinant of the size of the reentrant circuit. A decrease in conduction velocity results in a decrease in the wavelength and a lessening of the amount of tissue needed to sustain reentry. In contrast, an increase in conduction velocity will prolong the wavelength of excitation and, in this situation, a larger anatomical circuit will be necessary to sustain reentry. If a larger circuit is not possible, initiation or maintenance of tachycardia cannot occur.[56]

In some cardiac tissues (e.g., the AVN), slow conduction is normal physiology. Slow conduction also can be secondary to pathophysiological settings (e.g., MI) or caused by functional properties that can develop as a result of premature stimulation or evolve during a rapid transitional rhythm.[56]

Action potential propagation and conduction velocity in cardiac tissue are determined by source-sink relationships, which reflect the interplay between membrane factors (source) and tissue and structure factors (sink).[70] During action potential propagation, an excited cell serves as a source of electrical charge for depolarizing neighboring unexcited cells. The requirements of adjacent resting cells to reach the threshold membrane potential constitute an electrical sink (load) for the excited cell. For propagation to succeed, the excited cell must provide sufficient charge to the unexcited cells to bring their membrane to excitation threshold. Once threshold is reached and action potential generated, the load on the excited cell is removed, and the newly excited cell switches from being a sink to being a source for the downstream tissue, perpetuating the process of action potential propagation. Therefore, conduction velocity depends on how much capacitive current flows out of the cell at unexcited sites ahead of the propagating wavefront and also on the distance at which the capacitive current can bring membrane potential to threshold.

The safety factor for conduction predicts the success of action potential propagation and is based on the source-sink relationship. It can be defined as the ratio of the charge generated by the depolarizing ion channels of a cell to the charge consumed during the excitation cycle of a single cell in the tissue.[70,76] By this definition, conduction fails when the safety factor drops below 1 and becomes increasingly stable as it rises above 1.[77] This concept of propagation safety provides information about the dependence of propagation velocity on the state of the ion channels, cell-to-cell coupling, and tissue geometry. In essence, local source-sink relationships determine the formation of conduction heterogeneities and provide conditions for the development of slow conduction, unidirectional block, and reentry.[56,78]

Reduced Membrane Excitability

Conduction velocity depends, in part, on the rate of rise of phase 0 of the action potential (dV/dt) and the height to which it rises (V_{max}). These factors depend on the amount of the Na^+ inward current, which in turn is directly related to the membrane potential at the time of stimulation, the availability of Na^+ channels for stimulation, and the size of the Na^+ electrochemical potential gradient across the cell membrane. A reduction in the Na^+ inward current, leading to a reduction in the rate or amplitude of depolarization during phase 0 of the action potential, can decrease axial current flow (and therefore capacitive current) and slow conduction, and lead to conduction block.[56,79]

Reduced membrane excitability occurs in a number of physiological and pathophysiological conditions. The more negative the membrane potential, the more Na^+ channels are available for activation, the greater the influx of Na^+ into the cell during phase 0, and the greater the conduction velocity. In contrast, membrane depolarization to levels of −60 to −70 mV can inactivate half the Na^+ channels, and depolarization to −50 mV or less can inactivate all the Na^+ channels. Therefore, when stimulation occurs during phase 3 (e.g., during premature stimulation during the relative refractory period), before full recovery and at less negative potentials of the cell membrane, a portion of Na^+ channels will still be refractory and unavailable for activation. As a result, the Na^+ current and phase 0 of the next action potential will be reduced, and conduction of the premature stimulus will be slowed, facilitating reentry.[8,56]

Reduced membrane excitability can also be a consequence of genetic mutations that result in loss of Na^+ channel function, as occurs in the Brugada syndrome. Reduced membrane excitability is also present in cardiac cells with persistently low levels of resting potential caused by disease (e.g., during acute ischemia, tachycardia, certain electrical remodeling processes, and treatment with Class I antiarrhythmic agents).[42,56,78] At low resting potentials, the availability of excitable Na^+ channels is reduced because of inactivation of a significant percentage of the Na^+ channels and prolonged recovery of Na^+ channels from inactivation. With progressive reduction of excitability, less Na^+ source current is generated, and conduction velocity and the safety factor decrease monotonically. When the safety factor falls below 1, conduction can no longer be sustained and failure (conduction block) occurs.[80] Action potentials with reduced upstroke velocity resulting from partial inactivation of Na^+ channels are called depressed fast responses. These action potential changes are likely to be heterogeneous, with unequal degrees of Na^+ inactivation that create areas with minimally reduced velocity, more severely depressed zones, and areas of complete block. In addition, refractoriness in cells with reduced membrane potentials can outlast voltage recovery of the action potential; that is, the cell can still be refractory or partially refractory after the resting membrane potential returns to its most negative value.[78]

Thus, in a diseased region with partially depolarized fibers, there can be some areas of slow conduction and some areas of conduction block, depending on the level of resting potential and the number of Na^+ channels that are inactivated. This combination can cause reentry. The chance for reentry in such fibers is even greater during premature activation or during rhythms at a rapid rate, because slow conduction or the possibility of block is increased even further.

Reduced Cellular Coupling

Modification of cell-to-cell coupling occurs in a number of physiological and pathophysiological conditions.[56] Physiologically, cell-to-cell coupling can be reduced in atrial and ventricular myocardium in the transverse direction to the main fiber axis relative to the longitudinal direction (see later). Reduced intercellular coupling is also likely to contribute to slow impulse conduction in the AVN.[81,82] In pathophysiological settings (e.g., myocardial ischemia, ventricular hypertrophy, ventricular failure),[83-85] modification of cell-to-cell coupling can occur as a consequence of acute changes in the average conductance of gap junctions secondary to ischemia, hypoxia, acidification, or increase in intracellular Ca^{2+}, or it can be produced by changes in expression or cellular distribution patterns of gap junctions.[86,87]

Similar to its behavior during reduced membrane excitability, conduction velocity decreases monotonically with reduction in intercellular coupling. However, quantitatively, the slowing is more dramatic in the reduced coupling case, although a large reduction of intercellular coupling is required to cause major slowing of conduction velocity.[56,76] In contrast, the changes in safety factor with uncoupling are opposite to those observed with a reduction in membrane excitability. As cells become less coupled, there is greater confinement of depolarizing current to the depolarizing cell, with less electrotonic load and axial flow of charge to the downstream cells. As a result, individual cells depolarize with a high margin of safety, but conduction proceeds with long intercellular delays. At such low level of coupling, conduction is very slow but, paradoxically, very robust.[56,86,87]

Tissue Structure and Geometry

Tissue geometry can influence action potential propagation and conduction velocity. In contrast to an uncoupled cell strand, in which the high resistance junctions alternate with the low cytoplasmic resistance of the cells, a high degree of discontinuity can be produced by large tissue segments (consisting of a segment with side branches) alternating with small tissue segments having a small tissue mass (connecting segments without branches).[56]

When a small mass of cells has to excite the large mass (e.g., an impulse passing abruptly from a fiber of small diameter to one of large diameter, or propagating into a region where there is an abrupt increase in branching of the myocardium), transient slowing of the conduction velocity can be observed at the junction. This occurs because of sink-source mismatch, during which the current provided by the excitation wavefront (source) is insufficient to charge the capacity and thus excite the much larger volume of tissue ahead (sink).[56,88-91,77]

In a normal heart, abrupt changes in geometric properties are not of sufficient magnitude to provide sufficient sink-source mismatch and cause conduction block of the normal action potential because the safety factor for conduction is large; that is, there is a large excess of activating current over the amount required for propagation. However, when the action potential is abnormal, the unexcited area has decreased excitability (e.g., in the setting of acute ischemia), or both, anatomical impediments can result in conduction block.

Anisotropy and Reentry

The anisotropic cellular structure of the myocardium is important for the understanding of normal propagation and arrhythmogenesis. Structural anisotropy can relate to cell shape and to the cellular distribution pattern of proteins involved in impulse conduction, such as gap junction connexins and membrane ion channels. The anisotropic architecture of most myocardial regions, consisting of elongated cells that are forming strands and layers of tissue, leads to a dependence of propagation velocity on the direction of impulse spread.[56,92] In normal ventricular myocardium, conduction in the direction parallel to the long axis of the myocardial fiber bundles is approximately three times more rapid than that in the transverse direction. This is attributable principally to the lower resistivity of myocardium in the longitudinal versus the transverse direction. The gap junctions of the intercalated discs form a major source of intercellular resistance to current flow between fiber bundles. Therefore, the structure of the myocardium that governs the extent and distribution of these gap junctions has a profound influence on axial resistance and conduction.

Cellular Coupling: Gap Junctional Organization

Intercellular communication is maintained by gap junctional channels that connect neighboring cells and allow electrical and metabolic communication. In normal adult ventricular myocardium, gap junctions are confined almost exclusively to the intercalated discs, the sites of mechanical, metabolic, and electrical cellular coupling that facilitate coordinated interaction of the cells. Gap junctions form conduits between adjacent cells that are composed of connexin protein subunits and provide the pathways for intercellular current flow, enabling coordinated action potential propagation in cardiac tissue. Six connexin subunits form a hemichannel (connexon) in the plasma membrane that docks to another hemichannel in the plasma membrane of an adjacent cell to assemble a complete gap junctional channel.[93] In the mammalian heart, connexin 43 is the most abundant connexin, but connexin 40, also abundant in the atria, specialized conducting tissues, and subendocardial ventricular myocardium, and connexin 45 are the other connexins expressed by cardiac myocytes.[56,92]

The connexons in the abutting myocyte membranes align, and the pair forms a complete channel linking the cytoplasmic compartments, providing a relatively low-resistance pathway for the passage of ions and small molecules and for electrical propagation. However, the resistivity of the gap junctional membrane, although several orders of magnitude lower than the non–gap junctional plasma membrane, is several orders of magnitude higher than the cytoplasmic intracellular resistivity.

Under physiological conditions, a given cardiomyocyte in the adult working myocardium is electrically coupled to an average of approximately 11 adjacent cells, with gap junctions being predominantly localized at the intercalated discs. In normal atrial and ventricular myocardium, large intercalated discs exist at the ends of the myocytes, with smaller discs along the length of the cell. This particular subcellular distribution of gap junctions is a main determinant of anisotropic conduction in the heart; a wavefront will encounter more gap junctions in the transverse direction than over an equivalent distance in the longitudinal direction, because cell diameter is much smaller than cell length. Therefore, the wavefront must traverse more cells transversely, resulting in a greater resistance and slower conduction transversely than longitudinally.[56,93]

The anisotropic conductive properties of ventricular myocardium are dependent on the geometry of the interconnected cells and the number, size, and location of the gap junction plaques between them. Gap junctions vary in their molecular composition, degree of expression, and distribution pattern, whereby each of these variations can contribute to the specific propagation properties of a given tissue in a given species. Moreover, the permeability and conductance of each channel are determined by the physiological properties of the connexin isoform composing the channel. A reduction in the gap junctional conductance can increase the intercellular resistance, and the resulting reduction of conduction velocities is more than an order of magnitude larger than that observed during a reduction of excitability.[93] In almost all cardiac diseases predisposing to arrhythmias, changes in the distribution and number of gap junctions (gap junction remodeling) have been reported. Perhaps the most important influence on gap junctional resistance in pathological situations (e.g., during ischemia) is the level of intracellular Ca^{2+}. A significant rise of intracellular Ca^{2+} increases the resistance to current flow through the gap junctions and eventually leads to physiologic uncoupling of the cells.[92]

Myocyte Packing and Tissue Geometry

Discontinuities in myocardial architecture exist at several levels. In addition to discontinuities imposed by cell borders, microvessels and connective tissue sheets separating bundles of excitable myocytes can act as resistive barriers. A propagating impulse is expected to collide with such barriers and travels around them wherever it encounters excitable tissue.[75]

In some regions of the myocardium (e.g., the papillary muscles), connective tissue septa subdivide the myocardium into unit bundles composed of 2 to 30 cells surrounded by a connective tissue sheath.[8] Within a unit bundle, cells are tightly connected or coupled to each other longitudinally and transversely through intercalated discs that contain the gap junctions and are activated uniformly and synchronously as an impulse propagates along the bundle. Adjacent unit bundles also are connected to each other. Unit bundles are coupled better in the direction of the long axis of its cells and bundles, because of the high frequency of the gap junctions within a unit bundle, than in the direction transverse to the long axis, because of the low frequency of interconnections between the unit bundles. This is reflected as a lower axial resistivity in the longitudinal direction than in the transverse direction in cardiac tissues composed of many unit bundles. Additionally, anisotropy on a macroscopic scale can influence conduction at sites at which a bundle of cardiac fibers branches or separate bundles coalesce. Marked slowing can occur when there is a sudden change in the fiber direction, causing an abrupt increase in the effective axial resistivity. Conduction block, which sometimes can be unidirectional, can occur at such junction sites, particularly when membrane excitability is reduced.

Uniform Versus Nonuniform Anisotropy

Uniform anisotropy is characterized by smooth wavefront propagation in all directions and measured conduction velocity changes monotonically on moving from fast (longitudinal) to slow (transverse) axes, indicating relatively tight coupling between groups of fibers in all directions. However, this definition is based on the characteristics of activation at a macroscopic level, where the spatial resolution encompasses numerous myocardial cells and bundles, and therefore it describes the behavior of the myocardial syncytium. In contrast, when breaking down the three-dimensional network of cells into linear single-cell chains, gap junctions can be shown to limit axial current flow and induce saltatory conduction because of the recurrent increases in axial resistance at the sites of gap junctional coupling; that is, conduction is composed of rapid excitation of individual cells followed by a transjunctional conduction delay. In two- and three-dimensional tissue, these discontinuities disappear because of lateral gap junctional coupling, which serves to average local small differences in activation times of individual cardiomyocytes at the excitation wavefront.[77,94]

In multicellular tissue, saltatory conduction only reappears under conditions of critical gap junctional uncoupling, where it leads to a functional unmasking of the cellular structure and induces ultraslow and meandering conduction, which is well known to be a key ingredient in arrhythmogenesis.[77] Change in the characteristics of anisotropic propagation at the macroscopic scale from uniform to nonuniform strongly predisposes to reentrant arrhythmias. Nonuniform anisotropy has been defined as tight electrical coupling between cells in the longitudinal direction but uncoupling to the lateral gap junctional connections. Therefore, there is disruption of the smooth transverse pattern of conduction characteristic of uniform anisotropy, which results in a markedly irregular sequence or zigzag conduction, producing the fractionated extracellular electrograms characteristic of nonuniform anisotropic conduction (Fig. 1-16). In nonuniformly anisotropic muscle, there also can be an abrupt transition in conduction velocity from the fast longitudinal direction to the slow transverse direction, unlike the case with uniform anisotropic muscle, in which intermediate velocities occur between the two directions.

Nonuniform anisotropic properties can exist in normal cardiac tissues secondary to separation of the fascicles of muscle bundles in the transverse direction by fibrous tissue that proliferates with aging to form longitudinally oriented

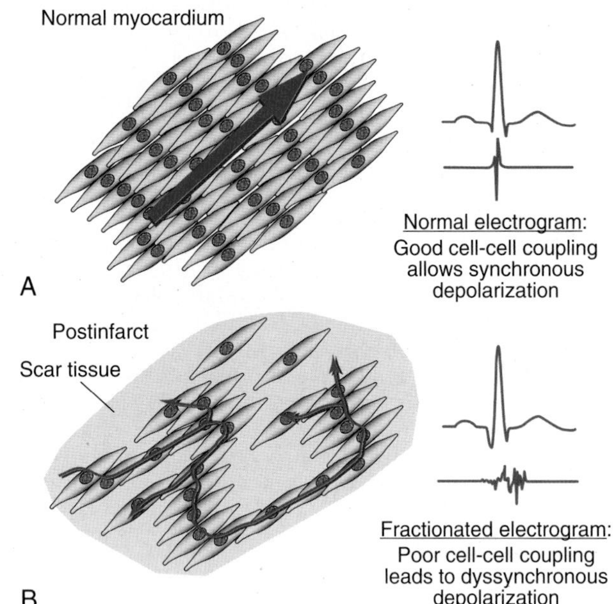

FIGURE 1–16 Effect of scar on electrical propagation. **A,** A homogeneous sheet of myocardium conducts an electrical wavefront rapidly, with synchronous activation of a large number of cells, leading to a sharp electrogram. **B,** Myocardial scarring produces disordered propagation, resulting in a low-amplitude electrogram, with multiple fragmented peaks.

insulating boundaries (e.g., crista terminalis, interatrial band in adult atria or ventricular papillary muscle). Similar connective tissue septa cause nonuniform anisotropy in pathological situations such as chronic ischemia or a healing MI, in which fibrosis in the myocardium occurs (see Fig. 1-16).[8,94]

Mechanism of Unidirectional Block in the Reentrant Circuit

Unidirectional block occurs when an impulse cannot conduct in one direction along a bundle of cardiac fibers but can conduct in the opposite direction. As mentioned earlier, this condition is necessary for the occurrence of classic reentrant rhythms. A number of mechanisms, involving active and passive electrical properties of cardiac cells, can cause unidirectional block.

Inhomogeneity of Membrane Excitability and Refractoriness

Unidirectional block develops when the activation wavefront interacts with the repolarization phase (tail) of a preceding excitation wave. There is a critical or vulnerable window during the relative refractory period of a propagating action potential within which unidirectional block occurs. When a premature stimulus is delivered outside this window, the induced action potential propagates or blocks in both directions; specifically, a stimulus delivered too early fails to induce a propagating action potential in either direction (bidirectional block), whereas a late stimulus results in bidirectional conduction (no block). In contrast, when a stimulus is applied within the vulnerable window, the induced action potential propagates incrementally in the retrograde direction, because the tissue is progressively more recovered as the distance from the window increases in this direction, but blocks in the anterograde direction following a short distance of decremental conduction, because the tissue is progressively less excitable as the distance from the window increases in this direction.[56]

The size of the vulnerable window provides an index of the vulnerability to the development of reentrant arrhythmias. Therefore, the probability that a premature stimulus will fall inside the window and induce reentry is high when the vulnerable window is large. In contrast, precise timing of a premature stimulus is required to induce reentry in a small window, and the probability of such an event is low. In normal tissue, the vulnerable window is very small and inducibility of unidirectional block and reentry is negligible.[89,95] The width of the vulnerable window can be affected by changes in the availability of Na^+ channels for depolarization, cell-to-cell coupling, and repolarizing K^+ currents. Additionally, the size of the vulnerable window can be widened (and reentry facilitated) by factors that increase the spatial inhomogeneity of refractoriness or decrease cellular coupling via gap junctions.[89,95]

Unidirectional conduction block in a reentrant circuit also can be persistent and independent of premature activation, in which case it often occurs in a region of depressed and heterogeneous excitability (as occurs in acute ischemia); this leads to a widening of the vulnerable window. Asymmetry in excitability, which can occur because of asymmetrical distribution of a pathological event, can lead to an abrupt rise in the threshold for excitation in one direction and to a more gradual rise in the other. Conduction fails when the wavefront encounters the least depressed site first and is successful in the direction at which it encounters the most depressed site first. Additionally, impulses are conducted more easily from a rapidly conducting tissue to a slowly conducting tissue than in the opposite direction.

Local dispersion of refractory periods is a normal feature of ventricular myocardium. Critical increases in the dispersion of refractoriness, the difference between the shortest and longest refractory periods, can result in the local widening of the vulnerability window and an increased probability for the generation of unidirectional block and reentry.[56,8] Increased heterogeneity of repolarization and dispersion of refractoriness can be caused by acute or prolonged ischemia, the long-QT syndrome, or electrical remodeling in the setting of ventricular hypertrophy and failure and in the setting of MI.[96,97] When differences in the duration of the refractory periods occur in adjacent areas, conduction of an appropriately timed premature impulse can be blocked in the region with the longest refractory period, which then becomes a site of unidirectional block, whereas conduction continues through regions with a shorter refractory period.[8]

Anisotropy and Unidirectional Block

The anisotropic properties of cardiac muscle can contribute to the occurrence of unidirectional block.[8] As mentioned earlier, in the anisotropic muscle, the safety factor for conduction is lower in the longitudinal direction of rapid than in the transverse direction of slow conduction. The low safety factor longitudinally is a result of a large current load on the membrane associated with the low axial resistivity and large membrane capacitance in the longitudinal direction. This low safety factor can result in a preferential conduction block of premature impulses in the longitudinal direction while conduction in the transverse direction continues. The site of block in the longitudinal direction can become a site of unidirectional block that leads to reentry.[8] In contrast to the propensity of premature impulses to block in the longitudinal direction in nonuniformly anisotropic myocardium because of the decreased depolarizing current and low safety factor, when coupling resistance between cells is increased, conduction of all impulses will block first in the transverse direction. Preferential block in this direction occurs because an increase in coupling resistance will reduce the safety factor below the critical level needed to maintain transverse conduction before the safety factor for longitudinal conduction is reduced to this critical level.[8,94]

Discontinuities in Tissue Structure and Geometry

Geometric factors related to tissue architecture also can influence impulse conduction and, under certain conditions, lead to unidirectional block.[56] Structural discontinuities exist in the normal heart in the form of trabeculations of the atrial and ventricular walls, sheets interconnected by small trabeculae, or myocardial fibers with different diameters packed in a connective tissue matrix. Structural discontinuities can also be secondary to pathophysiological settings, such as the connective tissue septa characteristic of aging, infarcted, hypertrophic, and failing myocardium. The propagating excitation wave is expected to interact with these normal and abnormal structural discontinuities. These structural features influence conduction by affecting the axial currents that flow ahead of the propagating wavefront.[56] Therefore, an impulse conducting in one direction can encounter a different sequence of changes in fiber diameter, branching, and frequency and distribution of gap junctions than it does when traveling in the opposite direction. The configuration of pathways in each direction is not the same.

REFERENCES

1. Peters NS, Cabo C, Wit AL: Arrhythmogenic mechanisms: Automaticity, triggered activity, and reentry. *In* Zipes DP, Jalife J (eds): Cardiac Electrophysiology: From Cell to Bedside, 3rd ed. Philadelphia, WB Saunders, 2000, pp 345-355.
2. Brown HF: Electrophysiology of the sinoatrial node. Physiol Rev 1982;62:505.
3. Zipes DP: Mechanisms of clinical arrhythmias. J Cardiovasc Electrophysiol 2003;14:902.
4. Dobrzynski H, Boyett MR, Anderson RH: New insights into pacemaker activity: promoting understanding of sick sinus syndrome. Circulation 2007;115:1921.
5. Couette B, Marger L, Nargeot J, Mangoni ME: Physiological and pharmacological insights into the role of ionic channels in cardiac pacemaker activity. Cardiovasc Hematol Disord Drug Targets 2006;6:169.
6. Barbuti A, Baruscotti M, DiFrancesco D: The pacemaker current: From basics to the clinics. J Cardiovasc Electrophysiol 2007;18:342.
7. DiFrancesco D: Funny channels in the control of cardiac rhythm and mode of action of selective blockers. Pharmacol Res 2006;53:399.
8. Waldo AL, Wit AL: Mechanisms of cardiac arrhythmias and conduction disturbances. *In* Fuster V, Alexander RW, O'Rourke RA (eds): Hurst's The Heart, 11th ed. Columbus, Ohio, McGraw-Hill, 2004, pp 787-816.
9. Mangoni ME, Marger L, Nargeot J: If current inhibition: Cellular basis and physiology. Adv Cardiol 2006;43:17-30.
10. Irisawa H, Giles WR: Sinus and atrioventricular node cells: Cellular electrophysiology. *In* Zipes DP, Jalife J (eds): Cardiac Electrophysiology: From Cell to Bedside. Philadelphia, WB Saunders, 1990, pp 95-102.
11. Watanabe Y, Nishimura M, Noda T: Atrioventricular junctional tachycardias. *In* Zipes DP, Jalife J (eds): Cardiac Electrophysiology: From Cell to Bedside. Philadelphia, WB Saunders, 1990, pp 564-570.
12. Haissaguerre M, Jais P, Shah DC, et al: Spontaneous initiation of atrial fibrillation by ectopic beats originating in the pulmonary veins. N Engl J Med 1998;339:659.
13. Swerdlow CD, Liem LB: Atrial and junctional tachycardias: Clinical presentation course and therapy. *In* Zipes DP, Jalife J (eds): Cardiac Electrophysiology: From Cell to Bedside. Philadelphia, WB Saunders, 1990, pp 742-755.
14. Zipes DP: Specific arrhythmias: Diagnosis and treatment. *In* Braunwald E (ed): Heart Disease: A Textbook of Cardiovascular Medicine. Philadelphia, WB Saunders, 1992, pp 667-725.
15. Qu J, Robinson RB: Cardiac ion channel expression and regulation: The role of innervation. J Mol Cell Cardiol 2004;37:439.
16. Zhang H, Vassalle M: Mechanisms of adrenergic control of sino-atrial node discharge. J Biomed Sci 2003;10:179.
17. Kohl P, Hunter P, Noble D: Stretch-induced changes in heart rate and rhythm: Clinical observations, experiments and mathematical models. Prog Biophys Mol Biol 1999;71:91.
18. Taggart P, Sutton PM: Cardiac mechano-electric feedback in man: Clinical relevance. Prog Biophys Mol Biol 1999;71:139.
19. Kohl P, Bollensdorff C, Garny A: Effects of mechanosensitive ion channels on ventricular electrophysiology: experimental and theoretical models. Exp Physiol 2006;91:301.
20. Venetucci LA, Trafford AW, O'Neill SC, Eisner DA: Na/Ca exchange: Regulator of intracellular calcium and source of arrhythmias in the heart. Ann N Y Acad Sci 2007;1099:315.
21. Grossman P, Kollai M: Respiratory sinus arrhythmia, cardiac vagal tone, and respiration: Within- and between-individual relations. Psychophysiology 1993;3:486.
22. Hoppe UC, Jansen E, Sudkamp M, Beuckelmann DJ: Hyperpolarization-activated inward current in ventricular myocytes from normal and failing human hearts. Circulation 1998;97:55.
23. Nuss HB, Kaab S, Kass DA, et al: Cellular basis of ventricular arrhythmias and abnormal automaticity in heart failure. Am J Physiol 1999;277(Pt 2):H801.
24. Chen YJ, Chen SA, Chang MS, Lin CI: Arrhythmogenic activity of cardiac muscle in pulmonary veins of the dog: Implication for the genesis of atrial fibrillation. Cardiovasc Res 2000;48:265.
25. Chen YJ, Chen YC, Yeh HI, et al: Electrophysiology and arrhythmogenic activity of single cardiomyocytes from canine superior vena cava. Circulation 2002;105:2679.
26. Ausma J, Wijffels M, Thone F, et al: Structural changes of atrial myocardium due to sustained atrial fibrillation in the goat. Circulation 1997;96:3157.
27. Calkins H, el-Atassi R, Leon A, et al: Effect of the atrioventricular relationship on atrial refractoriness in humans. Pacing Clin Electrophysiol 1992;15:771.
28. Jayachandran J, Arnett C, Antonuccio K: Short-term atrial electrical remodelling is prevented by inhibition of the Na^+/H^+ exchanger with HOE642. Pacing Clin Electrophysiol 1998;21:830.
29. Goette A, Honeycutt C, Langberg JJ: Electrical remodeling in atrial fibrillation. Time course and mechanisms. Circulation 1996;94:2968.
30. Jayachandran J, Zipes DP, Sih H: Acute ischemia mimics changes in atrial refractoriness and is inhibited by blockade of the Na^+/H^+ exchanger. Circulation 1998; 98:I210.
31. Zipes DP, Arbel E, Knope RF, Moe GK: Accelerated cardiac escape rhythms caused by ouabain intoxication. Am J Cardiol 1974;33:248.
32. Elvan A, Wylie K, Zipes DP: Pacing-induced chronic atrial fibrillation impairs sinus node function in dogs. Electrophysiologic remodeling. Circulation 1996;94:2953.
33. Gaspo R, Bosch RF, Talajic M, Nattel S: Functional mechanisms underlying tachycardia-induced sustained atrial fibrillation in a chronic dog model. Circulation 1997;96:4027.
34. Jayachandran J, Sih H, Hanish S: Heterogeneous sympathetic innervation of the atria in atrial fibrillation: Autonomic remodeling with rapid rates. Pacing Clin Electrophysiol 1998;21:831.
35. Sih H, Berbari E, Zipes DP, Olgin J: Organization of atrial fibrillation: Acute versus chronic atrial fibrillation in dogs. Pacing Clin Electrophysiol 1998;21:823.
36. Laitinen PJ, Brown KM, Piippo K, et al: Mutations of the cardiac ryanodine receptor (RyR2) gene in familial polymorphic ventricular tachycardia. Circulation 2001;103:485.
37. Marx SO, Reiken S, Hisamatsu Y, et al: PKA phosphorylation dissociates FKBP12.6 from the calcium release channel (ryanodine receptor): Defective regulation in failing hearts. Cell 2000;101:365.
38. Priori SG, Napolitano C, Tiso N, et al: Mutations in the cardiac ryanodine receptor gene (hRyR2) underlie catecholaminergic polymorphic ventricular tachycardia. Circulation 2001;103:196.
39. Priori SG, Napolitano C, Memmi M, et al: Clinical and molecular characterization of patients with catecholaminergic polymorphic ventricular tachycardia. Circulation 2002;106:69.
40. Wehrens XH, Lehnart SE, Huang F, et al: FKBP12.6 deficiency and defective calcium release channel (ryanodine receptor) function linked to exercise-induced sudden cardiac death. Cell 2003;113:829.
41. Leistad E, Aksnes G, Verburg E, Christensen G: Atrial contractile dysfunction after short-term atrial fibrillation is reduced by verapamil but increased by BAY K8644. Circulation 1996;93:1747.
42. Yue L, Feng J, Gaspo R, et al: Ionic remodeling underlying action potential changes in a canine model of atrial fibrillation. Circ Res 1997;81:512.
43. Wit AL, Tseng GN, Henning B, Hanna MS: Arrhythmogenic effects of quinidine on catecholamine-induced delayed afterdepolarizations in canine atrial fibers. J Cardiovasc Electrophysiol 1990;1:15.
44. January CT, Shorofsky S: Early afterdepolarizations: Newer insights into cellular mechanisms. J Cardiovasc Electrophysiol 1990;1:161.
45. Mendez C, Delmar M: Triggered activity: Its possible role in cardiac arrhythmias. *In* Zipes DP, Jalife J (eds): Cardiac Electrophysiology and Arrhythmias. Orlando, Fla, Grune & Stratton, 1985, pp 311-340.
46. Rubart M, Pressler ML, Pride HP, Zipes DP: Electrophysiologic mechanisms in a canine model of erythromycin-associated long QT syndrome. Circulation 1993;88(Pt 1):1832.
47. Christensen G, Leistad E: Atrial systolic pressure, as well as stretch, is a principal stimulus for release of ANF. Am J Physiol 1997;272(Pt 2):H820.
48. Ben-David J, Zipes DP, Ayers GM, Pride HP: Canine left ventricular hypertrophy predisposes to ventricular tachycardia induction by phase 2 early afterdepolarizations after administration of BAY K 8644. J Am Coll Cardiol 1992;20:1576.
49. Arakawa M, Miwa H, Kambara K, et al: Changes in plasma concentrations of atrial natriuretic peptides after cardioversion of chronic atrial fibrillation. Am J Cardiol 1992;70:550.
50. Bailie DS, Inoue H, Kaseda S, et al: Magnesium suppression of early afterdepolarizations and ventricular tachyarrhythmias induced by cesium in dogs. Circulation 1988;77:1395.
51. Ben-David J, Zipes DP: Alpha-adrenoceptor stimulation and blockade modulates cesium-induced early afterdepolarizations and ventricular tachyarrhythmias in dogs. Circulation 1990;82:225.
52. Antzelevitch C, Sicouri S: Clinical relevance of cardiac arrhythmias generated by afterdepolarizations. Role of M cells in the generation of U waves, triggered activity and torsade de pointes. J Am Coll Cardiol 1994;23:259.
53. Mines GR: On dynamic equilibrium in the heart. J Physiol 1913;46:349.
54. Mines GR: On circulating excitations in heart muscles and their possible relation to tachycardia and fibrillation. Trans R Soc Can 1914;IV:43.
55. Kall JG, Rubenstein DS, Kopp DE, et al: Atypical atrial flutter originating in the right atrial free wall. Circulation 2000;101:270.

56. Kleber AG, Rudy Y: Basic mechanisms of cardiac impulse propagation and associated arrhythmias. Physiol Rev 2004;84:431.
57. Allessie MA, Bonke FI, Schopman FJ: Circus movement in rabbit atrial muscle as a mechanism of tachycardia. II. The role of nonuniform recovery of excitability in the occurrence of unidirectional block, as studied with multiple microelectrodes. Circ Res 1976;39:168.
58. Allessie MA, Bonke FI, Schopman FJ: Circus movement in rabbit atrial muscle as a mechanism of tachycardia. III. The "leading circle" concept: A new model of circus movement in cardiac tissue without the involvement of an anatomic obstacle. Circ Res 1977;41:9.
59. Garrey W: Auricular fibrillation. Physiol Rev 1924;4:215.
60. Wit AL, Dillon SM: Anisotropic reentry. *In* Zipes DP, Jalife J (eds): Cardiac Electrophysiology: From Cell to Bedside. Philadelphia, WB Saunders, 1990, pp 353-364.
61. Peters NS, Coromilas J, Hanna MS, et al: Characteristics of the temporal and spatial excitable gap in anisotropic reentrant circuits causing sustained ventricular tachycardia. Circ Res 1998;82:279.
62. Antzelevitch C: Basic mechanisms of reentrant arrhythmias. Curr Opin Cardiol 2001;16:1.
63. Pertsov AM, Davidenko JM, Salomonsz R, et al: Spiral waves of excitation underlie reentrant activity in isolated cardiac muscle. Circ Res 1993;72:631.
64. Pertsov AM, Jalife J: Three-dimensional vortex-like reentry. *In* Zipes DP, Jalife J (eds): Cardiac Electrophysiology: From Cell to Bedside. Philadelphia, WB Saunders, 1995, pp 403-409.
65. Boersma L, Brugada J, Kirchhof C, Allessie M: Mapping of reset of anatomic and functional reentry in anisotropic rabbit ventricular myocardium. Circulation 1994;89:852.
66. Brugada J, Boersma L, Kirchhof CJ, et al: Reentrant excitation around a fixed obstacle in uniform anisotropic ventricular myocardium. Circulation 1991;84:1296.
67. Almendral JM, Rosenthal ME, Stamato NJ, et al: Analysis of the resetting phenomenon in sustained uniform ventricular tachycardia: Incidence and relation to termination. J Am Coll Cardiol 1986;8:294.
68. Kay GN, Epstein AE, Plumb VJ: Resetting of ventricular tachycardia by single extrastimuli. Relation to slow conduction within the reentrant circuit. Circulation 1990;81:1507.
69. Stevenson WG, Weiss JN, Wiener I, et al: Resetting of ventricular tachycardia: Implications for localizing the area of slow conduction. J Am Coll Cardiol 1988;11:522.
70. Josephson ME: Recurrent ventricular tachycardia. *In* Josephson M (ed): Clinical Cardiac Electrophysiology, 3rd ed. Philadelphia, Lippincott Williams, & Wilkins, 2002, pp 425-610.
71. Stamato NJ, Rosenthal ME, Almendral JM, Josephson ME: The resetting response of ventricular tachycardia to single and double extrastimuli: Implications for an excitable gap. Am J Cardiol 1987;60:5961.
72. Rosenthal ME, Stamato NJ, Almendral JM, et al: Resetting of ventricular tachycardia with electrocardiographic fusion: Incidence and significance. Circulation 1988;77:581.
73. Waldecker B, Coromilas J, Saltman AE, et al: Overdrive stimulation of functional reentrant circuits causing ventricular tachycardia in the infarcted canine heart. Resetting and entrainment. Circulation 1993;87:1286.
74. Almendral JM, Gottlieb CD, Rosenthal ME, et al: Entrainment of ventricular tachycardia: Explanation for surface electrocardiographic phenomena by analysis of electrograms recorded within the tachycardia circuit. Circulation 1988;77:569.
75. Kleber AG, Fast V: Molecular and cellular aspects of re-entrant arrhythmias. Basic Res Cardiol 1997;92(Suppl 1):111.
76. Shaw RM, Rudy Y: Ionic mechanisms of propagation in cardiac tissue. Roles of the sodium and L-type calcium currents during reduced excitability and decreased gap junction coupling. Circ Res 1997;81:727.
77. Rohr S: Role of gap junctions in the propagation of the cardiac action potential. Cardiovasc Res 2004;62:309.
78. Antzelevitch C: Cellular basis and mechanism underlying normal and abnormal myocardial repolarization and arrhythmogenesis. Ann Med 2004;36(Suppl 1):5.
79. Santana LF, Nunez-Duran H, Dilly KW, Lederer WJ: Sodium current and arrhythmogenesis in heart failure. Heart Fail Clin 2005;1:193.
80. Yan GX, Antzelevitch C: Cellular basis for the Brugada syndrome and other mechanisms of arrhythmogenesis associated with ST-segment elevation. Circulation 1999;100:1660.
81. Spach MS, Heidlage JF, Dolber PC, Barr RC: Electrophysiologic effects of remodeling cardiac gap junctions and cell size: Experimental and model studies of normal cardiac growth. Circ Res 2000;86:302.
82. Spach MS, Heidlage JF: The stochastic nature of cardiac propagation at a microscopic level. Electrical description of myocardial architecture and its application to conduction. Circ Res 1995;76:366.
83. Cooklin M, Wallis WR, Sheridan DJ, Fry CH: Changes in cell-to-cell electrical coupling associated with left ventricular hypertrophy. Circ Res 1997;80:765.
84. Peters NS, Wit AL: Gap junction remodeling in infarction: Does it play a role in arrhythmogenesis? J Cardiovasc Electrophysiol 2000;11:488.
85. Cascio WE, Yang H, Muller-Borer BJ, Johnson TA: Ischemia-induced arrhythmia: The role of connexins, gap junctions, and attendant changes in impulse propagation. J Electrocardiol 2005;38(Suppl 4):55.
86. van Rijen HV, van Veen TA, Gros D, et al: Connexins and cardiac arrhythmias. Adv Cardiol 2006;42:150.
87. Lee PJ, Pogwizd SM: Micropatterns of propagation. Adv Cardiol 2006;42:86.
88. Fast VG, Kleber AG: Cardiac tissue geometry as a determinant of unidirectional conduction block: Assessment of microscopic excitation spread by optical mapping in patterned cell cultures and in a computer model. Cardiovasc Res 1995;29:697.
89. Quan W, Rudy Y: Unidirectional block and reentry of cardiac excitation: a model study. Circ Res 1990;66:367.
90. Rohr S, Salzberg BM: Characterization of impulse propagation at the microscopic level across geometrically defined expansions of excitable tissue: Multiple site optical recording of transmembrane voltage (MSORTV) in patterned growth heart cell cultures. J Gen Physiol 1994;104:287.
91. Wang Y, Rudy Y: Action potential propagation in inhomogeneous cardiac tissue: safety factor considerations and ionic mechanism. Am J Physiol Heart Circ Physiol 2000;278:H1019.
92. Saffitz JE, Lerner DL, Yamada KA: Gap junction distribution and regulation in the heart. *In* Zipes DP, Jalife J (eds): Cardiac Electrophysiology: From Cell to Bedside. Philadelphia, WB Saunders, 2004, pp 181-191.
93. Sohl G, Willecke K: Gap junctions and the connexin protein family. Cardiovasc Res 2004;62:228.
94. Valderrabano M: Influence of anisotropic conduction properties in the propagation of the cardiac action potential. Prog Biophys Mol Biol 2007;94:144.
95. Shaw RM, Rudy Y: The vulnerable window for unidirectional block in cardiac tissue: characterization and dependence on membrane excitability and intercellular coupling. J Cardiovasc Electrophysiol 1995;6:115.
96. Kaab S, Dixon J, Duc J, et al: Molecular basis of transient outward potassium current downregulation in human heart failure: A decrease in Kv4.3 mRNA correlates with a reduction in current density. Circulation 1998;98:1383.
97. Priebe L, Beuckelmann DJ: Simulation study of cellular electric properties in heart failure. Circ Res 1998;82:1206.

CHAPTER 2

Electrophysiological Testing

PERIPROCEDURAL MANAGEMENT

Indications

Table 2-1 summarizes the American College of Cardiology/American Heart Association/ North American Society for Pacing and Electrophysiology (ACC/AHA/NASPE) recommendations for electrophysiology (EP) testing. Recommendations for specific clinical situations are discussed in subsequent chapters.[1]

Patient Preparation

Preprocedure Evaluation. Heart failure, myocardial ischemia, and electrolyte abnormalities should be treated and adequately controlled before any invasive EP testing is undertaken. Patients with critical aortic stenosis, severe hypertrophic cardiomyopathy, left main or severe three-vessel coronary artery disease, or decompensated heart failure are at high risk of complication. Induction of sustained tachyarrhythmias in these patients can cause severe deterioration. Anticoagulation for 4 weeks before the procedure, transesophageal echocardiography (to exclude the presence of intracardiac thrombus), or both, is required before studying patients who have persistent atrial fibrillation (AF) and atrial flutter (AFL).

Antiarrhythmic Drugs. Antiarrhythmic drugs are usually, but not always, stopped for at least five half-lives prior to EP testing. In selected cases, antiarrhythmic drugs can be continued if an arrhythmic event occurred while the patient was on a specific agent.

Consent. Patients generally are not as familiar with EP procedures as they are with other invasive cardiac procedures, such as cardiac catheterization. Therefore, patient education is an essential part of the procedure. The patient should be informed about the value of the EP study, its risks, and the expected outcome. Patients should also have a realistic idea of the benefit that they can derive from undergoing EP studies, including the possibility that the study result can be negative or equivocal.

Defibrillator Pads. A functioning cardioverter-defibrillator should be available at the patient's side throughout the EP study. Using preapplied adhesive defibrillator pads avoids the need to disrupt the sterile field in the event that electrical defibrillation or cardioversion is needed during the procedure. Biphasic devices are more effective than devices with monophasic waveforms.

Arterial Line. Arterial lines are used routinely in a minority of EP laboratories. Automated cuff blood pressure devices are usually adequate. However, invasive blood pressure monitoring is generally used in unstable patients and when transseptal left atrial access is planned.

Sedation. Many patients benefit from mild sedation. Longer procedures and ablations are now routinely performed using intravenous conscious sedation. The combination of a benzodiazepine (most commonly midazolam) and a narcotic (e.g., fentanyl) is typically used. Propofol is used in a minority of EP laboratories. Bispectral analysis of brain electrical activity is becoming more popular as a method of monitoring the depth and safety of sedation. In certain situations, especially when mapping and ablation of an automatic or triggered-activity tachycardia are expected, sedation can suppress the arrhythmic activity and delay or preclude the mapping-ablation procedure. In such cases, avoiding sedation is advisable until inducibility of the tachycardia is ensured.

Urinary Problems. Urinary retention can occur during lengthy EP procedures, particularly if combined with sedation, fluid administration, and a tachycardia-related diuresis. When such situations are anticipated, it is useful to insert a Foley catheter before the procedure.

Oxygen and Carbon Dioxide Monitoring. Monitoring of oxygen saturation is used routinely. Expired carbon dioxide monitors also can be useful in preventing hypercapnia in patients receiving supplemental oxygen, because oxygen saturation can be misleadingly high.

Complications

Risks and Complications

The complication rate of EP testing is relatively low when only right-heart catheterization is performed, with almost negligible mortality. Risk of complications increases

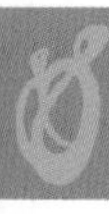

TABLE 2–1 Major Indications For Electrophysiology Testing

Indication	Class I	Class II	Class III
Evaluation of sinus node function	Symptomatic patients—SND suspected but unproved	Patients with documented SND in whom evaluation of AV or VA conduction can aid choice of pacing modality Sinus bradycardia—intrinsic versus autonomic or drug effects Symptomatic patients with sinus bradycardia, to rule out other causes of symptoms	Symptomatic patients with documented association between rhythm and symptoms; therapy would not change with EP testing Asymptomatic sinus bradycardia only with sleep, including sleep apnea
Acquired AV block	Symptomatic patients with HPS block suspected but unproved Paced patients with AV block who are still symptomatic and in whom another arrhythmia is suspected as cause of symptoms	Patients with second- or third-degree AV block in whom site of block or response to measures (e.g., drugs) could affect therapy Suspected concealed premature junctional depolarizations causing pseudo-AV block	Symptomatic patients with symptoms and AV block correlated by ECG findings Asymptomatic patients with transient AV block associated with sinus slowing (e.g., nocturnal type I second-degree AV block)
Chronic intraventricular conduction defects	Symptomatic patients, cause unknown	Asymptomatic patients with BBB in whom pharmacological therapy that could cause block is contemplated	Asymptomatic patients with intraventricular conduction defects Symptomatic patients in whom symptoms can be correlated with or excluded by ECG
Narrow QRS complex tachycardia	Patients with poorly tolerated tachycardia that does not respond adequately to drugs Patients who prefer ablation to pharmacological therapy	Patients with frequent episodes requiring drug treatment, in whom there is concern about proarrhythmia or drug effects on sinus node or AV conduction	Patients whose tachycardias are well controlled by vagal maneuvers or drugs, who are not candidates for nonpharmacological treatment
Wide QRS complex tachycardia	Correct diagnosis needed for treatment, but unclear on ECG	None	Definitive diagnosis of SVT or VT is made from ECG, and invasive EP data would not influence therapy
Prolonged QT interval syndrome	None	To identify proarrhythmic effects of a drug in patient with sustained VT or cardiac arrest while on the drug Patients with syncope or symptomatic arrhythmias and equivocal long-QT duration or TU wave configuration, in whom catecholamine effects can unmask distinct QT abnormality	Manifest congenital QT prolongation, with or without arrhythmias Acquired long-QT syndrome with symptoms closely correlated to identifiable cause or mechanism
WPW syndrome	Patients being evaluated for catheter ablation Patients with preexcitation who have had arrest or unexplained syncope Symptomatic patients in whom EP testing data could affect treatment	Asymptomatic patients with family history of sudden death or who engage in high-risk activities Patients with WPW pattern undergoing cardiac surgery for other reasons	Asymptomatic patients, except those in Class II
PVCs, couplets, nonsustained VT	None	Patients with other risk factors for future arrhythmic events (e.g., low ejection fraction, abnormal signal-averaged ECG, nonsustained VT on Holter) in whom EP testing will be used to guide treatment if sustained VT is inducible Highly symptomatic patients considered for catheter ablation	Asymptomatic or mildly symptomatic patients without other risk factors for sustained arrhythmias
Unexplained syncope	Patients with suspected structural heart disease and unexplained syncope	Patients with recurrent unexplained syncope, without structural heart disease and with negative tilt test	Patients with unexplained syncope whose treatment will not be altered by EP testing findings
Cardiac arrest survivors	Survivors without evidence of acute Q wave MI Cardiac arrest occurring > 48 hr after acute MI	Cardiac arrest caused by bradyarrhythmia Cardiac arrest possibly caused by congenital long-QT syndrome when results of noninvasive tests are equivocal	Cardiac arrest within first 48 hr after acute MI Cardiac arrest from clear cause (e.g., acute ischemia, aortic stenosis, long-QT syndrome)
Unexplained palpitations	Rapid pulse felt by medical personnel, without ECG documentation Palpitations followed by syncope	Patients with clinically significant palpitations in whom symptoms are sporadic and cannot be documented, for whom EP testing can help in diagnosis, risk assessment, treatment	Palpitations documented to have noncardiac cause (e.g., hyperthyroidism)

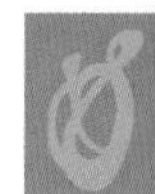

TABLE 2–1 Major Indications For Electrophysiology Testing—cont'd

Indication	Class I	Class II	Class III
Guiding drug therapy	Patients with sustained VT or cardiac arrest, especially those with prior MI Patients with AVNRT, AVRT, or AF with preexcitation in whom chronic drug therapy is involved	Sinus node reentrant tachycardia, AT, AF, or AFL, without preexcitation, in whom drug therapy is planned Patients with arrhythmias not inducible at baseline EP testing, for whom drug therapy is planned	Isolated PACs or PVCs VF with clearly identified reversible cause
Related to implantable devices	In patients with tachycarrhythmias, before and during device implantation and final (predischarge) programming to confirm performance Patients with prior ICD implant in whom changes in status or therapy may have altered the performance of the device Test interactions if two devices are to be used	In patients with documented indications for pacing, to optimize pacing mode and sites	Patients who are not device therapy candidates

AF = atrial fibrillation; AFL = atrial flutter; AT = atrial tachycardia; AV = atrioventricular; AVNRT = AV nodal reentry tachycardia; AVRT = AV reentrant tachycardia; BBB = bundle branch block; EP = electrophysiology; HPS = His-Purkinje system; ICD = implantable cardioverter-defibrillator; MI = myocardial infarction; PAC = premature atrial complex; PVC = premature ventricular complex; SND = sinus node dysfunction; SVT = supraventricular tachycardia; VA = ventricular-atrial; VT = ventricular tachycardia; WPW = Wolff-Parkinson-White.

From Zipes DP, DiMarco JP, Gillette PC, et al: Guidelines for clinical intracardiac electrophysiological and catheter ablation procedures. A report of the American College of Cardiology-American Heart Association Task Force on Practice Guidelines (Committee on Clinical Intracardiac Electrophysiologic and Catheter Ablation Procedures), developed in collaboration with the North American Society of Pacing and Electrophysiology. J Am Coll Cardiol 1995;26:555.

significantly in patients with severe or decompensated cardiac disease. Complications of EP testing include vascular injury (hematoma, pseudoaneurysm, and arteriovenous fistula), bleeding requiring transfusion, deep venous thrombosis and pulmonary embolism, systemic thromboembolism, infection at catheter sites, systemic infection, pneumothorax, cardiac perforation and tamponade, myocardial infarction (MI), stroke, complete atrioventricular (AV) block, and bundle branch block (BBB). Although potentially lethal arrhythmias such as rapid ventricular tachycardia (VT) or ventricular fibrillation (VF) can occur in the laboratory, they are not necessarily regarded as complications, but are often expected and anticipated.[2,3]

Iatrogenic Problems Encountered During EP Testing

Mechanical irritation from catheters during placement inside the heart, even when they are not being manipulated, can cause a variety of arrhythmias and conduction disturbances, including induction of atrial, junctional, and ventricular ectopic beats or tachyarrhythmias, BBB, and AV block. AV block can occur especially during right ventricle (RV) catheterization in patients with preexisting left bundle branch block (LBBB), and occasionally secondary to mechanical trauma of the compact AV node (AVN). Ventricular stimulation can also occur from physical movement of the ventricular catheter coincident with atrial contraction, producing patterns of ventricular preexcitation on the surface electrocardiogram (ECG). Recognition of all these iatrogenic patterns is important for avoiding misinterpretation of EP phenomena and determining the significance of findings in the laboratory.

AF and VF are to be avoided unless they are the subject of the study. AF will obviously not permit study of any other form of supraventricular tachycardia (SVT), and VF will require prompt defibrillation. If AF must be initiated for diagnostic purposes (e.g., to assess ventricular response over an AV bypass tract [BT]), it is preferably induced at the end of the study. Patients with a prior history of AF are more prone to the occurrence of sustained AF in the EP laboratory. Frequently, this will occur during initial placement of catheters; excessive manipulation of catheters in the atria should therefore be avoided.

Another iatrogenic problem is catheter trauma resulting in abolition of BT conduction, injury to the focus of a tachycardia or to the reentrant pathway, which can make the mapping and curative ablation difficult or impossible.

CATHETERIZATION TECHNIQUES

Electrode Catheters

Electrode catheters are used during EP testing for recording and pacing. These catheters consist of insulated wires; at the distal tip of the catheter, each wire is attached to an electrode, which is exposed to the intracardiac surface. At the proximal end of the catheter, each wire is attached to a plug, which can be connected to an external recording device. Electrode catheters are generally made of woven Dacron or newer synthetic materials, such as polyurethane. The Dacron catheters have the advantage of stiffness that helps maintain catheter shape with enough softness at body temperature that allows formation of loops. Catheters made of synthetic materials cannot be easily manipulated and change shapes within the body, but they are less expensive and can be made smaller.

Electrode catheters come in different sizes (3 to 8 Fr). In adults, sizes 5, 6, and 7 Fr catheters are the most commonly used. Recordings derived from electrodes can be unipolar (one pole) or bipolar (two poles). The electrodes are typically 1 to 2 mm in length. The interelectrode distance can range from 1 to 10 mm or more. The greater the interelectrode spacing on a conventional bipolar electrode, the more the recorded electrogram resembles a unipolar recording. Catheters with a 2- or 5-mm interelectrode distance are most commonly used.[4]

A large number of multipolar electrode catheters have been developed to facilitate placement of the catheter in the desired place and to fulfill various recording requirements. Bipolar or quadripolar electrode catheters are used to record and pace from specific sites of interest within the atria or ventricles. These catheters come with a variety of preformed distal curve shapes and sizes (Fig. 2-1). Multipolar recording electrode catheters are placed within the coronary sinus (CS) or along the crista terminalis in the right atrium (RA). The Halo catheter is a multipolar catheter used to map reentrant electrical activity around the tricuspid annulus during RA macroreentry (Fig. 2-2). A decapolar catheter with a distal ring configuration (Lasso catheter) is used to record electrical activity from the pulmonary vein (PV; Fig. 2-3).

Basket catheters capable of conforming to the chamber size and shape have also been used for mapping atrial and ventricular arrhythmias (Fig. 2-4). Special catheters are also used to record left atrium (LA) and left ventricle (LV) epicardial activity from the CS branches.[4]

Catheters can have a fixed or deflectable tip. Steerable catheters allow deflection of the tip of the catheter in one or two directions in a single plane; some of these catheters have asymmetrical bidirectional deflectable curves (Fig. 2-5).

Ablation catheters have tip electrodes that are conventionally 4 mm long and are available in sizes up to 10 mm in length (Fig. 2-6). The larger tip electrodes on ablation catheters reduce the resolution of a map obtained using recordings from the distal pair of electrodes.

Catheter Positioning

The percutaneous technique is used almost exclusively. RA, His bundle (HB), and RV electrograms are most commonly recorded using catheters inserted via a femoral vein. Some other areas (e.g., the CS) are more easily reached through the superior vena cava (SVC), although the femoral approach can be adequate in most cases. Insertion sites can also include the antecubital, jugular, and subclavian veins. Femoral arterial access can be required for mapping of the LV or mitral annulus or for invasive blood pressure monitoring. Rarely, an epicardial approach is required to map and ablate certain VTs. The epicardial surface is accessed via the CS and its branches or percutaneously (subxiphoid puncture).[5]

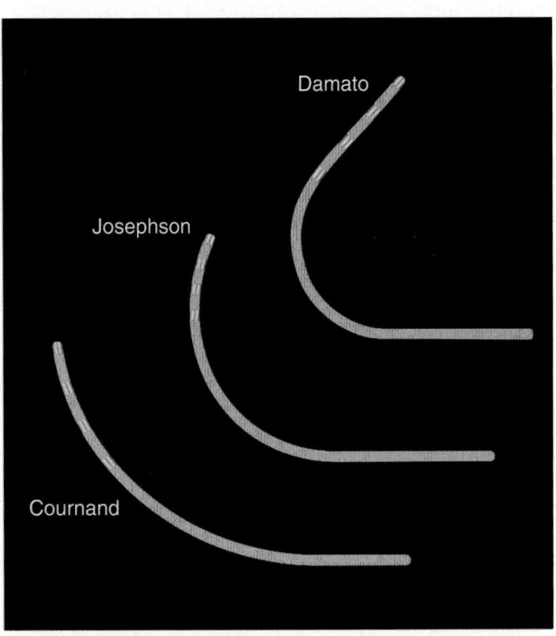

FIGURE 2-1 Multipolar electrode catheters with different preformed curve shapes. *(Courtesy of Boston Scientific, Boston.)*

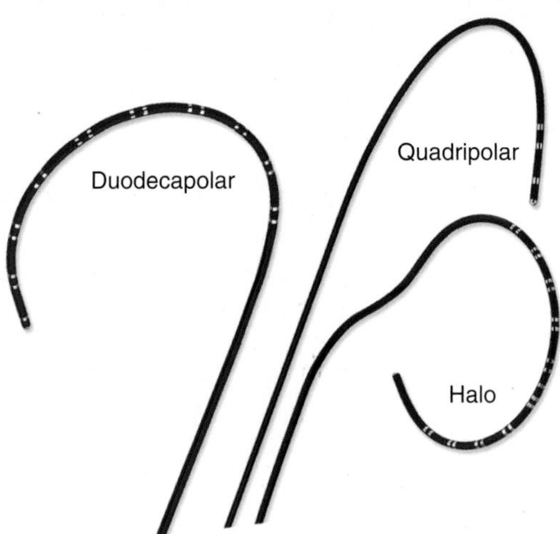

FIGURE 2-2 Multipolar electrode catheters with different electrode numbers and curve shape. **Left to right,** Duodecapolar catheter, quadripolar catheter, and Halo catheter. *(Courtesy of Boston Scientific, Boston.)*

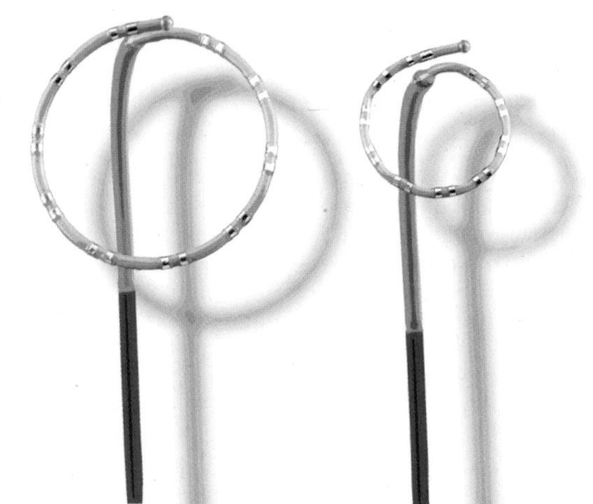

FIGURE 2-3 Lasso catheter with two different loop sizes. *(Courtesy of Biosense Webster, Inc., Diamond Bar, California; www.BiosenseWebster.com.)*

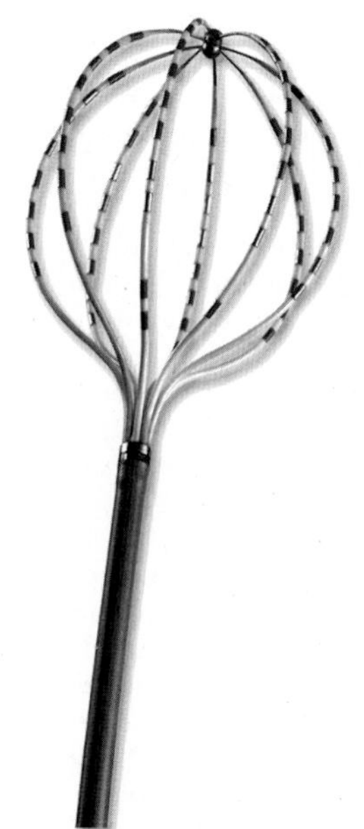

FIGURE 2-4 Basket catheter (Constellation). *(Courtesy of Boston Scientific, Boston.)*

Fluoroscopy is conventionally used to guide intracardiac positioning of the catheters. It is important to remember that catheters can be withdrawn without fluoroscopy, but should always be advanced under fluoroscopy guidance. More recently, new navigations systems have been tested to guide catheter positioning in an effort to limit radiation exposure (see Chap. 3).

Transcaval Approach

The modified Seldinger technique is used to obtain multiple venous accesses. The femoral approach is most common, but the subclavian, internal jugular, or brachial approaches may be used, most often for placement of a catheter in the CS.[5]

The femoral access should be avoided in patients with known or suspected femoral vein or inferior vena caval thrombosis, active lower extremity thrombophlebitis or postphlebitic syndrome, groin infection, bilateral leg amputation, extreme obesity, and/or severe peripheral vascular disease resulting in nonpalpable femoral arterial pulse.

Typically, the RA, HB, and RV catheters are introduced via the femoral veins. It is advisable to use the left femoral vein for diagnostic EP catheters and to save the right femoral vein for potential ablation or mapping catheter placement, which then would be easier to manipulate because it would be on the side closer to the operator. Multiple venous punctures and single vascular sheaths may be used for the different catheters. Alternatively, a single triport 12 Fr sheath can be used to introduce up to three EP catheters (usually the RA, HB, and RV catheters). The CS catheter is frequently introduced via the right internal jugular or subclavian vein, but also via the femoral approach.

Right Atrium Catheter. A fixed-tip, 5 or 6 Fr, quadripolar electrode catheter is typically used. The RA may be entered from the inferior vena cava (IVC) or SVC. The femoral veins are the usual entry sites. Most commonly, stimulation and recording from the RA is performed by placing the RA catheter tip at the high posterolateral wall at the SVC-RA junction in the region of the sinus node, or in the RA appendage (Fig. 2-7).

Right Ventricle Catheter. A fixed-tip, 5 or 6 Fr, quadripolar electrode catheter is typically used. All sites in the RV are accessible from any venous approach. The RV apex is most commonly chosen for stimulation and recording because of stability and reproducibility (see Fig. 2-7).

His Bundle Catheter. A fixed- or deflectable-tip, 6 Fr, quadripolar electrode catheter is typically used. The catheter is passed via the femoral vein into the RA and across the tricuspid annulus until it is clearly in the RV (under fluoroscopic monitoring, using the right anterior oblique [RAO] view; see Fig. 2-7). It is then withdrawn across the tricuspid orifice while maintaining a slight clockwise torque to maintain good contact with the septum until a His potential is recorded. Initially, a large ventricular electrogram can be observed and, as the catheter is withdrawn, the right bundle branch (RB) potential can appear (manifesting as a narrow spike less than 30 milliseconds before the ventricular electrogram). When the catheter is further withdrawn, the atrial electrogram appears and grows larger. The His potential

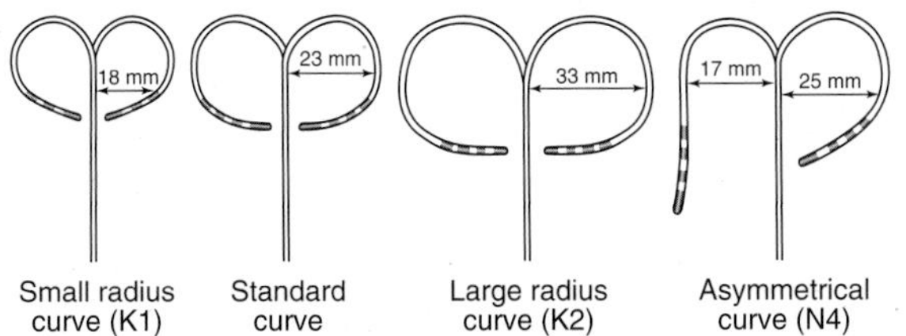

FIGURE 2–5 Deflectable multipolar electrode catheters with different curve sizes and shapes. *(Courtesy of Boston Scientific, Boston.)*

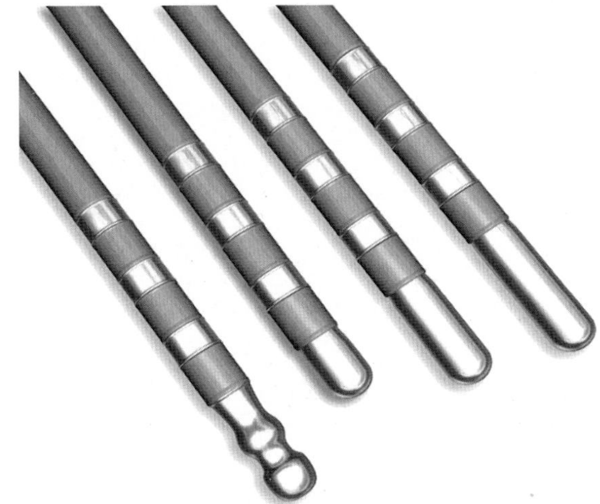

FIGURE 2–6 Ablation catheters with different tip electrode sizes and shapes. **Left to right,** Peanut 8-mm, 2-mm, 4-mm, and 8-mm tip electrodes. *(Courtesy of Boston Scientific, Boston.)*

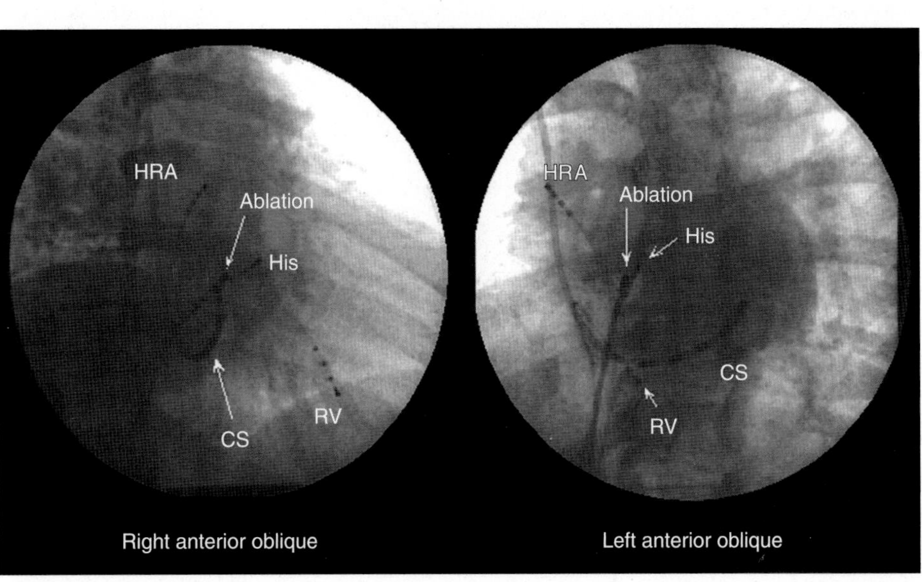

FIGURE 2–7 Fluoroscopic views of catheters in study for supraventricular tachycardia (SVT) (para-His accessory pathway ablation). Catheters are labeled HRA (high right atrium), right ventricle (RV), and coronary sinus (CS); the CS catheter was inserted from a jugular venous approach.

usually appears once the atrial and ventricular electrograms are approximately equal in size, and is manifest as a biphasic or triphasic deflection interposed between the local atrial and ventricular electrograms. If the first pass was unsuccessful, the catheter should be passed again into the RV and withdrawn with a slightly different rotation. If, after several attempts, a His potential cannot be recorded using a fixed-tip catheter, the catheter should be withdrawn and reshaped, or it may be exchanged with a deflectable-tip catheter. Once the catheter is in place, a stable recording can usually be obtained. Occasionally, continued clockwise torque on the catheter shaft is required to obtain a stable HB recording, which can be accomplished by looping the catheter shaft remaining outside the body and fixing the loop by placing a couple of towels on it, or by twisting the connection cable in the opposite direction so that it maintains a gentle torque on the catheter.

When access is from the SVC, it is more difficult to record the His potential because the catheter does not lie across the superior margin of the tricuspid annulus. In this case, a deflectable-tip catheter is typically used, advanced into the RV, positioned near the HB region by deflecting the tip superiorly to form a J shape, and then withdrawing the catheter so that it lies across the superior margin of the tricuspid annulus. Alternatively, the catheter can be looped in the RA ("figure-of-6"); then the body of the loop is advanced into the RV so that the tip of the catheter is pointing toward the RA and lying on the septal aspect of the RA. Gently withdrawing the catheter can increase the size of the loop and allow the catheter tip to rest on the HB location.

Recording of the HB electrogram can also be obtained via the retrograde arterial approach. Using this approach, the catheter tip is positioned in the noncoronary sinus of Valsalva (just above the aortic valve) or in the LV outflow tract (LVOT), along the interventricular septum (just below the aortic valve).

Coronary Sinus Catheter. A femoral, internal jugular, or subclavian vein may be used. It is easier to cannulate the CS using the right internal jugular or left subclavian vein versus the femoral vein because the CS valve is oriented anterosuperiorly and, when prominent, can prevent easy access to the CS from the femoral venous approach. A fixed-tip, 6 Fr, decapolar electrode catheter is typically used for access from the SVC, whereas a deflectable-tip catheter is preferred for CS access from the femoral veins.

When cannulating the CS from the SVC approach, the left anterior oblique (LAO) view is used, the catheter tip is directed to the left of the patient, and the catheter is advanced with some clockwise torque to engage the CS ostium (CS os); electrodes should resemble rectangles rather than ovals when the catheter tip is properly oriented to advance into the CS. Once the CS os is engaged, the catheter is further advanced gently into the CS, so that the most proximal electrodes lie at the CS os (see Fig. 2-7).

During cannulation of the CS from the IVC approach, the tip of the catheter is first placed into the RV, using the RAO view, and flexed downward toward the RV inferior wall. Subsequently, the catheter is withdrawn until it lies at the inferoseptal aspect of the tricuspid annulus. Using the LAO or RAO view, the catheter is then withdrawn gently with clockwise rotation until the tip of the catheter drops into the CS os. Afterward, the catheter is advanced into the CS concomitantly with gradual release of the catheter curve (Fig. 2-8). Alternatively, the tip of the catheter is directed toward the posterolateral RA wall and advanced with a tight curve to form a loop in the RA, using the LAO fluoroscopy view, with the tip directed toward the inferomedial RA. The tip is then advanced with gentle up-down, right-left manipulation using the LAO and RAO fluoroscopy views to cannulate the CS.

When attempting CS cannulation, the catheter can enter the RV and premature ventricular complexes (PVCs) or VT can be observed. Catheter position in the right ventricular outflow tract (RVOT) can be misleading and simulate a CS position. Confirming appropriate catheter positioning in the CS can be achieved by fluoroscopy and recorded electrograms. In the LAO view, further advancement in the CS will direct the catheter toward the left heart border, where it will curve toward the left shoulder. Conversely, advancement of a catheter lying in the RVOT will lead to an upward direction of the catheter toward the pulmonary artery. In the RAO view, the CS catheter is directed posteriorly, posterior to the AV sulcus, whereas the RVOT position is directed anteriorly. Recording from the CS catheter will show simultaneous atrial and ventricular electrograms, with the atrial electrogram falling in the later part of the P wave, whereas a catheter lying in the RVOT will record only a ventricular electrogram.

If used, the CS catheter should be placed first, because its positioning can be impeded by the presence of other catheters. It is also recommended that the CS catheter sheath be sutured to the skin to prevent displacement of the catheter during the course of the EP study.

Transaortic Approach

This approach is generally used for mapping the LV and mitral annulus (for VT and left-sided BTs). The right femoral

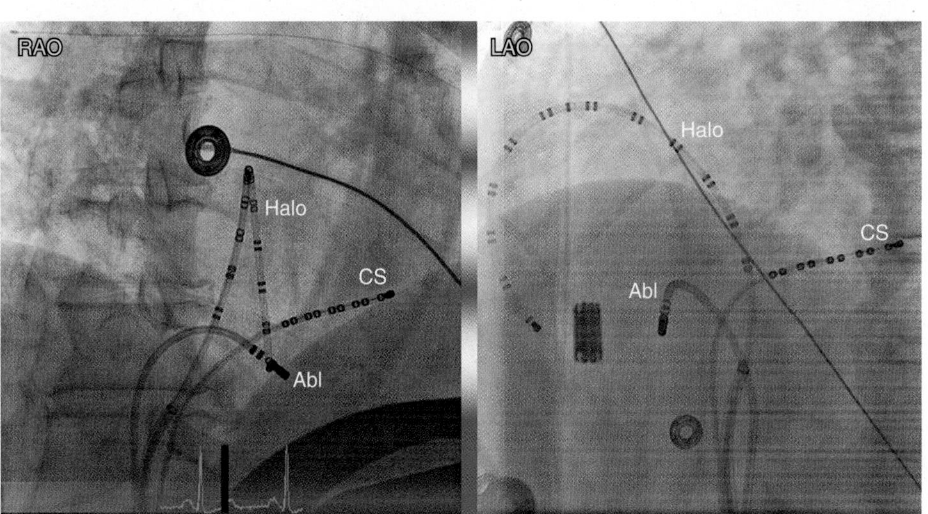

FIGURE 2–8 Left anterior oblique (LAO) and right anterior oblique (RAO) fluoroscopic views of catheters in a study of typical atrial flutter (AFL). A 20-pole halo catheter is positioned along the tricuspid annulus. The coronary sinus (CS) catheter was introduced from a femoral venous approach. The ablation catheter (Abl) is at the cavotricuspid isthmus.

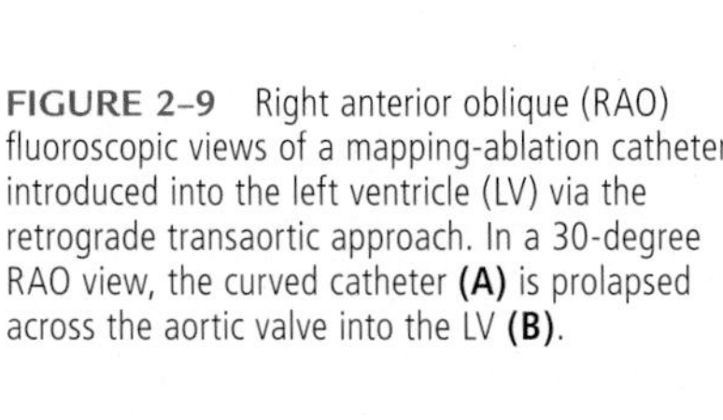

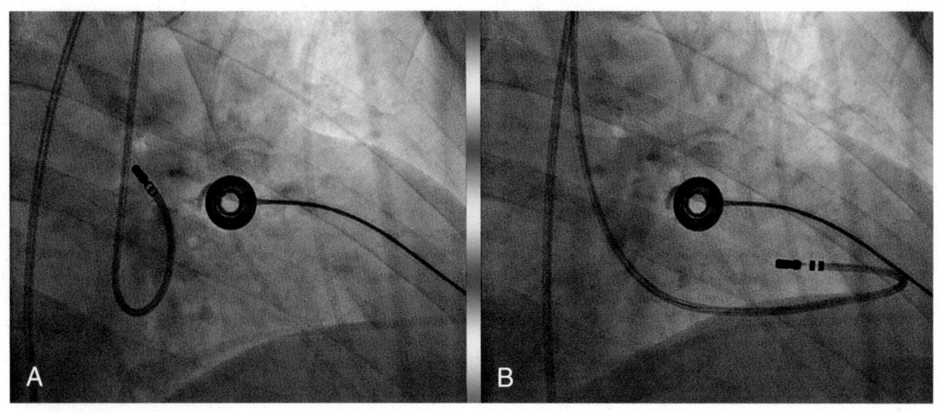

FIGURE 2–9 Right anterior oblique (RAO) fluoroscopic views of a mapping-ablation catheter introduced into the left ventricle (LV) via the retrograde transaortic approach. In a 30-degree RAO view, the curved catheter **(A)** is prolapsed across the aortic valve into the LV **(B)**.

artery is most commonly used. The mapping-ablation catheter is passed to the descending aorta and, in this position, a tight J curve is formed with the catheter tip before passage to the aortic root to minimize catheter manipulation in the arch. In a 30-degree RAO view, the curved catheter is advanced through the aortic valve with the J curve opening to the right, so the catheter passes into the LV oriented anterolaterally (Fig. 2-9). The straight catheter tip must never be used to cross the aortic valve because of the risk of leaflet damage or perforation, and also because the catheter tip can slip into the left or right coronary artery or a coronary bypass graft, mimicking entry to the LV and causing damage to these structures.

A long vascular sheath can provide added catheter stability. Anticoagulation should be started once the LV is accessed (IV heparin, 5000-unit bolus followed by a 1000-unit infusion is usually used), to maintain the activated clotting time (ACT) between 250 and 300 seconds.

Transseptal Approach

Anatomy of the Interatrial Septum

Mapping and ablation in the LA are performed through a transseptal approach. Multiple separate transseptal punctures can be required in AF ablation procedures, depending on the strategy used.

Knowledge of septal anatomy and its relationship to adjacent structures is essential to ensure safe and effective access to the LA.[6] Many apparent septal structures are not truly septal. The true interatrial septum is limited to the floor of the fossa ovalis, flap valve, and anteroinferior rim of the fossa.[7] Therefore, the floor of the fossa is the target for atrial septal crossing. The area between the superior border of the fossa and the mouth of the SVC is an infolding of the atrial wall filled with adipose tissue and, although often referred to as the septum secundum, it is not really a true septum and puncture in this region would lead to exiting of the heart.[6,7]

A search for a patent foramen ovale, which is present in 15% to 20% of normal subjects, is initially performed. If one is absent, atrial septal puncture is performed. The challenge for a successful atrial septal puncture is positioning the Brockenbrough needle at the thinnest aspect of the atrial septum, the membranous fossa ovalis, guided by fluoroscopy or intracardiac echocardiography (ICE).[8,9]

Although fluoroscopy provides sufficient information to allow safe transseptal puncture in the most cases, variations in septal anatomy, atrial or aortic root dilation, the need for multiple punctures, and the desired ability to direct the catheter to specific locations within the LA can make fluoroscopy an inadequate tool for complex LA ablation procedures. Intraoperative transesophageal echocardiography (TEE) allows identification of the fossa ovalis and its relation to surrounding structures and provides real-time evaluation of the atrial septal puncture procedure, with demonstration of tenting of the fossa prior to entry into the LA and visualization of the sheath advancing across the septum. However, the usefulness of TEE is limited by the fact that the probe obstructs the fluoroscopic field and is impractical in the nonanesthetized patient. Intracardiac echocardiography (ICE), which provides similar information on septal anatomy, can be used for the conscious patient and does not impede fluoroscopy. Radiofrequency (RF) ablation lesions have been used recently to aid perforation of an unusually thick or fibrotic atrial septum.

Fluoroscopy-Guided Transseptal Catheterization

Equipment required for atrial septal puncture include the following: a 62-cm, 8 Fr transseptal sheath for LA cannulation (SR0, SL1, or Mullins sheath, St. Jude Medical, Minnetonka, Minn), a 0.035-inch J guidewire, a 71-cm Brockenbrough needle (BRK, St. Jude Medical, Minnetonka, Minn), and a 190-cm, 0.014-inch guidewire (model 6724, Guidant, St. Paul, Minn).

Venous access is obtained via the femoral vein, preferably the right femoral vein because it is closer to the operator. The sheath, dilator, and guidewires are flushed with heparinized saline. The transseptal sheath and dilator are advanced over a 0.035-inch J guidewire into the SVC. The guidewire is then withdrawn, leaving the sheath and its dilator locked in place. The dilator within the sheath is flushed and attached to a syringe to avoid introduction of air into the RA.

Attention is then directed to preparing the transseptal needle. The Brockenbrough needle comes prepackaged with an inner stylet, which may be left in place to protect it as it is advanced within the sheath. Alternatively, the inner stylet may be removed and the needle connected to a pressure transducer line (pressure monitoring through the Brockenbrough needle will be required during the transseptal puncture); continuous flushing through the Brockenbrough needle is used while advancing the needle into the dilator. A third approach, when the use of contrast injection is planned, is to attach the Brockenbrough needle to a standard three-way stopcock via a freely rotating adapter. A 10-mL syringe filled with radiopaque contrast is attached to the other end of the stopcock while a pressure transducer line is attached to the third stopcock valve for continuous pressure monitoring.[10] The entire apparatus should be vigorously flushed to ensure that no air bubbles are present within the circuit.

The Brockenbrough needle is advanced into the dilator until the needle tip is within 1 to 2 cm of the dilator tip. The needle tip must be kept within the dilator at all times, except during transseptal puncture. The curves of the dilator, sheath, and needle should be aligned so that they are all in agreement and not contradicting each other. The sheath, dilator, and needle assembly is then rotated leftward and posteriorly toward the atrial septum, usually with the Brockenbrough needle arrow pointing at the 3 to 6 o'clock position relative to its shaft. By withdrawing the sheath, dilator, and needle assembly as a single unit, while maintaining the relative positions of its components, over the atrial septum under fluoroscopy guidance (30-degree LAO view), the dilator tip moves slightly leftward on entering the

RA and then leftward again while descending below the aortic root. A third abrupt leftward movement ("jump") below the aortic root indicates passage over the limbus into the fossa ovalis (Fig. 2-10). This latter jump generally occurs at the level of the HB catheter. If the sheath and dilator assembly is pulled back farther than intended (i.e., below the level of the fossa), the needle should be withdrawn and the guidewire placed through the dilator into the SVC. The sheath and dilator assembly is then advanced over the guidewire into the SVC and repositioning attempted, as described. The sheath and dilator assembly should never be advanced without the guidewire at any point during the procedure.

Several fluoroscopic markers are used to confirm the position of the dilator tip at the fossa ovalis.[8,9] An abrupt leftward movement (jump) of the dilator tip below the aortic knob is observed as the tip passes under the muscular atrial septum onto the fossa ovalis. In addition, the posterior extent of the aortic root is marked by a pigtail catheter positioned through the femoral artery in the noncoronary cusp or by the HB catheter (recording a stable proximal HB potential), which lies at the level of the fibrous trigone opposite and caudal to the noncoronary aortic cusp. When the dilator tip lies against the fossa ovalis, it is directed posteroinferiorly to the proximal HB electrode (or pigtail catheter) in the RAO view and to the left of the proximal HB electrode (or pigtail catheter) in the LAO view (see Fig. 2-10). Another method that can be used to ensure that the tip is against the fossa ovalis is injection of 3 to 5 mL of radiopaque contrast through the Brockenbrough needle to visualize the interatrial septum. The needle tip then can be seen tenting the fossa ovalis membrane with small movements of the entire transseptal apparatus.[10]

Once the position of the dilator tip is confirmed at the fossa ovalis, the needle is briskly advanced outside the dilator in the LAO view during continuous pressure monitoring. If excessive force is applied without a palpable "pop" to the fossa, then the Brockenbrough needle likely was not in proper position. After passage through the fossa ovale and before advancing the dilator and sheath, an intraatrial position of the needle tip within the LA, rather than the ascending aorta or posteriorly into the pericardial space, needs to be confirmed.[8,9] Recording an LA pressure waveform from the needle tip confirms an intraatrial location (Fig. 2-11). An arterial pressure waveform indicates intraaortic position of the needle. Absence of a pressure wave recording can indicate needle passage into the pericardial space or sliding up and not puncturing through the atrial septum. A second method is injection of contrast through the needle to assess the position of the needle tip. Alternatively, passing a 0.014-inch floppy guidewire through the Brockenbrough needle into a PV helps verify that needle tip position is within the LA. If the guidewire cannot be advanced beyond the cardiac silhouette or if it seems to follow the path of the aorta, contrast should be injected to assess the position of the Brockenbrough needle before advancing the transseptal dilator.[10]

Once the position of the needle tip is confirmed to be in the LA, both the sheath and dilator are advanced as a single unit over the needle using one hand while fixing the

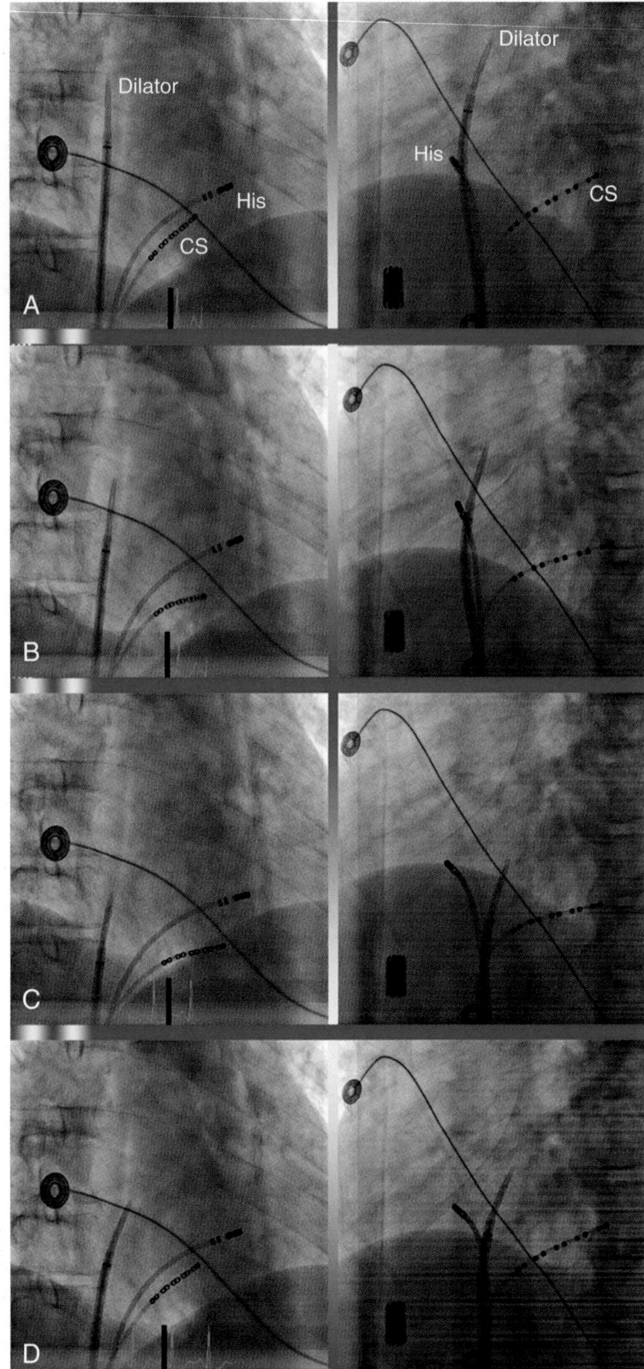

FIGURE 2–10 Right anterior oblique (RAO; **left**) and left anterior oblique (LAO; **right**) fluoroscopic views during transseptal catheterization. **A,** Initially, the transseptal sheath-dilator assembly is advanced into the superior vena cava. **B,** The transseptal assembly is withdrawn into the high right atrium. **C,** With further withdrawal, the dilator tip abruptly moves leftward, indicating passage over the limbus into the fossa ovalis at the level of the His bundle catheter. At the fossa ovalis, the dilator tip has an anteroposterior orientation in the RAO view and a leftward orientation in the LAO view. **D,** The transseptal assembly is advanced across the atrial septum. CS = coronary sinus.

Brockenbrough needle in position with the other hand (to prevent any further advancement of the needle). Once the dilator tip is advanced into the LA over the needle tip, the needle and dilator are firmly stabilized as a unit—to prevent any further advancement of the needle and dilator—and the sheath is advanced over the dilator into the LA. Once the transseptal sheath tip is within the LA, the dilator and

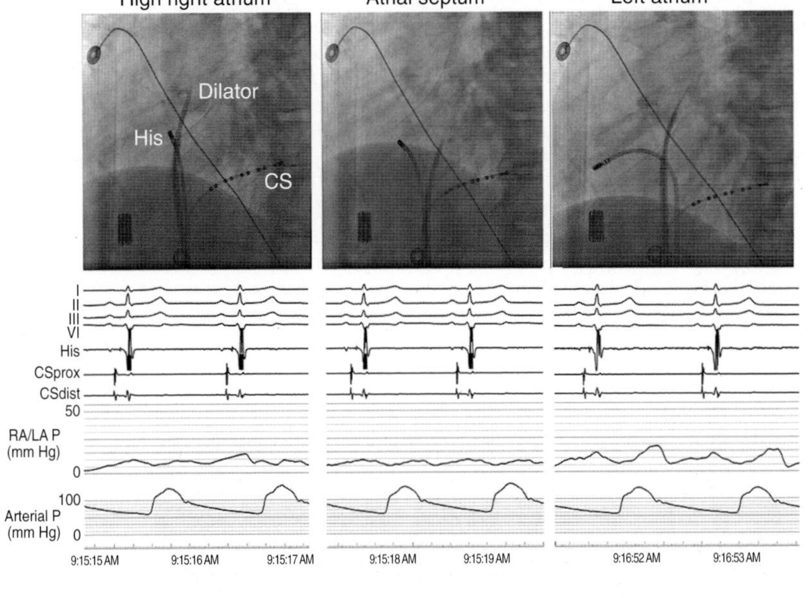

FIGURE 2–11 Left anterior oblique (LAO) fluoroscopic views and simultaneous electrical and pressure recordings during transseptal catheterization. **Left,** The transseptal assembly is in the right atrium (RA), indicated by typical A and V waves of right-heart pressure tracing. **Middle,** The pressure waveform is dampened somewhat as the catheter tip abuts the septum. **Right,** The needle is across the atrial septum and characteristic waves (V larger than A) are seen.

needle are withdrawn slowly during continuous flushing through the needle or while suction is maintained through a syringe placed on the sheath side port to minimize the risk of air embolism, and while fixing the sheath with the other hand to prevent dislodgment outside the LA. The sheath should be aspirated until blood appears without further bubbles; this usually requires aspiration of about 5 mL. The sheath is then flushed with heparinized saline at a flow rate of 3 mL/min during the entire procedure. The mapping-ablation catheter is advanced through the sheath into the LA. Flexing the catheter tip and applying clockwise and counterclockwise torque to the sheath help confirm free movement of the catheter tip within the LA, rather than possibly in the pericardium. It is important to recognize that merely recording LA electrograms does not confirm intracavitary catheter location because an LA recording can be obtained from the epicardial surface.

When two transseptal accesses are required, the second access can be obtained through a separate transseptal puncture performed in a fashion similar to that described for the first puncture. Alternatively, the first transseptal puncture can be used for the second sheath. This technique entails passing a guidewire or thin catheter through the first transseptal sheath into the LA, preferably into the left inferior or superior PV, and then the sheath is pulled back into the RA. Subsequently, a deflectable tip catheter is used through the second long sheath to interrogate the fossa ovalis and to try to access the LA through the initial puncture site. Once this is accomplished, the first sheath is advanced back into the LA, and the guidewire is replaced with the mapping catheter. Alternatively, instead of using a deflectable catheter, the needle, dilator, and sheath assembly is advanced into the SVC and pulled back and positioned at the fossa ovalis (as described earlier for the first transseptal puncture). Once the tip of the dilator falls into the fossa ovalis, gentle manipulation of the assembly under biplane fluoroscopy guidance is performed until the dilator tip passes along the guidewire through the existing transseptal puncture, without advancing the needle through the dilator. The assembly is then advanced as a single unit into the LA.[8]

After LA access is obtained and verified, an IV heparin bolus is administered followed by intermittent boluses or continuous infusion to maintain an elevated ACT (more than 250 to 300 seconds). Alternatively, heparin can be administered immediately prior to septal puncture.

Intracardiac Echocardiography–Guided Transseptal Catheterization

The intent of ICE-guided transseptal catheterization is to image intracardiac anatomy and identify the exact position of the distal aspect of the transseptal dilator along the atrial septum—in particular, to assess for tenting of the fossa ovalis with the dilator tip.[8,9]

Two types of ICE imaging systems are currently available, the electronic phased-array ultrasound catheter and the mechanical ultrasound catheter.[11,12] The electronic phased-array ultrasound catheter sector imaging system (AcuNav, Siemens Medical Solutions, Malvern, Pa) uses an 8 or 10 Fr catheter that has a forward-facing 64-element vector phased-array transducer scanning in the longitudinal plane. The catheter has a four-way steerable tip (160-degree anteroposterior or left-right deflections). The catheter images a sector field oriented in the plane of the catheter. The mechanical ultrasound catheter radial imaging system (Ultra ICE, EP Technologies, Boston Scientific, San Jose, Calif) uses a 9-MHz catheter-based ultrasound transducer contained within a 9 Fr (110-cm length) catheter shaft. It has a single rotating crystal ultrasound transducer that images circumferentially for 360 degrees in the horizontal plane. The catheter is not freely deflectable.

Using the mechanical radial ICE imaging system, a 9 Fr sheath, preferably a long preshaped sheath, for the ICE catheter is advanced via a femoral venous access. To enhance image quality, all air must be eliminated from the distal tip of the ICE catheter by flushing vigorously with 5 to 10 mL of sterile water. The catheter then is connected to the ultrasound console and advanced until the tip of the rotary ICE catheter images the fossa ovalis. Satisfactory imaging of the fossa ovalis for guiding transseptal puncture is viewed from the mid-RA (Fig. 2-12).[12]

The AcuNav ICE catheter is introduced under fluoroscopy guidance through a 23-cm femoral venous sheath. Once the catheter is advanced into the mid-RA with the catheter tension controls in neutral position (the ultrasound transducer oriented anteriorly and to the left), the RA, tricuspid valve, and RV are viewed. This is called the home view (Fig. 2-13A). Gradual clockwise rotation of a straight catheter from the home view allows sequential visualization of the aortic root and the pulmonary artery (see Fig. 2-13B), followed by the CS, the mitral valve, the LA append-

2

age orifice, and a cross-sectional view of the fossa ovalis (see Fig. 2-13C and D). The mitral valve and interatrial septum are usually seen in the same plane as the LA appendage. Posterior deflection or right-left steering of the imaging tip in the RA, or both, is occasionally required to optimize visualization of the fossa ovalis; the tension knob (lock function) can then be used to hold the catheter tip in position. Further clockwise rotation beyond this location will demonstrate images of the left PV ostia (see Fig. 2-13E). The optimal ICE image to guide transseptal puncture will demonstrate adequate space behind the interatrial septum on the LA side and clearly identify adjacent structures, but will not include the aortic root because it would be too anterior to be punctured safely. With an enlarged LA, a cross-sectional view that includes the LA appendage is also optimal if an adequate space exists behind the atrial septum on the LA side.[11,12]

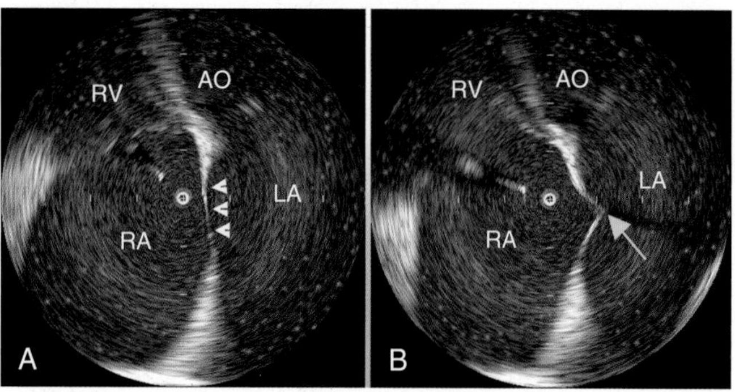

FIGURE 2–12 Intracardiac echocardiography (ICE)–guided transseptal puncture using the Ultra-ICE catheter. These ICE images, with the transducer placed in the right atrium (RA), show **(A)** the RA, fossa ovalis (arrowheads), left atrium (LA), and aorta (AO). **B,** The transseptal needle is properly positioned, with tenting (yellow arrow) against the midinteratrial septum at the fossa ovalis. RV= right ventricle.

The sheath, dilator, and needle assembly is introduced into the RA and the dilator tip is positioned against the fossa ovale, as described earlier. Before advancing the Brockenbrough needle, continuous ICE imaging should direct further adjustments in the dilator tip position until ICE confirms the tip is in intimate contact with the middle of the fossa, confirms proper lateral movement of the dilator toward the fossa, and excludes inadvertent superior displacement toward the muscular septum and aortic valve. With further advancement of the dilator, ICE demonstrates tenting of the fossa (see Figs. 2-12 and 2-14). If the distance from the tented fossa to the LA free wall is small, minor adjustments in the dilator tip position can be made to maximize the space. The Brockenbrough needle is then advanced. With successful transseptal puncture, a palpable "pop" is felt, and sudden collapse of the tented fossa is observed (Fig. 2-14). Advancement of the needle is then immediately stopped. With no change in position of the Brockenbrough needle, the transseptal dilator and sheath are advanced over the guidewire into the LA, as described earlier.

Complications of Atrial Transseptal Puncture

Injury to cardiac and extracardiac structures is the most feared complication. Because of its stiffness and large caliber, the transseptal dilator should never be advanced until the position of the Brockenbrough needle is confirmed with confidence. Advancing the dilator into an improper position can be fatal. Therefore, many operators recommend the use of ICE-guided transseptal puncture, especially for patients with normal atrial size.

When the aorta is advertently punctured by the Brockenbrough needle—an arterial waveform is recorded from the needle tip and dye injected through the needle is carried

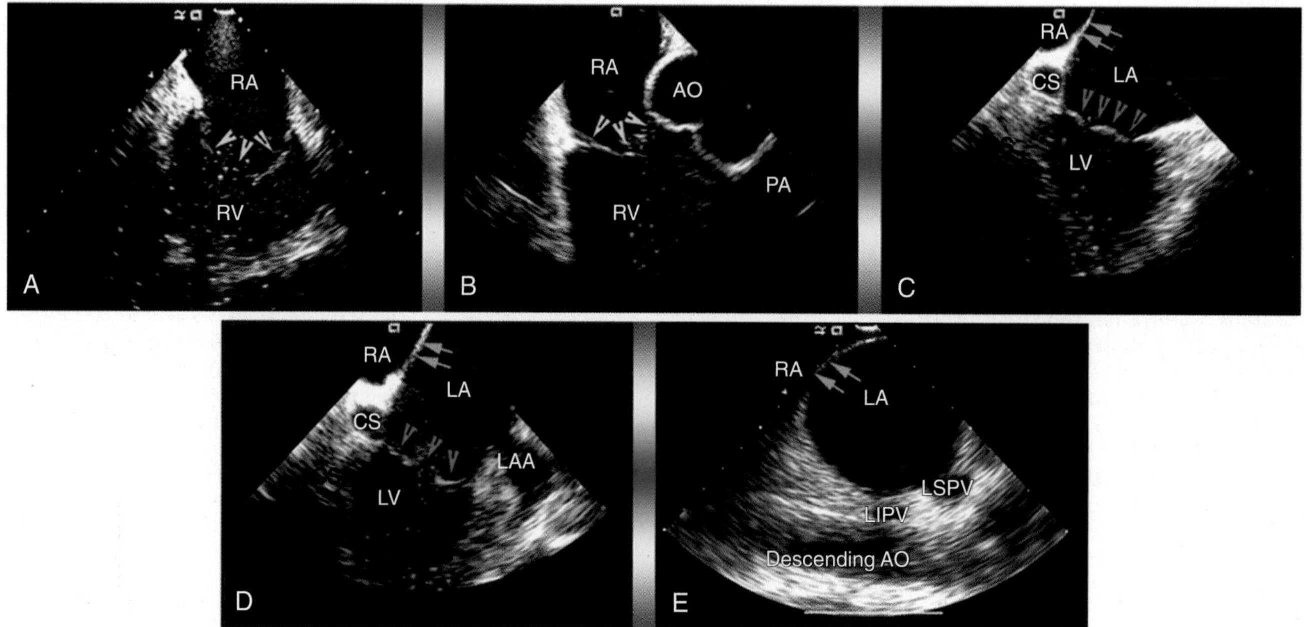

FIGURE 2–13 Phased-array intracardiac echocardiography (ICE) AcuNav serial images with the transducer placed in the mid-RA (right atrium) demonstrate serial changes in tomographic imaging views following clockwise rotation of the transducer. Each view displays a left-right (L-R) orientation marker to the operator's left side (i.e., craniocaudal axis projects from image right to left). **A,** Starting from the home view, the RA, tricuspid valve (yellow arrowheads) and right ventricle (RV) are visualized. **B,** Clockwise rotation brings the aorta (AO) into view. **C,** Further rotation allows visualization of the interatrial septum (green arrows), left atrium (LA), coronary sinus (CS), left ventricle (LV), and mitral valve (red arrowheads). **D,** Subsequently, the left atrium appendage (LAA) becomes visible. **E,** The ostia of the left superior pulmonary vein (LSPV) and left inferior PV (LIPV) can be visualized with further clockwise rotation. *(AcuNav, Siemens Medical Solutions, Malvern, Pa.)*

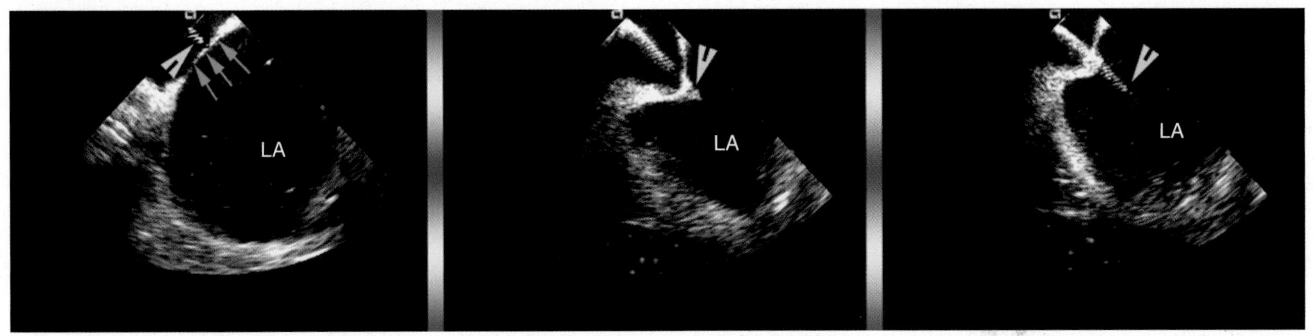

FIGURE 2–14 Phased-array intracardiac echocardiography (ICE)–guided transseptal puncture. **A,** These ICE images, with the transducer placed in the right atrium (RA), show a transseptal dilator tip (yellow arrowhead) lying against the interatrial septum (green arrows). **B,** With further advancement of the dilator, ICE demonstrates tenting of the interatrial septum at the fossa ovalis. **C,** Advancement of the transseptal needle is then performed, with the needle tip visualized in the left atrium (LA), and tenting of the interatrial septum is lost.

away from the heart—the needle can be withdrawn back into the dilator. If the patient remains stable for 15 minutes, another attempt at LA access can be made. Advancing the dilator and sheath assembly into the aorta can lead to catastrophic consequences.

It is important to recognize that a successful atrial septal puncture should be a painless procedure for the patient. If the patient experiences significant discomfort, careful assessment should be made of the catheter and sheath locations (pericardial space, aorta).

Another complication is embolism of thrombus or air. To avoid air emboli, catheters must be advanced and withdrawn slowly so as not to suck air. Thromboembolic complications can be avoided by flushing all sheaths and guidewire with heparinized saline and maintaining the ACT above 300 seconds. In addition, a guidewire should not be left in the LA for more than 1 minute, especially if no systemic heparin has been administered.

Epicardial Approach

Coronary veins can be used to perform epicardial mapping, but manipulation of the mapping catheter is limited by the anatomical distribution of these vessels. Therefore, the subxiphoid percutaneous approach to the epicardial space is the only technique currently available that allows extensive and unrestricted mapping of the epicardial surface of both ventricles, and has been used most commonly for VT mapping and ablation.[5,13-17]

The subxiphoid approach must be performed with the patient under general anesthesia, because of its high-risk nature and also because RF pulses applied in the epicardial surface are painful. Initially, a multipolar catheter is positioned in the CS and catheter in the RV apex through the femoral approach.[17] The pericardial space is reached using a spinal tap needle. The puncture must be performed at the angle between the left border of the subxiphoid process and the lower left rib. The needle must always point to the left shoulder; it must be introduced more horizontally if the target is the anterior portion of the ventricles and more vertically if the diaphragmatic portion of the heart is the area of interest. After crossing the subcutaneous tissue, the needle movement should be monitored under fluoroscopy in the 35- to 40-degree LAO view. The needle must be carefully moved toward the heart silhouette until heart movement can be detected. In general, with this technique, the needle will reach the midportion between the basal and apical areas of the heart (in the 35- to 40-degree RAO view). In the 40-degree LAO view, injection of a small amount of contrast (approximately 1 mL) demonstrates whether the needle tip is pushing or passing through the tissue. If the diaphragm has not been reached, the contrast will be seen in the subdiaphragmatic area. When the needle reaches the pericardial sac, the contrast will spread around the heart, restricted to its silhouette. In some cases, the needle will get close enough to the heart, but the contrast will not be clearly identified in the pericardial sac. In these cases, despite the needle being out of the pericardial sac, it is likely that a lesion has been created in the membrane, through which it is large enough to advance a guidewire and reach the pericardial sac. If the needle is not close enough to the pericardial membrane, the guidewire will move toward the subdiaphragmatic area. In these cases, the wire must be pulled back and small movements with the needle and the wire must be performed until the pericardial space is reached. The position of the guidewire is important to demonstrate that it is adequately inserted in the pericardial sac. It must be seen at the edge of the cardiac silhouette in the 35- to 40-degree LAO view and, when advanced, it should not induce PVCs.[5]

The percutaneous approach to the pericardial space can be difficult in patients with pericardial adhesions (e.g., following cardiac surgery or pericarditis). In postsurgical patients, the adhesions are mostly concentrated in the anterior portion of the heart; therefore, the puncture must be directed toward the diaphragmatic area. In postpericarditis patients, adhesion can be more diffuse than postsurgical patients.

After reaching the pericardial space with the guidewire, the needle must be withdrawn and a standard sheath must be introduced (generally 7 or 8 Fr). If it is necessary to insert another catheter, a second guidewire can be advanced through the sheath, which should be removed, leaving two wires inside the pericardial space. Subsequently, a separate sheath is introduced over each of the guidewires. Alternatively, a second puncture to the pericardial sac may be performed, using the same steps described for the first puncture. Before removing the dilator out of the sheath, the sheath must be pushed against the chest to guarantee that the tip of the sheath is placed inside the pericardial sac. The use of longer sheaths should be considered, especially in patients with a larger thorax.

Before introducing the mapping-ablation catheter, the sheath must be aspirated to check for bleeding. At this point, the anticoagulation should not have been administered; therefore, any bleeding should be self-limited and is generally considered a minor complication because it is not necessary to interrupt the procedure. Major bleeding is rare, and it can be related to the learning curve.[17]

When bleeding is under control, the mapping-ablation catheter can be introduced. Once it is inside the pericardial sac, the catheter can be easily moved, allowing the exploration of the entire epicardial surface. In patients with pericardial adhesions, the catheter can be used to perform blunt dissection of the adhesions. If the area of interest is too close to the tip of the sheath, a simple pull-back in the catheter can lead to the loss of pericardial access. Therefore, it is preferable to advance the catheter inside the pericardial space and return to the point of interest by deflecting the tip of the catheter back toward it.

Once in the pericardial space, atrial and ventricular surface mapping can be performed. Atrial surface mapping can be limited by the normal pericardial reflections and by the atrial irregular anatomy (RA and LA appendages). Ventricular surface mapping, however, can be performed more easily. During manipulation of the sheath, small amounts of air can reach the pericardial space, which can easily be detected by fluoroscopy. The presence of air can induce instability to the catheter secondary to the lack of contact between the parietal and visceral membranes of the pericardial sac. Aspiration of air will restore contact characteristic of the pericardial space.

To avoid coronary vessel damage, coronary angiography must be performed before the ablation procedure to select a safe area for RF applications. The base and the anterior and posterior septum areas are the more dangerous zones. In case of doubt, coronary angiography can be performed immediately before RF application, keeping the ablation catheter in the target site position.

At the completion of the mapping-ablation procedure, the catheter should be replaced by a pigtail catheter to check for bleeding. This catheter can be kept inside the pericardial sac for as long as it is considered necessary. Eventually, evaluation of the pericardial space can be performed using 2 to 3 mL of contrast, which should be aspirated before removing the sheath. After controlling the bleeding, monitoring the patient with serial transthoracic echocardiography 24 hours later is recommended.[17]

BASELINE MEASUREMENTS

Intracardiac Electrograms

Whereas the surface ECG records a summation of the electrical activity of the entire heart, intracardiac electrograms recorded by the electrode catheter represent only the electrical activity (phase 0 of the action potential) of the local cardiac tissue in the immediate vicinity of the catheter's electrodes. Cardiac electrograms are generated by the potential (voltage) differences recorded at two recording electrodes during the cardiac cycle. All clinical electrogram recordings are differential recordings from one source that is connected to the anodal (positive) input of the recording amplifier and a second source that is connected to the cathodal (negative) input.[18]

Recorded electrograms can provide three important pieces of information: (1) the local activation time—that is, the time of activation of myocardium immediately adjacent to the recording electrode relative to a reference; (2) the direction of propagation of electrical activity activation within the field of view of the recording electrode; and (3) the complexity of myocardial activation within the field of view of the recording electrode.

Analog Versus Digital Recordings

Intracardiac electrograms are recorded with amplifiers that have high-input impedances (more than 1010 Ω), to decrease unwanted electrical interference and ensure high-quality recordings.[18] Analog recording systems directly amplify the potential from the recording electrodes, plot the potential on a display oscilloscope and write it to recording paper, and/or store it on magnetic tape. Analog systems have largely been replaced by digital recording systems that use an analog to digital (A/D) converter that converts the amplitude of the potential recorded at each point in time to a number that is stored.

The quality of digital data is influenced by the sampling frequency and precision of the amplitude measurement.[18] The most common digital recording systems sample the signal approximately every 1 millisecond (i.e., 1000 Hz), which is generally adequate for practical purposes of activation mapping. However, higher sampling frequencies can be required for high-quality recording of high-frequency, rapid potentials that can originate from the Purkinje system or areas of infarction. The faster sampling places greater demands on the computer processor and increases the size of the stored data files.[18]

Unipolar Recordings

Unipolar recordings are obtained by positioning the exploring electrode in the heart and the second electrode (referred to as the indifferent electrode) distant from the heart so that it has little or no cardiac signal. The precordial ECG leads, for example, are unipolar recordings that use an indifferent electrode created by connecting the arm and left leg electrodes through high-impedance resistors.[18-20]

By convention, the exploring electrode in contact with the cardiac tissue is connected to the positive input of the recording amplifier. In this configuration, an approaching wavefront creates a positive deflection that quickly reverses itself as the wavefront passes directly under the electrode, generating an RS complex. In a normal homogeneous tissue, the maximum negative slope (dV/dt) of the signal coincides with the arrival of the depolarization wavefront directly beneath the electrode, because the maximal negative dV/dt corresponds to the maximum Na^+ channel conductance; Fig. 2-15). This is true for filtered and unfiltered unipolar electrograms.[18-20]

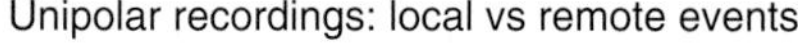

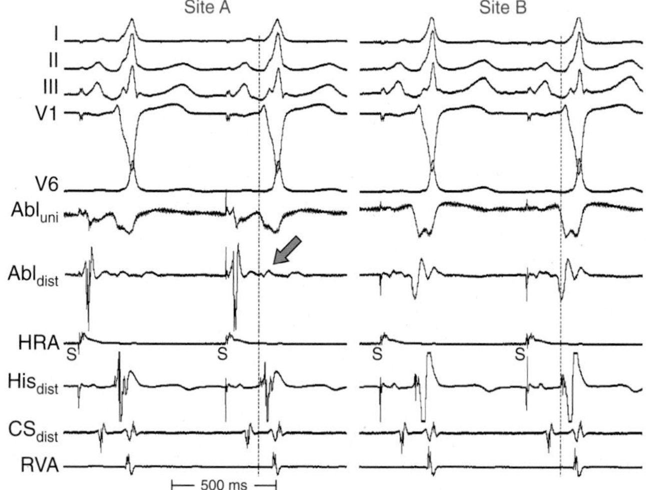

FIGURE 2–15 Unipolar and bipolar recordings. Two complexes from different sites are shown in a patient with Wolff-Parkinson-White syndrome. The dashed line denotes onset of the delta wave. **A,** At this site, the unfiltered unipolar recording shows a somewhat blunted "QS" complex and small atrial component, but the filtered (30- to 300-Hz) bipolar signal shows a very large atrial signal and very small ventricular signal (arrow), suggesting a poor choice for ablation site. **B,** This site shows a sharper "QS" in the unipolar signal, with a larger ventricular than atrial electrogram, and the initial nadir of bipolar recording coincides with the maximal negative dV/dt of the unipolar recording. Ablation at this site was successful.

The unfiltered unipolar recordings provide information about the direction of impulse propagation; positive deflections (R waves) are generated by propagation toward the recording electrode, and negative deflections (QS complexes) are generated by propagation away from the electrode. Unipolar recordings also allow pacing and recording at the same location while eliminating a possible anodal contribution to depolarization that is sometimes seen with bipolar pacing at high output.[18,19,21]

The unipolar electrograms are generally unfiltered (0.05 to 300 Hz or more), but are usually filtered at comparable settings to those of bipolar electrograms (10 to 40 to 300 Hz or more) when an abnormal tissue (scars or infarct areas) is studied, for which local electrograms can have very low amplitude and can be masked by larger far-field signals. Filtering the unipolar electrograms can help eliminate far-field signals; however, filtered unipolar recordings lose the ability to provide directional information.[18,19,21]

The major disadvantage of unipolar recordings is that they contain substantial far-field signals generated by depolarization of tissue remote from the recording electrode. Another disadvantage is the inability to record an undisturbed electrogram during or immediately after pacing.[20]

Bipolar Recordings

Bipolar recordings are obtained by connecting two electrodes that are exploring the area of interest to the recording amplifier. At each point in time, the potential generated is the sum of the potential from the positive input and the potential at the negative input. The potential at the negative input is inverted; this is subtracted from the potential at the positive input so that the final recording is the difference between the two.[18,21]

Unlike unipolar recordings, bipolar electrodes with short interpolar distances are relatively unaffected by far-field events. The bipolar electrogram is simply the difference between the two unipolar electrograms recorded at the two poles. Because the far-field signal is similar at each instant in time, it is largely subtracted out, leaving the local signal.[18,21] Therefore, compared with unipolar recordings, bipolar recordings provide an improved signal-to-noise ratio, and high-frequency components are more accurately seen.[5,20]

Although local activation is less precisely defined, in a homogeneous sheet of tissue the initial peak (or nadir) of a filtered (10 to 40 to 300 Hz or more) bipolar recording coincides with depolarization beneath the recording electrode and corresponds to the maximal negative dV/dt of the unipolar recording (see Fig. 2-15).

Several factors can affect bipolar electrogram amplitude and width, including conduction velocity (the greater the velocity, the higher the peak amplitude of the filtered bipolar electrogram), the mass of the activated tissue, the distance between the electrode and the propagating wavefront, the direction of propagation relative to the bipoles, the interelectrode distance, the amplifier gain, and other signal-processing techniques that can introduce artifacts.[18,21] To acquire true local electrical activity, a bipolar electrogram with an interelectrode distance less than 1 cm is desirable.[20]

The direction of wavefront propagation cannot be reliably inferred from the morphology of the bipolar signal. Moreover, bipolar recordings do not allow simultaneous pacing and recording from the same location. To pace and record simultaneously in bipolar fashion at endocardial sites as close together as possible, electrodes 1 and 3 of the quadripolar mapping catheter are used for bipolar pacing and electrodes 2 and 4 are used for recording.[5,20]

The differences in unipolar and bipolar recordings can be used to assist in mapping by simultaneously recording bipolar and unipolar signals from the mapping catheter.[18,19,21] Although bipolar recordings provide sufficient information for most mapping purposes in clinical EP laboratories, simultaneous unipolar recordings can provide an indication of the direction of wavefront propagation and a more precise measure of the timing of local activation.[20]

Signal Filtering

The surface ECG is usually filtered at 0.1 to 100.0 Hz. The bulk of the energy is in the 0.1- to 20.0-Hz range. Because of interference from alternating current (AC), muscle twitches, and similar relatively high-frequency interference, it is sometimes necessary to record the surface ECG over a lower frequency range or to use notch filters.[5,18]

Amplifiers are also used to filter the low- and high-frequency content of the intracardiac electrograms. Intracardiac electrograms are usually filtered to eliminate far-field noise, typically at 30 to 500 Hz. The range of frequencies not filtered out is frequently called the band pass. The high-pass filter allows frequencies above a limit to remain in the signal (i.e., it filters out lower frequencies) and the low-pass filter filters out frequencies above a certain limit.

High-Pass Filtering. High-pass filtering helps attenuate the frequencies that are slower than the specified cutoff (corner frequency) of the filter.[18] If intracardiac recordings were not filtered, the signal would wander up and down as this potential fluctuated with respiration, catheter movement, and variable catheter contact.

For bipolar electrograms, high-pass filters with corner frequencies between 10 and 50 Hz are commonly used. Filtering can distort the electrogram morphology and reduce its amplitude. The bipolar signal becomes more complex and additional peaks are introduced. In general, high-pass filtering can be viewed as differentiating the signal, so that the height of the signal is proportional to the rate of change of the signal rather than only the amplitude.[5]

Unipolar signals are commonly filtered at 0.05 to 0.5 Hz to remove baseline drift. Filtering at higher corner frequencies (e.g., 30 Hz) alters the morphology of the signal so that the morphology of the unipolar signal is no longer an indication of the direction of wavefront propagation and the presence or absence of a QS complex cannot be used to infer proximity to the site of earliest activation. However, filtering the unipolar signal does not affect its usefulness as a measure of the local activation time.[4,18] As mentioned earlier, during mapping of areas with infarcts or scars, where local electrograms can have very low amplitude and can be masked by larger far-field signals, high-pass filtering of a unipolar signal (at 30 Hz) can help reduce the far-field signal and improve detection of the lower amplitude local signals.[4,18]

Low-Pass Filtering. Low-pass filters attenuate frequencies that are faster than the specified corner frequency (usually 250 to 500 Hz). This is useful for reducing high-frequency noise and, at these frequencies, does not substantially affect electrograms recorded with clinical systems because most of the signal content is lower than 300 Hz.[18]

Band Pass Filtering. Defining a band of frequencies to record, such as setting the high-pass filter to 30 Hz and the low-pass filter to 300 Hz, defines a band of frequencies from 30 to 300 Hz that are not attenuated (i.e., band pass filtering). A notch filter is a special case of band pass filtering, with specific attenuation of frequencies at 50 or 60 Hz to reduce electrical noise introduced by the frequency of common AC current.

Timing of Local Events

As noted, with an unfiltered unipolar electrogram, a wavefront of depolarization that is propagating toward the exploring electrode generates a positive deflection (an R wave). As the wavefront reaches the electrode and propagates away, the deflection sweeps steeply negative. This rapid reversal constitutes the intrinsic deflection of the electrogram and represents the timing of the most local event (i.e., at the site of the electrode).[18] The maximum negative slope (dV/dt) of the signal coincides with the arrival of the depolarization wavefront directly beneath the electrode (see Fig. 2-15).[5]

Filtering the unipolar signal does not affect its usefulness as a measure of the local activation time. The slew rate or dV/dt of the filtered electrogram is so rapid in normal heart tissue that the difference between the peak and the nadir of the deflection is 5 milliseconds or less. Identification of the local event is therefore easy with filtered or unfiltered electrograms in normal tissue. On the other hand, diseased myocardium can conduct very slowly with fractionated electrograms, which makes local events harder to identify.

To acquire true local electrical activity, a bipolar electrogram with an interelectrode distance less than 1 cm is preferable. Smaller interelectrode distances record increasingly local events. In normal homogeneous tissue, the initial peak of a filtered (30 to 300 or more Hz) bipolar recording coincides with depolarization beneath the recording electrode and corresponds to the maximal negative dV/dt of the unipolar recording (see Fig. 2-15). However, in the case of complex multicomponent bipolar electrograms, such as those with marked fractionation and prolonged duration seen in regions with complex conduction patterns, determination of local activation time becomes problematic.[5]

When the intracardiac electrogram of interest is small relative to the size of surrounding electrograms (e.g., His deflection), and the gain must be markedly increased to produce a measurable deflection, clipping the signals can help eliminate the highly amplified surrounding signals to allow concentration on the deflection of interest (Fig. 2-16). It is important to recognize, however, that clippers eliminate the ability to determine the amplitude and timing of the intrinsic deflection (local timing) of the signals being limited.[4]

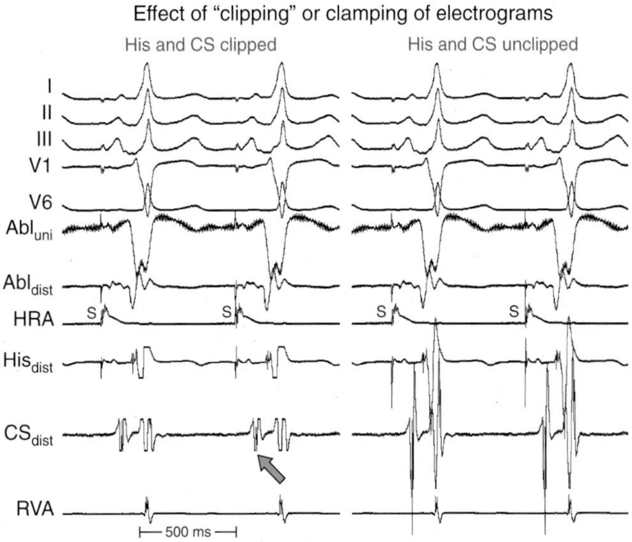

FIGURE 2–16 Effect of electronic clipping on recordings. The same two complexes are shown in both panels. **Left,** Both His and coronary sinus (CS) recordings are electronically attenuated (clipped) to reduce excursions on the display. The CS atrial and ventricular signals appear to have equal amplitude and the ventricular electrogram in the His recording is small. **Right,** Without clipping, the true signal amplitudes are seen, showing a very large ventricular signal in the His recording and a larger atrial than ventricular signal in the CS recording.

Choices of Surface and Intracardiac Signals

Baseline recordings obtained during a typical EP study include several surface ECG leads and several intracardiac electrograms, all of which are recorded simultaneously. Timing of events with respect to onset of the QRS complex or P wave on the surface ECG is often important during the EP study, but it is cumbersome to display all 12 leads of the regular surface ECG. It is more common to use leads I, II, aVF, V_1, and V_6, which provide most of the information required to determine the frontal plane axis, presence and type of intraventricular conduction abnormalities, and P wave morphology.

Intracardiac leads can be placed strategically at various locations within the cardiac chambers to record local events in the region of the lead. A classic display would include three to five surface ECG leads, high RA recording, HB recording, CS recording, and RV apex recording (Fig. 2-17). Depending on the type of study and information sought, stimulation and recording from other sites can be appropriate and can include RB recording, LV recording, transseptal LA recording, and atrial and ventricular mapping catheter tracings for EP mapping and ablation.[4,18]

The intracardiac electrograms are generally displayed in the order of normal cardiac activation. The first intracardiac tracing is a recording from the high RA close to the sinus node. The next intracardiac tracing is the HB recording, obtained from a catheter positioned at the HB, which shows low septal RA, HB, and high septal RV depolarizations. One to five recordings may be obtained from the CS, which reflects LA activation, followed by a recording from the RV catheter (see Fig. 2-17).[5]

High Right Atrium Electrogram. Depending on the exact location of the RA catheter, the high RA electrogram typically shows a local sharp, large atrial electrogram and a smaller, far-field ventricular electrogram. The catheter is usually positioned in the RA appendage because of stability and reproducibility. The recorded atrial electrogram will be earlier in the P wave when the catheter is positioned close to the sinus node. Recordings from this site also help determine the direction of atrial activation (e.g., high-low versus low-high, and right-left versus left-right). Pacing at this position allows evaluation of sinus node function and AV conduction as well as the induction of atrial arrhythmias.

Coronary Sinus Electrogram. Because the CS lies in the AV groove, in close contact to both the LA and LV, the CS catheter records both atrial and ventricular electrograms. However, the CS has a variable relationship to the mitral annulus. The CS lies 2 cm superior to the annulus as it crosses from the RA to the LA. More distally, the CS frequently overrides the LV. Consequently, the most proximal CS electrodes (located at the CS os) are closer to the atrium and typically show a local sharp, large atrial electrogram and a smaller, far-field ventricular electrogram. The more distal CS electrodes, lying closer to the LV than the LA, will record progressively smaller, less sharp, far-field atrial electrograms and larger, sharper, near-field ventricular electrograms (see Fig. 2-17).

During normal sinus rhythm (NSR), atrial activation sequence procedes from the CS os distally. However, if the CS catheter is deeply seated in the CS, so that the most proximal electrodes are distal to the CS os and the most distal electrodes are anterolateral on the mitral annulus, then both proximal and distal electrodes can be activated at the same time (Fig. 2-18).

His Bundle Electrogram. The HB catheter is positioned at the junction of the RA and RV. Therefore, it will record electrograms from local activation of the adjacent atrial, HB, and ventricular tissues (Fig. 2-19). Using a 5- to 10-mm bipolar recording, the His potential appears as a

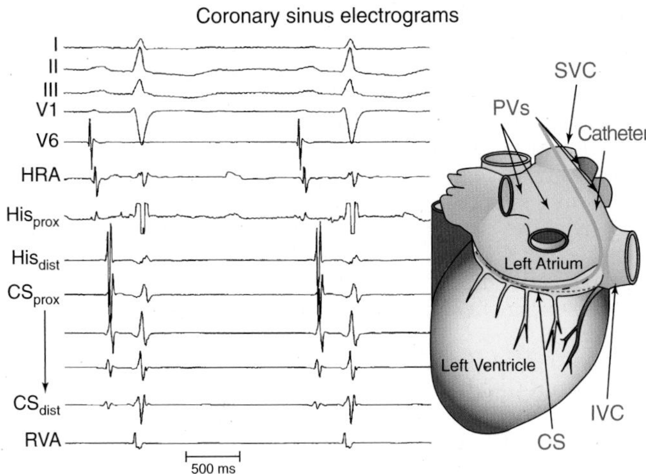

FIGURE 2–17 A classic display of surface ECG and intracardiac recordings during an electrophysiology study of supraventricular tachycardia. Included are four surface ECG leads, high right atrium (HRA) recording, two His bundle (HB) recordings (proximal and distal His), five coronary sinus (CS) recordings (in a proximal-to-distal sequence), and a right ventricle apex (RVA) recording. The relative amplitudes of atrial and ventricular electrograms in CS recordings are also shown. **Right,** The back of the heart is shown with a CS catheter in position. The distal portion of the CS is closer to the ventricle (originating as great cardiac vein on the anterior wall); the CS crosses the atrioventricular (AV) groove at the lateral margin and becomes an entirely atrial structure as it empties into the right atrium (RA). **Left,** Thus, proximal CS recordings show large atrial and small ventricular signals, whereas more distal recordings show small atrial, large ventricular signals. IVC = inferior vena cava; PV = pulmonary vein; SVC = superior vena cava.

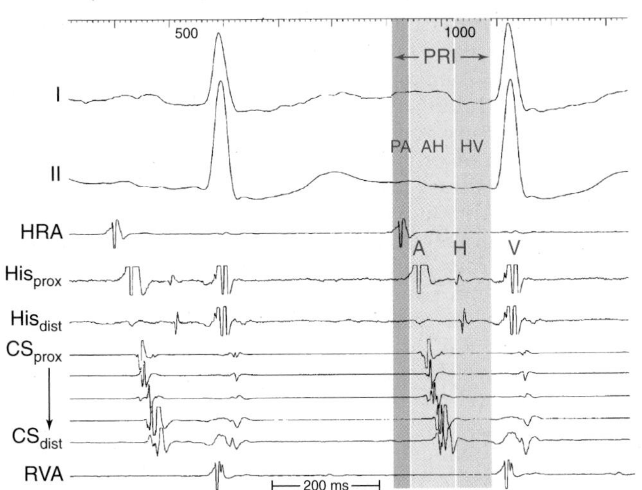

FIGURE 2–19 Intracardiac intervals. Shaded areas represent the pulmonary artery (PA) (blue), atrial–His bundle (AH) (pink), and His bundle–ventricular (HV) (yellow) intervals. It is important that the HV interval be measured from the onset of the His potential in the recording showing the most proximal (rather than the most prominent) His potential (His_{prox}) to the onset of the QRS on the surface ECG (rather than the ventricular electrogram on the His bundle [HB] recording). See text for details.

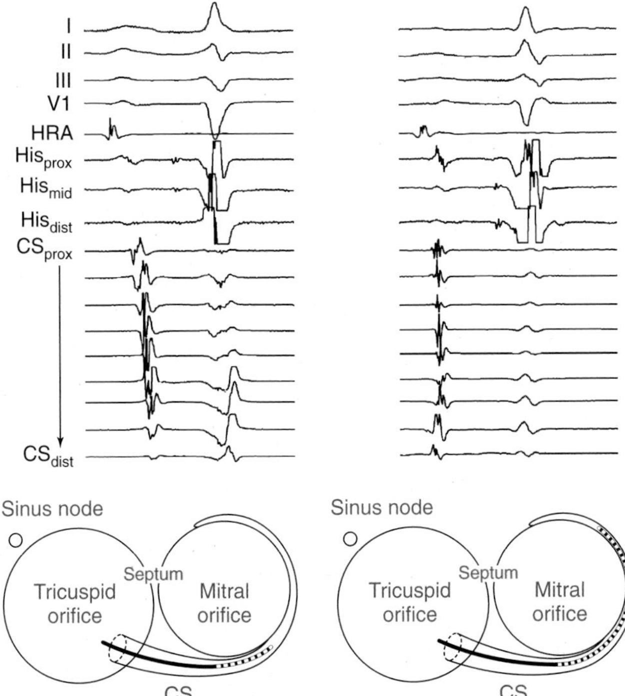

FIGURE 2–18 Influence of catheter position on coronary sinus (CS) atrial electrograms. Two different CS atrial activation sequences are shown from different patients. **Left,** A proximal-to-distal sequence is shown. **Right,** The latest activation is in the mid-CS electrodes. Diagrams at bottom show relative positions of CS catheter in each instance (atrioventricular grooves viewed from above). With more proximal CS position, propagation is proximal-distal, indicating relative distance from sinus node. With a more distal CS position, the mid-CS electrodes are furthest from the sinus node.

rapid biphasic spike, 15 to 25 milliseconds in duration, interposed between local atrial and ventricular electrograms. The use of a quadripolar catheter allows simultaneous recording of three bipolar pairs.[22]

Before measuring conduction intervals within the HB electrogram, it is important to verify that the spike recorded between the atrial and ventricular electrograms on the HB catheter actually represents activation of the most proximal HB and not the distal HB or RB. The most proximal electrodes displaying the His potential should be chosen, and a large atrial electrogram should accompany the proximal His potential. Anatomically, the proximal portion of the HB originates in the atrial side of the tricuspid annulus; thus, the most proximal HB deflection is the one associated with the largest atrial electrogram. Recording of His potential associated with a small atrial electrogram can reflect recording of the distal HB or RB, and therefore might miss important intra-His conduction abnormalities and falsely shorten the measured His bundle–ventricular (HV) interval (see Fig. 2-19). Even if a large His potential is recorded in association with a small atrial electrogram, the catheter should be withdrawn to obtain a His potential associated with a larger atrial electrogram. Using a multipolar (three or more) electrode catheter to record simultaneously proximal and distal HB electrogram (e.g., a quadripolar catheter records three bipolar electrograms over a 1.5-cm distance) can help evaluate intra-His conduction.[4]

Validation of HB recording can be accomplished by assessment of the HV interval and establishing the relationship between the His potential and other electrograms.[22] The HV interval should be 35 milliseconds or longer (in the absence of preexcitation). In contrast, the RB potential invariably occurs within 30 milliseconds before ventricular activation. Atrial pacing can be necessary to distinguish a true His potential from a multicomponent atrial electrogram. With a true His potential, the atrial–His bundle (AH) interval should increase with incremental pacing rates. HB pacing can also be a valuable means for validating HB recording. The ability to pace the HB through the recording electrode and obtain HB capture (i.e., QRS identical to that during NSR and S-QRS interval identical to the HV interval during NSR) provides the strongest evidence validating the His potential.[22] However, this technique is inconsistent in accomplishing HB capture, especially at low current output. Higher output can result in nonselective HB capture. The use of closely spaced electrodes and the reversal of current polarity (i.e., anodal stimulation) can facilitate HB capture. Failure to capture the HB selectively does not necessarily imply that the recorded potential is from the RB.

Other measures that can be used, although rarely required, to validate the HB recording include recording of pressure simultaneously with a luminal electrode catheter, which should reveal atrial pressure wave when the catheter

is at the proximal His electrogram position, and simultaneous left and right recording of the His potential. The His potential can be recorded in the noncoronary sinus of Valsalva (just above the aortic valve) or in the LVOT along the interventricular septum (just below the aortic valve). Because these sites are at the level of the central fibrous body, the proximal penetrating portion of the HB is recorded and can be used to time the His potential recorded via the standard venous route. Recording the HB from the noncoronary cusp (versus the LVOT) is preferred because only a true His potential can be recorded from that site.[27]

Right Ventricle Electrogram. The RV electrogram typically shows a local sharp and large ventricular electrogram and generally no atrial electrogram. The closer the RV catheter tip position to the apex, the closer it is to the RB myocardial insertion site and the earlier the ventricular electrogram timing to the onset of the QRS. The catheter is usually positioned in the RV apex because of stability and reproducibility.

Baseline Intervals

The accuracy of measurements made at a screen speed of 100 mm/sec is ±5 milliseconds, and at a speed of 400 mm/sec is ±1 millisecond.[22] In dealing with large intervals (e.g., sinus node function), a speed of 100 mm/sec is adequate. For refractory periods, a speed of 150 to 200 mm/sec is adequate, but for detailed mapping, a speed of 200 to 400 mm/sec is required.

P Wave-Atrial Interval. The P wave-atrial interval is measured from the first evidence of sinus node depolarization, whether on the intracardiac or surface ECG, to the atrial deflection as recorded in the HB lead. It represents conduction through the RA to the inferoposterior interatrial septum (in the region of the AVN and HB; see Fig. 2-19).

Although the PA interval is a reflection of internodal (sinus node to AVN) conduction, prolonged PA intervals suggest abnormal atrial conduction and can be a clue to the presence of biatrial disease or disease confined to the RA. The normal range of the PA interval is 20 to 60 milliseconds. Rarely, diseased atrial conduction can underlie first-degree AV block, indicated by a prolonged PA interval. A short PA interval suggests an ectopic source of atrial activation.

Interatrial Conduction. Normal atrial activation begins in the high or midlateral RA (depending on the sinus rate), spreads from there to the low RA and AV junction, and then spreads to the LA.

Activation of the LA is mediated by three possible routes. Superiorly, activation proceeds through the Bachman bundle; this can be seen in 50% to 70% of patients and can be demonstrated by CS os activation followed by distal CS and then mid-CS activation. Activation also propagates through the midatrial septum at the fossa ovalis and at the region of the central fibrous trigone at the apex of the triangle of Koch. The latter provides the most consistent amount of LA activation.

Interatrial conduction is measured by the interval between the atrial electrogram in the high RA lead to that in the CS lead. Left-to-right atrial activation during LA pacing appears to primarily cross the fossa and low septum and not the Bachman bundle, as reflected by relatively late high RA activation.

Normal retrograde atrial activation proceeds over the AVN. The earliest atrial activation is recorded in the AV junction (HB recording), then in the adjacent RA and CS os, and finally in the high RA and LA. More detailed mapping reveals atrial activation to start at the HB recording, with secondary breakthrough sites in the CS (reflecting activation over the LA extension of the AVN) and/or posterior triangle of Koch. At faster ventricular pacing rates, the earliest atrial activation typically shifts to the posterior portion of the triangle of Koch, the CS os, or within the CS itself.

Atrial–His Bundle Interval. The AH interval is measured from the first rapid deflection of the atrial deflection in the HB recording to the first evidence of HB depolarization in the HB recording (see Fig. 2-19). The AH interval is an approximation of the AVN conduction time, because it represents conduction time from the low RA at the interatrial septum through the AVN to the HB.

The AH interval can vary according to the site of atrial pacing. During LA or CS os pacing, the impulse can enter the AVN at a different site that bypasses part of the AVN, or it can just enter the AVN earlier in respect to the atrial deflection in the HB electrogram. Both mechanisms can give rise to a shorter AH interval.

The response of the AH interval to atrial pacing or drugs often provides more meaningful information about AVN function than an isolated measurement of the AH interval. Autonomic blockade with atropine (0.04 mg/kg) and propranolol (0.02 mg/kg) can be used to evaluate AVN function in the absence of autonomic influences. Not enough data, however, are available to define normal responses under these circumstances.[22]

The AH interval has a wide range in normal subjects (50 to 120 milliseconds) and is markedly influenced by the autonomic nervous system. Short AH intervals can be observed in cases of increased sympathetic tone, reduced vagal tone, enhanced AVN conduction, and preferential LA input into the AVN, as well as unusual forms of preexcitation (atrio-His BTs).

Long AH intervals are usually caused by negative dromotropic drugs such as digoxin, beta blockers, calcium channel blockers, and antiarrhythmic drugs; enhanced vagal tone; and intrinsic disease of the AVN. Artifactually prolonged AH intervals can result from an improperly positioned catheter and the incorrect identification of an RB potential as a His potential. This situation needs to be distinguished from true AH interval prolongation.

His Potential. His potential duration reflects conduction through the short length of the HB that penetrates the fibrous septum. Disturbances of the HB conduction can manifest as fractionation, prolongation (longer than 30 milliseconds), or splitting of the His potential.

His Bundle–Ventricular Interval. The HV interval is measured from the onset of the His potential to the onset of the earliest registered surface or intracardiac ventricular activation. It represents conduction time from the proximal HB through the distal His-Purkinje system (HPS) to the ventricular myocardium (see Fig. 2-19).[22]

The HV interval is not significantly affected by the autonomic tone, and usually remains stable. The range of HV intervals in normal subjects is narrow, 35 to 55 milliseconds. A prolonged HV interval is consistent with diseased distal conduction in all fascicles or in the HB itself. A validated short HV interval suggests ventricular preexcitation via a BT. A falsely shortened HV interval can occur during sinus rhythm with PVCs or an accelerated idioventricular rhythm that is isorhythmic with the sinus rhythm, or when an RB potential rather than a His potential is inadvertently recorded.

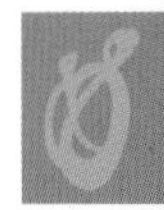

PROGRAMMED STIMULATION

Stimulators

Cardiac stimulation is carried out by delivering a pulse of electrical current through the electrode catheter from an external pacemaker (stimulator) to the cardiac surface. Such an electrical impulse depolarizes cardiac tissue near the pacing electrode, which then propagates through the heart. The paced impulses (stimuli) are introduced in predetermined patterns and at precise timed intervals using a programmable stimulator.

A typical stimulator has a constant current source and is capable of pacing at a wide range of CLs and variable current strengths (0.1 to 10 mA) and pulse widths (0.1 to 10 milliseconds). Additionally, current stimulators have at least two different channels of stimulation (preferably four) and allow delivery of multiple extrastimuli (three or more) and synchronization of the pacing stimuli to selected electrograms during intrinsic or paced rhythms.

Pacing Techniques

Pacing Output. Stimulation is usually carried out using an isolated constant current source that delivers a rectangular impulse. Pacing output at twice (2×) diastolic threshold is generally used. Pacing threshold is defined as the lowest current required for consistent capture determined in late diastole. The pacing threshold can be influenced by the pacing CL; therefore, the threshold should be determined at each pacing CL used. In general, refractory periods are somewhat longer when determined using 2× threshold (as opposed to higher outputs), and this can reduce the incidence of induction of nonclinical tachyarrhythmias.[22] Additionally, diastolic excitability can be influenced by drug administration; reevaluation of the pacing threshold and adjustment of the pacing output (2× threshold) is therefore required in such situations. A pulse duration of 1 or 2 milliseconds is generally used.

High current strength is generally used for determination of strength-interval curves to overcome drug-induced prolongation of refractoriness, assess the presence and mechanism of antiarrhythmic therapy, and overcome the effect of decreased tissue excitability (e.g., pace mapping in scar-related arrhythmias).

Cycle Length. During EP testing, CLs often change from beat to beat, so that these measures are more relevant than an overall rate expressed in beats per minute (beats/min). The use of rates in beats per minute is retained mostly to facilitate communication with physicians who are more comfortable with this terminology. Pacing rate is determined by dividing 60,000 by the CL (in milliseconds).

Incremental Versus Decremental. The terms *incremental* and *decremental* can have opposite meaning, depending on whether one is considering the pacing rate in beats per minute or pacing CL in milliseconds. The term *incremental pacing rate* is derived from stimulators controlled by an analog dial. Digitally controlled devices often increase the rate by choosing a sequence of CL decrements, but the term *incremental pacing* may still be used.

Overdrive Pacing (Straight Pacing). Pacing stimuli are delivered at a constant pacing rate (or pacing CL) throughout the duration of the stimulation. The pacing rate is faster than the rate of the baseline rhythm to ensure capture of the spontaneous rhythm.

Burst Pacing. Pacing stimuli are delivered at a constant rate for a relatively short duration, but at successively faster rates with each burst until a predetermined maximum rate (or minimum CL) has been reached. This technique is generally used for induction or termination of tachycardias.

Stepwise Rate-Incremental Pacing. After pacing at a given rate for a predetermined number of stimuli or seconds, the rate is increased (with intervening pauses) in a series of steps until predetermined endpoints are reached. It is important to maintain the pacing at any given rate for at least 15 seconds (period of accommodation) before increasing the pacing rate. Otherwise, the initial stimuli at any given rate can produce different effects than those observed several seconds later, because the ability of a tissue to conduct is affected by the baseline rate or CL of the preceding beats. A disadvantage for this technique is the prolonged pacing required at each rate, which is time-consuming.

Ramp Pacing. Ramp pacing implies a smooth change in the interval between successive stimuli, with gradual decrease of the pacing CL every several paced complexes (without intervening pauses). Ramps are often used as an alternative to the stepwise method for assessment of conduction. The pacing rate is slowly increased at 2 to 4 beats/min every several paced beats until block occurs. This method avoids prolonged rapid pacing at each pacing CL and is particularly useful when multiple assessments of conduction are planned (e.g., after therapeutic interventions) and in the assessment of retrograde conduction. Because each successive paced interval differs from its predecessor by only a few milliseconds, the interval at which block occurs can be determined more precisely using the ramp method. However, prolonged episodes of continuous high-rate pacing can provoke significant hypotension, and close monitoring of blood pressure is important while performing these maneuvers.

For tachycardia induction or termination, the ramp is decreased in duration, but the interstimulus intervals are decreased more rapidly. Ramp pacing is generally used in antitachycardia pacing algorithms in implantable cardioverter-defibrillators (ICDs). Programmed rate-incremental ramps are also known as autodecremental pacing.

Extrastimulus Technique

S1-S1 Drive Stimuli. The heart is paced, or driven, at a specified rate and duration (typically eight beats) after which a premature extrastimulus is delivered. The eight drive beats are each termed S_1 *stimulus*. The S_1-S_1 drive stimuli are sometimes called trains. These S_1 drive stimuli can be followed by first, second, third, and Nth premature extrastimuli, which are designated as S_2, S_3, S_4, and S_N. When the extrastimuli follow a series of sinus beats, the latter can also be designated as S_1.

S1, S2, S3, . . . SN. S_2 is the first extrastimulus, with the S_1-S_2 interval almost always shorter than the S_1-S_1 interval. S_3, S_4, . . . S_N are the second, third, . . . Nth extrastimuli. When stimulation is performed in the atrium, capture of S_1, S_2, S_3, . . . S_N results in atrial depolarizations, termed A_1, A_2, A_3, . . . A_N, respectively, and when stimulation is performed in the ventricle, they are termed V_1, V_2, V_3, . . . V_N, corresponding to the resultant ventricular depolarizations, respectively.

One or more extrastimuli (designated S_2, S_3, and S_N) are introduced at specific coupling intervals based on previous S_1 drive stimuli or spontaneous beats. Thereafter, the S_1-S_2 interval is altered, usually in 10- to 20-millisecond steps, until an endpoint is reached, such as tissue refractoriness or termination or induction of a tachycardia. It is usual to begin late in diastole and successively decrement the S_1-S_2 interval. A second extrastimulus (S_3) can then be introduced, with the S_2-S_3 interval altered similarly to that used for S_1-S_2.

Two methods are in common clinical use for decreasing the coupling intervals during delivery of multiple extrastimuli. In the simple sequential method, the S_1-S_2 coupling interval is decreased until it fails to capture, at which time the coupling interval is increased until it captures (usually within 10 to 20 milliseconds). The S_1-S_2 coupling interval is then held constant while the S_2-S_3 interval is decreased similarly to that used for S_1-S_2, and then the same for S_3-S_4. In the tandem method, the S_1-S_2 coupling interval is decreased until S_2 fails to capture, and then the S_1-S_2 coupling interval is increased by 40 to 50 milliseconds and held there. S_3 is then introduced and the S_2-S_3 interval decreased until S_3 fails to capture. At that point, the S_1-S_2 interval is decreased, and S_3 retested to see whether it captures. From that point on, the S_1-S_2 and S_2-S_3 are decreased in tandem until refractory. As compared with the simple sequential

method, the tandem method allows relatively longer intervals and provides a larger number of stimulation runs before moving on to the next extrastimulus. Prospective studies comparing the two methods have shown no differences between the two methods in any of the outcomes assessed.

Ultrarapid Train Stimulation. Pacing at very short CLs (10 to 50 milliseconds) is rarely performed, mainly for induction of VF (to test defibrillation threshold during ICD implantation).

TABLE 2–2	Definition of Refractory Periods
Period	**Definition**
Atrial ERP	Longest A_1-A_2 interval that fails to achieve atrial capture
Atrial FRP	Shortest A_1-A_2 interval recorded at a designated site (often the HB region) before failure of A_1-A_2 to capture the atrium
AVN ERP	Shortest H_1-H_2 in response to any A_1-A_2
HPS ERP	Longest H_1-H_2 not propagating to the ventricles
HPS FRP	Shortest V_1-V_2 interval before reaching the ERP of the HPS
Bundle branch ERP and FRP	Similar to those for the HPS but based on production of right or left BBB or fascicular block
Ventricular ERP	Longest V_1-V_2 interval that fails to achieve ventricular capture

AVN = atrioventricular node; BBB = bundle branch block; HB = His bundle; HPS = His-Purkinje system; ERP = effective refractory period; FRP = functional refractory period.

Conduction and Refractoriness

Definitions

Conduction. Conduction velocity refers to the speed of propagation of an electrical impulse through cardiac tissue; it reflects the rise of the depolarization phase (phase 0) of the action potential. Conduction can be assessed by observing the propagation of wavefronts during pacing at progressively incremental rates. Rate-incremental pacing is delivered to a selected site in the heart while propagation to a selected distal point is assessed. Conduction velocity is assessed by measuring the time it takes for an impulse to travel from one intracardiac location to another. During tests of conduction, it is usual for capture to be maintained at the site of stimulation and block to occur at a distal point.[5]

Refractoriness. The refractory period is the period after depolarization during which a cell cannot be depolarized again and is determined, in part, by the action potential duration and membrane potential. Capture of the heart by a paced stimulus can be assessed using tests of refractoriness. Refractoriness is defined by the response of a tissue to premature stimulation.[23,24]

Relative Refractory Period. The relative refractory period is defined as the longest premature coupling interval (S_1-S_2) that results in capture, generally at a prolonged conduction time (an increase in stimulus to distal response time) of the premature impulse relative to that of the basic drive. Conduction is slowed when a wavefront encounters tissue that is not completely repolarized. Thus, relative refractory period marks the end of the full recovery period, the zone during which conduction of the premature and basic drive impulses is identical.[5]

Absolute Refractory Period. During the absolute refractory period, the tissue cannot be depolarized, even by an extrastimulus of great amplitude.

Effective Refractory Period. The effective refractory period (ERP) is the longest premature coupling interval (S_1-S_2) at a designated stimulus amplitude (usually 2× diastolic threshold) that results in failure of propagation of the premature impulse through a tissue. ERP, therefore, must be measured proximal to the refractory tissue.

Functional Refractory Period. The minimum interval between two consecutively conducted impulses through a tissue is known as the functional refractory period (FRP). Because the FRP is a measure of output from a tissue, it is described by measuring points distal to that tissue. It is helpful to think of the FRP as a response-to-response measurement (in contrast, the ERP is a stimulus-to-stimulus measurement). Therefore, the FRP is a measure of refractoriness and conduction velocity of a tissue.

The definitions of anterograde ERP and FRP of the AV conduction system are given in Table 2-2.[22]

Measurements

Refractory periods are analyzed by the extrastimulus technique, with progressively premature extrastimuli delivered after a train of 8 to 10 paced beats at a fixed pacing CL to allow for reasonable (more than 95%) stabilization of refractoriness, which is usually accomplished after three or four paced beats. Several variables are considered in the assessment of refractory periods, including the stimulus amplitude and the drive rate or CL. Longer CLs are generally associated with longer refractory periods, but refractory periods of different parts of the conducting system do not respond comparably with changes in the drive CLs. Additionally, the measured ERP is invariably related to the current used. Thus, standardization of the pacing output is required. In most laboratories, it is arbitrarily standardized at 2× diastolic threshold.[5]

A more detailed method of assessing refractoriness (or, more appropriately, excitability) is to define the strength-interval curves at these sites. The steep portion of that curve defines the ERP of that tissue. The use of increasing current strengths to 10 mA usually shortens the measured ERP by approximately 30 milliseconds. However, such a method does not offer a useful clinical advantage except when the effects of antiarrhythmic drugs on ventricular excitability and refractoriness are to be characterized. Moreover, the safety of using high current strengths, especially when multiple extrastimuli are delivered, is questionable, because fibrillation is more likely to occur in such situations.

It is important that measurements of refractory periods be taken at specific sites. Measurements of atrial and ventricular ERP are taken at the site of stimulation. Measurements of AVN-ERP and HPS-ERP are taken from responses in the HB electrogram.[22]

Cycle Length Responsiveness of Refractory Periods

Normally, refractoriness of the atrial, HPS, and ventricular tissue is directly related to the basic drive CL (i.e., the ERP shortens with decreasing basic drive CL). This phenomenon is termed *peeling of refractoriness,* and is most marked in the HPS.[22,24] Abrupt changes in the CL also affect refractoriness of these tissues. A change from a long- to short-drive

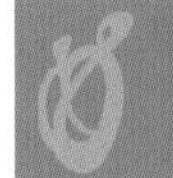

TABLE 2–3 Normal Refractory Periods in Adults (msec)

Study*	ERP Atrium	ERP AVN	FRP AVN	ERP HPS	ERP Ventricle
Denes et al (1974)	150-360	250-365	350-495	—	—
Akhtar et al (1975)	230-330	280-430	320-680	340-430	190-290
Josephson (2002)	170-300	230-425	330-525	330-450	170-290

*Studies performed at 2× threshold.

AVN = atrioventricular node; ERP = effective refractory period; FRP = functional refractory period; HPS = His-Purkinje system.

From Denes P, Wu D, Dhingra R, et al: The effects of cycle length on cardiac refractory periods in man. Circulation 1974;49:32; Akhtar M, Damato AN, Batsford WP, et al: A comparative analysis of antegrade and retrograde conduction patterns in man. Circulation 1975;52:766; Josephson ME: Electrophysiologic investigation: General aspects. *In* Josephson ME (ed): Clinical Cardiac Electrophysiology, 3rd ed. Lippincott, Williams & Wilkins, 2002, pp 19-67.

CL (e.g., with introduction of an extrastimulus [S_2] following a pacing drive [S_1] with a long CL) shortens the ERP of the HPS and atrium, whereas a change from a short- to long-drive CL markedly prolongs the HPS ERP but alters the ventricular ERP little, if at all. Refractoriness of the atrial, HPS, and ventricular tissue appears relatively independent of autonomic tone; however, data have shown that increased vagal tone reduces atrial ERP and increases ventricular ERP.[23]

In contrast, the AVN ERP increases with increasing basic drive CL because of the fatigue phenomenon, which most likely results because AVN refractoriness is time-dependent and exceeds its action potential duration (unlike HPS refractoriness). Additionally, AVN refractory periods are labile and can be markedly affected by the autonomic tone. On the other hand, the response of AVN FRP to changes in pacing CL is variable, but tends to decrease with decreasing pacing CL.[24] This paradox occurs because the FRP is not a true measure of refractoriness encountered by an atrial extrastimulus (AES; A_2); it is significantly determined by the AVN conduction time of the basic drive beat (A_1-H_1); the longer the A_1-H_1, the shorter the calculated FRP at any A_2-H_2.[22]

Limitations of Tests of Conduction and Refractoriness

It is unusual to be able to collect a complete set of measurements. With refractory period testing, the atrial ERP is often longer than the AVN ERP so that atrial refractoriness is encountered before AVN refractoriness, obviating the possibility of assessing the latter. Moreover, an AES cannot be used to test the HPS if conduction is blocked at the AVN level. This is a limitation that applies to most patients undergoing conduction or refractory period testing.[23] On the other hand, it is possible to assess anterograde conduction and refractoriness distal to the AVN by direct pacing of the HB. This is not part of the routine EP evaluation, however, and is reserved for cases in which the information is particularly desired.[5]

It is important to recognize that atrial conduction can materially affect the determination of refractory periods. Therefore, refractory periods should not be timed from the site of stimulation, but from the point in the conduction cascade that is being assessed. For example, if the high RA is stimulated in a patient with a left lateral BT, an early AES can encounter the relative refractory period of the atrium, so that intraatrial conduction time is prolonged. Thus, the timing of the S_1-S_2 stimuli in the high RA would be shorter than the timing of the propagated impulse when it arrives at the region of the BT as the local A_1-A_2 interval.

A wide range of normal values has been reported for refractory periods (Table 2-3). However, it is difficult to interpret these so-called normal values because they come from pooled data using different standards (different pacing CLs, stimulus strengths, and pulse widths).[22-24]

ATRIAL STIMULATION

Technical Aspects of Atrial Stimulation

Atrial stimulation provides a method for evaluation of the functional properties of the sinus node and AV conduction system and of the means of induction of different arrhythmias (supraventricular and, occasionally, ventricular arrhythmias). Atrial stimulation from different atrial sites can result in different patterns of AV conduction. Thus, stimulation should be performed from the same site if the effects of drugs and/or physiological maneuvers are to be studied. Atrial stimulation is usually performed from the high RA and CS.

Rate-incremental atrial pacing is usually started at a pacing CL just shorter than the sinus CL, with progressive shortening of the pacing CL (by 10- to 20-millisecond decrements) until 1:1 atrial capture is lost, Wenckebach AVN block develops, and/or a pacing CL of 200 to 250 milliseconds is reached. Ramp atrial pacing is equivalent to rate-incremental pacing if AVN Wenckebach CL is all that is required. Stepwise rate-incremental pacing, however, also allows evaluation of sinus node recovery time at each drive CL. Atrial pacing should always be synchronized because alteration of the coupling interval of the first paced beat of the pacing drive can affect subsequent AV conduction.

During stepwise rate-incremental pacing, pacing should be continued long enough (usually 15 to 60 seconds) at each pacing CL to ensure stability of conduction intervals and overcome two factors that significantly influence the development of a steady state—the phenomenon of accommodation and effects of autonomic tone. During rate-incremental pacing, if the coupling interval of the first beat of the drive is not synchronized, it can be shorter, longer, or equal to the subsequent pacing CL. Therefore, one can observe an increasing, decreasing, or stable AH interval pattern for several cycles, and the initial AH interval can be different from the steady-state AH interval. Oscillations of the AH interval, which dampen to a steady level, or AVN Wenckebach can occur under these circumstances. In regard to influence of the autonomic tone on AVN conduction, rapid pacing can produce variations in AVN conduction, depending on the patient's immediate autonomic state. Rapid pacing can also provoke symptoms or hypotension in patients who then produce neurohumoral responses that can alter results. Therefore, for assessment of AV conduction, ramp pacing is often an attractive alternative to the stepwise method. The pacing rate is slowly increased at 2 to 4 beats/min/sec until block occurs.[22]

Atrial extrastimulation (AES) is used for assessment of atrial and AVN refractory periods and for induction of arrhythmias. During programmed stimulation, a sequence of eight paced stimuli is delivered at a constant rate (the S_1 drive), which allows stable AVN conduction. Following these eight beats, an AES (S_2) is delivered. This stimulation sequence is repeated at progressively shorter S_1-S_2 coupling intervals, allowing the response of the sinus node and AVN to be recorded across a range of premature test stimuli.

Normal Response to Rate-Incremental Atrial Pacing

Sinus Node Response to Atrial Pacing. The sinus node is the prototype of an automatic focus. Automatic rhythms are characterized by spontaneous depolarization, overdrive suppression, and postoverdrive warm-up to baseline CL. Rapid atrial pacing results in overdrive suppression of the sinus rate, with prolongation of the return sinus CL following termination of the pacing train. Longer pacing trains and faster rates further prolong the return cycle. After cessation of pacing, the sinus rate resumes discharge at a slower rate and gradually speeds up (warms up) to return to the prepacing sinus rate.

Sinus node recovery time is the interval between the end of a period of pacing-induced overdrive suppression of sinus node activity and the return of sinus node function, manifested on the surface ECG by a post-pacing sinus P wave.

Atrioventricular Node Response to Atrial Pacing. The normal response to rate-incremental atrial pacing is for the PR and AH intervals to increase gradually as the pacing CL decreases, until AVN Wenckebach block appears (Fig. 2-20). With further decrease in the pacing CL, higher degrees of AV block (2:1 or 3:1) can appear.[22] Infranodal conduction (HV interval) generally remains unaffected.

Wenckebach block is frequently atypical; that is, the AH interval does not increase gradually in decreasing increments but stabilizes for several beats before the block, or it can show its greatest increment in the last conducted beat. The incidence of atypical Wenckebach block is highest during long Wenckebach cycles (more than 6.5). It is important to distinguish atypical Wenckebach periodicity from Mobitz II AV block. Additionally, it is important to ensure that the ventricular pauses observed during atrial pacing are not secondary to loss of atrial capture or occurrence of AVN echo beats ("pseudoblock"; see Fig. 2-20).

AVN Wenckebach CL is the longest pacing CL at which Wenckebach block in the AVN is observed. Normally, Wenckebach CL is 500 to 350 milliseconds, and it is sensitive to the autonomic tone. There is a correlation between the AH interval during NSR and the Wenckebach CL; patients with a long AH interval during NSR tend to develop Wenckebach block at longer pacing CL, and vice versa.

At short pacing CLs (less than 350 milliseconds), infranodal block can occasionally occur in patients with a normal baseline HV interval and QRS. This occurs especially when atrial pacing is started during NSR with the first or second paced impulses acting as a long-short sequence. The HPS can also show accommodation following the initiation of pacing. Prolongation of the HV interval or infranodal block at a pacing CL longer than 400 milliseconds is abnormal and indicates infranodal conduction abnormalities.

Atrial Response to Atrial Pacing. It is usually possible to maintain 1:1 atrial capture with rate-incremental pacing techniques to a pacing CL of 200 to 300 milliseconds. Pacing threshold normally tends to increase at faster rates. Rate-incremental pacing can result in prolongation of the intraatrial (P-A interval) and interatrial conduction. At rapid pacing rates, precipitation of AF is not rare and is not necessarily an abnormal response. Vagal tone and medications such as adenosine and edrophonium can slow the sinus rate, but they tend to shorten the atrial ERP, which makes the atrium more vulnerable to induction of AF.

Normal Response to Atrial Premature Stimulation

Sinus Node Response to Atrial Extrastimulation. Four zones of response of the sinus node to AES have been identified—zone of collision, zone of reset, zone of interpolation, and zone of reentry (Fig. 2-21).

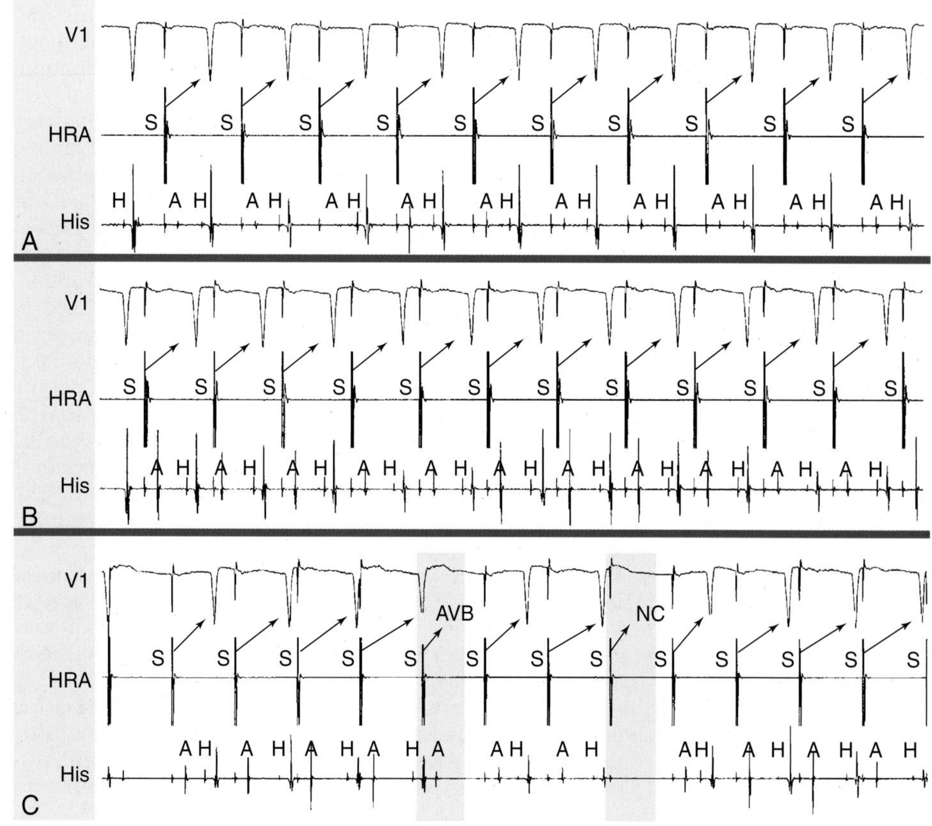

FIGURE 2–20 Normal atrioventricular node (AVN) response to rate-incremental atrial pacing. **A,** Fixed-rate high right atrial (HRA) pacing (S) at a cycle length (CL) of 600 milliseconds. **B,** Decreasing the pacing CL to 500 milliseconds results in prolongation of the atrial–His bundle (AH) interval, as illustrated in the His bundle recording (His). Infranodal conduction (His bundle–ventricular [HV] interval) remains unaffected. **C,** Further decrement of the pacing CL results in progressive prolongation of the AH interval until block occurs in the AVN (AVB), followed by resumption of conduction, indicating Wenckebach CL. The site of block is in the AVN because no HB deflection is present after the nonconducted atrial stimulus. Of note, apparent block of another atrial stimulus is observed (pseudoblock) because of failure of the atrial stimulus to capture (NC), which is confirmed by the absence of an atrial electrogram on the HB recording after the stimulus artifact.

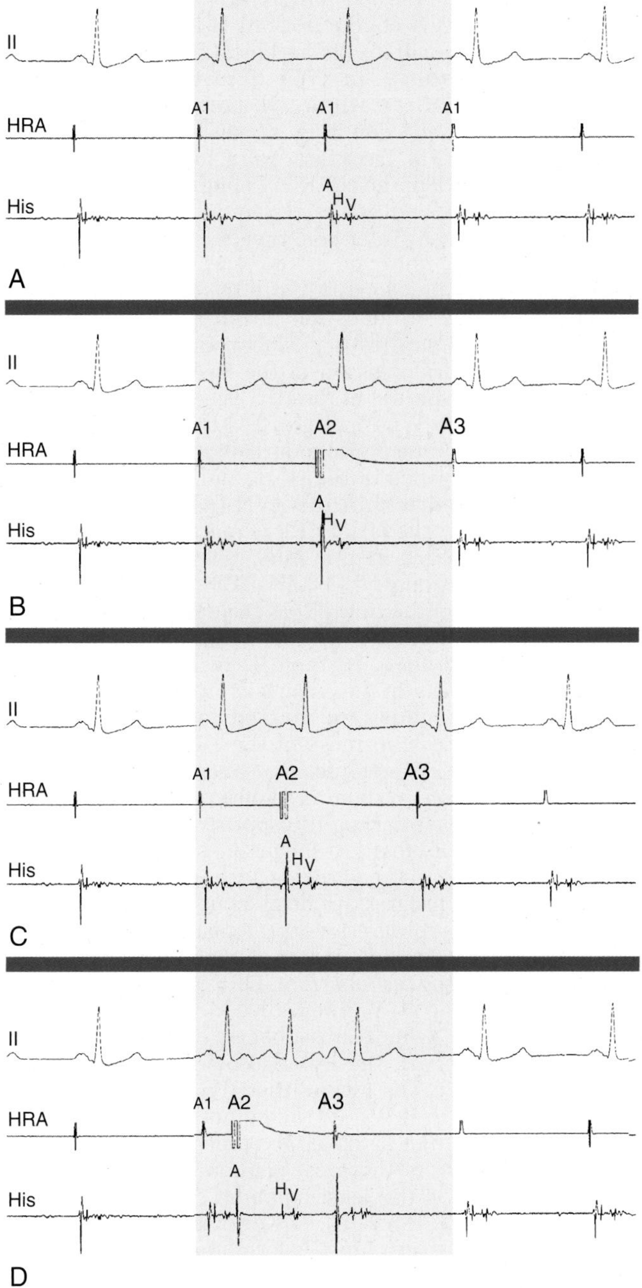

FIGURE 2–21 Normal sinus node and atrioventricular (AV) node response to atrial extrastimulation. **A,** Baseline sinus rhythm shown in surface ECG lead II, high right atrium (HRA) recording, and His bundle (His) recording. The shaded area represents two sinus cycle lengths (2×[A_1-A_1]). **B,** A late coupled atrial extrastimulus (AES) (A_2) collides with the exiting sinus impulse and therefore does not affect (or reset) the sinus pacemaker (zone of collision). The next sinus impulse (A_3) occurs at exactly twice the baseline sinus CL. **C,** An early coupled AES is able to penetrate and reset the sinus node (zone of resetting). **D,** An even earlier coupled AES reaches refractory tissue around the sinus node and is thus unable to penetrate the sinus node (entrance block); therefore, it does not affect sinus node discharge. The next spontaneous sinus beat (A_3) arrives exactly at the sinus interval (zone of interpolation). The atrial–His bundle (AH) interval progressively prolongs with progressively premature coupling intervals (**B** to **E**). In contrast, the His bundle–ventricular (HV) interval remains constant.

Zone I. A late-coupled AES with very long A_1-A_2 intervals (with A_2 falling in the last 20% to 30% of the sinus CL) collides with the impulse already emerging from the sinus node, resulting in fusion of atrial activation (fusion between the AES [A_2] with the spontaneous sinus impulse [A_1]) or paced-only atrial activation sequence; it fails to affect the timing of the next sinus beat, producing a fully compensatory pause. This zone, also known as the zone of collision, zone of interference, and nonreset zone, is defined by the range of A_1-A_2 at which A_2-A_3 is fully compensatory (see Fig. 2-21).[22]

Zone II. An earlier coupled AES results in penetration of the sinus node with resetting so that the resulting pause is less than compensatory (i.e., A_1-A_3 is less than 2×[A_1-A_1]), but without changing sinus node automaticity. The range of A_1-A_2 at which resetting of the sinus pacemaker occurs, resulting in a less than compensatory pause, defines zone II, also known as the the zone of reset (see Fig. 2-21). This zone is typically of long duration (40% to 50% of the sinus CL). In most patients, A_2-A_3 remains constant throughout zone II, producing a plateau in the curve because, while A_2 penetrates and resets the sinus node, it does so without changing the sinus pacemaker automaticity. Hence, A_2-A_3 should equal the spontaneous sinus CL (A_1-A_1) plus the time it takes the AES (A_2) to enter and exit the sinus node. The difference between A_2-A_3 and A_1-A_1, therefore, has been taken as an estimate of total sinoatrial conduction time.[22]

Zone III. A very early-coupled AES encounters a refractory sinus node (following the last sinus discharge) and fails to enter or reset the sinus node. The next sinus discharge will be on time because the atrium is already fully recovered following that early AES. The range of A_1-A_2 coupling intervals at which A_2-A_3 is less than A_1-A_1, and A_1-A_3 is less than 2×(A_1-A_1) defines zone III, also known as the zone of interpolation (see Fig. 2-21).[22] The A_1-A_2 coupling intervals at which incomplete interpolation is first observed define the relative refractory period of the perinodal tissue. Some refer to this as the sinus node refractory period. In this case, A_3 represents delay of A_1 exiting the sinus node, which has not been affected.[25] The A_1-A_2 coupling interval at which complete interpolation is observed probably defines the ERP of the most peripheral of the perinodal tissue, because the sinus impulse does not encounter refractory tissue on its exit from the sinus node. In this case, (A_1-A_2) + (A_2-A_3) = A_1-A_1 and sinus node entrance block is said to exist.[25]

Zone IV. This zone, also know as the zone of reentry, is defined as the range of A_1-A_2 at which A_2-A_3 is less than A_1-A_1, (A_1-A_2) + (A_2-A_3) is less than A_1-A_1, and the atrial activation sequence and P wave morphology are identical to those of the sinus. The incidence of single beats of sinus node reentry is approximately 11% in the normal population.

Atrioventricular Node Response to AES. Progressively premature AES results in prolongation of PR and AH intervals, with inverse relationship between the AES coupling interval (A_1-A_2) and the AH interval (A_2-H_2). The shorter the coupling interval of the AES, the longer the A_2-H_2 interval (see Fig. 2-21). More premature AES can block in the AVN with no conduction to the ventricle (defining AVN ERP). Occasionally, conduction delay and block occur in the HPS, especially when the AES is delivered following long basic drive CLs, because HPS refractoriness frequently exceeds the AVN FRP at long pacing CLs.[22]

The patterns of AV conduction can be expressed by plotting refractory period relating A_1-A_2 interval to the responses of the AVN and HPS. Plotting the A_1-A_2 interval versus H_1-H_2 and V_1-V_2 intervals illustrates the functional input-output relationship between the basic drive beat and the AES, and provides an assessment of the FRP of the AV conduction system. In contrast, plotting the A_2-H_2 interval (AVN conduction time of the AES) and the H_2-V_2 interval (HPS conduction time of the AES) versus the A_1-A_2 interval (the AES coupling interval) allows determination of the conduction times through the various components of the AV conduction system.[22]

Type I Response. In this type, the progressively premature AES encounters progressive delay in the AVN without any changes in the HPS. Therefore, refractoriness of the AVN determines the FRP of the entire AV conduction, and the ERP of the AV conduction system is determined at the atrial or AVN level. This response is characterized by initial shortening of the H_1-H_2 and V_1-V_2 intervals as the AES coupling interval (A_1-A_2) shortens, while AVN conduction (A_2-H_2) and HPS conduction (H_2-V_2) remain stable (Fig. 2-22). With further shortening of the A_1-A_2 interval, the relative refractory period of the AVN is encountered, resulting in progressive delay in AVN conduction (manifesting as progressive prolongation of the A_2-H_2 interval) accompanied by

a stable HPS conduction (H_2-V_2) and a progressive but identical prolongation of both the H_1-H_2 and V_1-V_2 intervals, until the AES is blocked within the AVN (AVN ERP) or until the atrial ERP is reached. The minimum H_1-H_2 and V_1-V_2 intervals attained define the FRP of the AVN and entire AV conduction system. AVN conduction (A_2-H_2) usually increases by 2 to 3× baseline values before block.[22]

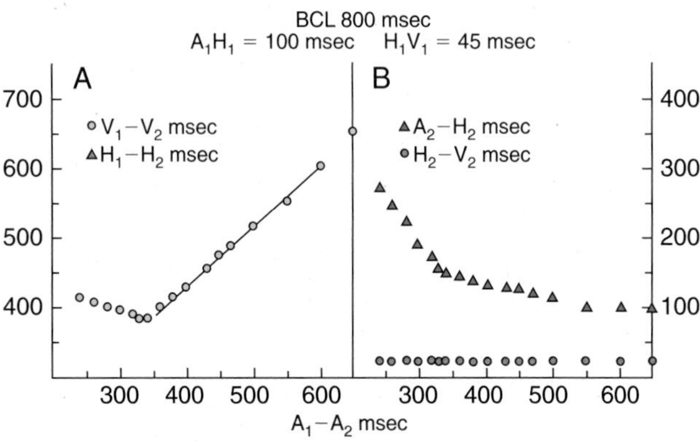

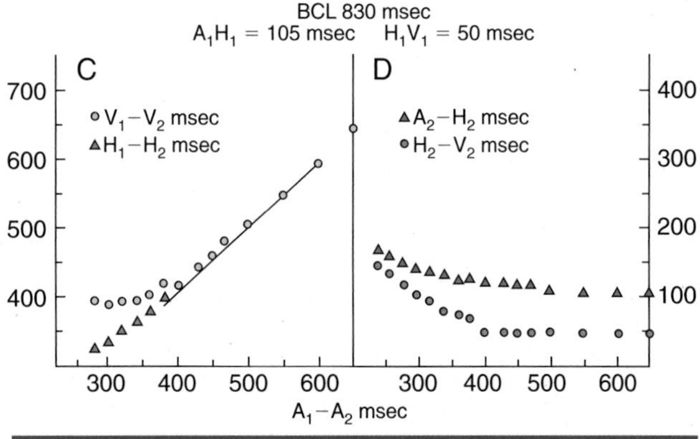

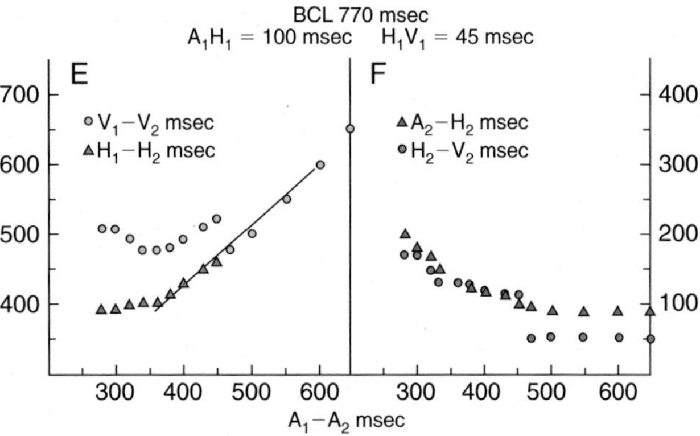

FIGURE 2–22 **A, B,** Type I pattern of atrioventricular node (AVN) response to atrial extrastimulation (AES). **C, D,** Type II pattern of response to AES. **E, F,** Type III pattern of response to AES. See text for details. BCL = basic cycle length. *(Reproduced with permission from Josephson ME: Electrophysiologic investigation: General aspects. In Josephson ME [ed]: Clinical Cardiac Electrophysiology, 3rd ed. Philadelphia, Lippincott, Williams & Wilkins, 2004, pp 19-67.)*

Type II Response. In type II response, conduction delay occurs initially in the AVN; however, with further shortening of the AES coupling interval, progressive delay develops in the HPS. Therefore, refractoriness of the HPS determines the FRP of the entire AV conduction system, and the ERP of the AV conduction system is determined at any level. At longer A_1-A_2 intervals, type II response is similar to type I response; however, as the A_1-A_2 interval shortens, conduction delay develops initially in the AVN (manifesting as progressive prolongation of the A_2-H_2 interval) but then in the HPS (manifesting as aberrant QRS conduction and progressive prolongation of the H_2-V_2 interval) as the relative refractory period of the HPS is encountered. Therefore, in contrast to type I response, both A_2-H_2 and H_2-V_2 intervals prolong in response to progressively shorter A_1-A_2, resulting in divergence in the H_1-H_2 and V_1-V_2 curves until the AES is blocked within the AVN (AVN ERP), the HPS (HPS ERP) or until the atrial ERP is reached (see Fig. 2-22). Block usually occurs in the AVN, but can occur in the atrium and occasionally in the HPS (modified type II response). AVN conduction (A_2-H_2) usually increases only modestly (by less than 2× baseline values before block).[22]

Type III Response. In type III response, conduction delay occurs initially in the AVN; however, at a critical AES coupling interval, sudden and marked delay develops in the HPS. Therefore, refractoriness of the HPS determines the FRP of the entire AV conduction system, and the ERP of the AV conduction system is determined at any level. However, in contrast to type II response, the HPS is invariably the first site of block. At longer A_1-A_2 intervals, type II response is similar to type I response; however, as the A_1-A_2 interval shortens, progressive delay is noted initially in the AVN (manifest as progressive prolongation in the A_2-H_2 interval), but then a sudden delay of conduction in the HPS occurs (manifesting as aberrant QRS conduction and a sudden jump in the H_2-V_2 interval). This results in a break in the V_1-V_2 curve, which subsequently descends until, at a critical A_1-A_2 interval, the impulse blocks in the AVN or HPS (see Fig. 2-22). The FRP of the HPS occurs just before the marked jump in H_2-V_2. AVN conduction (A_2-H_2) usually increases by less than 2× baseline values before block.[22]

Type I response is the most common pattern, whereas type III response is the least common. The pattern of AV conduction (type I, II, or III), however, is not fixed in any patient. Drugs (e.g., atropine, isoproterenol) or changes in CL can alter the refractory period relationship between different tissues so that one type of response can be switched to another. For example, atropine can decrease the FRP of the AVN and allow the impulse to reach the HPS during its relative refractory period, changing type I response to type II or III.

The ERP of the atrium is not infrequently reached earlier than that of the AVN, especially when the basic drive is slow (which increases atrial ERP and decreases AVN ERP) or when the patient is agitated, which increases sympathetic tone and decreases AVN ERP. The first site of block is in the AVN in most patients (45%), in the atrium in 40%, and in the HPS in 15%.[23]

Atrial Response to Atrial Extrastimulation. Early AESs can impinge on atrial relative refractory period, resulting in local latency (i.e., long interval between the pacing artifact and the atrial electrogram on the pacing electrode).[22] A very early AES delivered during the atrial ERP will fail to capture the atrium. The atrial ERP can be longer or shorter than the AVN ERP, especially at long basic drive CLs or in cases of enhanced AVN conduction secondary to autonomic influences.

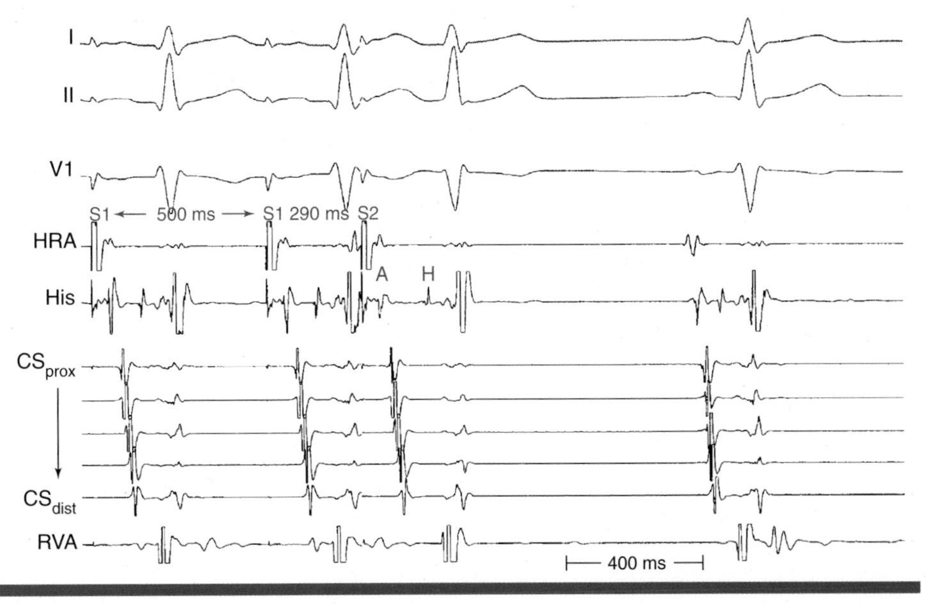

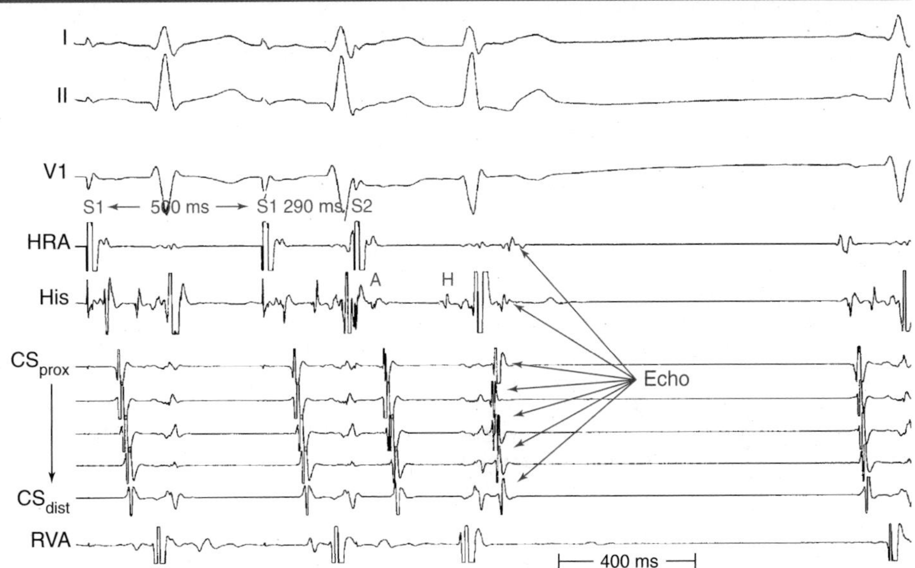

FIGURE 2–23 Anterograde dual atrioventricular nodal pathways. **Top panel,** A single extrastimulus is introduced from the high right atrium (RA; S_2) at 290 milliseconds after the last afterdrive stimulus (S_1). This results in an atrial–His bundle (AH) interval of 140 milliseconds. **Bottom panel,** An extrastimulus is delivered 10 milliseconds earlier than above (280 milliseconds), resulting in marked prolongation of the AH interval to 202 milliseconds and an atrial echo.

As with rate-incremental pacing, AES can result in prolongation of intraatrial and interatrial conduction, which is more pronounced in patients with a history of atrial arrhythmias. Development of a fractionated atrial electrogram is more often observed in patients who have a history of AF. Intraatrial block in response to AES is unusual. Occasionally, double or triple AESs induce AF in patients with no history of such arrhythmia. Such episodes usually terminate spontaneously and are not clinically relevant in the absence of a history of known or suspected atrial arrhythmias.

Repetitive Atrial Responses

Atrial stimulation can trigger extra atrial complexes or echo beats. Those complexes can be caused by different mechanisms; the most common are intraatrial reentrant beats and AVN echo beats.

Intraatrial reentrant beats usually occur at short coupling intervals. They can originate anywhere in the atrium, and atrial activation sequence depends on the site of origin of the beat. The incidence of these responses increases with increasing the number of AESs, increasing the number of drive-pacing CLs and stimulation sites used.

Repetitive atrial responses can also be caused by reentry in the AVN. These patients have anterograde dual AVN physiology, and the last paced beat conducts slowly down the slow AVN pathway and then retrogradely up the fast pathway to produce the echo beat (Fig. 2-23). Atrial activation sequence is consistent with retrograde conduction over the fast AVN pathway, earliest in the HB catheter recording. Atrial and ventricular activations occur simultaneously.

VENTRICULAR STIMULATION

Technical Aspects of Ventricular Stimulation

Ventricular stimulation is used to assess retrograde (ventricular-atrial, VA) conduction and refractory periods, retrograde atrial activation patterns, including sequences that can indicate the presence of a BT, and vulnerability to inducible ventricular arrhythmias.[23]

Stepwise rate-incremental ventricular pacing or ramp pacing is used in the assessment of VA conduction. It is unusual to provoke ventricular arrhythmias with these tests, even in patients with known ventricular arrhythmia.

Rate-incremental ventricular pacing is usually started at a pacing CL just shorter than the sinus CL, and the pacing CL is then gradually decreased (in 10- to 20-millisecond decrements) down to 300 milliseconds. Shorter pacing CL may be used to assess rapid conduction in patients with SVTs or to induce VT. With ramp pacing, the pacing rate is slowly increased at 2 to 4 beats/min/sec until VA block occurs.

Ventricular extrastimulus (VES) testing is used to assess ventricular, HPS, and AVN refractory periods and to induce arrhythmias.[23] During programmed stimulation, a sequence

of eight paced stimuli is delivered at a constant rate (the S_1 drive), which allows stable VA conduction. Following these eight beats, a VES (S_2) is delivered. This stimulation sequence is repeated at progressively shorter S_1-S_2 intervals, allowing the response of the HPS and AVN to be recorded across a range of premature test stimuli.

During ventricular stimulation, the HB electrogram will show a retrograde His potential in 85% of patients with a normal QRS during NSR.[22] Ventricular pacing at the base of the heart opposite the AV junction facilitates recording a retrograde His potential, because it allows the ventricles to be activated much earlier relative to the HB (Fig. 2-24). The ventricular–His bundle (VH) or stimulus–His bundle (S-H) interval always exceeds the anterograde HV interval by the time it takes for the impulse to travel from the stimulation site to the ipsilateral bundle branch. In patients with normal HV intervals, a retrograde His potential can usually be seen before the ventricular electrogram in the HB recording during RV apical pacing. In contrast, when ipsilateral BBB is present, especially with long HV intervals, a retrograde His potential is less usually seen and, when it is seen, it is usually inscribed after the QRS when pacing from the ipsilateral ventricle (Fig. 2-25).[22]

Ventricular stimulation is relatively safe; however, induction of clinically irrelevant serious arrhythmias, including VF, can occur in patients with normal hearts and those who have not had spontaneous ventricular arrhythmias. The induction of these arrhythmias is directly related to the aggressiveness of the ventricular stimulation protocol. Thus, the stimulation protocol is usually limited to single or double VES in patients without a clinical history consistent with malignant ventricular arrhythmias.[22] The use of high pacing output can also increase the risk of such arrhythmias. Therefore, ventricular stimulation at 2× diastolic threshold and 1-millisecond pulse width is preferable.

Normal Response to Rate-Incremental Ventricular Pacing

Ventricular pacing provides information about VA conduction, which is present in 40% to 90% of patients, depending on the population studied. Absence of VA conduction at any paced rate is common and normal. There is no difference in the capability of VA conduction regarding the site of ventricular stimulation in patients with a normal HPS. When present, normal VA conduction uses the normal AV conduction system, with the earliest atrial activation site usually in the septal region in proximity to the AVN. In some cases, the slow posterior pathway is preferentially engaged so that the earliest atrial activation site is somewhat posterior to the AVN, closer to the CS os.[22]

The normal AVN response to rate-incremental ventricular pacing is a gradual delay of VA conduction (manifest as gradual prolongation of the HA interval) as the pacing CL decreases. Retrograde VA Wenckebach block and a higher degree of block appear at shorter pacing CLs. Occasionally, VA Wenckebach cycles are terminated with ventricular echo beats secondary to retrograde dual AVN physiology. When a retrograde His potential is visible, a relatively con-

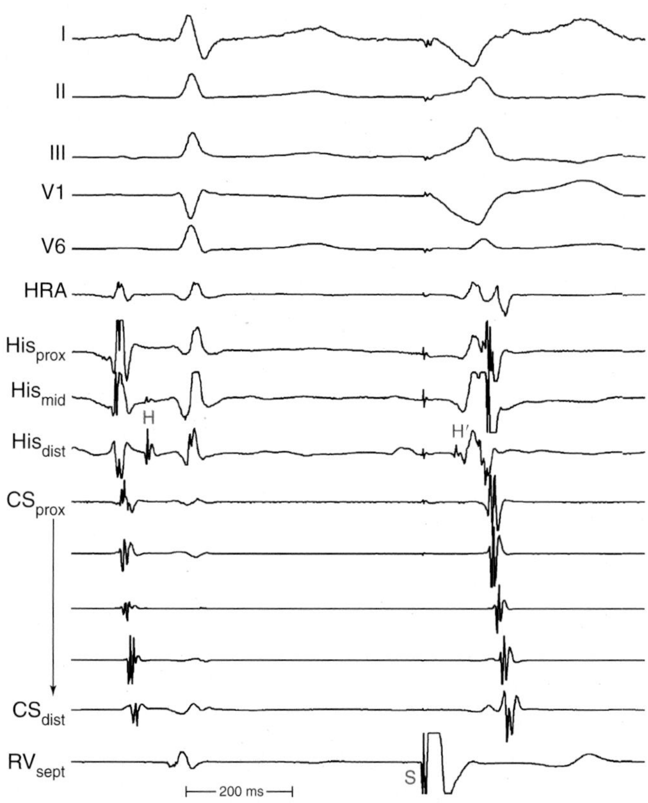

FIGURE 2–24 Retrograde activation with right ventricular (RV) septal stimulation. Sinus and RV septal stimulated complexes (S) are shown. Retrograde atrial activation is concentric, following a retrograde His potential (H′).

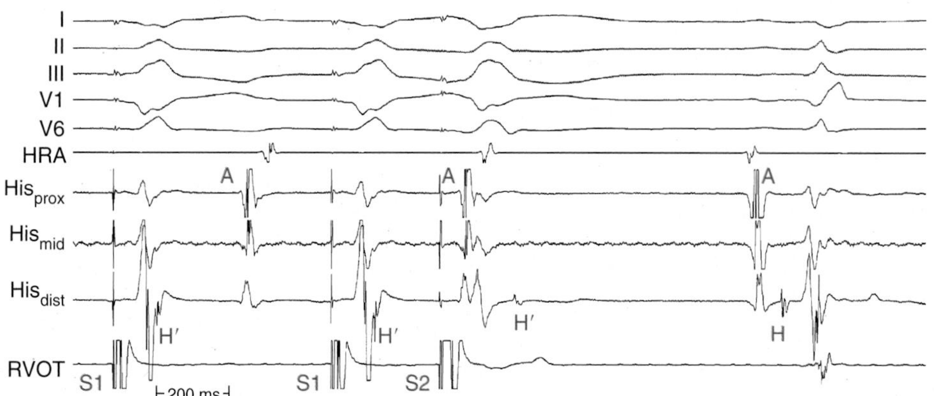

FIGURE 2–25 His recordings in presence of right bundle branch block (RBBB). Two right ventricular drive complexes (S_1) and an extrastimulus (S_2) are shown, with a subsequent sinus complex with typical RBBB. Retrograde His activation (H′) cannot traverse the blocked right bundle branch and must occur over the left bundle branch following transseptal ventricular activation, resulting in a long S-H′ interval. The S-H′ interval prolongs further following the extrastimulus (S_2). Of note, S_2 is associated with retrograde ventricular-atrial (VA) block in the atrioventricular node (AVN).

stant VH interval at a rapid pacing rate, despite the development of retrograde VA block, localizes the site of block to the AVN (Fig. 2-26). When a retrograde His potential is not visible during ventricular pacing, the site of VA block, when it occurs, must be inferred from the effect of paced impulses on conduction of spontaneous or stimulated atrial beats (i.e., by analyzing the level of retrograde concealment; see Fig. 2-26).[22] If the AH interval of the atrial beat is independent of the time relationship of the paced impulse, the site of block is in the HPS (infranodal). On the other hand, if the AH interval varies according to the coupling interval of the atrial beat to the paced QRS, or if the atrial beat fails to depolarize the HB, the site of block is in the AVN. Moreover, drugs that enhance AVN (but not HPS) conduction (e.g., atropine) improve VA conduction if the site of block is in the AVN, but do not affect VA conduction if the site of block is in the HPS.

At comparable pacing CLs, anterograde AV conduction is better than retrograde VA conduction in most patients (62%).[23] AVN conduction is the major determinant of retrograde VA conduction. Patients with prolonged PR intervals are much less likely to demonstrate retrograde VA conduction.[23] Furthermore, patients with prolonged AVN conduction are less capable of VA conduction than patients with infranodal conduction delay. Anterograde AV block in the AVN is almost universally associated with retrograde VA block. On the other hand, anterograde AV block in the HPS is associated with some degree of VA conduction in up to 40% of cases. However, the exact comparison between anterograde and retrograde AVN conduction can be limited by the absence of a visible retrograde His potential during ventricular stimulation and, consequently, localization of the exact site of conduction delay or block (AVN versus HPS) may not be feasible. The response to rate-incremental pacing at two different pacing CLs may differ because of the opposite effects of the pacing CL on AVN and HPS refractoriness.[22]

Rapid ventricular pacing can result in ipsilateral retrograde BBB, with subsequent impulse propagation across the septum, retrogradely up the contralateral bundle branch, and then to the HB. Such an event can manifest as sudden prolongation of the HV interval during pacing. This can be followed by resumption of VA conduction after a period of VA block in the AVN when the VH interval is short, because the delay in the HPS will allow recovery of the AVN (the gap phenomenon). This occurrence can permit better visualization of the His potential and, by comparing the ventricular electrogram in the HB recording when the His potential is clearly delayed to that with normal retrograde ipsilateral bundle branch conduction, a previously unappreciated His potential within that electrogram can now be visualized (see Fig. 2-26).

To exclude the presence of a nondecremental retrogradely conducting BT, the VES technique is usually more effective than rate-incremental ventricular pacing for demonstrating normal prolongation of the VA interval. If uncertainty continues to exist, adenosine can be extremely helpful, which is much more likely to block AVN conduction than BT.

Normal Response to Ventricular Premature Stimulation

Because a retrograde His potential may not be visible in 15% to 20% of patients during ventricular pacing, evaluation of the HPS, and consequently VA conduction, is often incomplete. Additionally, in the absence of a visible His potential during ventricular pacing, the FRP of the HPS (theoretically, the shortest H_1-H_2 interval at any coupling interval) must be approximated by the S_1-H_2 interval (S_1 being the stimulus artifact of the basic drive CL), so that the S_1-H_2 interval approximates the H_1-H_2 interval, but exceeds it by a fixed amount, the S_1-H_1 interval.[23] Retrograde AVN conduction time (H_2-A_2) is best measured from the end of the His potential to the onset of the atrial electrogram on the HB tracing.

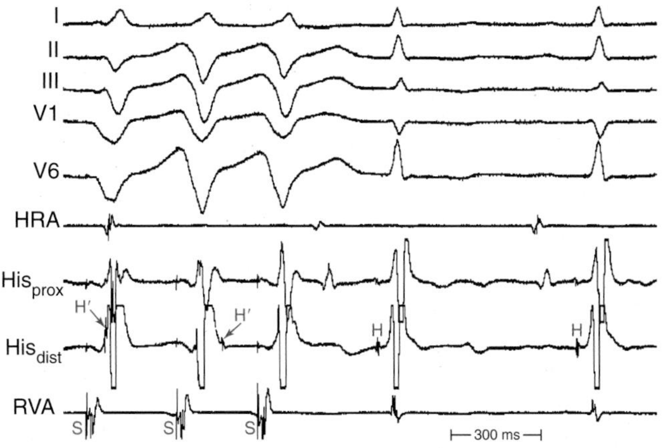

FIGURE 2–26 Complete retrograde ventricular-atrial (VA) block in the atrioventricular node (AVN). Three ventricular paced complexes are shown, the first two of which have a clear retrograde His potential (H′) and no retrograde atrial activation (sinus rhythm in atria), suggesting the AVN as the site of VA block. However, the site of VA block (AVN versus His-Purkinje system [HPS]) following the third ventricular complex is not obvious because there is no His potential visible following that ventricular stimulus. The site of VA block, however, can be inferred from the effect of paced impulses on conduction of the sinus complex after cessation of pacing. The atrial–His bundle (AH) interval of the conducted sinus complex after the last paced ventricular complex is longer than the baseline AH interval (at right), consistent with retrograde penetration of the AVN by the ventricular stimulus (resulting in concealed conduction) and, therefore, suggesting the AVN as the site of VA block.

Typically, VA conduction proceeds over the RB or LB, and then to the HB, AVN, and atrium. With a progressively premature VES, the initial delay occurs in the HPS, and the most common site of retrograde VA block is in the HPS. Delay or block in the AVN can occur but is less common.[23]

The typical response can be graphically displayed by plotting the S_1-S_2 interval versus S_2-H_2, S_2-A_2, and H_2-A_2 intervals, as well as the S_1-S_2 interval versus S_1-H_2 and A_1-A_2 intervals.[22,23] At long S_1-S_2 intervals, no delay occurs in the retrograde conduction (S_2-A_2). Further shortening of the S_1-S_2 intervals results in prolongation in the S_2-A_2 intervals, and localization of the exact site of S_2-A_2 delay may not be feasible unless a retrograde His potential is visible (Fig. 2-27A and B). During RV pacing, the initial delay usually occurs in retrograde RB conduction. At a critical coupling interval (S_1-S_2), block in the RB occurs and retrograde conduction proceeds over the LB. A retrograde His potential (H_2) eventually becomes visible after the ventricular electrogram in the HB recording (see Fig. 2-27D). Once a retrograde His potential is seen, progressive prolongation in the S_2-H_2 interval (HPS conduction delay) occurs as the S_1-S_2 interval shortens, and the VA conduction time (S_2-A_2) is determined by the HPS conduction delay (S_2-H_2), as demonstrated by parallel S_2-A_2 and S_2-H_2 curves. The degree of prolongation of the S_2-H_2 interval varies, but it can exceed 300 milliseconds.[22]

In patients with preexistent BBB, retrograde block in the same bundle is common. This is suggested by a prolonged VH interval during a constant paced drive CL or late VES from the ventricle ipsilateral to the BBB, so that a retrograde His potential is usually seen after the ventricular electrogram in the HB tracing (see Fig. 2-25).

In most cases, once a retrograde His potential is visible, the S_1-H_2 curve becomes almost horizontal because the

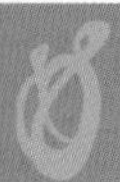

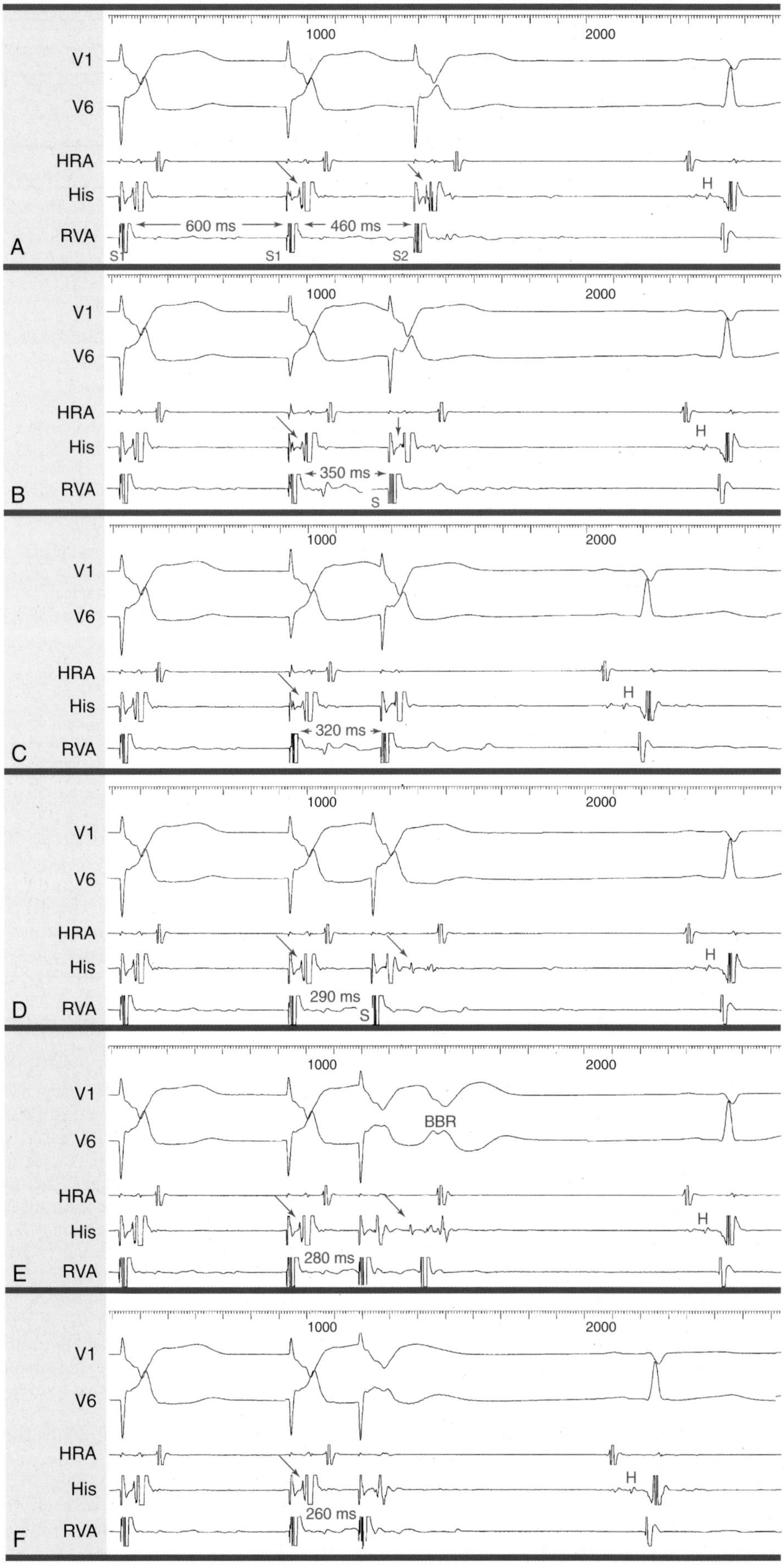

2

FIGURE 2–27 Normal response to progressively premature ventricular stimulation. Following a drive stimulus (S_1) at a cycle length (CL) of 600 milliseconds, a progressively premature ventricular extrastimulus (VES; S_2) is delivered from the right ventricular apex (RVA). **A,** At a VES coupling interval of 460 milliseconds, retrograde His potential (arrow) is visible just before the local ventricular electrogram on the His bundle (HB) tracing, and ventricular-atrial (VA) conduction is intact. **B,** An earlier VES is followed by some delay in VA conduction and prolongation of the His bundle–atrial (HA) interval. **C,** A short coupled VES is followed by VA block. A retrograde His potential is not clearly visible. **D,** An earlier VES is associated with retrograde block in the right bundle branch (RB), followed by transseptal conduction and retrograde conduction up the left bundle branch (LB) to the HB (the retrograde His potential is now visible well after the local ventricular electrogram). VA conduction now resumes because of proximal delay (in the His-Purkinje system [HPS]), allowing distal recovery in the atrioventricular node (AVN; the gap phenomenon). **E,** Further decrement in the VES coupling interval results in progressive delay in retrograde HPS conduction (and further prolongation of the S_2-H_2 interval), allowing for anterograde recovery of the RB, so that the impulse can return down the initially blocked RB, producing a QRS with a typical left bundle branch block pattern (bundle branch reentrant beat, BBR). **F,** A very early ventricular extrastimulus (VES) is followed by ventricular-atrial (VA) block secondary to retrograde block in both the RB and LB; therefore, no His potential is visible.

increase in the S_2-H_2 interval is similar to the decrease in the S_1-S_2 interval. This response results in a relatively constant input to the AVN (as determined by measuring the S_1-H_2 interval) and consequently a fixed H_2-A_2 interval. Occasionally, the increase in the S_2-H_2 interval greatly exceeds the decrease in the S_1-S_2 interval, giving rise to an ascending limb on the curve, with a subsequent decrease in the AVN conduction time (H_2-A_2) because of decreased input to the AVN. As the S_1-S_2 interval is further shortened, block within the HPS appears or ventricular ERP is reached.[22]

HPS refractoriness depends markedly on the CL, and shortening of the basic drive CL will shorten the FRP and ERP of the HPS and ventricle. The general pattern, however, remains the same, with an almost linear increase in the S_2-H_2 interval as the S_1-S_2 interval is shortened. The curves for S_2-H_2 versus S_1-S_2 are shifted to the left, and the curves for S_1-S_2 versus S_1-H_2 are shifted down.

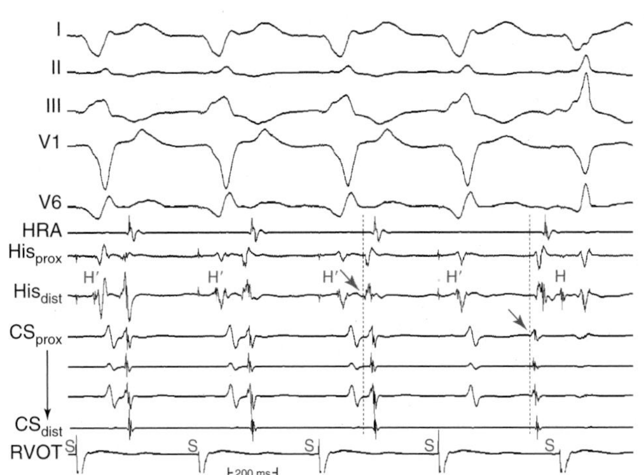

FIGURE 2–28 Retrograde dual atrioventricular pathways. Fixed-rate ventricular pacing results in retrograde conduction; retrograde His potential is labeled H′. The first three complexes are conducted over a fast AVN pathway; with the fourth complex, the fast AVN pathway conduction is blocked and retrograde conduction proceeds up the slow pathway (longer VA interval), followed by a fused QRS complex, partially paced and partially conducted to the His bundle (HB) anterogradely over the fast pathway. The two AVN pathways have different earliest atrial activation sites, indicated by colored arrows and dashed lines.

Repetitive Ventricular Responses

Ventricular stimulation can trigger extra ventricular beats. Those beats can be caused by different mechanisms; the most common are bundle branch reentrant beats, ventricular echo beats, and intraventricular reentrant beats. Multiple mechanisms may be responsible for repetitive responses in the same patient. Almost always, one of these responses will be BBR.

Bundle Branch Reentry Beats. This is the most common response, and can occur in up to 50% of normal individuals.[22] In patients with normal hearts, bundle branch reentry (BBR) is rarely sustained and is usually self-limiting in one or two complexes. The occurrence of nonsustained BBR in patients with or without structural heart disease is not related to the presence of spontaneous ventricular arrhythmias.

The longest refractory periods in the HPS are found most distally, at or near the Purkinje-myocardial junction. This creates a distal gate that inhibits retrograde conduction of early VES. Thus, when an early VES is delivered to the RV apex, the nearby distal gate of the RB can still be refractory, resulting in progressive retrograde conduction delay and block occurring in the distal RB with subsequent transseptal conduction of the impulse to the LV, resulting in retrograde conduction up the LB to the HB (see Fig. 2-27D). At this point, the His potential usually follows the local ventricular electrogram in the HB recording, and retrograde atrial stimulation, if present, follows the His potential. Further decrease in the VES coupling interval produces progressive delay in retrograde HPS conduction. When a critical degree of HPS delay (S_2-H_2) is attained, the impulse can return down the initially blocked RB, producing a QRS with a typical LBBB pattern and left-axis deviation, because ventricular activation originates solely from conduction over the RB (see Fig. 2-27E). This beat is called a BBR beat or V_3 phenomenon.[22]

The HV interval of the BBR beat usually approximates that during anterograde conduction; however, it can be shorter or longer, depending on the site of HB recording relative to the turnaround point and on anterograde conduction delay down the RB.

Ventricular Echo Beats. This is the second most common response and can occur in 15% to 30% of normal individuals.[22] It is caused by reentry in the AVN, and it appears when a critical degree of retrograde AVN delay is achieved. These patients have retrograde dual AVN physiology, and the last paced beat conducts slowly retrogradely up the slow AVN pathway and then anterogradely down the fast pathway to produce the echo beat (Fig. 2-28). In most cases, this delay is achieved before the appearance of a retrograde His potential beyond the local ventricular electrogram. At a critical H_2-A_2 interval (or V_2-A_2 interval, when the His potential cannot be seen), an extra beat with a normal anterograde QRS morphology results. Atrial activity also precedes the His potential before the echo beat.[22]

This phenomenon can occur at long or short coupling intervals and depends only on the degree of retrograde AVN conduction delay. The presence of block within the HPS will prevent its occurrence, as will block within the AVN. If a retrograde His potential can be seen throughout the zone of coupling intervals, a reciprocal relationship between the H_2-A_2 and A_2-H_3 intervals can often be seen.

Intraventricular Reentrant Beats. This response usually occurs in the setting of a cardiac pathological condition, especially coronary artery disease (CAD) with a prior MI. It usually occurs at short coupling intervals and can have any morphology, but more often RBBB than LBBB in patients with a prior MI.[22] Such beats occur in less than 15% of normal patients with a single VES at 2× diastolic threshold, and in 24% with a double VESs. In contrast, intraventricular reentrant beats occur following single or double VESs in 70% to 75% of patients with prior VT or VF and cardiac disease. The incidence of this response increases with increasing the number of VESs, basic drive CLs, and stimulation sites used.[22] These responses are usually nonsustained (1 to 30 complexes) and typically polymorphic. In patients without prior clinical arrhythmias, such responses are of no clinical significance.

MISCELLANEOUS ELECTROPHYSIOLOGICAL PHENOMENA

Concealed Conduction

Concealed conduction can be defined as the propagation of an impulse within the specialized conduction system of the heart that can be recognized only from its effect on the subsequent impulse, interval, or cycle.[26] This phenomenon can occur in any portion of the AV conduction system. As long as the cardiac impulse is traveling in the specialized conduction system, the amount of electrical current generated is too small to be recorded on the surface ECG. However, if this impulse travels only a limited distance—incomplete anterograde or retrograde penetration—within the system, it can interfere with the formation or propagation of another impulse. When this interference can be recognized in the tracing because of an unexpected behavior of the subsequent impulse, unexpected in the sense that the event cannot be explained on the basis of readily apparent physiological or pathophysiological processes, it is known as concealed conduction.[26-28]

The effect on subsequent events is an important part of the definition of concealed conduction, because it differentiates the concept of concealed conduction from other forms of incomplete conduction, such as block of conduction at the level of the AVN or HPS. Ideally, a diagnosis of concealed conduction is supported by evidence in other areas of the same tracing where, given the opportunity and proper physiological setting, an impulse that is occasionally concealed can be conducted. However, this condition cannot always be satisfied, nor is it absolutely necessary for the diagnosis of concealed conduction. Following are descriptions of the most frequent clinical circumstances in which concealed conduction can be observed.

Ventricular Response During Atrial Fibrillation. Repetitive concealed conduction is the mechanism of a slow ventricular rate during AF and AFL, with varying degrees of penetration into the AVN.[26-28] During AF, the irregular ventricular response is due to varying depth of penetration of the numerous wavefronts approaching the AVN. Although the AVN would be expected to conduct whenever it recovers excitability after the last conducted atrial impulse, which would then be at regular intervals, the ventricular response is irregularly irregular because some fibrillatory impulses penetrate the AVN incompletely and block, leaving it refractory in the face of subsequent atrial impulses.

Unexpected Prolongation or Failure of Conduction. Prolongation of the PR (and AH) interval or AVN block can occur secondary to a nonconducted premature depolarization of any origin (atrium, ventricle, or HB). The premature impulse incompletely penetrates the AVN (anterogradely or retrogradely), resets its refractoriness, and can make it fully or partially refractory in the face of the next sinus beat, which may then be blocked or may conduct with longer PR interval (see Fig. 2-26). For example, concealed junctional (HB) impulses can manifest as isolated PR interval prolongation, pseudo–type I AV block, or pseudo–type II AV block. ECG clues to concealed junctional extrasystoles causing such unexpected events include abrupt unexplained prolongation of the PR interval, the presence of apparent type II AV block in the presence of a normal QRS, the presence of types I and II AV block in the same tracing, and the presence of manifest junctional extrasystoles elsewhere in the tracing.

Unexpected Facilitation of Conduction. When a premature impulse penetrates the AV conduction system, it can result in facilitation of AV conduction and normalization of a previously present AV block or BBB by one of two mechanisms: (1) preexciting parts of the conduction system so that its refractory period ends earlier than expected (i.e., peeling back the refractory period of that tissue, allowing more time to recover excitability); or (2) causing CL-dependent shortening of refractoriness of tissues (i.e., atria, HPS, and ventricles) by decreasing the CL preceding the subsequent spontaneous impulse.[26-28] Abrupt normalization of the aberration by a PVC, the finding of which proves retrograde concealment as the mechanism for perpetuation of aberration, is based on these principles.

Perpetuation of Aberrant Conduction During Supraventricular Tachycardias. The most common mechanism (70%) of perpetuation of aberrant conduction during tachyarrhythmias is retrograde penetration of the blocked bundle branch subsequent to transseptal conduction.[29] For example, a PVC from the LV during an SVT can activate the LB early and then conduct transseptally and later penetrate the RB retrogradely. Subsequently, the LB recovers in time for the next SVT impulse, whereas the RB remains refractory. Therefore, the next SVT impulse travels to the LV over the LB (with an RBBB pattern, phase 3 aberration). Conduction subsequently propagates from the LV across the septum to the RV. By this time, the distal RB has recovered, allowing for retrograde penetration of the RB by the transseptal wavefront, thereby rendering the RB refractory to each subsequent SVT impulse. This scenario is repeated and RBBB continues until another, well-timed PVC preexcites the RB (and either peels back or shortens its refractoriness), so that the next impulse from above finds the RB fully recovered and conducts without aberration.

Gap Phenomenon

The term *gap* in AVN conduction was originally used to define a zone in the cardiac cycle during which PACs failed to evoke ventricular responses while PACs of greater or lesser prematurity conducted to the ventricles. The physiological basis of the gap phenomenon depends on a distal area with a long refractory period and a proximal site with a shorter refractory period. During the gap phenomenon, initial block occurs distally. With earlier impulses, proximal conduction delay is encountered, which allows the distal site of early block to recover excitability and resume conduction.[26,28,30,31]

The gap phenomenon is not an abnormality, but reflects the interplay between conduction velocity and refractory periods at two different levels in the AV conduction system. Demonstration of the gap phenomenon can be enhanced or eliminated by any intervention that alters the relationship between the EP properties of those structures (e.g., changes in the neurohumoral tone created by drugs or changes in the heart rate by pacing).

An example of the most common type of gap phenomenon is an AES (A_2) conducting with modest delay through the AVN that finds the HB still refractory, causing block. With increasing prematurity of the AES, the AES travels more slowly through the AVN (i.e., the A_2-H_2 interval prolongs further) so that the H_1-H_2 interval now exceeds the refractory period of the HB. By the time the impulse traverses the AVN, the HB has completed its ERP and conduction resumes (Fig. 2-29).

Other types of the gap phenomenon are described in which the required conduction delay is in the HB, proximal AVN, or atria. The gap phenomenon depends on the relationship between the EP properties of two sites; any pair of structures in the AV conduction system that have the appropriate physiological relationship can exhibit gap phenomenon (e.g., AVN-HB, HB-HPS, atrium-AVN, atrium-HPS, proximal AVN–distal AVN, proximal HPS–distal HPS), and gap can occur during anterograde or retrograde stimulation. Therefore, there are almost endless possibilities for gaps, all based on the fundamental precept of "proximal delay allows distal recovery" (see Fig. 2-27C and D).[26,28]

Supernormality

Supernormal conduction implies conduction that is better than anticipated or conduction that occurs when block is expected. Electrocardiographically, however, supernormal conduction is not better than normal conduction, only better than expected. Conduction is better earlier in the cycle than later and occurs when block is expected. When an alteration in conduction can be explained in terms of known physio-

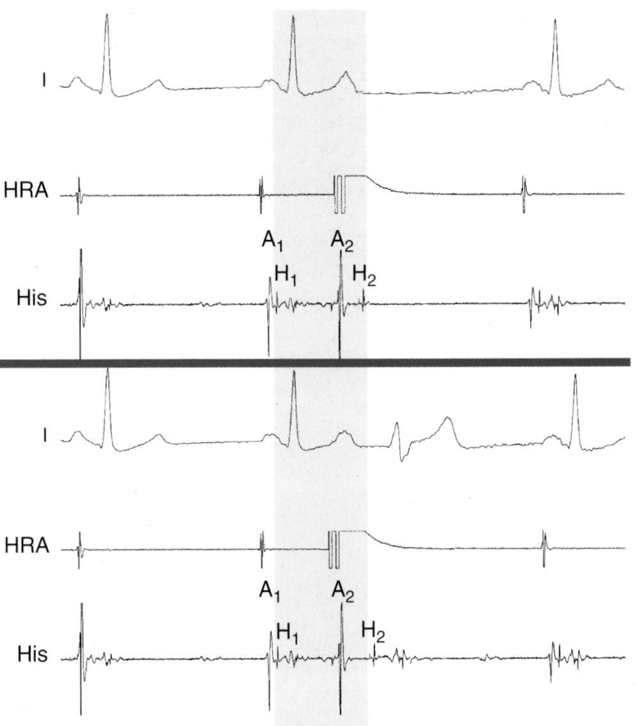

FIGURE 2–29 Anterograde atrioventricular (AV) gap phenomenon. **Upper panel,** An atrial extrastimulus (AES; A_2) conducting with modest delay through the AV node (AVN) finds the His bundle (HB) still refractory, causing AV block. **Lower panel,** An earlier AES results in further prolongation of the A_2-H_2 interval and the subsequent H_1-H_2 interval (shaded area). The longer H_1-H_2 interval now exceeds the refractory period of the HB and, by the time the impulse traverses the AVN, the HB has completed its effective refractory period (ERP) and conduction resumes; however, the conducted QRS has a left bundle branch block (LBBB) morphology and a longer HV interval because the LB is still refractory.

logical events, true supernormal conduction need not be invoked.[26]

Supernormal conduction is dependent on supernormal excitability, a condition that exists during a brief period of repolarization, at the end of phase 3. During the supernormal period, excitation is possible in response to an otherwise subthreshold stimulus; that same stimulus fails to elicit a response earlier or later than the supernormal period.[26,28,32] Two factors are responsible for supernormality, the availability of fast Na^+ channels and the proximity of the membrane potential to threshold potential. During the supernormal phase of excitability, the cell has recovered enough to respond to a stimulus; however, because the membrane potential is still reduced, it requires only a little additional depolarization to bring the fiber to threshold; thus, a smaller stimulus than is normally required elicits an action potential. Supernormality has been demonstrated in the HPS, Bachmann bundle in the dog, and working myocardium of the atrium and ventricle, but not in the AVN.

Supernormal excitability is diagnosed when the myocardium responds to a stimulus that is ineffective when applied earlier or later in the cycle. Some ECG manifestations of supernormality include the following:

1. Paradoxical normalization of bundle branch conduction at an R-R interval shorter than that with BBB. This can occur with a premature atrial complex (PAC) conducting with a normal QRS during baseline NSR with BBB, or with acceleration-dependent BBB that normalizes at even faster rates.
2. Intermittent AV conduction during periods of high-degree AV block. Only the P waves falling on or just after the terminal part of the T wave are conducted, whereas other timed P waves fail to conduct.
3. A failing pacemaker that captures just at the end of the T wave, but not elsewhere in the cardiac cycle.

Although supernormal conduction is a proven property of the HPS and has been demonstrated in vitro, it is uncertain whether true supernormal conduction is a clinically important phenomenon. Other physiological mechanisms can be invoked to explain almost all reported examples of supernormal conduction in humans. Causes of apparent or pseudosupernormal conduction include the gap phenomenon (the most common mechanism of pseudosupernormal conduction), peeling back of refractoriness, shortening of refractoriness by changing the preceding CL, Wenckebach phenomena in the bundle branches, bradycardia-dependent (phase 4) block, summation, dual AVN physiology, reentry with ventricular echo beats, and concealed junctional extrasystoles.[26,28,32]

REFERENCES

1. Zipes DP, DiMarco JP, Gillette PC, et al: Guidelines for clinical intracardiac electrophysiological and catheter ablation procedures. A report of the American College of Cardiology-American Heart Association Task Force on Practice Guidelines (Committee on Clinical Intracardiac Electrophysiologic and Catheter Ablation Procedures), developed in collaboration with the North American Society of Pacing and Electrophysiology. J Am Coll Cardiol 1995;26:555.
2. Scheinman MM, Huang S: The 1998 NASPE prospective catheter ablation registry. Pacing Clin Electrophysiol 2000;23:1020.
3. Wellens HJ: Catheter ablation of cardiac arrhythmias: Usually cure, but complications may occur. Circulation 1999;99:195.
4. Josephson ME: Electrophysiologic investigation: Technical aspects. *In* Josephson ME (ed): Clinical Cardiac Electrophysiology, 3rd ed. Philadelphia, Lippincott, Williams & Wilkins, 2002, pp 1-18.
5. Markides V, Segal O, Tondato F, Peters N: Mapping. *In* Zipes D, Jalife J (eds): Cardiac Electrophysiology: From Cell to Bedside, 4th ed. Philadelphia, WB Saunders, 2004, pp 858-868.
6. McGavigan AD, Kalman JM: Atrial anatomy and imaging in atrial fibrillation ablation. J Cardiovasc Electrophysiol 2006;17(Suppl 3):S8.
7. Anderson RH, Brown NA, Webb S: Development and structure of the atrial septum. Heart 2002;88:104.
8. Daoud EG: Transseptal catheterization. Heart Rhythm 2005;2:212.
9. Johnson SB, Seward JB, Packer DL: Phased-array intracardiac echocardiography for guiding transseptal catheter placement: Utility and learning curve. Pacing Clin Electrophysiol 2002;25(4 Pt 1):402.
10. Cheng A, Calkins H: A conservative approach to performing transseptal punctures without the use of intracardiac echocardiography: Stepwise approach with real-time video clips. J Cardiovasc Electrophysiol 2007;18:686.
11. Fisher WG: Transseptal catheterization. *In* Huang SKS, Wilber DH (eds): Catheter Ablation of Cardiac Arrhythmias. Philadelphia, WB Saunders, 2006, pp 635-648.
12. Ren JF, Callans DJ: Utility of intracardiac echocardiographic imaging for catheterization. *In* Ren J-F, Marchlinski FE, Callans DJ, Schwartsman D (eds): Practical Intracardiac Echocardiography in Electrophysiology. Malden, Mass, Wiley-Blackwell, 2006, pp 56-73.
13. Brugada J, Berruezo A, Cuesta A, et al: Nonsurgical transthoracic epicardial radiofrequency ablation: An alternative in incessant ventricular tachycardia. J Am Coll Cardiol 2003;41:2036.
14. Hsia HH, Marchlinski FE: Characterization of the electroanatomic substrate for monomorphic ventricular tachycardia in patients with nonischemic cardiomyopathy. Pacing Clin Electrophysiol 2002;25:1114.
15. Schweikert RA, Saliba WI, Tomassoni G, et al: Percutaneous pericardial instrumentation for endo-epicardial mapping of previously failed ablations. Circulation 2003;108:1329.
16. Soejima K, Stevenson WG, Sapp JL, et al: Endocardial and epicardial radiofrequency ablation of ventricular tachycardia associated with dilated cardiomyopathy: The importance of low-voltage scars. J Am Coll Cardiol 2004;43:1834.
17. Sosa E, Scanavacca M: Epicardial mapping and ablation techniques to control ventricular tachycardia. J Cardiovasc Electrophysiol 2005;16:449.
18. Stevenson WG, Soejima K: Recording techniques for clinical electrophysiology. J Cardiovasc Electrophysiol 2005;16:1017.
19. Delacretaz E, Soejima K, Gottipaty VK, et al: Single catheter determination of local electrogram prematurity using simultaneous unipolar and bipolar recordings to replace the surface ECG as a timing reference. Pacing Clin Electrophysiol 2001;24(4 Pt 1):441.
20. Arora R, Kadish A: Fundamental of intracardiac mapping. *In* Huang SKS, Wilber DH (eds): Catheter Ablation of Cardiac Arrhythmias. Philadelphia, WB Saunders, 2006, pp 107-134.
21. DeBakker JMT, Haner RNW, Simmers TA: Activation mapping: Unipolar versus bipolar recording. *In* Zipes DP, Jalife J (eds): Cardiac Electrophysiology. From Cell to Bedside. Philadelphia, WB Saunders, 1995, pp 1068.

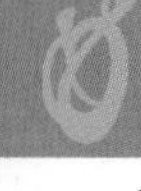

22. Josephson ME: Electrophysiologic investigation: General aspects. *In* Josephson ME (ed): Clinical Cardiac Electrophysiology, 3rd ed. Lippincott, Williams & Wilkins, 2002, pp 19-67.
23. Akhtar M, Damato AN, Batsford WP, et al: A comparative analysis of antegrade and retrograde conduction patterns in man. Circulation 1975;52:766.
24. Denes P, Wu D, Dhingra R, et al: The effects of cycle length on cardiac refractory periods in man. Circulation 1974;49:32.
25. Josephson ME: Sinus node function. *In* Josephson ME (ed): Clinical Cardiac Electrophysiology, 3rd ed. Lippincott, Williams & Wilkins, 2002, pp 19-67.
26. Josephson ME: Miscellaneous phenomena related to atrioventricular conduction. *In* Josephson ME (ed): Clinical Cardiac Electrophysiology, 3rd ed. Lippincott, Williams & Wilkins, 2002, pp 140-154.
27. Fisch C, Knoebel SB: Concealed conduction. *In* Fisch C, Knoebel SB (eds): Electrocardiography of Clinical Arrhythmias. Armonk, New York, Futura, 2000, pp 153-172.
28. Kilborn MF, McGuire MA: Electrocardiographic manifestations of supernormal conduction, concealed conduction, and exit block. *In* Zipes DP, Jalife J (eds): Cardiac Electrophysiology: From Cell to Bedside. Philadelphia, WB Saunders, 2004, pp 733-738.
29. Wellens HJ: Functional bundle branch block during supraventricular tachycardia in man: Observations on mechanisms and their incidence. *In* Zipes DP, Jalife J (eds): Cardiac Electrophysiology and Arrhythmias. New York, Grune & Stratton, 1995, pp 435-440.
30. Fisch C, Knoebel SB: Atrioventricular and ventriculoatrial conduction and blocks, gap, and overdrive suppression. *In* Fisch C, Knoebel SB (eds): Electrocardiography of Clinical Arrhythmias. Futura, 2000, pp 315-344.
31. Toeda T, Suetake S, Tsuchida K, et al: Exercise-induced atrioventricular block with gap phenomenon in atrioventricular conduction. Pacing Clin Electrophysiol 2000;23(4 Pt 1):527.
32. Fisch C, Knoebel SB: Supernormal conduction and excitability. *In* Fisch C, Knoebel SB (eds): Electrocardiography of Clinical Arrhythmias. Armonk, New York, Futura, 2000, pp 237-252.

CHAPTER 3

Mapping and Navigation Modalities

Cardiac mapping refers to the process of identifying the temporal and spatial distributions of myocardial electrical potentials during a particular heart rhythm. Cardiac mapping is a broad term that covers several modes of mapping such as body surface, endocardial, and epicardial mapping. Cardiac mapping during a tachycardia aims at elucidation of the mechanism(s) of the tachycardia, description of the propagation of activation from its initiation to its completion within a region of interest, and identification of the site of origin or a critical site of conduction to serve as a target for catheter ablation.

Conventional radiofrequency (RF) ablation has revolutionized the treatment of many supraventricular tachycardias (SVTs) as well as ventricular tachycardias (VTs). Success in stable arrhythmias with predictable anatomical locations or characteristics identifying endocardial electrograms, such as idiopathic VT, atrioventricular nodal reentrant tachycardia (AVNRT), or typical atrial flutter (AFL), has approached 90% to 99%. However, as interest has turned to a broad array of more complex arrhythmias, including some atrial tachycardias (ATs), many forms of intraatrial reentry, most VTs, and atrial fibrillation (AF), ablation of such arrhythmias continues to pose a major challenge. This stems in part from the limitations of fluoroscopy and conventional catheter-based mapping techniques to localize arrhythmogenic substrates that are removed from fluoroscopic landmarks and lack characteristic electrographic patterns.

Newer mapping systems have revolutionized the clinical electrophysiology (EP) laboratory in recent years to overcome the limitations of conventional mapping, and have offered new insights into arrhythmia mechanisms. They are aimed at improving the resolution, three-dimensional (3-D) spatial localization, and/or rapidity of acquisition of cardiac activation maps. These systems use novel approaches to determine the 3-D location of the mapping catheter accurately, and local electrograms are acquired using conventional, well-established methods. Recorded data of the catheter location and intracardiac electrogram at that location are used to reconstruct in real time a representation of the 3-D geometry of the chamber, color-coded with relevant electrophysiological information.

The application of these various techniques for mapping of specific arrhythmias is described elsewhere in this text, as are the details involved in the diagnosis, mapping, and treatment of specific arrhythmias.

ACTIVATION MAPPING

Fundamental Concepts

Essential to the effective management of any cardiac arrhythmia is a thorough understanding of the mechanisms of its initiation and maintenance. Conventionally, this has been achieved by careful study of the surface electrocardiogram (ECG) and correlation of the changes therein with data from intracardiac electrograms recorded by catheters at various key locations within the cardiac chambers (i.e., activation mapping). A record of these electrograms documenting multiple sites simultaneously is studied to determine the mechanisms of an arrhythmic event.

The main value of intracardiac and surface ECG tracings is the timing of electrical events and determining the direction of impulse propagation. Additionally, electrogram morphology can be of significant importance during mapping. Interpretation of recorded electrograms is fundamental to the clinical investigation of arrhythmias during EP studies. Establishing electrogram criteria, which permits accurate determination of the moment of myocardial activation at the recording electrode, is critical for construction of an area map of the activation sequence. Bipolar recordings are generally used for activation mapping. Unipolar recordings are used to supplement the information obtained from bipolar recordings. The differences in unipolar and bipolar recordings can be used to assist in mapping by simultaneously recording bipolar and unipolar signals from the mapping catheter.[1-3]

Unipolar Recordings

Timing of Local Activation. The major component of the unipolar electrogram allows determination of the local

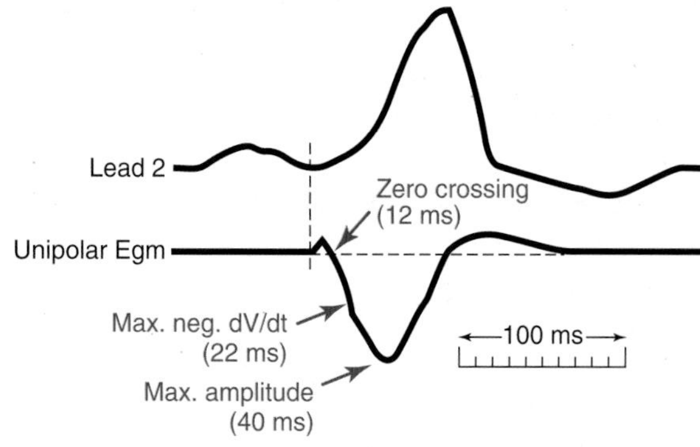

3 FIGURE 3–1 Unipolar electrogram activation times. A lead 2 electrocardiogram and a unipolar electrogram (Egm) from the ventricle of a patient with Wolff-Parkinson-White (WPW) syndrome are shown. The vertical dashed line denotes the onset of the delta wave; the horizontal dotted line is the baseline of the unipolar recording. Several candidates for the timing of unipolar activation are labeled with corresponding activation times relative to delta wave onset.

activation time, although there are exceptions. The point of maximum amplitude, the zero crossing, the point of maximum slope (maximum first derivative), and the minimum second derivative of the electrogram have been proposed as indicators for underlying myocardial activation (Fig. 3-1). The maximum negative slope (i.e., maximum change in potential, dV/dt) of the signal coincides best with the arrival of the depolarization wavefront directly beneath the electrode because the maximal negative dV/dt corresponds to the maximum sodium channel conductance. Using this fiducial point, errors in determining the local activation time as compared with intracellular recordings have typically been less than 1 millisecond.[1-3] This is true for filtered and unfiltered unipolar electrograms.

Direction of Local Activation. The morphology of the unfiltered unipolar recording indicates the direction of wavefront propagation. By convention, the mapping electrode that is in contact with the myocardium is connected to the positive input of the recording amplifier. In this configuration, positive deflections (R waves) are generated by propagation toward the recording electrode, and negative deflections (QS complexes) are generated by propagation away from the electrode (Figs. 3-2 and 3-3). If a recording electrode is at the source from which all wavefronts propagate (at the site of initial activation), depolarization produces a wavefront that spreads away from the electrode, generating a monophasic QS complex. It is also important to recognize that a QS complex can be recorded when the mapping electrode is not in contact with the myocardium, but is floating in the cavity. In that situation, the initial negative slope of the recording is typically slow, suggesting that the electrogram is a far-field signal, generated by tissue some distance from the recording electrode.[2] Filtering at higher corner frequencies (e.g., 30 Hz) alters the morphology of the signal, so that the morphology of the unipolar signal is no longer an indication of the direction of wavefront propagation and the presence or absence of a QS complex cannot be used to infer proximity to the site of earliest activation (Fig. 3-4).[1-3]

Advantages of Unipolar Recordings. One important value of unipolar recordings is that they provide a more precise measure of local activation. This is true for filtered and unfiltered unipolar electrograms. In addition, unfiltered unipolar recordings provide information about the direction of impulse propagation. Using the unipolar configuration also eliminates a possible anodal contribution to depolarization and allows pacing and recording at the same

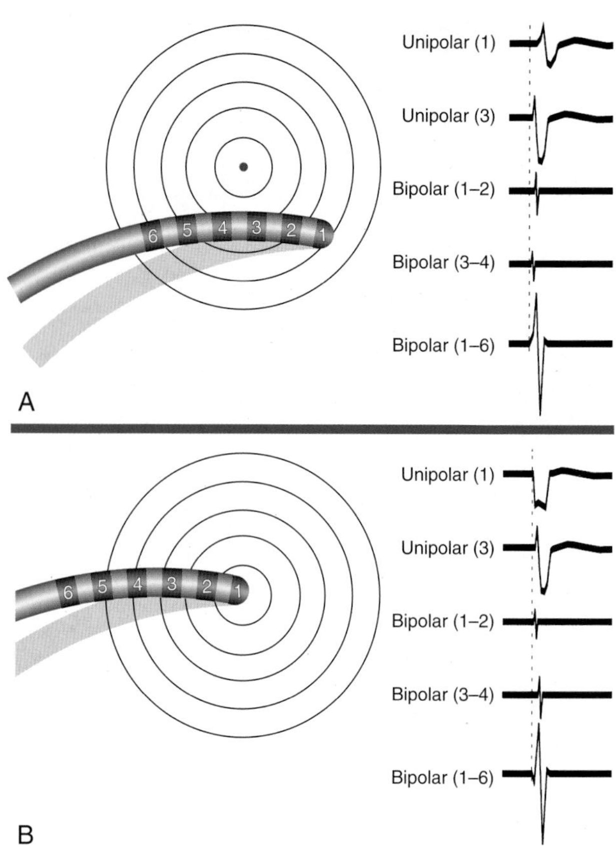

FIGURE 3–2 Hypothetical recordings from a multipolar electrode catheter. **A,** The electrodes are near a point source of activation (red dot in center of concentric rings). Note the timing and shape of the resultant electrogram patterns based on distance from point source, unipolar or bipolar recording, and width of bipole. **B,** The tip electrode (1) is at the point source of activation. Note differences in timing and shape of electrograms compared with **A**.

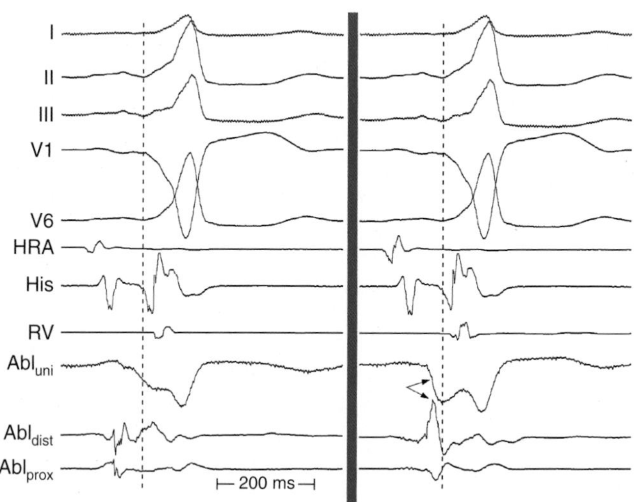

FIGURE 3–3 Unipolar and bipolar recordings from a patient with Wolff-Parkinson-White (WPW) syndrome. The dashed line denotes onset of QRS complex (delta wave). **Right panel,** Recordings at the successful ablation site, characterized by QS in the unipolar recording. The most rapid component precedes the delta wave onset by 22 milliseconds, has the same timing as the peak of the ablation distal electrode recording, and precedes the ablation proximal electrode recording (*arrows*). **Left panel,** Recordings from a poorer site, with an rS in the unipolar recording; most of the bipolar recordings are atrial.

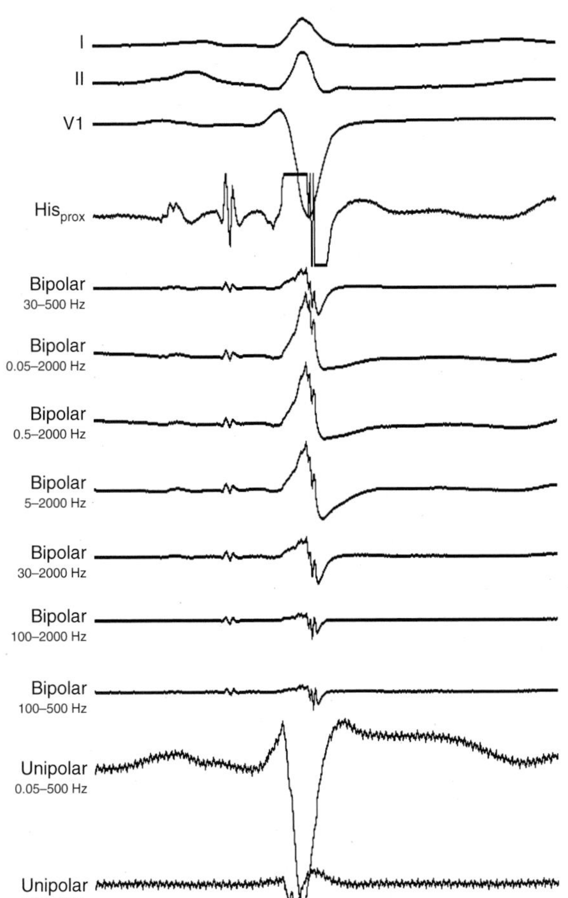

FIGURE 3–4 Effect of filtering on intracardiac recordings. The signal labeled "Bipolar 30-500 Hz" is the same signal as the His_{prox} above it, displayed at lower gain. All signals beneath this are of the same gain but different filter bandwidths, illustrating progressive loss of signal amplitude as bandwidth is narrowed. Unipolar signals below are of the same gain.

location. This generally facilitates the use of other mapping modalities, namely pace mapping.

Disadvantages of Unipolar Recordings. The major disadvantage of unipolar recordings is that they have poor signal-to-noise ratio and contain substantial far-field signal generated by depolarization of tissue remote from the recording electrode. Therefore, distant activity can be difficult to separate from local activity. This is especially true when recording from areas of prior myocardial infarction (MI), where the fractionated ventricular potentials are ubiquitous and it is often impossible to select a rapid negative dV/dt when the entire QS potential is slowly inscribed—that is, cavity potential.[1,3] Another disadvantage is the inability to record an undisturbed electrogram during or immediately after pacing. This is a significant disadvantage when entrainment mapping is to be performed during activation mapping, because recording of the return tachycardia complex on the pacing electrode immediately after cessation of pacing is required to interpret entrainment mapping results.[2]

Bipolar Recordings

Timing of Local Activation. Algorithms for detecting local activation time from bipolar electrograms have been more problematic, partly because of generation of the bipolar electrogram by two spatially separated recording poles. In a homogeneous sheet of tissue, the initial peak of a filtered (30 to 300 or more Hz) bipolar signal, the absolute maximum electrogram amplitude, coincides with depolarization beneath the recording electrode, appears to correlate most consistently with local activation time, and corresponds to the maximal negative dV/dt of the unipolar recording (see Fig. 3-3).[1-3] However, in the case of complex multicomponent bipolar electrograms, such as those with marked fractionation and prolonged duration seen in regions with complex conduction patterns (e.g., in regions of slow conduction in macroreentrant AT or VT), determination of local activation time becomes problematic, and the decision of which activation time is most appropriate needs to be made in the context of the particular rhythm being mapped. To acquire true local electrical activity, a bipolar electrogram with an interelectrode distance less than 1 cm is desirable. Smaller interelectrode distances record increasingly local events (as opposed to far-field). Elimination of far-field noise is usually accomplished by filtering the intracardiac electrograms, typically at 30 to 500 Hz.[1-3]

Direction of Local Activation. The morphology and amplitude of bipolar electrograms are influenced by the orientation of the bipolar recording axis to the direction of propagation of the activation wavefront. A wavefront that is propagating in the direction exactly perpendicular to the axis of the recording dipole produces no difference in potential between the electrodes, and hence no signal.[1-3] However, the direction of wavefront propagation cannot be reliably inferred from the morphology of the bipolar signal, although a change in morphology can be a useful finding.[1-3] For example, when recording from the lateral aspect of the cavotricuspid isthmus during pacing from the coronary sinus (CS), a reversal in the bipolar electrogram polarity from positive to negative at the ablation line indicates complete isthmus block. Similarly, if bipolar recordings are obtained with the same catheter orientation parallel to the atrioventricular (AV) annulus during retrograde bypass tract (BT) conduction, an RS configuration electrogram will be present on one side of the BT, where the wavefront is propagating from the distal electrode toward the proximal electrode, and a QR morphology electrogram on the other side, where the wavefront is propagating from the proximal electrode toward the distal electrode (Fig. 3-5).

Advantages of Bipolar Recordings. Bipolar recordings provide an improved signal-to-noise ratio, and high-frequency components are more accurately seen, which facilitates identification of local depolarization, especially in abnormal areas of infarction or scar.

Disadvantages of Bipolar Recordings. In contrast to unipolar signals, the direction of wavefront propagation cannot be reliably inferred from the morphology of the bipolar signal. Furthermore, bipolar recordings do not allow simultaneous pacing and recording from the same location. To pace and record simultaneously in bipolar fashion at endocardial sites as close together as possible, electrodes 1 and 3 of the mapping catheter are used for bipolar pacing and electrodes 2 and 4 are used for recording.[2] The precision of locating the source of a particular electrical signal depends on the distance between the recording electrodes, because the signal of interest can be beneath the distal or proximal electrode (or both) of the recording pair.[2]

Mapping Procedure

Prerequisites for Activation Mapping. Several factors are important for the success of activation mapping, including inducibility of tachycardia at the time of EP testing, hemodynamic stability of the tachycardia, and stable tachycardia morphology. In addition, determination of an electrical reference point, determination of the mechanism of the tachycardia (focal versus macroreentrant) and, subsequently, the goal of mapping are essential prerequisites.

3

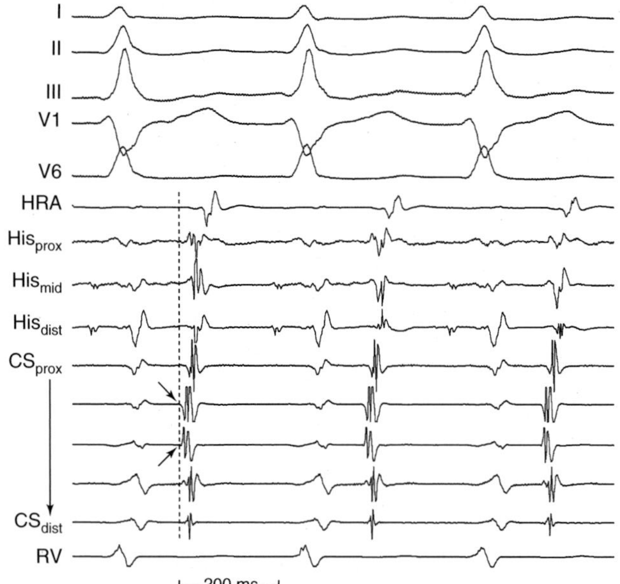

FIGURE 3–5 Recordings from a patient with a left lateral bypass tract during supraventricular tachycardia showing electrogram inversion at mid–coronary sinus (*arrows*), where earliest retrograde atrial activation occurs (*dashed line*).

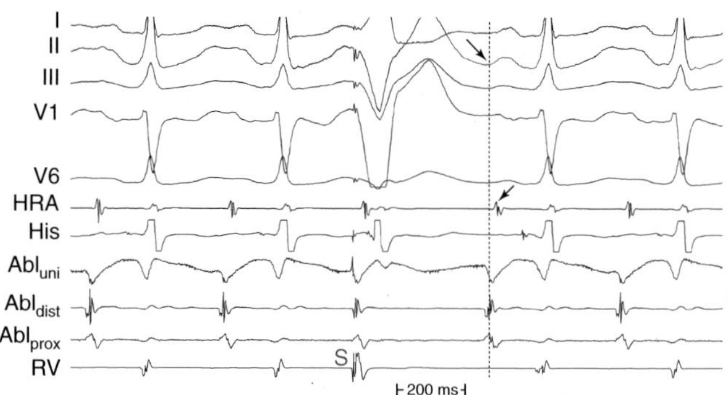

FIGURE 3–6 Use of ventricular extrastimulus (VES) to clarify onset of P wave during atrial tachycardia (AT). A single VES (S) delivered during AT advances the timing of ventricular activation to show P wave (*long arrow*) by itself without overlying ST segment and T wave, which made it difficult to determine P wave onset during ongoing tachycardia. Dashed line denotes onset of the P wave; timing of reference electrogram (HRA; *short arrow*) can thereafter be used as surrogate for P wave onset.

Selection of the Electrical Reference Point. Local activation times must be relative to some external and consistent fiducial marker, such as the onset of the P wave or QRS complex on the surface ECG or a reference intracardiac electrode. For VT, the QRS complex onset should be assessed using all surface ECG leads to search for the lead with the earliest QRS onset. This lead should then be used for subsequent activation mapping. Similarly, the P wave during AT should be assessed using multiple ECG leads and choosing the one with the earliest P onset. However, determining the onset of the P wave can be impossible if the preceding T wave or QRS is superimposed. To facilitate visualization of the P wave, a ventricular extrastimulus (VES) or a train of ventricular pacing can be delivered to advance (create premature) ventricular activation and repolarization and permit careful distinction of the P wave onset (Fig. 3-6). After determining the P wave onset, a surrogate marker, such as a right atrium (RA) or CS electrogram indexed to the P wave onset, where it is clearly seen, can be used rather than the P wave onset.

Defining the Goal of Mapping. Determination of the mechanism of the tachycardia (focal versus macroreentrant) is essential to define the goal of activation mapping. For focal tachycardias, activation mapping entails localizing the site of origin of the tachycardia focus. This is reflected by the earliest presystolic activity that precedes the onset of the P wave (during focal AT) or QRS (during focal VT) by an average of 10 to 40 millliseconds, because only this short amount of time is required after the focus discharges to activate enough myocardium and begin generating a P wave or QRS complex (Fig. 3-7). For mapping macroreentrant tachycardias, the goal of mapping is identification of the critical isthmus of the reentrant circuit, as indicated by finding the site with a continuous activity spanning diastole or with an isolated mid-diastolic potential (see Fig. 3-7).

Epicardial Versus Endocardial Mapping. Activation mapping is predominantly performed endocardially. Occasionally, epicardial mapping can be required because of an inability to ablate some VTs or AV BTs using the endocardial approach. Epicardial mapping can be performed with special recording catheters that can be steered in the branches of the CS. This technique has been used for

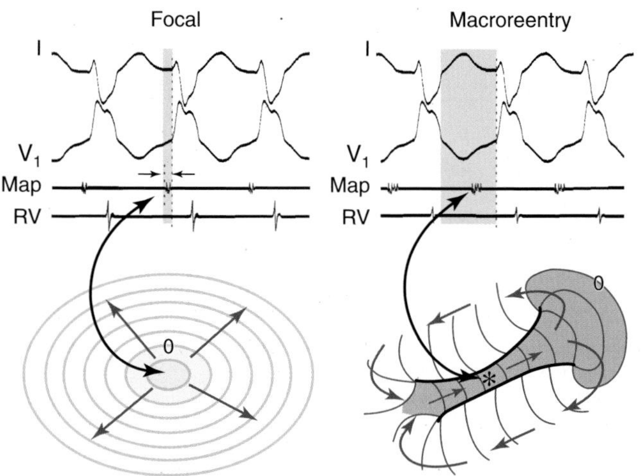

FIGURE 3–7 Focal versus macroreentrant ventricular tachycardia (VT). **Top,** Electrocardiogram (ECG) and intracardiac electrograms from the mapping and right ventricle (RV) catheters. **Bottom,** Depictions of events at sites where mapped electrograms are obtained. **Left,** VT focus fires and activation spreads to normal myocardium within 30 to 40 milliseconds, generating a QRS complex. Thus, the electrogram at the site of the focus will generally be 40 milliseconds or less prior to the QRS onset. **Right,** In contrast, in a macroreentrant VT, some myocardium is being activated at each instant in the cardiac cycle. During surface ECG diastole, only a few cells are activating (too few to cause surface ECG deflections). The area of a protected diastolic corridor, often cordoned off by scar, contains mid-diastolic recordings and is an attractive ablation site. The 0 isochrone indicates the time at which the QRS begins.

mapping ischemic VT and AV BTs, but its scope is limited by the anatomy of the coronary venous system.[4] Another epicardial mapping technique using a subxyphoid percutaneous approach for accessing the epicardial surface has been used to map VT in patients with Chagas' disease and after failed endocardial ablation of other VTs. A wider application of this technique may be possible, but it is currently performed at only a few centers.[5,6] The same fundamental principles of activation mapping are used for both endocardial and epicardial mapping.[7]

Mapping Catheters. The simplest form of mapping is achieved by moving the mapping catheter sequentially to sample various points of interest on the endocardium to measure local activation. The precision of locating the source of a particular electrical signal depends on the distance between the recording electrodes on the mapping catheter. For ablation procedures, recordings between adjacent electrode pairs are commonly used (e.g., between electrodes 1-2, 2-3, and 3-4), with 1 to 5 mm between electrodes (i.e., interelectrode spacing). In some studies, wider bipolar recordings (e.g., between electrodes 1-3 and 2-4) have been used to provide an overlapping field of view. For bipolar recordings, the signal of interest can be beneath the distal or proximal electrode (or both) of the recording pair. As noted, this is germane in that ablation energy can be delivered only from the distal (tip) electrode.

Mapping Focal Tachycardias

The goal of activation mapping of focal tachycardias (automatic, triggered activity, or microreentrant) is identifying the site of origin, defined as the site with the earliest presystolic bipolar recording in which the distal electrode shows the earliest intrinsic deflection and QS unipolar electrogram configuration (Figs. 3-8 and 3-9). Local activation at the site of origin precedes the onset of the tachycardia complex on the surface ECG by an average of 10-40 milliseconds. Earlier electrograms occurring in mid-diastole, as in the case of macroreentrant tachycardias, are not expected and do not constitute a target for mapping.[2]

Endocardial activation mapping of focal tachycardias can trace the origin of activation to a specific area, from where it spreads centrifugally. There is generally an electrically silent period in the tachycardia CL that on the surface ECG is reflected by an isoelectric line between tachycardia complexes. Intracardiac mapping will show significant portions of the tachycardia cycle length (CL) without recorded electrical activity, even when recording from the entire cardiac chamber of tachycardia origin. However, in the presence of complex intramyocardial conduction disturbances, activation during focal tachycardias can extend over a large proportion of the tachycardia CL, and conduction spread may follow circular patterns suggestive of macroreentrant activation.[1-3,7]

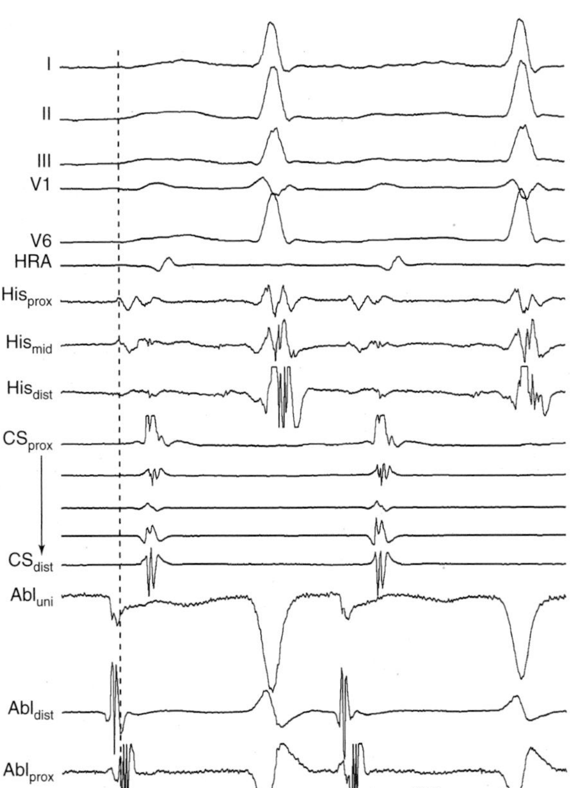

FIGURE 3-8 Focal atrial tachycardia. The unipolar electrogram recorded by the distal ablation electrode (Abl$_{uni}$) show a QS configuration and its timing coincides with the Abl$_{dist}$ recording at the site of successful ablation.

Technique of Activation Mapping of Focal Tachycardias. Initially, one should seek the general region of the origin of the tachycardia as indicated by the surface ECG. In the EP laboratory, additional data can be obtained by placing a limited number of catheters within the heart in addition to the mapping catheter(s); these catheters are frequently placed at the right ventricular apex, His bundle (HB) region, high RA, and CS. During initial arrhythmia evaluation, recording from this limited number of sites allows rough estimation of the site of interest. Mapping simultaneously from as many sites as possible greatly enhances the precision, detail, and speed of identifying regions of interest.[2]

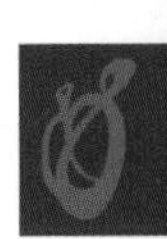

Subsequently, a single mapping catheter is moved under the guidance of fluoroscopy over the endocardium of the chamber of interest to sample bipolar signals. Using standard equipment, mapping a tachycardia requires recording and mapping performed at a number of sites based on the ability of the investigator to recognize the mapping sites of interest from the morphology of the tachycardia on the surface ECG and baseline intracardiac recordings.

Local activation time is then determined from the filtered (30 to 300 or more Hz) bipolar signal recorded from the distal electrode pair on the mapping catheter; this time is determined and compared with the timing reference (fiducial point). The distal pole of the mapping catheter should be used for mapping earliest activation site, because it is the pole through which RF energy is delivered. Activation times are generally measured from the onset of the first rapid deflection of the bipolar electrogram to the onset of the tachycardia complex on the surface ECG or surrogate marker (see Fig. 3-6). Using the onset of a local bipolar electrogram is preferable because it is easier to determine reproducibly when measuring heavily fractionated, low-amplitude local electrograms.[7]

Once an area of relatively early local activation is found, small movements of the catheter tip in the general target region are undertaken until the site is identified with the earliest possible local activation relative to the tachycardia complex. Recording from multiple bipolar pairs from a multipolar electrode catheter is helpful in that if the proximal pair has a more attractive electrogram than the distal, the

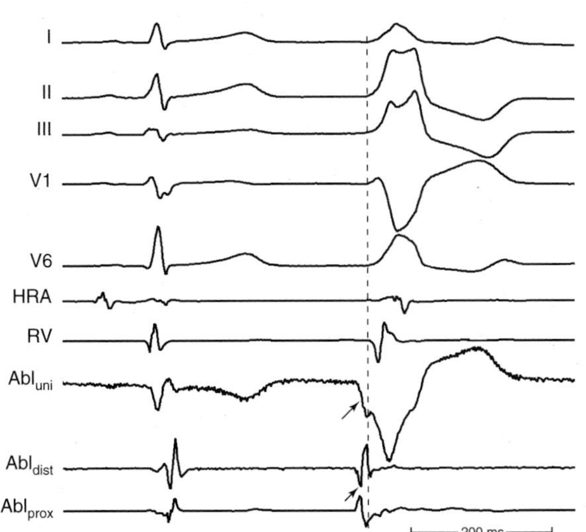

FIGURE 3-9 Sinus rhythm and a single premature ventricular complex from a patient with focal ventricular tachycardia. Abl$_{uni}$ show a QS configuration, the most rapid slope of which times with the initial peak in the Abl$_{dist}$ recording (*arrows*) at the site of successful ablation.

catheter may be withdrawn slightly to achieve the same position with the distal electrode.

Once the site with the earliest bipolar signal is identified, the unipolar signal from the distal ablation electrode should be used to supplement bipolar mapping.[1-3] The unfiltered (0.05 to 300 or more Hz) unipolar signal morphology should show a monophasic QS complex with a rapid negative deflection if the site was at the origin of impulse formation (see Figs. 3-8 and 3-9). However, the size of the area with a QS complex can be larger than the tachycardia focus, exceeding 1 cm in diameter. Thus, a QS complex should not be the only mapping finding used to guide ablation. Successful ablation is unusual, however, at sites with an RS complex on the unipolar recording, because these are generally distant from the focus (see Fig. 3-2). Concordance of the timing of the onset of the bipolar electrogram with that of the filtered or unfiltered unipolar electrogram (with the rapid downslope of the S wave of the unipolar QS complex coinciding with the initial peak of the bipolar signal) helps ensure that the tip electrode, which is the ablation electrode, is responsible for the early component of the bipolar electrogram. The presence of ST elevation on the unipolar recording and the ability to capture the site with unipolar pacing are used to indicate good electrode contact.[7]

Mapping Macroreentrant Tachycardias

The main goal of activation mapping of macroreentrant tachycardias (e.g., post-MI VT, macroreentrant AT) is identification of the isthmus critical for the macroreentrant circuit.[8-10] The "site of origin" of a tachycardia is the source of electrical activity producing the tachycardia complex. Although this is a discrete site of impulse formation in focal rhythms, during macroreentry it represents the exit site from the diastolic pathway (i.e., from the critical isthmus of the reentrant circuit) to the myocardium giving rise to the ECG deflection. During macroreentry, an isthmus is defined as a corridor of conductive myocardial tissue bounded by nonconductive tissue (barriers) through which the depolarization wavefront must propagate to perpetuate the tachycardia. These barriers can be scar areas or naturally occurring anatomical or functional (present only during tachycardia) obstacles. The earliest presystolic electrogram closest to mid-diastole is the most commonly used definition for the site of origin of the reentrant circuit; however, recording a continuous diastolic activity and/or bridging of diastole at adjacent sites or mapping a discrete diastolic pathway is more specific. Therefore, the goal of activation mapping during macroreentry is finding the site(s) with continuous activity spanning diastole or with an isolated mid-diastolic potential. Unlike focal tachycardias, a presystolic electrogram preceding the tachycardia complex by 10 to 40 milliseconds is not adequate in defining the site of origin of a macroreentrant tachycardia (Figs. 3-10 and 3-11; see also Fig. 3-7).[1-3,7]

However, identification of critical isthmuses is often challenging. The abnormal area of scarring, where the isthmus is located, is often large and contains false isthmuses (bystanders) that confound mapping. Additionally, multiple potential reentry circuits can be present, giving rise to multiple different tachycardias in a single patient. Furthermore, in abnormal regions such as infarct scars, the tissue beneath the recording electrode can be small relative to the surrounding myocardium outside the scar; thus, a large far-field signal can obscure the small local potential. For this reason, despite the limitations of bipolar recordings, they are preferred in scar-related VTs because the noise is removed and high-frequency components are more accurately seen. Unipolar recordings are usually of little help when mapping arrhythmias associated with regions of scar, unless they are filtered to remove far-field signal. Much

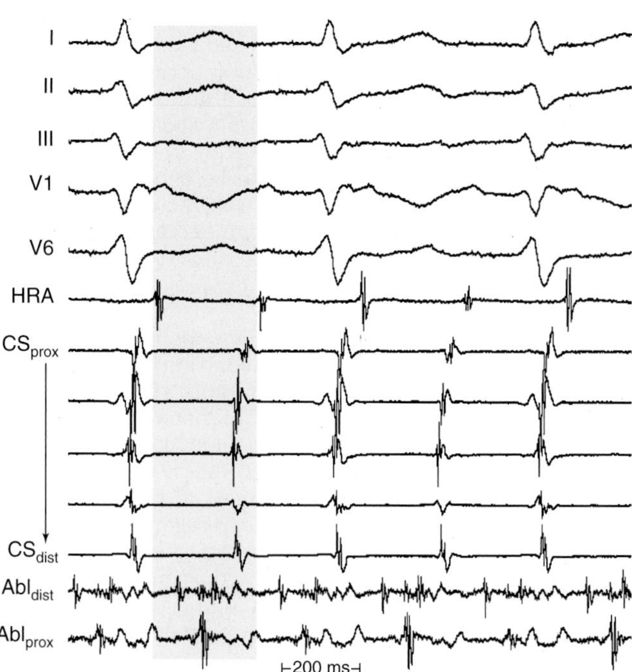

FIGURE 3–10 Macroreentrant atrial tachycardia. Electrical activity spans the tachycardia cycle length (*shaded*); thus, a merely presystolic electrogram is a poor indicator of optimal ablation site.

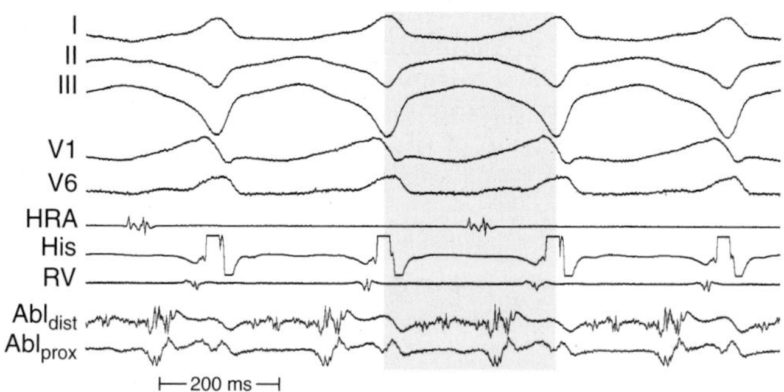

FIGURE 3–11 Macroreentrant post–myocardial infarction ventricular tachycardia. Electrical activity spans diastole and nearly the tachycardia cycle length (*shaded*); thus, a simply presystolic electrogram is a poor indicator of the optimal ablation site.

of the far-field signal in a unipolar recording is comprised of lower frequencies than the signal generated by local depolarization because the high-frequency content of a signal diminishes more rapidly with distance from the source than the low-frequency content. Therefore, high-pass filtering of unipolar signals (at 30 or 100 Hz) is generally used when mapping scar-related arrhythmias to reduce the far-field signal and improve detection of lower amplitude local signals from abnormal regions.[1-3]

Although activation mapping alone is usually inadequate for defining the critical isthmus of a macroreentrant tachycardia, it can help guide other mapping modalities (e.g., entrainment or pace mapping, or both) to the approximate region of the isthmus.[7,8,10]

Continuous Activity. Theoretically, if reentry were the mechanism of the tachycardia, electrical activity should occur throughout the tachycardia cycle. For example, in macroreentrant AT, the recorded electrical activity at different locations in the atrium should span the tachycardia CL (see Fig. 3-10).[9]

For macroreentrant VT, conduction during diastole is extremely slow and is in a small enough area so that it is not recorded on the surface ECG. The QRS complex is caused by propagation of the wavefront from the exit of the circuit from that isthmus to the surrounding myocardium. After leaving the exit of the isthmus, the circulating reentry wavefront can propagate through a broad path (loop) along the border of the scar, back to the entrance of the isthmus (see Fig. 3-7).[8,10] Continuous diastolic activity is likely to be recorded only if the bipolar pair records a small circuit; if a large circuit is recorded (i.e., the reentrant circuit is larger than the recording area of the catheter, the catheter is not covering the entire circuit, or both), nonholodiastolic activity will be recorded. In such circuits, repositioning of the catheter to other sites may allow visualization of what is termed *bridging of diastole*; electrical activity in these adjacent sites spans diastole.[1-3,7]

All areas from which diastolic activity is recorded are not necessarily part of the reentrant circuit. Such sites can reflect late activation and may not be related to the tachycardia site of origin. Analysis of the response of these electrograms to spontaneous or induced changes in tachycardia CL is critical in deciding their relationship to the tachycardia mechanism. Electrical signals that come and go throughout diastole should not be considered continuous (Fig. 3-12). For continuous activity to be consistent with reentry, it must be demonstrated that such electrical activity is required for initiation and maintenance of the tachycardia, so that termination of the continuous activity, either spontaneously or following stimulation, without affecting the tachycardia, would exclude such continuous activity as requisite for sustaining the tachycardia. Additionally, it is important to verify that an electrogram that extends throughout diastole is not just a broad electrogram whose duration equals the tachycardia CL. This can be achieved by analyzing the local electrogram during pacing at a CL comparable to tachycardia CL; if pacing produces a continuous diastolic activity in the absence of tachycardia, the continuous electrogram has no mechanistic significance. Furthermore, the continuous activity should be recorded from a circumscribed area, and motion artifact should be excluded.[7,10]

Mid-Diastolic Activity. An isolated mid-diastolic potential is defined as a low-amplitude, high-frequency diastolic potential separated from the preceding and subsequent electrograms by an isoelectric segment (Fig. 3-13). Sometimes, these discrete potentials provide information that defines a diastolic pathway, which is believed to be generated from a narrow isthmus of conduction critical to the reentrant circuit. Localization of this pathway is critical for guiding catheter-based ablation.[10]

Detailed mapping will usually reveal more than one site of presystolic activity, and mid-diastolic potentials can be recorded from a bystander site attached to the isthmus. Therefore, regardless of where in diastole the presystolic electrogram occurs (early, mid, or late), its position and appearance on initiation of the tachycardia, although necessary, does not confirm its relevance to the tachycardia mechanism. One must always confirm that the electrogram is required to maintain, and cannot be dissociated from, the tachycardia.[10] Thus, during spontaneous changes in the tachycardia CL or those produced by programmed stimulation, the electrogram, regardless of its position in diastole, should show a fixed relationship to the subsequent tachycardia complex (and not the preceding one). Very early diastolic potentials, in the first half of diastole, can represent an area of slow conduction at the entrance of a protected isthmus. These potentials will remain fixed to the prior tachycardia complex (exit site from the isthmus) and delay between it and the subsequent tachycardia complex would reflect delay entering or propagating through the protected diastolic pathway.[7]

If, after very detailed mapping, the earliest recorded site is not at least 50 milliseconds presystolic, this suggests that the map is inadequate (most common), the mechanism of tachycardia is not macroreentry, or the diastolic corridor is deeper than the subendocardium (in the midmyocardium or subepicardium).

Limitations

Standard transcatheter endocardial mapping, as performed in the EP laboratory, is limited by the number, size, and type of electrodes that can be placed within the heart. Therefore, these methods do not cover a vast area of the endocardial surface. Time-consuming, point by point maneuvering of the catheter is required to trace the origin of an arrhythmic event and its activation sequence in the neighboring areas.

The success of roving point mapping depends on the sequential beat by beat stability of the activation sequence being mapped and the ability of the patient to tolerate sustained arrhythmia. Therefore, it can be difficult to perform activation mapping in poorly inducible tachycardias, in hemodynamically unstable tachycardias, and in tachycardias with unstable morphology. Sometimes, poorly tolerated rapid tachycardias can be slowed by antiarrhythmic agents to allow for mapping. Alternatively, mapping can be facilitated by starting and stopping the tachycardia after data acquisition at each site. Additionally, newer techniques (e.g., basket catheter and noncontact mapping) can facilitate activation mapping in these cases by simultaneous multipoint mapping.

Although activation mapping is adequate for defining the site of origin of focal tachycardias, it is deficient by itself in defining the critical isthmus of macroreentrant tachycardias, and adjunctive mapping modalities (e.g., entrainment mapping, pace mapping) are required. Moreover, the labori-

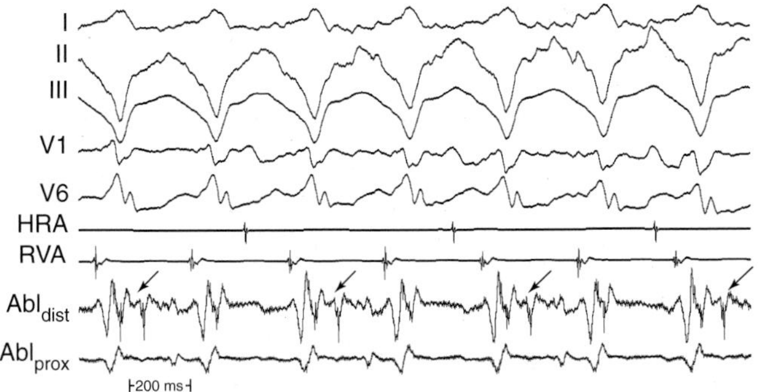

FIGURE 3–12 Diastolic recordings during ventricular tachycardia that have 2:1 conduction ratio (*arrows*). Cells causing these recordings are clearly not integrally involved in the ongoing arrhythmia. They are not atrial, because atrial ventricular dissociation is evident in the high right atrium recording.

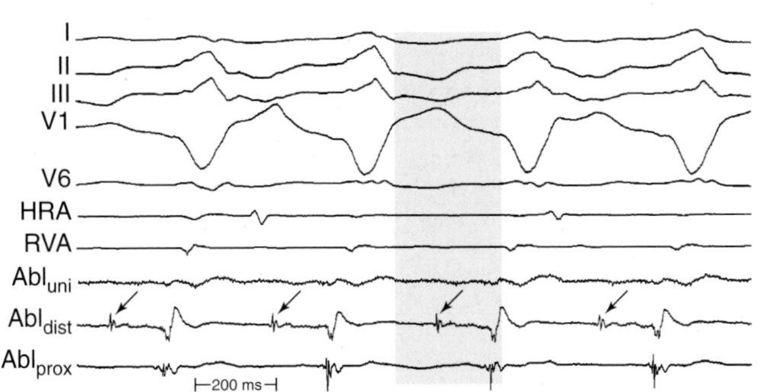

FIGURE 3–13 Mid-diastolic potential during ventricular tachycardia (VT)—duration of diastole (*shaded area*); isolated mid-diastolic potential from site at which ablation eliminated VT (*arrows*).

ous process of precise mapping with conventional techniques can expose the electrophysiologist, staff, and patient to undesirable levels of radiation from the extended fluoroscopy time.

Using conventional activation mapping techniques, it is difficult to conceive the 3-D orientation of cardiac structures because a limited number of recording electrodes guided by fluoroscopy is used. Although catheters using multiple electrodes to acquire data points are available, the exact location of an acquired unit of EP data is difficult to ascertain because of inaccurate delineation of the location of anatomical structures. The inability to associate the intracardiac electrogram with a specific endocardial site accurately also limits the reliability with which the roving catheter tip can be placed at a site that was previously mapped. This results in limitations when the creation of long linear lesions is required to modify the substrate, and when multiple isthmuses or channels are present. This inability to identify, for example, the site of a previous ablation increases the risk of repeated ablation of areas already dealt with and the likelihood that new sites can be missed.

ENTRAINMENT MAPPING

Fundamental Concepts

To help understand the concept of entrainment, a hypothetical reentrant circuit is shown in Figure 3-14. This reentrant circuit has several components—a common pathway, an exit site, an outer loop, an inner loop, an entry site, and bystander sites. The reentrant wavefront propagates through the common pathway (protected critical isthmus) during electrical diastole. Because this zone is usually composed of a small amount of myocardium and is bordered by anatomical or functional barriers preventing spread of the electrical signal except in the orthodromic direction, propagation of the wavefront in the protected isthmus is electrocardiographically silent. The exit site is the site at which the reentrant wavefront exits the protected isthmus to start activation of the rest of the myocardium, including the outer loop. Activation of the exit site corresponds to the onset of the tachycardia complex on the surface ECG. The outer loop is the path through which the reentrant wavefront propagates while at the same time activating the rest of the myocardium. Activation of the outer loop corresponds to electrical systole (P wave during AT and QRS during VT) on the surface ECG. An inner loop can serve as an integral part of the reentrant circuit or function as a bystander pathway. If conduction through the inner loop is slower than conduction from the exit to entrance sites (through the outer loop), the inner loop will serve as a bystander and the outer loop will be the dominant. If conduction through the inner loop is faster than conduction through the outer loop, it will form an integral component of the reentrant circuit. The entry site is where the reentrant wavefront enters the critical isthmus. Bystander sites are sites that are activated by the reentrant wavefront but are not an essential part of the reentrant circuit. These sites can be remote, adjacent, or attached to the circuit. Elimination of these sites does not terminate reentry.[7,10]

Understanding the concepts associated with resetting is critical to understanding entrainment. When a premature stimulus is delivered to sites remote from the reentrant circuit, it can interact with the circuit in different ways.[10] When the stimulus is late-coupled, it can reach the circuit after it has just been activated by the reentrant wavefront. Consequently, although the extrastimulus may have resulted in activation of part of the myocardium, it fails to affect the reentrant circuit, and the reentrant wavefront continues to propagate in the critical isthmus and through the exit site to result in the next tachycardia complex on time. To reset a reentrant tachycardia, the paced wavefront must reach the reentrant circuit (entry site, critical isthmus, or both), encounter excitable tissue within the circuit (i.e., enter the excitable gap of the reentrant circuit), collide in the antidromic (retrograde) direction with the previous tachycardia complex, and propagate in the orthodromic (anterograde) direction through the same tachycardia reentrant path (critical isthmus) to exit at an earlier than expected time and perpetuate the tachycardia (see Fig. 1-13). If the extrastimulus encounters a fully excitable tissue, which commonly occurs in reentrant tachycardias with large excitable gaps, the tachycardia is advanced by the extent that the paced wavefront arrives at the entrance site prematurely. If the tissue is partially excitable, which can occur in reentrant

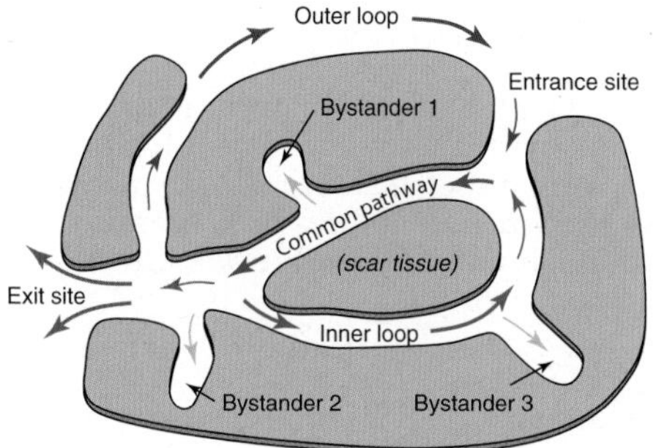

FIGURE 3–14 Representation of a ventricular tachycardia (VT) circuit, showing common diastolic pathway, entrance and exit sites, inner and outer loops, and bystander dead-end paths in three locations. The accompanying table describes the behavior of each of these locations during VT, as well as pacing during VT and sinus rhythm.

Site	Electrogram timing in VT	Entrainment with concealed fusion	Entrained stimulus-QRS	(S-QRS) VTCL	Post-pacing interval	Sinus rhythm pacemap	
						QRS vs VT	Stimulus-QRS
Common pathway	diastolic	present	≈Egm−QRS	<0.7	≈TCL	Same †	≈Egm−QRS †
Inner loop	systolic	present	<Egm−QRS	>0.7	≈TCL	Same †	≈Egm−QRS †
Outer loop	systolic	absent	<Egm−QRS	>0.7	≈TCL	Different	<Egm−QRS
Entrance site	early diastolic	present*	≈Egm−QRS	<0.7	≈TCL	Different	<Egm−QRS
Exit site	late diastolic	present	>Egm−QRS	>0.7	>TCL	Same	≈Egm−QRS
Bystander 1	mid-diastolic*	present	>Egm−QRS	>0.7	>TCL	Same	>Egm−QRS
Bystander 2	late diastolic*	present	>Egm−QRS	>0.7	>TCL	Same	>Egm−QRS
Bystander 3	early diastolic*	present*	>Egm−QRS	>0.7	>TCL	Same †	>Egm−QRS

* variable † depends on whether captured orthodromically or antidromically

tachycardias with small or partially excitable gaps, or even in circuits with large excitable gaps when the extrastimulus is very premature, the stimulated wavefront will encounter some conduction delay in the orthodromic direction within the circuit. Consequently, the degree of advancement of the next tachycardia complex will depend on both the degree of prematurity of the extrastimulus and the degree of slowing of its conduction within the circuit. Therefore, the reset tachycardia complex may be early, on time, or later than expected.[7,10]

Termination of the tachycardia occurs when the extrastimulus collides with the preceding tachycardia impulse antidromically and blocks in the reentrant circuit orthodromically. This occurs when the premature impulse enters the reentrant circuit early enough in the relative refractory period, as it fails to propagate in the anterograde direction because it encounters absolutely refractory tissue (see Fig 1-13). In the retrograde direction, it encounters increasingly recovered tissue and is able to propagate until it meets the circulating wavefront and terminates the arrhythmia.[7,10]

Entrainment is the continuous resetting of a reentrant circuit by a train of capturing stimuli. However, following the first stimulus of the pacing train that penetrates and resets the reentrant circuit, the subsequent stimuli interact with the reset circuit, which has an abbreviated excitable gap. The first entrained complex results in retrograde collision between the stimulated and tachycardia impulse, whereas in all subsequent beats, the collision occurs between the presently stimulated wavefront and that stimulated previously. Depending on the degree that the excitable gap is preexcited by that first resetting stimulus, subsequent stimuli fall on fully or partially excitable tissue. Entrainment is said to be present when two consecutive extrastimuli conduct orthodromically through the circuit with the same conduction time, while colliding antidromically with the preceding paced wavefront.[7,10]

During entrainment, each pacing impulse creates two activation wavefronts, one in the orthodromic and the other in the antidromic direction. The wavefront in the antidromic direction collides with the existing tachycardia wavefront. The wavefront that enters the reentrant circuit in the orthodromic direction (i.e., the same direction as the spontaneous tachycardia wavefront), conducts through the critical isthmus, resets the tachycardia, and emerges through the exit site to activate the myocardium and collide with the antidromically paced wavefront from the next paced stimulus. This sequence continues until cessation of pacing or development of block somewhere within the reentrant circuit. Because all pacing impulses enter the tachycardia circuit during the excitable gap, each paced wavefront advances and resets the tachycardia. Thus, when pacing is terminated, the last paced impulse will continue to activate the entire tachycardia reentrant circuit orthodromically at the pacing CL, and also will activate the entire myocardium orthodromically on exiting the reentrant circuit.

Entrainment of reentrant tachycardias by external stimuli was originally defined in the clinical setting as an increase in the rate of a tachycardia to a faster pacing rate, with resumption of the intrinsic rate of the tachycardia on either abrupt cessation of pacing or slowing of pacing beyond the intrinsic rate of the tachycardia, and taken to indicate an underlying reentrant mechanism. The ability to entrain a tachycardia also establishes that the reentrant circuit contains an excitable gap.[7,10]

Entrainment does not require that the pacing site be located in the reentrant circuit. The closer the pacing site to the circuit, however, the less premature a single stimulus needs to be to reach the circuit and, with pacing trains, the fewer the number of stimuli required before a stimulated wavefront reaches the reentrant circuit without being extinguished by collision with a wave emerging from the circuit. Overdrive pacing at relatively long CLs (i.e., 10 to 30 milliseconds shorter than the tachycardia CL) can almost always entrain reentrant tachycardias. However, the number of pacing stimuli required to entrain the reentrant circuit depends on the tachycardia CL, duration of the excitable gap of the tachycardia, refractoriness at the pacing site, and conduction time from the stimulation site to the reentrant circuit.[7,10]

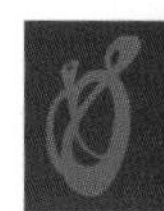

During constant-rate pacing, entrainment of a reentrant tachycardia will result in the activation of all myocardial tissue responsible for maintaining the tachycardia at the pacing CL, with the resumption of the intrinsic tachycardia morphology and rate after cessation of pacing. Unfortunately, it is almost impossible to document the acceleration of all tissue responsible for maintaining the reentrant circuit to the pacing CL. Therefore, a number of surface ECG and intracardiac electrogram criteria have been proposed for establishing the presence of entrainment (Fig. 3-15): (1) fixed fusion of the paced complexes at a constant pacing rate; (2) progressive fusion or different degrees of fusion at different pacing rates (i.e., the surface ECG and intracardiac morphology progressively look more like the purely paced configuration and less like the pure tachycardia beat in the course of pacing at progressively shorter pacing CLs; Fig. 3-16); and (3) resumption of the same tachycardia morphology following cessation of pacing with the first post-pacing complex displaying no fusion but occurring at a return cycle equal to the pacing CL.[7,10]

Fusion During Entrainment

A stimulated impulse is said to be fused when its morphology is a hybrid between that of a fully paced complex and a tachycardia complex. Fusion can be observed on the surface ECG, intracardiac recordings, or both.[10] For fusion to be observed on the surface ECG, the tachycardia and stimulated wavefronts must collide within the reentrant circuit after the tachycardia wavefront has exited from the circuit. This requires the paced wavefront to have access to an entrance site of the reentrant circuit that is anatomically distinct from the exit site. If the antidromically stimulated wavefront penetrates into the reentrant circuit and collides with the tachycardia wavefront (or previously stimulated orthodromic wavefront) before the point at which the tachycardia wavefront would be exiting to the mass of the myocardium, then no fusion will be evident on the surface ECG and the surface ECG will appear entirely paced.[7,10]

The ability to demonstrate surface ECG fusion requires a significant mass of myocardium be depolarized by the extrastimulus and the tachycardia. The degree of fusion represents the relative amounts of myocardium depolarized by the two separate wavefronts.[10] The relative degree of myocardium antidromically activated by the paced wavefront depends on the site of pacing relative to the reentrant circuit, pacing CL, and degree of conduction delay within the reentrant circuit. With a single extrastimulus, the farther the stimulation site from the reentrant circuit, the less likely ECG fusion will occur, because the extrastimulus must be delivered at a shorter coupling interval, well before the tachycardia wavefront exits the circuit, so as to reach the circuit with adequate prematurity. Therefore, by the time the tachycardia wavefront exits the circuit, most of the myocardium has already been activated by the paced wavefront, and consequently the stimulated impulse will have a purely paced morphology with no ECG fusion. Nevertheless, continuous pacing at a slow CL at a site remote from the exit site affords the best opportunity to demonstrate fusion, whereas pacing closer to the presumed exit site will show less fusion. Presystolic electrograms in the reentrant circuit that are activated orthodromically can be used to demonstrate the presence of intracardiac (local) fusion when the

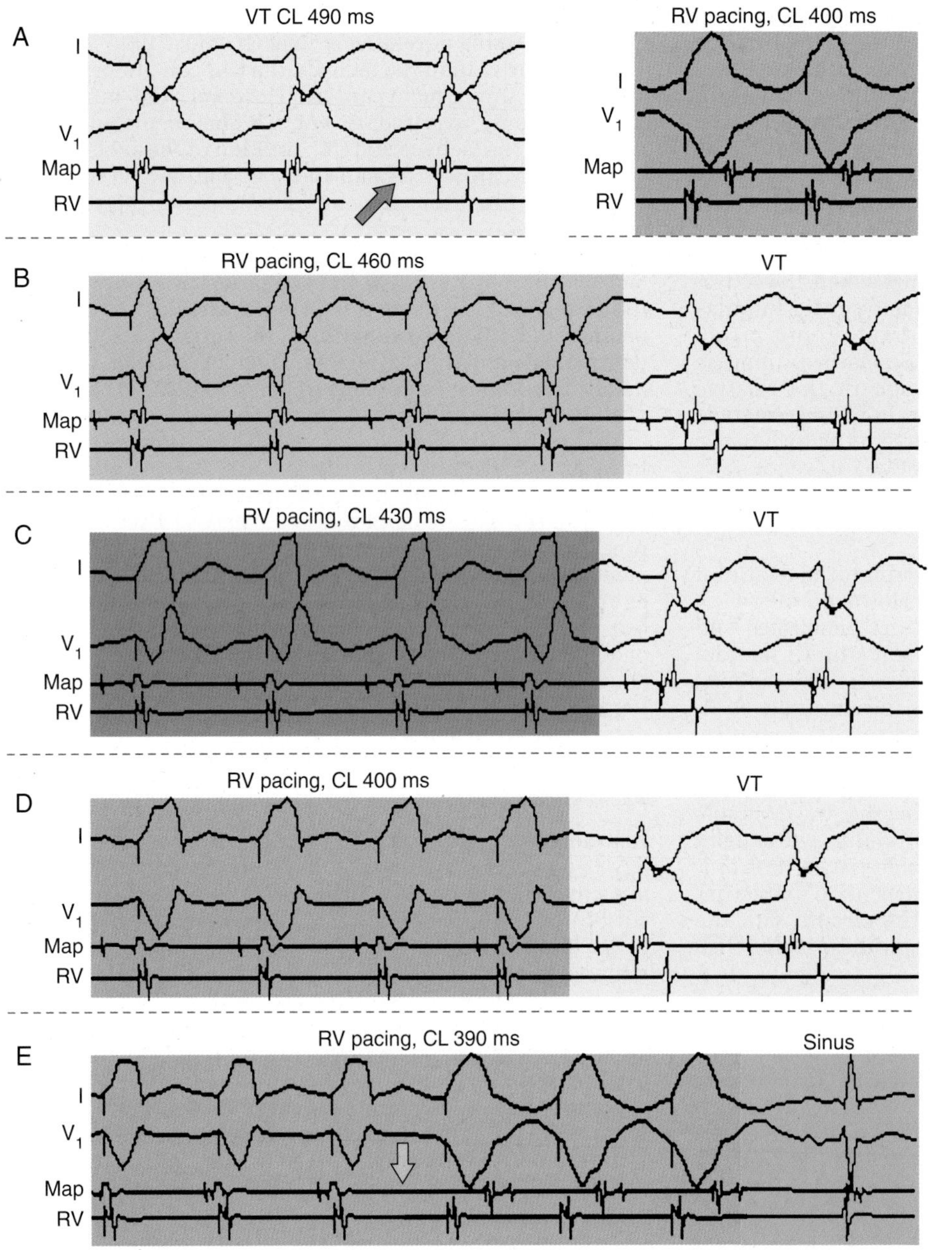

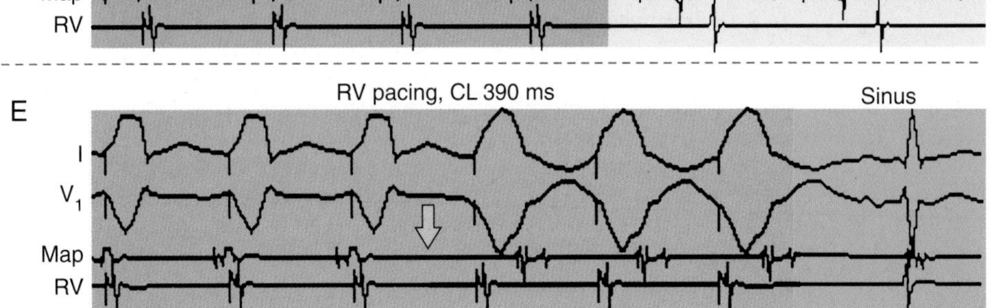

FIGURE 3–15 Entrainment of ventricular tachycardia (VT). **A,** Pure VT is shown in yellow (right bundle branch block, right axis), pure right ventricle (RV) pacing in red (left bundle branch block, left axis). A mid-diastolic potential during VT (*arrow*) is recorded by the mapping catheter. **B,** Pacing the RV at 460 milliseconds (30 milliseconds faster than VT), each paced complex is a stable blend of pacing and VT (orange). This illustrates fixed fusion. After cessation of pacing, VT resumes. **C,** Pacing the RV faster (430 milliseconds), all complexes are again identical to each other but different than with pacing at 460 milliseconds; they look slightly more like pure RV pacing (deeper orange shading). **D,** Pacing the RV faster still (400 milliseconds), QRS complexes again are identical to each other (fixed fusion) but look progressively more like fully paced (progressive fusion). **E,** Finally, with pacing rapidly enough, an antidromic wavefront captures the diastolic potential, QRS complexes become fully paced and, when pacing ceases, sinus rhythm resumes. This figure demonstrates all established entrainment criteria (fixed fusion at a given paced cycle length (CL), progressive fusion over a range of paced CLs, and antidromic capture of critical circuit elements leading to termination of the tachycardia).

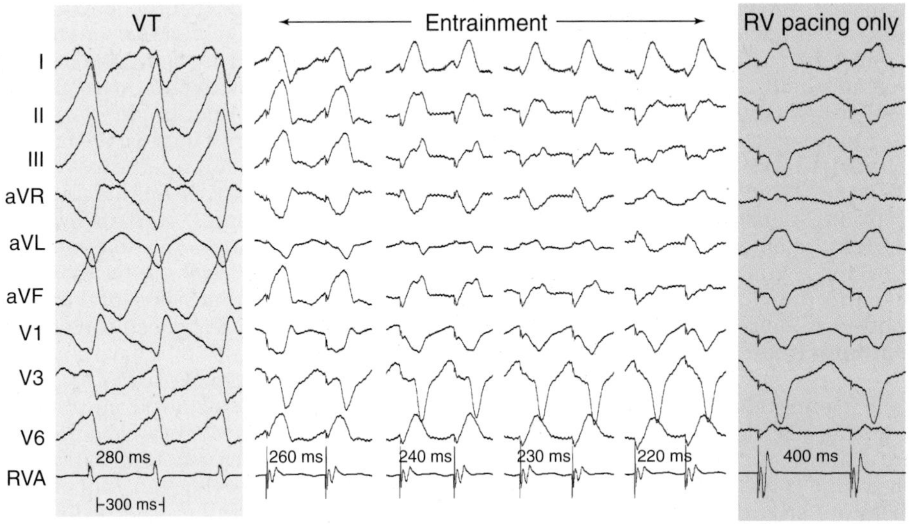

FIGURE 3–16 QRS fusion during entrainment of ventricular tachycardia VT. Progressive ECG fusion is shown over a range of paced CLs. Pure tachycardia complexes are shown at right; fully paced complexes are shown at right. As the paced CL shortens, complexes gradually appear more like fully paced.

ECG is insufficiently sensitive. This is particularly helpful with ATs because the P waves are small and often obscured by QRS complex, ST segments, and T waves.[7]

Once stability in collision sites of the antidromic and orthodromic wavefronts occurs, constant surface ECG fusion will be achieved. Fixed fusion in the surface ECG is said to be present during entrainment if the following criterion is met: (1) the surface ECG complex is of constant morphology, representing a hybrid of the complex morphology of the tachycardia and that observed during pacing during normal sinus rhythm (NSR; see Figs. 3-15 and 3-16), or (2) the onset of the surface ECG complex precedes the stimulus artifact of each paced beat by a fixed interval (see Figs. 9-5 and 10-6). It is worth noting that to be certain that a hybrid or blended ECG complex is present, one must know the configurations of both pure tachycardia and pure pacing (Fig. 3-17; see also Figs. 3-15 and 3-16).

Focal tachycardias (automatic, triggered activity, or microreentrant) cannot manifest fixed fusion during overdrive pacing. However, overdrive pacing of a tachycardia of any mechanism can result in a certain degree of fusion, especially when the pacing CL is only slightly shorter than the tachycardia CL. Such fusion, however, is unstable during the same pacing drive at a constant CL, because pacing stimuli fall on a progressively earlier portion of the tachycardia cycle, producing progressively less fusion and more fully paced morphology. Such phenomena should be distinguished from entrainment, and sometimes this requires pacing for long intervals to demonstrate variable degrees of fusion. Moreover, overdrive pacing frequently results in suppression (automatic) or acceleration (triggered activity) of focal tachycardias rather than resumption of the original tachycardia with an unchanged tachycardia CL.[7]

Varying degrees of fusion at different pacing rates is caused by a progressive increase in the amount of myocardium activated by the antidromic wavefront at progressively shorter pacing CLs (see Figs. 3-15 and 3-16).[10] At slower pacing CLs, a larger amount of the myocardium is activated by the orthodromic wavefront exiting from the reentrant circuit prior to its intracardiac collision, with the subsequent antidromic wavefront traveling outward from the pacing site. With a faster pacing rate, more myocardium will be antidromically activated because the orthodromic wavefront must continue to traverse the zone of slow conduction within the reentrant circuit, thus creating progressive fusion with changing pacing CLs. In the extreme situation, the antidromic wavefront can capture the exit site of the reentrant circuit, producing a fully paced complex. Once this occurs, pacing at shorter pacing CLs will not cause further progressive fusion, although entrainment is still

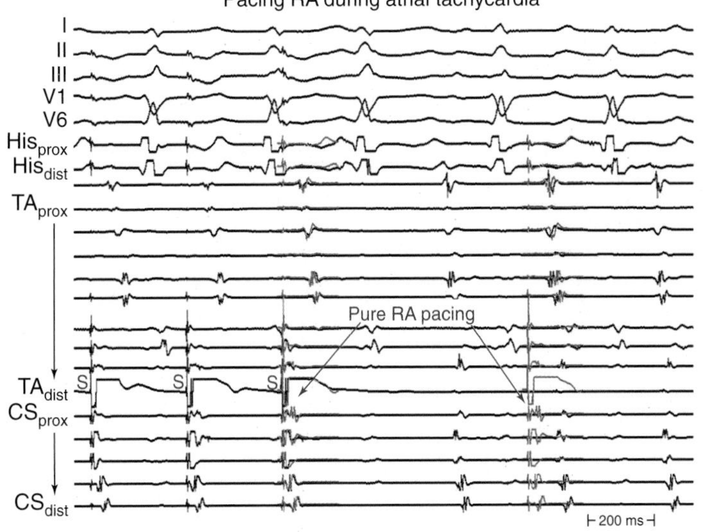

FIGURE 3–17 Overdrive pacing during focal atrial tachycardia (AT). **Top,** The last three complexes of pacing (S) from the high right atrium (RA) are shown, following which AT resumes. Red overlay is recordings of pure high RA pacing that perfectly match the electrogram sequence of high RA pacing during AT; thus, fusion is absent. **Bottom,** Similar findings with pacing from distal coronary sinus (CS). Red overlay of pure CS pacing perfectly matches the electrogram sequence of CS pacing during AT; thus, there is no fusion.

present. Progressive fusion at decreasing pacing CLs during entrainment of tachycardia excludes the possibility of automaticity or triggered activity as the mechanism of the tachycardia. In those cases, overdrive pacing would yield solely the morphology of the pacing stimulus for a nonprotected focus or would yield varying (not progressive) degrees of fusion for a protected focus with entrance block. Of note, a microreentrant circuit with entrance block could also yield variable fusion during overdrive pacing; thus, this latter finding would not exclude reentry as the underlying mechanism.[7,10]

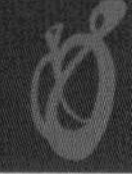

On cessation of pacing, the last paced wavefront traverses the protected isthmus and exits the circuit to produce a normal (nonfused) tachycardia complex at the pacing CL, because there is no paced antidromic wavefront with which to fuse. The wavefront continues around the reentrant circuit to maintain the tachycardia. Constant fusion of the surface ECG can occur, however, without the first nonpaced beat occurring at the pacing CL. When surface ECG fusion occurs, the initial portion of the ECG complex usually reflects activation of the myocardium by the paced wavefront, whereas the terminal portion represents the orthodromically activated wavefront exiting from the tachycardia circuit. The point at which this wavefront exits the circuit can be late in the surface ECG complex. The degree to which the first ECG post-pacing interval (PPI) exceeds the pacing CL is primarily a reflection of the time from the onset of the paced surface ECG complex to the exit of the orthodromic wavefront from the reentrant circuit. This represents the period of time during which the myocardium is depolarized by the stimulated wavefront before the activation of any portion of the myocardium by the tachycardia wavefront. Thus, constant fusion occurring in the absence of the first ECG PPI being equal to the pacing CL can be a valid manifestation of entrainment. In this situation, appropriate placement of intracardiac electrodes will demonstrate orthodromic entrainment of some intracardiac recording sites occurring at the pacing CL, despite the last entrained ECG complex occurring at an interval longer than the pacing CL. Alternatively, decremental conduction within the reentrant circuit can explain a first PPI that exceeds the pacing CL.[7]

Entrainment with antidromic capture is also associated with a return cycle longer than the pacing CL. When pacing is performed at a CL significantly shorter than the tachycardia CL, the paced impulse can penetrate the circuit antidromically and retrogradely capture the presystolic electrogram so that no exit from the tachycardia circuit is possible. When pacing is stopped, the impulse that conducts antidromically also conducts orthodromically to reset the reentrant circuit with orthodromic activation of the presystolic electrogram. When antidromic (retrograde) capture of the local presystolic electrogram occurs, the return cycle, even when measured at the site of the presystolic electrogram, will exceed the pacing CL by the difference in time from when the electrogram is activated retrogradely (i.e., preexcited antidromically) and when it would have been activated orthodromically.[7,10]

Entrainment with Manifest Fusion. Entrainment with manifest fusion demonstrates surface ECG evidence of constant fusion at a constant pacing rate and progressive fusion with incremental-rate pacing (see Fig. 3-16).[10] When entrainment is manifest, the last captured wave is entrained at the pacing CL but does not demonstrate fusion.

Entrainment with Inapparent, Local, or Intracardiac Fusion. Entrainment with inapparent fusion (also referred to as local or intracardiac fusion) is said to be present when a fully paced morphology with no ECG fusion results, even when the tachycardia impulse exits the reentrant circuit (orthodromic activation of the presystolic electrogram present). Fusion is limited to a small area and does not produce surface ECG fusion, and only intracardiac (local) fusion is recognized (Fig. 3-18; see also Fig. 10-6).[10] Local fusion can only occur when the presystolic electrogram is activated orthodromically. Collision with the last paced impulse must occur distally to the presystolic electrogram, either at the exit from the circuit or outside the circuit. In such cases, the return cycle measured at this local electrogram will equal the pacing CL. Therefore, a stimulus delivered after the onset of the tachycardia complex on the surface ECG during entrainment will always demonstrate local fusion. This is to be distinguished from entrainment with antidromic capture. As noted, when antidromic (retrograde) capture of the local presystolic electrogram occurs, the return cycle, even when measured at the site of the presystolic electrogram, will exceed the pacing CL.[10]

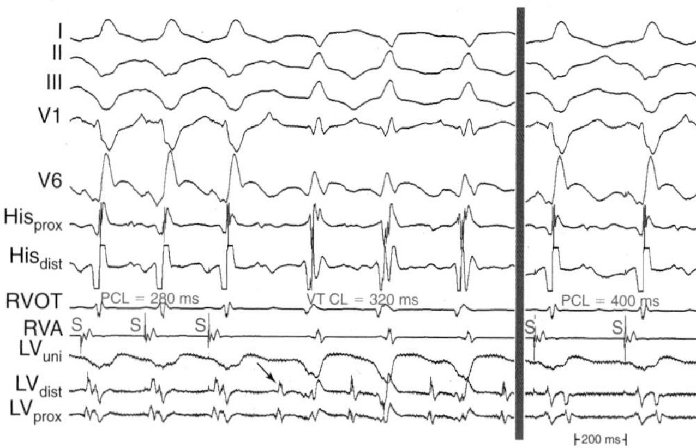

FIGURE 3–18 Inapparent fusion. The last three complexes paced from the right ventricular apex during ventricular tachycardia (VT) are shown; VT resumes on cessation of pacing. Fusion is not evident on the surface electrocardiogram because these complexes are identical to fully paced QRS complexes at the far right, yet fusion is present on the Abl_{dist} recording (mid-diastolic potential at arrow seen during pacing as well). CL = cycle length; PCL = pacing cycle length.

Entrainment with Concealed Fusion. Entrainment with concealed fusion (also called concealed entrainment or exact entrainment) is defined as entrainment with orthodromic capture and a surface ECG complex identical to that of the tachycardia (see Figs. 9-5 and 10-6).[10] Entrainment with concealed fusion suggests that the pacing site is within a protected isthmus inside or outside but attached to the reentrant circuit (i.e., the pacing site can be in, attached to, or at the entrance to a protected isthmus that forms the diastolic pathway of the circuit; see Fig. 3-14). In this case, the stimulated and tachycardia wavefronts collide in or near the reentry circuit—hence, no evidence of fusion. Entrainment with concealed fusion may occur by pacing from bystander pathways, such as a blind alley, alternate pathway, or inner loop, that are not critical to the maintenance of reentry. In this case, activation proceeds from the main circuit loop but is constrained by block lines having the shape of a cul-de-sac; ablation there does not terminate reentry.[7,10]

Post-Pacing Interval

The PPI is the time interval from the last pacing stimulus that entrained the tachycardia to the next nonpaced recorded electrogram at the pacing site (Fig. 3-19). During entrainment from sites within the reentrant circuit, the orthodromic wavefront from the last stimulus propagates through the reentry circuit and returns to the pacing site, following the same path as the circulating reentry wavefronts. The conduction time required is the revolution time through the circuit. Thus, the PPI (measured from the pacing site recording) should be equal (within 30 milliseconds) to the tachy-

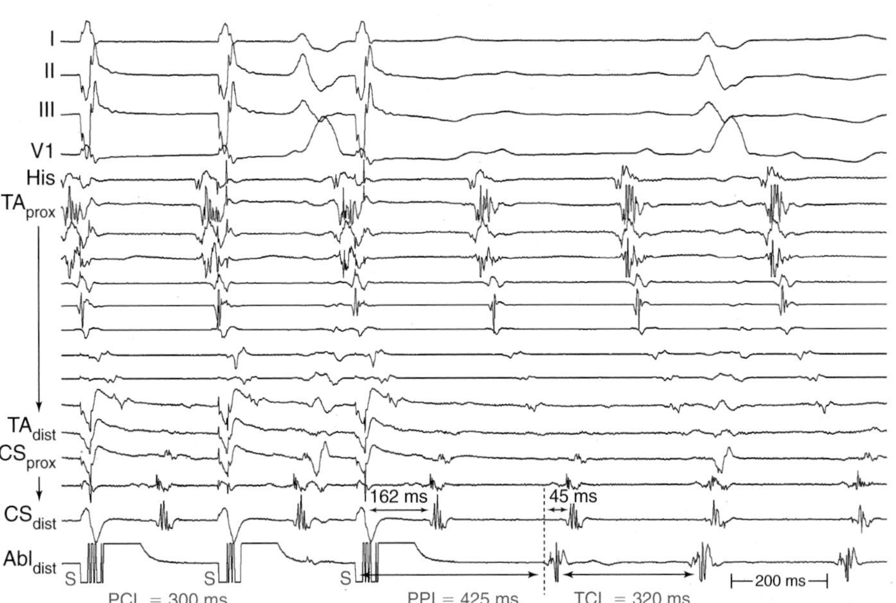

FIGURE 3–19 Bystander site during atypical left atrial (LA) flutter. The last three complexes of pacing from the posterior LA are shown in a patient with LA macroreentry. Although the timing of the electrogram at the pacing site is in early mid-diastole and the paced activation sequence is similar to tachycardia, thereby giving the appearance of an attractive ablation site, the results of entrainment indicate otherwise, with a large difference between the stimulus-CS electrogram interval (162 milliseconds) and ablation recording–CS electrogram interval (45 milliseconds), as well as a large difference between the post-pacing interval (PPI) (425 milliseconds) and tachycardia cycle length (TCL, 320 milliseconds). PCL = pacing CL.

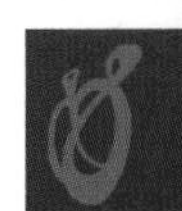

cardia CL (if the conduction velocities and the reentrant path did not change during pacing; see Fig. 3-14).[11] At sites remote from the circuit, stimulated wavefronts propagate to the circuit, then through the circuit, and finally back to the pacing site. Thus, the PPI should equal the tachycardia CL plus the time required for the stimulus to propagate from the pacing site to the tachycardia circuit and back. The greater the difference between the PPI and the tachycardia CL, the longer the conduction time between the pacing site and reentry circuit (see Figs. 9-5 and 10-6).

Several factors have to be considered when evaluating the PPI. The PPI should be measured to the near-field potential that indicates depolarization of tissue at the pacing site. In regions of scar, electrode catheters often record multiple potentials separated in time, some of which are far-field potentials that result from depolarization of adjacent myocardium. This potential is obscured by capture during pacing, whereas far-field potentials can be undisturbed during pacing.[11] Furthermore, when pacing artifacts obscure recordings from the pacing site, preventing assessment of the PPI, the electrograms from the proximal electrodes of the mapping catheter can be used, provided such electrograms are also present in the distal electrode recordings. When the electrograms from the pacing site are not discernible because of stimulus artifact, relating the timing of the near-field potential to a consistent intracardiac electrogram or surface ECG wave can be used to determine the PPI.[7]

Conduction Time from the Pacing Site to the Circuit Exit Site

During entrainment of reentrant tachycardia, the interval between the pacing stimulus and the onset of the tachycardia complex on the surface ECG (QRS or P wave) reflects conduction time from the pacing site to the exit of the reentrant circuit (stimulus-exit interval), regardless of whether the pacing site is inside or outside the reentrant circuit, because activation starts at the pacing site and propagates in sequence to the circuit exit site. On the other hand, during tachycardia, the interval between the local electrogram at a given site and circuit exit (electrogram-exit interval) may reflect the true conduction time between those two sites if they are activated in sequence (which occurs when that particular site is located within the reentrant pathway), or may be shorter than the true conduction time if those two sites are activated in parallel (which occurs when that particular site is located outside the reentrant circuit) (see Figures 3.14, 3.19).[7,10]

Therefore, at any given pacing site, electrogram-exit interval that is equal (±20 milliseconds) to the stimulus-exit interval indicates that the pacing site lies within the reentry circuit and excludes the possibility that the site is a dead-end pathway attached to the circuit (i.e., not a bystander). On the other hand, pacing sites outside the reentrant circuit will have an electrogram-exit interval significantly (more than 20 milliseconds) shorter than the stimulus-exit interval. However, the electrogram-exit interval may not be exactly equal to the stimulus-exit interval at sites within the reentrant circuit. Several factors can explain this. One potential factor is decremental conduction properties of the zone of slow conduction, producing lengthening of the stimulus-exit interval during pacing; however, this appears to occur rarely. Therefore, the stimulus-exit interval should be measured during pacing at the slower CL that reliably entrains the tachycardia. Moreover, stimulus latency in an area of diseased tissue can account for a delay in the stimulus-exit interval compared with the electrogram-QRS interval. Additionally, failure of the recording electrodes to detect low-amplitude depolarizations at the pacing site can account for a mismatch of the stimulus-exit and electrogram-exit intervals.[7,10]

Mapping Procedure

Before attempting to use entrainment methods for mapping, it is necessary to show that the tachycardia can be entrained, providing strong evidence that it is caused by reentry rather than by triggered activity or automaticity. Potential ablation sites are sought by pacing at sites thought to be related to the reentrant circuit, based on other mapping modalities, such as activation mapping and pace mapping. The areas of slow conduction can be identified by endocardial mapping revealing fractionated electrograms, mid-diastolic electrograms, or long delays between the pacing stimulus and the captured surface ECG complex (see Fig. 3-14). These sites are then targeted by entrainment mapping. However, proof of entrainment is best obtained by pacing from sites remote from the circuit, which will most readily demonstrate fusion.[7]

Entrainment mapping can be reliably carried out only if one can record and stimulate from the same area (e.g., for 2-5-2 mm spacing catheters, record from the second and fourth poles and stimulate from the first and third poles). Pacing is usually started at a CL just shorter (10 to 20 milliseconds) than the tachycardia CL. Pacing should be continued for a long enough duration to allow for entrainment. Short pacing trains are usually not helpful. Pacing is then repeated at progressively shorter pacing CLs.[10]

After cessation of each pacing drive, the presence of entrainment should be verified by demonstrating the presence of fixed fusion of the paced complexes at a given pacing CL, progressive fusion at faster pacing CLs, and resumption of the same tachycardia morphology following cessation of pacing with a nonfused complex at a return cycle equal to the pacing CL. The mere acceleration of the tachycardia to the pacing rate and then resumption of the original tachycardia after cessation of pacing does not establish the presence of entrainment. Evaluation of the PPI or other criteria are meaningless when the presence of true entrainment has not been established. Moreover, it is important to verify the absence of termination and reinitiation of the tachycardia during the same pacing drive.[7]

Once the presence of entrainment is verified, several criteria can be used to indicate the relation of the pacing site to the reentrant circuit. The first entrainment criterion to be sought is concealed fusion. Entrainment with concealed fusion indicates that the pacing site is in a protected isthmus located within or attached to the reentrant circuit. Whether this protected isthmus is crucial to the reentrant circuit or just a bystander site needs to be verified by other criteria, mainly comparing the PPI with the tachycardia CL and the stimulus-exit interval with the electrogram-exit interval. Features of entrainment when pacing from different sites are listed in Table 3-1 (see also Figs. 3-14, 3-18, and 3-19).

Clinical Implications

Entrainment mapping is the gold standard for ablation of reentrant circuits generating hemodynamically well-tolerated tachycardias. Achievement of entrainment of tachycardia establishes a reentrant mechanism of that tachycardia, and excludes triggered activity and abnormal automaticity as potential mechanisms. Entrainment may also be used to estimate how far the reentrant circuit is from the pacing site qualitatively. For example, entrainment of an AT from multiple sites in the RA with a PPI significantly longer than the tachycardia CL can help identify a left atrial origin of the AT before attempting LA access (see Fig. 10-6). In addition, pacing at multiple sites and measuring the difference between the PPI and tachycardia CL provides an indication as to how far or near the pacing site is from the circuit (Fig. 3-20).[7,10]

Entrainment mapping has been useful to identify the critical isthmus in patients with macroreentrant VT or AT. Focal ablation of all sites defined as in the reentrant circuit may not result in a cure of reentrant tachycardia. Cure requires ablation of an isthmus bordered by barriers on either side, which is critical to the reentrant circuit. Entrainment mapping helps identify this critical part of the reentrant circuit, which serves as the target of ablation.[11-13] Sites demonstrating entrainment with concealed fusion are initially sought. Once these sites are identified, their relationship to the reentrant circuit is verified using the PPI or stimulus-exit interval (see earlier). Sites demonstrating concealed fusion, PPI equal to the tachycardia CL (±30 milliseconds), and stimulus-exit interval equal to the electrogram-exit interval (±20 milliseconds) have a very high positive predictive value for successful ablation.[7]

TABLE 3–1 Entrainment Mapping of Reentrant Tachycardias

Pacing from Sites *Outside* the Reentrant Circuit · Manifest fusion on surface ECG and/or intracardiac recordings · PPI-tachycardia CL > 0 msec · Stimulus-exit interval > electrogram-exit interval
Pacing from Sites *Inside* the Reentrant Circuit · Manifest fusion on surface ECG and/or intracardiac recordings · PPI-tachycardia CL < 30 msec · Stimulus-exit interval = electrogram-exit interval (±20 msec)
Pacing from a Protected Isthmus Inside the Reentrant Circuit · Concealed fusion · PPI-tachycardia CL < 30 msec · Stimulus-exit interval = electrogram-exit interval (±20 msec)

CL = cycle length; ECG = electrocardiogram; PPI = post-pacing interval.

Limitations

Entrainment mapping requires the presence of sustained, hemodynamically well-tolerated tachycardia of stable morphology and CL. Overdrive pacing can result in termination, acceleration, or transformation of the index tachycardia into a different one, making further mapping challenging. Bipolar pacing at relatively high stimulus strengths used during entrainment can result in capture of an area larger than the local area. Additional errors can be introduced by the decremental conduction properties of the zone of slow conduction that might cause a rate-dependent lengthening of the PPI. This is more likely to occur at rapid pacing rates.[7,10]

Pacing and recording from the same area are required for entrainment mapping. This is usually satisfied by pacing from electrodes 1 and 3 and recording from electrodes 2 and 4 of the mapping catheter. However, this technique has several limitations:

1. There are differences, albeit slight, of the area from which the second and fourth electrodes record as compared with the first and third. When the local electrogram is not recorded from the same pair of electrodes used for pacing, errors can be introduced when comparing the PPI with the tachycardia CL.
2. The bipolar pacing technique has the potential of anodal contribution to local capture.
3. The total area affected by the pacing stimulus can exceed the local area, especially when high currents (more than 10 mA) are required for stimulation.
4. The pacing artifact can obscure the early part of the captured local electrogram. In such a case, a comparable

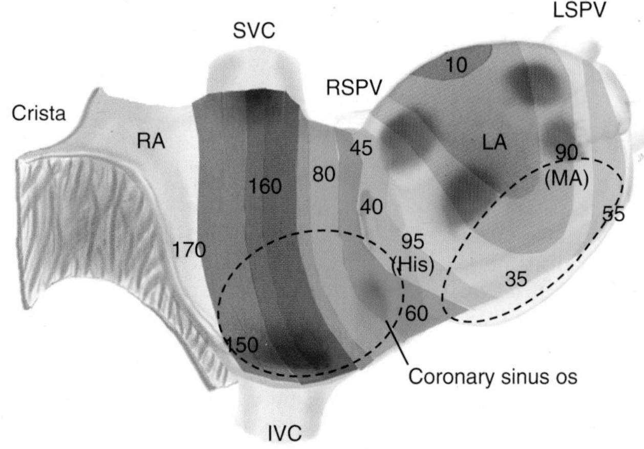

FIGURE 3–20 The post-pacing interval (PPI)–tachycardia cycle length (TCL) interval as indicator of distance from pacing site to circuit (in dome of the left atrium [LA], near 10). In this representation of both atria viewed from the front, colors indicate isochrones of the difference between PPI and TCL in milliseconds at various pacing sites (indicated by numbers). IVC = inferior vena cava; LSPV = left superior pulmonary vein; MA = mitral annulus; Os = ostium; RA = right atrium; RSPV = right superior pulmonary vein; SVC = superior vena cava.

component of the electrogram can be used to measure the PPI.

5. Far-field electrical signals generated by depolarization of adjacent tissue can cause false-positive entrainment criteria at some sites.[7,10]

PACE MAPPING

Fundamental Concepts

Pace mapping is a technique designed to help locate tachycardia sources by pacing at different endocardial sites to reproduce the ECG morphology of the tachycardia. Pace mapping is based on the principle that pacing from the site of origin of a focal tachycardia at a pacing CL similar to the tachycardia CL will result in the same activation sequence as that during the tachycardia.[7]

When myocardial activation originates from a point-like source, such as during focal tachycardia or during pacing from an electrode catheter, ECG configuration of the resultant tachycardia or paced complex (QRS or P wave) is determined by the sequence of myocardial activation, which is largely determined by the initial site of myocardial depolarization, assuming no conduction abnormalities from that site. Analysis of specific surface ECG configurations in multiple leads allows estimation of the pacing site location to within several square centimeters, and comparing the paced complex configuration with that of tachycardia can be used to locate the arrhythmia focus (Fig. 3-21).[14,15]

On the other hand, reentry circuits in healed infarct scars (e.g., post-MI VT) often extend over several square centimeters and can have various configurations. In many circuits, the excitation wave proceeds through surviving myocytes in the scarred region, depolarization of which is not detectable in the standard surface ECG. The QRS complex is then inscribed after the reentry wavefront activates a sufficient amount of muscle outside the dense scar area. At sites at which the reentrant wavefront exits the scar, pace mapping is expected to produce a QRS configuration similar to that of VT. Pace mapping at sites more proximally located in the isthmus of the reentrant circuit should also produce a similar QRS complex, but with a longer stimulus-to-QRS (S-QRS) interval.[16]

Interpretation of Pace Mapping

Pace maps with identical or near-identical matches of the tachycardia morphology in all 12 surface ECG leads are indicative of the site of origin of the tachycardia (Fig. 3-22). Differences in the morphology between pacing and spontaneous tachycardia in a single lead can be critical. For VT, pacing at a site 5 mm from the index pacing site results in minor differences in QRS configuration (e.g., notching, new small component, change in amplitude of individual component, or overall change in QRS shape) in at least one lead in most patients. In contrast, if only major changes in QRS morphology are considered, pacing sites separated by as much as 15 mm can produce similar QRS morphologies.

Although qualitative comparison of the 12-lead ECG morphology between a pace map and clinical tachycardia is frequently performed, there are few objective criteria for quantifying the similarity between two 12-lead ECG waveform morphologies. Such comparisons are frequently completely subjective or semiquantitative, such as a 10/12 lead match. Unsuccessful ablation can result, in part, from subjective differences in the opinion of a pace map match to the clinical tachycardia. Furthermore, criteria for comparing the similarity in 12-lead ECG waveforms from one labo-

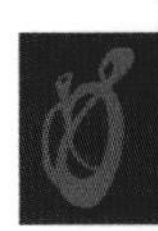

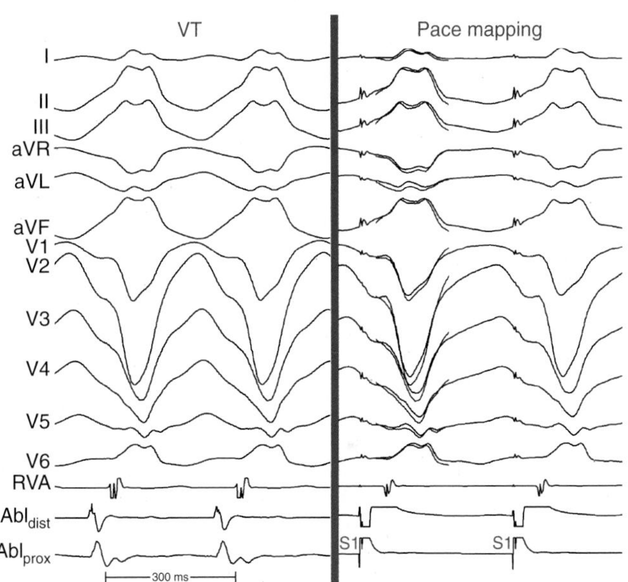

FIGURE 3–21 Pace-mapping of ventricular tachycardia (VT). At left, 12 ECG leads and intracardiac recordings during idiopathic right ventricular outflow tract VT are shown (cycle length [CL], 280 milliseconds). At right, pace mapping from the site of earliest ventricular activation at CL 350 milliseconds produces an identical 12-lead ECG configuration (gray image is a VT complex superimposed on a paced complex).

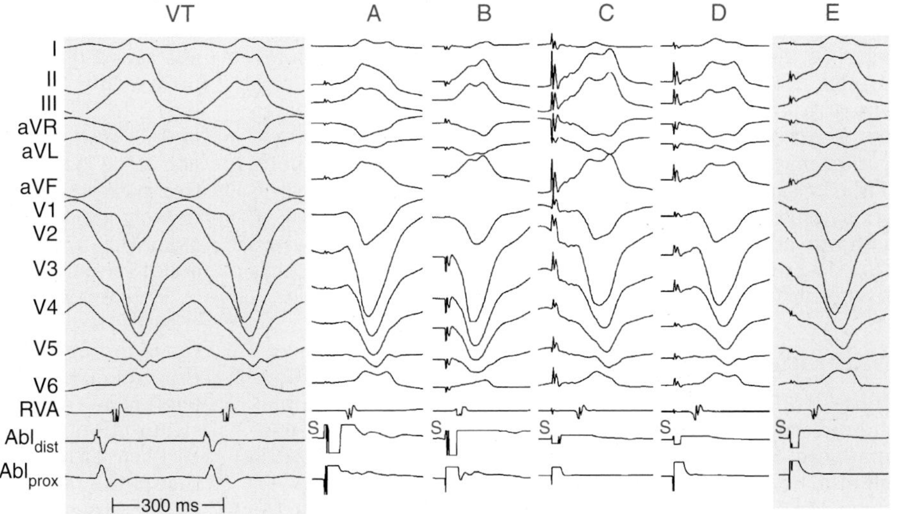

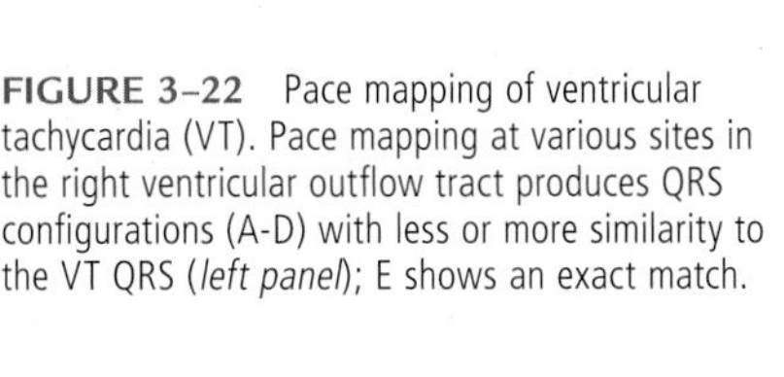

FIGURE 3–22 Pace mapping of ventricular tachycardia (VT). Pace mapping at various sites in the right ventricular outflow tract produces QRS configurations (A-D) with less or more similarity to the VT QRS (*left panel*); E shows an exact match.

ratory with another or for describing such comparisons in the literature are lacking.[17] Two waveform comparison metrics, the correlation coefficient (CORR) and the mean absolute deviation (MAD), have been recently evaluated to quantify the similarity of 12-lead ECG waveforms during VT and pace mapping objectively, and it has been suggested that an automated objective interpretation can have some advantage to qualitative interpretation.[17] Although CORR is more commonly used, MAD is more sensitive to differences in waveform amplitude. The most common human error is not appreciating subtle amplitude or precordial lead transition differences between two ECG patterns. It is important to note that such subtle differences in multiple leads can be reflected in a single quantitative number.[17]

The MAD score grades 12-lead ECG waveform similarity as a single number ranging from 0% (identical) to 100% (completely different). A MAD score of 12% or less was 93% sensitive and 75% specific for a successful ablation site. It is not surprising that the MAD score is more sensitive than specific; characteristics other than a 12-lead ECG match are necessary for a successful ablation, including catheter-tissue contact, catheter orientation, and tissue heating. MAD scores more than 12%, and certainly more than 15% (100% negative predictive value), suggest sufficient dissimilarity between the pace map and clinical tachycardia to dissuade ablation at that site. MAD scores of 12% or less should be considered an excellent match, and ablation at these sites is warranted if catheter contact and stability are adequate.[17]

S-QRS Interval During Pace Mapping

Ventricular pacing in normal myocardium is associated with an S-QRS interval less than 40 milliseconds. On the other hand, an S-QRS interval more than 40 milliseconds is consistent with slow conduction from the pacing site, and is typically associated with abnormal fractionated electrograms recorded from that site. Thus, pace mapping can provide a measure of slow conduction, as indicated by the S-QRS interval.[16,18] For post-MI VTs, at sites at which the reentrant wavefront exits the scar, pace mapping is expected to produce a QRS configuration similar to that of the VT. Pace mapping at sites more proximally located in the isthmus should also produce a similar QRS complex, but with a longer S-QRS interval. The S-QRS interval lengthens progressively as the pacing site is moved along the isthmus, consistent with pacing progressively further from the exit. Therefore, parts of VT reentry circuit isthmuses can be traced during NSR by combining both the QRS morphology and the S-QRS delay from pace mapping in anatomical maps. This works well when pacing is performed during tachycardia, at which time wavefront propagation is constrained in one direction through a corridor bounded by barriers that can be anatomically or functionally determined. However, pace mapping at the same sites during sinus rhythm can yield different results because the barriers may not exist then, the preferential direction of propagation may not be the same as during tachycardia, or both. This is especially true of entrance sites (Fig. 3-23). It is likely that pacing sites with long S-QRS delays are in an isthmus adjacent to regions of conduction block. However, this isthmus can be part of the reentrant circuit or a bystander.[7]

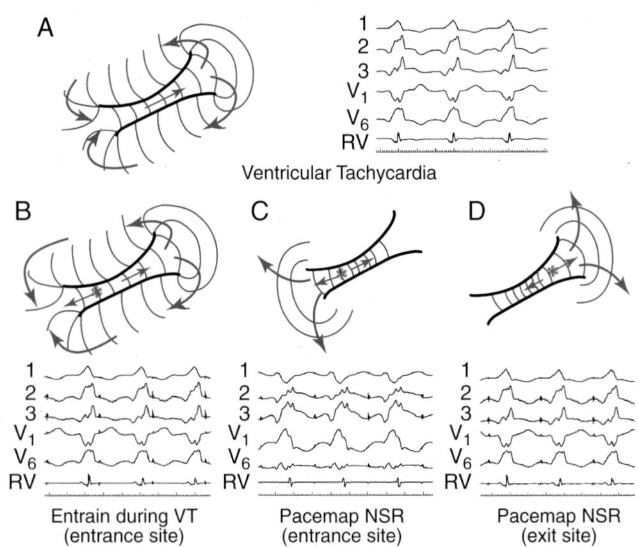

FIGURE 3–23 Pacing to verify ablation sites in reentrant ventricular tachycardia (VT). **A,** Five ECG leads of VT are shown with a figure-of-8 circuit with propagation of the reentrant wavefront (*arrows*); the protected diastolic corridor is also shown (*short straight arrow*). **B,** Pacing is performed during VT from a site near the entrance to the diastolic corridor (*asterisk*); the impulse must traverse a significant slow conduction zone before exiting to generate a QRS complex, resulting in a long S-QRS as shown. **C,** Pacing is performed at the same site as in **B**, but during sinus rhythm; the impulse exits in the opposite direction from **B**, because it takes less time to propagate in this direction (short S-QRS). The resulting QRS complex is completely different, despite pacing at the same site. **D**, Pacing is performed during sinus rhythm from a site closer to the exit of the diastolic corridor. The QRS is the same as VT because the path taken is the same as in VT, and the S-QRS is short. NSR = normal sinus rhythm.

Mapping Procedure

Initially, the exact morphology of the tachycardia complex should be determined and used as a template for pace mapping. For VT, QRS morphology during the tachycardia should be inspected in all 12 surface ECG leads. For AT, determining the morphology of the P wave during the tachycardia can be challenging, and proper interpretation of discrete changes in P wave shape is limited by its low voltage and distortion or masking by the preceding ST segment and T wave. Therefore, the P wave during AT should be assessed using multiple ECG leads in addition to an intracardiac electrogram activation sequence. Delivery of a VES (or a train of ventricular pacing) to advance ventricular activation and repolarization can allow careful distinction of the P wave onset and morphology. Using multiple intraatrial catheters (e.g., Halo catheter during right AT) can provide more intracardiac atrial electrograms that are useful for comparing the paced and tachycardia atrial activation sequence.[7]

Pace mapping during tachycardia (at a pacing CL 20 to 40 milliseconds shorter than the tachycardia CL) is preferable whenever possible, because it facilitates rapid comparison of tachycardia and paced complexes at the end of the pacing train in a simultaneously displayed 12-lead ECG. If sustained tachycardia cannot be induced, mapping is performed during spontaneous nonsustained runs or ectopic beats. In this case, the pacing CL and coupling intervals of extrastimulus should match those of spontaneous ectopy. For atrial pace mapping, it is unclear whether the conduction pattern of an atrial stimulus depends on the pacing CL; in fact, some have suggested that it is not mandatory to pace exactly at the same tachycardia CL to reproduce a similar atrial sequence.[19]

Pace mapping is preferably performed with unipolar stimuli (10 mA, 2 milliseconds) from the distal electrode of the mapping catheter (cathode) and an electrode in the inferior vena cava (IVC) (anode), or with closely spaced bipolar pacing at twice diastolic threshold to eliminate far-field stimulation effects.

The resulting 12-lead ECG morphology is compared with that of the tachycardia. ECG recordings should be reviewed at the same gain and filter settings and at a paper-sweep speed of 100 mm/sec. It is often helpful to display all 12 ECG leads side by side in review windows on screen as well as a printout of regular 12-lead ECGs for side by side comparison on paper. The greater the degree of concordance between the morphology during pacing and tachycardia, the closer the catheter is to the site of origin of the tachycardia. Concordance occurring in 12 of 12 leads on the surface ECG is indicative of the site of origin of the tachycardia.

For mapping macroreentrant VT circuits, evaluation of the S-QRS interval, the interval from the pacing stimulus to the onset of the earliest QRS on the 12-lead ECG, is of value.[16,18] The reentry circuit exit, which is more likely to be at the border of the infarct and close to the normal myocardium, often has no delay during pace mapping during NSR even though it is a desirable target for ablation. A delay between the pacing stimulus and QRS onset is consistent with slow conduction away from the pacing site; this can indicate a greater likelihood that the pacing site is in a reentry circuit. This can be a useful method for initially screening sites during NSR.

Clinical Implications

Pace mapping is typically used to confirm the results of activation mapping. It can be of great help, especially when the tachycardia is difficult to induce. The highest benefit of pace mapping has been found in focal tachycardias, especially in idiopathic VT.[14]

For macroreentrant VT, pace mapping remains at best a corroborative method of localizing the isthmus critical to the reentrant circuit.[16] It can be used to focus initial mapping efforts to regions likely to contain the reentrant circuit exit or abnormal conduction but may not be sufficiently specific or sensitive to be the sole guide for ablation. Pace mapping can also be used in conjunction with substrate mapping when other mapping techniques are not feasible, so that it can provide information on where ablation can be directed. Pace mapping has advantages over activation mapping in that induction of VT is not required; thus, it allows identification of the site of origin when the induced VT is poorly tolerated or when VT is not inducible by EP techniques but the QRS morphology from a prior 12-lead ECG is available.[7]

Limitations

Pacing at two different endocardial sites may produce similar surface ECG or intracardiac recordings. An optimal spatial pace mapping resolution requires a short maximum distance between two points generating a similar ECG configuration. Usually, the spatial resolution of unipolar stimulation is 5 mm or less. Spatial resolution deteriorates with wide electrodes, bipolar stimulation, and pacing at pathological areas. Spatial resolution worsens with bipolar stimulation by inducing electrical capture at both electrodes with variable contribution of the proximal electrode (generally anode) to depolarization. Such changes in paced ECG morphology potentially induced by bipolar pacing can be minimized by low pacing outputs and small inter-electrode distance (5 mm or less).[16]

The morphology of single paced complexes can vary, depending on the coupling interval, and the paced complex morphology during overdrive pacing is affected by the pacing CL. Therefore, the coupling interval or CL of the template arrhythmia should be matched during pace mapping, especially during mapping of VTs. Similarly, spontaneous couplets from the same focus can have slight variations in QRS morphology that must be considered when seeking a pace match.

Pace mapping during post-MI VT has several other limitations. Some areas of conduction block are not anatomically determined, but can be functional. Therefore, pacing within the diastolic corridor of the VT circuit during NSR can generate a completely different QRS complex than that of the VT (see Fig. 3-23). During pace mapping, consequently, a QRS configuration different from VT does not reliably indicate that the pacing site is distant from the reentry circuit.[16] At best, a pace map that matches the VT would only identify the exit site to the normal myocardium, and can be distant from the critical sites of the circuit required for ablation. On the other hand, pacing during NSR from sites attached to the reentrant circuit but not part of the circuit can occasionally produce QRS morphology identical to that of the VT, because the stimulated wavefront can be physiologically forced to follow the same route of activation as the VT as long as pacing is carried out between the entrance and exit of the protected isthmus.

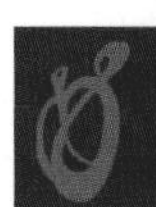

BASKET CATHETER MAPPING

Fundamental Concepts

The basket catheter mapping system consists of a basket catheter (Constellation, EPT, Inkster, Mich), a conventional ablation catheter, the Astronomer (Boston Scientific, Natick, Mass) which is used for navigation inside the basket catheter, and a mapping system.

The basket catheter consists of an open-lumen catheter shaft with a collapsible, basket-shaped, distal end.[20,21] Currently, baskets are composed of 64 platinum-iridium ring electrodes mounted on eight equidistant, flexible, self-expanding nitinol splines (metallic arms; see Fig. 2-4). Each spline contains eight 1.5-mm electrodes equally spaced at 4 or 5 mm apart, depending on the size of the basket catheter used. Each spline is identified by a letter (from A to H) and each electrode by a number (distal 1 to proximal 8). The basket catheter is constructed of a superelastic material to allow passive deployment of the array catheter and optimize endocardial contact. The size of the basket catheter used depends on the dimensions of the chamber to be mapped, requiring antecedent evaluation (usually by echocardiogram) to ensure proper size selection.

The Astronomer is used for navigation with the ablation-mapping catheter inside the basket catheter. This system consists of a switching-locating device and a laptop computer with proprietary software. The device and the laptop communicate on a standard RS-232 interface. The device delivers AC current (32 kHz, 320 μA) between the ablation catheter tip electrode and a reference electrode (skin patch), and the resulting electrical potentials are sensed at each basket catheter electrode. On the basis of the sensed voltages at each of the basket catheter electrodes, the Astronomer device determines whether the roving electrode is in close proximity to a basket catheter electrode and lights the corresponding electrodes on a representation of the basket catheter displayed on the laptop.

The mapping system consists of an acquisition module connected to a computer, which is capable of simultaneously processing bipolar electrograms from the basket catheter, 16 bipolar-unipolar electrograms signals, a 12-lead ECG, and a pressure signal. Color-coded activation maps are reconstructed on-line. The color-coded animation images simplify the analysis of multielectrode recordings and help establish the relation between activation patterns and anatomical structures (Fig. 3-24). The electrograms and activation maps are displayed on a computer monitor and the acquired signals can be stored on optical disk for off-line analysis. Activation marks are generated automatically with a peak or slope (dV/dt) algorithm, and the activation times are then edited manually as needed.

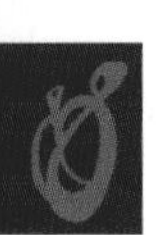

3

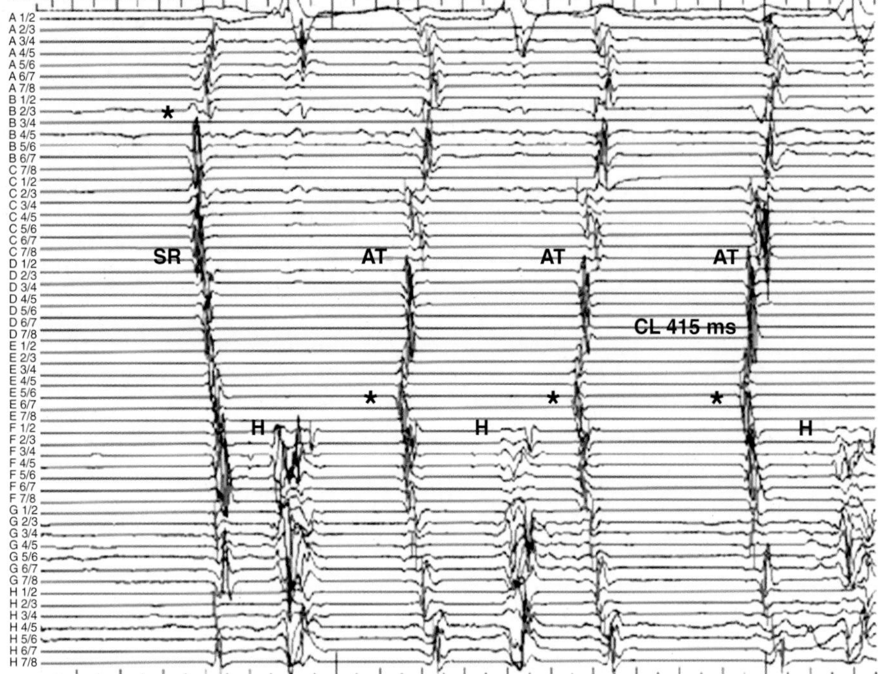

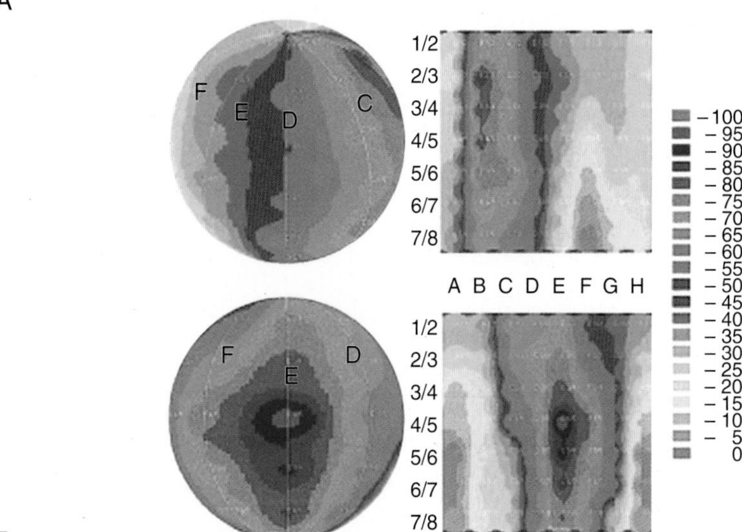

FIGURE 3–24 Basket catheter mapping during focal atrial tachycardia (AT). **A,** Simultaneous recordings of the surface ECG leads I and aVF, and 56 bipolar electrograms from the basket catheter in a patient with focal AT. The first beat is a sinus beat. The next three beats are tachycardia beats. His bundle (HB) potential is recorded in electrode pairs F2-3 and F3-4. The earliest spot of activation during sinus rhythm (SR) and AT is shown (*asterisks*). Spline A was located in the anterolateral right atrium (RA), splines B and C in the lateral region, splines D and E in the posterior region, and splines G and H across the tricuspid valve. The activation times are marked with red bars. **B, Upper panel,** Animated map of the SR beats. **Lower panel,** Animated map of the AT beats. Planar and 3-D options are shown. During SR, the impulse emerged in the high lateral area (spline B1-2) and propagated rapidly down the lateral wall. The complete activation of the RA took 85 milliseconds. During focal AT, the earliest activity emerged in the midposterior wall (spline E4-5). The activation sequence of the RA was entirely different from that of SR. The complete activation of the RA took 95 milliseconds. CL = cycle length. (From Zrenner B, Ndrepepa G, Schneider M, et al: Computer-assisted animation of atrial tachyarrhythmias recorded with a 64-electrode basket catheter. J Am Coll Cardiol 1999;34:2051.)

Mapping Procedure

The size of the cardiac chamber of interest is initially evaluated, usually with echocardiography, to help select the appropriate size of the basket catheter. The collapsed basket catheter is advanced under fluoroscopic guidance through a long sheath into the chamber of interest; the catheter is then expanded (Fig. 3-25). Electrical-anatomical relations are determined by fluoroscopically identifiable markers (spline A has one marker and spline B has two markers located near the shaft of the basket catheter), and by the electrical signals recorded from certain electrodes (e.g., ventricular, atrial, or HB electrograms), which can help identify the location of those particular splines.

From the 64 electrodes, 64 unipolar signals and 32 to 56 bipolar signals can be recorded (by combining electrodes 1-2, 3-4, 5-6, 7-8, or 1-2, 2-3 until 7-8 electrodes on each spline). Color-coded activation maps can be reconstructed (see Fig. 3-24). The concepts of activation mapping discussed earlier are then used to determine the site of origin of the tachycardia.

The Astronomer navigation system permits precise and reproducible guidance of the ablation catheter tip electrode to targets identified by the basket catheter. Without the use of this navigation system, it is often difficult to identify the alphabetical order of the splines by fluoroscopic guidance.

The electrograms recorded from the basket catheter can be used to monitor changes in the activation sequence in real time and thereby indicate the effects of ablation as lesions are created. The capacity of pacing from most basket electrodes allows the evaluation of activation patterns, pace mapping, and entrainment mapping.

Clinical Implications

The multielectrode endocardial mapping system allows simultaneous recording of electrical activation from multi-

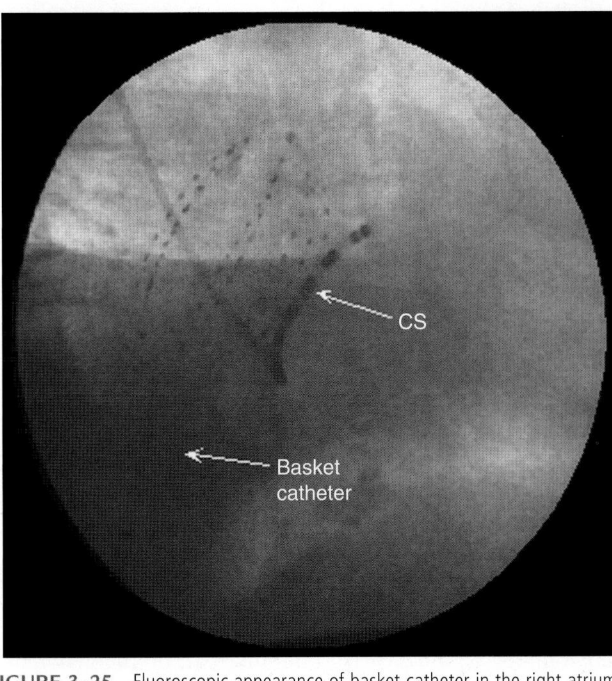

FIGURE 3–25 Fluoroscopic appearance of basket catheter in the right atrium (right anterior oblique view). Note the radiopaque electrodes on splines of basket catheter. CS = coronary sinus.

ple sites and fast reconstruction of endocardial activation maps. This can limit the time endured in tachycardia compared with single point mapping techniques without the insertion of multiple electrodes. It also facilitates endocardial mapping of hemodynamically unstable or nonsustained tachycardias. Importantly, the recording of only a single beat can be sufficient to enable analysis of the arrhythmogenic substrate.

Endocardial mapping with a multielectrode basket catheter has been shown to be feasible and safe for various arrhythmias, including AT, AFL, VT, and pulmonary vein (PV) isolation. However, in view of more advanced mapping systems, and because of significant limitations of the current basket catheters, its use has been limited.[20,21]

Limitations

Because of its poor spatial resolution, the basket catheter in its current iteration has demonstrated only limited clinical useulness for guiding ablation of reentrant atrial or ventricular arrhythmias. The relatively large interelectrode spacing in available catheters prevents high-resolution reconstruction of the tachycardia and is generally not sufficient for a catheter-based ablation procedure, given the small size and precise localization associated with RF lesions. The quality of recordings is critically dependent on proper selection of the basket size. Resolution is limited to the proportion of electrodes in contact with the endocardium and by unequal deployment and spacing of the splines. Unfortunately, the electrode array does not expand to provide adequate contact with the entire cardiac chamber; therefore, good electrode contact at all sites on the endocardium is difficult to ensure because of irregularities in the cardiac chamber surface, so that areas crucial to arrhythmia circuit or focus may not be recorded. Moreover, regions such as the RA appendage, LA appendage, and cavotricuspid isthmus are incompletely covered by the basket catheter. As a result, arrhythmia substrates involving these structures are not recorded by the basket catheter.

Voltage, duration, and late potential maps are not provided by this mapping approach. Additionally, basket catheter mapping does not permit immediate correlation of activation times to precise anatomical sites, and a second mapping-ablation catheter is still required to be manipulated to the site identified for more precise mapping and localization of the target for ablation, as well as for RF energy delivery. Basket catheters also have limited torque capabilities and limited maneuverability, which hampers correct placement, and they can abrade the endocardium.[20]

Carbonizations are occasionally observed after ablation on the splines of the basket catheter, which can potentially cause embolism. Carbonizations, which appear as dark material attached to the basket catheter electrodes or splines, are thought to be caused by the concentration of RF energy on the thin splines, which results in very high local temperatures that induce denaturization of proteins. Carbonization can be greatly diminished with the use of an irrigated tip catheter as opposed to conventional ablation catheters.[20]

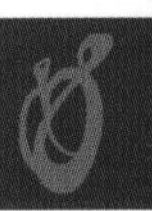

High-Density Mapping Catheter

A recent study has evaluated a new mapping approach for AT using a novel high-density multielectrode mapping catheter (PentaRay, Biosense Webster, Diamond Bar, Calif).[22] This 7 Fr steerable catheter (180 degrees of unidirectional flexion) has 20 electrodes distributed over five soft radiating spines (1-mm electrodes separated by 4-4-4 or 2-6-2 mm interelectrode spacing), allowing splaying of the catheter to cover a surface diameter of 3.5 cm. The spines have been given alphabetical nomenclature (A to E), with spines A and B being recognized by radiopaque markers (Fig. 3-26).[22]

Localization of the atrial focus can be performed during tachycardia or atrial ectopy.[22] Guided by the ECG appearance, the catheter is sequentially applied to the endocardial surface in various atrial regions to allow rapid activation mapping. By identifying the earliest site of activation around the circumference of the high-density catheter, vector mapping is performed, moving the catheter and applying it to the endocardium in the direction of earliest activation (outer bipoles) to identify the tachycardia origin and bracket activation—that is, demonstrating later activation in all surrounding regions.

The high-density mapping catheter can offer several potential advantages.[22] In contrast to the basket catheter, which provides a global density of mapping but limited localized resolution, the high-density mapping catheter allows splaying of the spines against the endocardial surface to achieve high-density contact mapping and better localized resolution.[22]

ENSITE NONCONTACT MAPPING SYSTEM

Fundamental Concepts

The noncontact mapping system (EnSite 3000, Endocardial Solutions, St. Paul, Minn) consists of a catheter-mounted multielectrode array (MEA), which serves as the probe, a custom-designed amplifier system, a computer workstation used to display 3-D maps of cardiac electrical activity, and a conventional ablation catheter.[7,21,23]

The MEA catheter consists of a 7.5-mL ellipsoid balloon mounted on a 9 Fr catheter around which is woven a braid of 64 insulated 0.003-mm diameter wires (Fig. 3-27). Each wire has a 0.025-mm break in insulation that serves as a noncontact unipolar electrode.[21,23] The system acquires more than 3000 noncontact unipolar electrograms from all points in the chamber simultaneously. The unipolar signals are recorded using a ring electrode located on the shaft of

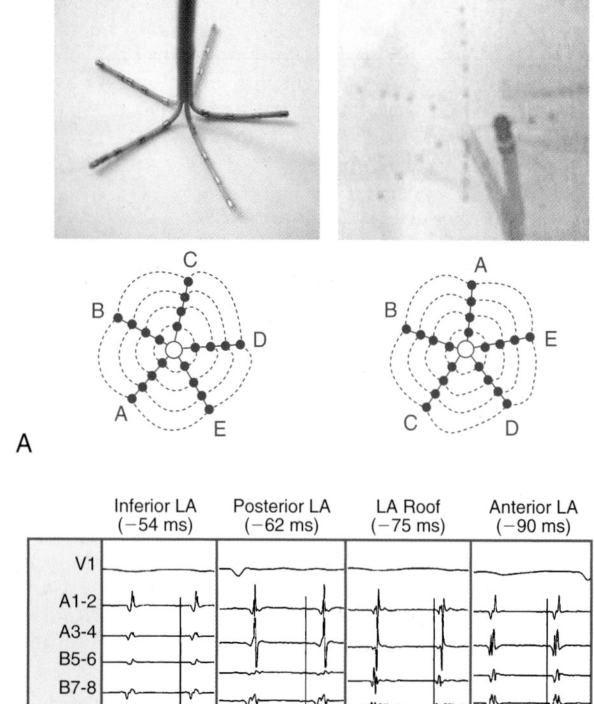

FIGURE 3–26 The high-density mapping catheter. **A,** Picture and a fluoroscopic image of the high-density mapping catheter. Below each figure is a schematic representation indicating the orientation of the catheter spines. Note that the marker band on spine A is between electrodes 1 to 2, and on spine B between electrodes 2 to 3. **B,** Vector mapping using the high-density mapping catheter to identify the earliest site of activation of focal atrial tachycardia. Shown is the catheter in four distinct locations within the left atrium (LA). Mapping is commenced along the inferior LA, where the earliest activation is 54 milliseconds ahead of the coronary sinus (CS). The catheter is moved in the direction of the spine demonstrating the earliest activation (spine D). In the midposterior LA, activation precedes the coronary sinus (CS) by 62 milliseconds. Again, the catheter is moved in the earliest direction (spine D) to a more cranial location on the LA roof. At this site, activation precedes the CS by 75 milliseconds. At this site, spine B, which is slightly anterior, is the earliest. Moving the catheter in the direction of spine B to the anterior-superior LA demonstrates the site with the earliest endocardial activation (90 milliseconds ahead of the CS, which was 40 milliseconds ahead of the P-wave). (From Sanders P, Hocini M, Jais P, et al: Characterization of focal atrial tachycardia using high-density mapping. J Am Coll Cardiol 2005;46:2088.)

the array catheter as a reference. The raw far-field EP data acquired by the array catheter are fed into a multichannel recorder and amplifier system that also has 16 channels for conventional contact catheters, 12 channels for the surface ECG, and pressure channels. Using data from the 64-electrode array catheter suspended in the heart chamber, the computer uses sophisticated algorithms to compute an inverse solution to determine the activation sequence on the endocardial surface.

The EnSite 3000 mapping system is based on the premise that endocardial activation creates a chamber voltage field that obeys the Laplace equation. Therefore, when one 3-D surface of known geometry is placed within another of

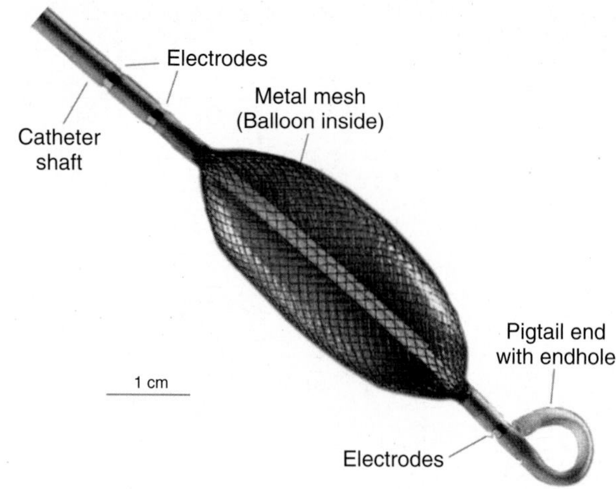

FIGURE 3–27 The multielectrode array for noncontact endocardial mapping.

known geometry, if the electrical potential on one surface is known, the potential on the other can be calculated.[21,23] Because the geometry of the balloon catheter is known, and the geometry of the cardiac chamber can be reconstructed during the procedure (see later), endocardial surface potential can then be determined once the potentials over the balloon catheter are recorded. Using this concept, the raw far-field EP data acquired by the array catheter, which are generally lower in amplitude and frequency than the source potential of the endocardium itself and therefore have limited usefulness, are mathematically enhanced and resolved using an inverse solution to the Laplace equation to reconstruct electrograms at endocardial sites in the absence of physical electrode contact at those locations (virtual electrograms). Once the potential field has been established, over 3000 activation points can be displayed as computed electrograms or as isopotential maps.

The system can locate any conventional mapping-ablation catheter in space with respect to the array catheter (and thus with respect to the cardiac chamber being mapped).[21,23] A low current (5.68 kHz) locator signal is passed between the contact catheter electrode being located and reference electrodes on the noncontact array. This creates a potential gradient across the array electrodes, which is then used to position the source. This locator system is also used to construct the 3-D computer model of the endocardium (virtual endocardium) that is required for the reconstruction of endocardial electrograms and isopotential maps. This model is acquired by moving a conventional contact catheter around the endocardial surface of the cardiac chamber; the system collects the location information, building up a series of coordinates for the endocardium, and generating a patient-specific, anatomically contoured model of its geometry. During geometry creation, only the most distant points visited by the roving catheter are recorded to ignore those detected when the catheter is not in contact with the endocardial wall. Using mathematical techniques to process potentials recorded from the array, the system is able to reconstruct more than 3000 unipolar electrograms simultaneously and superimpose them onto the virtual endocardium, producing isopotential maps with a color range representing voltage amplitudes. Additionally, the locator signal can be used to display and track the position of any catheter on the endocardial model (virtual endocardium) and allows marking of anatomical locations identified using fluoroscopy and electrographic characteristics. During catheter ablation procedures, the locator system is used in real time to navigate the catheter to sites of interest identified from the isopotential color maps, catalogue the position of

RF energy applications on the virtual endocardium, and facilitate revisitation of sites of interest by the ablation catheter.[7]

In addition, the most recent version of the EnSite software provides the capability of point by point contact mapping, allowing the creation of activation and voltage maps by acquiring serial contact electrograms and displaying them on the virtual endocardium (see later). This is useful for adding detail, familiarity, and validation of the information obtained by the noncontact method.[24]

Mapping Procedure

The EnSite 3000 system requires placing a 9 Fr multielectrode array and a 7 Fr mapping-ablation catheter.[21,23,25-27] To create a map, the balloon catheter is advanced over a 0.035-inch guidewire under fluoroscopic guidance into the cardiac chamber of interest. The balloon is then deployed and can be filled with contrast dye, permitting it to be visualized fluoroscopically (Fig. 3-28). The balloon is positioned in the center of the cardiac chamber of interest and does not come in contact with the walls of the chamber being mapped. In addition, the position of the array in the chamber must be secured to avoid significant movement that would invalidate the electrical and anatomical information. The array must be positioned as closely as possible (and in direct line of sight through the blood pool) to the endocardial surface being mapped, because the accuracy of the map is sensitive to the distance between the center of the balloon and the endocardium being mapped.[7,24]

During the use of this mapping modality, systemic anticoagulation is critical to avoid thromboembolic complications. Intravenous heparin is usually given to maintain the activated clotting time longer than 250 seconds for right-sided and longer than 300 seconds for left-sided mapping.

A conventional (roving) deflectable mapping catheter is also positioned in the chamber being mapped and used to collect geometry information. The mapping catheter is initially moved to known anatomical locations, which are tagged. A detailed geometry of the chamber is then reconstructed by moving the mapping catheter and tracing the contour of the endocardium (using the locator technology). To create a detailed geometry, attempts must be made to make contact with as much endocardium as possible. This requires maneuvering on all sides of the array, which can be challenging and can require decreasing the profile of the balloon by withdrawing a few milliliters of fluid. This results in the rapid formation of a relatively accurate 3-D geometric model of the cardiac chamber. Creation of chamber geometry can be performed during NSR or tachycardia.[7,24]

Once the chamber geometry has been delineated, tachycardia is induced and mapping is started. The data acquisition process is performed automatically by the system, and all data for the entire chamber are acquired simultaneously. Following this, the segment must be analyzed by the operator to find the early activation or diastolic pathway of the reentry circuit (Fig. 3-29).

The noncontact mapping system is capable of simultaneously reconstructing more than 3360 unipolar electrograms over the virtual endocardium. From these electrograms, isopotential or isochronal maps can be reconstructed (Fig. 3-30).[21,23,25-27] Because of the high density of data, color-coded isopotential maps are used to depict graphically regions that are depolarized, and wavefront propagation is displayed as a user-controlled 3-D "movie." The color range represents voltage or timing of onset. The highest chamber voltage is at the site of origin of the electrical impulse. Although the electrode closest to the origin of the impulse is influenced the most, all the electrodes on the array catheter are influenced, the degree of influence diminishing with the distance between the electrode and each endocardial point.

In addition, the system can simultaneously display as many as 32 electrograms as waveforms (see Fig. 3-29). Unipolar or bipolar electrograms (virtual electrograms) can be selected at any given interval of the tachycardia cycle using the mouse from any part of the created geometry and displayed as waveforms as if from point, array, or plaque electrodes. The reconstructed electrograms are subject to the same electrical principles as contact catheter electrograms, because they contain far-field electrical information from the surrounding endocardium as well as the underlying myocardium signal vector, and distance from measurement may affect the contribution to the electrogram. These selected unipolar waveforms are used to augment information obtained from the 3-D map by demonstrating the slope of depolarization, presence of double potentials or fractionation, and differentiation of far-field signals from more relevant endocardial activation.[24]

Clinical Implications

The multielectrode array has been successfully deployed in all four cardiac chambers using a transvenous, transseptal, or retrograde transaortic approach to map atrial and ventricular tachyarrhythmias.[21,25-27]

The biggest advantage of noncontact endocardial mapping is its ability to recreate the endocardial activation sequence

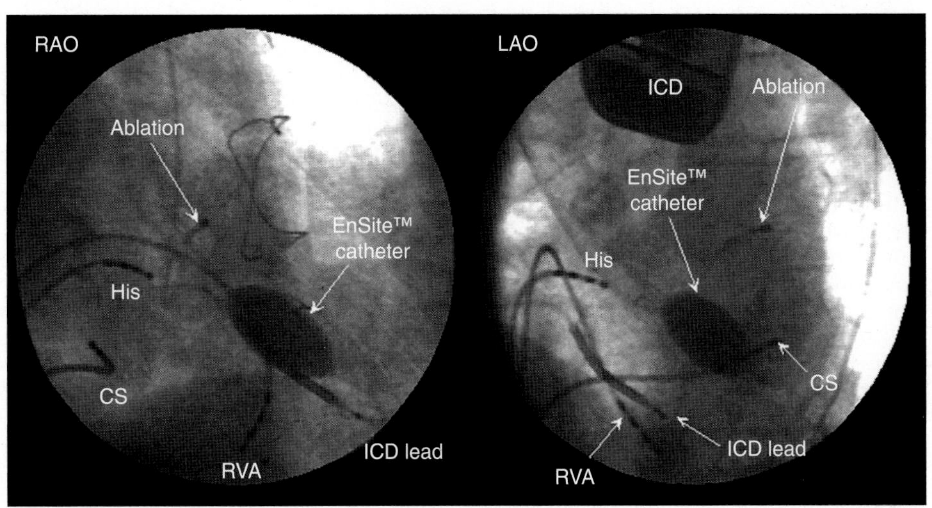

FIGURE 3–28 Fluoroscopic views of noncontact mapping catheter (EnSite 3000, Endocardial Solutions, St. Paul, Minn) situated in the left ventricle (LV). CS = coronary sinus; ICD = implantable cardioverter-defibrillator; LAO = left anterior oblique; RAO = right anterior oblique; RVA = right ventricular apex.

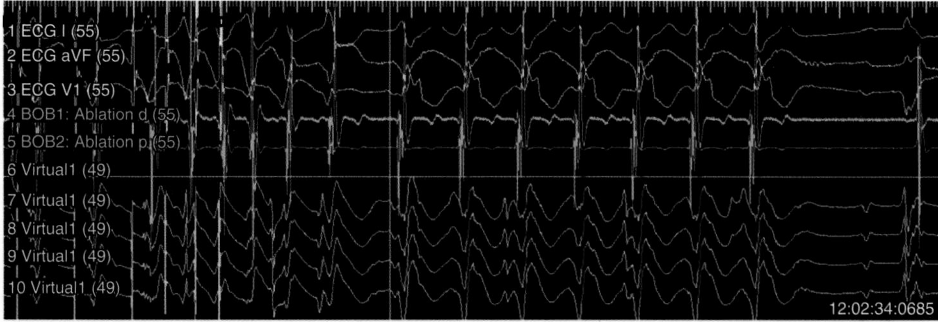

FIGURE 3–29 Noncontact mapping data during an episode of hemodynamically unstable ventricular tachycardia (VT). Surface electrocardiographic and intracardiac contact (blue) and virtual noncontact (yellow) electrograms are shown during nonsustained VT; such short episodes would be difficult to map with conventional methods.

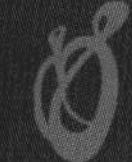

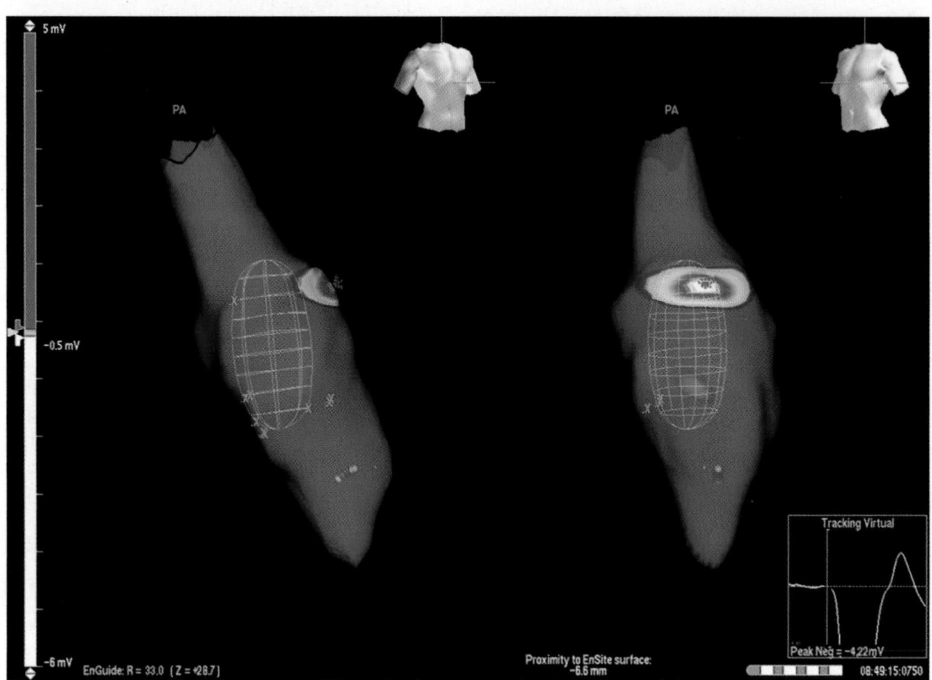

FIGURE 3–30 Noncontact mapping of idiopathic right ventricular outflow tract (RVOT) tachycardia. Shown are right anterior oblique and left anterior oblique views of color-coded isopotential map of RVOT activation during a single premature ventricular complex. **Inset,** Virtual electrograms at the site of earliest activation (note QS pattern).

from simultaneously acquired multiple data points over a few (theoretically one) tachycardia beats, without requiring sequential point-to-point acquisitions, obviating the need for prolonged tachycardia episodes that the patient might tolerate poorly. It can be used to map nonsustained arrhythmias, premature atrial complexes (PACs) or premature ventricular complexes (PVCs), irregular rhythms such as AF or polymorphic VT, and rhythms that are not hemodynamically stable, such as very rapid VT (see Fig. 3-30).[25-27]

The system generates isopotential maps of the endocardial surface at successive cross sections of time and, when these are animated, the spread of the depolarization wave can be visualized. These maps are particularly useful for identifying slowly conducting macroreentrant pathways, such as the critical slow pathways in ischemic VT and rapid breakthrough points or reentrant AT in patients with surgically corrected congenital heart disease. In macroreentrant tachycardias such as typical AFL or VT, the reentry circuit can be fully identifiable, along with other aspects, such as the slowing, narrowing, and splitting of activation wavefronts in the isthmus.[25-27]

The system can also map multiple cardiac cycles in real time, which discloses changes in the activation sequence from one beat to the next. Because mapping data are acquired without conventional electrode catheters being in direct contact with the endocardium, the use of noncontact mapping can help avoid the mechanical induction of ectopic activity that is frequently seen during conventional mapping. An additional advantage of this system is that any catheter from any manufacturer can be used in conjunction with this mapping platform. Other useful features include radiation-free catheter navigation, revisitation of points of interest, and cataloguing ablation points on the 3-D model.[7]

In complex substrate-related arrhythmias, the use of activation mapping alone may not be sufficient for rhythm analysis or identifying ablation targets. Substrate mapping based on scar or diseased tissue is of value in these cases. Although substrate mapping used to be relatively limited with the noncontact mapping technology (very low-amplitude signals may not be detected, particularly if the distance between the center of the balloon catheter and endocardial surface exceeds 4 cm), dynamic substrate mapping, which has been recently introduced, allows the creation of voltage maps from a single cardiac cycle and provides the capability of identifying low-voltage areas, as well as fixed and functional block, on the virtual endocardium through noncontact methodology. When combined with the activation sequence, substrate mapping provides essential information for guiding ablation, even when the arrhythmia is nonsustained.[24]

Limitations

Because the geometry of the cardiac chamber is contoured at the beginning of the study during NSR, changes of the chamber size and contraction pattern during tachycardia or administration of medications (e.g., isoproterenol) can adversely affect the accuracy of the location of the endocardial electrograms. Moreover, because isopotential maps are predominantly used, ventricular repolarization must be distinguished from atrial depolarization and diastolic activity. Early diastole can be challenging to map during VT.[21,28]

The overall accuracy of the reconstructed electrograms decreases with distance of the area mapped from the array catheter, thus creating problems in mapping large cardiac chambers. Virtual electrogram quality deteriorates at a distance of more than 4 cm from the array catheter and at polar regions. Therefore, the array must be positioned as closely as possible to the endocardial area of interest, and at times it can be necessary to reposition the array catheter to acquire adequate isopotential maps.

Only data segments up to a maximum of 10 seconds in length can be stored retroactively by the EnSite system once the record button has been pushed. Thus, continuous recording and storage of all segments of an arrhythmia is not possible at the time of evaluation of the arrhythmia maps. Therefore, some isolated PACs or PVCs that can be of interest during evaluation and mapping could be missed. In addition, the acquired geometry with the current version of software is somewhat distorted, requiring multiple set points to establish the origin and shape of complicated structures such as the LA appendage or PVs clearly. Otherwise, these structures can be lost in the interpolation between several neighboring points. Also, synchronized mapping of multiple chambers requires multiple systems, and maps are highly sensitive to changes in filtering frequencies used in postprocessing analysis.

Sometimes it is difficult to manipulate the ablation catheter around the outside of the balloon, especially during mapping in the LA. Special attention and care also are necessary during placement of the large balloon electrode in a relatively small cardiac chamber. Although the risk of complications is low, aggressive anticoagulation measures because of balloon deployment in the cardiac chamber expose patients to potential bleeding complications.

CARTO ELECTROANATOMICAL MAPPING SYSTEM

Fundamental Concepts

The CARTO mapping system (Biosense Webster, Diamond Bar, Calif) consists of an ultralow magnetic field emitter, a magnetic field generator locator pad (placed beneath the operating table), an external reference patch (fixed on the patient's back), a deflectable 7 Fr quadripolar mapping-ablation catheter with a 4- or 8-mm tip and proximal 2-mm ring electrodes, location sensors inside the mapping-ablation catheter tip (the three location sensors are located orthogonally to each other and lie just proximal to the tip electrode, totally embedded within the catheter), a reference catheter (placed intracardially), a data-processing unit, and a graphic display unit to generate the electroanatomical model of the chamber being mapped.

CARTO is a nonfluoroscopic mapping system that uses a special catheter to generate 3-D electroanatomical maps of the heart chambers. This system uses magnetic technology to determine the location and orientation of the mapping-ablation catheter accurately while simultaneously recording local electrograms from the catheter tip. By sampling electrical and spatial information from different endocardial sites, the 3-D geometry of the mapped chamber is reconstructed in real time and analyzed to assess the mechanism of arrhythmia and the appropriate site for ablation.[7]

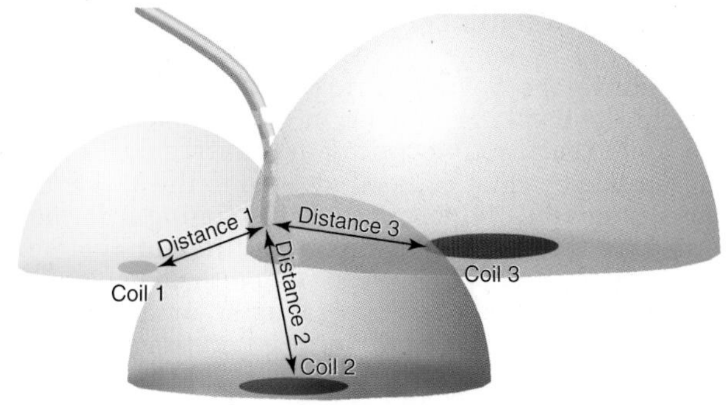

FIGURE 3–31 CARTO electroanatomical map setup. The three hemispheres represent fields from three different electromagnets situated beneath the patient; the catheter tip contains an element that is sensed by these fields and this triangulating information is used to monitor the location and orientation of the catheter tip in the heart.

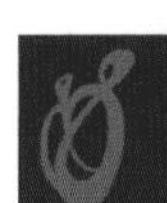

Electroanatomical mapping is based on the premise that a metal coil generates an electrical current when placed in a magnetic field. The magnitude of the current depends on the strength of the magnetic field and the orientation of the coil in it. The CARTO mapping system uses a triangulation algorithm similar to that used by a global positioning system (GPS). The magnetic field emitter, mounted under the operating table, consists of three coils that generate a low-intensity magnetic field, approximately 0.05 to 0.2 Gauss, which is a very small fraction of the magnetic field intensity inside a magnetic resonance (MR) machine (Fig. 3-31).

The sensor in the catheter tip detects the intensity of the magnetic field generated by each coil, allowing for determination of its distance from each coil. These distances determine the area of theoretical spheres around each coil and the intersection between these three spheres determines the location of the tip of the catheter. The accuracy of determination of the location is highest in the center of the magnetic field; therefore, it is important to position the location pad under the patient's chest. In addition to the x, y, and z coordinates of the catheter tip, the CARTO system can determine three orientation determinants—roll, yaw, and pitch—for the electrode at the catheter tip. The position and orientation of the catheter tip can be seen on the screen and monitored in real time as it moves within the electroanatomical model of the chamber mapped. The catheter icon has four color bars (green, red, yellow, and blue), enabling the operator to view the catheter as it turns clockwise or counterclockwise. In addition, because the catheter always deflects in the same direction, each catheter will always deflect toward a single color. Hence, to deflect the catheter to a specific wall, the operator should first turn the catheter so that this color faces the desired wall.[7]

The unipolar and bipolar electrograms recorded by the mapping catheter at each endocardial site are archived within that positional context. Using this approach, local tissue activation at each successive recording site produces activation maps within the framework of the acquired surrogate geometry.

When mapping the heart, the system can deal with four types of motion artifacts—cardiac motion (the heart is in constant motion; thus the location of the mapping catheter changes throughout the cardiac cycle), respiratory motion (intrathoracic change in the position of the heart during the respiratory cycle), patient motion, and system motion. Several steps are taken by the CARTO mapping system to compensate for these possible motion artifacts and to ensure that the initial map coordinates are appropriate, including using a reference electrogram and an anatomical reference.

Electrical Reference. This is the fiducial marker on which the entire mapping procedure is based. The timing of the fiducial point is used to determine the activation timing in the mapping catheter in relation to the acquired points and to ensure collection of data during the same part of the cardiac cycle; it is therefore vital to the performance of the system. All the local activation timing information recorded by the mapping catheter at different anatomical locations during mapping (displayed on the completed 3-D map) will be relative to this fiducial point, with the acquisition being gated so that each point is acquired during the same part of the cardiac electrical signal. It is important that the rhythm being mapped is monomorphic and the fiducial point is reproducible at each sampled site. The fiducial point is defined by the user by assigning a reference channel and an annotation criterion. The system has a great deal of flexibility in terms of choosing the reference electrogram and gating locations. Any ECG lead or intracardiac electrogram in bipolar or unipolar mode can serve as a reference electrogram. For the purpose of stability when intracardiac electrograms are selected, CS electrograms are usually chosen for mapping of supraventricular rhythms, and a right ventricle (RV) electrode or surface ECG lead is commonly chosen as the electrical reference during mapping of ventricular rhythms. Care must be taken to ensure that automatic sensing of the reference is reproducible and is not subject to oversensing in the case of annular electrograms (e.g., oversensing of a ventricular electrogram on the CS reference electrode during mapping an atrial rhythm). Automated sensing of mapping and reference electrograms is accomplished by detecting peak amplitude or peak slope.[29]

Anatomical Reference. Once the mapping catheter is placed inside the heart, its location in relation to the fixed magnetic field sensors placed under the patient can be determined. However, several of the factors mentioned earlier, including a change in the patient's position during the procedure, can result in loss of orientation of the structures. To overcome the effect of motion artifacts, a reference catheter with a sensor similar to that of the mapping catheter is used. This reference catheter is fixed in its location inside the heart or on the body surface. The anatomical reference (location sensor) is typically placed in an adhesive reference patch secured on the patient's back. The fluoroscopic (anteroposterior view) location of the anatomical reference should be close to the cardiac chamber being mapped. Movement of the anatomical reference indicates movement of the patient's chest, which must be corrected to prevent distortion of the electroanatomical map. The CARTO mapping system continuously calculates the position of the mapping catheter in relation to the anatomical reference, thus solving the problem of any possible motion artifacts. An intracardiac reference catheter has the advantage of moving with the patient's body and with the heart during the phases of respiration. However, the intracardiac reference catheter can change its position during the course of the procedure, especially during manipulation of the other catheters. It is therefore better to use an externally positioned reference catheter strapped to the back of the patient's chest in the interscapular area. The movement of the ablation catheter is then tracked relative to the position of this reference catheter.[7]

Window of Interest. Defining an electrical window of interest is a crucial aspect in ensuring the accuracy of the initial map coordinates. The window of interest is defined as the time interval relative to the fiducial point during which the local activation time is determined (Fig. 3-32). Within this window, activation is considered early or late relative to the reference. The total length of the window of interest should not exceed the tachycardia CL (usually 90% of the tachycardia CL). The boundaries are set relative to the reference electrogram. Thus, the window is defined by two intervals, one extending before the reference electrogram and the other after it. For macroreentrant circuits, the sensing window should approximate the tachycardia CL, and designating activation times in a circuit as early or late is arbitrary. In theory, a change in the window or reference would not change a macroreentrant circuit but only result in a phase shift of the map. If the activation window spans two adjacent beats of an arrhythmia, the resulting map can be ambiguous, lack coherency, and give rise to a spurious pattern of adjacent regions of early and late activation (see Fig. 3-32).[29]

Another important concept in CARTO mapping is determination of the local activation time. Once the reference electrogram, anatomical reference, and window of interest have been chosen, the mapping catheter is moved from point to point along the endocardial surface of the cardiac chamber being mapped (Fig. 3-33). These points can be acquired in a unipolar or bipolar configuration. These electrograms are analyzed using the principles of activation mapping discussed above. The local activation time at each sampled site is calculated as the time interval between the fiducial point on the reference electrogram and the corresponding local activation determined from the unipolar or bipolar local electrogram recorded from that site.[7]

The newer versions of CARTO (CARTO Merge) incorporate the use of computed tomography (CT) or MR imaging to allow verification of the anatomical landmarks and cardiac geometry and to help guide the ablation catheter precisely to the different areas of interest. CARTO Merge allows for images from a preacquired CT angiogram or MR scan to be integrated on the electroanatomical imaging created with the CARTO system (Fig. 3-34).[30-32]

QwikMapping has been introduced as a means of mapping multiple sites simultaneously. The QwikMap catheter is a multipolar catheter with six quadripolar, orthogonally arranged electrode sets located on the shaft. This allows simultaneous, direct multipoint mapping from multiple locations along the catheter to create chamber geometry and activation maps. Additionally, the QwikMap catheter is equipped with two magnetic field sensors on the shaft, which enable the precise calculation of catheter location, orientation, and trajectory by the CARTO system during the mapping procedure, which could reduce the need for fluoroscopy.

Mapping Procedure

Following selection of the reference electrogram, positioning of the anatomical reference and determination of the window of interest, the mapping catheter is positioned in the mapping chamber under fluoroscopic guidance. The 7 Fr quadripolar, deflectable catheter is initially positioned (using fluoroscopy) at known anatomical points that serve as landmarks for the electroanatomical map. For example, to map the RA, points such as the superior vena cava (SVC), inferior vena cava (IVC), HB, tricuspid annulus, and coronary sinus ostium (CS os) are marked. The catheter is then advanced slowly around the chamber walls to sample multiple points along the endocardium, sequentially acquiring the location of its tip together with the local electrogram.[7]

Points are selected only when the catheter is in stable contact with the wall. The system continuously monitors the quality of catheter-tissue contact and local activation time stability to ensure validity and reproducibility of each local measurement. The stability of the catheter and contact is evaluated at every site by examining the following: (1) local activation time stability, defined as a difference between the local activation calculated from two consecutive beats of less than 2 milliseconds; (2) location stability,

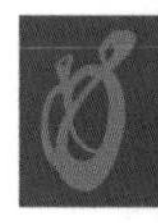

Atrial flutter, CL 268 ms

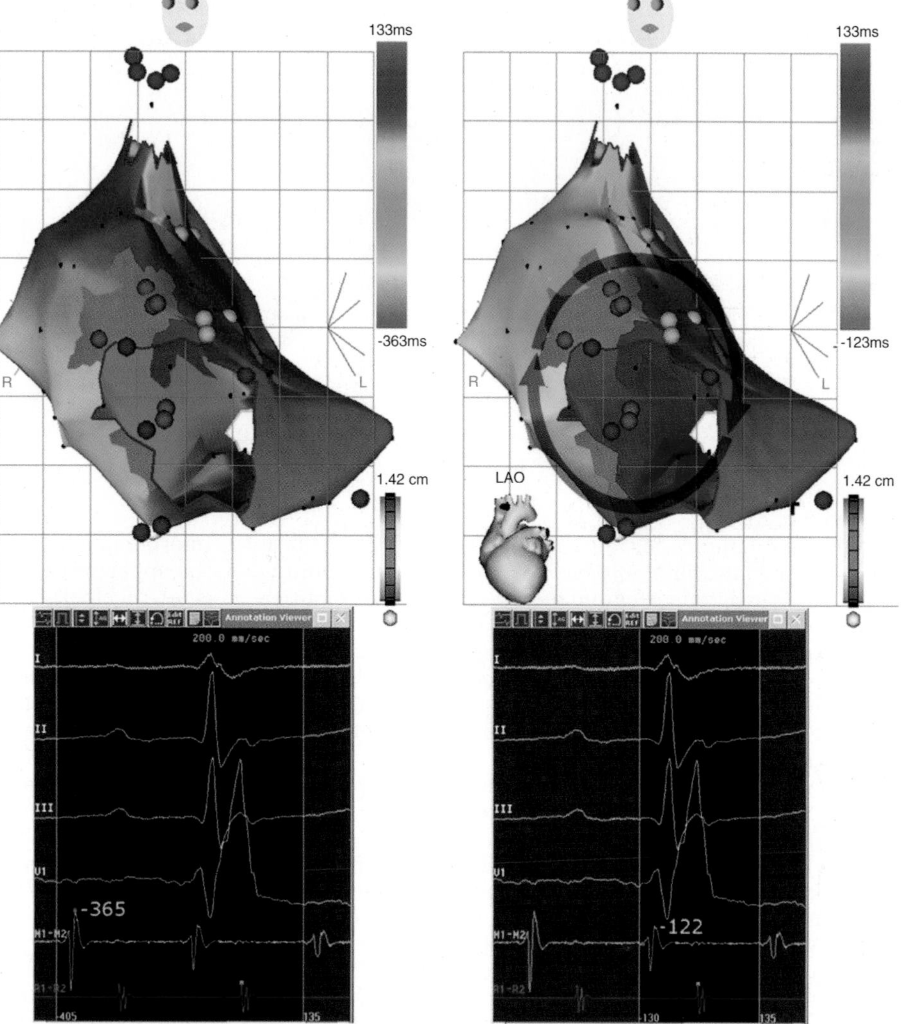

FIGURE 3–32 CARTO window of interest and influence on activation map. **Top,** Activation maps of macroreentrant typical atrial flutter, AFL (cycle length [CL], 270 milliseconds, with "clockwise" rotation around tricuspid annulus). **Bottom,** So-called window of interest for the AFL. Figures on left half show results of having the window too wide (spanning more than one tachycardia cycle); computer picks inappropriately "early" activation time (–365 milliseconds, more than the flutter CL) yielding a map (*above*) that makes little sense. When the same site has correct activation time (–123 milliseconds) assigned by narrowing the window (*lower right*), the color activation map clearly reveals peritricuspid reentry.

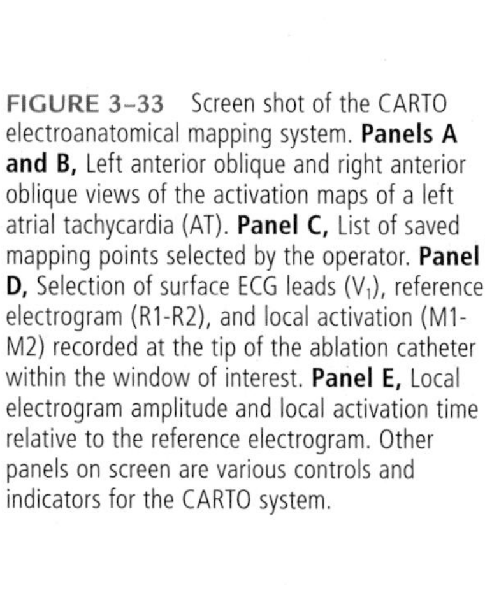

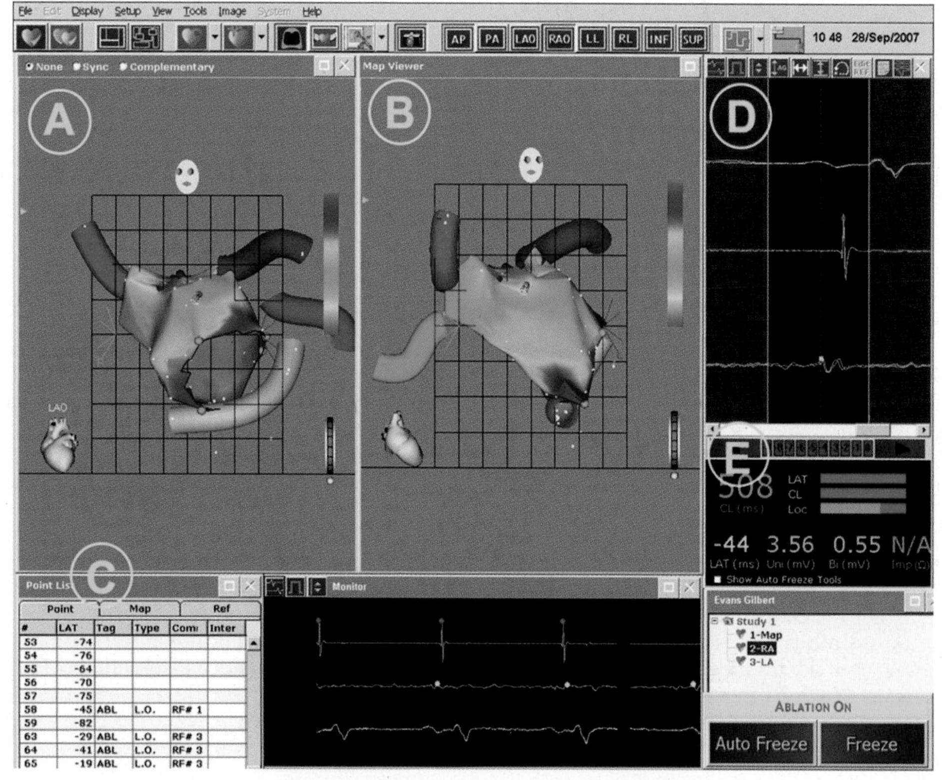

#	LAT	Tag	Type	Comm	Inter
53	-74				
54	-76				
55	-64				
56	-70				
57	-75				
58	-45	ABL	L.O.	RF# 1	
59	-82				
63	-29	ABL	L.O.	RF# 3	
64	-41	ABL	L.O.	RF# 3	
65	-19	ABL	L.O.	RF# 3	

FIGURE 3–33 Screen shot of the CARTO electroanatomical mapping system. **Panels A and B,** Left anterior oblique and right anterior oblique views of the activation maps of a left atrial tachycardia (AT). **Panel C,** List of saved mapping points selected by the operator. **Panel D,** Selection of surface ECG leads (V_1), reference electrogram (R1-R2), and local activation (M1-M2) recorded at the tip of the ablation catheter within the window of interest. **Panel E,** Local electrogram amplitude and local activation time relative to the reference electrogram. Other panels on screen are various controls and indicators for the CARTO system.

3

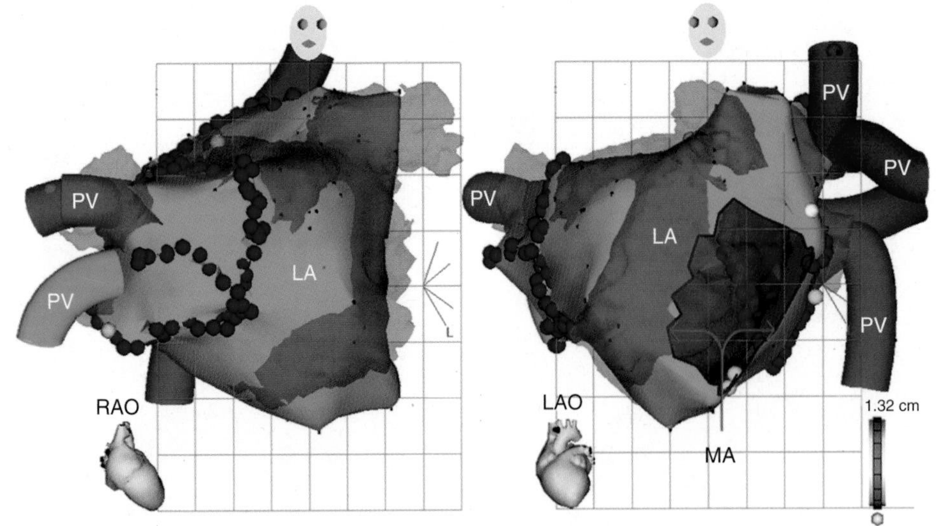

FIGURE 3–34 Integration of computed tomography (CT) and electroanatomical (EA) mapping data. Shown are right anterior oblique (RAO) and left anterior oblique (LAO) views of the electroanatomical contour acquired with catheter manipulation in the left atrium (LA) during atrial fibrillation (AF) ablation is shown overlaid on a CT image of the LA acquired several days earlier. Small red circles are tagged sites at which radiofrequency energy was applied to isolate the pulmonary vein (PV) antra. MA = mitral annulus.

defined as a distance between two consecutive gated locations of less than 2 mm; (3) morphological superpositioning of the intracardiac electrogram recorded on two consecutive beats; and (4) CL stability, defined as the difference between the CL of the last beat and the median CL during the procedure. Respiratory excursions that can cause significant shifts in apparent catheter location can be addressed by visually selecting points during the same phase of the respiratory cycle.

Each selected point is tagged on the 3-D map. The local activation time at each site is determined from the intracardiac bipolar electrogram and is measured in relation to the fixed reference electrogram. Lines of block (manifest as double potentials) are tagged for easy identification, because they can serve as boundaries for subsequent design of ablation strategies. Electrically silent areas, defined as an endocardial potential amplitude less than 0.05 mV, which is the baseline noise in the CARTO system and the absence of capture at 20 mA, and surgically related scars are tagged as "scar" and therefore appear in gray on the 3-D maps and are not assigned an activation time (see Figs. 10-1 and 10-2). The map can also be used to catalogue sites at which pacing maneuvers are performed during assessment of the tachycardia.

Sampling the location of the catheter together with the local electrogram is performed from a plurality of endocardial sites. The points sampled are connected by lines to form several adjoining triangles in a global model of the chamber. Next, gated electrograms are used to create an activation map, which is superimposed on the anatomical model. The acquired local activation times are then color-coded and superimposed on the anatomical map with red indicating early-activated sites, blue and purple late-activated areas, and yellow and green intermediate activation times (see Figs. 8-9, 8-11, and 9-6). Between these points, colors are interpolated and the adjoining triangles are colored with these interpolated values. However, if the points are widely apart, no interpolation is done. The degree to which the system will interpolate activation times is programmable (as the triangle fill threshold) and can be modified if necessary. As each new site is acquired, the reconstruction is updated in real time to create a 3-D chamber geometry color progressively encoded with activation time.[7]

Sampling an adequate number of homogeneously distributed points is necessary. If a map is incomplete, bystander sites can be mistakenly identified as part of a reentrant circuit. Regions that are poorly sampled will have activation interpolated between widely separated points. This can give the appearance of conduction, but critical features such as lines of block can be missed. In addition, low-resolution mapping can obscure other interesting phenomena, such as the second loop of a dual-loop tachycardia. Some arrhythmias, such as complex reentrant circuits, require more than 80 to 100 points to obtain adequate resolution. Other tachycardias can be mapped with fewer points, including focal tachycardias and some less complex reentrant arrhythmias, such as isthmus-dependent AFL.[29]

It is also important to identify areas of scar or central obstacles to conduction; failure to do so can confuse an electroanatomical map because interpolation of activation through areas of conduction block can give the appearance of wavefront propagation and confuse the reentrant circuit. This occurrence precludes identification of a critical isthmus in reentrant arrhythmias to target for ablation. A line of conduction block can be inferred if there are adjacent regions with wavefront propagation in opposite directions separated by a line of double potentials or dense isochrones.[29]

The electroanatomical model, which can be seen in a single view or in multiple views simultaneously and freely rotated in any direction, forms a reliable road map for navigation of the ablation catheter. Any portion of the chamber can be seen in relation to the catheter tip in real time, and points of interest can easily be revisited even without fluoroscopy. The electroanatomical maps can be presented in two or three dimensions as activation, isochronal, propagation, or voltage maps.

Activation Map. The activation maps display the local activation time color-coded overlaid on the reconstructed 3-D geometry (see Fig. 3-32; also see Figs. 8-9, 8-11, and 9-6). Activation mapping is performed to define the activation sequence. A reasonable number of points homogenously distributed in the chamber of interest have to be recorded. The selected points of local activation time are color-coded—red for the earliest electrical activation areas; orange, yellow, green, blue, and purple for progressively delayed activation areas. The electroanatomical maps of focal tachycardias demonstrate radial spreading of activation, from the earliest local activation site (red) in all directions and, in these cases, activation time is markedly shorter than tachycardia CL (see Figs. 8-9 and 8-11). On the other hand, a continuous progression of colors (from red to purple) around the mapped chamber with close proximity of earliest and latest local activation, suggests the presence of a macroreentrant tachycardia (see Figs. 9-6, 10-1, and 10-2). It is important to recognize that if an insufficient number of points is obtained in this early meets late zone, it might be falsely concluded through the interpolation of activation times that the wavefront propagates in the wrong direction.[7,29]

Isochronal Map. The system can generate isochrones of electrical activity as color-coded static maps. The isochronal map depicts all the points with an activation time within a specific range (e.g., 10 milliseconds) with the same color. Depending on conduction velocity, each color layer will be of variable width; isochrones are narrow in areas of slow conduction and broad in areas of fast conduction. Displaying information as an isochronal map helps demonstrate the direction of wavefront propagation, which is perpendicular to the isochronal lines. Furhtermore, isochronal crowding indicating a conduction velocity of 0.033 cm/msec (slower than 0.05 cm/msec) is considered a zone of slow conduction, whereas a collision of two wavefronts traveling in different directions separated temporally by 50 milliseconds is defined as a region of local block. Spontaneous zones of block or slow conduction (less than 0.033 cm/msec) may have a major role in the stabilization of certain arrhythmias.[7]

Propagation Map. The CARTO system also can generate color-coded animated dynamic maps of activation wavefront (propagation maps). This is a two-colored map, in which the whole chamber is blue and electrical activation waves are seen in red, spreading throughout the chamber as a continuous animated loop (see Figs. 8-11 and 9-6). Propagation of electrical activation is visualized superimposed on the 3-D anatomical reconstruction of the cardiac chamber in relation to the anatomical landmarks and barriers. Analysis of the propagation map can allow estimation of the conduction velocity along the reentrant circuit and identification of areas of slow conduction.

Voltage Map. The voltage map displays the peak-to-peak amplitude of the electrogram sampled at each site. This value is color-coded and superimposed on the anatomical model, with red as the lowest amplitude and orange, yellow, green, blue, and purple indicating progressively higher amplitudes (Fig. 3-35). The gain on the 3-D color display allows the user to concentrate on a narrow or wide range of potentials. By diminishing the color scale, as might be required to see a fascicular potential or diastolic depolarization during reentry, larger amplitude signals will be eliminated. To visualize the broad spectrum of potentials present during a tachycardia cycle, the scale would be opened up to include an array of colors representing a spectrum of voltages. Local electrogram voltage mapping during sinus, paced, or any other rhythm can help define anatomically correct regions of no voltage (presumed scars or electrical scars), low voltage, and normal voltage, although the true range of normal is often difficult to define, especially with bipolar recordings, and different criteria have been used. Myocardial scars are seen as low voltage, and their delineation can help in understanding the location of the arrhythmia.

Clinical Implications

The capability of the CARTO system to associate relevant EP information with the appropriate spatial location in the heart and the ability to study activation patterns with high spatial resolution (less than 1 mm) during tachycardia in relation to normal anatomical structures and areas of scar significantly facilitate the mapping and ablation procedure. This mapping system facilitates defining the mechanism(s) underlying the arrhythmia, rapid distinction between a focal origin and macroreentrant tachycardia, precise description of macroreentrant circuits and sequence of activation during the tachycardia, understanding of the reentrant circuit in relation to native barriers and surgical scars, identification of all slow-conducting pathways, rapid visualization of the activation wavefront (propagation maps), and identification of appropriate sites for entrainment and pace mapping.[18,33-35]

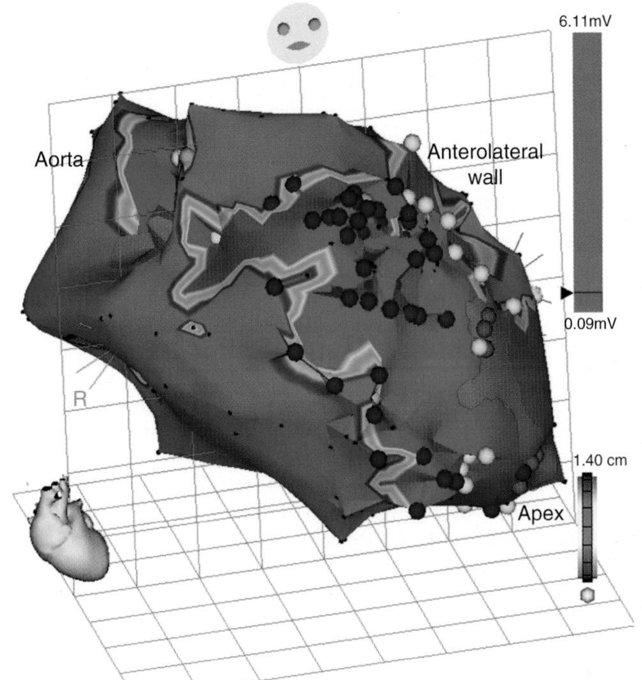

FIGURE 3–35 Electroanatomical (CARTO) voltage map of the left ventricle in a patient with ventricular tachycardia after anteroapical myocardial infarction. An adjusted voltage scale is shown at right; all sites with voltage less than 0.5 mV are colored red on the map, and those with voltage more than 0.6 mV are purple, with interpolation of color for intermediate amplitudes. The gray area denotes no detectable signal (scar). A large anteroapical infarction is clearly evident. Red circles denote ablation sites.

The CARTO system provides a highly accurate geometric rendering of a cardiac chamber with a straightforward geometric display having the capability to determine the 3-D location and orientation of the ablation catheter accurately. The position of the mapping tip at any point in time is readily apparent from a tip icon, providing that the tip is at or beyond the rendered chamber geometry. The catheter can anatomically and accurately revisit a critically important recording site (e.g., sites with double potentials or those with good pace maps) identified previously during the study, even if the tachycardia is no longer present or inducible and map-guided catheter navigation is no longer possible. This accurate repositioning provides significant advantages over conventional techniques and is of great value in ablation procedures. Ablation lesions can be tagged, facilitating creation of lines of block with considerable accuracy by serial RF lesion placement and allowing verification of the continuity of ablation line (see Fig. 3-34). This is of particular value after incomplete ablations caused by catheter dislocation or early coagulum formation, especially if these ablations had caused interruption of the target tachycardia. Extra RF applications can be delivered closely around an apparently successful ablation site to ensure elimination of the arrhythmogenic area.[7]

Voltage maps can help define the arrhythmogenic substrate when the arrhythmia arises in the setting of cardiac structural abnormalities, which is of particular value during mapping of hemodynamically unstable or nonsustained arrhythmias. Additionally, fluoroscopy time can be reduced via electromagnetic catheter navigation, and the catheter can be accurately guided to positions removed from fluoroscopic markers. Although fluoroscopy is always needed for initial orientation, an experienced operator can usually generate an extensive endocardial activation map with substantially reduced radiation exposure for himself or herself and for the patient and laboratory staff.[7]

Limitations

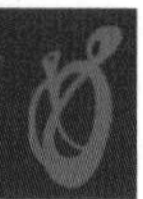

The sequential data acquisition required for map creation remains very time-consuming, because the process of creation of an electroanatomical map requires tagging many points, depending on the spatial details needed to analyze a given arrhythmia. Because the acquired data are not coherent in time, multiple beats are required and stable, sustained, or frequently repetitive arrhythmia is usually needed for creation of the activation map. Because these points do not provide real-time, constantly updated information, more time can be needed for making new maps to see a current endocardial activation sequence, detect a change in arrhythmia, or fully visualize multiple tachycardias. In addition, rapidly changing or transient arrhythmias are not easily recorded, and may only be mapped if significant substrate abnormalities are present. Variation of the tachycardia CL of more than 10% can prevent complete understanding of a circuit, and decreases the confidence in the CARTO map. Single PVCs or PACs or nonsustained events may be mapped, although at the expense of an appreciable amount of time.

If highly fractionated and wide potentials are present, it can be difficult to assign an activation time. In some macroreentrant circuits, large percentages of the tachycardia CL are occupied by fractionated low-amplitude potentials. If these potentials are dismissed or assigned relatively late activation times, a macroreentrant tachycardia might mimic a focal arrhythmia, and it will appear as if substantially less than 90% of the tachycardia CL is mapped.

The patient or the intracardiac reference catheter can move, thus necessitating remapping. Additionally, a change in rhythm can alter cardiac geometry to the extent that anatomical points acquired during one rhythm cannot be relied on after a change in rhythm.

Another limitation of the CARTO system is the requirement of a special Biosense Webster catheter. No other catheter types may be used with this system, and bidirectional steerable catheters are not available. Furthermore, the magnetic signal necessary for the CARTO system can create interference with other EP laboratory recording systems. Implantable cardioverter-defibrillators (ICDs) and pacemakers are safe with the system but the magnetic field can prevent device communication with its programmer, and the magnetic field may need to be disabled temporarily to allow device programming.

The QwikMap catheter approach has been suggested as a means of mapping multiple sites simultaneously. The surface geometries so created may be somewhat distorted if the chamber under examination distends with the mapping catheter. When including both tip points and shaft points, the chamber geometries tend to be artificially large. Annotation of the location of specific ablative sites on the surface geometry with this new software may be a laborious process.

ENSITE NAVX NAVIGATION SYSTEM

Fundamental Concepts

The EnSite NavX system (St. Jude Medical, Austin, Tex) consists of a set of three pairs of skin patches, a data module, a system reference patch, ten ECG electrodes, and a display workstation. The EnSite NavX combines catheter location and tracking features of the LocaLisa system (Medtronic, Minneapolis, Minn) with the ability to create an anatomical model of the cardiac chamber using only a single conventional EP catheter and skin patches.[28,36]

This mapping modality is based on currents across the thorax, developed as originally applied in the LocaLisa system. In contrast to the NavX system, LocaLisa does not allow generation of 3-D geometry of the heart cavity because catheters and desired anatomical landmarks are displayed in a Cartesian frame of reference.[7] This technology has undergone substantial additional development in the NavX iteration. When an electrical current is externally applied through the thorax, a voltage drop occurs across internal organs like the heart. The resulting voltage can be recorded via standard catheter electrodes and potentially can be used to determine electrode position. Analogous to the Frank lead system, three orthogonal electrode pairs (skin patches) positioned on the body surface are used to send three independent, alternating, low-power currents of 350 μA at a frequency of 5.7 kHz through the patient's chest in three orthogonal (x, y, and z) directions, with slightly different frequencies of approximately 30 kHz used for each direction. The mixture of the 30-kHz signals, recorded from each catheter electrode, is digitally separated to measure the amplitude of each of the three frequency components. The three electrical field strengths are calculated automatically by use of the difference in amplitudes measured from neighboring electrode pairs with a known interelectrode distance for three or more different spatial orientations of that dipole. The 3-D position of each electrode is then calculated by dividing each of the three amplitudes (V) by the corresponding electrical field strength (V/cm). The specific position of a catheter tip within the chamber can then be established, based on the three resulting potentials measured in the recording tip with respect to a reference electrode seen over the distance from each patch set to that recording tip. The NavX system allows real-time visualization of the position and motion of up to 64 electrodes on both ablation and standard catheters positioned elsewhere in the heart (Fig. 3-36).

The NavX system also allows for rapid creation of detailed models of cardiac anatomy (see Fig. 3-36). Sequential positioning of a catheter at multiple sites along the endocardial surface of a specific chamber establishes that chamber's geometry. The system automatically acquires points from a nominated electrode(s) at a rate of 96 points/sec. Chamber geometry is created by several thousand points. The algorithm defines the surface by using the most distant points in any given angle from the geometry center, which can be chosen by the operator or defined by the system. In addition, the operator is able to specify fixed points that represent contact points during geometry acquisition; these points cannot be eliminated by the algorithm that calculates the surface. In addition to mapping at specific points, there is additional interpolation, providing a smooth surface, onto which activation voltages and times can be registered. To control for variations related to the cardiac cycle, acquisition can be gated to any electrogram.

Activation and voltage mapping was not possible with the previous version of NavX; however, a recent software upgrade has been released, permitting these mapping techniques (see Fig. 3-36). Additionally, the EnSite Digital Image Fusion (DIF) allows for simultaneously displaying 3-D maps side by side with CT or MR segmented cardiac scans to confirm cardiac structures and guide therapy.

Mapping Procedure

NavX-guided procedures are performed using the same catheter setup as conventional approaches. Any electrode

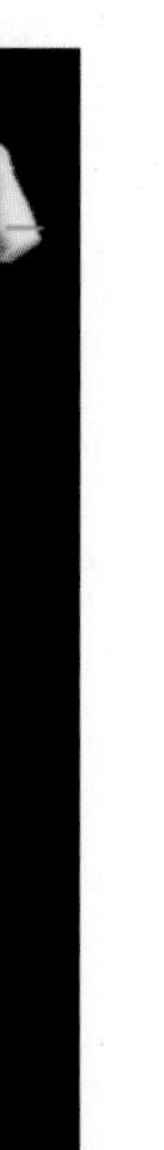

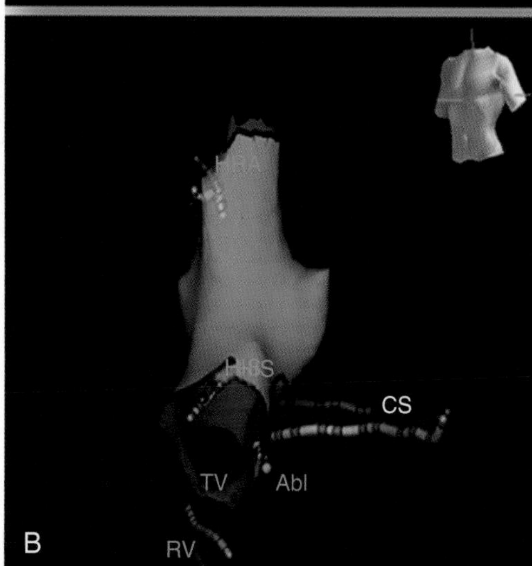

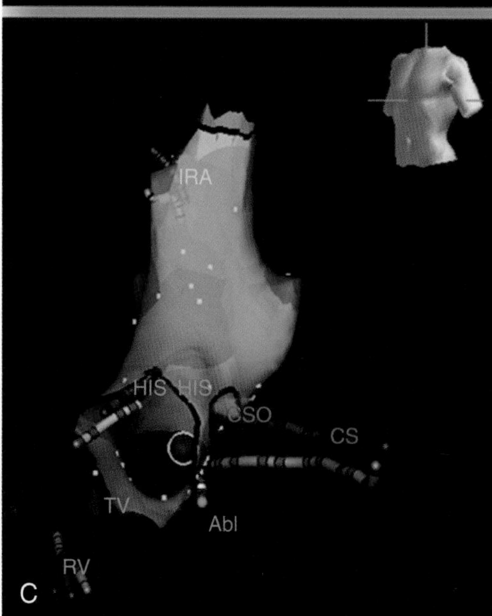

FIGURE 3-36 The NavX system. **A,** Left anterior oblique view of four standard diagnostic catheters (positioned in the high right atrium [HRA], His bundle [His], right ventricular (RV) apex, and coronary sinus [CS]) and a standard ablation catheter (Abl) as visualized by the NavX system during mapping of a focal atrial tachycardia. Note the shadows placed over the four diagnostic catheters to record their original position and recognize displacement during the procedure. **B,** A virtual anatomical geometry of the RA is acquired by moving the catheter in all directions throughout the chamber of interest. Any electrode catheter (not just the mapping catheter) can be used to create the 3-D geometry. **C,** Color-coded activation map superimposed on the RA 3-D geometry localizing the origin of the atrial tachycardia to the triangle of Koch between the His bundle, coronary sinus ostium (CSO), and tricuspid valve (TV).

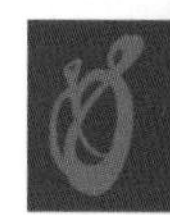

can be used to gather data, create static isochronal and voltage maps, and perform ablation procedures. Standard EP catheters of choice are introduced into the heart; up to 12 catheters and 64 electrodes can be viewed simultaneously. The system can locate the position of the catheters from the moment that they are inserted in the vein. Therefore, all catheters can be navigated to the heart under guidance of the EnSite NavX system and the use of fluoroscopy can be minimized for preliminary catheter positioning. However, interrupted fluoroscopy has to be used repeatedly when an obstacle to catheter advancement is encountered. Once in the heart, one intracardiac catheter is used as reference for geometry reconstruction. A shadow (to record original position) is placed over this catheter to recognize displacement during the procedure, in which case the catheter can be returned easily to its original location under the guidance of NavX. A shadow can also be displayed on each of the other catheters to record the catheter's spatial position (see Fig. 3-36).

Subsequently, 3-D intracardiac geometry is obtained. Characteristic anatomical landmarks in the chamber of interest are initially acquired and marked. The locations of veins are established and readily displayed by the juxtaposition of multiple mapping markers, or sphere stacking, spheres along the length of that vein. The size of each marker is based on size selection rather than actual vessel dimensions. The system is then allowed to create the geometry automatically. A virtual anatomical geometry is acquired by moving the catheter in all directions throughout the chamber of interest, keeping contact with the endocardial wall.[37,38]

Additional tagging of sites of interest and ablation points can be done during the procedure. Point-to-point activation mapping is carried out to create static isochronal, voltage, and activation maps (see Fig. 3-36). Standard catheters are used to sample voltage and activation timing at various locations during a sustained rhythm. The system collects and visually organizes activation timing and voltage data and permanently saves 10 beats with every collected point for later review. An unlimited number of maps can be created per procedure. The system works with most manufacturers' ablation catheters and RF or cryogenerators. Ablation lesions can be tagged, facilitating creation of lines of block with considerable accuracy by serial RF lesion placement, and allowing verification of the continuity of ablation line.[37]

Clinical Implications

NavX is a novel mapping and navigation system with the ability to visualize and navigate a complete set of intracardiac catheters in any cardiac chamber for diagnostic and therapeutic applications.[28] It enables electrophysiologists to display in real time up to 64 electrodes simultaneously on

12 catheters with almost every commercially available catheter, including pacemaker leads. Earlier versions of NavX permitted the creation of 3-D cardiac geometry by using all these catheters, without visualization of electrical activity. Thus, they are particularly suitable for ablation of arrhythmias with well-known substrates that can be treated by an anatomical approach, such as AFL and linear LA ablation for AF.[37-40] A recent software upgrade allowing point-to-point activation mapping for the NavX system has also been introduced. This is a substantial improvement, permitting the same type of activation mapping and display as is possible with other systems, with the similar advantage of specified voltage mapping as well. This point-to-point mapping, however, is only suited for sustained arrhythmias

or frequently recurrent PACs, PVCs, or nonsustained arrhythmias. This can be augmented by the addition of noncontact mapping to the procedure.[28]

NavX technology has an important advantage in reducing the operator's and patient's radiation exposure. The fact that catheters can be positioned for ablation without the use of fluoroscopy is important, because NavX allows the display of catheters from the puncture site to the final destination in the heart. Indeed, this nonfluoroscopic navigation system allows real-time assessment of wall contact and catheter stability as well as assessment of the anatomical position and the relation between the ablation catheter and other intracardiac catheters. Because of these capabilities, catheter displacement and insufficient wall contact are readily recognized without the use of fluoroscopy, resulting in reduction of radiation exposure, procedure duration, and the trend to reduced RF energy delivery.

The ablation procedure is also facilitated by NavX.[28,37,39,40] The system works with most manufacturers' ablation catheters and RF or cryogenerators. The ablation lesions can be tagged, facilitating creation of lines of block with considerable accuracy by serial RF lesion placement, and allowing verification of the continuity of the ablation line and anatomical visualization of the remaining gaps, where additional RF applications can be delivered. It also helps avoid repeated ablations at the same location. The catheter can anatomically and accurately revisit a critically important recording site identified previously during the study.

In contrast to CARTO, NavX allows simultaneous visualization of all catheters and permits use of a wide selection of catheter types.[28] The NavX system acquires points at a speed of 96 points/sec, much faster than the CARTO system. Also, chamber geometry created by the NavX system can identify and tag anatomical landmarks with a much higher resolution than that created by the CARTO system. This is because in the CARTO system, the manually acquired points are limited, only up to a total of 50 to 100 points, whereas in the NavX system the points are acquired automatically and the geometry is created by several thousand points.

Limitations

The point-to-point activation mapping required while using the NavX system is only suited for sustained arrhythmias or frequently recurrent ectopy or nonsustained arrhythmias. Additionally, in the NavX system, the algorithm defines the surface by using the most distant points in any given angle from the geometric center, and the catheter can protrude out against the wall of the cardiac chamber when acquiring points; thus, chamber geometry of the NavX system is oversized. Furthermore, with individual interpolation schemes, significant anatomical distortions in complex structures can occur unless a family of fixed points is incorporated into the geometry to preserve critical junctions between those structures. Appropriate filtering has decreased this problem.

REAL-TIME POSITION MANAGEMENT SYSTEM

Fundamental Concepts

The Real-time Position Management (RPM) system (Boston Scientific, Natick, Mass) combines full EP recording functionality with advanced mapping, navigation, and catheter visualization.[28] For this system, two reference catheters and one mapping-ablation catheter are used. This 3-D mapping system uses ultrasound ranging techniques to determine the position of a mapping-ablation catheter relative to the two reference catheters. One reference catheter is positioned in the CS and the other in the RV apex.[28] The mapping-ablation catheter is a 7 Fr, 4-mm tip bidirectional steerable catheter. The reference catheters have a 6 Fr fixed curve distal shaft. The shaft of the CS reference catheter contains nine 1-mm ring electrodes and one 2-mm tip electrode (interelectrode distance, 1 mm), whereas the RV reference and ablation catheters contain three 1-mm ring electrodes and one 4-mm tip electrode (interelectrode distance, 1 mm).[7]

The ultrasound transmitter device sends a continuous cycle of ultrasound pulses (558.5 kHz) to the transducers of the reference and ablation catheters.[28] By measuring the time delay from the departure of a transmitted ultrasound pulse and the reception of this pulse at the other transducers, assuming a speed of sound in blood of 1550 m/sec, the distance between the individual transducers can be calculated. These data are used to define the location of the catheter(s) within the reference frame. Once the 3-D reference frame is established, triangulation can be used to track the position of additional transducers. Because dimensional and structural characteristics of the catheter are known, it is possible to construct a real-time 3-D graphic representation of the catheters, including the position of the electrodes and transducer. As one of the transducers is positioned distally to the deflection point of the shaft of the catheter, it is possible to display the curvature of the catheter as well. Furthermore, the RPM system graphically displays the beat-to-beat movement of the tip of the catheters.[7]

The geometry generated with this approach is built with point-to-point sequential catheter positioning. Because of multiorder interpolation for establishing the surface geometry, critical fixed or snap points must be specified and incorporated into the chamber geometry to prevent interpolation obliteration from obscuring intersections of uniquely shaped structures, such as PVs.

Clinical Implications

The RPM system provides both nonfluoroscopic visualization and navigation plus the ability to recall displays of the catheter positions associated with previously recorded electrogram events. The RPM system displays the ablation catheter and the reference diagnostic catheters. Furthermore, the catheter images show the full, real-time, nonfluoroscopic display of catheter curves (not just the tip electrode) for up to seven catheters (ablation and diagnostic). The original position of the reference catheters can be displayed on the real-time window, thereby allowing repositioning of catheters after displacement.[7]

The RPM system can simultaneously process and display 24 bipolar or 48 unipolar electrograms and a 12-lead ECG. The system allows synchronous recording of catheter positions and electrograms and the creation and display of local or global isochronal maps. The real-time display of the catheter tip and the possibility of on-line retrieval of previous positions and curves of a catheter facilitate repositioning of a catheter at previously marked sites. Hence, use of this system can potentially reduce fluoroscopy time. Additionally, there is a fully integrated functionality for conventional recording system. A recent upgrade has allowed the system to reconstruct color-coded activation maps.[7]

Routine application of the RPM system requires only the use of special catheters; no additional catheters or skin electrodes are needed. Because any type of catheter containing ultrasound transducers can be tracked within the reference frame and used to locate positions, it is possible to position, for example, two catheters simultaneously in the RA and the LA to create lesions using this guidance system. This can be useful in case of the creation of linear lesions in AF patients. The ability to create lesions within a defined area will allow systematic ablation of endocardial zones of slow conduction critical for the perpetuation of reentrant VT.

Limitations

The RPM system requires the use of specified catheters fitted with the ultrasound transducers. Moreover, failure of ultrasound transducers, requiring replacement of a catheter, occurs occasionally. In addition, a voltage map cannot be obtained.[7]

STEREOTAXIS MAGNETIC NAVIGATION SYSTEM

Fundamental Concepts

Catheter navigation by magnetic force was initially introduced in the early 1990s for diagnostic studies in neonates. However, the development of conventional steerable electrodes with integrated pull wires to deflect the catheter tip was pursued, and this constitutes the current technique for catheter ablation. The conventional technique is limited by the fixed maximal catheter deflection and relies mostly on the skill of the investigator to ensure stable catheter positioning. A novel magnetic navigation system (MNS; 0.15 T, Telstar, Stereotaxis, St. Louis, Mo) has recently been introduced to clinical practice. It has proven to be a safe and feasible tool for catheter ablation, although it did not allow remote catheter ablation. The second-generation MNS (Niobe, Stereotaxis) now allows, for the first time, complete, remote RF catheter ablation.[41-43]

The Niobe MNS consists of two permanent neodymium-iron-boron magnets; their positions, relative to each other, are computer-controlled inside a fixed housing and positioned on either side of the single-plane fluoroscopy table.[41-43] While positioned in the "navigate" position, the magnets create a 360-degree omnidirectional rotation of the device by a uniform magnetic field (0.08 T) within an approximately spherical navigation volume 20 cm in diameter (NaviSphere), sufficient to encompass the heart when the patient is properly positioned. The combination of rotation, translation, and tilt movements of the magnets adjusts the magnetic field to any desired orientation within the NaviSphere.[41-43]

The mapping and ablation catheters are extremely flexible distally, especially the distal shaft of the ablation catheters, and have tiny magnets (single or multiple, in various configurations) inserted in their distal portion. The latest catheters have three tiny magnets distributed along the distal shaft and tip of the catheter to increase responsiveness of the catheter to the magnetic field generated (Fig. 3-37). The catheter magnets align themselves with the direction of the externally controlled magnetic field to enable the catheter tip to be steered effectively. By changing the orientation of the outer magnets relative to each other, the orientation of the magnetic field changes, thereby leading to deflection of the catheter.[41-43]

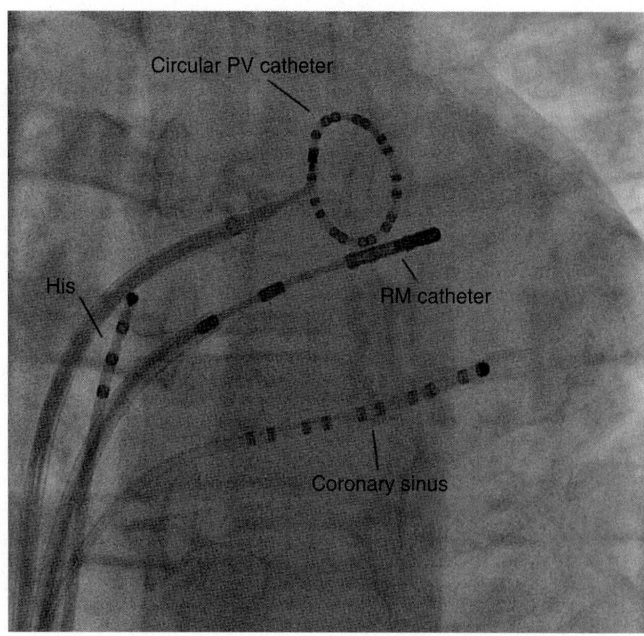

FIGURE 3–37 Stereotaxis catheters (Stereotaxis, St. Louis, Mo). Anteroposterior fluoroscopic view of the Stereotaxis remote magnetic (RM) catheter in the left atrium. A multipolar circular mapping catheter, coronary sinus, and His bundle catheters are also shown. The RM catheter has a large distal mapping and ablation electrode; this, as well as three other opaque regions more proximally on the catheter shaft, contain magnetic elements that conform to changes in direction of an externally applied magnetic field.

The system is integrated with a modified C-arm digital x-ray system, mainly a single-plane unit because of the limitations imposed by the magnets, although a biplane system can be installed for use when the magnets are stowed and not in use. Because of the magnets, the rotation of the imaging system is limited to approximately 30 degrees right anterior oblique (RAO) and left anterior oblique (LAO) in Niobe I and almost 45 degrees with Niobe II. In the Niobe I iteration, the magnets can only be swung in (active navigation) or stowed, whereas in the Niobe II the magnets have a different housing and can also be tilted to allow for more angulation of the single-plane C-arm imaging system.[41-43]

It is important to emphasize that the external magnetic field does not pull or push the tiny magnets and the catheters or guidewires in which they are contained. The position of the magnetic catheter within the heart is controlled by manual advancement or retraction of the catheter through the vascular sheath. A computer-controlled catheter advancer system (Cardiodrive unit, Stereotaxis) is used to allow truly remote catheter navigation without the need for manual manipulation. The operator is positioned in a separate control room, at a distance from the x-ray beam and the patient's body. The graphic workstation (Navigant II, Stereotaxis), in conjunction with the Cardiodrive unit, allows precise orientation of the catheter by 1-degree increments and by 1-mm steps in advancement or retraction. The system is controlled by a joystick or mouse and allows remote control of the ablation catheter from inside the control room. Additionally, the x-ray image data can be transferred from the x-ray system to the user interface of the magnetic navigation system to provide an anatomical reference.[41-43]

Directional catheter navigation is accomplished by drawing a desired magnetic field vector on orthogonal fluoroscopic views with a digitization tablet (Fig. 3-38).[41,43] A control computer then calculates the appropriate currents to each of the superconducting electromagnets. The resultant composite magnetic field interacts with a permanent

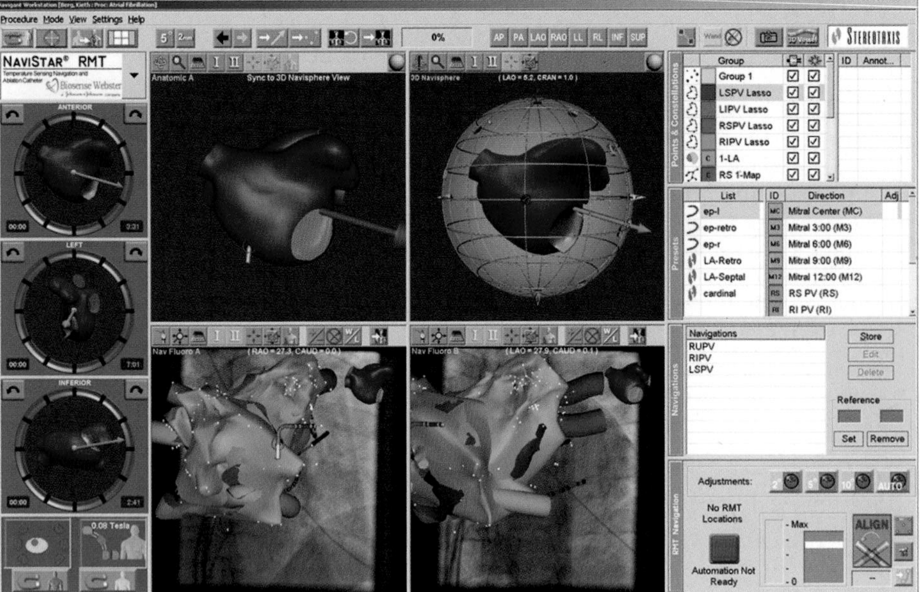

FIGURE 3-38 Stereotaxis monitor—screen shot of the remote magnetic guidance system (Stereotaxis, St. Louis, Mo). **Top two central panels,** Representation of idealized left atrium shells with a green arrow ("vector") that can be pointed in any direction with a computer mouse, commanding the magnetic steering mechanism to deflect the catheter tip in that direction. **Bottom two central panels,** shell generated by electroanatomical mapping, integrated with the images on the Stereotaxis unit. These overlie the patient's initial right anterior oblique and left anterior oblique fluoroscopic images. Tubular structures are the pulmonary veins and coronary sinus (pink). Other panels on the screen are various controls and indicators for the Stereotaxis manipulation.

magnet in the tip of the magnetic ablation catheter and deflects the catheter to align parallel to the magnetic field. Magnetic field orientations corresponding to specific map points can be stored on the MNS and reapplied to return repeatedly and accurately to previously visited locations on the map. Navigation to a particular target often requires two or three manipulations of the magnetic field to refine the catheter position. Each magnetic field manipulation requires less than 20 seconds to activate. By changing the orientation of the outer magnets, the orientation of the magnetic field changes, thereby leading to the deflection of the catheter in parallel.[41-43]

More recently, the MNS has become integrated with a newly developed electroanatomical mapping system, the CARTO RMT system (Biosense Webster, Diamond Bar, Calif). The CARTO RMT system is able to send real-time catheter tip location and orientation data to the magnetic navigation system. It also sends target locations, groups of points, and anatomical surface information from the electroanatomical map to the magnetic navigation system.

Mapping Procedure

All the components of the MNS, as well as the x-ray, ablator, and stimulator, can be operated from the control room. Therefore, after initial placement of sheaths and catheters, the entire ablation procedure can be performed remotely from the control room. The Navigant system is the computerized graphical user interface system. It includes the software used for image integration and for control of the magnetic fields that orient the catheter within the heart, which allows the operator to direct the movement of the tip of the catheter to access the region of interest (see Fig. 3-38).[41-43]

After synchronizing with respiratory and cardiac cycles, such as inspiration and end-diastolic period, a pair of best-matched RAO-LAO images are transferred and kept in the Navigant screen as background references for orientation and navigation (see Fig. 3-38). Thus, the real-time catheter location information can be displayed on the Navigant reference x-ray images, enabling continuous real-time monitoring of the catheter tip position, even without acquiring a fresh x-ray image.[41-43]

The operator can access an area of interest using vector-based or target-based navigation. In vector-based navigation the operator tells the system, by drawing a vector in virtual 3-D space on the computer, what orientation of the magnetic field is required. In target-based navigation a target is placed on a specified point using the stored orthogonal fluoroscopic views; the user marks the support or base of the catheter (the distal portion of the sheath) on the pair of x-ray images. This provides Navigant with the data needed to compute field orientations corresponding to particular targets. Each time a vector is selected or a target is marked, the computer sends information to the magnets, which changes their relative orientation, and with it the orientation of the uniform magnetic field in the chest, so that catheter orientation is then changed within a few seconds (see Fig. 3-38). A target can also be defined by selecting a preset magnetic field vector based on a selected study protocol from the list on the Navigant. The software contains a number of preset vectors selected by the manufacturer, after careful appraisal of multiple CT images and reconstructions, for positioning the catheter at various anatomical landmarks. When a preset vector is applied, it can steer the catheter near the approximate region indicated. In addition, the software can be used to map various chambers of the heart automatically.[41-43]

The magnetic catheter is advanced to target positions in the cardiac chamber of interest and guided by using the x-ray system, user interface monitors, and catheter advancer (Cardiodrive) system, which allows precise orientation of the catheter in extremely small increments (1-degree increments, by 1-mm steps) within the heart and vessels in advancement or retraction, making mapping more accurate. All vectors and targets selected can be saved, as can relative positions of the catheter advancer system, allowing specific areas in the heart or side branches of vessels to be revisited reproducibly.

CARTO RMT has also been integrated with the MNS and has been specifically redesigned to work in the magnetic environment of Stereotaxis. CARTO RMT includes all the latest updates such as CARTO Merge, in which a 3-D reconstruction of a CT or MR image can be integrated into the electroanatomical map. With the CARTO integration, there is communication between the two systems, allowing for real-time catheter orientation and positioning data to be sent from CARTO to the Stereotaxis system, and for the catheter tip to be displayed on the saved images stored on the Navigant system. This permits tracking of the ablation catheter without having to update the radiographic image as often.

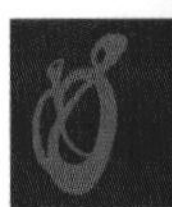

Magnetic vectors can also be applied from the CARTO screen. A feature called "design line" can be used to send a line of points—either for mapping a specific area, or potentially as a line of ablation points. "Click and go" is a tool allowing for an area of the map to be clicked on to set a target and have the system guide the catheter to this point. Because Stereotaxis and CARTO have feedback integration, the CARTO system can feed back to the Stereotaxis system if the exact point is not reached, allowing for further automatic compensation by the software until the desired point is reached. The combined system has the capability of automatically mapping chambers (anatomy and activation times) using predetermined scripts. The accuracy of such automaps is highly dependent on the anatomy, as well as where in the heart the operator designates the starting point for mapping. At present, 4- and 8-mm tip and irrigated tip RF catheters are available.

Clinical Implications

Precise target localization and catheter stability are prerequisite for successful RF applications and to minimize risks of potential complications. Stiff, manually deflectable catheters, with a unidirectional or bidirectional deflection radius, which deflect in a single plane, have several inherent limitations, because stable wall contact can be difficult to achieve, particularly in regions of complex cardiac anatomy. In contrast, the promise of the current MNS lies in the precision of catheter movement and the ability to steer the flexible distal portion of the catheter in any direction in 3-D space.[41-43]

The MNS is being increasingly used for ablation of AVNRT, AV BTs, idiopathic outflow tract VTs, and especially AF. Intracardiac electrograms and stimulation thresholds are not significantly different from those recorded with a standard, manually deflected ablation catheter, and the safety of standard EP procedures has not been compromised by use of the MNS.[41-43]

Although the current MNS does not offer a distinct advantage over conventional catheters for navigation to targets that are easily reached, it has potential advantages for complex catheter maneuvers and navigation to sites that are exceptionally difficult to reach with a standard catheter. In addition, catheter mobility and endocardial stability can be superior by virtue of the compliance of the distal catheter and lack of constraints on the magnetic vector used to steer the catheter. Cardiac and respiratory motion can be buffered by the catheter compliance, thereby contributing to endocardial contact stability.

After the diagnostic catheters are positioned, the EP study and ablation process can be performed completely from inside the control room. This offers several potential advantages, including reducing fluoroscopic exposure time for the operator, reducing the strain from standing next to the bed for long periods wearing a lead apron, and facilitating simultaneous catheter navigation and electrogram analysis.

A unique feature of the current MNS is that the magnetic vector coordinates used to navigate the magnetic catheter to a particular site can be stored and reused later in the study to return to a site of interest. The integration of a stable magnetic catheter with the CARTO electroanatomical mapping system is useful to reconstruct an accurate electroanatomical map by acquiring many more points than are possible manually for successful ablation, even of challenging areas.[43]

The maximum tissue force that can be applied by the flexible catheter used in the MNS is less than the average, and significantly less than the maximum that can be applied using a standard catheter. Because of the flexibility of the catheters, cardiac perforation is extremely unlikely and has not been reported to date.

Limitations

A potential limitation of the MNS is the interference induced by the magnetic field in the surface ECG.[41-43] The origin of the induced potentials is thought to be attributable to blood flow within the magnetic field. Blood is an electrolyte solution that can induce the potential because of motion within the magnetic field. The magnetic field strength used for catheter manipulation is about one order of magnitude less than that associated with MR imaging. The interaction of the magnetic field with the surface ECG is, therefore, less in magnitude compared to MR and is restricted to the ST segment, and the temporal distribution of the interfering signal component probably would not compromise cardiac rhythm analysis, or analysis of the P wave or QRS morphology. However, interpretation of changes in the ST segment would be predictably compromised by this interference. Whether this distortion will affect arrhythmia analysis is currently being investigated.

Claustrophobia and morbid obesity are contraindications for using the MNS because of the restricted space within the MNS. The next generation of the MNS features an open design that is more comfortable for obese patients and those with claustrophobia.[41-43] Patients with pacemakers or defibrillators are also excluded because of electromagnetic interference. Further study is required to determine whether the magnetic field strength is compatible with pacemakers or defibrillators.[41-43] Additionally, the MNS requires monitoring instruments that are compatible with magnetic fields.

The angulation of the fluoroscopic system is limited to 30 to 45 degrees for both LAO and RAO projections when the magnets are in the "navigate" position. Although this may not be important in simple ablations, addressing more complex substrates can be more challenging.[41-43]

The MNS is an evolving technology. Further technical development through the availability of additional catheter designs (e.g., number of recording electrodes) is necessary to address more complex arrhythmias in the future.

BODY SURFACE POTENTIAL MAPPING

Fundamental Concepts

Although extensively used, the limitations of the conventional 12-lead ECG for optimal detection of cardiac abnormalities are widely appreciated. The main deficiency in the 12-lead approach is the fact that only six chest electrodes are incorporated, which cover a relatively constrained area of the precordium. The main reason for the choice of the location of the conventional precordial electrodes, suggested by Wilson over 70 years ago, was the need to adopt some standard, which to this day has remained relatively unchallenged. In the years since then, the growing appreciation for the limitations of the conventional precordial electrode positions and the increase in understanding of the localization of various cardiac abnormalities on the body surface has led to the suggestion of various alternatives.[44,45]

One of the most widely studied alternatives to the 12-lead ECG in clinical and experimental electrocardiology has been body surface potential mapping (BSPM). In this approach, anywhere from 32 to 219 electrodes are used in an attempt to sample all electrocardiographic information as projected onto the body's surface. The merits of this enhanced spatial sampling are obvious, in that localized abnormalities that might be difficult to detect using the 12-

lead approach can readily be picked up with the additional electrodes.[44]

BSPM is defined as the temporal sequence of potential distributions observed on the thorax throughout one or more electrical cardiac cycles. BSPM is an extension of conventional ECG aimed at refining the noninvasive characterization and use of cardiac-generated potentials. The improved characterization is accomplished by increased spatial sampling of the body surface ECG, recorded as tens or even hundreds of unipolar ECGs, simultaneously or individually, with subsequent time alignment.[45]

BSPMs provide much more electrical and diagnostic information than the 12-lead ECG. They contain all the electrical information that can be obtained from the surface of the body, and they reveal diagnostically significant electrical features in areas that are not sampled by the 12-lead ECG systems. In addition, BSPMs often show distinct electrical manifestations of two or more events simultaneously evolving in the heart; they make it possible to compute any ECG that would be obtained from any pair or combination of body surface electrodes—that is, from any current or future lead system. Also, the recorded data can be displayed as a sequence of contour maps, allowing isolation of significant electrocardiographic events in both space and time.[44]

BSPMs can be used to reconstruct epicardial and, in some cases, endocardial potential distributions, excitation times, and electrograms noninvasively, by means of inverse procedures, which help transform the ECG into an imaging method of electrical activity. This yields 3-D images that depict anatomical features with superimposed activation isochrones or excitation and recovery potentials, isochrones, and electrograms.[45]

In BSPM measurements, unipolar potentials of single heartbeats are acquired simultaneously at more than 60 locations covering the whole thorax. A Wilson central terminal is used as a reference for the unipolar leads. Lead sites in the array are arranged in columns and rows, and the electrodes are attached to flexible plastic strips, attached to dozens of thoracic sites vertically, with the highest electrode density at the left anterior thorax. Recordings are band pass–filtered at 0.16 to 300 Hz, digitized with a sampling frequency of 1 kHz, and stored on a CD.[45]

BSPMs depict the spatial distribution of heart potentials on the surface of the torso. Initially, all lead tracings are visually screened to reject poor-quality signals. The amplitude of every electrogram is measured at a given time instant during the cardiac cycle and plotted on a chart representing the torso surface. Several analytical procedures are used to convert the grid of data points into map contours. The time interval between successive instantaneous maps (frames) is generally 1 to 2 milliseconds. A sequence of 400 to 800 frames shows the evolution of the potential pattern during the cardiac cycle. Often, 20 to 50 properly selected maps are sufficient to show the essential features of the time-varying surface field.[45]

Localization of the site of origin of focal tachycardia, pacing site, or myocardial insertion site of a BT relates to the thoracic site of greatest negativity in the isointegral map. An activation wavefront moving away from such sites yields a negative body surface identifier because of the dominant effect of activating the remainder of the myocardial mass away from the stimulus site.

Clinical Implications

BSPM has been used for patients with conditions such as pulmonary embolism, aortic dissection, and acute coronary syndromes. It has also been used for diagnosing an old MI, localizing the BT in Wolff-Parkinson-White (WPW) syndrome, recognizing ventricular hypertrophy, and ascertaining the location, size, and severity of the infarcted area in acute MI and the effects of different interventions designed to reduce the size of the infarct.[45] From an EP standpoint, BSPM has been studied for the discrimination of clockwise and counterclockwise AFL, localization of the earliest retrograde atrial activation site in dogs with simulated WPW and orthodromic AVRT, localization of the ventricular insertion site of BTs during preexcitation, localization of sites of origin of ATs and VTs, and localization of endocardial or epicardial pacing sites.

Although ongoing research continues to address the role of BSPM, and how BSPM addresses many of the inadequacies associated with the conventional 12-lead approach, the clinical effectiveness of this procedure has not been established. BSPM is mostly used as a research tool rather than a routine diagnostic method because of significant limitations.[44]

Limitations

The main limitation of BSPM is the complexity of the recording, which requires many leads from each patient, sophisticated instrumentation, and dedicated personnel.[44] Complexity of the interpretation is another limitation, because it is mostly based on pattern recognition and knowledge of variability in normal subjects and patients, which are difficult to memorize. Therefore, visual inspection and measurement of BSPMs cannot result, per se, in direct localization of single or multiple electrical events as they occur in the heart.[46] Furthermore, BSPMs do not offer a picture of the heart but show an attenuated and distorted projection of epicardial and intracardiac events on the body surface. Additionally, the method of interpolating maps from acquired data is vulnerable to the precision of localization of the electrode sites and to the assurance that each electrode is receiving a true signal.[44]

ELECTROCARDIOGRAPHIC IMAGING

Fundamental Concepts

Electrocardiographic imaging (ECGI) has three main components—a multielectrode electrocardiographic vest, a multichannel mapping system for ECG signal acquisition, and an anatomical imaging modality to determine the heart-torso geometry. ECGI is a cardiac functional imaging modality that noninvasively reconstructs epicardial potentials, electrograms, and isochrones (activation maps) from multichannel body surface potential recordings using geometrical information from CT and a mathematical algorithm.[47-51]

ECGI has two requirements, electrocardiographic unipolar potentials measured over the entire body surface and the heart-torso geometrical relationship. The body surface electrocardiographic unipolar potentials are measured using a multielectrode electrocardiographic vest. The prototype electrocardiographic vest has 224 electrodes arranged in rows and columns on strips, with Velcro attachments at the sides to secure the vest to the torso (Fig. 3-39). The vest is connected to a multichannel mapping system, which measures electrocardiographic unipolar potentials over the entire body surface and facilitates simultaneous signal acquisition and amplification from all channels. Body surface potentials are monitored to ensure proper contact and gain adjustment, and then signals are recorded over several heartbeats.[47-51]

After signal acquisition, the exact geometry of the epicardial and torso surfaces and vest electrode positions is obtained by anatomical imaging modalities, such as thoracic CT or MR imaging. Scans are usually set to an axial resolution between 0.6 and 1 mm, and are typically gated at

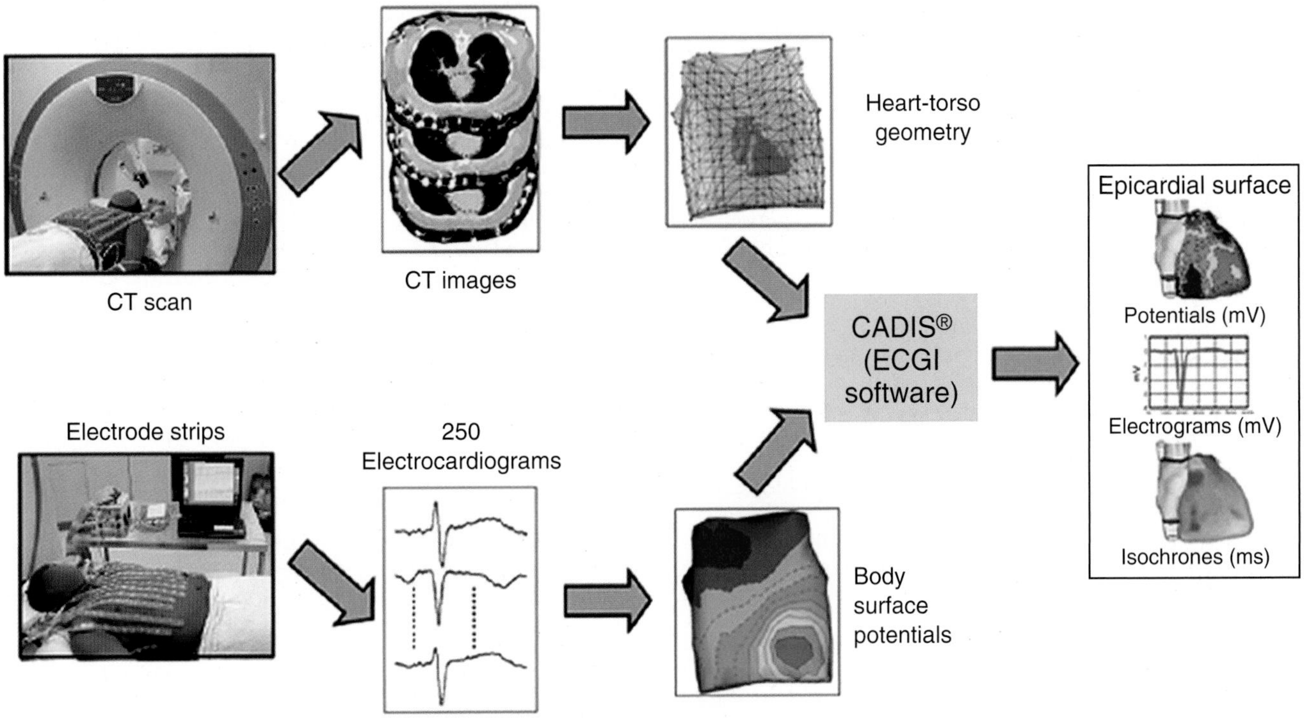

FIGURE 3–39 Electrocardiographic imaging (ECGI) procedure. Body surface potential mapping (BSPM) is recorded using a multichannel (256-electrode) mapping system. Noncontrast CT images with the body surface ECGI electrodes applied simultaneously record the locations of the electrodes (*shining dots in CT images*) and the geometry of the heart surface. By combining the BSPM and heart-torso geometry information, ECGI reconstructs potential maps, electrograms, and isochrones (activation patterns) on the epicardial surface of the heart. (From Wang Y, Cuculich PS, Woodard PK, et al: Focal atrial tachycardia after pulmonary vein isolation: Noninvasive mapping with electrocardiographic imaging (ECGI). Heart Rhythm 2007;4:1081.)

the R wave of the ECG to obtain diastolic volume (geometry for reconstruction of activation). Systolic volume, gated during the T wave of the ECG, is also measured to obtain suitable geometry for reconstruction during the repolarization phase. The transverse slices are segmented slice by slice to obtain heart geometry (as epicardial contours on each slice) and torso geometry (described by body surface electrode positions, seen as bright dots on the images; see Fig. 3-39). The geometry of the heart and torso surfaces is then assembled in a common x-y-z coordinate system to provide the geometrical heart-torso relationship.[47-51]

ECGI noninvasively computes potentials on the heart surface by solving the Laplace equation within the torso volume, using torso surface potentials and the geometric relationship between the epicardial and torso surfaces as inputs. The potential and geometry data are processed through CADIS, the ECGI software package (see Fig. 3-39). The software has four modules. The preprocessing module preprocesses the acquired electrocardiographic signals by noise filtration, baseline correction, elimination of bad signals (poor contact), and interpolation of missing signals. The geometry module includes image segmentation algorithms for heart and body surface segmentation and meshing of heart and torso surfaces. The numerical module includes boundary element algorithms to derive the transfer matrix relating body surface potentials to epicardial potentials, and epicardial potential reconstruction algorithms that use Tikhonov regularization and the generalized minimal residual algorithm to compute unipolar epicardial potentials from the transfer matrix and body surface potentials. The fourth module is the postprocessing module, which includes tools to analyze reconstructed epicardial data and formats for efficient visualization and analysis.[47-51]

Four modes of display are typically used. Epicardial potential maps depict the spatial distributions of potentials on the epicardium (see Fig. 3-39). Each map depicts one instant of time; maps are computed at 1-ms intervals during the entire cardiac cycle. The electrograms depict the variation of potential with respect to time at a single point on the epicardium. The electrograms are computed at many points (typically 400-900 sites) around the epicardium. Isochrone maps depict the sequence of epicardial activation based on local activation time, taken as the point of maximum negative derivative ($-dV/dt_{max}$) of the QRS segment in each electrogram (intrinsic deflection). Recovery times are assigned as the point of maximum derivative (dV/dt_{max}) of the T wave segment. Activation times are determined as the time of maximum negative derivative in the epicardial electrograms. Information from neighboring electrograms is used to edit activation times in electrograms with multiple large negative derivatives. Lines of block are drawn to separate sites with activation time differences more than 30 milliseconds.[47-51]

Clinical Implications

Noninvasive diagnosis of arrhythmias is currently based on the standard 12-lead ECG, BSPMs, or paced body surface QRS integral mapping. Standard diagnostic techniques such as the ECG provide only low-resolution projections of cardiac electrical activity on the body surface and cannot provide detailed information on regional electrical activity in the heart, such as the origin of arrhythmogenic activity, sequence of arrhythmic activation, or existence and location of an abnormal EP substrate.

A noninvasive imaging modality for cardiac EP is much needed for the following: (1) screening people with genetic predisposition or altered myocardial substrate (such as post-MI) for risk of life-threatening arrhythmias, to take prophylactic measures; (2) specific diagnosis of the arrhythmia mechanism to determine the most suitable intervention; (3) determination of cardiac location for optimal localized intervention (e.g., ablation, pacing, targeted drug delivery, or targeted gene transfer); (4) evaluation of efficacy and guidance of therapy over time; and (5) studying the mechanisms and properties of cardiac arrhythmias in humans, in whom the EP substrate is different from that in experimental animal models used thus far for this purpose.

ECGI images potentials, electrograms, and activation sequences (isochrones) on the epicardium and combines established technologies (BSPMs and CT scans) in a unique fashion to generate noninvasive images of cardiac electrical activity. Studies in animals and humans have demonstrated the ability of ECGI to image human cardiac electrophysiology noninvasively, including imaging of activation and repolarization during normal excitation, pacing, focal tachycardias, and reentrant circuits.[47-51] ECGI can image the reentry pathway and its key components, including the critical isthmus, its entry and exit sites, lines of block, and regions of slow and fast conduction. Although clinical reentry usually occurs in the endocardium, the subepicardium plays an important role in the maintenance of reentry in a small proportion of patients undergoing ablation therapy.[47-51]

Furthermore, in the case of transmural MI, ECGI can be used to characterize the electrophysiology of the infarct substrate and identify sites of epicardial breakthrough during reentrant activation. Interpretation of intramural arrhythmogenic activity can be further enhanced by direct catheter mapping or noncontact catheter reconstruction of EP information on the endocardial surface simultaneously with noninvasive epicardial ECGI. The combination of epicardial and endocardial EP information, with knowledge of the intramural anatomical organization of the myocardium, can provide an unprecedented ability to localize arrhythmogenic activity within the myocardial depth using only noninvasive or minimally invasive procedures.[47-51]

ECGI's ability to detect abnormal EP substrates can provide a noninvasive procedure for identifying patients at a high risk of life-threatening arrhythmias. After screening, prophylactic measures (e.g., implantable defibrillators, ablation, drug therapy, or genetic or molecular modification) can be instituted before sudden cardiac death occurs. Implementing ECGI in the clinical setting will require additional validation in patients with known activation sequences.

Limitations

ECGI provides EP information about the heart's epicardial surface; it does not directly reconstruct intramural information in the 3-D myocardium. Nevertheless, in contrast to BSPMs, epicardial potentials provide high-resolution reflection of underlying intramural activity.[51] Also, ECGI can have limited success in defining components of arrhythmia pathways that involve small volumes of tissue, such as microreentry. Furthermore, the need to use CT limits the clinical application of ECGI during intervention in the EP laboratory, where CT is not available. A recently developed method uses biplane x-ray images that can be acquired routinely in the EP laboratory for estimating the epicardial surface geometry.

INTRACARDIAC ECHOCARDIOGRAPHY

Catheter Design

Two types of intracardiac echocardiographic (ICE) imaging systems are currently available, the mechanical ultrasound catheter radial imaging system and the electronic phased-array catheter sector imaging system.

Mechanical Ultrasound Catheter Radial Imaging System

In the mechanical ultrasound catheter (Ultra ICE) radial imaging system (EP Technologies, Boston Scientific, San Jose, Calif), the ultrasound transducer is mounted at the end of a nonsteerable 9 Fr (110-cm length) catheter and has a single, rotating, crystal ultrasound transducer. An external motor drive unit rotates the crystal at 1800 rpm within the catheter to provide an imaging plane that is 360 degrees circumferential and perpendicular to the long axis of the catheter, with the catheter located centrally. Mechanical ICE uses imaging frequencies of 9 to 12 MHz, which provide near-field clarity (within 5 to 7 cm of the transducer) but poor tissue penetration and far-field resolution. As a result, these systems have not allowed clear imaging of the LA and PV, except when introduced directly into the LA (transseptally). This technology lacks Doppler capability, and the catheter is not freely deflectable.[52,53]

Electronic Phased-Array Catheter Sector Imaging System

In the electronic phased-array ultrasound catheter (AcuNav) sector imaging system (Acuson Corporation, Siemens Medical Solutions, Malvern, Pa), the ultrasound transducer is mounted on the distal end of an 8 Fr or 10 Fr (90-cm length) catheter and has a forward-facing 64-element vector phased-array transducer scanning in the longitudinal plane. The catheter has a four-way steerable tip (160 degrees anteroposterior and left-right deflections). The catheter images a sector (wedge-shaped) field in a plane in line with the catheter shaft and oriented in the plane of the catheter. Imaging capabilities include 90-degree sector two-dimensional, M-mode, and Doppler imaging (pulse-wave, continuous-wave, color, and tissue Doppler), with tissue penetration up to 16 cm, and variable ultrasound frequency (5.5, 7.5, 8.5, and 10 MHz).[52,53]

Imaging Technique

Using the Mechanical Radial Intracardiac Echocardiographic Catheter

Initially, all air must be eliminated from the distal tip of the ICE catheter by flushing vigorously with 5 to 10 mL of sterile water to optimize the ultrasound image. The ICE catheter is introduced through a long femoral venous sheath. Because the catheter is not deflectable, preshaped angled long sheaths are preferred to allow some steerability.[52,53] The mechanical radial ICE catheter generates a panoramic 360-degree image perpendicular to the catheter, with the tip as a central reference point. The catheter is connected to the ultrasound console and advanced until the tip of the rotary ICE catheter image is in the RA.[52,53]

When the transducer is advanced into the SVC, the ascending aorta, the right pulmonary artery and, occasionally, the right superior PV are viewed.[54] Withdrawing the the catheter into the mid-RA brings the fossa ovalis and LA in view; the crista terminalis and aortic valve are usually visible in this view (Fig. 3-40). The LA, left PV orifices, and aortic root are imaged by positioning the transducer at the fossa ovalis. However, visualization of the LA and PV ostia is limited because of limited penetration depth. Withdrawing the catheter to the low RA allows visualization of the eustachian valve, lateral crista terminalis, and CS os (see Fig. 3-40).[52,54] When the transducer is placed in the RV through the tricuspid valve and further advanced into the RV outflow tract (RVOT), both ventricles and the pulmonary artery can be visualized.

Using the AcuNav Catheter

A femoral venous approach is used for the insertion of the ICE catheter. The catheter is advanced to the RA under

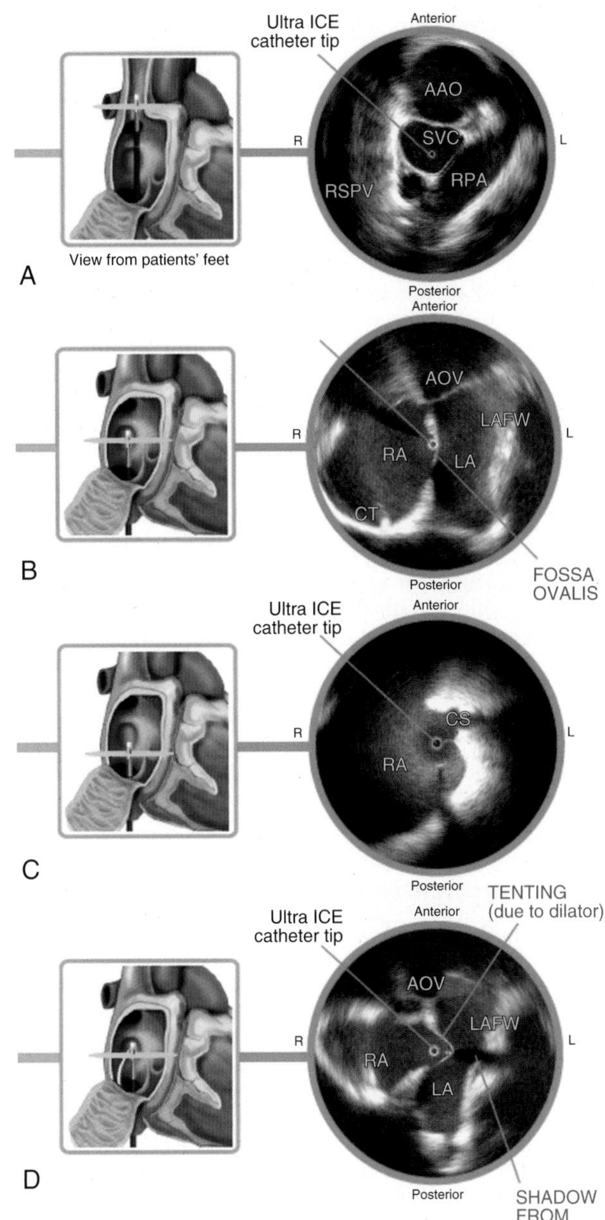

FIGURE 3–40 Mechanical radial implantable cardioverter-defibrillator intracardiac echocardiographic (ICE) images from different levels in the right atrium (RA) and superior vena cava (SVC). **A,** With the transducer tip in the SVC, typical structures visible in this plane are the ascending aorta (AAO), right pulmonary artery (RPA), and right superior pulmonary vein (RSPV). **B,** Withdrawing the ICE catheter into the mid-RA brings the fossa ovalis into view. Typical structures visible in this plane are the left atrium (LA), LA free wall (LAFW), aortic valve (AOV), and crista terminalis (CT). **C,** Withdrawing the ICE catheter down to the RA floor visualizes the coronary sinus (CS) and inferior vena cava (IVC). **D,** During transseptal puncture, tenting of the fossa is observed on the ICE. (Courtesy of Boston Scientific, San Jose, Calif.)

fluoroscopy guidance. The ICE two-dimensional 90-degree sector scanning demonstrates a cross-sectional anatomical view oriented from the tip to the shaft of the imaging catheter's active face.[52,53] The left-right (L-R) orientation marker indicates the catheter's shaft side. When the L-R orientation marker is set to the operator's right, the craniocaudal axis projects left to right from the image and the posterior to anterior axis projects from the image top to bottom. Changing the L-R marker to the left side inverts the image but does not change top to bottom image orientation.[52,53] Image orien-

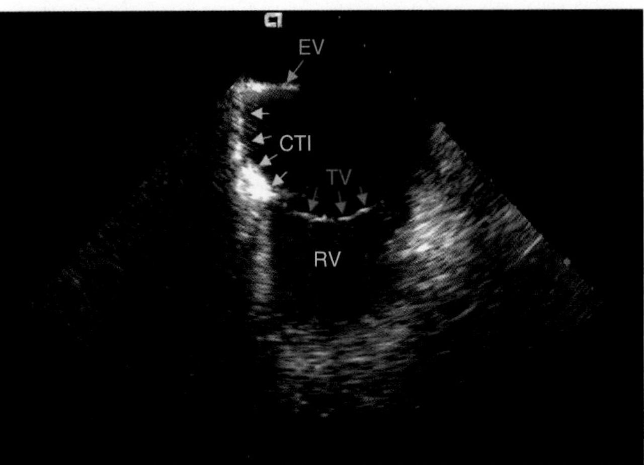

FIGURE 3–41 Intracardiac echocardiographic (ICE) image of the cavotricuspid isthmus (CTI, yellow arrows) between the eustachian valve (EV, green arrow) and tricuspid valve (TV, red arrows). RV = right ventricle.

tation can be adjusted to visualize targeted structures by simple catheter advancement or withdrawal, by tip deflection in four directions (anterior-posterior and left-right), or by catheter rotation.

The AcuNav ICE catheter includes variable ultrasound frequency (5.5, 7.5, 8.5, and 10 MHz). Increasing ultrasound frequency improves axial image resolution; however, tissue penetration decreases, resulting in decreased imaging depth. An ultrasound frequency of 7.5 MHz is useful for imaging most cardiac structures. Frequency can then be increased (to 8.5 or 10 MHz) for imaging near-field structures, or decreased (to 5.5 MHz) for imaging far-field structures.[52,53]

Right Atrial Targets. All RA targets are visualized by advancing or withdrawing the ICE catheter to an appropriate level within the RA and rotating the catheter to bring the target into view. The best resolution of near- and mid-field structures is obtained at an 8.5-MHz frequency. Once the catheter is advanced into the mid-RA with the catheter tension controls in neutral position (the ultrasound transducer oriented anteriorly and to the left), the RA, tricuspid valve, and RV are viewed. This is called the home view (see Fig. 2-13), and can serve as a starting point; whenever one gets lost, he or she can go back to the home view and start over. From the home view, counterclockwise rotation of the catheter brings the RA appendage into view, whereas anterior deflection of the catheter tip toward the RV allows visualization of the tricuspid valve and cavotricuspid isthmus (Fig. 3-41). The superior crista terminalis is visualized when the catheter is advanced to the RA-SVC junction in an anterior direction.[54]

Interatrial Septum. Gradual clockwise rotation of a straight catheter from the home view allows sequential visualization of the aortic root and the pulmonary artery, followed by the CS, mitral valve, LA appendage orifice, and a cross-sectional view of the fossa ovalis (see Fig. 2-13). The mitral valve and interatrial septum are usually seen in the same plane as the LA appendage. Posterior deflection, right-left steering, or both, of the imaging tip in the RA is occasionally required to optimize visualization of the fossa ovalis; the tension knob (lock function) can then be used to hold the catheter tip in position. Further clockwise rotation beyond this location will demonstrate images of the left PV ostia (see Fig. 2-13). The optimum ICE image to guide transseptal puncture will demonstrate adequate space behind the interatrial septum on the LA side and clearly identify adjacent structures (see Fig. 2-14).[52]

Left Atrial Structures. A 7.5- or 8.5-MHz imaging frequency optimizes visualization of LA structures and PVs beyond the interatrial septum. PV imaging is possible by first visualizing the membranous fossa from a mid to low RA catheter tip position. With clockwise catheter rotation, the LA appendage can be visualized, followed by long-axis views of the left superior and inferior PVs (Fig. 3-42; see also Fig. 2-13). Further clockwise rotation of the catheter brings the orifices of the right superior and inferior PVs into view. The ostia of these veins are typically viewed en face, yielding an owl's eyes appearance at the vein's orifice. The LA appendage can also be visualized with the transducer positioned in the CS.

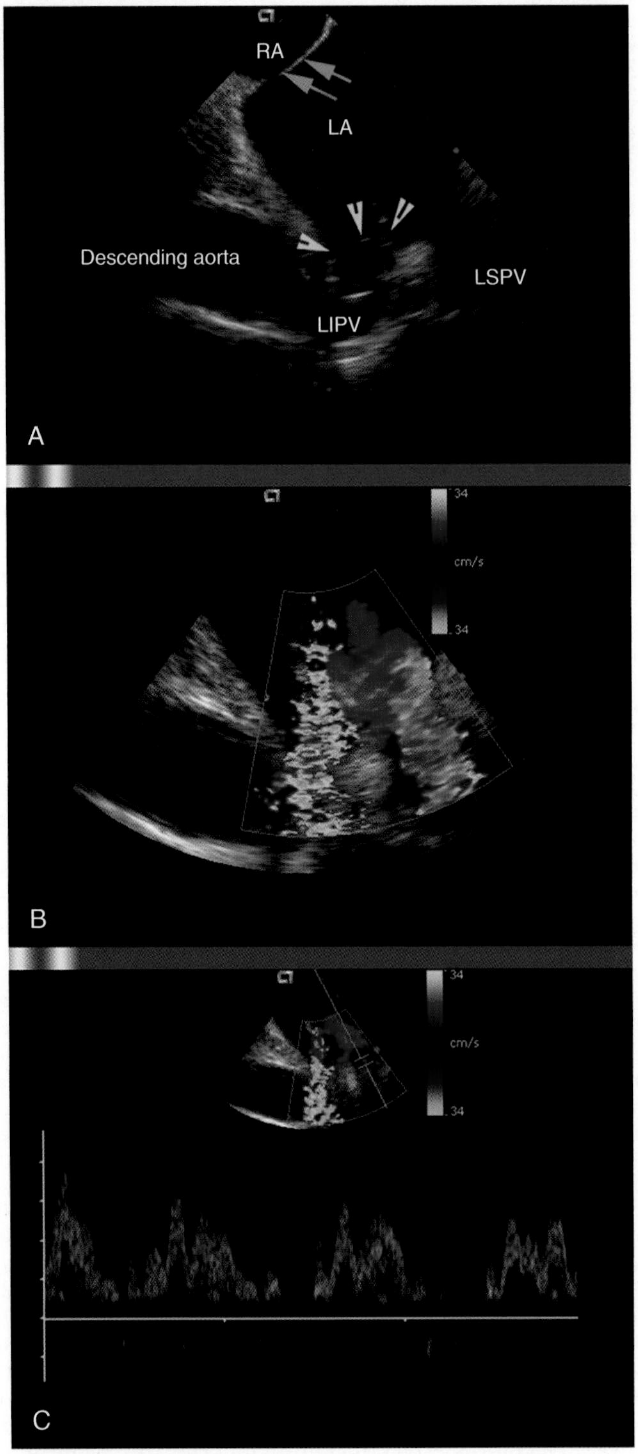

Left and Right Ventricular Targets. Imaging of each targeted LV structure at depths of 6 to 15 cm is accomplished with the catheter tip in a low RA position. When the catheter transducer is placed near the fossa and oriented anteriorly and to the left, the LVOT and truncated LV are imaged. With clockwise rotation and slight adjustment of the transducer level, the mitral valve and LV apex can be viewed. To image the mitral valve in a long-axis, two-chamber view (LA, mitral valve, and LV), a mild degree of apically directed catheter tip deflection can be required. The RVOT, LVOT, and aortic root with coronary artery ostia can be imaged by advancing the catheter in the RA to the level of the outflow tracts (mid-RA), with an appropriate deflection to the right. The aortic valve can also be imaged in its cross-section from this region (Fig. 3-43). A long-axis of the LV can also be visualized by advancing the catheter with its anteriorly deflected tip into the RV with clockwise rotation against the interventricular septum (Fig. 3-44). Further clockwise rotation or right-left steering of the catheter tip allows a short-axis view of the LV, as well as the mitral valve (see Fig. 3-44). Pericardial effusions usually can be readily identified from these views. Withdrawing the catheter back to the base of the RVOT and rotating the shaft allows the RVOT to be visualized in its long axis, with a cross-sectional view of the pulmonic valve.[52,53]

FIGURE 3–42 Intracardiac echocardiographic (ICE) images of the left pulmonary veins with transducer placed in the right atrium (RA). **A,** The RA, interatrial septum (green arrows), left inferior pulmonary vein (LIPV), left superior pulmonary vein (LSPV), and descending aorta are visualized. The Lasso catheter (yellow arrowheads) is visualized at the ostium of the LIPV. Color Doppler images of both LIPV and LSPV **(B)**, and pulsed wave Doppler tracing **(C)** obtained from the LSPV are shown.

Clinical Implications

Transesophageal imaging has been used to guide ablation of VT and BTs, as well as transseptal catheterization, and for the closure of atrial septal defects or cardiac biopsy. This approach, however, has been limited in the interventional arena by aspiration risk and patient discomfort accompanying prolonged esophageal intubation, and requires a second ultrasound operator to complete the study.

Previous human applications of intracardiac ultrasound have been limited to those generated by the mechanical rotation of a single piezoelectric element in 6 to 10 Fr catheters. Miniaturization of these elements required the use of higher 10- to 20-MHz transducer frequencies, limiting ultra-

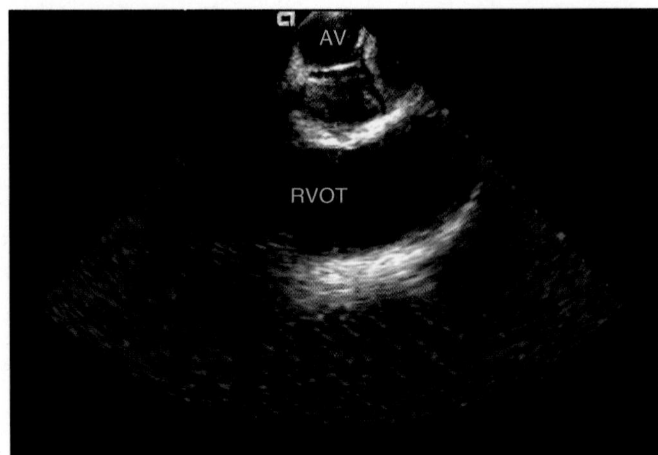

FIGURE 3–43 Short-axis view of the aortic valve (AV) cusps with the intracardiac echocardiographic (ICE) transducer placed in the mid–right atrium deflected near the posterior wall of the aortic root. RVOT = right ventricular outflow tract.

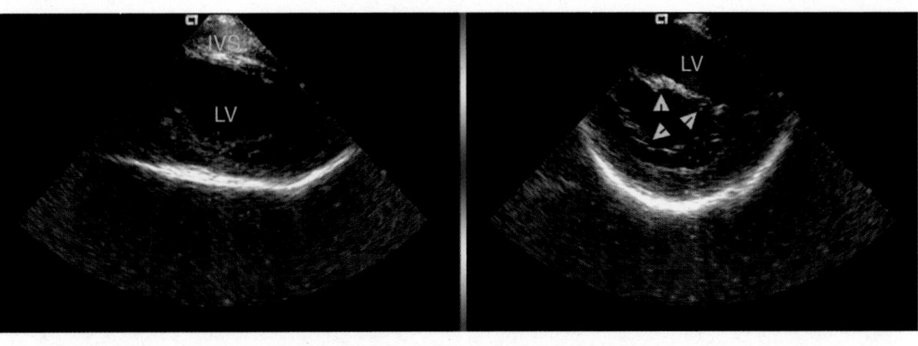

FIGURE 3–44 Intracardiac echocardiographic (ICE) images of the left ventricle (LV), with transducer placed in the right ventricle (RV) against the interventricular septum (IVS). **Left,** Long-axis view of the LV. **Right,** Short-axis view of the LV at the level of the mitral valve (*arrowheads*).

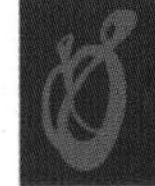

sound penetration to surrounding cardiac tissues. This technology has been applied for the imaging of RA structures in humans and animals, membranous fossa ovalis, crista terminalis, eustachian ridge, tricuspid annulus, and SVC-RA junction in the region of the sinus node. However, visualization of the LA and PV ostia is limited using this system because of limited penetration depth, except when introduced directly into the LA (transseptally).

The electronic phased-array ultrasound system offers deeper field, standard intracardiac visualization of specific right- and left-sided cardiac structures, as well as color flow and pulsed and continuous-wave Doppler imaging by a single operator. This has been of significant value for PV isolation procedures and LA linear ablation for AF.

Several practical uses for ICE have emerged in the setting of EP procedures, including the following: (1) assessment of catheter contact with cardiac tissues; (2) determination of catheter location relative to cardiac structures (specifically useful in otherwise difficult to localize areas, such as the PVs)[52,55]; (3) guidance of transseptal puncture, particularly in the setting of complex or unusual anatomy[56]; (4) facilitation of deployment of mapping or ablation systems, such as PV encircling devices, noncontact mapping systems, and basket technologies; (5) visualization of evolving lesions during RF energy delivery; both changing tissue echogenicity and microbubbles reflect tissue heating, with the latter providing a signal for energy termination[55]; (6) evaluation of cardiac structures before and after intervention (e.g., cardiac valves and PVs); (7) assessment of PV anatomy, dimensions, and function via 2-D anatomical imaging and Doppler physiological measurements; (8) assessment of complications (e.g., tamponade, electromechanical dissociation, or thrombus formation)[57]; and (9) identification of the anatomical origin of certain arrhythmias—for example, ICE can facilitate ablation of inappropriate sinus tachycardia or sinus nodal reentrant tachycardia.

COMPUTED TOMOGRAPHY AND MAGNETIC RESONANCE IMAGING

Fundamental Concepts

During catheter ablation procedures, catheters are usually manipulated under the guidance of fluoroscopy. However, fluoroscopy does not provide adequate depiction of cardiac anatomy because of its poor soft tissue contrast and the 2-D projective nature of the formed image, which hinders its application for complex ablation procedures such as AF ablation. On the other hand, CT and MR images offer anatomical detail in 3-D. However, images are presented out of the context of the ablation catheter, thus greatly diminishing their potential value. An optimal strategy would therefore be to integrate the 3-D images generated by CT or MR with the electrical and navigational information obtained with an interventional system. This can be achievd through the process of integration. Image integration refers to the process of aligning the pre-procedural cardiac CT and MR images with the real-time 3-D electroanatomical maps reconstructed from multiple endocardial locations. The process of image integration consists of three steps—preprocedural CT and MR imaging, image segmentation and extraction, and image registration.

Image Acquisition. Cross-sectional or axial CT or MR images are acquired at sufficient resolution to delineate cardiac structures less than 1 to 2 mm in thickness. Images at 0.625-mm thickness can be reconstructed from images obtained at 1.25-mm intervals with currently available multirow helical scanners. A simultaneous ECG is recorded to assign the source images retrospectively to the respective phases of cardiac cycle. MR images are similarly obtainable, although at slightly lower spatial resolution. Rendering a volume or reconstructing any cardiac chamber in 3-D from the axial images is a straightforward process using any one of various software packages.

Image Segmentation. Image segmentation refers to the process of extraction of the 3-D anatomy of individual cardiac structures from its surrounding structures. The volume of cardiac structures is extracted from the whole-volume data set using a computerized algorithm that differentiates the boundary between the blood pool (which is high in contrast) and the endocardium (which is not contrast-enhanced). This allows for clear differentiation between the chamber lumen and endocardial wall (Fig. 3-45). Subsequently, the volumes of individual cardiac structures are separated from each other with the use of another algorithm capable of detecting their boundaries (see Fig. 3-45). Using a third algorithm, the segmented volumes for individual cardiac structures are extracted as 3-D surface reconstructions (see Fig. 3-45). The segmented volumes can be viewed from an external perspective or from within the chamber using virtual endoscopic or cardioscopic displays. These images, in addition to providing a road map for ablation, can also be used for registration (see Fig. 3-45).

Image Registration. Although the segmented structures are highly useful for visualizing the cardiac structures and characteristics of the tissue forming that structure, they do not convey the physiology of an arrhythmia. Integrating that physiology, as captured by electroanatomical or noncontact mapping, with the spatial information contained in the CT or MR images requires registration of activation or voltage data to an appropriate location on a 3-D representation of a chamber. This is of critical importance in that it establishes the relationship between anatomy and physiology as required for the structure- and activity-based understanding of arrhythmias and for enabling image-guided intervention.

Image registration refers to superimposing the 3-D CT and MR surface reconstructions onto the real-time electroanatomical maps derived from catheter mapping (see Fig. 3-34). During registration, the assumption is made that the

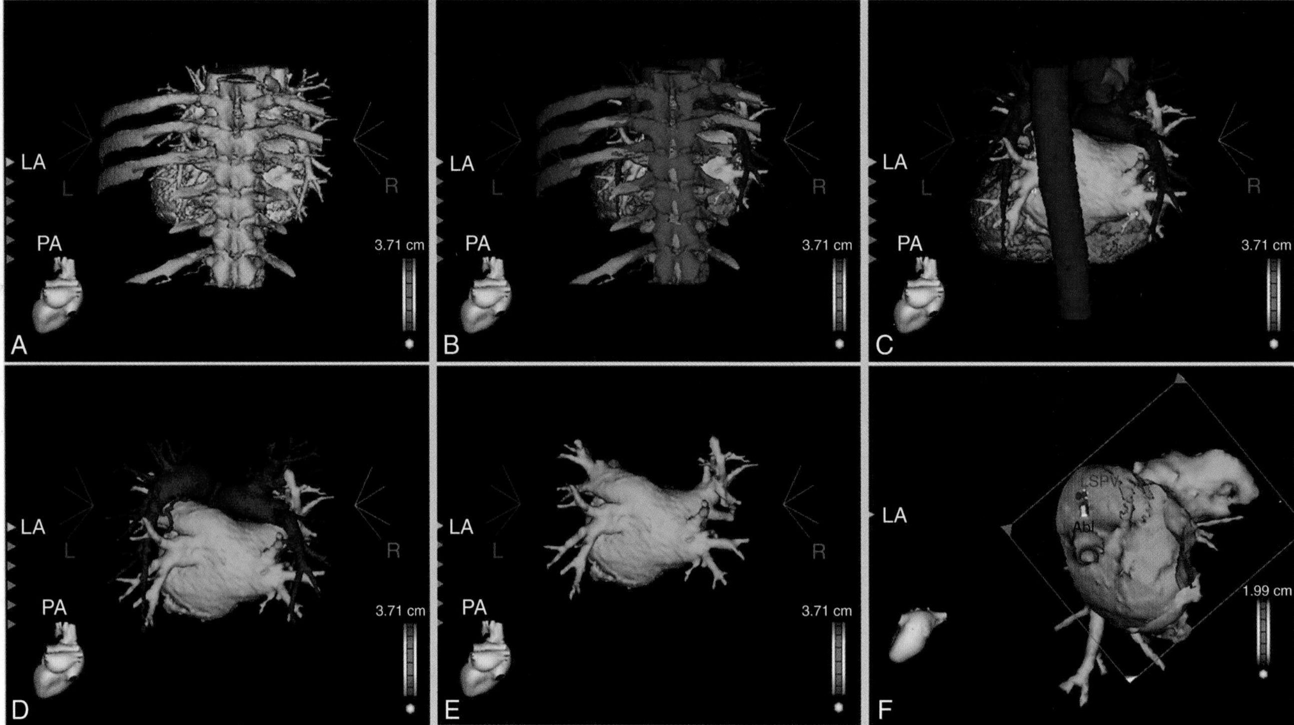

FIGURE 3–45 CT image segmentation and integration with electroanatomical mapping (CARTO) data. **A,** 3-D reconstruction of the heart and part of the spine from the 2-D CT image (posteroanterior view). **B and C,** Individual cardiac chambers are segmented from each other using computerized algorithms capable of detecting their boundaries (aorta, red; left atrium [LA], yellow; left ventricle, green; pulmonary artery, blue; right atrium, orange). **D and E,** The cardiac chamber is selected (LA in this case) and others are deleted. **F,** Integration of CT and electroanatomical mapping (CARTO) data. Shown is a left lateral cardioscopic view of the ostia of the left pulmonary veins (PVs) during PV electrical isolation. Radiofrequency applications (small red circles) were deployed at the posterior aspect of the ostium of the left superior PV (LSPV). The ablation catheter tip is positioned at the inferior aspect of the LSPV.

anatomy of the organ being registered has not changed. Two computerized algorithms are used to accomplish the image registration process, landmark registration and surface registration. Landmark registration aligns the 3-D CT and MR image reconstructions with corresponding electroanatomical maps through linking a set number of points on both images that are easily identifiable. Using fluoroscopy, ICE guidance, or both, at least three landmark pairs are created by real-time catheter tip locations on the interventional system being used for registration and then placed on their estimated locations on the 3-D CT and MR image reconstructions. Using more landmark points increases the accuracy of the registration process. Surface registration is an algorithm that attaches the acquired endocardial points to the closest CT and MR surface to compose the best fit of the two sets of images by minimizing the average distance between the landmarks, and the distance from multiple endocardial locations, to the surface of 3-D CT and MR image reconstructions. Surface registration complements landmark registration to improve the registration accuracy. However, because of surface indentation and potentially missed areas during mapping, the acquired electroanatomical map does not represent the perfect anatomy of the cardiac chamber.

Clinical Implications

CT and MR imaging approaches have already been of significant benefit in AF catheter ablation procedures, providing critical information regarding the number, location, and size of PVs, as needed for planning the ablation and selecting appropriately sized ablation devices.[58] Resulting images also identify branching patterns of potentially arrhythmogenic PVs, disclose the presence of fused superior and inferior veins into antral structures, and clarify the potentially confounding origins of far-field electrograms that masquerade as PV potentials. CT has also been used for postablation evaluation for PV stenosis.

The last several years have also seen the rapid development of integrated, anatomy-based mapping and ablation. This has been driven by a realization of both the critical coupling and dependence of arrhythmias on their underlying anatomy and the limitations of surrogate geometries of contemporary mapping systems for reflecting that anatomy. Over this same time frame, rapid CT and MR imaging systems have emerged as the mainstays of imaging in the EP laboratory and have been used to plan or guide ablation. Each company is actively working on image incorporation into its system.[30-32,59,60] Helical 16- to 64-row CT and MR studies provide a broad anatomy library of an individual patient at one point in time. Segmented CT volumes can be downloaded on the CARTO and NavX platforms, with similar integration work underway for the RPM system. A novel version of an electroanatomical mapping system (CARTO XP, Biosense Webster) has been equipped with image integration software (CARTO Merge Image Integration Module). This system is able to register the surrogate map fully onto actual CT and MR anatomy; it also enables integration of electroanatomical mapping with preacquired CT and MR images and allows real-time visualization of the location and orientation of the catheter tip within the registered CT anatomical framework (see Figs. 3-34 and 3-45).[24,61]

The use of registered CT and MR images to guide catheter ablation presents a significant advantage over the less detailed surrogate geometry created by previously available

3-D mapping systems. Because it provides detailed anatomical information on the catheter tip location in relation to the true cardiac anatomy, the image integration technique has the potential to affiliate many ablation procedures, especially those anatomically based ablation strategies, such as AF ablation, nonidiopathic VT ablation, and ablation of intraatrial reentrant tachycardias following corrective surgery for congenital heart diseases. Initial experience has shown that the registered CT and MR of LA reconstructions can provide accurate information on the catheter tip location in relation to the important LA structures, such as PV ostium and LA appendage. The real-time update of the catheter tip location and the marking of ablation lesions on the detailed 3-D image can potentially improve quality of lesion sets, reduce complications, and shorten procedure and fluoroscopy times.

Limitations

Although CT and MR imaging provide exquisite images of the underlying structures relevant in arrhythmogenesis, they are limited by the requirement of off-line generation of the CT and MR libraries and inability to reflect all phases of the cardiac cycle during an arrhythmia. As CT and MR imaging is performed prior to the ablation procedure, registration error can arise from interval changes in the heart size because of differences in rhythm, rate, contractility, or fluid status. Performing image registration and ablation procedures within 24 hours after CT and MR scans and CT and MR image acquisition and image registration during the same rhythm can help limit interval changes.

In addition, the static images of the registered CT and MR reconstructions provide little information on true catheter-tissue contact. Furthermore, as the initial landmark points are picked up by the operator using fluoroscopy, ICE, or both, the exact location of these points in the 3-D space can be deceptive. Also, because multiple points are needed for surface registration, the accuracy of the chamber reconstruction is therefore directly dependent on the number of points taken and the position of the catheter, thus adding a significant amount of time and a manual component to the process.[24,59]

To overcome some of these limitations, fusion of real-time ICE images with those generated by CT and MR scans is becoming available and can provide a more real-time interactive display, as well as real-time information on catheter-tissue contact and RF lesion formation. Also, it is highly likely that subsequent generations of CT or MR scanners will be sufficiently fast to permit real-time or almost real-time imaging for interventional guidance. Recent studies have demonstrated the ability to merge the 3-D CT and MR images with real-time 2-D fluoroscopy images for navigation on a virtual anatomy, because the images can be corrected against the background of real-time fluoroscopy as needed.[24,59,62]

The accuracy of registration remains the subject of investigation. 3-D image integration aims at improving the operator's perception of the catheter spatial location in relation to the patient's cardiac structures. However, the success of this approach is primarily dependent on the accuracy of the image integration process. Even if the 3-D cardiac chamber image provides an accurate model of a matched phase of the chamber volume at the time of the procedure, it needs to be accurately registered to the procedural chamber orientation to provide reliable navigation. Current registration algorithms depend on accurate catheter geometry; this requires an accurate update of 3-D coordinates of the catheter tip, which is recorded and displayed on the computer image. Movement of the catheter tip is complex and is affected by wall motion and respiration. Point collection should therefore be gated to the same phase of the cardiac and respiratory cycle as the CT or MR scan. Additionally, catheter tip pressure can cause tenting of the chamber wall, thereby distorting the chamber geometry. Stability of catheter contact with the endocardial wall should also be optimized. Catheter contact can vary with the type of ablation catheter and introducer sheath, as well as the degree of regional wall motion; for example, the mitral annulus and appendage are more dynamic than the posterior atrial wall. Ideally, geometry points should be collected from stable catheter positions. The operator may then accept good points or delete bad points. This process can be aided by fluoroscopy, electrogram morphology, and confirmation of the catheter tip location on ICE. However, the process still remains a subjective art.

Several studies of AF catheter ablation have reported success using different integration modalities with CT or MR, either by using noncontact mapping or fluoroscopy as a second integrated image. The registration technique has also varied, including three- or four-point registration or surface registration. Alternatively, a single point and the surface have been used as well (visual alignment). Different techniques for point localization have been reported, including fluoroscopy alone, angiography, or ICE for direct visualization of the catheter at the designated site. The mean error for surface registration in most studies varied between 1.8 and 2.7 mm; one study that compared the landmark registration with and without surface registration has found that surface registration increases the accuracy of image integration. On the other hand, a recent study found the most accurate landmark registration is achieved when posterior points are acquired at the PV-LA junction, whereas points acquired on the anterior wall, LA appendage, or other structures outside the LA, such as the CS or SVC, afford less accuracy. In addition, surface registration usually results in shifting the landmark points away from the initially acquired position on the corresponding PVs using ICE.[63] Furthermore, an accurate surface registration does not guarantee an accurate alignment with the important anatomical structures. Another report has found that serious inaccuracies of the CARTO Merge image intergration algorithims still exist, depite using the precautions discussed earlier.[64]

CONCLUSIONS

Recording and analyzing extracellular electrograms form the basis for cardiac mapping. More commonly, cardiac mapping is performed with catheters introduced percutaneously into the heart chambers that sequentially record the endocardial electrograms with the purpose of correlating local electrogram to cardiac anatomy. These EP catheters are navigated and localized with the use of fluoroscopy.

However, the use of fluoroscopy for these purposes can be problematic for a number of reasons, including the following: (1) the inability to associate intracardiac electrograms accurately with their precise location within the heart; (2) the endocardial surface is invisible using fluoroscopy and target sites may only be approximated by their relationship with nearby structures, such as ribs, blood vessels, and the position of other catheters; (3) because of the limitations of 2-D fluoroscopy, navigation is not exact, it is time-consuming, and requires multiple views to estimate the 3-D location of the catheter; (4) the inability to return the catheter accurately and precisely to a previously mapped site; and (5) exposure of the patient and medical team to radiation.

The limitations of conventional mapping are being overcome with the introduction of sophisticated mapping systems that integrate 3-D catheter localization with sophisticated complex arrhythmia maps. The choice of a specific mapping system for a particular interventional case is shaped by the importance of a specific characteristic in the mapping process. Advanced mapping systems have a limited role in the ablation of typical AFL, AVNRT, or BTs, given the high success rate of the conventional approach. However, for more complex arrhythmias, such as macroreentrant AT, AF, and unstable VT, advanced mapping modalities offer a clear advantage. Additionally, advanced mapping systems can potentially shorten procedural time, reduce radiation exposure, and enhance the success rate for the ablation of typical AFL, idiopathic outflow tract VT, and sustained, stable macroreentrant VT.

In cases for which an undistorted anatomical rendering,

with high spacial accuracy, is required, the CARTO system is of advantage; it has fewer problems with interstructure delineation and requires fewer fixed or snap points to preserve the anatomy. The CARTO, NavX, and RPM systems all work well for mapping sustained, stable arrhythmias. Mapping nonsustained arrhythmias, PACs, or PVCs can be tedious with each of these three approaches. With these arrhythmias, the noncontact mapping array works well, although the maps can be filter frequency–dependent. The noncontact approach provides a quick snapshot of activation during unstable VTs, obviating the need for long periods of tachycardia. Substrate mapping, such as scar or voltage mapping, is a useful alternative to noncontact mapping. CARTO performs very well in this regard. NavX also works reasonably well with its dynamic substrate mapping capabilities.

In some cases, the choice of mapping system depends on the skill and experience of the operator. The user interfaces of the CARTO and NavX systems are acceptably straightforward. The noncontact system requires more steps in the creation of a user-friendly working geometry. Each of these systems is currently in the development stage, and their various capabilities can change substantially over the next couple of years.

REFERENCES

1. Delacretaz E, Soejima K, Gottipaty VK, et al: Single catheter determination of local electrogram prematurity using simultaneous unipolar and bipolar recordings to replace the surface ECG as a timing reference. Pacing Clin Electrophysiol 2001;24:441.
2. Josephson M: Electrophysiologic investigation: Technical aspects. *In* Josephson ME (ed): Clinical Cardiac Electrophysiology, 3rd ed. Philadelphia, Lippincott Williams & Wilkins. 2002, pp 1-18.
3. Stevenson WG, Soejima K: Recording techniques for clinical electrophysiology. J Cardiovasc Electrophysiol 2005;16:1017.
4. Morady F: Catheter ablation of supraventricular arrhythmias: State of the art. J Cardiovasc Electrophysiol 2004;15:1249.
5. Soejima K, Stevenson WG, Sapp JL, et al: Endocardial and epicardial radiofrequency ablation of ventricular tachycardia associated with dilated cardiomyopathy: the importance of low-voltage scars. J Am Coll Cardiol 2004;43:1834.
6. Sosa E, Scanavacca M: Epicardial mapping and ablation techniques to control ventricular tachycardia. J Cardiovasc Electrophysiol 2005;16:449.
7. Markides V, Segal O, Tondato F, Peters N: Mapping. *In* Zipes DP, Jalife J (eds): Cardiac Electrophysiology: From Cell to Bedside. Philadelphia, WB Saunders, 2004, pp 858-868.
8. Arenal A, Glez-Torrecilla E, Ortiz M, et al: Ablation of electrograms with an isolated, delayed component as treatment of unmappable monomorphic ventricular tachycardias in patients with structural heart disease. J Am Coll Cardiol 2003;41:81.
9. Cosio FG, Martin-Penato A, Pastor A, et al: Atypical flutter: A review. Pacing Clin Electrophysiol 2003;26:2157.
10. Josephson M: Recurrent Ventricular Tachycardia. *In* Josephson ME (ed): Clinical Cardiac Electrophysiology, 3rd ed. Philadelphia, Lippincott Williams & Wilkins. 2002, pp 425-610.
11. Tung S, Soejima K, Maisel WH, et al: Recognition of far-field electrograms during entrainment mapping of ventricular tachycardia. J Am Coll Cardiol 2003;42:110.
12. Brunckhorst CB, Stevenson WG, Jackman WM, et al: Ventricular mapping during atrial and ventricular pacing. Relationship of multipotential electrograms to ventricular tachycardia reentry circuits after myocardial infarction. Eur Heart J 2002;23:1131.
13. Morton JB, Sanders P, Deen V, et al: Sensitivity and specificity of concealed entrainment for the identification of a critical isthmus in the atrium: relationship to rate, anatomical location and antidromic penetration. J Am Coll Cardiol 2002;39:896.
14. Azegami K, Wilber DJ, Arruda M, et al: Spatial resolution of pacemapping and activation mapping in patients with idiopathic right ventricular outflow tract tachycardia. J Cardiovasc Electrophysiol 2005;16:823.
15. Brunckhorst CB, Delacretaz E, Soejima K, et al: Identification of the ventricular tachycardia isthmus after infarction by pace mapping. Circulation 2004;110:652.
16. Brunckhorst CB, Stevenson WG, Soejima K, et al: Relationship of slow conduction detected by pace-mapping to ventricular tachycardia re-entry circuit sites after infarction. J Am Coll Cardiol 2003;41:802.
17. Gerstenfeld EP, Dixit S, Callans DJ, et al: Quantitative comparison of spontaneous and paced 12-lead electrocardiogram during right ventricular outflow tract ventricular tachycardia. J Am Coll Cardiol 2003;41:2046.
18. Soejima K, Suzuki M, Maisel WH, et al: Catheter ablation in patients with multiple and unstable ventricular tachycardias after myocardial infarction: Short ablation lines guided by reentry circuit isthmuses and sinus rhythm mapping. Circulation 2001;104:664.
19. Perez-Castellano N, Almendral J, Villacastin J, et al: Basic assessment of paced activation sequence mapping: implications for practical use. Pacing Clin Electrophysiol 2004;27:651.
20. Arentz T, von RJ, Blum T, et al: Feasibility and safety of pulmonary vein isolation using a new mapping and navigation system in patients with refractory atrial fibrillation. Circulation 2003;108:2484.
21. Friedman PA: Novel mapping techniques for cardiac electrophysiology. Heart 2002;87:575.
22. Sanders P, Hocini M, Jais P, et al: Characterization of focal atrial tachycardia using high-density mapping. J Am Coll Cardiol 2005;46:2088.
23. Schilling RJ, Friedman PA, Stanton MS: Mathematical Reconstruction Of Endocardial Potentials With Non-Contact Multielectrode Array. Field Clinical Training Manual. St. Paul, Minn, Endocardial Solutions, 2006.
24. Chinitz LA, Sethi JS: How to perform noncontact mapping. Heart Rhythm 2006;3:120.
25. Chow AW, Schilling RJ, Davies DW, Peters NS: Characteristics of wavefront propagation in reentrant circuits causing human ventricular tachycardia. Circulation 2002;105:2172.
26. Gasparini M, Mantica M, Coltorti F: The use of advanced mapping systems to guide right linear lesions in paroxysmal atrial fibrillation. Eur Heart J 2001; 3:41.
27. Higa S, Tai CT, Lin YJ, et al: Focal atrial tachycardia: new insight from noncontact mapping and catheter ablation. Circulation 2004;109:84.
28. Packer DL: Three-dimensional mapping in interventional electrophysiology: Techniques and technology. J Cardiovasc Electrophysiol 2005;16:1110.
29. Markowitz SM, Lerman BB: How to interpret electroanatomical maps. Heart Rhythm 2006;3:240.
30. Dickfeld T, Calkins H, Zviman M, et al: Anatomical stereotactic catheter ablation on three-dimensional magnetic resonance images in real time. Circulation 2003 11;108:2407.
31. Dickfeld T, Calkins H, Zviman M, et al: Stereotactic magnetic resonance guidance for anatomically targeted ablations of the fossa ovalis and the left atrium. J Interv Card Electrophysiol 2004;11:105.
32. Sra J, Krum D, Hare J, et al: Feasibility and validation of registration of three-dimensional left atrial models derived from computed tomography with a noncontact cardiac mapping system. Heart Rhythm 2005;2:55.
33. Hoffmann E, Reithmann C, Nimmermann P, et al: Clinical experience with electroanatomical mapping of ectopic atrial tachycardia. Pacing Clin Electrophysiol 2002;25:49.
34. Reithmann C, Hoffmann E, Dorwarth U, et al: Electroanatomical mapping for visualization of atrial activation in patients with incisional atrial tachycardias. Eur Heart J 2001;22:237.
35. Wetzel U, Hindricks G, Schirdewahn P, et al: A stepwise mapping approach for localization and ablation of ectopic right, left, and septal atrial foci using electroanatomical mapping. Eur Heart J 2002;23:1387.
36. Kirchhof P, Loh P, Eckardt L, et al: A novel nonfluoroscopic catheter visualization system (LocaLisa) to reduce radiation exposure during catheter ablation of supraventricular tachycardias. Am J Cardiol 2002;90:340.
37. Earley MJ, Showkathali R, Alzetani M, et al: Radiofrequency ablation of arrhythmias guided by non-fluoroscopic catheter location: A prospective randomized trial. Eur Heart J 2006;27:1223.
38. Novak PG, Macle L, Thibault B, Guerra PG: Enhanced left atrial mapping using digitally synchronized NavX three-dimensional nonfluoroscopic mapping and high-resolution computed tomographic imaging for catheter ablation of atrial fibrillation. Heart Rhythm 2004;1:521.
39. Essebag V, Baldessin F, Reynolds MR, et al: Non-inducibility post-pulmonary vein isolation achieving exit block predicts freedom from atrial fibrillation. Eur Heart J 2005;26:2550.
40. Takahashi Y, Rotter M, Sanders P, et al: Left atrial linear ablation to modify the substrate of atrial fibrillation using a new nonfluoroscopic imaging system. Pacing Clin Electrophysiol 2005;28(Suppl 1):S90.
41. Ernst S, Ouyang F, Linder C, et al: Initial experience with remote catheter ablation using a novel magnetic navigation system: Magnetic remote catheter ablation. Circulation 2004;109:1472.
42. Ernst S, Ouyang F, Linder C, et al: Modulation of the slow pathway in the presence of a persistent left superior caval vein using the novel magnetic navigation system Niobe. Europace 2004;6:10.
43. Pappone C, Vicedomini G, Manguso F, et al: Robotic magnetic navigation for atrial fibrillation ablation. J Am Coll Cardiol 2006;47:1390.
44. Finlay DD, Nugent CD, McCullagh PJ, Black ND: Mining for diagnostic information in body surface potential maps: A comparison of feature selection techniques. Biomed Eng Online 2005;4:51.

45. Taccardi B, Punske B: Body surface potential mapping. *In* Zipes DP, Jalife J (eds): Cardiac Electrophysiology: From Cell to Bedside. Philadelphia, WB Saunders, 2004, pp 803-811.
46. Lopez JA, Nugent CD, Van HG, et al: Visualization of body surface electrocardiographic features in myocardial infarction. J Electrocardiol 2004;37:149.
47. Ghanem RN, Jia P, Ramanathan C, et al: Noninvasive electrocardiographic imaging (ECGI): Comparison to intraoperative mapping in patients. Heart Rhythm 2005 April;2(4):339-354.
48. Intini A, Goldstein RN, Jia P, et al: Electrocardiographic imaging (ECGI), a novel diagnostic modality used for mapping of focal left ventricular tachycardia in a young athlete. Heart Rhythm 2005;2:1250.
49. Jia P, Ramanathan C, Ghanem RN, et al: Electrocardiographic imaging of cardiac resynchronization therapy in heart failure: Observation of variable electrophysiologic responses. Heart Rhythm 2006;3:296.
50. Ramanathan C, Ghanem RN, Jia P, et al: Noninvasive electrocardiographic imaging for cardiac electrophysiology and arrhythmia. Nat Med 2004;10:422.
51. Zhang X, Ramachandra I, Liu Z, et al: Noninvasive three-dimensional electrocardiographic imaging of ventricular activation sequence. Am J Physiol Heart Circ Physiol 2005;289:H2724.
52. Morton JB, Wilber DJ, Kalman JM: Role of intracardiac echocardiography in clinical and experimental electrophysiology. *In* Huang SKS, Wood MA (eds): Catheter Ablation of Cardiac Arrhythmias. Philadelphia, WB Saunders, 2006, pp 163-180.
53. Ren JF, Marchlinski FE: Intracardiac echocardiography: Basic concepts. *In* Ren JF, Marchlinski FE, Callans DJ, Schwartzman D (eds): Practical Intracardiac Echocardiography in Electrophysiology. Malden, Mass, Blackwell Futura, 2006, pp 1-4.
54. Ren JF, Weiss JP: Imaging technique and cardiac structures. *In* Ren JF, Marchlinski FE, Callans DJ, Schwartzman D (eds): Practical Intracardiac Echocardiography in Electrophysiology. Malden, Mass, Blackwell Futura, 2006, pp 18-40.
55. Marrouche NF, Martin DO, Wazni O, et al: Phased-array intracardiac echocardiography monitoring during pulmonary vein isolation in patients with atrial fibrillation: Impact on outcome and complications. Circulation 2003;107:2710.
56. Johnson SB, Seward JB, Packer DL: Phased-array intracardiac echocardiography for guiding transseptal catheter placement: Utility and learning curve. Pacing Clin Electrophysiol 2002;25(4 Pt 1):402.
57. Ren JF, Marchlinski FE: Monitoring and early diagnosis of procedural complications. *In* Ren JF, Marchlinski FE, Callans DJ, Schwartzman D (eds): Practical Intracardiac Echocardiography in Electrophysiology. Malden, Mass, Blackwell Futura, 2006, pp 180-207.
58. Kato R, Lickfett L, Meininger G, et al: Pulmonary vein anatomy in patients undergoing catheter ablation of atrial fibrillation: Lessons learned by use of magnetic resonance imaging. Circulation 2003;107:2004.
59. Sra J, Krum D, Malloy A, et al: Registration of three-dimensional left atrial computed tomographic images with projection images obtained using fluoroscopy. Circulation 2005;112:3763.
60. Triedman J: Virtual reality in interventional electrophysiology. Circulation 2005;112:3677.
61. Malchano ZJ, Neuzil P, Cury RC, et al: Integration of cardiac CT/MR imaging with three-dimensional electroanatomical mapping to guide catheter manipulation in the left atrium: Implications for catheter ablation of atrial fibrillation. J Cardiovasc Electrophysiol 2006;17:1221.
62. Sra J, Narayan G, Krum D, et al: Computed tomography-fluoroscopy image integration-guided catheter ablation of atrial fibrillation. J Cardiovasc Electrophysiol 2007;18:409.
63. Fahmy TS, Mlcochova H, Wazni OM, et al: Intracardiac echo-guided image integration: optimizing strategies for registration. J Cardiovasc Electrophysiol 2007;18:2762.
64. Zhong H, Lacomis JM, Schwartzman D: On the accuracy of CartoMerge for guiding posterior left atrial ablation in man. Heart Rhythm 2007;4:595.

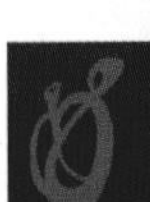

CHAPTER 4

Ablation Energy Sources

RADIOFREQUENCY ABLATION

Biophysics of Radiofrequency Energy

Radiofrequency (RF) refers to the portion of the electromagnetic spectrum in which electromagnetic waves can be generated by alternating current fed to an antenna.[1] Electrosurgery ablation currently uses hectomeric wavelengths found in band 6 (300 to 3000 kHz), which are similar to those used for broadcast radio; however, the RF energy is electrically conducted, not radiated, during catheter ablation. The RF current is similar to low-frequency alternating current or direct current with regard to its ability to heat tissue and create a lesion, but it oscillates so rapidly that cardiac and skeletal muscles are not stimulated, thereby avoiding induction of arrhythmias and decreasing the pain perceived by the patient. RF current rarely induces rapid polymorphic arrhythmias; such arrhythmias can be observed in response to low-frequency (60 Hz) stimulation. Frequencies higher than 1000 kHz are also effective in generating tissue heating; however, such high frequencies are associated with considerable energy loss along the transmission line. Therefore, frequencies of the RF current commonly used are in the range of 300 to 1000 kHz, which combines efficacy and safety.[2-4]

Radiofrequency Energy Delivery

Delivery of RF energy depends on the establishment of an electric circuit involving the human body as one of its in-series elements. The RF current is applied to the tissue via a metal electrode at the tip of the ablation catheter and is generally delivered in a unipolar fashion between the tip electrode and a large dispersive electrode (indifferent electrode, or ground pad) applied to the patient's skin. The polarity of connections from the electrodes to the generator is not important because the RF current is an alternating current. Bipolar RF systems also exist, in which current flows between two closely apposed small electrodes, limiting the current flow to small tissue volumes interposed between the metal conductors. Bipolar systems, partly because of their relative safety, are now the preferred tools in electrosurgery (oncology, plastic surgery, and ophthalmology). Their clinical application for catheter-based ablation has not yet been evaluated.[2-4]

The system impedance comprises the impedance of the generator, transmission lines, catheter, electrode-tissue interface, dispersive electrode-skin interface, and interposed tissues. As electricity flows through a circuit, every point of that circuit represents a drop in voltage, and some energy gets dissipated as heat. The point of greatest drop in line voltage represents the area of highest impedance and is where most of that electrical energy becomes dissipated as heat. Therefore, with excessive electrical resistance in the transmission line, the line will actually warm up and power will be lost. Current electrical conductors from the generator all the way through to the patient and from the dispersive electrode back to the generator have low impedance, so as to minimize power loss.[2,3]

With normal electrode-tissue contact, only a fraction of all power is effectively applied to the tissue. The rest is dissipated in the blood pool and the rest of the patient. With an ablation electrode in contact with the endocardial wall, part of the electrode will contact tissue and the rest will contact blood, and the RF current flows through both the myocardium and the blood pool in contact with the electrode. The distribution between both depends on the impedance of both routes and also on how much electrode surface contacts blood versus endocardial wall. Whereas tissue heating is the target of power delivery, the blood pool is the most attractive route for RF current because blood is a better conductor and has significantly lower impedance than tissue, and because the contact between electrode and blood will often be better than with tissue. Therefore, with normal electrode-tissue contact, much more power will generally be delivered to blood than to cardiac tissue.[2-5]

After leaving the electrode-blood-tissue interface, the current flows through the thorax to the indifferent electrode. Part of the RF power is lost in the patient's body, including the area near the patch. Dissipation of energy can occur at the dispersive electrode site (at the contact point between that ground pad and the skin) to a degree that can limit lesion formation. In fact, if ablation is performed with a high-amplitude current (more than 50 W) and skin contact by the dispersive electrode is poor, it is possible to cause skin burns.[1] Nevertheless, because the surface area of the ablation electrode (approximately 12 mm^2) is much smaller than that of the dispersive electrode (approximately 100 to 250 cm^2), the current density is higher at the ablation site, and heating occurs preferentially at that site, with no significant heating occurring at the dispersive electrode.[6]

The dispersive electrode may be placed on any convenient skin surface. The geometry of the RF current field is defined by the geometry of the ablation electrode and is relatively uniform in the region of volume heating. Thus, the position of the dispersive electrode (on the patient's back or thigh) has little effect on impedance, voltage, current delivery, catheter tip temperature, or geometry of the resulting lesion.[2,3,6]

The size of the dispersive electrode, however, is of importance. Sometimes it is advantageous to increase the surface area of the dispersive electrode, which leads to lower impedance, higher current delivery, increased catheter tip temperatures, and more effective tissue heating. This is especially true in patients with baseline system impedance more than 100 Ω. Moreover, when the system is power-limited, as with a 50-W generator, heat production at the catheter tip will vary with the proportion of the local electrode-tissue interface impedance to the overall system impedance. If the impedance at the skin-dispersive electrode interface is high, then a smaller amount of energy is available for tissue heating at the electrode tip. Therefore, when ablating certain sites, the addition of a second dispersive electrode or optimizing the contact between the dispersive electrode and skin should result in relatively more power delivery to the target tissue.[6,7]

Tissue Heating

During alternating current flow, charged carriers in tissue (ions) attempt to follow the changes in the direction of the alternating current, thus converting electromagnetic (current) energy into molecular mechanical energy or heat. This type of electric current-mediated heating is known as ohmic (resistive) heating. Using Ohm's law, with resistive heating, the amount of power (= heat) per unit volume equals the square of current density times the specific impedance of the tissue. With a spherical electrode, the current flows outward radially and current density therefore decreases with the square of distance from the center of the electrode. Consequently, power dissipation per unit volume decreases with the fourth power of distance. The thickness of the electrode, however, eliminates the first steepest part of this curve and the decrease in dissipated power with distance is therefore somewhat less dramatic.[2,3]

Approximately 90% of all power that is being delivered to the tissue is absorbed within the first 1 to 1.5 mm from the electrode surface. Therefore, only a thin rim of tissue in immediate contact with the RF electrode is directly heated (within the first 2 mm of depth from the electrode). The remainder of tissue heating occurs as a result of heat conduction from this rim to the surrounding tissues.[5] On initiation of fixed-level energy application, the temperature at the electrode-tissue interface rises monoexponentially to reach steady state within a few seconds ($t_{\{1/2\}}$ = 7 to 10 seconds), and the steady state is usually maintained between 80° and 90°C. However, whereas resistive heating starts immediately with the delivery of RF current, conduction of heat to deeper tissue sites is relatively slow and requires 1 to 2 minutes to equilibrate (thermal equilibrium).[5] Therefore, the rate of tissue temperature rise beyond the immediate vicinity of the RF electrode is much slower, resulting in a steep radial temperature gradient as tissue temperature decreases radially in proportion to the distance from the ablation electrode; however, deep tissue temperatures continue to rise for several seconds after interruption of RF delivery (the so-called *thermal latency phenomenon*).[5] Therefore, RF ablation requires at least 30 to 60 seconds to create full-grown lesions. In addition, when temperature differences between adjacent areas develop because of differences in local current density or local heat capacity, heat will conduct from hotter to colder areas, causing the temperature of the former to decrease and that of the latter to increase. Furthermore, heat loss to the blood pool at the surface and to intramyocardial vessels determines the temperature profile within the tissue.[2,3,8]

At steady state, the lesion size is proportional to the temperature measured at the interface between the tissue and the electrode as well as to the RF power amplitude. By using higher powers and achieving higher tissue temperatures, the lesion size can be increased. However, once the peak tissue temperature exceeds the threshold of 100°C, boiling of the plasma at the electrode-tissue interface can ensue. When boiling occurs, denatured serum proteins and charred tissue form a thin film that adhere to the electrode, forming an electrically insulating coagulum, which is accompanied by a sudden increase in electrical impedance preventing further current flow into the tissue and further heating.[2,3]

The range of tissue temperatures used for RF ablation is 50° to 90°C. Within this range, smooth desiccation of tissue can be expected. If the temperature is less than 50°C, no or only minimal tissue necrosis results. Because the rate of temperature rise at deeper sites within the myocardium is slow, a continuous energy delivery of at least 60 seconds is often warranted to maximize depth of lesion formation.

Convective Cooling

The dominant factor opposing effective heating of myocardium is the convective heat loss into the circulating blood pool. Because the tissue surface is cooled by the blood flow, the highest temperature during RF delivery occurs slightly below the endocardial surface. Consequently, the width of the endocardial lesion matures earlier than the intramural lesion width (20 versus 90 to 120 seconds). Therefore, the maximum lesion width is usually located intramurally, and the resultant lesion is usually teardrop-shaped, with less necrosis of the superficial tissue.[2,3]

As the magnitude of convective cooling increases (e.g., unstable catheter position, poor catheter-tissue contact, or high blood flow in the region of catheter position), there is decreased efficiency of heating because of more energy being carried away in the blood and less energy delivered to the tissue. When RF power is limited, lesion size is reduced by such convective heat loss. On the other hand, when RF power delivery is not limited, convective cooling allows for more power to be delivered into the tissue and higher tissue temperatures can be achieved (despite low temperatures measured by the catheter tip sensors), resulting in larger lesion size, without the risk of overheating and coagulum formation.[2-4]

The concept of convective cooling can explain why there are few coronary complications with conventional RF ablation. Coronary arteries act as a heat sink; substantive heating of vascular endothelium is prevented by heat dissipation in the high-velocity coronary blood flow, even when the catheter is positioned close to the vessel. Although this is advantageous, because coronary arteries are being protected, it can limit success of the ablation lesion if a large perforating artery is close to the ablation target.[6,9]

The effects of convective cooling have been exploited to increase the size of catheter ablative lesions. To eliminate the risk of overheating at the electrode-tissue contact point but increase the magnitude of power delivery and the depth of volume heating, investigators have used porous-tipped electrodes for open irrigation of the electrode tip or closed irrigation systems for electrode tip cooling.[10]

Catheter Tip Temperature

Ablation catheter tip temperature depends on tissue temperature, convective cooling by the surrounding blood, tissue contact of the ablation electrode, electrode material and its heat capacity, and type and location of the temperature sensor.[2,11]

Catheter tip temperature is measured by a sensor located in the ablation electrode. There are two different types of temperature sensors, thermocouples and thermistors. Thermistors require a driving current and the electrical resistance changes as the temperature of the electric conductor changes. More frequently used are thermocouples, which consist of copper and constantan wires and are incorporated in the center of the ablation electrode. Thermocouples are based on the so-called Seebeck effect; when two different metals are connected (sensing junction), a voltage can be measured at the reference junction that is proportional to the temperature difference between the two metals.[2,3,11]

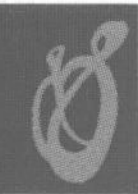

4

The electrode temperature rise is an indirect process—the ablation electrode is not heated by RF energy, but it heats up because it happens to touch heated tissue. Consequently, the catheter tip temperature is always lower than, or ideally equal to, the superficial tissue temperature. Conventional electrode catheters with temperature monitoring only report the temperature from the center of the electrode mass with one design or from the apex of the tip of the catheter with another design, and it is likely that the measured temperature underestimates the peak tissue temperature; it can be significantly lower than the tissue temperature. With a thermosensor placed approximately 1 mm beneath a 4-mm electrode, the temperature within the tissue is on average 42° ± 6°C higher than at the electrode tip after 30 seconds of RF delivery, with a preset target temperature of 70°C.

Several other factors can increase the disparity between catheter tip temperature and tissue temperature, including catheter tip irrigation, large ablation electrode size, and poor electrode-tissue contact. Catheter tip irrigation increases the disparity between tissue temperature and electrode temperature because it results in cooling of the ablation electrode, but not the tissue. With a large electrode tip, a larger area of the electrode tip is exposed to the cooling effects of the blood flow than with standard tip lengths, resulting in lower electrode temperatures. Similarly, with poor electrode-tissue contact, less electrode material is in contact with the tissue and heating of the tip by the tissue occurs at a lower rate, resulting in relatively low tip temperatures.[3,7,11,12]

Pathophysiology of Lesion Formation by Radiofrequency Ablation

Cellular Effects of Radiofrequency Ablation

The primary mechanism of tissue injury by RF ablation is likely to be thermally mediated. Hyperthermic injury to the myocyte is both time- and temperature-dependent, and it can be caused by changes in the cell membrane, protein inactivation, cytoskeletal disruption, nuclear degeneration, or a number of other potential mechanisms.[2,3]

Experimentally, the resting membrane depolarization is related to temperature.[8] In the low hyperthermic range (37° to 45°C), little tissue injury occurs, and a minor change may be observed in the resting membrane potential and action potential amplitude. However, the action potential duration shortens significantly and conduction velocity becomes greater than at baseline. In the intermediate hyperthermic range (45° to 50°C), progressive depolarization of the resting membrane potential occurs and the action potential amplitude decreases. Also, abnormal automaticity is observed, reversible loss of excitability occurs, and conduction velocity progressively decreases. In the high temperature ranges (more than 50°C), marked depolarization of the resting membrane potential occurs and permanent loss of excitability is observed. Temporary (at temperatures of 49.5° to 51.5°C) and then permanent (at 51.7° to 54.4°C) conduction block develops, and a fairly reliable irreversible myocardial injury occurs with a short hyperthermic exposure.[2,3,8]

In the clinical setting, the success of ablation is related to the mean temperature measured at the electrode-tissue interface. Block of conduction in an atrioventricular (AV) bypass tract (BT) usually occurs at 62° ± 15°C. During ablation of the AV junction, an accelerated junctional rhythm, which is probably caused by thermally or electrically induced cellular automaticity or triggered activity, is observed at temperatures of 51° ± 4°C, whereas reversible complete AV block occurs at 58° ± 6°C and irreversible complete AV block occurs at 60° ± 7°C.

RF ablation typically results in high temperatures (70° to 90°C) for a short time (up to 60 seconds) at the electrode-tissue interface, but significantly lower temperatures at deeper tissue sites. This leads to rapid tissue injury within the immediate vicinity of the RF electrode but relatively delayed myocardial injury with increasing distance from the RF electrode. Therefore, although irreversible loss of EP function can usually be demonstrated immediately after successful RF ablation, this finding can be delayed because tissue temperatures continue to rise somewhat after termination of RF energy delivery (thermal latency phenomenon). This effect can account for the observation that patients undergoing atrioventricular node (AVN) modification procedures who demonstrate transient heart block during RF energy delivery can progress to persisting complete heart block, even if RF energy delivery is terminated immediately. Reversible loss of conduction can be demonstrated within seconds of initiating the RF application, which can be caused by an acute electrotonic effect. On the other hand, there can be late recovery of electrophysiological (EP) function after an initial successful ablation.[2,6]

In addition to the dominant thermal effects of RF ablation, some of the cellular injury has been hypothesized to be caused by a direct electrical effect, which can result in dielectric breakdown of the sarcolemmal membrane with creation of transmembrane pores (electroporation), resulting in nonspecific ion transit, cellular depolarization, calcium overload, and cell death. Such an effect has been demonstrated with the use of high-voltage electrical current. However, it is difficult to examine the purely electrical effects in isolation of the dominant thermal injury.

Tissue Effects of Radiofrequency Ablation

Changes in myocardial tissue are apparent immediately on completion of the RF lesion. Pallor of the central zone of the lesion is attributable to denaturation of myocyte proteins (principally myoglobin) and subsequent loss of the red pigmentation. Slight deformation, indicating volume loss, occurs at the point of catheter contact in the central region of lesion formation. The endocardial surface is usually covered with a thin fibrin layer and occasionally, if a temperature of 100°C has been exceeded, with char and thrombus. Also, a coagulum (an accumulation of fibrin, platelets, and other blood and tissue components) can form at the ablation electrode because of the boiling of blood and tissue serum.[2,3]

On sectioning, the central portion of the RF ablation lesion shows desiccation, with a surrounding region of hemorrhagic tissue and then normal-appearing tissue. The histology of an acute lesion shows typical coagulation necrosis with basophilic stippling consistent with intracellular calcium overload. Immediately surrounding the central lesion is a region of hemorrhage and acute monocellular and neutrophilic inflammation. The progressive changes seen in the evolution of an RF lesion are typical of healing after any acute injury. Within 2 months of the ablation, the lesion shows fibrosis, granulation tissue, chronic inflammatory infiltrates, and significant volume contraction. The lesion border is well demarcated from the surrounding viable myocardium without evidence of a transitional zone. This likely accounts for the absence of proarrhythmic side effects of RF catheter ablation. As noted, because of the high-velocity blood flow within the epicardial coronary arteries, these vessels are continuously cooled and are typically spared from injury, despite nearby delivery of RF energy. However, high RF power delivery in small hearts, such as in pediatric patients, or in direct contact with the vessel can potentially cause coronary arterial injury.[2,3]

The border zone around the acute pathological RF lesion accounts for several phenomena observed clinically. The border zone is characterized by marked ultrastructural abnormalities of the microvasculature and myocytes acutely, and a typical inflammatory response later. The most thermally sensitive structures appear to be the plasma membrane and gap junctions, which show morphological changes as far as 6 mm from the edge of the pathological lesion. The border zone accounts for documented effects of RF lesion formation well beyond the acute pathological lesion. The progression of the EP effects after completion of the ablation procedure can be caused by further inflammatory injury and necrosis in the border zone region, resulting in late progression of physiological block and a delayed cure in some cases. On the other hand, initial stunning and then early or late recovery of function can be demonstrated in the border zone, accounting for the recovery of EP function after successful catheter ablation in the clinical setting, which can be caused by healing of the damaged, but surviving, myocardium.[2,3]

Determinants of Lesion Size

Lesion size is defined as the total volume or dimensions (width and depth) of the lesion. The size of the lesion created by RF power is determined by the amount of tissue heated above the critical temperature for producing irreversible myocardial damage (50°C). Higher tissue temperatures result in larger lesions. However, temperatures higher than 100°C are associated with coagulum formation on the RF ablation electrode and electrical impedance rise, which potentially limits lesion size.

Electrode Tip Temperature. It is important to understand that it is the amount of RF power delivered effectively into the tissue that determines tissue heating and thus lesion size, and that the catheter tip temperature is poorly correlated with lesion size. As noted, catheter tip temperature is always lower than the superficial tissue temperature. With good contact between catheter tip and tissue and low cooling of the catheter tip, the target temperature can be reached with little power, resulting in fairly small lesions although a high catheter tip temperature is being measured. In contrast, a low catheter tip temperature can be caused by a high level of convective cooling, allowing a higher amount of RF power to be delivered to the tissue (because it is no longer limited by temperature rise of the ablation electrode) and yielding relatively large lesions. This is best illustrated with active cooling of the ablation electrode using irrigation during RF energy delivery; the tip temperature is usually below 40° C, which allows the application of high-power output for longer durations.

Radiofrequency Duration. The RF lesion is predominantly generated within the first 10 seconds of target energy delivery and tissue temperatures and it reaches a maximum after 30 seconds. Further extension of RF delivery during power controlled RF delivery does not seem to increase lesion size further.

Electrode-Tissue Contact. Energy transfer to the myocardium largely depends on electrode-tissue contact. An improvement in tissue contact leads to a higher amount of RF power that can be effectively delivered to the tissue. Consequently, the same tissue temperatures and lesion size can be reached at a much lower power level. However, at a certain moderate contact force, further increase in contact firmness results in progressively smaller lesions because a lesser amount of RF power is required to reach target temperature.[5]

Additionally, the surface area at the electrode-tissue interface influences the lesion size. When the catheter is wedged—that is, between ventricular trabeculae or under a valvular leaflet—the electrode surface area exposed to tissue can be much higher. With half the electrode in contact with blood and the other half in contact with (twice) more resistive tissue, the amount of power delivered to blood will be two times higher than to tissue (as compared to six times with 25% contact). This will result in a more than twofold increase in tissue heating. In practice, however, power output will rarely reach 50 W in these situations; temperature rise of the ablation electrode will signal excessive tissue heating and limit power delivery.[5,13]

Close monitoring of the changes in temperature and impedance provides information regarding the degree of electrode-tissue contact. Increased contact results in increased initial impedance levels (by a mean of 22%) and an increase in the rate and level of impedance reduction and the plateau is reached later. Additionally, increased electrode-tissue contact results in higher tissue temperatures, and the plateau is achieved later. Beat-to-beat stability of electrograms and pacing threshold also provide some information about tissue contact.[5,13]

Electrode Orientation. When the catheter tip is perpendicular to the tissue surface, a much smaller surface area is in contact with the tissue (versus that exposed to the cooling effect of blood flow) than if the catheter electrode tip is lying on its side. Clinically, perpendicular electrode orientation yields larger lesion volumes using less power than parallel electrode orientation. However, if the RF power level is adjusted to maintain a constant current density, lesion size increases proportionally to the electrode-tissue contact area, which is larger with parallel tip orientation.[13] Lesion depth is only slightly affected by catheter tip orientation using 4-mm long tip catheters, but lesions are slightly longer in the parallel orientation as compared with the perpendicular orientation. Moreover, the character of the lesion created with temperature control depends on the placement of the temperature sensor(s) relative to the portion of the electrode in contact with tissue. Thus, the orientation of the electrode and its temperature sensors will determine the appropriate target temperature required to create maximal lesions while avoiding coagulum formation caused by overheating at any location within the electrode-tissue interface.[2,3]

Electrode Length. Ablation catheters have tip electrodes that are conventionally 4 mm long and are available in sizes up to 10 mm long (see Fig. 2-6). An increased electrode size reduces the interface impedance with blood and tissue, but the impedance through the rest of the patient remains the same. The ratio between interface impedance

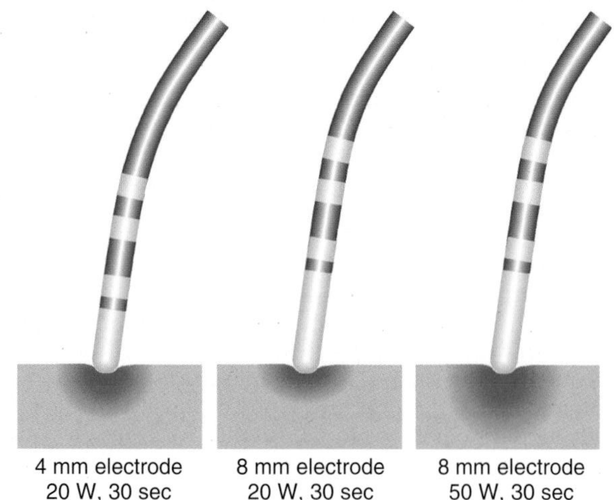

4 **FIGURE 4–1** Effect of electrode size and power delivery on lesion size. The effect of 20 W delivered for 30 sec is shown for a 4-mm electrode (*left*) and 8-mm electrode (*center*). The larger electrode dissipates more of the energy into the blood pool and thus paradoxically creates a smaller lesion. Because of electrode cooling from its larger surface area, the same 8-mm electrode can deliver more power than the 4-mm electrode and could create a larger lesion (*right*).

and the impedance through the rest of the patient is thus lower with an 8-mm electrode than with a 4-mm electrode, which reduces the efficiency of power transfer to the tissue. Thus, with the same total power, lesions with a larger electrode will always be smaller than with a smaller electrode (Fig. 4-1). A larger electrode size also creates a greater variability in power transfer to the tissue because of greater variability of tissue contact, and tissue contact becomes much more dependent on catheter orientation with longer electrodes. Consequently, an 8-mm electrode may require a 1.5 to 4 times higher power level than a 4-mm electrode to create the same lesion size.[5]

When the power is not limited, however, catheters with large distal electrodes create larger lesions, both by increasing the ablation electrode surface area in contact with bloodstream, resulting in augmented convective cooling effect, and by increasing the volume of tissue directly heated because of an increased surface area at the electrode-tissue interface (see Fig. 4-1). However, this assumes that the electrode-tissue contact, tissue heat dissipation, and blood flow are uniform throughout the electrode-tissue interface. As the electrode size increases, the likelihood that these assumptions are true diminishes because of variability in cardiac chamber trabeculations and curvature, tissue perfusion, and intracardiac blood flow, which will affect the heat dissipation and tissue contact. These factors will result in unpredictable lesion size and uniformity for electrodes more than 8 mm long.[2,3]

There is a potential safety concern with the use of long ablation electrodes because of nonuniform heating, with maximal heating occurring at the electrode edges. Thus, large electrode-tipped catheters with only a single thermistor can underestimate maximal temperature, allowing char formation and potential thromboembolic complications. Catheter tips with multiple temperature sensors at the electrode edges may be preferable for temperature feedback. In addition, the greater variation in power delivered to the tissue and the greater discrepancy between electrode and tissue temperature make it hard to avoid intramural gas explosions and blood clot formation. Another point of concern is that the formation of blood clots may only minimally affect electrode impedance by covering a much smaller part of the electrode surface. Therefore, the lower electrode temperature and the absence of any impedance rise may erroneously suggest a safer ablation process.[5]

The two principal limitations of a large ablation electrode (8 to 10 mm in length) are the reduction in mobility and flexibility of the catheter, which can impair positioning of the ablation electrode, and a reduction in the resolution of recordings from the ablation electrode, making it more difficult to identify the optimal ablation site. A larger electrode dampens the local electrogram, especially that of the distal electrode. With an 8- or 10-mm long distal and a 1-mm short proximal ring electrode, the latter can be the main source for the bipolar electrogram; this then confuses localization of the optimal ablation site. In contrast, a smaller electrode improves mapping accuracy and feedback of tissue heating. Its only drawback is the limited power level that can be applied to the tissue.[5]

Ablation Electrode Material. Although platinum electrodes have been the standard for most RF ablation catheters, gold electrodes have four times the thermal conductivity of platinum and, therefore, allow for greater power delivery to create deeper lesions at a given electrode temperature without impedance increases.[14] Heat generated in the tissue will be conducted more easily to the bulk of the gold electrode and therefore more easily to the blood pool. Enhanced electrode cooling allows for the delivery of somewhat higher RF power levels. Consequently, a larger lesion can be created at the same electrode target temperature.[5] However, the higher thermal conductivity of gold electrodes is no longer an advantage in areas of low blood flow (e.g., among myocardial trabeculae), where convective cooling at the electrode tip is minimal. Under these circumstances, electrode materials with a low thermal conductivity can produce larger lesions.[3]

Reference Patch Electrode Location and Size. The RF current path and skin reference electrode interface present significant impedance for the ablation current flow, therefore dissipating part of the power. Increasing patch size (or using two patches) provides for increased heating at the electrode-endocardium interface and thus increases ablation efficiency and increases lesion size. On the other hand, the position of the dispersive electrode (on the patient's back or thigh) has little effect on the size of the resulting lesion.[6]

Blood Flow. The ablation electrode temperature is dependent on the opposing effects of heating from the tissue and cooling by the blood flowing around the electrode. Because lesion size is primarily dependent on the RF power delivered to the tissue, lesion size will vary with the magnitude of local blood flow. At any given electrode temperature, the RF power delivered to the tissue is significantly reduced in areas of low local blood flow (e.g., deep pouch in the cavotricuspid isthmus, dilated and poorly contracting atria, and dilated and poorly contracting ventricles). The reduced cooling associated with low blood flow causes the electrode to reach the target temperature at lower power levels and, if the ablation lesion is temperature-controlled, power delivery will be limited. In these locations, increasing electrode temperature to 65° or 70°C only minimally increases RF power and increases the risk of thrombus formation and impedance rise. In contrast, increasing local blood flow is associated with increased convective cooling of the ablation electrode. Consequently, more power is delivered to the tissue to reach and maintain target temperature, resulting in larger lesion volumes.[2,3,11]

Radiofrequency System Polarity. Most RF lesions are created by applying energy in a unipolar fashion between an ablating electrode touching the myocardium and a grounded reference patch electrode placed externally on the skin. The unipolar configuration creates a highly localized lesion, with the least amount of surface injury. Energy can also be applied in a bipolar mode between two endocardial electrodes. Bipolar energy delivery produces larger lesions than unipolar delivery. Multiple bipolar RF power applications (between proximal, middle, and distal pairs of electrodes on a catheter with four 2-mm electrodes) result in much larger lesions than those created by single applications. This method is under investigation and may prove to be useful in increasing the efficiency of creating long linear ablation lesions.[2,3]

Monitoring Radiofrequency Energy Delivery

The goal of optimizing RF ablation is to create an adequate-sized lesion while minimizing the chance of an impedance increase because of coagulum formation at the electrode itself, or steam formation within the tissue. Lesion creation is influenced by many factors, some of which can be controlled, whereas others are variable and can be unpredictable. With standard RF, power delivery is titrated to electrode temperature, typically at 55° to 65°C. Higher temperatures can increase the chance of reaching 100°C at edges of the ablation electrode, resulting in coagulum formation. An increase in tissue temperature is accompanied by a decrease in impedance, also a reliable marker of tissue heating. Impedance reduction and temperature rise correlate with both lesion width and depth; maximum temperature rise is best correlated with lesion width, and maximum impedance reduction is best correlated with lesion depth.[3,4,11]

The efficiency of tissue heating (i.e., the temperature per watt of applied power) is dependent on several variables, including catheter stability, electrode-tissue contact pressure, electrode orientation relative to the endocardium, effective electrode contact area, convective heat loss into the blood pool, and target location. Thus, applied energy, power, and current are poor indicators of the extent of lesion formation, and the actual electrode-tissue interface temperature remains the only predictor of the actual lesion size. Currently, although less than ideal, monitoring temperature and impedance are used to help ensure adequate but not excessive heating at the electrode-tissue interface. Newer technologies may be implemented in the future to monitor tissue temperatures during RF delivery, including infrared sensors and ultrasound transducers.

In addition to impedance and catheter tip temperature monitoring, reduction in amplitude and steepness of the local electrogram is an important indicator to monitor lesion growth. This, however, only applies to the unipolar distal electrogram. With a bipolar recording, the signal from the ring electrode may dominate the electrogram and the bipolar amplitude may theoretically even rise during ablation, because of a greater difference between the signals from both electrodes.[5]

Impedance Monitoring

The magnitude of the current delivered by the RF generator used in ablation is largely determined by the impedance between the ablation catheter and the dispersive electrode, which is influenced by several factors, including intrinsic tissue properties, catheter contact pressure, catheter electrode size, dispersive electrode size, presence of coagulum, and body surface area. Impedance measurement does not require any specific catheter-based sensor circuitry and can be performed with any catheter designed for RF ablation. Larger dispersive electrodes and larger ablation electrodes result in lower impedance.[3,11]

Typically, the impedance associated with firm catheter contact (before tissue heating has occurred) is 90 to 120 Ω. When catheter contact is poor, the initial impedance is 20% to 50% less, because of the lower resistivity of blood. Moreover, larger electrodes have larger contact area and, consequently, lower impedance.

The impedance drop during RF ablation is mainly because of a reversible phenomenon, such as tissue temperature rise, rather than an irreversible change in tissues secondary to ablation of myocardial tissue. Therefore, impedance provides a useful qualitative assessment of tissue heating; however, it does not correlate well with lesion size.[5] A 5- to 10-Ω reduction in impedance is usually observed in clinically successful RF applications, correlates with a tissue temperature of 55° to 60°C, and is rarely associated with coagulum formation. Larger decrements in impedance are noted when a coagulum formation is imminent. Once a coagulum is formed, an abrupt rise in impedance to more than 250 Ω is usually observed.[3,11]

To titrate RF energy using impedance monitoring alone, the initial power output is set at 20 to 30 W and is then gradually increased to target a 5- to 10-Ω decrement in impedance. When target impedance is reached, power output should be manually adjusted throughout the RF application, as needed, to maintain the impedance in the target range. A larger decrement of impedance should prompt reduction in power output.

The drop in impedance as a monitoring tool has several limitations. When blood flow rates are low, blood can also be heated and electrode impedance will drop accordingly. Moreover, a large rise in tissue temperature at a small contact area and a smaller rise with better tissue contact can result in a similar drop in impedance. Inversely, similar tissue heating with different tissue contact can result in a different change in impedance. Also, resistive heating nearby is fast, whereas conductive heating to deeper layers is relatively slow. The former, at close distance, will have a much greater effect on impedance than the latter, which occurs at greater distance. Like electrode temperature rise, the drop in impedance during RF application, therefore, is not a reliable parameter for estimating tissue heating and lesion growth.[3,5,11]

Although coagulum formation is usually accompanied by an abrupt rise in impedance, the absence of impedance rise during ablation does not guarantee the absence of blood clot formation on the tissue contact site, which can unnoticeably be created on the lesion surface. Also, as noted, with large ablation electrodes, formation of blood clots may only minimally affect electrode impedance by covering a much smaller part of the electrode surface.

Temperature Monitoring

Monitoring catheter tip temperature and closed-loop control of power output are useful to avoid excessive heating at the tissue surface, which can result in coagulum formation, and to accomplish effective heating at the target area. However, catheter tip temperature is affected by cooling effects and electrode-tissue contact and thus poorly correlates with lesion size. Tissue temperature can be markedly higher than catheter tip temperature; a higher target temperature can increase the incidence of tissue overheating associated with crater formation and coagulum formation. In high-flow areas the tip is cooled and more RF power is delivered to the tissue to reach target temperature, resulting in relatively large lesions and vice versa.[3,11,15]

As mentioned earlier, temperature monitoring requires a dedicated sensor within the catheter. Two types of sensors are available, thermistor and thermocouple. No catheter or thermometry technology has been demonstrated to be superior in clinical use; however, closed-loop control of power output is easier to use than manual power titration. Conventional electrode catheters with temperature monitoring only report the temperature from the center of the electrode mass with one design or from the apex of the tip of the catheter with another design, and it is likely that the measured temperature underestimates the peak tissue temperature. Therefore, it is best if target temperatures no higher than 70° to 80°C are selected in the clinical setting.[3,11]

Titration of RF energy using temperature monitoring is usually done automatically by a closed-loop temperature monitoring system. When manual power titration is directed by temperature monitoring, the power initially is set to 20 to 30 W and then gradually increased until the target temperature is achieved. With both manual and automatic power titration, change in power output is frequently required throughout the RF application to maintain the target temperature. Application of RF energy is continued if the desired clinical effect is observed within 5 to 10 seconds after the target temperature or impedance is achieved. If the desired endpoint does not occur within this time, the failed application is probably because of inadequate mapping. If the target temperature or impedance is not achieved with maximum generator output within 20 seconds, the time it takes to achieve subendocardial steady-state temperature, the RF application can be terminated, and catheter adjustment should be considered to obtain better tissue contact.[3,11]

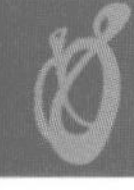

The target ablation electrode temperature varies according to the arrhythmia substrate. For atrioventricular nodal reentrant tachycardia (AVNRT), target temperature is usually 50° to 55°C. For BT, AV junction, atrial tachycardia (AT), and ventricular tachycardia (VT), a higher temperature (55° to 60°C) is usually targeted.

When using 4-mm tip catheters, the target temperature should be less than 80°C. In high-flow areas in the heart, the disparity between tip temperature and tissue temperature is large and a lower target temperature should be considered (e.g., 60°C), whereas in low flow areas the tissue temperature is much better reflected by the tip temperature and a higher target temperature can be considered (e.g., 70° to 80°C). The duration of RF application can be limited to 30 seconds for nonirrigated 4-mm tip electrodes. The lesion is predominantly formed within the first 30 seconds. A longer duration does not create larger lesions.

When using 8-mm tip catheters, a larger portion of the ablation electrode is exposed to the blood and thus cooled by blood flow, and a relatively large difference between catheter tip temperature and tissue temperature can be expected. Consequently, a moderate target temperature (e.g., 60°C) should be chosen; the RF power may be limited to 50 to 60 W to avoid tissue overheating and coagulum formation.[3,11]

It is important to recognize that prevention of coagulum formation is difficult, even with temperature and impedance monitoring. The clot will first adhere to the tissue because that is the site with the highest temperature and may only loosely attach to the cooler electrode. The denaturized proteins probably have higher electrical impedance than blood, but the contact area with the electrode can be small and RF impedance may not rise noticeably. The absence of flow inside the clot and its presumed higher impedance accelerate local heating and, because of some contact with the electrode, also accelerate heating of the electrode. Desiccation and adherence to the electrode then lead to coagulum formation on the metal electrode and impedance rise. Automatic power reduction by temperature-controlled RF ablation will compensate for the reduction of electrode cooling and may prevent desiccation and impedance rise. The clot, however, can still be formed as demonstrated by experimental in vivo studies, and this can remain unnoticeable until it detaches from the tissue. Therefore, the absence of thermal and electrical phenomena does not imply that the ablation has been performed safely.[3,11]

Clinical Applications of Radiofrequency Ablation

RF is the most frequently used mode of ablation energy and has become a widely accepted treatment for most atrial and ventricular arrhythmias. Studies have demonstrated the effectiveness of RF current in producing precise and effective lesions.

Although RF energy for catheter- and surgical-based treatment of cardiac arrhythmias has been proven to be effective and relatively safe, several limitations exist. Many of these limitations center on how RF creates the tissue lesion. Current flow and energy delivery are critically dependent on a low-impedance electrode-tissue junction, but tissue desiccation, coagulation, and charring around the electrode can result in marked falls in conductivity.

A major limitation of RF ablation is the relatively small depth of tissue injury produced by this technique. This can be attributed to the precipitous falloff of direct tissue heating (volume heating) by the RF energy as the distance from the electrode-tissue interface increases. Deeper tissue layers can be ablated by heat conduction from the volume-heated source, but the maximum lesion depth is limited.

Because the success of RF catheter ablation in the clinical setting is sometimes limited by the relatively small size of the lesion, attempts have been made to increase the size of those lesions reliably and safely. One approach is to increase the size and surface area of the electrode. The RF power needs to be increased comparably to achieve a similar current density and temperature at the electrode-tissue interface, and the result is a greater depth of volume heating and a larger lesion.[13] Modifications to the RF energy delivery mechanism, including cooled catheters and pulsed energy, have also helped address some of these limitations.[10] Moreover, investigation into alternative energy sources appears to be more promising, including microwave, ultrasound, laser, and cryoablation.[2,3]

Complications of Radiofrequency Ablation

In a report of 1050 patients who underwent RF catheter ablation using a temperature-controlled system, a major complication occurred in 3% and a minor complication in 8.2%. Complications include death (approximately 0.1% to 0.3%), heart block requiring permanent pacemaker (1% to 2%), thromboembolism, including stroke, systemic embolism, pulmonary embolism (less than 1%), complications related to vascular access (2% to 4%), including bleeding, infection, hematoma and vascular injury, cardiac trauma, including myocardial perforation, tamponade, infarction, and valvular damage (1% to 2%). The frequency of valvular complications is slightly higher with left-sided ablation using a retrograde aortic technique. Radiation exposure is another complication and can result in skin burns and increased risk of malignancy. After ablation for atrial fibrillation (AF), pulmonary hypertension can develop because of pulmonary vein (PV) stenosis occurring near the junction with the left atrium (LA). Late stenosis of the right coronary artery has been observed in children with Ebstein's anomaly of the tricuspid valve who undergo ablation of a right-sided AV BT.[16] Predictors for a complication included structural heart disease and the presence of multiple targets for ablation.[3,17]

Theoretically, the RF lesions themselves can serve as arrhythmogenic foci but occurrence of new arrhythmias following RF ablation has not been a clinical problem. Although new AF can occur in patients undergoing ablation for atrial flutter (AFL), it is possible that this occurs primarily in patients predisposed to AF. New catheter ablation techniques for AF, however, have been associated with occurrence of atypical LA flutters related to RF ablation lines. Inappropriate sinus tachycardia may occur in some patients after posteroseptal BT or AVN ablation, suggesting disruption of the parasympathetic and/or sympathetic inputs into the sinus node and AVN. Ventricular fibrillation (VF) has been reported in up to 6% of patients with chronic AF after AVN ablation when the ventricular pacing rate is lower than 70 beats/min. This complication can be minimized by postablation pacing for 3 months at a higher rate—that is, 90 beats/min. A possible mechanism for postablation ventricular arrhythmia is activation of the sympathetic nervous system and a prolongation in action potential duration.[17]

Myocardial injury indicated by elevated troponin I occurs in up to 68% of patients undergoing ablation, and it correlates with the number of RF lesions applied, the site of lesions (ventricular more than atrial more than annular), and the approach to the left side (transaortic more than transseptal). The prognostic significance of asymptomatic elevations of troponin I remains unclear. Similarly, mild elevations of brain natriuretic peptide, also of uncertain clinical significance, have been noted following ablation procedures. This rise correlates closely with modest troponin I elevations, as well as with the duration of ventricular stimulation and total RF energy application.[17]

COOLED RADIOFREQUENCY ABLATION

Biophysics of Cooled Radiofrequency Ablation

Mechanism

Excessive surface heating invites coagulum formation, carbonization, and steam popping. These adverse effects may limit the depth of RF lesions, making it difficult to produce lesions of sufficient depth in scar tissue or thickened ventricular walls. Such limitations of conventional RF systems have stimulated the evaluation of modified electrode systems. One important modification involves cooling of the ablation electrode, which was designed to prevent overheating of the endocardium while allowing sufficient energy delivery to achieve a larger lesion size and depth.[18]

There are two methods of active electrode cooling by irrigation: internal and external (Fig. 4-2). With the internal (closed-loop) system (Chilli, Boston Scientific, Natick, Mass), cooling of the ablation electrode is performed by circulating fluid within the electrode.[19-22] In contrast, with the external (open-loop) system (ThermoCool, Biosense Webster, Diamond Bar, Calif), electrode cooling is performed by flushing saline through openings in the porous-tipped electrode (showerhead-type system).[22,23] Another cooling system is sheath-based open irrigation, which uses a sheath around the ablation catheter for open irrigation. The latter system was found to provide the best results,[24] but this type of catheter tip cooling is not clinically available.

Active electrode cooling by irrigation can produce higher tissue temperatures and create larger lesions, compared with standard RF ablation catheters, because of a reduction in overheating at the tissue-electrode interface, even at sites with low blood flow. Thus, this allows the delivery of higher amounts of RF power for a longer duration to create relatively large lesions with greater depth but without the risk of coagulum and char formation.[10] Unlike with standard RF ablation, the area of maximum temperature with cooled ablation is within the myocardium rather than at the electrode-myocardial interface. Higher power results in greater depth of volume heating but, if the ablation is power limited, power dissipation into the circulating blood pool can actually result in decreased lesion depth (Fig. 4-3).[22] Compared with large-tip catheters, active cooling has been shown to produce equivalent lesions with energy delivery via smaller electrodes, with less dependence on catheter tip orientation and extrinsic cooling, whereas larger electrodes have significant variability in their electrode-tissue interface, depending on catheter orientation (see Fig. 4-3).[13]

Lesion depth seems to be similar between closed-loop and open-irrigation electrodes. However, open irrigation appears to be more effective in cooling the electrode-tissue interface, as reflected by lower interface temperature, lower incidence of thrombus, and smaller lesion diameter at the surface (with the maximum diameter produced deeper in the tissue). These differences between the two electrodes are greater in low blood flow, presumably because the flow of saline irrigation out of the electrode provides additional cooling of the electrode-tissue interface (external cooling). Ablation with the closed-loop electrode, with irrigation providing only internal cooling, in low blood flow frequently results in high electrode-tissue interface temperature (despite low electrode temperature) and thrombus formation.[18,22]

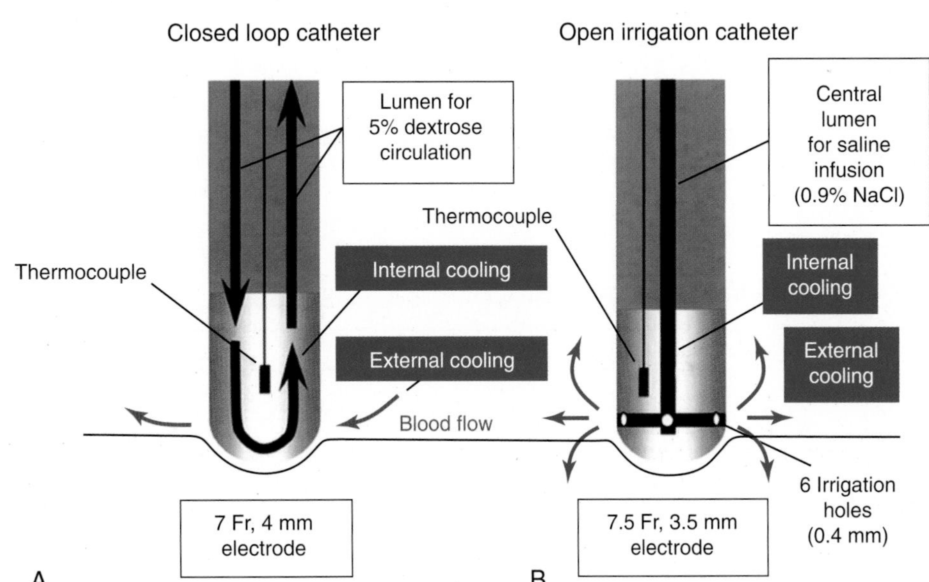

FIGURE 4–2 Schematic representation of irrigated electrode catheters. **A,** Closed-loop irrigation catheter has a 7 Fr, 4-mm tip electrode with an internal thermocouple. **B,** Open-irrigated catheter has a 7.5 Fr, 3.5-mm tip electrode with an internal thermocouple and six irrigation holes (0.4-mm diameter) located around the electrode, 1.0 mm from the tip. (From Yokoyama K, Nakagawa H, Wittkampf FH, et al: Comparison of electrode cooling between internal and open irrigation in radiofrequency ablation lesion depth and incidence of thrombus and steam pop. Circulation 2006;113:11.)

Risk of Larger Lesions

Although creation of larger ablation lesions can improve the efficacy of ablation for some patients, particularly when the targeted arrhythmia originates deep to the endocardium and when large areas require ablation, it is associated with increased risk of damage to tissue outside the target region (Table 4-1).[17,18]

Higher power can be used with convective cooling, but higher power can cause superheating within the tissue (with subendocardial tissue temperatures exceeding 100°C), which can result in boiling of any liquids under the electrode. Consequently, evaporation and rapid steam expansion can occur intramurally, and a gas bubble can develop in the tissue under the electrode. Continuous application of RF energy causes the bubble to expand and its pressure to increase, which can lead to eruption of the gas bubble (causing a popping sound) through the path with the least mechanical resistance, leaving behind a gaping hole (the so-called pop lesion). This is often toward the heat-damaged endocardial surface (crater formation) or, more rarely, across the myocardial wall (myocardial rupture).[20,22] This is often associated with sudden impedance rise and catheter dislodgment and can cause significant tissue damage.[17,18]

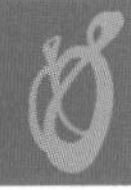

4

Consequently, increasing power delivery and convective cooling can create large lesions, but lesion production is somewhat difficult to control. Surface cooling does reduce the risk of boiling and coagulum formation; however, it does not allow the temperature at the tip to be monitored, and thus some feedback about lesion formation is lost.[7,20,22]

These concerns can be more pronounced with internal cooling as compared with open irrigation. Open irrigation cools the electrode and its direct environment, blood and tissue surface. In contrast, with internal cooling, the main parameter affected by cooling is the temperature of the electrode. There can be minimal cooling of the direct electrode-tissue interface, but only at the true contact site between metal and tissue. Blood flow around the electrode makes it highly unlikely that there will be any noticeable cooling of the tissue surface at a distance of a few millimeters from the contact site. Consequently, one would not expect much effect of internal electrode cooling on the surface area or depth of the lesion. Electrode cooling does, however, enable larger lesions (at higher power levels) because the ablation process is no longer limited by electrode temperature rise. This can also be dangerous; in cases with good tissue contact, power delivery to the tissue can be much higher than average. With standard electrodes, this situation is signaled by an excessive electrode temperature rise but, without this warning, tissue overheating can occur. Blood clots can also be formed, but they will not adhere to a cool electrode and will not cause an impedance rise.[5,18]

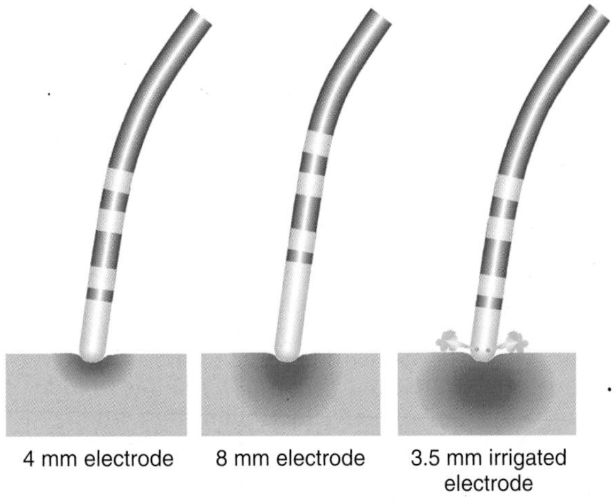

4 mm electrode | 8 mm electrode | 3.5 mm irrigated electrode

FIGURE 4–3 Effect of electrode type on lesion size. Representative blocks of myocardium are shown with lesions (*dark shading*) resulting from optimal radiofrequency energy delivery for each electrode type. A 4-mm electrode makes a small shallow lesion (*left*). An 8-mm electrode makes a larger, deeper lesion (*center*). The open-irrigated electrode makes a larger, deeper lesion, with a maximum width at some tissue depth (*right*).

Monitoring Radiofrequency Energy Delivery

There is significant discrepancy between monitored electrode temperature and tissue temperature during cooled RF ablation.[7,12] The thermal effects on the electrode temperature are dependent on electrode heating from the tissue, internal cooling by the irrigation fluid, and external cooling from blood flow or open irrigation. With high irrigation flow rates, catheter tip temperature is not representative of tissue temperature and therefore feedback cannot be used to guide power output. The difference between the electrode temperature and interface temperature is greater with the closed-loop electrode than with the open-irrigation electrode. The discrepancy is likely to be increased in areas of high blood flow by increasing the irrigation flow rate or by cooling the irrigant.[7,25] Saline-irrigated catheters cause peak tissue heating several millimeters from the electrode-tissue interface. Because maximum tissue heating does not occur at the electrode-tissue interface, the value of temperature and impedance monitoring is limited with this type of catheter.[18]

TABLE 4–1 Comparison of Features of Ablation Electrodes

Feature	4-mm RF	8-mm RF	4-mm Cooled RF (Closed)	4-mm Cooled RF (Open)	6-mm Cryoablation
Electrogram resolution	+++	+	++++	++++	++
Lesion depth	+	+++	+++	+++	++
Lesion surface area	++	++++	++++	++++	+++
Usefulness of temperature monitoring	+++	++	0	0	0
Risk of steam pop	+	++	+++	+++	0
Thrombus risk	++	++++	+++	+	0
Time efficiency of ablation*	++	++++	++++	++++	+

*Inverse function of duration of energy application for effective lesion (higher efficiency = best).
0 = none, + = least/worst, ++ = minimal, +++ = moderate, ++++ = most, best.
RF = radiofrequency.

Therefore, it has been challenging to monitor lesion formation and optimize power delivery during cooled RF ablation.[7] Appropriate energy titration is important to allow greater power application and produce large lesions, while avoiding overheating of tissue with steam formation leading to "pops." Moreover, the inability to assess tissue heating, and hence to titrate power to an objective endpoint, prevents the operator from determining whether unsuccessful applications are caused by inadequate mapping or inadequate heating.[18]

Electrode-tissue contact and orientation and the cooling effect of blood flow around the electrode and within the tissue are not as easily adjusted, and also influence tissue heating. However, a number of other factors can be potentially manipulated to adjust ablation with saline-irrigated catheters, including flow rate, irrigant temperature, and RF power and duration.[18] The most easily controllable factors are the power and duration of RF application. Instead of increasing the power to achieve the desired effect, which increases the likelihood of crater formation, the duration may be increased. A moderate power of 20 to 35 W with a relatively long RF duration of 60 to 300 seconds should be considered to achieve relatively large lesions, with a limited risk of crater formation.[7]

The flow rate of the irrigant determines the degree of cooling. Faster flow rates would likely allow greater power application without impedance rises, increase the difference between tissue and electrode temperature, and thereby potentially increase the risk of steam pops if temperature is used to guide ablation. With the internally irrigated ablation system, the approved flow rate is fixed at 36 mL/min and is not presently manipulated.[7] With the externally irrigated ablation system, an irrigation flow rate of 10 to 17 mL/min during RF application (and 2 to 3 mL/min during all other times) may be selected in a power-ontrolled mode with a delivered power of up to 30 W. The irrigation flow rate should be increased to 20 to 30 mL/min when more than 30 W are delivered to avoid excessive heat development at the superficial tissue layers.[7] Additionally, the temperature of the irrigant can potentially be manipulated. Cooling the irrigant can allow power delivery to be increased without coagulum formation. The cooled irrigant is warmed as it passes through the tubing to reach the catheter, and through the length of the catheter.[7] The impact of cooling the irrigant has not been well studied. In most studies, the irrigant that enters the catheter is at room temperature.[18]

Several indicators of tissue heating may be monitored, including catheter tip temperature, EP effects of RF, and the use of intracardiac echocardiography (ICE). As noted, with cooled RF, the discrepancy between measured electrode temperature and tissue temperature is greater than during standard RF ablation.[7,12] With the internally irrigated system, the room temperature irrigant flowing at 36 mL/min typically cools the measured electrode temperature to 28° to 30°C. During RF application, the temperature increases; temperatures of 50°C can indicate that cooling is inadequate or has stopped, which warrants termination of RF application. The measured impedance typically decreases during cooled RF ablation by 5 to 10 Ω, in a manner similar to that observed during standard RF ablation.[7]

Evidence of tissue heating from an effect on recorded electrograms or the arrhythmia can be used to guide ablation energy.[7] The termination of VT, AFL, or supraventricular tachycardia (SVT) during the process of ablating provides immediate feedback about the disruption of tissue integrity. Thus, interruption of tachycardia is one marker of tissue damage. An increase in pacing threshold may also be used as an indication that a lesion has been created. A decrease in electrogram amplitude also indicates tissue damage. These factors are not easily monitored during the RF application, however, particularly the change in pacing threshold. Also, the decrease in electrogram amplitude is often not visible during RF application because of superimposed electrical artifact.[7,26]

Ultrasound imaging can allow assessment of tissue heating and pops. The presence of microbubbles on intracardiac or transesophageal echocardiography is typically associated with a tissue temperature higher than 60°C and increased lesion size, and continued RF application after the appearance of the bubbles is usually followed by an increase in impedance. Moreover, pops are not always audible but can be seen well on ultrasound, often with a sudden explosion of echocardiographic contrast.[7] Microbubble formation, however, is not a straightforward surrogate for tissue heating. The absence of microbubble formation clearly does not indicate that tissue heating is inadequate or that the power level should be increased, nor does the presence of scattered microbubbles indicate safe tissue heating. This marker is fairly specific for tissue heating as judged by tissue temperatures but is not a routinely sensitive one.[7] Specifically, scattered microbubbles are noted to occur over the entire spectrum of tissue temperatures, whereas dense showers of microbubbles occurred only at tissue temperatures higher than 60°C. Scattered microbubbles may represent an electrolytic phenomenon, whereas dense showers of microbubbles suggest steam formation, with associated tissue disruption and impedance rises.[7]

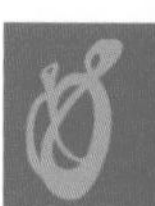

The optimal method for adjusting power during saline-irrigated RF ablation is not yet clearly defined, but some useful guidelines have emerged. One approach is to perform ablation in a power-controlled mode, typically starting at 20 to 30 W and gradually increasing power to achieve evidence of tissue heating or damage.[7] An impedance fall likely indicates tissue heating, similar to that observed with conventional RF. When catheter temperature is between 28° and 31°C, power can be ramped up watching for a 5- to 10-Ω impedance fall. Measured electrode temperature will generally increase. A measured electrode temperature of 37° to 40°C is commonly achieved. Temperatures exceeding 40°C with power greater than 30 W may be associated with a greater risk of steam pops and impedance rises, particularly during long RF applications, exceeding 60 seconds. Temperatures higher than 40°C achieved with low power (less than 20 W) may indicate that the electrode is in a location with little or no cooling from the surrounding circulating blood, or that there is a failure of the catheter cooling system that requires attention.[7] Steam pops are often, but not always, audible. A sudden decrease in temperature, sudden catheter movement (as a consequence of the pop blowing the catheter out of position), and a sudden change in impedance are all potential indications that a pop has occurred. The consequence of a steam pop depends on the area of the heart being ablated. The risk of cardiac perforation is low in regions of ventricular scar. The risk is likely to be higher for ablation in the thin-walled RV outflow tract and in the atria. Therefore, it may be reasonable to take a more conservative approach to power application in these areas. A second approach is irrigated temperature-controlled RF delivery, which yields relatively large lesions without crater formation if a moderate target temperature between 60° and 70°C and a low irrigation flow rate of 1 mL/min are chosen. A target temperature of greater than 70°C can result in tissue overheating and crater formation.[7]

Clinical Applications of Cooled Radiofrequency Ablation

Cooled tip catheters have several advantages. First, they allow the desired power to be delivered independent of local blood flow, which results in increased lesion size. Second, they reduce the temperature of the ablation electrode as well as the temperature at the tissue interface, especially with the open irrigation system, which helps spare the endocardium and reduce the risk of clots and charring. Third, when compared with standard 8-mm tip ablation catheters, a 3.5- to 4-mm irrigated electrode offers higher mapping accuracy while providing comparable ablation lesion size.[18]

Cooled tip catheters are preferred for long linear ablations (in the RA or LA), complex atrial arrhythmias (AFL or AF), targets resistant to previous conventional ablation (focal tachycardias or BTs), and specific areas with low local blood flow, including the coronary sinus (CS), particularly CS aneurysms. Clinical trials have found irrigated tip catheters to be more effective than and as safe as conventional catheters for AFL ablation, facilitating the rapid achievement of bidirectional isthmus block.[27,28] Irrigated tip catheters also were found to be safe and effective in eliminating BT conduction resistant to conventional catheters, irrespective of the location,[23] and they have been successfully used for PV isolation for treatment of AF.[28,29] Irrigated tip catheters also offer an advantage over conventional RF catheters in the case of some post–myocardial infarction (MI) VTs, facilitating creation of larger and deeper lesions which can help eliminate intramyocardial or subepicardial reentrant pathways necessary for VT circuit.[28]

Power levels typically used during open irrigation ablation depend on the site of ablation—25 to 30 W in the left atrial (LA) and right atrial (RA) free wall, 35 to 40 W for cavotricuspid isthmus and mitral isthmus ablation, 50 W in the left ventricle (LV), and 20 W in the CS. At low power levels, the irrigation flow rate may be set lower than at higher levels; 17 mL/min is used below 30 W whereas 30 mL/min is used above that level. Using a lower irrigation flow rate (10 mL/min) in the LA can help maintain some temperature feedback, with a cutoff temperature of 43°C. Lesion formation is monitored via attenuation of the local unipolar electrogram. Because of the very limited or absent temperature feedback, tissue overheating (pops) is a potential risk, especially in thin-walled chambers. This, however, most frequently occurs with perpendicular (high-pressure) tissue contact that one should try to avoid, especially at higher power levels. The temperature is usually set at 40° to 45°C. If the temperature at the tip is less than 40°C, the flow rate may be reduced. If the desired power is not met because the target temperature is reached at a lower power, the irrigation flow rate may be increased to a maximum of 60 mL/min.[5,30]

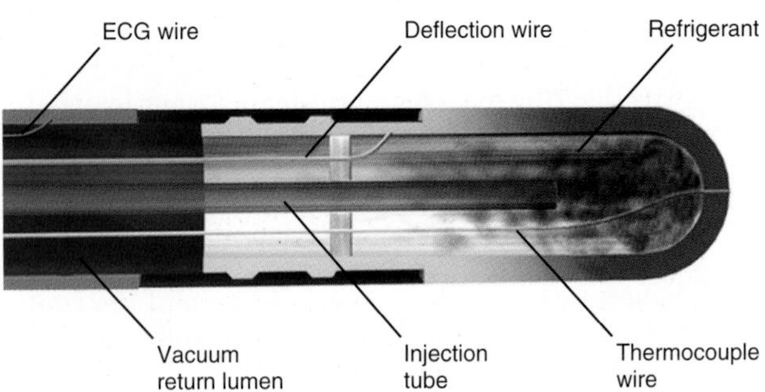

FIGURE 4–4 Schematic diagram demonstrating the CryoCath Freezor cryocatheter internal design. (Courtesy of CryoCath Technologies, Montreal.)

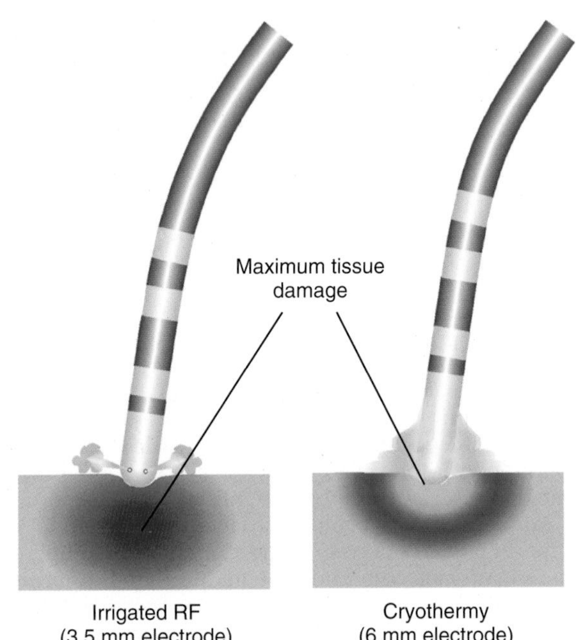

FIGURE 4–5 Depth of maximum tissue injury with irrigated-tip radiofrequency (RF) versus cryothermy. With irrigated RF (*left*), the maximum tissue heating occurs at some tissue depth because of cooling at the surface. With cryothermy (*right*), the maximum effect is at the endocardial surface.

CRYOABLATION

Biophysics of Cryothermal Energy

Cryoablation uses a steerable catheter and a dedicated console, which are connected by a coaxial cable used to deliver fluid nitrous oxide to the catheter and to remove the gas from the catheter separately.[31] A tank of fluid nitrous oxide is located inside the console; the gas removed from the catheter to the console is evacuated through a scavenging hose into the vacuum line of the EP laboratory. The system has several sensors to avoid inadvertent leaks of nitrous oxide into the patient body and to check connections of the different cables to the console.

Cryoablation catheters have a terminal segment whose temperature can be lowered to −75°C or less by delivery of precooled compressed liquid refrigerant (N_2O argon) across a sudden luminal widening at the end of the catheters' refrigerant circulation system (Fig. 4-4). Decompression and expansion of the refrigerant (liquid to gas phase change) achieves cooling based on the Joule-Thompson effect.[32]

The effect produced by cryothermal ablation is secondary to tissue freezing, the result of a temperature gradient occurring at the electrode-tissue interface (i.e., local heat absorption by the cooled catheter tip); it greatly depends on the minimum temperature reached, the duration of energy application, and the temperature time constant. The latter value indicates the course of the descent of temperature to the target temperature and a shorter value (expressed in seconds) identifies a more effective application. Important modulatory variables that can affect tissue damage produced by cryoablation include firmness of the catheter-tissue contact, tip temperature, freeze duration, and blood flow.[32]

At the electrode-tissue interface, the coldest area is the one adjacent to the catheter tip, where functional effects of energy delivery are observed earlier (Fig. 4-5). Conversely, the less cooled area is the one at the periphery of the cryolesion, whose dimensions can also vary according to the duration of freezing. Because of limited cooling of the outer limit of the lesion (both in time and temperature), this region is less likely to suffer irreversible damage. As a consequence, the effects obtained late during cryothermal energy application are likely to be reversible early on rewarming and, therefore, any expected functional modification induced by cryoenergy should occur early (usually within the first 30 seconds of the application) to obtain a successful and permanent ablation of a given arrhythmogenic substrate.[32]

Currently, two different systems of catheter cryoablation are available for clinical and experimental use, the CryoCath system (CryoCath Technologies, Montreal) and CryoCor system (CryoCor, San Diego, Calif). The CryoCath uses 7 or 9 Fr steerable catheters with 4-, 6-, or 8-mm-long tip electrodes. The ablation catheter is connected to a dedicated console, which has two algorithms available. The first is for cryomapping with a slow decrease of temperature to −30°C for up to 80 seconds, and the second is for cryoablation with a faster decrease of temperature to −75°C for up to 480 seconds. Additionally, the target temperature can be manually preset on the console at any value between −30° and −75°C. The CryoCor system has 10 Fr steerable catheters with 6.5- or 10-mm-long tip electrodes. The console has a built-in closed loop precooler for the fluid nitrous oxide, whose flow at the catheter tip is adjusted during the application to maintain a temperature of −80°C.[32]

Pathophysiology of Lesion Formation by Cryoablation

Mechanism of Tissue Injury

The mechanisms underlying lesion formation by cryoenergy are twofold, direct cell injury and vascular-mediated tissue injury. The mechanisms of cellular death associated with tissue freezing involve immediate cellular effects as well as late effects that determine the lesion produced.[32]

Direct Cell Injury

Extracellular Ice (Solution Effect Injury). Direct cellular injury results from ice formation. Ice forms only extracellularly when the tissue is cooled to mild temperatures (0° to −20°C) and results in hypertonic stress (the extracellular environment becomes hyperosmotic), with consequent shift of water from the intracellular to the extracellular space, ultimately causing cell shrinkage and damage to the plasma membrane cellular constituents. These effects are reversible when rewarming is achieved within a short period (30 to 60 seconds); however, extended periods of extracellular freezing result in cellular death and rewarming then results in cellular swelling, sufficient to disrupt cellular membranes.[31]

Intracellular Ice. When the tissue is cooled to −40°C or lower, especially if cooled at rapid rates, ice forms extracellularly and intracellularly. Intracellular ice results in major and irreversible disruption of organelles and cell membranes, with cellular death.[31] Furthermore, intracellular ice can propagate from one cell to another via intercellular channels, potentially resulting in lesion growth. Cellular injury, disruption of membranous organelles in particular, is importantly enhanced on cellular thawing, and the injury can be extended by repeated freeze-thaw cycles. Final rewarming evokes an inflammation response to released cellular constituents and reperfusional hemorrhage, leading to tissue repair and eventual dense scarring.[31,32]

Vascular-Mediated Tissue Injury. Tissue freezing results in vasoconstriction, hypoperfusion, and ischemic necrosis.[31] Subsequent tissue rewarming produces a hyperemic response with increased vascular permeability and edema formation. Endothelial disruption within the frozen tissue is also observed, which results in platelet aggregation, microthrombi, and microcirculatory stagnation within the lesion. Cryolesions, however, are associated with substantially less degree of endothelial damage and overlying thrombus formation than standard RF lesions. Extensive surgical experience has shown that cryolesions result in dense homogenous fibrosis, with a well-demarcated border zone. They are nonarrhythmogenic and preserve the underlying extracellular matrix and tensile strength.[32]

Determinants of Lesion Size

During cryoablation, lesion size and tissue temperature are related to convective warming, electrode orientation, electrode contact pressure, electrode size, refrigerant flow rate, and electrode temperature.[33] Lesion sizes during catheter cryoablation can be maximized by use of larger ablation electrodes with higher refrigerant delivery rates. A horizontal electrode orientation to the tissue and firm contact pressure also enhance lesion size. For a given electrode size, electrode temperature may be a poor predictor of tissue cooling and lesion size. In contrast to RF ablation, cryoablation in areas of high blood flow can result in limited tissue cooling and smaller lesion sizes because of convective warming. Conversely, cryoablation lesion size can be maximized in areas of low blood flow.[32,33]

Technical Aspects of Cryoablation

The intervention is often performed in two steps. First, "cryomaps" are obtained by moderate reversible cooling of tissue (electrode-tissue interface temperature approximately −28° to −32°C). Second, "cryoablation" cools the selected cryomapped pathways to much lower temperatures (electrode-tissue interface temperature below −68°C) and produces ice formation inside and outside of cells, a mechanism of irreversible cellular injury.[32]

"Cryomapping"

"Cryomapping" is designed to verify that ablation at the chosen site will have the desired effect and to reassure the absence of complications (i.e., to localize electric pathways to be destroyed or spared). This is generally performed using various pacing protocols that can be performed during cryomapping (or ice mapping) at −30°C. At this temperature, the lesion is reversible (for up to 60 seconds) and the catheter is stuck to the adjacent frozen tissue because of the presence of an ice ball that includes the tip of the catheter (cryoadherence). This permits programmed electrical stimulation to test the functionality of a potential ablation target during ongoing ablation and prior to permanent destruction; it also allows ablation being performed during tachycardia without the risk of catheter dislodgment on termination of the tachycardia.[34-39]

In the cryomapping mode, the temperature is not allowed to drop below −30°C, and the time of application is limited to 60 seconds. Formation of an ice ball at the catheter tip and adherence to the underlying myocardium are signaled by the appearance of electrical noise recorded from the ablation catheter's distal bipole. Once an ice ball is formed, programmed stimulation is repeated to verify achievement of the desired effect. If cryomapping does not yield the desired result within 20 to 30 seconds or results in unintended effect (e.g., AV conduction delay or block), cryomapping is interrupted, allowing the catheter to thaw and become dislodged from the tissue; after a few seconds, the catheter may be moved to a different site and cryomapping repeated.[32]

"Cryoablation"

When sites of successful cryomapping are identified by demonstrating the desired effect with no adverse effects, the cyoablation mode is activated, in which a target temperature below –75°C is sought (a temperature of –75° to –80° is generally achieved). The application is then continued for 4 to 8 minutes, creating an irreversible lesion.[34-39] If the catheter tip is in close contact with the endocardium, a prompt drop in catheter tip temperature should be observed as soon as the cyoablation mode is activated. A slow decline in catheter tip temperature or very high flow rates of refrigerant during ablation suggests poor electrode-tissue contact and, in such case, cryoablation is interrupted and the catheter is repositioned.[32]

Advantages of Cryoablation

The use of cryoablation in the EP laboratory provides some distinct advantages not seen with conventional RF ablation. The slow development of the cryolesion (approximately 240 seconds), although time-consuming, enables the creation of reversible lesions and modulation of lesion formation in critical areas. As noted, cryomapping allows functional assessment of a putative ablation site during ongoing ablation and prior to permanent destruction. This offers a safety advantage when ablation is performed close to critical structures such as the AVN or His bundle (HB).[34-39]

Compared with standard RF lesions, cryolesions are associated with a substantially lower degree of endothelial disruption, less platelet activation, and lower thrombogenic tendency; therefore, the risk of coagulum formation, charring, and steam popping is less than with RF ablation (see Table 4-1). Furthermore, cryoablation results in dense homogenous fibrotic lesions with well-demarcated border zone, and does not cause collagen denaturation or contracture related to hyperthermic effects. Therefore, cryothermal energy application in close proximity to the coronary arteries (e.g., during epicardial ablation) or in venous vessels (CS, middle cardiac vein, and PVs) does not result in damage, perforation, or chronic stenosis of their lumen.[32,40]

The cryoadherence effect results in the formation of a very focal lesion because of fixed and stable tip electrode contact to adjacent frozen tissue throughout the whole application. This has a particular safety advantage, especially for ablation in the proximity of critical areas, such as the AVN and HB. In addition, cryoadherence augments catheter stability throughout the energy application, even when sudden changes in heart rhythm that can potentially displace the ablation catheter (e.g., tachycardia termination) occur. At the same time, cryoadherence does not compromise safety; on discontinuation of cryothermal application, the defrost phase is fast (within 3 seconds) and the catheter can be immediately disengaged from the ablation position.

Cryothermal energy application is characterized by the absence of pain perception in nonsedated patients. In fact, cryoablation can be performed without analgesia. Occasionally, a light sense of cold or headache is perceived as minor discomfort. This characteristic can be particularly useful in younger and pediatric patients.[32]

Clinical Applications of Cryoablation

Catheter-based cryothermal ablation is relatively new. However, it has quickly been adapted for specific arrhythmogenic substrates in which RF has limitations and cryothermy has specific safety advantages. It is unlikely that cryoablation will replace standard RF ablation in unselected cases. Nevertheless, for the above-mentioned peculiarities, cryothermal ablation has proven effective and safe for the ablation of arrhythmogenic substrates close to the normal conduction pathways, becoming the first-choice method to ablate superoparaseptal and midseptal BTs and difficult cases of AVNRT because of its widely demonstrated safety profile. As the technology evolves and further iterations of the catheter proceed, the role for this technology is likely to grow.[32]

Atrioventricular Nodal Reentrant Tachycardia. So far, slow pathway ablation for AVNRT by cryothermal energy represents the larger experience in the clinical application of this new technology.[31,37-39,41,42] According to current data, cryothermal energy is a valuable and useful alternative to RF energy to treat patients with AVNRT. Absence of permanent inadvertent damage of AV conduction makes this new technology particularly useful for cases with difficult anatomy, unsuccessful prior standard ablation procedure, pediatric patients, and in all cases in whom even the small risk of AV block associated with RF ablation is considered unacceptable. Cryoablation can be of particular advantage in several situations, including posterior displacement of the fast pathway or AVN, small space in the triangle of Koch between the HB and the coronary sinus ostium (CS os), and when ablation must be performed in the midseptum. However, given the high success rate and low risk of RF slow pathway ablation, it can be difficult to demonstrate a clinical advantage of cryoablation over RF ablation in unselected AVNRT cases.[32]

Bypass Tracts. Cryothermal ablation of BTs in the superoparaseptal and midseptal areas, both at high risk of complete permanent AV block when standard RF energy is applied, is highly safe and successful.[34-36,41,42] Cryoablation can be also successfully and safely used to ablate selected cases of epicardial left-sided BTs within the CS, well beyond the middle cardiac vein, once attempts using the transseptal and transaortic approaches have failed.[31] The experience with cryoablation in unselected BTs is more limited and less satisfactory; this can be related to multiple factors, including the learning curve and the smaller size of the lesion produced by cryoablation. In addition, all the peculiarities of cryothermal energy, which are optimal for septal ablation, are less important or even useless for ablation of BTs located elsewhere.[31]

Focal Atrial Tachycardia. Occasionally, successful cryoablation of focal AT has been reported. Its safety has also been confirmed for ablation of atrial foci located close to the AVN.

Typical Atrial Flutter. Studies have reported cryoablation of the cavotricuspid isthmus for typical AFL with acute and long-term success comparable to those of RF ablation.[43,44] The major advantage of using cryothermal energy for the ablation of typical AFL is the absence of pain perception related to energy application. However, the procedural time is significantly longer with cryoablation as compared with RF ablation.[43,44]

Pulmonary Vein Isolation. For the characteristics mentioned above, cryothermal energy ablation can be considered an ideal and safer energy source for PV isolation, and the incidence of PV stenosis and thromboembolic events is expected to be dramatically reduced compared with RF ablation.[40,45-49] On the other hand, cryothermal injury is sensitive to surrounding thermal conditions. The high flow of the PVs can present a considerable heat load to cryothermal technologies, which can limit the size and depth of the lesion produced by cryothermal energy at the ostium of the PV. Moreover, the longer time required to produce a permanent lesion can relevantly reflect on procedure duration, limiting the clinical use of this theoretically optimal energy source. Therefore, complete and permanent PV isolation with cryothermy in the presence of substantial heat load can be challenging. Technological evolution is now aimed at developing new catheter designs for circumferential ostial ablation of the PVs, with the option of deploying an inflatable balloon in the PVs to reduce the heat load related to blood flow (Fig. 4-6).[31,40,47,48,50]

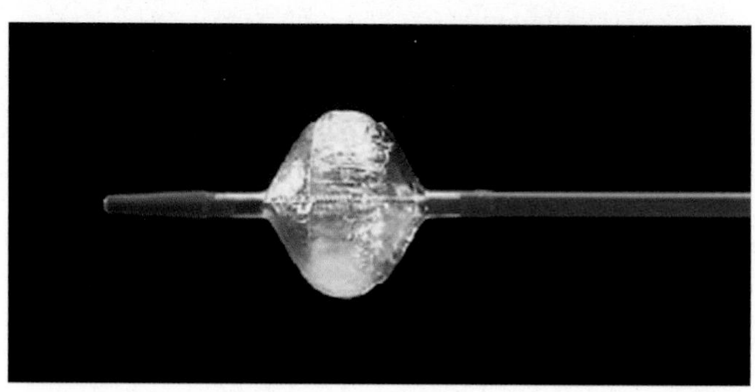

FIGURE 4–6 Cryothermal balloon catheter. (From Sarabanda AV, Bunch TJ, Johnson SB, et al: Efficacy and safety of circumferential pulmonary vein isolation using a novel cryothermal balloon ablation system. J Am Coll Cardiol 2005;46:1902.)

Ventricular Tachycardia. Cryothermal energy can be of potential advantage in percutaneous subxiphoid epicardial ablation of VT because of less potential damage to the epicardial coronary arteries.[51] The reduced heat load in the pericardial space related to the absence of blood flow limits RF energy delivery but can be to the advantage of cryoablation, with the possibility of producing larger transmural lesions.[32,52]

MICROWAVE ABLATION

Biophysics of Microwave Energy

Microwaves are the portion of the electromagnetic spectrum between 0.3 and 300 GHz. For the ablation of cardiac arrhythmias, microwave energy has been used at frequencies of 0.915 and 2.450 GHz.[53,54] Similar to RF, microwave energy produces thermal cell necrosis; however, in contrast to heating by electrical resistance as observed during RF ablation, the mechanism of heating from a high-frequency microwave energy source is dielectrics. Dielectric heating occurs when high-frequency electromagnetic radiation stimulates the oscillation of dipolar molecules (e.g., water molecules) in the surrounding medium at a very high speed, thereby converting electromagnetic energy into kinetic energy. This high-speed vibration favors friction between water molecules within the myocardial wall, which results in an increase of myocardial tissue heat.[1,55] This mode of heating lends microwave ablation the potential for a greater depth of volume heating than RF ablation and should theoretically result in a larger lesion size.[15,53,56]

Microwave energy is not absorbed by blood and can propagate through blood, desiccated tissue, or scar, and it can be deposited directly into the myocardial tissue at a distance, regardless of the intervening medium. The microwave energy field generated around the ablation catheter antenna can create myocardial lesions up to 6 to 8 mm in depth without overheating the endocardial surface, which can potentially limit the risk of charring, coagulum formation, and intramyocardial steam explosions. Penetration depth achieved with microwave energy depends on a number of factors—dielectric properties of the tissue, frequency of the microwave energy, antenna design, and composition and thickness of the cardiac layers.

The effectiveness of microwave ablation depends on the radiating ability of the microwave antenna that directs the electric field and determines the amount transmitted into the myocardium, which is critical for heating. An end-firing monopolar antenna has been used to produce lesions at depths of 1 cm without disruption of the endocardium in porcine ventricles. The depth of these lesions increased exponentially over time as compared with standard nonirrigated RF energy, which had minimal lesion expansion after 60 seconds of ablation.[1] To concentrate more of the energy distribution near the electrode tip, circularly polarized coil antennas have been developed. Other configurations of the microwave antenna include helical, dipole, and whip designs; these have a large effect on the magnetic field created. However, many of these catheters are still under clinical investigation.[1,15]

Pathophysiology of Lesion Formation by Microwave Ablation

Microwave energy produces thermal cell necrosis and transmural damage, with foci of coagulation necrosis of myocytes in the central part of the lesion. Hyperthermia (more than 56°C) causes protein denaturation and changes in myocardial cellular EP properties, resulting from movement of mobile ions within the aqueous biological medium, altering membrane permeability. The acute myocyte changes include architectural disarray, loss of contractile filaments, and focal interruption of the plasma membrane, which are signs of irreversible injury. Additionally, occlusion of the lumen of the small intramyocardial vessels and severe disruption of endothelial and/or adventitial layers are observed.[53,56] Carbonization does not occur on tissue surfaces because of the good penetration of microwave energy. Fibrotic tissue eventually replaces the necrotic muscle, which typically becomes sharply demarcated from normal myocardium.[15,54,56]

In vitro and in vivo experiments have demonstrated good uniformity in the distribution of the electromagnetic energy throughout the tissue and excellent penetration depth, with no areas of discontinuity over the length of the ablating probe. Energy distribution is maximal near the center of the ablating element, indicating that depth of ablation is relatively deeper at the midpoint of a lesion. There is no indication of edge effect along the ablating tip, which can potentially produce overheating of the tissue surface and induce charring. The temperature at the tissue surface typically remains below 100°C over the time required to produce a 6-mm-deep lesion. This is a critical finding because the ability to raise the tissue temperature to 50°C while maintaining one less than 100°C is paramount to effective and safe hyperthermic ablation.

Ablation depth can be predictably controlled by modifying microwave energy power or ablation time. Ablation depth obtained after 25 seconds is significantly greater than depth achieved after 10 seconds; however, ablation depths achieved after 25 and 40 seconds do not differ significantly. This phenomenon can be explained by the fact that with a progressively increased duration of microwave energy application, a quasistatic state is reached in which lesion growth essentially plateaus. In the absence of a feedback mechanism, the reliable ablation depth demonstrated with microwave is important to ensure safety and reproducibility in the clinical setting.[15]

Clinical Applications of Microwave Ablation

Microwave ablation has been applied clinically only in the last few years, and can be a promising technique that is potentially capable of treating a wide range of ventricular and supraventricular arrhythmias. The physics of the microwave energy source can be particularly useful for transmural ablation lesions of atrial tissue, as well as the treatment of tachyarrhythmias arising from deep foci of ventricular myocardium.[53,56]

A hypothetical advantage of microwave energy is that it provides sufficient lesions, independent of contact. However, experimental data have shown that penetration of electromagnetic fields into tissue declines exponentially and the decline is steep when using frequencies in the microwave range; therefore, distance is still an important consideration. Nevertheless, this theoretical advantage can potentially improve the versatility of microwave ablation, especially in areas where muscular ridges and valleys may pose problems for conventional RF ablation.[1,15]

Currently, microwave ablation has been increasingly used intraoperatively (epicardially or endocardially) during surgical maze procedures. The ability to make microwave antennas into flexible linear applicators and place them parallel to the endocardium by means of clamps has increased the effectiveness of microwave as a tool in open chest and in minimally invasive surgery.[54,55,57-59]

On the other hand, the application of microwave energy for catheter ablation has been slow to develop because of the difficulty in designing flexible catheters. Only a few case reports have described the successful use of transvenous catheter microwave ablation of the AV junction and cavotricuspid isthmus.[60,61] Currently, only one transvenous microwave catheter system (MedWaves, San Diego, Calif) is available for investigational use. This system includes a 10 Fr helical coil antenna with temperature monitoring, bipolar electrode recording, and a generator delivering microwave at 900 to 930 MHz. Clinical studies on the use of transvenous catheter microwave ablation for AF and AFL ablation are currently underway to investigate the safety and feasibility of this technique.[60,61]

ULTRASOUND ENERGY

Sound is a propagation of cyclical (oscillatory) displacements of atoms and molecules around their average position in the direction of propagation. When the cyclical events occur at frequencies of more than 20,000 Hz (i.e., above the average threshold of the human hearing), the sound is defined as ultrasound.[1,60]

Ultrasound beams can be treated in a manner analogous to light beams, including focusing (ultrasonic lens) and minimization of convergence and divergence (collimation). These optical geometric manipulations allow for ultrasound to be directed toward confined distant (deep) tissue volumes. This is a pivotal capability of therapeutic ultrasound.[4,15]

Ultrasound energy transmission is subject to attenuation with distance and medium, especially with air. The amount of ultrasound energy transferred to tissue is proportional to the intensity of the wave and the absorption coefficient of the tissue. Because of this property, ultrasound ablation does not require direct contact with the myocardium, in contrast to RF ablation. Ultrasound energy decreases proportionally with the distance (1/r), whereas RF ablation electrical conduction decreases with the square of the distance ($1/r^2$). This feature allows ultrasound energy to create deeper and transmural lesions. The duration of application and acoustic power used have a direct relationship with the lesion depth.[15,60]

Tissue injury caused by ultrasound is mediated by two mechanisms, thermal and mechanical energy. Ultrasound waves can propagate through living tissue and fluids without causing any harm to the cells; however, by focusing highly energetic ultrasound waves (high-intensity focused ultrasound, HIFU) to a well-defined volume, a local heat increase (usually more than 56°C and up to 80°C) occurs and causes rapid tissue necrosis by coagulative necrosis. Thermal energy results from the energy transported by an ultrasound beam becoming attenuated as it propagates through viscous (viscoelastic) media, such as human soft tissue. The attenuation partly represents a conversion of ultrasound energy into heat. Fortunately, a steep temperature gradient is observed between the focus and the surrounding tissue, allowing for the production of sharply demarcated lesions and reducing collateral damage. Another major mechanism by which HIFU destroys tissue is mechanical energy, which results from pressure waves (sound waves) propagating in gas-containing tissues as they cyclically expand (explode) and shrink (implode) microbubbles in the tissue (i.e., oscillation and collapse of gas microbubbles), a process known as microcavitation. This process of vibration of cellular structures causes local hyperthermia and mechanical stress by bubble formation because of rapid changes in local pressure, leading to cell death.[1,15]

Preliminary studies with a 10-MHz transducer have been performed in canine hearts. Lesion depth increased with longer duration of energy delivery from 15 to 60 seconds, and there was a linear relationship between increasing power and depth of lesions.[1]

Because it can be focused at specific depths, ultrasound can be advantageous when considering epicardial ablation. The presence of epicardial fat makes the use of standard RF current difficult, both with catheter-based epicardial ablation and minimally invasive surgical ablation.[1,62,63]

The ability of ultrasound to be collimated through echolucent fluid medium (e.g., water, blood) makes it ideal for a balloon delivery system.[1,50] An 8-MHz cylindrical transducer mounted within a saline-filled balloon has been designed for PV isolation. The ablation system (Atrionix, Palo Alto, Calif) consists of a 0.035-inch diameter luminal catheter with a distal balloon (maximum diameter, 2.2 cm) housing a centrally located ultrasound transducer. The system is advanced over a guidewire into the target PV. Tissue surface temperature monitoring is achieved by thermocouples on the balloon and the ultrasound transducer. Despite initial enthusiasm, the long-term report including 33 patients was disappointing, with a chronic cure of about 30%, although electrical isolation was acutely achieved in all but one of the PVs targeted. Surprisingly, several applications were required to achieve PV isolation. The variability of the PV anatomy was the main culprit for the system failure. In larger PV orifices, it was difficult to achieve adequate heating. The system delivered a narrow band of ultrasound energy radially from a centrally located transducer, and it was at times challenging to place the catheter in all PVs at the proximal portion. Therefore, foci at the most proximal lip of a PV may not be ablated successfully.[15]

More recently, a forward-projecting HIFU balloon catheter (ProRhythm, Ronkonkoma, NY) has been developed for circumferential PV isolation outside the PV ostia (to limit the risk of PV stenosi). Radially emitted ultrasound is reflected from the back of the balloon, resulting in forward projection of ultrasound energy, with a focal point at the balloon-endocardial interface (Fig. 4-7). This system has two noncompliant balloons. A 9-MHz ultrasound crystal is located in the distal balloon filled with contrast and water. The proximal balloon, filled with carbon dioxide, forms a parabolic interface with the distal balloon to reflect the ultrasound energy in the forward direction, focusing a 360-degree ring (sonicating ring) of ultrasound energy 2 to 6 mm in front of the distal balloon surface. The distal balloon has three sizes, 24, 28, or 32 mm in diameter, producing sonicating rings of 20, 25, or 30 mm in diameter. The acoustic power of the system is 45 W for all three balloons, with negligible loss of power in the balloon. The distal balloon is irrigated with contrast and water at 20 mL/min during

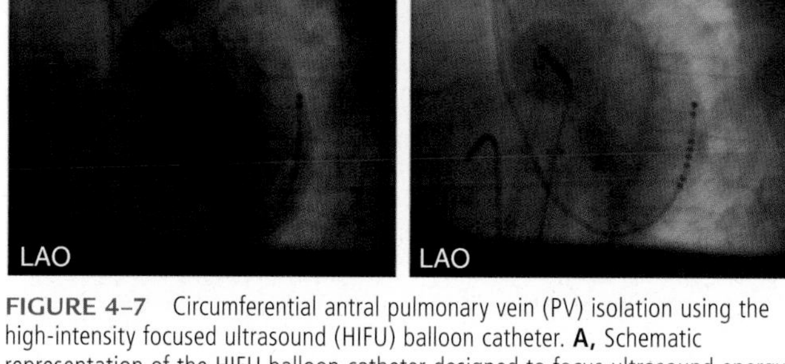

FIGURE 4–7 Circumferential antral pulmonary vein (PV) isolation using the high-intensity focused ultrasound (HIFU) balloon catheter. **A,** Schematic representation of the HIFU balloon catheter designed to focus ultrasound energy circumferentially outside the PV (PV antrum). **B,** HIFU balloon. **C,** right anterior oblique and left anterior oblique fluoroscopic views of the angiograms (*right*) and HIFU balloon positioning (*left*) in the right superior PV (RSPV). (From Schmidt B, Antz M, Ernst S, et al: Pulmonary vein isolation by high-intensity focused ultrasound: First-in-man study with a steerable balloon catheter. Heart Rhythm 2007;4:575.)

ablation to keep the balloon cool (lower than 42°C). Clinical application of this system has recently been evaluated, with successful electrical isolation of 87% of targeted PVs, elimination of symptomatic AF at 12-month follow-up in 59% of 27 patients with paroxysmal or persistent AF, and no occurrence of PV stenosis or atrioesophageal fistula.[64-66]

A potential advantage of ultrasound is that it does not rely on extensive heating on the vein surface and heat is not conducted to the cardiac tissue, as it is with RF. This can potentially prevent PV stenosis seen with RF ablation. If catheter design limitations are addressed, PV isolation using through the balloon ultrasound can add significantly to the tools available for AF catheter ablation. However, patients with common PV ostia with diameters more than 30 mm may not be eligible, because the maximal available balloon size is only 30 mm. Currently, no HIFU catheters are available that can be used for linear (instead of circular) ablation. Thus, if additional linear lesions are required, as proposed for patients with permanent AF, RF catheter ablation should be considered.[64-66]

LASER ENERGY

*L*ight ***a***mplification by ***s***timulated ***e***mission of ***r***adiation (laser) produces a monochromatic (narrow-frequency range) phase-coherent beam at a specific wavelength. This beam can be directed for a specific duration and intensity and, as it penetrates into the tissue, it is absorbed and scattered. The photothermal effect occurs with the absorption of photon energy, producing a vibrational excited state in molecules (chromophores). By absorbing this energy, the tissue is heated and a lesion is created (i.e., tissue injury is thermally mediated).[1,4,15]

Laser energy can be delivered in a continuous or a pulsed mode. Laser energy is selectively absorbed by the tissues over several millimeters and it decays exponentially as it passes through the tissue secondary to absorption and scatter. The extent of absorption and scatter of laser energy depends on laser beam diameter and the optical properties of the tissue. Lesion size is determined by the extent of light diffusion and heat transport.[4,15]

Three major laser systems are used—argon laser, Nd:YAG laser, and diode laser.[1]

Argon Laser. This system uses a gaseous lasing medium (argon), which emits light at a wavelength of 500 nM. With this system, the light energy is absorbed rapidly in the first few millimeters of tissue, resulting in surface vaporization with crater formation.

Nd:YAG Laser. This system uses a solid lasing medium (neodymium-yttrium-aluminum-garnet), which emits energy at a wavelength of 1060 to 2000 nM in the infrared spectrum. This system is associated with significant scatter in tissue, causing more diffuse and deeper tissue injury and resulting in photocoagulation necrosis.

Diode Laser. This system uses semiconductors and emits energy at a wavelength of 700 to 1500 nM (near-infrared).[4]

Early studies of laser ablation used a high-energy laser that carried a high risk of crater formation and endothelial damage. These studies focused on the intraoperative use of lasers in the ultraviolet and visible range (308- to 755-nm wavelength), and appeared to show effectiveness of the lesions placed. More recently, studies have demonstrated the feasibility of delivering precisely located lesions from a sharp-tipped linear optical fiber diffuser advanced into the midmyocardium from the tip of an endocardial catheter. The lesions were precise, with well-defined edges and no evidence of endocardial damage. This approach can be ideal for subepicardial foci without entering the pericardial space; it would decrease the risk of pericarditis and eliminate the difficulty posed by epicardial fat.[4,15]

Laser energy can also be delivered along the entire length of a linear diffuser, which provides uniform linear laser ablation and a superior transmural lesion when compared with previous end-firing optical delivery systems. The use of the linear diffuser in combination with lasers in the infrared or near-infrared wavelength (800 to 1100 nm) is currently under investigation.[1,67] Additionally, laser balloons designed for PV isolation have been developed using a beam splitter, which provides circumferential laser ablation at the PV ostium. However, as with other balloon technologies, the efficacy of the laser balloon ablation depends on good contact around the balloon circumference; fiberoptic technology is being developed to facilitate establishment of contact once the balloon is deployed and to improve the performance of such systems.[1]

Laser-delivered energy has several potential advantages, including short application time and easy control of the amount of energy delivered. However, if catheter laser ablation is to be developed, several issues have to be evaluated, including tissue contact, the ability to focus the laser on the specific target, and the homogeneity of the target tissue, which can absorb laser energy to variable degrees.[15]

REFERENCES

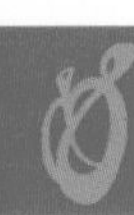

1. Cummings JE, Pacifico A, Drago JL, et al: Alternative energy sources for the ablation of arrhythmias. Pacing Clin Electrophysiol 2005;28:434.
2. Haines DE: Biophysics of radiofrequency lesion formation. *In* Huang SKS, Wood MA (eds): Catheter Ablation of Cardiac Arrhythmias. Philadelphia, WB Saunders, 2006, pp 3-20.
3. Haines DE: The biophysics and pathyophysiology of lesion formation during radiofrequency catheter ablation. *In* Zipes DP, Jalife J (eds): Cardiac Electrophysiology: From Cell to Bedside. Philadelphia, WB Saunders, 2004, pp 1018-1027.
4. Josephson M: Catheter and surgical ablation in the therapy of arrhythmias. *In* Josephson M (ed): Clinical Cardiac Electrophysiology, 3rd ed. Philadelphia, Lippincott, Williams & Wilkins, 2002, pp 710-836.
5. Wittkampf FH, Nakagawa H: RF catheter ablation: Lessons on lesions. Pacing Clin Electrophysiol 2006;29:1285.
6. Haines D: Biophysics of ablation: application to technology. J Cardiovasc Electrophysiol 2004;15(Suppl 10):S2.
7. Stevenson WG, Cooper J, Sapp J: Optimizing RF output for cooled RF ablation. J Cardiovasc Electrophysiol 2004;15(Suppl 10):S24.
8. Nath S, Haines D: Pathophysiology of lesion formation by radiofrequency catheter ablation. *In* Huang SKS, Wilber DJ (eds): Radiofrequency Catheter Ablation of Cardiac Arrhythmias: Basic Concepts and Clinical Applications, 2nd ed. Armonk, NY: Futura, 2000, pp 25-46.
9. Fuller IA, Wood MA: Intramural coronary vasculature prevents transmural radiofrequency lesion formation: implications for linear ablation. Circulation 2003;107:1797.
10. Dorwarth U, Fiek M, Remp T, et al: Radiofrequency catheter ablation: Different cooled and noncooled electrode systems induce specific lesion geometries and adverse effects profiles. Pacing Clin Electrophysiol 2003;26(Pt 1):1438.
11. Demazumder D, Schwartzman D: Titration of radiofrequency energy during endocardial catheter ablation. *In* Huang SKS, Wood MA (eds): Philadelphia, WB Saunders, 2006, pp 21-34.
12. Bruce GK, Bunch TJ, Milton MA, et al: Discrepancies between catheter tip and tissue temperature in cooled-tip ablation: Relevance to guiding left atrial ablation. Circulation 2005;112:954.
13. Chan RC, Johnson SB, Seward JB, Packer DL: The effect of ablation electrode length and catheter tip to endocardial orientation on radiofrequency lesion size in the canine right atrium. Pacing Clin Electrophysiol 2002;25:4.
14. Lewalter T, Bitzen A, Wurtz S, et al: Gold-tip electrodes—a new "deep lesion" technology for catheter ablation? In vitro comparison of a gold alloy versus platinum-iridium tip electrode ablation catheter. J Cardiovasc Electrophysiol 2005;16:770.
15. Doshi S, Keane D: Catheter microwave, laser, and ultrasound: Biophysics and applications. Catheter Ablation of Cardiac Arrhythmias. Philadelphia, WB Saunders, 2006, pp 69-82.
16. Lickfett L, Mahesh M, Vasamreddy C, et al: Radiation exposure during catheter ablation of atrial fibrillation. Circulation 2004;110:3003.
17. Chowdhry T, Calkins H: Complications associated with radiofrequency catheter ablation of cardiac arrhythmias. *In* Huang SKS, Wood MA (eds): Catheter Ablation of Cardiac Arrhythmias. Philadelphia, WB Saunders, 2006, pp 619-634.
18. Lin K, Chen SA, Lin Y, Chang KHS: Irrigated and cooled-tip radiofrequency catheter ablation. *In* Huang SKS, Wood MA (eds): Catheter Ablation of Cardiac Arrhythmias. Philadelphia, WB Saunders, 2006, pp 35-48.
19. Calkins H, Epstein AE, Packer DL, et al: Catheter ablation of ventricular tachycardia in patients with structural heart disease using cooled radiofrequency energy. J Am Coll Cardiol 2000;35:1905.
20. Cooper JM, Sapp JL, Tedrow U, et al: Ablation with an internally irrigated radiofrequency catheter: learning how to avoid steam pops. Heart Rhythm 2004;1:329.
21. Marrouche NF, Martin DO, Wazni O, et al: Phased-array intracardiac echocardiography monitoring during pulmonary vein isolation in patients with atrial fibrillation: Impact on outcome and complications. Circulation 2003;107:2710.
22. Yokoyama K, Nakagawa H, Wittkampf FH, et al: Comparison of electrode cooling between internal and open irrigation in radiofrequency ablation lesion depth and incidence of thrombus and steam pop. Circulation 2006;113:11.
23. Yamane T, Jais P, Shah DC, et al: Efficacy and safety of an irrigated-tip catheter for the ablation of accessory pathways resistant to conventional radiofrequency ablation. Circulation 2000;102:2565.
24. Demazumder D, Mirotznik MS, Schwartzman D: Comparison of irrigated electrode designs for radiofrequency ablation of myocardium. J Interv Card Electrophysiol 2001;5:391.
25. Cooper JM, Sapp JL, Robinson D: Blood flow plays an important role in cooled radiofrequency ablation. Circulation 2003;108:422.
26. Delacretaz E, Soejima K, Brunckhorst CB, et al: Assessment of radiofrequency ablation effect from unipolar pacing threshold. Pacing Clin Electrophysiol 2003; 26:1993.
27. Atiga WL, Worley SJ, Hummel J, et al: Prospective randomized comparison of cooled radiofrequency versus standard radiofrequency energy for ablation of typical atrial flutter. Pacing Clin Electrophysiol 2002;25:1172.
28. Calkins H: Cooled ablation. J Cardiovasc Electrophysiol 2004;15(Suppl 10):S12.
29. Marrouche NF, Dresing T, Cole C, et al: Circular mapping and ablation of the pulmonary vein for treatment of atrial fibrillation: impact of different catheter technologies. J Am Coll Cardiol 2002;40:464.
30. Tanner H, Lukac P, Schwick N, et al: Irrigated-tip catheter ablation of intraatrial reentrant tachycardia in patients late after surgery of congenital heart disease. Heart Rhythm 2004;1:268.
31. Skanes AC, Klein G, Krahn A, Yee R: Cryoablation: Potentials and pitfalls. J Cardiovasc Electrophysiol 2004;15(Suppl 10):S28.
32. Novak P, Dubuc M: Catheter cryoablation: biophysics and applications. *In* Huang SKS, Wood MA (eds): Catheter Ablation of Cardiac Arrhythmias. Philadelphia, WB Saunders, 2006, pp 49-68.
33. Wood MA, Parvez B, Ellenbogen AL, et al: Determinants of lesion sizes and tissue temperatures during catheter cryoablation. Pacing Clin Electrophysiol 2007;30:644.
34. Ali FI, Green MS, Tang AS, Lemery R: A cool ablation. J Cardiovasc Electrophysiol 2002;13:299.
35. Atienza F, Arenal A, Torrecilla EG, et al: Acute and long-term outcome of transvenous cryoablation of midseptal and parahisian accessory pathways in patients at high risk of atrioventricular block during radiofrequency ablation. Am J Cardiol 2004;93:1302.
36. Gaita F, Haissaguerre M, Giustetto C, et al: Safety and efficacy of cryoablation of accessory pathways adjacent to the normal conduction system. J Cardiovasc Electrophysiol 2003;14:825.
37. Kimman GP, Theuns DA, Szili-Torok T, et al: CRAVT: A prospective, randomized study comparing transvenous cryothermal and radiofrequency ablation in atrioventricular nodal re-entrant tachycardia. Eur Heart J 2004;25:2232.
38. Skanes AC, Dubuc M, Klein GJ, et al: Cryothermal ablation of the slow pathway for the elimination of atrioventricular nodal reentrant tachycardia. Circulation 2000;102:2856.
39. Zrenner B, Dong J, Schreieck J, et al: Transvenous cryoablation versus radiofrequency ablation of the slow pathway for the treatment of atrioventricular nodal re-entrant tachycardia: A prospective randomized pilot study. Eur Heart J 2004;25:2226.
40. Tse HF, Reek S, Timmermans C, et al: Pulmonary vein isolation using transvenous catheter cryoablation for treatment of atrial fibrillation without risk of pulmonary vein stenosis. J Am Coll Cardiol 2003;42:752.
41. Friedman PL, Dubuc M, Green MS, et al: Catheter cryoablation of supraventricular tachycardia: Results of the multicenter prospective "frosty" trial. Heart Rhythm 2004;1:129.
42. Lowe MD, Meara M, Mason J, et al: Catheter cryoablation of supraventricular arrhythmias: A painless alternative to radiofrequency energy. Pacing Clin Electrophysiol 2003;26(Pt 2):500.
43. Manusama R, Timmermans C, Limon F, et al: Catheter-based cryoablation permanently cures patients with common atrial flutter. Circulation 2004;109: 1636.
44. Rodriguez LM, Geller JC, Tse HF, et al: Acute results of transvenous cryoablation of supraventricular tachycardia (atrial fibrillation, atrial flutter, Wolff-Parkinson-White syndrome, atrioventricular nodal reentry tachycardia). J Cardiovasc Electrophysiol 2002;13:1082.
45. Dill T, Neumann T, Ekinci O, et al: Pulmonary vein diameter reduction after radiofrequency catheter ablation for paroxysmal atrial fibrillation evaluated by contrast-enhanced three-dimensional magnetic resonance imaging. Circulation 2003; 107:845.
46. Ernst S, Ouyang F, Goya M, et al: Total pulmonary vein occlusion as a consequence of catheter ablation for atrial fibrillation mimicking primary lung disease. J Cardiovasc Electrophysiol 2003;14:366.
47. Hoyt R, Wood MA, Daoud E: Transvenous catheter cryoblation for treatment of AF. Pacing Clin Electrophysiol 2005;28:S78.
48. Sarabanda AV, Bunch TJ, Johnson SB, et al: Efficacy and safety of circumferential pulmonary vein isolation using a novel cryothermal balloon ablation system. J Am Coll Cardiol 2005;46:1902.
49. Skanes AC, Jensen SM, Papp R, et al: Isolation of pulmonary veins using a transvenous curvilinear cryoablation catheter: Feasibility, initial experience, and analysis of recurrences. J Cardiovasc Electrophysiol 2005;16:1304.
50. Saliba W, Wilber D, Packer D, et al: Circumferential ultrasound ablation for pulmonary vein isolation: Analysis of acute and chronic failures. J Cardiovasc Electrophysiol 2002;13:957.
51. Atienza F, Arenal A, Ormaetxe J, Almendral J: Epicardial idiopathic ventricular tachycardia originating within the left main coronary artery ostium area: Identification using the LocaLisa nonfluoroscopic catheter navigation system. J Cardiovasc Electrophysiol 2005;16:1239.
52. Reek S, Geller JC, Schildhaus HU, et al: Feasibility of catheter cryoablation in normal ventricular myocardium and healed myocardial infarction. Pacing Clin Electrophysiol 2004;27:1530.
53. Manasse E, Colombo PG, Barbone A, et al: Clinical histopathology and ultrastructural analysis of myocardium following microwave energy ablation. Eur J Cardiothorac Surg 2003;23:573.
54. van Brakel TJ, Bolotin G, Salleng KJ, et al: Evaluation of epicardial microwave ablation lesions: histology versus electrophysiology. Ann Thorac Surg 2004;78: 1397.
55. Erdogan A, Grumbrecht S, Neumann T, et al: Microwave, irrigated, pulsed, or conventional radiofrequency energy source: Which energy source for which catheter ablation? Pacing Clin Electrophysiol 2003;26(Pt 2):504.
56. Climent V, Hurle A, Ho SY, et al: Early morphological changes following microwave endocardial ablation for treatment of chronic atrial fibrillation during mitral valve surgery. J Cardiovasc Electrophysiol 2004;15:1277.

57. Iwasa A, Storey J, Yao B, et al: Efficacy of a microwave antenna for ablation of the tricuspid valve—inferior vena cava isthmus in dogs as a treatment for type 1 atrial flutter. J Interv Card Electrophysiol 2004;10:191.
58. Hurle A, Ibanez A, Parra JM, Martinez JG: Preliminary results with the microwave-modified maze III procedure for the treatment of chronic atrial fibrillation. Pacing Clin Electrophysiol 2004;27:1644.
59. Khargi K, Hutten BA, Lemke B, Deneke T: Surgical treatment of atrial fibrillation: a systematic review. Eur J Cardiothorac Surg 2005;27:258.
60. Yiu K, Lau C, Lee KL, Tse H: Emerging energy sources for catheter ablation of atrial fibrillation. J Cardiovasc Electrophysiol 2006;17(Suppl 3):S56.
61. Chan JY, Fung JW, Yu CM, Feld GK: Preliminary results with percutaneous transcatheter microwave ablation of typical atrial flutter. J Cardiovasc Electrophysiol 2007;18:286.
62. Schweikert RA, Saliba WI, Tomassoni G, et al: Percutaneous pericardial instrumentation for endo-epicardial mapping of previously failed ablations. Circulation 2003;108:1329.
63. Soejima K, Stevenson WG, Sapp JL, et al: Endocardial and epicardial radiofrequency ablation of ventricular tachycardia associated with dilated cardiomyopathy: The importance of low-voltage scars. J Am Coll Cardiol 2004;43:1834.
64. Nakagawa H, Antz M, Wong T, et al: Initial experience using a forward directed, high-intensity focused ultrasound balloon catheter for pulmonary vein antrum isolation in patients with atrial fibrillation. J Cardiovasc Electrophysiol 2007;18:136.
65. Schmidt BM, Chun KJM, Kuck K-HM, Antz MM: Pulmonary vein isolation by high-intensity focused ultrasound. Indian Pacing Electrophysiol J 2006;7:126.
66. Schmidt B, Antz M, Ernst S, et al: Pulmonary vein isolation by high-intensity focused ultrasound: first-in-man study with a steerable balloon catheter. Heart Rhythm 2007;4:575.
67. Fried NM, Lardo AC, Berger RD, et al: Linear lesions in myocardium created by Nd:YAG laser using diffusing optical fibers: in vitro and in vivo results. Lasers Surg Med 2000;27:295.

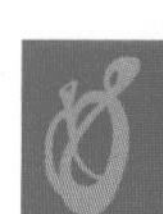

CHAPTER 5

Sinus Node Dysfunction

GENERAL CONSIDERATIONS

Anatomy and Physiology of the Sinus Node

The sinus node is the dominant pacemaker of the heart. Its pacemaker function is determined by its low maximum diastolic membrane potential and steep phase 4 spontaneous depolarization.[1]

The sinus node is located laterally in the epicardial groove of the sulcus terminalis. The sinus node in adults measures 10 to 20 mm long and 2 to 3 mm wide and thick, tending to narrow caudally toward the inferior vena cava (IVC). Starting epicardially in the right atrial (RA) sulcus terminalis at the junction of the superior vena cava (SVC) and RA, it courses downward and to the left, to end subendocardially. The sinus node is a spindle-shaped structure with a central body and tapering ends. The head extends toward the interatrial groove, and the tail extends toward the orifice of IVC.[1-4] The sinus node is not insulated from the adjacent atrial myocardium, although it consists of densely packed specialized myocytes in a connective tissue matrix and it often surrounds the nodal artery.[4]

The sinus node is in reality a region, which is functionally larger and less well-defined than initially believed. It is composed of nests of principal pacemaker cells (referred to as P cells because of their relatively pale appearance on electron micrography), which spontaneously depolarize. In addition to this principal nest of cells, other nests contain cells with slower intrinsic depolarization rates and serve as backup pacemakers in response to changing physiological and pathological conditions. The pacemaker activity is not confined to a single cell in the sinus node; rather, sinus nodal cells function as electrically coupled oscillators that discharge synchronously because of mutual entrainment. In fact, sinus rhythm may result from impulse origin at widely separated sites, with two or three individual wavefronts created that merge to form a single, widely disseminated wavefront.[5] Additionally, the pacemaker locus can shift within the sinus node to cells discharging faster or more slowly. Mapping of activation indicates that at faster rates, the sinus impulse originates in the superior portion of the sinus node, whereas at slower rates it arises from a more inferior portion.[6] The sinus node can be insulated from the surrounding atrial myocytes, except at a limited number of preferential exit sites. Shifting pacemaker sites can select different exit pathways to the atria. Normal conduction velocities within the sinus node are slow (2 to 5 cm/sec), increasing the likelihood of intranodal conduction block.[1]

The blood supply to the sinus node region is variable, making it vulnerable to damage during operative procedures. The blood supply predominantly comes from a large central artery, the sinus nodal artery, which is a branch of the right coronary artery in 55% to 60% of patients and from the circumflex artery in 40% to 45%. The sinus nodal artery is disproportionately large in size, which is considered physiologically important in that its perfusion pressure can affect the sinus rate. Distention of the artery slows the sinus rate, whereas collapse causes an increase in rate.[1,3]

The sinus node is densely innervated with postganglionic adrenergic and cholinergic nerve terminals (threefold greater density of beta-adrenergic and muscarinic cholinergic receptors than adjacent atrial tissue), both of which influence the rate of spontaneous depolarization in pacemaker cells and can cause a shift in the principal pacemaker site within the sinus node region, which is often associated with subtle changes in P wave morphology. Enhanced vagal activity can produce sinus bradycardia, sinus arrest, and sinoatrial exit block, whereas increased sympathetic activity can increase the sinus rate and reverse sinus arrest and sinoatrial exit block. Sinus node responses to brief vagal bursts begin after a short latency and dissipate quickly; in contrast, responses to sympathetic stimulation begin and dissipate slowly. The rapid onset and offset of responses to vagal stimulation allow dynamic beat-to-beat vagal modulation of the heart rate, whereas the slow temporal response to sympathetic stimulation precludes any beat-to-beat regulation by sympathetic activity.[1]

Periodic vagal bursting (as may occur each time a systolic pressure wave arrives at the baroreceptor regions in the aortic and carotid sinuses) induces phasic changes in the sinus cycle length (CL) and can entrain the sinus node to discharge faster or slower at periods identical to those of the vagal burst.[3] Because the peak vagal effects on sinus rate and atrioventricular node (AVN) conduction occur at different times in the cardiac cycle, a brief vagal burst can slow the sinus rate without affecting AVN conduction or can prolong AVN conduction time and not slow the sinus rate.[1]

Pathophysiology of Sinus Node Dysfunction

The cause of sinus node dysfunction (SND) can be classified as intrinsic (secondary to a pathological condition involving the sinus node proper) or extrinsic (caused by depression of sinus node function by external factors such as drugs or autonomic influences).

Causes of Intrinsic Sinus Node Dysfunction

Idiopathic degenerative disease is probably the most common cause of intrinsic SND.[2] Ischemic heart disease can be responsible for one third of cases of SND. Transient slowing of the sinus rate or sinus arrest can complicate acute myocardial infarction (MI), which is usually seen with acute inferior wall MI, and is caused by autonomic influences. Cardiomyopathy, long-standing hypertension, infiltrative disorders (e.g., amyloidosis and sarcoidosis), collagen vascular diseases, and surgical trauma can also result in SND.[7,8]

Orthotropic cardiac transplantation with atrial-atrial anastomosis is associated with a high incidence of SND in the donor heart (likely because of sinus nodal artery damage). Musculoskeletal disorders such as myotonic dystrophy or Friedreich's ataxia are rare causes of SND. Congenital heart disease can be associated with SND, such as sinus venosus and secundum atrial septal defects, even though no surgery has been performed.[9] Surgical trauma is responsible for most cases of SND in the pediatric population. Most commonly associated with this complication is Mustard's procedure for transposition of the great arteries and repair of atrial septal defects, especially of the sinus venosus type.[9]

Causes of Extrinsic Sinus Node Dysfunction

In the absence of structural abnormalities, the predominant causes of SND are drug effects and autonomic influences. Drugs can alter sinus node function by direct pharmacological effects on nodal tissue or indirectly by neurally mediated effects.[10] Drugs known to depress sinus node function include beta blockers, calcium channel blockers (verapamil and diltiazem), digoxin, sympatholytic antihypertensive agents (e.g., clonidine), and antiarrhythmic agents (types IA, IC, and III).[11]

SND can sometimes result from excessive vagal tone in individuals without intrinsic sinus node disease. Hypervagotonia can be seen in carotid sinus syndrome and neurocardiogenic syncope.[12] Well-trained athletes with increased vagal tone can require some deconditioning to help prevent symptomatic bradyarrhythmias.[13,14] Less common extrinsic causes of SND include electrolyte abnormalities such as hyperkalemia, hypothermia, intracranial hypertension, hypoxia, hypercapnia, hypothyroidism, advanced liver disease, typhoid fever, brucellosis, and sepsis.

Clinical Presentation

The symptoms reported by patients with SND are varied and often nonspecific, and the intermittent nature of these symptoms makes documentation of the associated arrhythmia difficult at times. More than 50% of the patients affected are older than 50 years. Patients with SND commonly present with paroxysmal dizziness, presyncope, or syncope, which are predominantly related to prolonged sinus pauses. The highest incidence of syncope associated with SND probably occurs in patients with tachycardia-bradycardia syndrome, in whom syncope typically occurs secondary to a long sinus pause following cessation of the supraventricular tachycardia (SVT) (usually atrial fibrillation [AF]). Occasionally, a stroke can be the first manifestation of SND in patients presenting with paroxysmal AF and thromboembolism.[3,10,15]

Patients with sinus bradycardia or chronotropic incompetence can present with decreased exercise capacity or fatigue. Chronotropic incompetence is estimated to be present in 20% to 60% of patients with SND.[16-18]

Natural History of Sinus Node Dysfunction

The natural history of SND can be variable, but slow progression (over 10 to 30 years) is expected. The prognosis largely depends on the type of dysfunction and the presence and severity of the underlying heart disease. The worst prognosis is associated with the tachycardia-bradycardia syndrome (mostly because of the risk for thromboembolic complications), whereas sinus bradycardia is much more benign. The incidence of new-onset AF in patients with SND is 5.2% per year. New atrial tachyarrhythmias occur with less frequency in patients who are treated with atrial pacing (3.9%) compared with a greatly increased incidence of similar arrhythmias in those with only ventricular pacing (22.3%).[19,20] Furthermore, thromboembolism occurs in 15.2% among unpaced patients with SND versus 13% among patients treated with only ventricular pacing versus 1.6% among those treated with atrial pacing.[10,15,21]

The incidence of advanced AV conduction system disease in patients with SND is low and, when present, its progression is slow. At the time of diagnosis of SND, approximately 17% of the patients have some degree of AV conduction system disease (PR interval more than 240 milliseconds, bundle branch block, His bundle–ventricular (HV) interval prolongation, AV Wenckebach rate less than 120 beats/min, and/or second- or third-degree AV block). New AV conduction abnormalities develop at a rate of approximately 2.7% per year. The incidence of advanced AV block during long-term follow-up is low (approximately 1% per year).[15]

Diagnostic Evaluation of Sinus Node Dysfunction

Generally, the noninvasive methods of ECG monitoring, exercise testing, and autonomic testing are used first. However, if symptoms are infrequent and noninvasive evaluation is unrevealing, invasive electrophysiological (EP) testing may be pursued.

Electrocardiogram and Ambulatory Monitoring. A 12-lead electrocardiogram (ECG) needs to be obtained in symptomatic patients. However, the diagnosis of SND as the cause of the symptoms is rarely made from the ECG. In patients with frequent symptoms, 24- or 48-hour ambulatory Holter monitoring can be useful. Cardiac event monitoring or implantable loop recorders may be necessary in patients with less frequent symptoms. Documentation of symptoms in a diary by the patient while wearing the cardiac monitor is essential for correlation of symptoms with the heart rhythm at the time. In some cases, the ambulatory monitoring can exclude SND as the cause of symptoms, if normal sinus rhythm (NSR) is documented at the time of symptoms occurrence. In contrast, sinus pauses recorded may not be associated with symptoms.[22]

Autonomic Modulation. An abnormal response to carotid sinus massage (pause longer than 3 seconds) can indicate SND, but this response can also occur in asymptomatic older individuals. Heart rate response to the Valsalva maneuver (normally decreased) or upright tilt (normally increased) can also be used to verify that the autonomic nervous system itself is intact.[23] Complete pharmacological autonomic blockade is used to determine the intrinsic heart rate (see later).[3]

Exercise Testing. Exercise testing to assess chronotropic incompetence is of value in patients with exertional symptoms (see later).

Electrophysiological Testing. Noninvasive testing is usually adequate in establishing the diagnosis of SND and guiding subsequent therapy. However, invasive EP testing can be of value in symptomatic patients in whom SND is suspected but cannot be documented in association with symptoms. In addition to assessing SND, EP testing can be of value in evaluation of other potential causes for symptoms of syncope and palpitations (e.g., AV block, SVT, and ventricular tachycardia [VT]).[10,15]

ELECTROCARDIOGRAPHIC FEATURES

Sinus Bradycardia. Sinus bradycardia (less than 60 beats/min) is considered abnormal when it is persistent, unexplained, and inappropriate for physiological circumstances. Sinus bradycardia less than 40 beats/min (not associated with sleep or physical conditioning) is generally considered abnormal.[3]

Sinus Pauses. Sinus arrest and sinoatrial exit block can result in sinus pauses, and are definite evidence of SND.

Sinus Arrest. The terms "sinus arrest" and "sinus pause" are often used interchangeably; sinus arrest is a result of total cessation of impulse formation within the sinus node. The pause is not an exact multiple of the preceding P-P interval but is random in duration (Fig. 5-1). Although asymptomatic pauses of 2 to 3 seconds can be seen in up to 11% of normal individuals and in one third of trained athletes, pauses longer than 3 seconds are rare in normal individuals and may or may not be associated with symptoms, but are usually caused by SND.[3]

Sinoatrial Exit Block. Sinoatrial exit block results when a normally generated sinus impulse fails to conduct to the atria because of delay in conduction or block within the sinus node itself or perinodal tissue. Sinoatrial exit block produces a pause that is eventually terminated by a delayed sinus beat or an atrial or junctional escape beat.[24] In theory, sinoatrial exit block can be distinguished from sinus arrest because the exit block pause is an exact multiple of the baseline P-P interval. However, sinus arrhythmia causing normal beat-to-beat variations in the sinus rate often makes the distinction impossible.[3]

Exit block is classified into three types, analogous to those of AV block—first-degree, second-degree, and third-degree exit block.[24] First-degree sinoatrial exit block is caused by abnormal prolongation of the sinoatrial conduction time. It occurs every time a sinus impulse reaches the atrium, but is conducted with a delay at a fixed interval. This type of sinoatrial exit block is concealed on the surface ECG and can only be diagnosed by direct sinus node recording or indirect measurement of sinoatrial conduction time during an EP study. Second-degree sinoatrial exit block is marked by intermittent failure of the sinus impulse to exit the sinus node. Type I block is viewed as Wenckebach periodicity of the P wave on the surface ECG, and manifests as progressive delay in conduction of the sinus-generated impulse through the sinus node to the atrium, finally resulting in a nonconducted sinus impulse and absence of a P wave on the surface ECG. Because the sinus discharge is a silent event on the surface ECG, this arrhythmia can be inferred only because of a dropped P wave and the signs of Wenckebach periodicity seen with this type of arrhythmia. The increment in delay in impulse conduction through the sinus node tissue is progressively less; thus, the P-P intervals become progressively shorter until a P wave fails to occur. The pauses associated with this type of sinoatrial exit block are less than twice the shortest sinus cycle. Type II block manifests as an abrupt absence of one or more P waves because of failure of the atrial impulse to exit the sinus node, without previous progressive prolongation of sinoatrial conduction time (and without progressive shortening of the P-P intervals). Sometimes, two or more consecutive sinus impulses are blocked within the sinus node, which creates considerably long pauses. The sinus pause should be an exact multiple of the immediately preceding P-P interval. However, normal variations in the sinus rate caused by sinus arrhythmia can obscure this measurement. Third-degree or complete sinoatrial exit block manifests as absence of P waves, with long pauses resulting in lower pacemaker escape rhythm. This type of block is impossible to distinguish from sinus arrest with certainty without invasive sinus node recordings.[15,25,26]

Tachycardia-Bradycardia Syndrome. Tachycardia-bradycardia syndrome, frequently referred to as sick sinus syndrome, is a common manifestation of SND, and it refers to the presence of intermittent sinus or junctional bradycardia alternating with atrial tachyarrhythmias (Fig. 5-2). The atrial tachyarrhythmia is most commonly paroxysmal AF, but atrial tachycardia (AT), atrial flutter (AFL), and occasionally atrioventricular nodal reentrant tachycardia (AVNRT) or atrioventricular reentrant tachycardia (AVRT) can also occur.[3,27]

Apart from an underlying sinus bradycardia of varying severity, these patients often experience prolonged sinus arrest and asystole on termination of the atrial tachyarrhythmia, resulting from suppression of the sinus node and secondary pacemakers. Long sinus pauses that occur following electrical cardioversion of AF are another manifestation of SND. Therapeutic strategies to control tachyarrhythmias often result in the need for pacemaker therapy. On the other hand, atrial tachyarrhythmias can be precipitated by prolonged sinus pauses.[2,3,28,29]

Persistent Atrial Fibrillation. Persistent AF with a slow ventricular response in the absence of AVN blocking drugs is often present in patients with SND. These patients can demonstrate very slow ventricular rates at rest or during

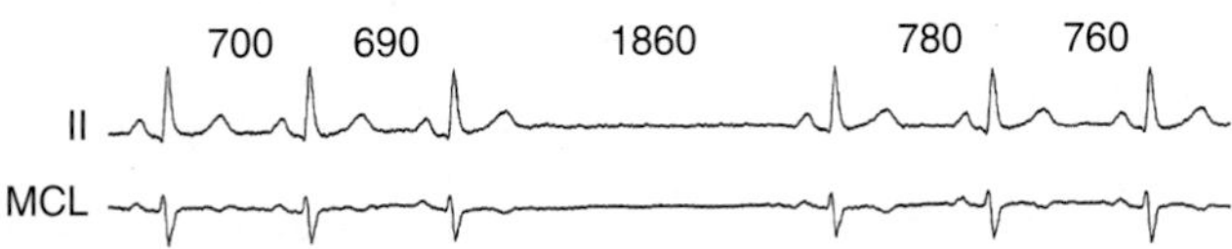

FIGURE 5-1 Sinus pause is shown in two monitor leads. Although the sinus rate is slightly irregular, the pause significantly exceeds any two P-P intervals (excluding sinus exit block).

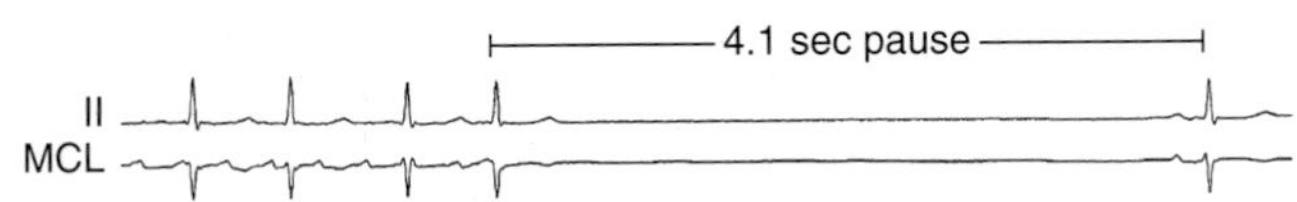

FIGURE 5-2 Tachycardia-bradycardia syndrome. Two surface ECG leads are shown during an atrial tachyarrhythmia that suddenly terminates, followed by a 4.1-second pause before sinus rhythm resumes. The patient became lightheaded during this period.

sleep and occasionally have long pauses. Occasionally, they can develop complete AV block with a junctional or ventricular escape rhythm. They can also conduct rapidly and develop symptoms caused by tachycardia during exercise. In some cases, cardioversion results in a long sinus pause or junctional escape rhythm before the appearance of sinus rhythm. Although a combination of sinus node and AV conduction disease can be present in many cases, examples of rapid ventricular responses during atrial tachyarrhythmias can frequently be found.[2,27]

Persistent Atrial Standstill. Atrial standstill is a rare clinical syndrome in which there is no spontaneous atrial activity and the atria cannot be electrically stimulated. The surface ECG usually reveals junctional bradycardia without atrial activity. The atria are generally fibrotic and without any functional myocardium. Lack of mechanical atrial contraction poses a high risk for thromboembolism in these patients.[30,31]

Chronotropic Incompetence. Treadmill exercise testing can be of substantial value in assessing the chronotropic response ("competence") to increases in metabolic demands in patients with sinus bradycardia who are suspected of having SND. Although the resting heart rate can be normal, these patients can have the inability to increase their heart rate during exercise or have unpredictable fluctuations in the heart rate during activity. Some patients can initially experience a normal increase in the heart rate with exercise, which then plateaus or decreases inappropriately.[16,17,25,26]

The definition of chronotropic incompetence is not agreed on, but it is reasonable to designate it as an abnormally low heart rate response to exercise manifesting as a less than normal increase in the sinus rate at each stage of exercise, with a plateau at less than 70% to 75% of the age-predicted maximum heart rate (220 − age) or inability to achieve a sinus rate of 100 to 120 beats/min at maximum effort. Irregular (and nonreproducible) increases, and even decreases, in the sinus rate during exercise, can also occur but are rare. Other patients with SND can achieve an appropriate peak heart rate during exercise but may have slow sinus rate acceleration in the initial stage or rapid deceleration of heart rate in the recovery stage.[16-18]

Carotid Sinus Hypersensitivity. An abnormal response to carotid sinus massage (pause longer than 3 seconds) can indicate SND, but this response may also occur in asymptomatic older individuals (Fig. 5-3).[1,24-26]

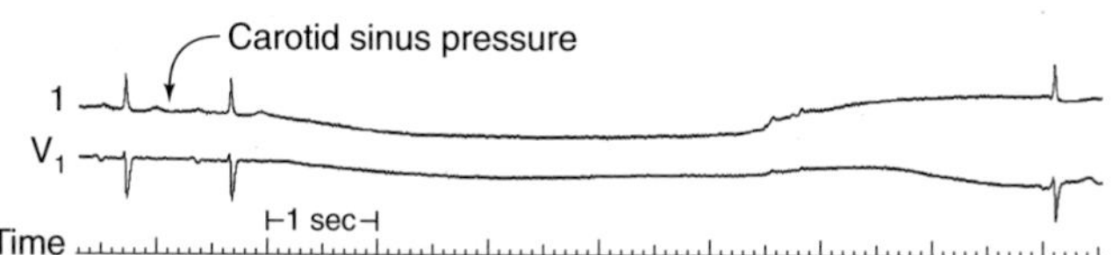

FIGURE 5–3 Carotid sinus hypersensitivity. Two surface ECG leads are shown during carotid sinus pressure, as indicated. The PR interval is prolonged, followed by a 7.5-second sinus pause ended by a P wave and probable junctional escape complex. The patient was near-syncopal during this period.

Sinus Arrhythmia. Respiratory sinus arrhythmia, in which the sinus rate increases with inspiration and decreases with expiration, is not an abnormal rhythm and is most commonly seen in young healthy subjects. Sinus arrhythmia is present when the P wave morphology is normal and consistent and the P-P intervals vary by more than 160 milliseconds. Nonrespiratory sinus arrhythmia, in which phasic changes in sinus rate are not related to the respiratory cycle, may be accentuated by the use of vagal agents such as digitalis and morphine; its mechanism is unknown. Patients with nonrespiratory sinus arrhythmia are likely to be older and to have underlying cardiac disease, although the arrhythmia is not a marker for structural heart disease. None of the sinus arrhythmias (respiratory or nonrespiratory) indicates SND. Additionally, respiratory variation in the sinus P wave contour can be seen in the inferior leads and should not be confused with wandering atrial pacemaker, which is unrelated to breathing and therefore is not phasic.[25,26]

Ventriculophasic sinus arrhythmia is an unusual rhythm that occurs when sinus rhythm and high-grade or complete AV block coexist; it is characterized by shorter P-P intervals when they enclose QRS complexes and longer P-P intervals when no QRS complexes are enclosed (Fig. 5-4). The mechanism is uncertain but may be related to the effects of the mechanical ventricular systole itself: the ventricular contraction increases the blood supply to the sinus node, thereby transiently increasing its firing rate. Ventriculophasic sinus arrhythmia is not a pathological arrhythmia and should not be confused with premature atrial complexes (PACs) or sinoatrial block.

ELECTROPHYSIOLOGICAL TESTING

Role of Electrophysiological Testing

The diagnosis of SND usually can be made based on clinical and ECG findings, which is typically adequate for deciding subsequent treatment. Once symptoms and SND are correlated by ECG findings, further documentation by invasive studies is not required. Similarly, asymptomatic patients with evidence of SND need not be tested, because no therapy is indicated. However, EP testing can be important to test sinus node function in patients who have had symptoms compatible with SND and in whom no documentation of the arrhythmia responsible for these symptoms has been obtained by prolonged monitoring. In these cases, EP testing can yield information that may be used to guide appropriate therapy. The most useful measures of the overall sinus node function are a combination of the responses to atropine and exercise, and the sinus node recovery time (SNRT).[24]

Sinus Node Recovery Time

The sinus node is the archetype of an automatic focus. Automatic rhythms are characterized by spontaneous depolarization, overdrive suppression, and postoverdrive warm-up or gradual return to baseline CL. SNRT is the

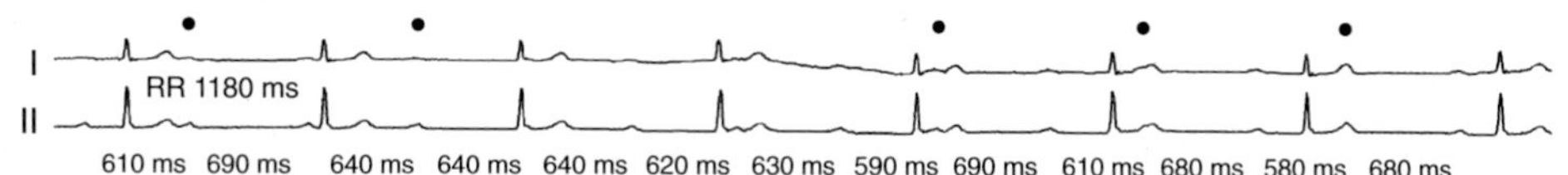

FIGURE 5–4 Ventriculophasic sinus arrhythmia. Two monitor leads are shown during sinus rhythm with complete atrioventricular (AV) block and junctional escape rhythm (cycle length, 1180 milliseconds). Dissociated sinus P waves occur at different times in the ventricular cycle (numbers below the tracing indicate P-P intervals). Black dots above the tracing denote P waves that surround a QRS complex and occur earlier than anticipated (ventriculophasic arrhythmia).

interval between the end of a period of pacing-induced overdrive suppression of sinus node activity and the return of sinus node function, manifest on the surface ECG by a postpacing sinus P wave. Clinically, SNRT is used to test sinus node automaticity.[25,26,32]

Technique

Pacing Site. Pacing is performed in the high RA at a site near the sinus node, so as to decrease the conduction time to and from the sinus node.[24]

Pacing Cycle Length. SNRT is preferably measured after pacing at multiple CLs. Pacing is started at a CL just shorter than the sinus CL. After a 1-minute rest, pacing is repeated at progressively shorter CLs (with 50- to 100-millisecond decrements) down to a pacing CL of 300 milliseconds.[24]

Pacing Duration. Pacing is continued for 30 or 60 seconds at a time. Although pacing durations beyond 15 seconds usually have little effect on the SNRT in healthy subjects, patients with SND can have marked suppression after longer pacing durations. It is also preferable to perform pacing at each CL for different durations (30, 60, and/or 120 seconds) to ensure that sinus entrance block has not obscured the true SNRT.[24]

Measurements

Several intervals have been used as a measure of SNRT.

Sinus Node Recovery Time. SNRT is the longest pause from the last paced beat to the first sinus return beat at a particular pacing CL. Normally, the SNRT is less than 1500 milliseconds, with a scatter on multiple tests of less than 250 milliseconds (Fig. 5-5). SNRT tends to be shorter with shorter baseline sinus CLs, and therefore a variety of corrections have been introduced.[25,26,32]

Corrected Sinus Node Recovery Time. Corrected SNRT equals SNRT minus the baseline sinus CL. Normal values of corrected SNRT have been reported from 350 to 550 milliseconds, with 500 milliseconds being most commonly used (see Fig. 5-5). However, the use of corrections at slow sinus rates can produce odd results. For example, a patient with symptomatic bradycardia at 1500-millisecond CL and SNRT of 2000 milliseconds, the corrected SNRT will be 500 milliseconds. For cases of severe bradycardia, an abnormal uncorrected SNRT of 2000 milliseconds is more accurate; in fact, one does not need SNRT to make the clinical diagnosis.

Maximum Sinus Node Recovery Time. Maximum SNRT is the longest pause from the last paced beat to the first sinus return beat at any pacing CL.

Ratio of Sinus Node Recovery Time to Sinus Cycle Length. The ratio of

$$(\text{SNRT}/\text{sinus CL}) \times 100\%$$

is lower than 160% in normal subjects.

Total Recovery Time. On cessation of atrial pacing, the pattern of subsequent beats returning to the basic sinus CL should be analyzed. Various patterns exist.[24] Total recovery time equals the time to return to basic sinus CL (normal total recovery time is less than 5 seconds, usually by the fourth to sixth recovery beat).

Secondary Pauses. Normally, following cessation of overdrive pacing, a gradual shortening of the sinus CL is observed until the baseline sinus CL is reached, typically within a few beats. Limited oscillations of recovery CLs before full recovery can be observed, especially at shorter pacing CLs.[24] Secondary pauses are identified when there is an initial shortening of the sinus CL after the SNRT, followed by an unexpected lengthening of the CL (see Fig. 5-5). Sudden and marked secondary pauses occurring during sinus recovery are abnormal. Sinoatrial exit block of variable duration is the primary mechanism of prolonged pauses, with a lesser component of depression of automaticity. Both may, and often do, coexist. However, secondary pauses can be a normal reflex following hypotension induced by pacing at rapid rates, or in response to pressure overshoot in the first recovery beat because of the prolonged filling time. Because these secondary pauses represent SND and because they occur more frequently following rapid atrial pacing, pacing should be performed at rates up to 200 beats/min.[24,25,32,33]

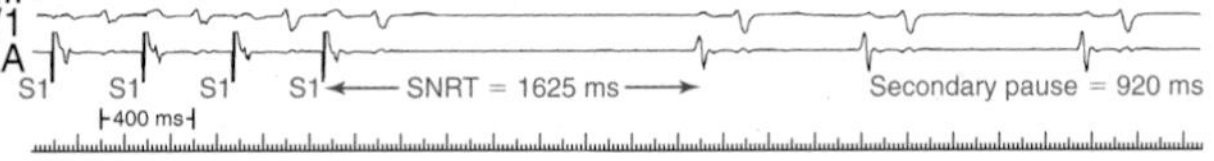

Limitations of Sinus Node Recovery Time

Many factors in addition to automaticity are involved in the measurement of SNRT, including proximity of the pacing site to the sinus node and conduction time from the pacing site to sinus node and vice versa, conduction time in and out the sinus node, and sinus node entrance block during rapid atrial pacing, which can lead to a shorter SNRT, whereas sinus node exit block after cessation of pacing can result in marked prolongation of the SNRT.[24] Moreover, sometimes SNRT cannot be measured because of atrial ectopic or junctional escape beats that preempt the sinus beat.[25,26]

Despite these limitations, SNRT is probably the best and most widely used test for sinus node automaticity. Pacing at rates near the baseline sinus CL causes no overdrive suppression so that the interval between the last paced beat and the next sinus beat is comparable with the baseline CL. If the SNRT after pacing at 500 milliseconds is shorter than after 600 milliseconds, or there is marked variation (more than 250 milliseconds) in the SNRTs when multiple tests are performed after pacing at 500 milliseconds, this can imply that some impulses have not penetrated the sinus node (i.e., some degree of atrial-nodal block exists). At pacing CLs shorter than 500 milliseconds, there is usually little further prolongation of the SNRT; on the contrary, changes in neurohumoral tone may result in shorter SNRTs.[25,32]

The duration of the maximum SNRT and corrected SNRT are independent of age. Evaluation of corrected SNRT following pharmacological denervation (see later) may increase the sensitivity of the test.[33]

Sinus Node Recovery Time in Patients with Sinus Node Dysfunction

The sensitivity of a single SNRT measurement is approximately 35% in patients with SND. This rises to more than 85% when multiple SNRTs at different rates are recorded, along with scatter and total recovery time, with a specificity of more than 90%. Prolonged SNRT or corrected SNRT is found in 35% to 93% of patients suspected of having SND (depending on the population studied). The incidence is lowest in patients with sinus bradycardia. Marked abnormalities in corrected SNRT usually occur in symptomatic patients with clinical evidence of sinoatrial block or bradycardia-tachycardia syndrome.[24,33]

FIGURE 5–5 Sinus node recovery time (SNRT). Surface ECG leads and high right atrial (HRA) recordings are shown at the end of a burst of atrial pacing, suppressing sinus node automaticity. The interval at which the first sinus complex returns (SNRT) is abnormally long at 1625 milliseconds. With a baseline sinus cycle (CL) equals 720 milliseconds, the corrected SNRT (1625 – 720 = 905 milliseconds) is also prolonged. In addition, there is a secondary pause after the first two sinus complexes.

The pacing CL at which maximum suppression occurs in patients with SND is unpredictable and, unlike healthy subjects, tends to be affected by the rate and duration of pacing. However, if sinus entrance block is present, the greatest suppression is likely to occur at relatively long pacing CLs. If the longest SNRT occurs at pacing CLs more than 600 milliseconds, a normal value can reflect the presence of entrance block. In such cases, a normal SNRT is an unreliable assessment of sinus node automaticity. The fact that the longest SNRT occurs at pacing CLs longer than 600 milliseconds is in itself a marker of SND.[24]

Marked secondary pauses are another manifestation of SND and can occasionally occur in the absence of prolongation of SNRT, in which case sinoatrial block is the mechanism. Approximately 69% of patients with secondary pauses have clinical evidence of sinoatrial exit block, and 92% of patients with sinoatrial exit block demonstrate marked secondary pauses.[24]

Sinoatrial Conduction Time

Although the sinus node is the dominant cardiac pacemaker, neither sinus node impulse initiation nor conduction is visible on the surface ECG or on the standard intracardiac recordings because depolarization within the sinus node is of very low amplitude. The sinus node function, therefore, has usually been assessed indirectly. Normal sinus node function is assumed when the atrial musculature is depolarized at a normal rate and in a normal temporal sequence—so-called normal sinus rhythm. In NSR, the atrial rate is assumed to correspond to the rate of impulse formation within the sinus node; however, the time of impulse conduction from the sinus node to the atrium cannot be ascertained. Several methods have been developed for the assessment of sinoatrial conduction time (SACT), either indirectly (the Strauss and Narula methods) or by directly recording the sinus node electrogram. Signal-averaging techniques have also been used to measure SACT noninvasively.[25,26,33]

Direct Recordings

Sinus node depolarization can be recorded directly using high-gain unfiltered electrograms in approximately 50% of patients.[24] A catheter with a 0.5- to 1.5-mm interelectrode distance is used. The catheter is placed directly at the SVC-RA junction or a loop is formed in the RA and the tip of the catheter is then placed at the SVC-RA junction. Optimizing filter setting can help reduce baseline drift (0.1 to 0.6 Hz to 20 to 50 Hz), with signal gain at 50 to 100 μV/cm.[33]

SACT is measured as the interval between the pacemaker prepotential on the local electrogram and the onset of the rapid atrial deflection (Fig. 5-6). When SACT is normal, a smooth upstroke slope merges into the atrial electrogram. When SACT is prolonged, an increasing amount of sinus node potential becomes visible before the rapid atrial deflection. Sinoatrial block is said to occur when the entire sinus node electrogram is seen in the absence of a propagated response to the atrium.[24]

Sinus node electrogram can be validated by the ability to record the electrogram in only a local area, and loss of the upstroke potential during overdrive atrial pacing. Additionally, persistence of the sinus node electrogram following carotid sinus massage, following induced pauses, or during pauses following overdrive suppression is an important method for validation.

Strauss Technique

The Strauss technique uses atrial premature stimulation to assess SACT. Baseline sinus beats are designated A_1. Progressively premature atrial extrastimuli (AESs; A_2) are delivered after every eighth to tenth A_1, and the timing of the recovery beat (A_3) is measured.[24] The Strauss method is useful as part of an overall EP study when information is also sought on conduction system refractoriness or possible dual AVN physiology or bypass tracts (BT)s during sinus rhythm. Four zones of response of the sinus node to AES have been identified. SACT can be measured only in the zone of reset (Fig. 5-7).[25,26,32]

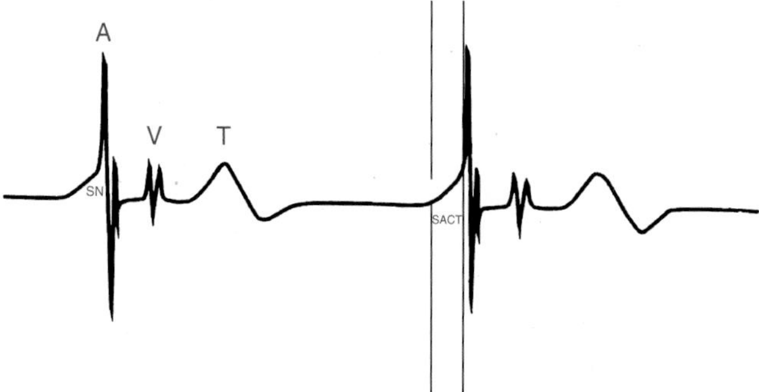

FIGURE 5–6 Schematic illustration showing the direct measurement of sinoatrial conduction time (SACT). A schematic copy of a sinus node electrogram is shown. On the sinus node electrogram, high right atrial depolarization (A), ventricular depolarization (V), T wave (T), and the sinus node potential (SN) are identified. In the second beat, reference lines are drawn through the point at which the SN potential first becomes evident and the point at which atrial activation begins. SACT is the interval between these two reference lines. (From Reiffel JA: The human sinus node electrogram: A transvenous catheter technique and a comparison of directly measured and indirectly estimated sinoatrial conduction time in adults. Circulation 1980;62:1324.)

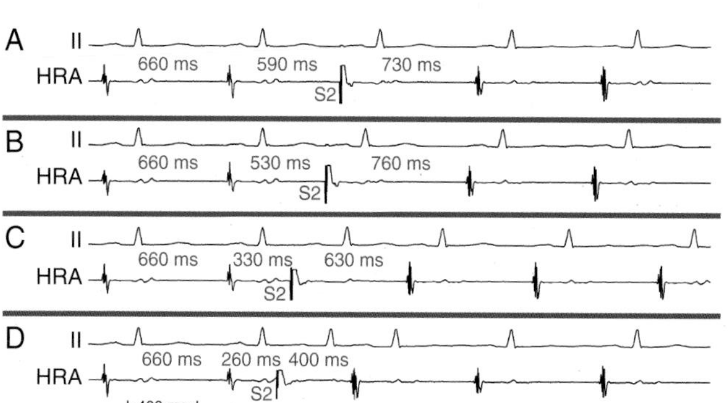

FIGURE 5–7 Strauss sinoatrial conduction time zones. Leads 2 and recording from the high right atrium (HRA) are shown, with a single extrastimulus (S) delivered during sinus rhythm (cycle length, 660 milliseconds) at progressively shorter coupling intervals as indicated relative to the preceding sinus complex. The timing of the subsequent sinus P wave relative to when it would be expected if there were no extrastimulus determines the zone of effect: A = collision; B = reset; C = interpolation; D = reentry. See text for details.

1. Zone I: Zone of Collision, Zone of Interference, Nonreset Zone. This zone is defined by the range of A_1-A_2 intervals at which the A_2-A_3 interval is fully compensatory (see Fig. 5-7). Very long A_1-A_2 intervals (with A_2 falling in the last 20% to 30% of the sinus CL) generally result in collision of the AES (A_2) with the spontaneous sinus impulse (A_1). The sinus pacemaker and the timing of the subsequent sinus beat (A_3) are therefore unaffected by A_2—that is, A_1-A_3 = 2 × (A_1-A_1), a complete compensatory pause.

2. Zone II: Zone of Reset. The range of A_1-A_2 intervals at which reset of the sinus pacemaker occurs, resulting in a less than compensatory pause, defines the zone of reset (see Fig. 5-7). Shorter A_1-A_2 intervals result in penetration of the sinus node with resetting so that the resulting pause is less than compensatory—A_1-A_3 < 2 × (A_1-A_1)—but without changing sinus node automaticity. This zone typically occupies a long duration (40% to 50% of the sinus CL). In most patients, the A_2-A_3 interval remains constant throughout zone II, producing a plateau in the curve because, while A_2 penetrates and resets the sinus node, it does so without changing the sinus pacemaker automaticity. Hence, the A_2-A_3 interval should equal the spontaneous sinus CL (A_1-A_1) plus the time it takes the AES (A_2) to enter and exit the sinus node. The difference between the A_2-A_3 and A_1-A_1 intervals, therefore, has been taken as an estimate of total SACT (Fig. 5-8).[33]

Conventionally, it is assumed that the conduction times into and out of the sinus node are equal (i.e., SACT = $[A_2\text{-}A_3 - A_1\text{-}A_1]/2$). Data, however, suggest that the conduction time into the sinus node is shorter than that out of the sinus node (see Fig. 5-8). The Strauss method for assessment of SACT can be affected by the site of stimulation; the farther the site of stimulation from the sinus node, the greater the overestimation of SACT (because conduction through more intervening atrial and perinodal tissue will be incorporated in the measurement). The value of SACT can also be affected by the prematurity of the AES (A_2)—the more premature is an A_2, the more likely it will encroach on perinodal and/or atrial refractoriness, which will slow conduction into the sinus node. In addition, an early AES commonly causes pacemaker shift to a peripheral latent pacemaker, which can exit the atrium earlier because of its proximity to the tissue, thus shortening conduction time out of the sinus node.[24,25,33]

Despite those limitations, for practical purposes, the Strauss method is a reasonable estimate of functional SACT, provided that stimulation is performed as closely as possible to the sinus node and the measurement is taken when a true plateau is present in zone II.[24] SACT appears to be independent of the spontaneous sinus CL. However, marked sinus arrhythmia invalidates the calculation of SACT, because it is impossible to know whether the return cycle is a result of spontaneous oscillation or is a result of the AES. To eliminate the effects of sinus arrhythmia, multiple tests need to be performed at each coupling interval. Alternatively, atrial pacing drive at a rate just faster than the sinus rate is used instead of delivery of AES during NSR (Narula method; see later). However, this latter method can result in depression of sinus node automaticity, pacemaker shifts, sinus entrance block, sinus acceleration (if the drive pacing CL is within 50 milliseconds of sinus CL), and shortening of sinus action potential, leading to earlier onset of phase IV, each of which can yield misleading results.[32,33]

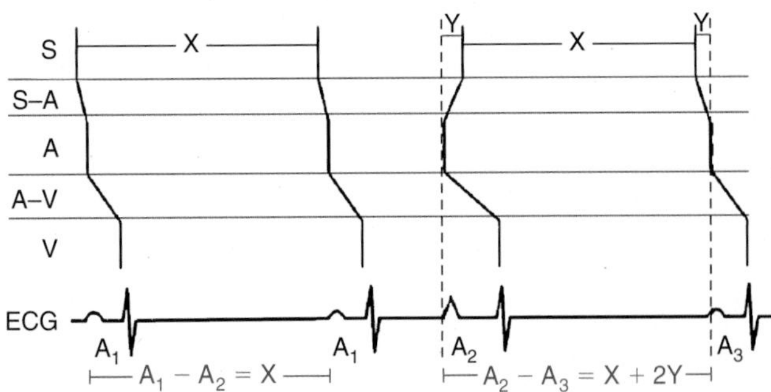

FIGURE 5–8 Calculation of sinoatrial conduction time (SACT) using the Strauss method. The baseline sinus cycle length (A_1-A_2) equals X. The third P wave represents an atrial extrastimulus AES (A_2) that reaches and discharges the sinoatrial (SA) node, which causes the next sinus cycle to begin at that time. Therefore, the A_2-A_3 interval = X + 2Y milliseconds, assuming no depression of sinus node automaticity. Consequently, SACT = Y = ($[A_2\text{-}A_3] - [X]$)/2. (From Olgin JE, Zipes DP: Specific arrhythmias: Diagnosis and treatment. *In* Libby P, Bonow RO, Mann DL, and Zipes DP (eds): Braunwald's Heart Disease: A Textbook of Cardiovascular Medicine, 8th ed. Philadelphia, Saunders, 2008, p 869.)

In an occasional patient, in response to progressively premature AESs, the A_2-A_3 interval either continuously prolongs or does so after a brief plateau (in both cases, the pause remains less than compensatory). This progressive prolongation of the A_2-A_3 interval during zone II can be caused by suppression of sinus node automaticity, a shift to a slower latent pacemaker, or an increase in conduction time into the sinus node because of A_2 encroaching on perinodal tissue refractoriness. Thus, it is recommended to use the first third of zone II to measure SACT, because it is less likely to introduce such errors.[24] Analysis of the A_3-A_4 interval may provide insights into changes in sinus node automaticity or pacemaker shift. If the A_3-A_4 interval is longer than A_1-A_1 interval, depression of sinus node automaticity is suggested and, therefore, the calculated SACT will overestimate the true SACT, and correction of SACT is necessary (in which case the A_3-A_4 interval is used as the basic sinus CL to which the A_2-A_3 interval is compared).[24]

3. Zone III: Zone of Interpolation. This zone is defined as the range of A_1-A_2 intervals at which the A_2-A_3 interval is less than the A_1-A_1 interval and the A_1-A_3 interval is less than twice the A_1-A_1 interval (see Fig. 5-7).[24] The A_1-A_2 coupling intervals at which incomplete interpolation is first observed define the relative refractory period of the perinodal tissue. Some refer to this as the sinus node refractory period. In this case, A_3 represents delay of A_1 exiting the sinus node, which has not been affected.[24] The A_1-A_2 coupling interval at which complete interpolation is observed probably defines the effective refractory period of the most peripheral of the perinodal tissue, because the sinus impulse does not encounter refractory tissue on its exit from the sinus node. In this case, (A_1-A_2) + (A_2-A_3) = A_1-A_1 and sinus node entrance block is said to exist.[24,33]

4. Zone IV: Zone of Reentry. This zone is defined as the range of A_1-A_2 intervals at which the A_2-A_3 interval is less than the A_1-A_1 interval and (A_1-A_2) + (A_2-A_3) is less than A_1-A_1, and the atrial activation sequence and P wave morphology are identical to sinus beats. The incidence of single beats of sinus node reentry is approximately 11% in the normal population.[25,26,32]

Narula Method

The Narula method for measuring SACT is simpler than the Strauss technique. Instead of atrial premature stimulation, atrial pacing at a rate slightly faster (10 beats/min or more) than the sinus rate is used as A_2. It is assumed that such atrial pacing will depolarize the sinus node without significant overdrive suppression. The SACT is then calculated using the same formula as the Strauss method. The Narula method is the quickest and easiest to perform but gives only SACT and does not provide information about the AV conduction system.[25,26,32]

Kirkorian-Touboul Method

In contrast to the Strauss method that uses progressively premature AESs delivered during NSR to evaluate SACT, the Kirkorian-Touboul method uses progressively premature AESs delivered following an eight-beat pacing train at a fixed rate. This method was designed to determine SACT independently of baseline sinus CL, which can normally be somewhat variable. It can have several advantages, especially for the study of drug effects at identical basic rate, but it is less widely used than the other methods.

Sinoatrial Conduction Time in Patients with Sinus Node Dysfunction

The normal SACT = 45 to 125 milliseconds. There is a good correlation between direct and indirect measurements of SACT in a patient with or without SND. However, SACT is an insensitive indicator of SND, especially in patients with isolated sinus bradycardia. SACT is prolonged in only 40% of patients with SND, and more frequently (78%) in patients with sinoatrial exit block and/or bradycardia-tachycardia syndrome.[24] In patients with sinus pauses, corrected SNRT is more commonly abnormal than SACT (80% versus 53%). SACT appears to be directly related to the baseline sinus CL, and sinus node refractory period is directly related to the drive CL.[33]

Effects of Drugs

Autonomic Blockade (Intrinsic Heart Rate)

Autonomic blockade is the most commonly used pharmacological intervention, and is used to determine the intrinsic heart rate (i.e., the rate independent of autonomic influences). Complete autonomic blockade is accomplished by administering atropine, 0.04 mg/kg, and propranolol, 0.2 mg/kg (or atenolol, 0.22 mg/kg). The resulting intrinsic heart rate represents sinus node rate without autonomic influences. The normal intrinsic heart rate is age-dependent and can be calculated using the following equation: intrinsic heart rate (beats/min) = 118.1 – (0.57 × age); normal values are ±14% for age younger than 45 years and ±18% for age older than 45. A low intrinsic heart rate is consistent with intrinsic SND. A normal intrinsic heart rate in a patient with known SND suggests extrinsic SND caused by abnormal autonomic regulation. Autonomic blockade with atropine and propranolol also results in shortening of corrected SNRT, as well as sinus CL and SACT.[33]

Atropine. The normal sinus node response to atropine is an acceleration of heart rate to more than 90 beats/min and an increase over the baseline rate by 20% to 50%. Atropine-induced sinus rate acceleration is usually blunted in patients with intrinsic SND. Failure to increase the sinus rate to above the predicted intrinsic heart rate following 0.04 mg/kg of atropine is diagnostic of impaired sinus node automaticity. Atropine (1 to 3 mg) markedly shortens SNRT and, in most cases, corrected SNRT. Atropine also abolishes the marked oscillations frequently observed following cessation of rapid pacing. Atropine occasionally results in the appearance of a junctional escape rhythm on cessation of pacing before sinus escape beats in normal subjects (especially in young men with borderline slow sinus rate) and, more commonly, in patients with SND. When this occurs, the junctional escape rhythm is usually transient (lasting only a few beats). Persistence of junctional rhythm and failure of the sinus rate to increase is indicative of SND.[24] Atropine with or without propranolol shortens SACT (unrelated to its effects on the sinus rate).[32,33]

Propranolol. Propranolol (0.1 mg/kg) produces a 12% to 22.5% increase in sinus CL in normal subjects. Patients with SND have a similar chronotropic response to propranolol, suggesting that sympathetic tone and/or responsiveness is intact in most patients with SND. Propranolol increases SNRT by 160% in approximately 40% of patients with SND and increases SACT in most patients with SND. The mechanism of these effects is unclear. Effects are minimal in normal subjects.[24]

Isoproterenol. Isoproterenol (1 to 3 μg/min) produces sinus acceleration of at least 25% in normal subjects. An impaired response to isoproterenol correlates well with a blunted chronotropic response to exercise observed in some patients with SND.[24]

Digoxin. Digoxin shortens SNRT and/or corrected SNRT in some patients with clinical SND, probably because of increased perinodal tissue refractoriness with consequent sinus node entrance block.[24]

Verapamil and Diltiazem. Verapamil and diltiazem have minimal effects on SNRT and SACT in normal persons. Effects in patients with SND have not been studied, but worsening of the SND is expected.[24]

Antiarrhythmic Agents. Procainamide, quinidine, mexilitine, and amiodarone can adversely affect sinus node function in patients with SND. Severe sinus bradycardia and sinus pauses are the most common problems encountered. Amiodarone is the worst offender and has even caused severe SND in patients without prior evidence of SND.[11] In general, other drugs have minimal effects on sinus node function in normal persons.[25,33]

PRINCIPLES OF MANAGEMENT

Correlation of symptoms with ECG evidence of SND is an essential part of the diagnostic strategy. Because of the episodic nature of symptomatic arrhythmias, ambulatory monitoring is often required. For the patient with asymptomatic bradycardia or sinus pauses, no treatment is necessary. For symptomatic patients with SND, pacing is the mainstay of treatment (Table 5-1). SND is currently the most common reported diagnosis for pacemaker implantation, accounting for 40% to 60% of new pacemaker implants. However, before instituting permanent pacing, the possibility of a reversible cause of the SND should be investigated. Any offending drug should be withdrawn, if possible. For symptomatic patients with tachycardia-bradycardia syndrome, pacing may be required to prevent symptomatic bradycardia and allow the use of drug therapy for control of the tachycardia. These patients are at increased risk for thromboembolism and the issue of long-term anticoagulation for stroke prevention should be addressed.[21,25,26]

Once the decision to pace is made, choosing the optimal pacemaker prescription is essential. For those patients with SND who have normal AV conduction, a single-

TABLE 5–1 Guidelines for Permanent Pacing in Sinus Node Dysfunction
Class I
With documented symptomatic bradycardia Symptomatic chronotropic incompetence Symptomatic sinus bradycardia that results from required drug therapy for medical conditions
Class IIa
With heart rate <40 beats/min when a clear association between significant symptoms consistent with bradycardia and the actual presence of bradycardia has not been documented With syncope of unexplained origin when clinically significant abnormalities of sinus node function are discovered or provoked in electrophysiological studies
Class IIb
Minimally symptomatic patients with chronic heart rate <40 beats/min while awake
Class III
Asymptomatic patients In patients whose symptoms suggestive of bradycardia have been clearly documented to occur in the absence of bradycardia With symptomatic bradycardia caused by nonessential drug therapy

From Epstein AE, DiMarco JP, Ellenbogen KA, et al: ACC/AHA/HRS 2008 Guidelines for Device-Based Therapy of Cardiac Rhythm Abnormalities: a report of the American College of Cardiology/American Heart Association Task Force on Practice Guidelines (Writing Committee to Revise the ACC/AHA/NASPE 2002 Guideline Update for Implantation of Cardiac Pacemakers and Antiarrhythmia Devices): developed in collaboration with the American Association for Thoracic Surgery and Society of Thoracic Surgeons. Circulation 2008;117:e350-408.

chamber atrial pacemaker is a reasonable consideration, although in the United States, a dual-chamber pacemaker is usually implanted, largely because of the 1% to 3% annual risk of developing AV block.[20,34,35] The use of rate-adaptive pacing is important for patients with chronotropic incompetence. For patients with intermittent atrial tachyarrhythmias, atrial pacing has been shown to greatly decrease the incidence of AF and thromboembolism, whereas those who are only ventricular-paced have not seen a similar benefit.[19] Current pacemakers used to treat the tachycardia-bradycardia syndrome use a special algorithm to switch from a DDD or DDDR mode of operation to a VVI, VVIR, DDI, or DDIR mode on sensing an atrial tachyarrhythmia, and back again to DDD or DDDR mode when a normal atrial rate is sensed.[34] For patients with permanent AF, implantation of a single-chamber ventricular pacemaker is appropriate.[3,21,25,26]

REFERENCES

1. Rubart M, Zipes DP: Genesis of cardiac arrhythmias: Electrophysiological considerations. *In* Zipes DP, Libby P, Bonow R, Braunwald E (eds): Braunwald's Heart Disease: A Textbook of Cardiovascular Medicine, 7th ed. Philadelphia, WB Saunders, 2004, pp 653-688.
2. Dobrzynski H, Boyett MR, Anderson RH: New insights into pacemaker activity: Promoting understanding of sick sinus syndrome. Circulation 2007;115:1921.
3. Line D, Callans D: Sinus rhythm abnormalities. *In* Zipes D, Jalife J (eds): Cardiac Electrophysiology: From Cell to Bedside. Philadelphia, WB Saunders, 2004, pp 479-484.
4. Sanchez-Quintana D, Cabrera JA, Farre J, et al: Sinus node revisited in the era of electroanatomical mapping and catheter ablation. Heart 2005;91:189.
5. Boullin J, Morgan JM: The development of cardiac rhythm. Heart 2005;91:874.
6. Boyett MR, Honjo H, Kodama I: The sinoatrial node, a heterogeneous pacemaker structure. Cardiovasc Res 2000;47:658.
7. Sanders P, Kistler PM, Morton JB, et al: Remodeling of sinus node function in patients with congestive heart failure: Reduction in sinus node reserve. Circulation 2004;110:897.
8. Kistler PM, Sanders P, Fynn SP, et al: Electrophysiological and electroanatomic changes in the human atrium associated with age. J Am Coll Cardiol 2004;44:109.
9. Walsh EP: Interventional electrophysiology in patients with congenital heart disease. Circulation 2007;115:3224.
10. Wolbrette D, Naccarelli G: Bradycardias: Sinus nodal dysfunction and atrioventricular conduction disturbances. *In* Topol E (ed): Textbook of Cardiovascular Medicine, 2nd ed. Philadelphia, Lippincott Williams & Wilkins, 2002, pp 1385-1402.
11. Essebag V, Hadjis T, Platt RW, et al: Effect of amiodarone dose on the risk of permanent pacemaker insertion. Pacing Clin Electrophysiol 2004;27:1519.
12. Shirayama T, Hadase M, Sakamoto T, et al: Swallowing syncope: Complex mechanisms of the reflex. Intern Med 2002;41:207.
13. Schuchert A, Wagner SM, Frost G, Meinertz T: Moderate exercise induces different autonomic modulations of sinus and AV node. Pacing Clin Electrophysiol 2005;28:196.
14. Stein R, Medeiros CM, Rosito GA, et al: Intrinsic sinus and atrioventricular node electrophysiological adaptations in endurance athletes. J Am Coll Cardiol 2002;39:1033.
15. Sakai Y, Imai S, Sato Y, et al: Clinical and electrophysiological characteristics of binodal disease. Circ J 2006;70:1580.
16. Brubaker PH, Kitzman DW: Prevalence and management of chronotropic incompetence in heart failure. Curr Cardiol Rep 2007;9:229.
17. Kitzman DW: Exercise intolerance. Prog Cardiovasc Dis 2005;47:367.
18. Gentlesk PJ, Markwood TT, Atwood JE: Chronotropic incompetence in a young adult: Case report and literature review. Chest 2004;125:297.
19. Ellenbogen KA: Pacing therapy for prevention of atrial fibrillation. Heart Rhythm 2007;4(Suppl 3):S84.
20. Castelnuovo E, Stein K, Pitt M, et al: The effectiveness and cost-effectiveness of dual-chamber pacemakers compared with single-chamber pacemakers for bradycardia due to atrioventricular block or sick sinus syndrome: Systematic review and economic evaluation. Health Technol Assess 2005;9:iii, xii,246.
21. Sweeney M: Sinus node dysfunction. *In* Zipes D, Jalife J (eds): Cardiac Electrophysiology: From Cell to Bedside. Philadelphia, WB Saunders, 2004, pp 879-883.
22. Kennedy H: Use of long-term (Holter) electrocardiographic recordings. *In* Zipes D, Jalife J (eds): Cardiac Electrophysiology: From Cell to Bedside. Philadelphia, WB Saunders, 2004, pp 772-792.
23. Benditt D, Ermis C, Lu F: Head-up tilt table testing. *In* Zipes D, Jalife J (eds): Cardiac Electrophysiology: From Cell to Bedside. Philadelphia, WB Saunders, 2004, pp 812-822.
24. Josephson ME: Sinus node function. *In* Josephson ME (ed): Clinical Cardiac Electrophysiology, 3rd ed. Philadelphia, Lippincott Williams & Wilkins, 2002, pp 19-67.
25. Miller JM, Zipes DP: Diagnosis of cardiac arrhythmias. *In* Zipes D, Libby P, Bonow R, Braunwald E (eds): Braunwald's Heart Disease: A Textbook of Cardiovascular Medicine, 7th ed. Philadelphia, WB Saunders, 2004, pp 697-712.
26. Benditt DG, Sakaguchi S, Lurie K, Lu F: Sinus node dysfunction. *In* Willerson J, Cohn J, Wellens Jr H, Holmes D (eds): Cardiovascular Medicine. New York, Springer, 2007, pp 1925-1941.
27. Manios EG, Kanoupakis EM, Mavrakis HE, et al: Sinus pacemaker function after cardioversion of chronic atrial fibrillation: Is sinus node remodeling related with recurrence? J Cardiovasc Electrophysiol 2001;12:800.
28. Hocini M, Sanders P, Deisenhofer I, et al: Reverse remodeling of sinus node function after catheter ablation of atrial fibrillation in patients with prolonged sinus pauses. Circulation 2003;108:1172.
29. Hadian D, Zipes DP, Olgin JE, Miller JM: Short-term rapid atrial pacing produces electrical remodeling of sinus node function in humans. J Cardiovasc Electrophysiol 2002;13:584.
30. Disertori M, Marini M, Cristoforetti A, et al: Enormous bi-atrial enlargement in a persistent idiopathic atrial standstill. Eur Heart J 2005;26:2276.
31. Fazelifar AF, Arya A, Haghjoo M, Sadr-Ameli MA: Familial atrial standstill in association with dilated cardiomyopathy. Pacing Clin Electrophysiol 2005;28:1005.
32. Fisher J: Electrophysiological testing. *In* Topol E (ed): Textbook of Cardiovascular Medicine, 2nd ed. Philadelphia, Lippincott Williams & Wilkins, 2002, Chapter 62.
33. Masood A: Techniques of electrophysiological evaluation. *In* Fuster V, Alexander R, O'Rourke R (eds): Hurst's The Heart, 11th ed. Columbus, Ohio, McGraw-Hill, 2004, pp 935-948.
34. Schwaab B, Kindermann M, Schatzer-Klotz D, et al: AAIR versus DDDR pacing in the bradycardia tachycardia syndrome: A prospective, randomized, double-blind, crossover trial. Pacing Clin Electrophysiol 2001;24:1585.
35. Lamas GA, Lee KL, Sweeney MO, et al: Ventricular pacing or dual-chamber pacing for sinus-node dysfunction. N Engl J Med 2002;346:1854.

CHAPTER 6

Atrioventricular Conduction Abnormalities

GENERAL CONSIDERATIONS

Anatomy and Physiology of the Atrioventricular Junction

Internodal and Intraatrial Conduction

Evidence indicates the presence of preferential impulse propagation from the sinus to the atrioventricular node (AVN)—that is, higher conduction velocity between the nodes in some parts of the atrium than in other parts. However, whether preferential internodal conduction is caused by fiber orientation, size, or geometry, or by the presence of specialized preferentially conducting pathways located between the nodes has been controversial.[1-4]

Anatomical evidence indicates the presence of three intraatrial pathways. The anterior internodal pathway begins at the anterior margin of the sinus node and curves anteriorly around the superior vena cava (SVC) to enter the anterior interatrial band, called the Bachmann bundle. This band continues to the left atrium (LA), with the anterior internodal pathway entering the superior margin of the AVN. The Bachmann bundle is a large muscle bundle that appears to conduct the cardiac impulse preferentially from the right atrium (RA) to the LA. The middle internodal tract begins at the superior and posterior margins of the sinus node, travels behind the SVC to the crest of the interatrial septum, and descends in the interatrial septum to the superior margin of the AVN. The posterior internodal tract starts at the posterior margin of the sinus node and travels posteriorly around the SVC and along the crista terminalis to the eustachian ridge, and then into the interatrial septum above the coronary sinus (CS), where it joins the posterior portion of the AVN. Some fibers from all three tracts bypass the crest of the AVN and enter its more distal segment. These groups of internodal tissue are best referred to as internodal atrial myocardium, not tracts, because they do not appear to be histologically discrete specialized tracts, only plain atrial myocardium.[1]

Atrioventricular Node

The AVN lies beneath the RA endocardium at the apex of the triangle of Koch, which is formed by the tendon of Todaro and the septal leaflet of the tricuspid valve. The compact AVN lies anterior to the cornary sinus ostium (CS os), and directly above the insertion of the septal leaflet of the tricuspid valve, where the tendon of Todaro merges with the central fibrous body. Slightly more anteriorly and superiorly is where the His bundle (HB) penetrates the AV junction through the central fibrous body and the posterior aspect of the membranous AV septum.[1,5]

The normal AV junctional area can be divided into distinct regions: the transitional cell zone (which represents the approaches from the working atrial myocardium to the AVN), the compact AVN, and the penetrating part of the HB.[6,7] The AVN and perinodal area are comprised of at least three electrophysiologically distinct cells: the atrionodal (AN), nodal (N), and nodal-His (NH) cells. The AN region corresponds to the cells in the transitional region, which are activated shortly after the atrial cells. The N region corresponds to the region where the transitional cells merge with midnodal cells. The N cells represent the most typical of the nodal cells and appear to be responsible for the major part of AV conduction delay, because they have slow rising and longer action potentials and exhibit decremental properties in response to premature stimulation. The NH region corresponds to the lower nodal cells. Sodium channel density is lower in the midnodal zone of the AVN than in the AN and NH cell zones, and the inward L-type Ca^{2+} current is the basis of the upstroke of the N cell action potential. Therefore, conduction is slower through the compact AVN than the AN and NH cell zones.[1,8,9]

The AVN is the only normal electrical connection between the atria and the ventricles. The main function of the AVN is modulation of atrial impulse transmission to the ventricles, thereby coordinating atrial and ventricular contractions. A primary function of the AVN is to limit the number of impulses conducted from the atria to the ventricles, which is particularly important during fast atrial rates (e.g., atrial fibrillation [AF] or atrial flutter [AFL]) when only a fraction of impulses are conducted to the ventricles, whereas the remainder are blocked in the AVN. Additionally, fibers in the lower part of the AVN can exhibit automatic impulse formation, and the AVN may serve as a subsidiary pacemaker.[1,8]

The AVN region is innervated by a rich supply of cholinergic and adrenergic fibers. Sympathetic stimulation shortens AVN conduction time and refractoriness, whereas vagal stimulation prolongs AVN conduction time and refractoriness. The negative dromotropic response of the AVN to vagal stimulation is mediated by activation of the inwardly rectifying K^+ current $I_{K(Ach,Ado)}$, which results in hyperpolarization and action potential shortening of AVN cells, increased threshold of excitation, depression of action potential amplitude, and prolonged conduction time. The positive dromotropic effect of sympathetic stimulation arises as a consequence of activation of the L-type Ca^{2+} current.[1,5]

The blood supply to the AVN predominantly comes from a branch of the right coronary artery in 85% to 90% of patients and from the circumflex artery in 10% to 15%.

His Bundle

The HB connects with the distal part of the compact AVN, perforates the central fibrous body, and continues through the annulus fibrosis, where it is called the nonbranching portion as it penetrates the membranous septum, along the crest of the left side of the interventricular septum, for 1 to 2 cm and then divides into the right and left bundle branches. Proximal cells of the penetrating portion are heterogeneous and resemble those of the compact AVN; distal cells are similar to cells in the proximal bundle branches. Connective tissue of the central fibrous body and membranous septum encloses the penetrating portion of the HB, which can send out extensions into the central fibrous body.[1] The HB has a dual blood supply from branches of the anterior and posterior descending coronary arteries, which makes the conduction system at this site less vulnerable to ischemic damage unless the ischemia is extensive.[1]

The AVN and HB region are innervated by a rich supply of cholinergic and adrenergic fibers, with a density exceeding that found in the ventricular myocardium. Although neither sympathetic nor vagal stimulation affects normal conduction in the HB, either can affect abnormal AV conduction.[1]

Pathophysiology of Atrioventricular Block

Block or delay of a cardiac impulse can take place anywhere in the heart, or even within a single cell. AV block can be defined as a delay or interruption in the transmission of an impulse from the atria to the ventricles caused by an anatomical or functional impairment in the conduction system. The conduction disturbance can be transient or permanent.

Congenital Atrioventricular Block

Congenital complete AV block is thought to result from embryonic maldevelopment of the AVN (and, much less frequently, the His-Purkinje system [HPS]). The incidence of congenital complete AV block varies from 1 in 15,000 to 1 in 22,000 live births. The defect usually occurs proximal to the HB and the QRS duration is less than 120 milliseconds.[10] Neonatal lupus, caused by maternal antibodies targeting intracellular ribonucleoproteins that cross the placenta to affect the fetal heart but not the maternal heart, is responsible for 60% to 90% of cases of congenital complete AV block.[11,12] Approximately 50% of patients with congenital AV block have concurrent congenital heart disease (e.g., congenitally corrected transposition of the great vessels, atrioventricular discordance, ventricular septal defects, atrioventricular canal defect, and Ebstein's anomaly of the tricuspid valve).[13]

Acquired Atrioventricular Block

Drugs. A variety of drugs can impair conduction and cause AV block. Digoxin and beta blockers act indirectly on the AVN through their effects on the autonomic nervous system. Calcium channel blockers and other antiarrhythmic drugs, such as amiodarone, act directly to slow conduction in the AVN. Type I and III antiarrhythmic drugs can also affect conduction in the HPS, resulting in infranodal block. These effects, however, typically occur in patients with preexisting conduction abnormalities. Patients with normal conduction system function rarely develop complete heart block as a result of using antiarrhythmic agents.[14]

Acute Myocardial Infarction. AV block occurs in 12% to 25% of all patients with acute myocardial infarction (MI); first-degree AV block occurs in 2% to 12%, second-degree AV block in 3% to 10%, and third-degree AV block in 3% to 7%. First-degree and type 1 second-degree (Wenckebach) AV block occur more commonly in inferior MI, usually caused by increased vagal tone, and usually associated with other signs of vagotonia, such as sinus bradycardia and responsiveness to atropine and catecholamine stimulation. Wenckebach AV block in the setting of acute inferior MI is usually transient (resolving within 48 to 72 hours of MI) and asymptomatic, and rarely progresses to high-grade or complete AV block. Wenckebach AV block occurring later in the course of an acute inferior MI is less responsive to atropine and probably is associated with ischemia of the AVN or the release of adenosine during acute MI. In this setting, Wenckebach AV block rarely progresses to more advanced block and commonly resolves within 2 to 3 days of onset. The site of conduction block is usually in the AVN. Type 2 second-degree (Mobitz type II) AV block occurs in only 1% of patients with acute MI (more commonly in anterior than inferior MI) and has a worse prognosis than type 1 second-degree block. Type 2 second-degree AV block occurring during an acute anterior MI is typically associated with HB or bundle branch ischemia or infarction and frequently progresses to complete heart block. Complete AV block occurs in 8% to 13% of patients with acute MI. It can occur with anterior or inferior acute MI. In the setting of acute inferior MI, the site of the block is usually at the level of the AVN, resulting in a junctional escape rhythm with a narrow QRS complex and a rate of 40 to 60 beats/min. The block tends to be reversed by vagolytic drugs or catecholamines and usually resolves within several days. Development of complete AV block with anterior MI, however, is associated with a higher risk of ventricular tachycardia (VT) and ventricular fibrillation (VF), hypotension, pulmonary edema, and in-hospital mortality. In the setting of acute anterior MI, the block is usually associated with ischemia or infarction of the HB or bundle branches, and is often preceded by bundle branch block (BBB), fascicular block, or type 2 second-degree AV block. The escape rhythm usually originates from the bundle branch and Purkinje system, with a rate less than 40 beats/min and a wide QRS complex. It is less likely to be reversible. In general, patients who develop transient or irreversible AV block are older and have a larger area of damage associated with their acute MI.[10,15,16]

Chronic Ischemic Heart Disease. Chronic ischemic heart disease can result in persistent AV block. Transient AV block can occur during angina pectoris and Prinzmetal's angina.

Degenerative Diseases. Fibrosis and sclerosis of the conduction system is the most common cause of acquired conduction system disease, accounting for about half of cases of AV block, and can be induced by several different conditions, which often cannot be distinguished clinically.

Lev's disease is a result of proximal bundle branch calcification or fibrosis. It is postulated as a hastening of the aging process by hypertension and arteriosclerosis of the blood vessels supplying the conduction system. Lenègre's disease is a sclerodegenerative process that occurs in a younger population and involves the more distal portions of the bundle branches. Calcification of the aortic or (less commonly) mitral valve annulus can extend to the nearby conduction system and produce AV block.[10,15]

Rheumatic Diseases. AV block can occur in association with collagen vascular diseases such as scleroderma, rheumatoid arthritis, Reiter's syndrome, systemic lupus erythematosus, ankylosing spondylitis, and polymyositis.

Infiltrative Processes. Infiltrative cardiomyopathies such as amyloidosis, sarcoidosis, hemochromatosis, and tumors can be associated with AV block.

Neuromyopathies. A number of neuromuscular diseases are associated with AV block, including Becker muscular dystrophy, peroneal muscular dystrophy, Kearns-Sayre syndrome, Erb's dystrophy, and myotonic muscular dystrophy.[17]

Infectious Diseases. Infective endocarditis (especially of the aortic valve) and myocarditis with various viral, bacterial, and parasitic causes (including Lyme disease, rheumatic fever, Chagas' disease, tuberculosis, measles, and mumps) result in varying degrees of AV block. Complete AV block occurs in 3% of cases.[14]

Iatrogenic. Cardiac surgery can be complicated by varying degrees of AV block caused by trauma and ischemic damage to the conduction system. AV block is most frequently associated with aortic valve replacement and, less commonly, following coronary artery bypass grafting. Repair of congenital heart defects in the region of the conduction system, such as endocardial cushion malformations, ventricular septal defects, and tricuspid valve abnormalities, can lead to transient or persistent AV block.[13,18] The block is usually temporary and is thought to be secondary to postoperative local inflammation. However, AV block can appear years later, usually in those who had transient block just after the operation.[19,20] Intracardiac catheter manipulation can inadvertently produce varying degrees of heart block, which is usually temporary. Complete heart block can occur during right-sided heart catheterization in a patient with preexisting left bundle branch block (LBBB), or during LV catheterization (LV angiography or ablation procedures) in a patient with preexisting right bundle branch block (RBBB). AV block can also complicate radiofrequency (RF) catheter ablation of atrioventricular nodal reentrant tachycardia (AVNRT) or bypass tracts in the AVN vicinity.[21]

Vagally Mediated Atrioventricular Block. Vagally induced AV block can occur in otherwise normal patients, in those with cough or hiccups, and during swallowing or micturition when vagal discharge is enhanced.[22] Vagally mediated AV block occurs in the AVN, is associated with a narrow QRS complex, and is generally benign. The block is characteristically paroxysmal and is often associated with clearly visible sinus slowing on the electrocardiogram (ECG), because the vagal surge can cause simultaneous sinus slowing and AVN block. Additionally, transient AV block can occur secondary to enhanced vagal tone caused by carotid sinus massage, hypersensitive carotid sinus syndrome, or neurocardiogenic syncope. AV block in athletes is typically type 1 second-degree block, probably an expression of hypervagotonia related to physical training, and it resolves after physical deconditioning.[23] This form of AV block may or may not be associated with sinus bradycardia because the relative effects of sympathetic and parasympathetic systems on the AVN and sinus node can differ.[24]

Long-QT Syndrome. In long-QT syndrome (LQTS) with a very long QT interval (e.g., in LQT2, LQT3, LQT8, and LQT9), functional block between the HB and ventricular muscle caused by prolonged ventricular refractoriness can lead to 2:1 AV block and severe bradycardia. Conduction abnormalities of the HPS, including PQ prolongation and RBBB or LBBB, occur in some patients with LQTS.

Clinical Presentation

Symptoms in patients with AV conduction abnormalities are generally caused by bradycardia and loss of AV synchrony. Individuals with first-degree AV block are usually asymptomatic; however, patients with marked prolongation of the PR interval (longer than 300 milliseconds) can experience symptoms similar to those with pacemaker syndrome caused by loss of AV synchrony and atrial contraction against closed AV valves, and patients with left ventricular (LV) dysfunction can experience worsening of heart failure.[25] Symptoms caused by more advanced AV block can range from exercise intolerance, easy fatigability, dyspnea on exertion, angina, mental status changes, dizziness, and near-syncope to frank syncope.[10,15]

In patients with paroxysmal or intermittent complete heart block, symptoms are episodic and routine ECGs may not be diagnostic. Congenital AV block can be apparent in utero or at birth; however, many individuals have few or no symptoms and reach their teens or young adulthood before the diagnosis is made. Because of the presence of reliable subsidiary HB pacemakers with adequate rates (especially in the presence of catecholamines), syncope is rare with congenital complete AVN block. Some patients become symptomatic only when aging produces chronotropic incompetence of the HB rhythm.[10,15]

Natural History of Atrioventricular Block

The natural history of patients with AV block depends on the underlying cardiac condition; however, the site of the block and the resulting rhythm disturbances themselves contribute to the prognosis. Patients with first-degree AV block have an excellent prognosis, even when associated with chronic bifascicular block, because the rate of progression to third-degree AV block is low.[25] Type 1 second-degree AV block is generally benign; however, when type 1 AV block occurs in association with bifascicular block, the risk of progression to complete heart block is significantly increased because of probable infranodal disease. Type 2 second-degree AV block, usually seen with BBB, carries a high risk of progression to advanced or complete AV block. The prognosis of 2:1 AV block depends on whether the site of block is within or below the AVN.[10]

The prognosis for patients with symptomatic complete heart block is very poor in the absence of pacing, regardless of the extent of underlying heart disease. Once appropriate pacing therapy has been established, however, the prognosis depends on the underlying disease process.[14] Complete heart block secondary to anterior MI carries a poor prognosis because of the large area of damage associated with the MI. In contrast, complete heart block secondary to idiopathic bundle branch fibrosis in the absence of additional cardiac disease carries a more benign prognosis.[10]

Congenital complete heart block generally carries a more favorable prognosis than the acquired form when not associated with underlying heart disease. Patients with concomitant structural heart disease, wide QRS complex, LQTS, or complete heart block discovered at an early age are more likely to develop symptoms early and are at an increased risk for sudden death.

Diagnostic Evaluation of Atrioventricular Block

Because the prognosis and, in some cases, the treatment of AV block differ depending on whether the block is within the AVN or infranodal, determining the site of block is important. In most cases, this can be achieved noninvasively.

Electrocardiography

The QRS duration, PR interval, and ventricular rate on the surface ECG can provide important clues in localizing the level of block (see later).

Autonomic Modulation

Whereas the AVN is richly innervated and highly responsive to both sympathetic and vagal stimuli, the HPS is influenced minimally by the autonomic nervous system. Carotid sinus massage increases vagal tone and worsens second-degree AVN block, whereas exercise and atropine improve AVN conduction because of sympathetic stimulation and/or parasympatholysis. In contrast, carotid sinus massage may improve second-degree infranodal block by slowing the sinus rate and allowing HPS refractoriness to recover. However, exercise and atropine worsen infranodal block because of the increased rate of impulses conducted to the HPS.[10,15]

Exercise Testing

Vagolysis and increased sympathetic drive that occur with exercise enhance AVN conduction. Thus, patients with first-degree AV block can have shorter PR intervals during exercise, and patients with type 1 second-degree AV block can develop higher AV conduction ratios (e.g., 3:2 at rest becoming 6:5 during exercise).

Exercise testing can be a useful tool to help confirm the level of block in second- or third-degree AV block associated with a narrow or wide QRS complex. Patients with presumed type 1 block or congenital complete heart block and a normal QRS complex usually have an increased ventricular rate with exercise. On the other hand, patients with acquired complete heart block and a wide QRS complex usually show minimal or no increase in ventricular rate. Additionally, patients with 2:1 AV block in whom the site of conduction block is uncertain can benefit from exercise testing by observing whether the AV conduction ratio increases in a Wenckebach-like manner (e.g., to 3:2 or 4:3) or decreases (e.g., to 3:1 or 4:1). In the latter case, the increase in the sinus rate finds the HPS refractory, causing the higher degrees of block. This response is always abnormal and it indicates intra- or infra-Hisian block, which will require permanent cardiac pacing.

Electrophysiological Testing

Electrophysiological (EP) testing is usually not required for the diagnosis or treatment of AV block, because the above noninvasive measures are usually adequate. On the other hand, EP testing can be of value in symptomatic patients in whom AV conduction abnormalities are suspected but cannot be documented or those with equivocal ECG findings.

ELECTROCARDIOGRAPHIC FEATURES

First-Degree Atrioventricular Block (Delay)

First-degree AV block manifests on the surface ECG as a PR interval more than 200 milliseconds following a normally timed (nonpremature) P wave. All P waves are conducted, but with delay. Each P wave is followed by a QRS complex with a constant, prolonged PR interval.

Site of Block. The degree of PR interval prolongation and QRS duration can help predict the site of conduction delay: Very long (more than 300 milliseconds) or highly variable PR intervals indicate involvement of the AVN. Normal QRS duration also suggests involvement of the AVN.[14,26]

Atrioventricular Node. Although the conduction delay can be anywhere along the AVN-HPS, the AVN is the most common site of delay (87% when the QRS complex is narrow, and more than 90% when the PR interval is more than 300 milliseconds; Fig. 6-1).

His-Purkinje System. Intra-Hisian conduction delay or HPS disease can cause first-degree AV block. First-degree AV block in the presence of BBB is caused by infranodal conduction delay in 45% of cases. A combination of delay within the AVN and in the HPS must also be considered (Fig. 6-2).

Atrium. First-degree AV block caused by intra- or interatrial conduction delay is not uncommon. Left atrial enlarge-

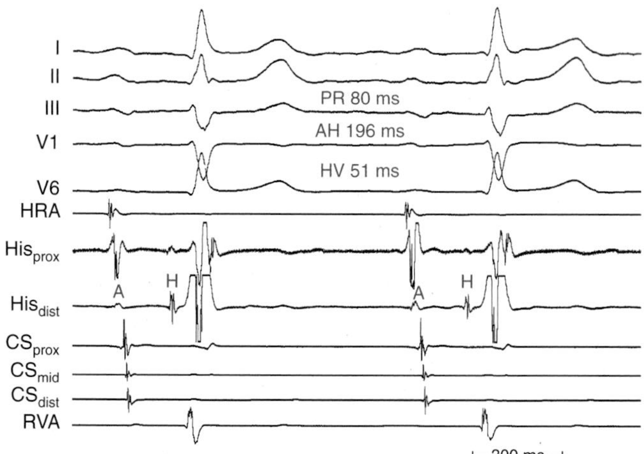

FIGURE 6–1 First-degree atrioventricular block caused by intranodal conduction delay, as indicated by the prolonged atrial–His bundle (AH) and normal PA and His bundle–ventricular (HV) intervals.

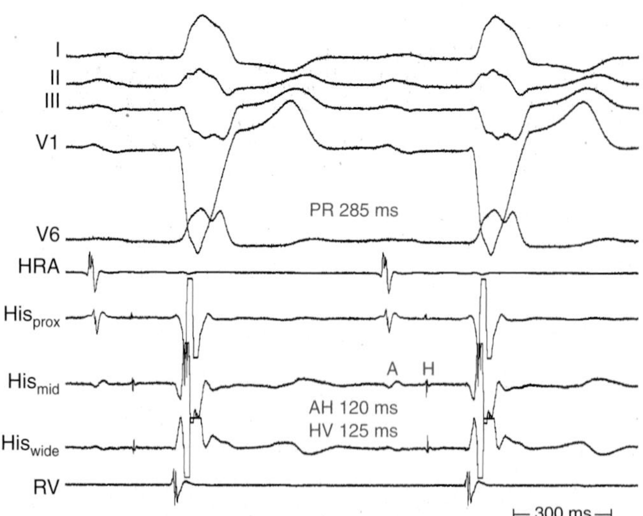

FIGURE 6–2 First-degree atrioventricular block secondary to His-Purkinje system (HPS) disease. The atrial–His bundle interval (AH) is normal but the His bundle–ventricular interval (HV) is markedly prolonged and associated with complete left bundle branch block.

ment pattern on the ECG (i.e., prolonged P wave duration) reflects the presence of interatrial conduction delay. Right atrial enlargement can prolong the PR interval (Fig. 6-3). In certain cases of congenital structural heart disease, such as Ebstein's anomaly of the tricuspid valve or endocardial cushion defects, intraatrial conduction delay can cause first-degree AV block.

Second-Degree Atrioventricular Block

The term *second-degree AV block* is applied when intermittent failure of AV conduction is present (one or more atrial impulses that should be conducted fail to reach the ventricles). This term encompasses several conduction patterns. Types 1 and 2 AV block are ECG patterns that describe the behavior of the PR intervals (in sinus rhythm) in sequences (with at least two consecutively conducted PR intervals) in which a *single* P wave fails to conduct to the ventricles. The anatomical site of block should not be characterized as either type 1 or type 2 because type 1 and type 2 designations refer only to ECG patterns.[10,24]

1. Type 1 Second-Degree Atrioventricular Block

Type 1 second-degree AV block (Wenckebach or Mobitz type I block) manifests on the surface ECG as progressive prolongation of the PR interval before failure of an atrial impulse to conduct to the ventricles. The PR interval immediately after the nonconducted P wave returns to its baseline value and the sequence begins again.

The behavior of Wenckebach block can be simplified by relating it to an abnormally long relative refractory period of the AVN. With a long AVN relative refractory period, the rate of AVN conduction depends on the time that the impulse arrives at the AVN. The earlier it arrives at the AVN, the longer it takes to propagate through the AVN, and the longer the PR interval; the later it arrives, the shorter the conduction time, and the shorter the PR interval. Thus, Wenckebach periodicity develops because each successive atrial impulse arrives earlier and earlier in the relative refractory period of the AVN, resulting in longer and longer conduction delay and PR interval, until one impulse arrives during the absolute refractory period and fails to conduct, resulting in a ventricular pause. In other words, the shorter the RP interval, the longer the PR interval; and the longer the RP interval, the shorter the PR interval. This is referred to as RP-PR reciprocity or RP-dependent PR interval. Using this concept, it is easy to explain the behavior of the PR interval during the Wenckebach periodicity. The first atrial impulse conducting after the pause has an unusually long RP interval, whereas with the following atrial impulse the RP interval dramatically shortens, resulting in prolongation of the PR interval. With the following atrial impulses, although having shorter RP intervals, such shortening is not as dramatic, and consequently the progressive prolongation of the PR interval is of lesser degree.[24] In other words, while each successive PR interval prolongs, it does so at a decreasing increment. So, for example, if the PR interval following the first conducted P wave in the cycle increased by 100 milliseconds, the PR interval of the next beat would increase by 50 milliseconds, and so forth.

Features of typical Wenckebach periodicity include the following: (1) progressive lengthening of the PR interval throughout the Wenckebach cycle; (2) lengthening of the PR interval occurring at progressively decreasing increments, resulting in progressively shorter R-R intervals; (3) a pause between QRS complexes encompassing the nonconducted P wave that is less than the sum of R-R intervals of any two consecutively conducted beats; (4) shortening of the PR interval postblock, compared with the PR interval just preceding the blocked cycle; and (5) group beating, which offers a footprint that identifies Wenckebach periodicity (Fig. 6-4). It is important to recognize that, during Wenckebach periodicity, the atrial impulse conducted to the ventricles is not always represented by the P wave that immediately pre-

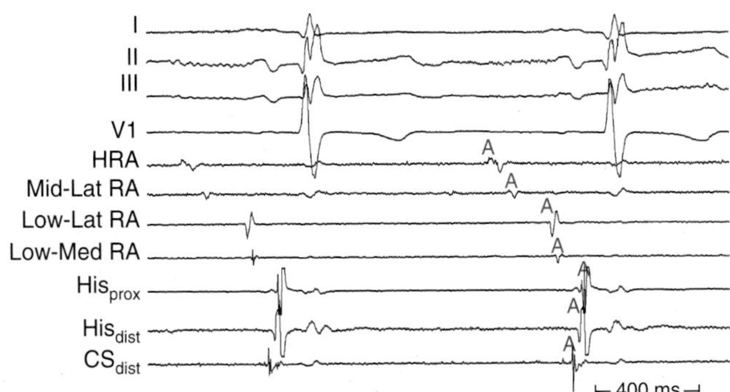

FIGURE 6–3 First-degree atrioventricular block caused by intraatrial conduction delay. The long PR interval (240 milliseconds) is caused by prolonged conduction in the RA (prolonged PA interval) in a patient who has undergone Fontan repair for complex congenital heart disease.

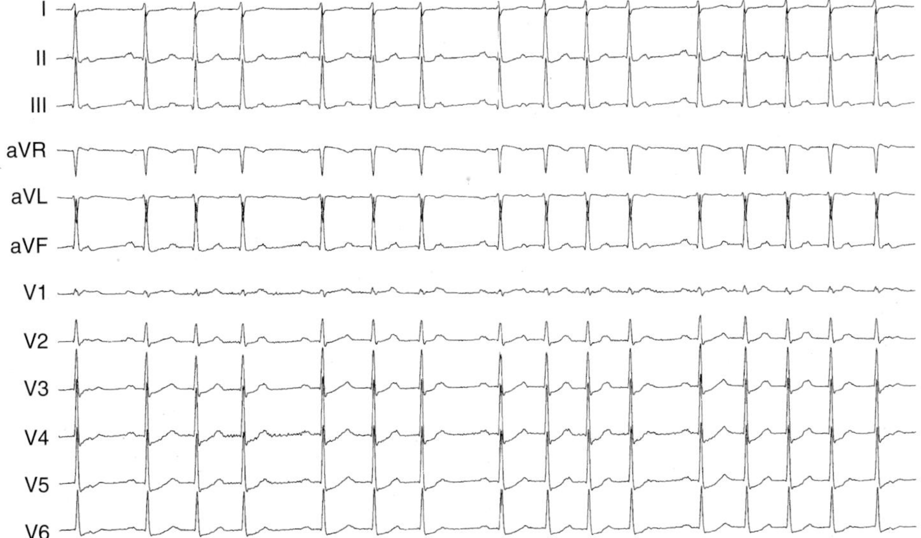

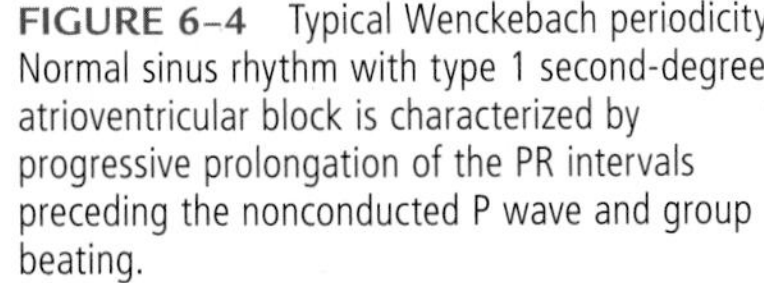

FIGURE 6–4 Typical Wenckebach periodicity. Normal sinus rhythm with type 1 second-degree atrioventricular block is characterized by progressive prolongation of the PR intervals preceding the nonconducted P wave and group beating.

cedes the QRS complex; the PR interval can be very long and exceed the P-P interval.[10,15,24]

Less than 50% of type 1 AV block cases follow this typical pattern. Typical Wenckebach periodicity is more frequently observed during pacing-induced AV block. Atypical patterns are more likely found with longer Wenckebach periods (more than 6:5). In patients with dual AVN physiology, Wenckebach cycles are almost always atypical; the greatest increment in the AH interval occurs when block occurs in the fast pathway, whichever beat this may be. Differentiating atypical from typical patterns is of little clinical significance. However, an atypical pattern can be misdiagnosed as type 2 second-degree AV block. Some possible atypical features of Wenckebach periodicity include the following (Fig. 6-5): (1) the second (conducted) PR interval (after the pause) often fails to show the greatest increment, and the increment may actually increase for the PR interval of the last conducted beat in the cycle (Fig. 6-6); (2) very little incremental conduction delay and no discernible change in the duration of the PR intervals for a few beats just before termination of a sequence (this is seen most often during long Wenckebach cycles and in association of increased vagal tone, and is usually accompanied by slowing of the sinus rate; see Fig. 6-5); (3) the PR interval can actually shorten and then lengthen in the middle of a Wenckebach sequence; and (4) a junctional escape beat can end the pause following a nonconducted P wave, resulting in an apparent shortening of the PR interval.[24,26,27]

AVN block can usually be reversed completely or partially by altering autonomic tone (e.g., with atropine). However, occasionally, these measures fail, especially in the presence of structural damage (congenital heart disease or inferior wall MI) to the AVN. In such cases, progression to complete AV block can occur, although such an event is more likely to occur with block in the HPS.

Site of Block. The degree of PR interval prolongation and QRS duration can help predict the site of block. A normal QRS duration usually indicates AVN involvement, whereas the presence of BBB suggests (but does not prove) HPS involvement. Furthermore, short baseline PR interval and small PR interval increments preceding the block suggest HPS involvement.[24,26,27]

Atrioventricular Node. Wenckebach block is almost always within the AVN (and rarely intra-Hisian) when a narrow QRS complex is present.

His-Purkinje System. When type 1 block is seen with the presence of BBB, the block is still more likely to be in the AVN (Fig. 6-7), but it can also be localized within or below the HPS (Fig. 6-8). In this case, a very long PR interval is more consistent with AVN block.[24,26,27]

2. Type 2 Second-Degree Atrioventricular Block

Type 2 second-degree (Mobitz type II) AV block is characterized on the surface ECG by a constant (normal or prolonged) PR interval of *all* conducted P waves, followed by sudden failure of a P wave to be conducted to the ventricles (Fig. 6-9). The RP-PR reciprocity, the hallmark of type 1 block, is absent in type 2 block. Consequently, the PR interval following a long RP interval (immediately following the pause) is identical to that following a short RP interval (immediately preceding the nonconducted P wave). Type 2 block cannot be diagnosed if the first P wave after a blocked beat is absent or if the PR interval following the pause is shorter than all the other PR intervals of the conducted P waves, regardless of the number of constant PR intervals before the block. The P-P intervals remain constant, and the pause encompassing the nonconducted P wave equals twice the P-P interval.[24]

A true Mobitz type II block in conjunction with a narrow QRS complex is relatively rare and occurs without sinus slowing and without associated type 1 sequences. Atypical forms of Wenckebach block with only minimal PR interval variation should be excluded (see Fig. 6-5). Apparent Mobitz type II AV block can be observed under the influence of increased vagal tone during sleep, in which case, a type 1 block without discernible or measurable increments in the PR intervals is the actual diagnosis; sinus slowing with AV block essentially rules out type 2 block.[26] When a narrow QRS type 2-like pattern occurs with intermittent type 1 sequences (as in Holter recordings), a true type 2 block can be safely excluded because narrow QRS type 1 and type 2 blocks almost never coexist within the HB. Sustained advanced second-degree AV block is far more common in

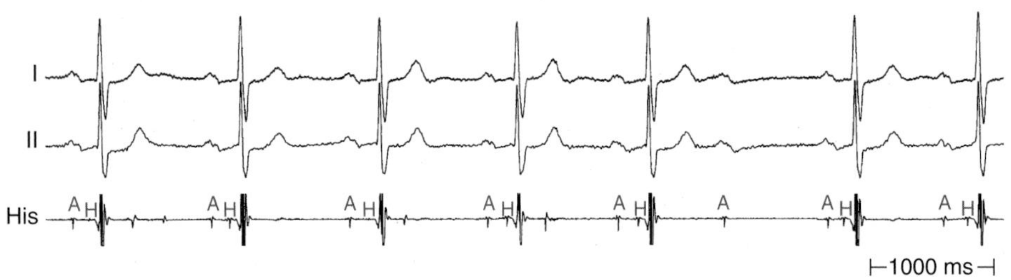

FIGURE 6–5 Atypical Wenckebach periodicity (type 1 second-degree atrioventricular block). Note the very small increments in the duration of the PR intervals for a few beats just before termination of a sequence. The first conducted P wave after the pause, however, is associated with obvious shortening of the PR interval.

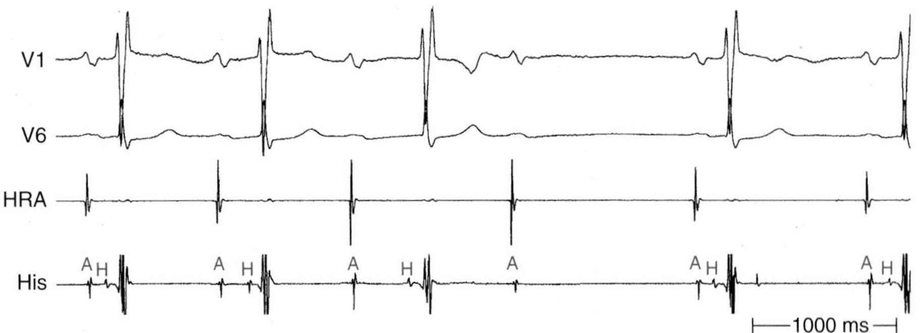

FIGURE 6–6 Atypical Wenckebach periodicity (type 1 second-degree atrioventricular [AV] block) caused by heightened vagal tone. Note the greatest increment occurs in the PR interval of the last conducted beat in the cycle and not in the second PR interval after the pause. Also the slowing in the sinus rate coinciding with significant increase in the PR interval and then AV block, suggesting that increased vagal tone is responsible for both slowing of the sinus rate and atrioventricular nodal block.

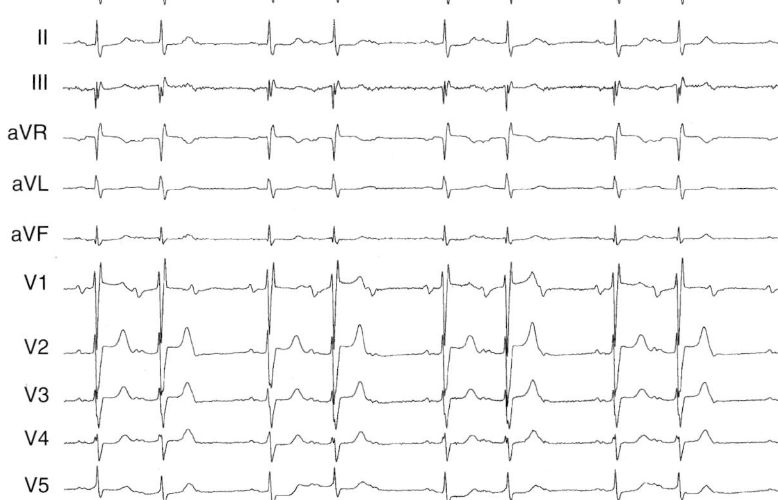

FIGURE 6–7 Typical Wenckebach periodicity. Normal sinus rhythm with type 1 second-degree atrioventricular (AV) block is characterized by progressive prolongation of the PR intervals preceding the nonconducted P wave and group beating. Despite the presence of His-Purkinje system disease (as indicated by incomplete right bundle branch block), Wenckebach AV block is more common in the AV node (AVN). At right, the last four P waves encountered 2:1 AV block.

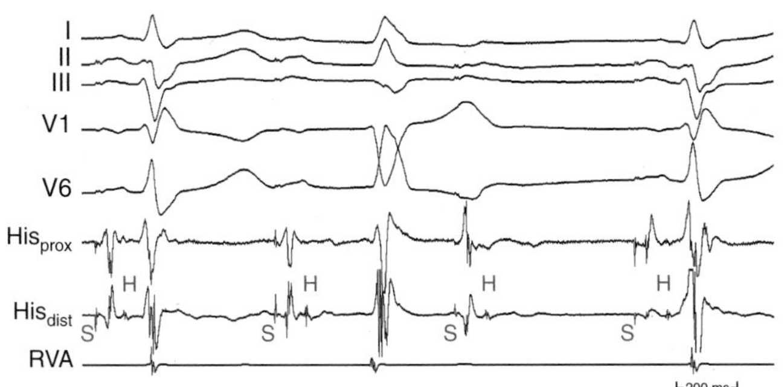

FIGURE 6–8 Infra-Hisian second-degree Wenckebach atrioventricular (AV) block. Atrial pacing in a patient with a normal prolonged atrial–His bundle interval (AH) but prolonged His bundle–ventricular interval (HV) and right bundle branch block (RBBB). On the second complex, the HV is dramatically prolonged and left bundle branch block is present, suggesting very slow conduction over the right bundle branch. With the third paced complex, AV block occurs below the His bundle recording, and on the fourth complex, conduction with RBBB resumes, suggesting a Wenckebach cycle in the His-Purkinje system.

association with true type 2 block than with type 1 block or its variant.[24]

Apparent Mobitz type II AV block can also be caused by concealed junctional extrasystoles (confined to the specialized conduction system and not propagated to the myocardium) and junctional parasystole. Exercise-induced second-degree AV block is most commonly infranodal and rarely is secondary to AVN disease or cardiac ischemia.[24]

Site of Block

His-Purkinje System. Type 2 second-degree AV block is almost always below the AVN, occurring in the HB in about 30% of cases and in the bundle branches in the remainder. Infrequently, type 2 second-degree AV block is found with a narrow QRS complex and is caused by intra-Hisian block (Fig. 6-10; see Fig. 6-9).[24]

Atrioventricular Node. Type 2 second-degree AV block has not yet been convincingly demonstrated in the body of the AVN or the N zone. Although multiple reports have described the occurrence of type 2 second-degree AV block in the AVN, in each case either the block could have been localized to the HPS rather than the AVN or the block probably was atypical Wenckebach block.[24,26]

3. 2:1 Atrioventricular Block

When only alternate beats are conducted, resulting in 2:1 ratio, the PR interval is constant for the conducted beats, provided that the atrial rhythm is regular (Fig. 6-11). A 2:1 AV block cannot be classified as type 1 or type 2; using the term *type 1* to describe 2:1 AV block when the lesion is in the AVN or when there is evidence of decremental conduction, and using the term *type 2* to describe 2:1 AV block when it is infranodal or when there is evidence of all-or-none conduction should be discouraged, because this practice violates the well-accepted traditional definitions of types 1 and 2 block based on ECG patterns, not on the anatomical site of block. Both types 1 and 2 block can progress to a 2:1 AV block, and a 2:1 AV block can regress to a type 1 or 2 block.[24]

Site of Block. Fixed 2:1 AV block poses a diagnostic dilemma because it can be difficult to localize the site of block by the surface ECG alone. Several ECG features can help in the differential diagnosis:

1. 2:1 AV block associated with a narrow QRS complex is likely to be intranodal, whereas that associated with a wide QRS complex is likely to be infranodal, but could still be at the level of the AVN (Fig. 6-12; see Fig. 6-11).
2. Fixed 2:1 AV block with PR intervals less than 160 milliseconds indicates intra- or infra-Hisian block, whereas very long PR intervals (more than 300 milliseconds) suggest AVN block.
3. If the PR interval of all the conducted complexes is constant despite a varying RP interval, infranodal block is likely.
4. Presence of Wenckebach block before or after episodes of 2:1 AV block is highly suggestive of block at the AVN level (see Fig. 6-7).
5. Improvement of block with atropine or exercise suggests AVN block; however, the absence of such response does not exclude intranodal block.[26]

4. High-Grade Atrioventricular Block

Failure of conduction of two or more consecutive P waves when AV synchrony is otherwise maintained is sometimes termed *high-grade AV block* or *advanced second-degree AV block* (Fig. 6-13).[14] This block must happen because of the existing block itself, and not because of retrograde concealment in the AVN or HPS resulting from junctional or ventricular escape complexes that prevent conduction.

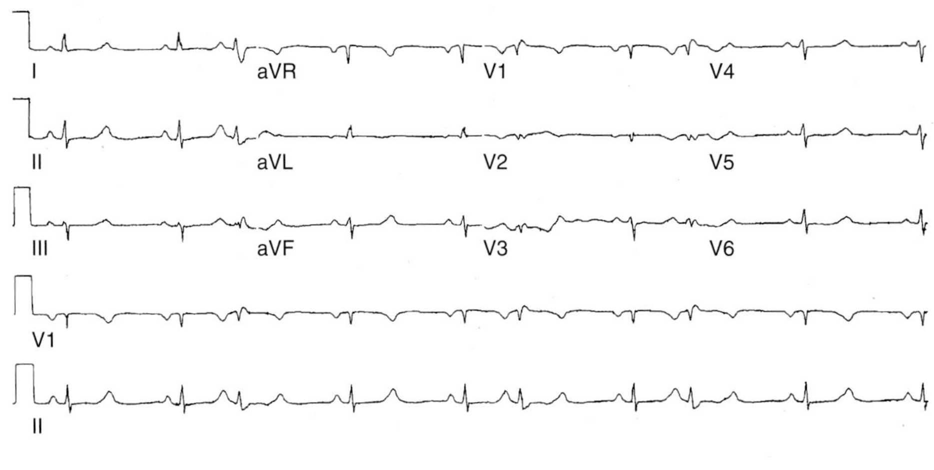

FIGURE 6–9 Second-degree atrioventricular block. Despite the presence of narrow QRS complexes, the block is likely secondary to be intra-Hisian, as suggested by the short PR intervals on conducted beats and no increment in the PR intervals on 3 : 2 cycles.

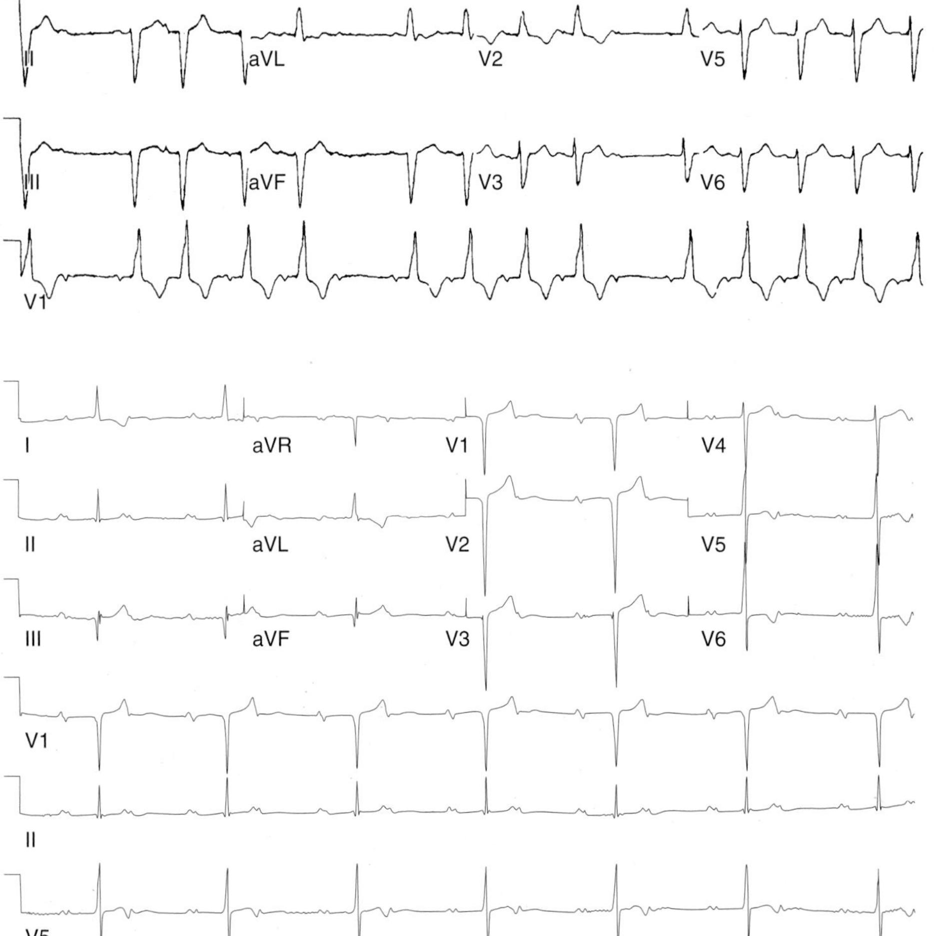

FIGURE 6–10 Second-degree infranodal atrioventricular block. Bifascicular block (right bundle branch block and left anterior fascicular block) and normal, constant PR intervals (196 milliseconds) are observed during conducted beats, consistent with infranodal block.

FIGURE 6–11 Second-degree 2 : 1 atrioventricular block. Note the long PR interval during conducted complexes and the narrow QRS complexes, suggesting intranodal block. Q waves are observed in the inferior leads, indicating prior myocardial infarction.

Site of Block. The level of block can be at the AVN or the HPS. When high-degree AV block is caused by block in the AVN, QRS complexes of the conducted beats are usually narrow. Wenckebach periodicity can also be seen, and atropine administration produces lesser degrees of AV block. Features indicating block in the HPS are conducted beats with BBB and no improvement in block with atropine.

Third-Degree (Complete) Atrioventricular Block

AV block is termed *complete* when all P waves fail to conduct, despite having ample opportunity for conduction. Therefore, if there is less than optimal opportunity for the AVN-HPS to conduct, it cannot be regarded as a failure if

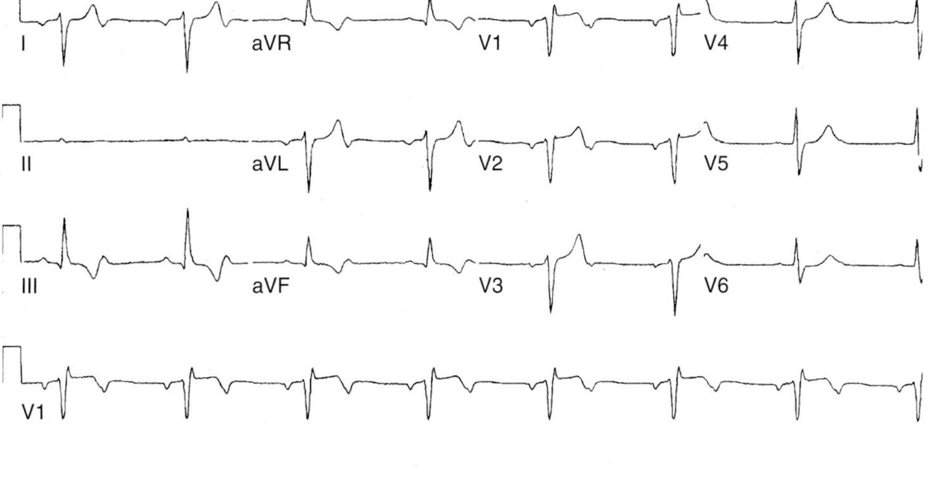

FIGURE 6–12 Second-degree 2:1 atrioventricular block. Note the short PR interval during conducted complexes and the wide QRS complexes, suggesting block in the His-Purkinje system.

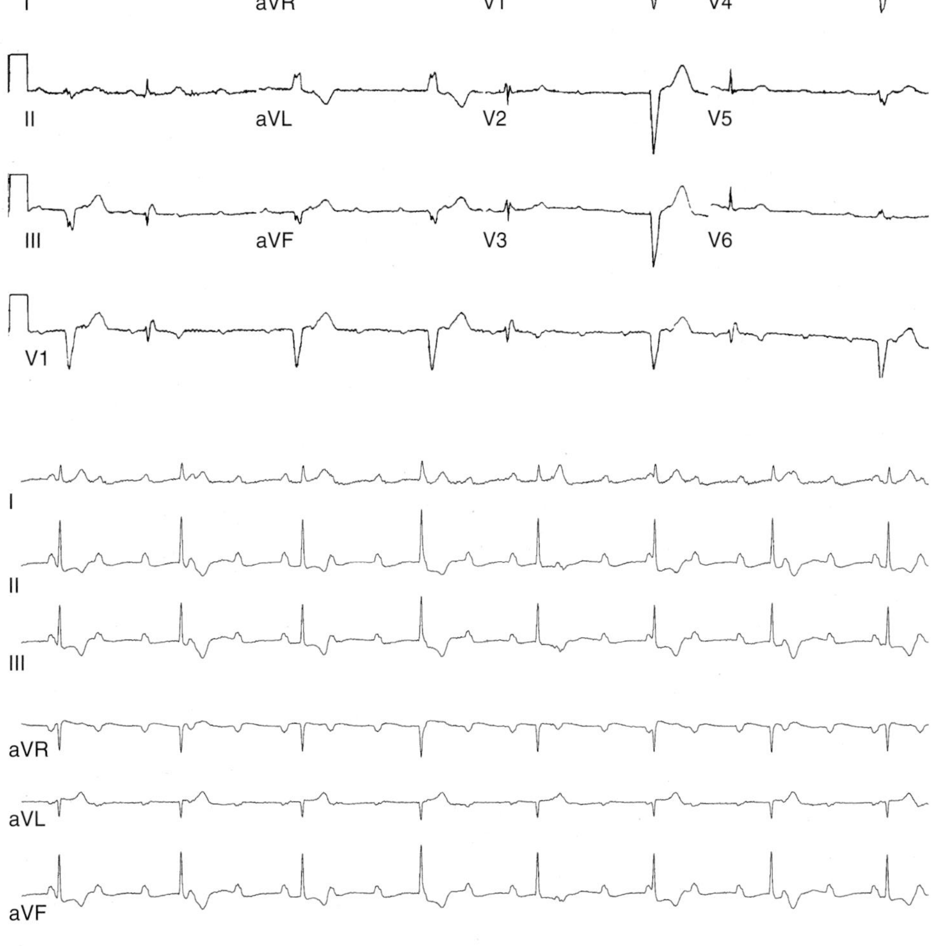

FIGURE 6–13 High-grade atrioventricular block. Note that only three P waves conducted to the ventricle in the whole tracing. Conducted P waves were associated with normal PR intervals and right bundle branch block, suggesting infranodal block. All other P waves were blocked, and ventricular escape rhythm with a left bundle branch block pattern is observed. Note that the block is not caused by retrograde concealment in the atrioventricular node or His-Purkinje system from the ventricular escape complexes, because the conducted P waves occurred at a short cycle following the escape complexes.

FIGURE 6–14 Congenital third-degree atrioventricular (AV) block. Sinus rhythm with complete AV block and junctional escape rhythm with a narrow QRS is seen, consistent with intra-nodal block.

it does not conduct. Third-degree AV block is seen on the surface ECG as completely dissociated P waves and QRS complexes, each firing at its own pacemaker rate, with continuously changing P-R relationship as the P waves march through all phases of the ventricular cycle in the presence of a regular ventricular rhythm (Fig. 6-14). Every possible chance for conduction is afforded, with the P waves occurring at every conceivable RP interval, but the atrial impulse is never conducted to the ventricles. The atrial rate is always faster than the ventricular rate.[26,27]

Site of Block

Atrioventricular Node. Most cases of congenital third-degree AV block are localized to the AVN (see Fig. 6-14), as is transient AV block associated with acute inferior wall MI, beta blockers, calcium channel blockers, and digitalis toxicity. Complete AVN block is characterized by a junctional escape rhythm with a narrow QRS complex and a rate of 40 to 60 beats/min, which tends to increase with exercise or atropine. However, in 20% to 50% of patients with chronic AV block, a wide QRS escape rhythm may occur. Rhythms

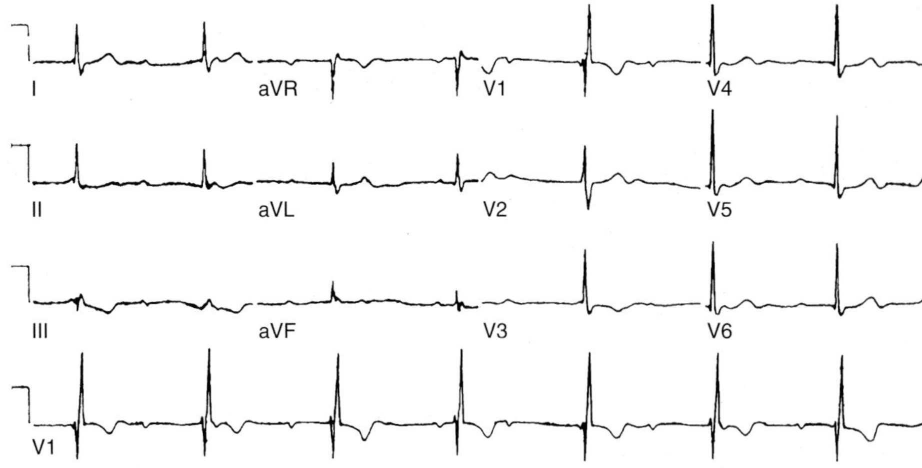

FIGURE 6–15 Complete infranodal atrioventricular (AV) block. Complete AV dissociation is observed and all the P waves fail to conduct, despite having ample opportunity for conduction. Note the slow ventricular escape rhythm with a wide QRS complex and a rate of 40 beats/min, consistent with block in the His-Purkinje system.

originating in the distal HB may have a wide QRS. Those rhythms are usually slower and nonresponsive to atropine.[26]

His-Purkinje System. Acquired complete heart block is usually associated with block in the HPS, resulting in an
6 escape rhythm with a wide QRS complex with a rate of 20 to 40 beats/min (Fig. 6-15).

Paroxysmal Atrioventricular Block

Paroxysmal AV block is characterized by abrupt and persistent AV block in the presence of a preexisting, otherwise normal, conduction system.[27] The block usually starts following a conducted or nonconducted premature atrial complex (PAC) or premature ventricular complex (PVC), and persists until another PAC or PVC terminates it. Episodes of AV block are commonly associated with prolonged periods of ventricular asystole. Paroxysmal AV block is believed to be caused by intra-Hisian disease. The exact mechanism of the block is unclear, although phase 4 depolarization producing block has been suggested.

ELECTROPHYSIOLOGICAL TESTING

Role of Electrophysiological Testing

ECG diagnosis of AV block is usually adequate for deciding subsequent treatment and, once symptoms and AV block are correlated by electrocardiography, further documentation by invasive studies is not required, unless additional information is needed. Similarly, asymptomatic patients with transient Wenckebach block associated with increased vagal tone should not undergo EP testing.

However, EP testing can help diagnose an equivocal ECG pattern or delineate the site of conduction abnormality, if that is required for decision-making. EP testing is indicated in a patient with suspected high-grade AV block as the cause of syncope or presyncope when documentation cannot be obtained noninvasively. Similarly, in patients with coronary artery disease, it can be unclear whether symptoms are secondary to AV block or ventricular tachycardia (VT); therefore, EP testing can be useful in establishing the diagnosis. Some patients with known second- or third-degree block can benefit from an invasive study to localize the site of AV block to help determine therapy or assess prognosis.[26,27]

Normal Atrioventricular Conduction

The normal PR interval is 120 to 200 milliseconds. This interval reflects the conduction time from the high RA to the point of ventricular activation (i.e., QRS onset), and includes activation of the atrium, AVN, HB, bundle branches and fascicles, and terminal Purkinje fibers. To measure the different components of the conduction system that the PR interval includes, intracardiac tracings from the high RA and HB region are required (see Fig. 2-19).

The PA interval, measured from the high RA electrogram to the low RA deflection in the HB recording, gives an indirect approximation of the intraatrial conduction time. The normal PA interval is 20 to 60 milliseconds.

The atrial–His bundle (AH) interval is measured from the first rapid deflection of the atrial deflection in the HB recording to the first evidence of HB depolarization in the HB recording. The AH interval is an approximation of the AVN conduction time, because it represents conduction time from the low RA at the interatrial septum through the AVN to the HB. The AH interval has a wide range in normal subjects (50 to 120 milliseconds) and is markedly influenced by the autonomic nervous system.

His potential duration reflects conduction through the short length of the HB that penetrates the fibrous septum. Disturbances of the HB conduction can manifest as fractionation, prolongation (more than 30 milliseconds), or splitting of the His potential.

The His bundle–ventricular (HV) interval is measured from the onset of the His potential to the onset of the earliest registered surface or intracardiac ventricular activation, and it represents conduction time from the proximal HB through the distal HPS to the ventricular myocardium. The most proximal electrodes displaying the His potential should be chosen, and a large atrial electrogram should accompany the proximal His potential. The HV interval is not significantly affected by the autonomic tone, and usually remains stable. The range of HV intervals in normal subjects is narrow, 35 to 55 milliseconds.

Localization of the Site of Atrioventricular Block

EP testing allows analysis of the HB electrogram, as well as providing atrial and ventricular pacing to uncover conduction abnormalities. A markedly prolonged HV interval (100 milliseconds or longer) is associated with a high incidence of progression to complete heart block. In addition, a His potential 30 milliseconds or longer in duration or that is frankly split into two deflections is indicative of intra-Hisian conduction delay.

When the His potential is recorded during atrial pacing at progressively shorter cycle lengths (CLs), the AH interval normally gradually lengthens until Wenckebach block develops. The HV interval normally remains constant, despite different pacing rates. Abnormal AVN conduction produces Wenckebach block at slower atrial pacing rates than what is normally seen (i.e., at a pacing CL more than 500 milliseconds). To determine whether AVN disease is truly present or just under the influence of excessive vagal tone, atropine or isoproterenol can be administered to evaluate for improvement in conduction. Infranodal block is present when the atrial deflection is followed by the His potential but no ventricular depolarization is seen. Block below the HB is abnormal unless associated with short pacing CLs (350 milliseconds or less). Block in the HB can be masked by prolonged AVN conduction time or refractoriness. When block in the AVN develops at slow pacing rate, atropine can be administered to improve AVN conduction and allow evaluation of the HPS at faster pacing rates.

Site of First-Degree Atrioventricular Block

Atrioventricular Node. An AH interval more than 130 milliseconds with a normal HV interval indicates intranodal conduction delay (see Fig. 6-1). Dual AVN physiology can produce transient, abrupt, or alternating first-degree block caused by block in the fast AVN pathway and conduction down the slow pathway. The change in the PR interval seen on the surface ECG corresponds with a jump in the AH interval viewed on the HB electrogram.[26]

His-Purkinje System. As long as at least one fascicle conducts normally, the HV interval should not exceed 55 milliseconds (or 60 milliseconds in the presence of LBBB). A prolonged HV interval (more than 55-60 milliseconds) with or without prolonged His potential duration (>30 milliseconds) or split His potential is diagnostic for HPS disease, even in the presence of a normal PR interval (Fig. 6-16; see Fig. 6-2). A prolonged HV interval is almost always associated with an abnormal QRS, because the impairment of intra-Hisian conduction is not homogeneous. Most patients have an HV interval of 60 to 100 milliseconds, and occasionally more than 100 milliseconds. With pure intra-Hisian conduction delay, the atrial-to-proximal His (AH) interval and the distal His-to-ventricular (H′-V) interval are normal, while the duration of the His potential is more than 30 milliseconds, with a notched, fragmented, or split His potential. In this case, verification of the origin of the "split H" from the HB (and not part of the atrial or ventricular electrograms) is critical. This can be achieved by dissociation of the His potential from atrial activation with atrial pacing, adenosine, or vagal stimulation, and dissociation of the His potential from ventricular activation by documenting that the HV interval is longer than 30 milliseconds.[26]

Atrium. A prolonged PA interval with normal AH and HV intervals indicates intraatrial conduction delay (see Fig. 6-3).

Site of Type 1 Second-Degree Atrioventricular Block

Atrioventricular Node. Wenckebach block in the AVN is characterized by progressive prolongation of the AH interval, until an atrial deflection is not followed by His and ventricular deflections (see Figs. 6-5 and 6-6).[24]

His Bundle. Prolonged His potential duration or split His potential is indicative of intra-Hisian disease. Intra-Hisian Wenckebach block can occur between the two His deflections, characterized by progressive conduction delay until the first His deflection is not followed by the second one.

Bundle Branches. In type 1 block secondary to block below the HB, progressive prolongation of the HV interval is followed by a His deflection without an associated ventricular activation (see Fig. 6-8).

Site of Type 2 Second-Degree Atrioventricular Block (Mobitz Type II Block)

His-Purkinje System. The blocked cycle features atrial and HB deflections without ventricular depolarization (Fig. 6-17). The conducted beats usually show evidence of infranodal conduction system disease, with prolonged HV interval, or even split His potential, and BBB.[24]

Site of Third Degree (Complete) Atrioventricular Block

Atrioventricular Node. Complete heart block at the AVN level is usually seen on the intracardiac tracings as His potentials consistently preceding each ventricular electrogram. The atrial electrograms are dissociated from the HV complexes (Fig. 6-18). Most often, the escape rhythm originates in the HB (with normal QRS preceded by a His potential and normal HV interval); however, in 20% to 50% of patients with chronic AV block, a wide QRS escape rhythm can occur. Rhythms originating in the distal HB can have a QRS preceded by a retrograde His potential or no His potential at all. Those rhythms are usually slower and nonresponsive to atropine. The stability of the HB rhythm can be assessed by noting the effects of overdrive suppression

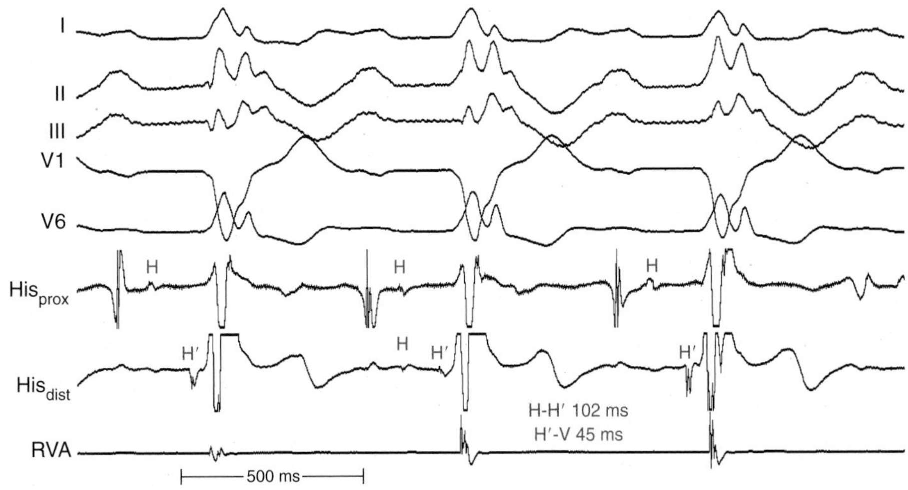

FIGURE 6–16 Split His potentials in a patient with cardiomyopathy and left bundle branch block. Recording only the distal His signal (H′) would give the false impression of normal infranodal conduction (H′V = 42 milliseconds).

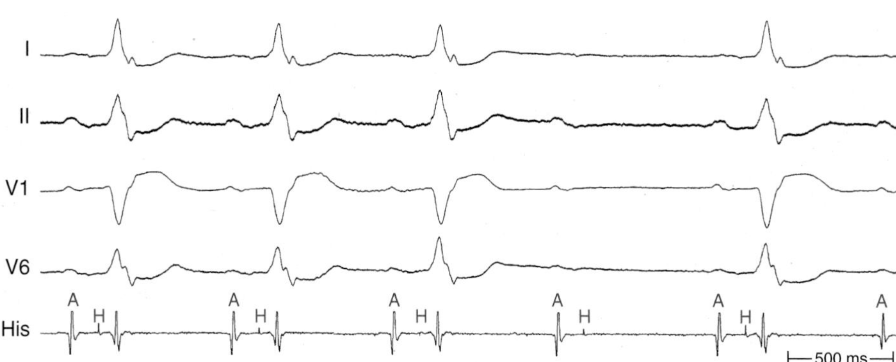

FIGURE 6–17 Type 2 second-degree (Mobitz type II) atrioventricular (AV) block. Sinus rhythm is observed with a wide QRS complex. The PR interval of all conducted P waves is constant and slightly prolonged (224 milliseconds). The fourth P wave fails to conduct to the ventricle, but is followed by a His potential, suggesting the level of AV block is infra-Hisian.

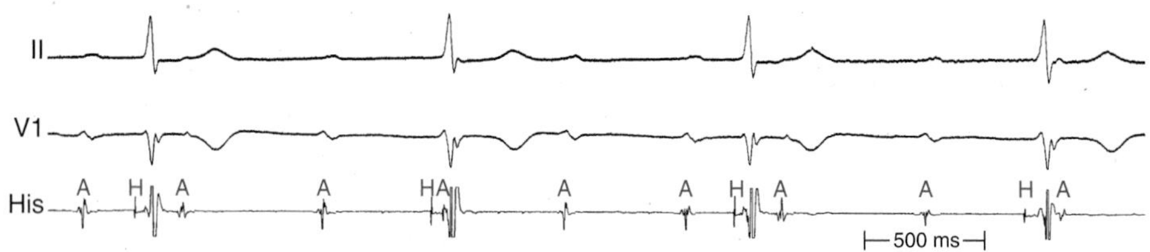

FIGURE 6–18 Complete atrioventricular (AV) block. Complete AV dissociation is observed and all the P waves fail to conduct, despite having ample opportunity for conduction. Note the junctional escape rhythm with a narrow QRS complex and a rate of 45 beats/min, consistent with block in the AVN. Note that the P waves surrounding a QRS complex occur at a faster rate when compared with the P waves that occur sequentially without an intervening QRS complex (ventriculophasic arrhythmia).

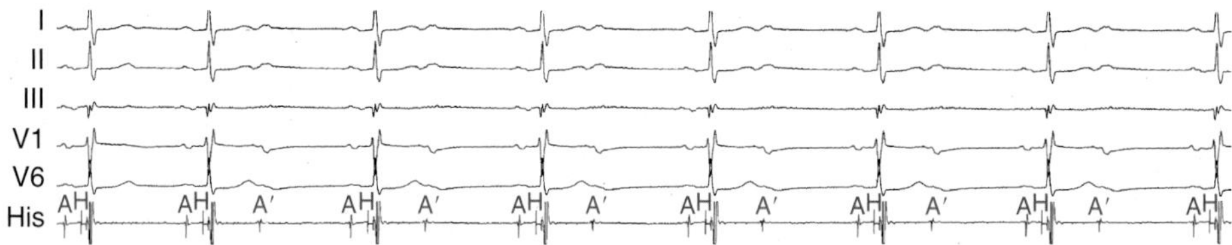

FIGURE 6–19 Sinus rhythm with normal atrioventricular (AV) conduction. Frequent premature atrial complexes (PACs; A′) are observed in a bigeminal pattern. The PACs arrive at the atrioventricular node during the absolute refractory period and fail to conduct to the ventricle, mimicking 2:1 AV block. In contrast to 2:1 AV block, the nonconducted P waves are premature (compare with the first A-A interval, which is not interrupted by a PAC) and have different morphology than the conducted sinus P waves.

produced by ventricular pacing (in a manner analogous to testing sinus node function); prolonged pauses (i.e., the lack of HB escapes) herald failure of the escape rhythm.[26]

His-Purkinje System. The intracardiac electrogram shows HB deflections consistently following atrial electrograms, but ventricular depolarizations are completely dissociated from the AH complexes. Block below the HB is thus demonstrated.[14,27]

Exclusion of Other Phenomena

Nonconducted Premature Atrial Complexes

Early PACs can arrive at the AVN during the absolute refractory period and fail to conduct to the ventricle. This can be misdiagnosed as type 1 or type 2 second-degree AV block. Similarly, atrial bigeminy, with failure of conduction of the PACs, can be misinterpreted as 2:1 AV block (Fig. 6-19). In type 2 second-degree AV block, the atrial rhythm is regular and the P-P interval is constant, and the nonconducted P wave occurs on time as expected, and P wave morphology is constant. On the other hand, with nonconducted PACs, the P wave occurs prematurely and usually has a different morphology from that of the baseline atrial rhythm. Nonconducted PACs can often be hidden in the preceding T wave. Additionally, the mere occurrence of PACs in a trigeminal or quadrigeminal pattern can produce a periodicity mimicking Wenckebach periodicity (Fig. 6-20).

Concealed Junctional Ectopy

Ectopic beats arising from the HB that fail to conduct to both the atria and ventricles, with retrograde concealment in the AVN, slowing or blocking conduction of the following sinus P wave, can manifest as type 2 second-degree AV block. Such a phenomenon can be difficult to differentiate from actual block without EP testing. ECG clues to concealed junctional extrasystoles causing such unexpected events include (1) abrupt, unexplained prolongation of the PR interval, (2) the presence of apparent Mobitz type II block in the presence of a normal QRS, (3) the presence of types 1 and 2 AV block in the same tracing, and (4) the presence of manifest junctional extrasystoles elsewhere in the tracing.

Atrioventricular Dissociation

The distinction between AV dissociation and complete AV block is important. AV dissociation is present when the atria and ventricles depolarize independent of each other. The ventricles are activated by a nonatrial source and are uninfluenced by atrial activity. By definition, there is no retrograde conduction from the ventricles to the atria.[14] AV dissociation can occur secondary to complete AV block, atrial bradycardia with a faster independent junctional-

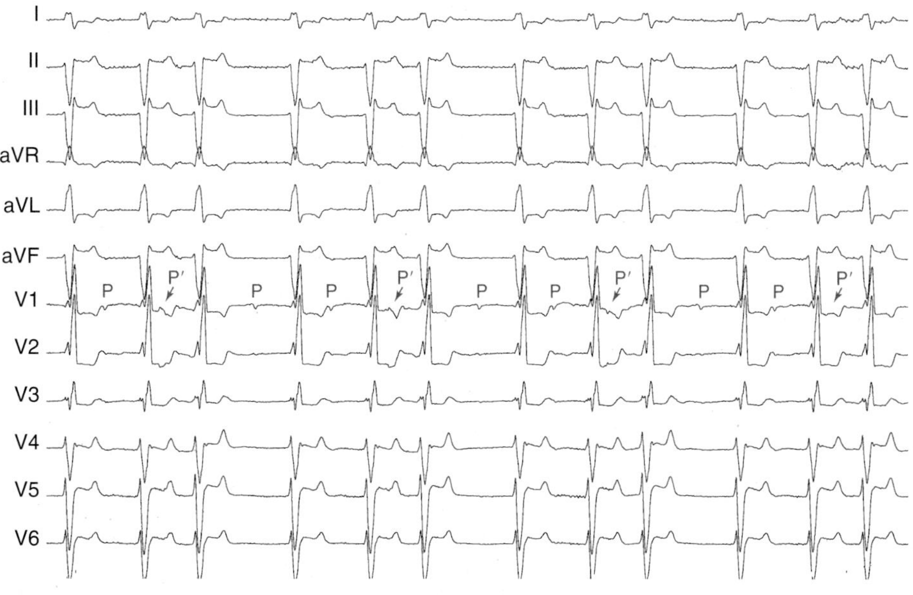

FIGURE 6–20 Sinus rhythm with marked first-degree atrioventricular (AV) block and bifascicular block (right bundle branch block and left anterior fascicular block). Frequent premature atrial complexes (PACs; P′) are observed in a trigeminal pattern. The PACs are conducted to the ventricles; however, they produce a periodicity, mimicking Wenckebach AV block. Note that no P waves fail to conduct to the ventricle. Despite the presence of marked His-Purkinje system disease, the marked prolongation of the PR intervals (420 milliseconds) suggests the atrioventricular node as the site of AV conduction delay.

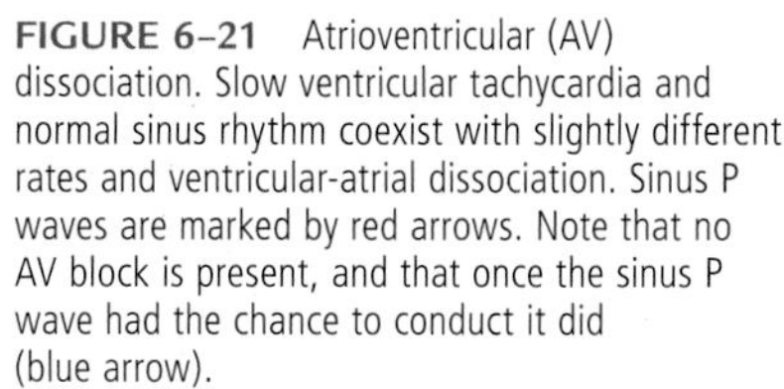

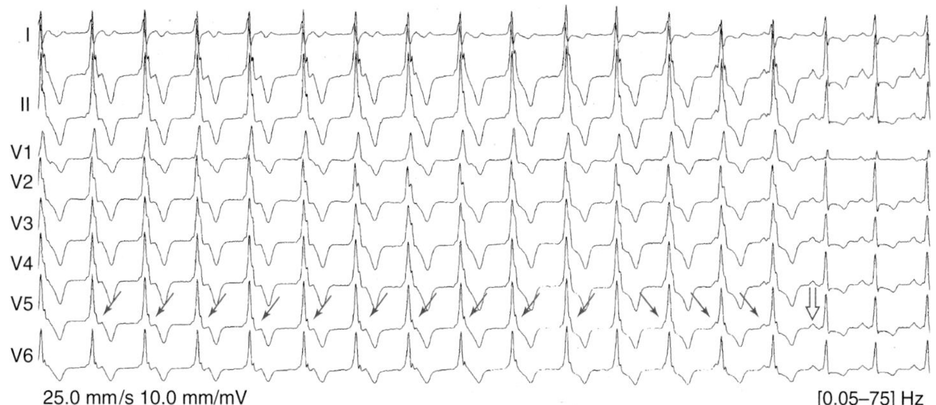

FIGURE 6–21 Atrioventricular (AV) dissociation. Slow ventricular tachycardia and normal sinus rhythm coexist with slightly different rates and ventricular-atrial dissociation. Sinus P waves are marked by red arrows. Note that no AV block is present, and that once the sinus P wave had the chance to conduct it did (blue arrow).

ventricular escape rhythm, or increased discharge rate of a subsidiary pacemaker that takes control of the ventricular rhythm.[10,28]

In complete AV block, the atrial rate is faster than the ventricular rate. For AV block to be diagnosed, the P waves must fail to conduct, given every opportunity for optimal conduction. Thus, failure of conduction of all the P waves, even those occurring at long RP intervals and throughout the phases of the ventricular cycle, has to be documented. Occasionally, the rate of the junctional or ventricular rhythm during AV dissociation is only slightly different from that of the atrial rhythm. In this case, the standard ECG may not provide a recording opportunity long enough to verify failure of conduction, because all the P waves recorded on a single ECG recording may not occur at an appropriate time to allow conduction. Thus, obtaining ECG recording for an adequate length of time is important (Fig. 6-21). Regularity of both the atrial and ventricular rhythm with constantly changing P-R relationships, despite that fact that the P wave falls at every conceivable RP interval, and an independent ventricular rate 40 beats/min or less (faster in congenital complete AV block), is diagnostic of complete AV block. On the other hand, some irregularity of the ventricular rhythm should immediately draw attention to the possibility of intermittent conduction of P waves, which may reflect lesser degrees of AV block or incomplete AV dissociation. Moreover, with complete AV block, the ventricular rate is almost always slower than the atrial rate, whereas in other forms of AV dissociation, the reverse is true.[10,28] Therefore, complete AV block with a junctional or ventricular escape rhythm is one form of AV dissociation. However, AV dissociation (complete or incomplete) can occur in the absence of AV block.

In the case of atrial bradycardia, the atrial rate can become slower than a subsidiary escape focus from the AV junction or ventricle. When the faster junctional or ventricular escape rhythm is associated with VA block, it results in failure of the atrial impulses to conduct anterogradely secondary to retrograde concealment by the escape rhythm impulses.

An increase in the discharge rate of a subsidiary pacemaker, such as accelerated junctional rhythm, accelerated idioventricular rhythm, or VT, which then exceeds the normal sinus rate, can result in a competing junctional or ventricular rhythm, in which case the atrial rate is always slower than the ventricular rate (see Fig. 6-21).

AV dissociation can be complete or incomplete. In complete AV dissociation, both the atrial and ventricular rates remain constant and, therefore, the PR interval varies, with none of the atrial complexes being conducted to the ventricles. In incomplete AV dissociation, ventricular capture beats occur because some of the atrial impulses arrive at the AV junction when the AV junction is no longer refractory.

This phenomenon is common in advanced AV block with periodic capture beats.

Echo Beats

AVN echo beats can manifest as "group beating" and be misdiagnosed as Wenckebach block. Verification of constant P-P intervals and P wave morphology during the Wenckebach cycle can avoid such misinterpretation. On the other hand, in the presence of dual AVN physiology, not infrequently Wenckebach AV block can result in AVN echo beats.

Atrial Tachyarrhythmias

Failure of the AVN to conduct during fast atrial tachyarrhythmias (atrial tachycardia [AT] or atrial flutter [AFL]) should not be considered as pathological AV block. One of the main physiological roles of the AVN is to safeguard the ventricles from rapid atrial rates. Therefore, failure of the AVN to conduct every atrial impulse occurring at a fast rate should be considered as normal physiology caused by normal refractoriness. In such situations, terms such as *3:2 or 2:1 AV conduction* are more appropriate than *3:2 or 2:1 AV block.*

Atrial Fibrillation with Slow Ventricular Rate

AF with slow ventricular response can be misinterpreted as complete AV block. Verification of the regularity of the slow ventricular rhythm is critical. When AV block is present, the escape rhythm is regular, whereas in AF associated with very slow ventricular response, the ventricular rhythm is a result of conducted atrial beats and is irregular (Fig. 6-22).

Ventriculophasic Sinus Arrhythmia

A ventriculophasic sinus arrhythmia can be observed whenever there is second- or third-degree AV block, and is manifest as intermittent differences in the P-P intervals based on their relationship to the QRS complex. The two P waves surrounding a QRS complex have a shortened interval or occur at a faster rate when compared with two P waves that occur sequentially without an intervening QRS complex (see Fig. 6-18). The mechanism of this phenomenon is not certain; however, it has been suggested that ventricular contractions enhance sinus node automaticity by increasing the pulsatile blood flow through the sinus nodal artery and by mechanical stretch on the sinus node.

PRINCIPLES OF MANAGEMENT

Pacing is the mainstay of treatment for symptomatic AV block (Table 6-1). Identifying transient or reversible causes for AV conduction disturbances is the first step in management. Withdrawal of any offending drugs, correction of any electrolyte abnormalities, or treatment of any infectious processes should be considered prior to permanent pacing therapy. Pharmacological therapy (atropine, isoproterenol) is only effective as a short-term emergency measure until pacing can be accomplished. Temporary percutaneous or transvenous pacing is necessary in patients with hemodynamically significant AV block and bradycardia to provide immediate stabilization prior to permanent pacemaker placement or to provide pacemaker support when the block is precipitated by what is presumed to be a transient event, such as ischemia or drug toxicity.[29]

A key point in the decision to provide permanent pacing in AV block is the presence of symptoms. Intermittent block can make correlating bradycardia with symptoms difficult. Patients with complete heart block and syncope have clearly been shown to have an improved survival with permanent pacing. Most patients with acquired complete heart block are symptomatic and require pacing. Patients with congenital complete heart block are more likely to be asymptomatic, but prophylactic pacemaker implantation can be an appropriate consideration. Block in the AVN is less likely to be associated with slow ventricular rates, progression to complete heart block, and symptoms than infranodal block.[29]

Permanent pacemaker implantation is indicated in most patients with symptomatic advanced heart block, regardless of the site of block. Permanent pacemakers are also indicated in asymptomatic patients with complete heart block and infra-Hisian second-degree AV block, especially those with documented ventricular pauses longer than 3.0 seconds or a ventricular escape rhythm less than 40 beats/min.[29]

In children with congenital heart block, permanent pacing is recommended in those with exercise intolerance, abrupt pauses in the intrinsic rate, or inappropriately slow average ventricular rate, and also in asymptomatic patients with a wide complex escape rhythm, complex congenital heart disease, ventricular dysfunction, significant ventricular ectopy, or a long-QT interval.[29]

Dual-chamber pacing can be beneficial in some patients with marked first-degree AV block (more than 200 millisec-

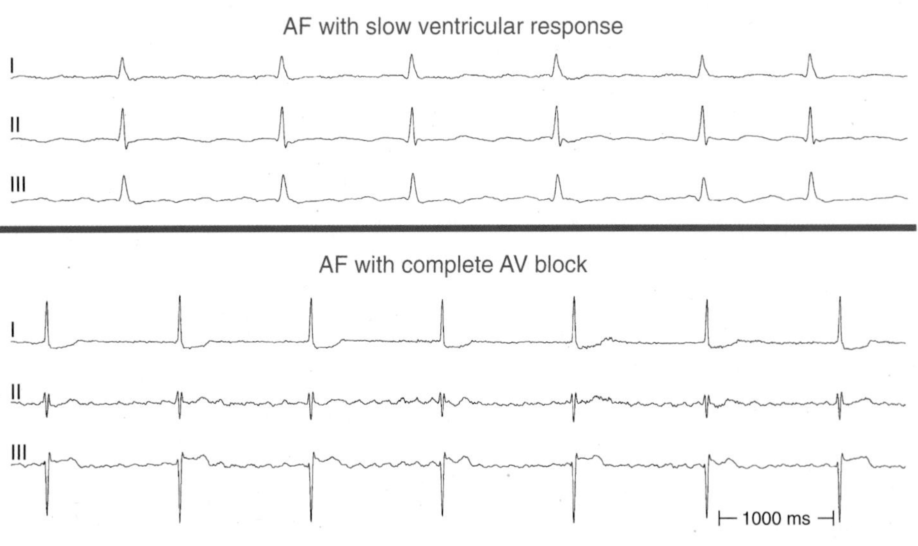

FIGURE 6–22 Atrial fibrillation (AF) with slow ventricular rate. **Upper panel,** The ventricular rhythm is irregular, indicating that it is the result of conducted atrial beats. **Lower panel,** The ventricular rhythm is regular, consistent with the presence of complete AV block and a regular junctional escape rhythm.

TABLE 6–1 Guidelines for Permanent Pacing in Acquired Atrioventricular Block in Adults

Class I
Third-degree and advanced second-degree AV block at any level, associated with any one of the following: · Symptomatic bradycardia · Ventricular arrhythmias presumed to be due to AV block · Arrhythmias and other conditions that require drugs that result in symptomatic bradycardia · Asymptomatic patients with documented periods of asystole ≥3.0 sec or any escape rate <40 beats/min, or with an escape rhythm that is below the AVN · After catheter ablation of the AV junction · Postoperative AV block that is not expected to resolve · Neuromuscular diseases, such as myotonic muscular dystrophy, Kearns-Sayre syndrome, Erb dystrophy (limb-girdle muscular dystrophy), and peroneal muscular atrophy, with or without symptoms · Awake, symptom-free patients with atrial fibrillation and bradycardia with 1 or more pauses of at least 5 sec · Average awake ventricular rates of 40 beats/min or faster if cardiomegaly or left ventricular dysfunction is present or if the site of block is below the AVN Second-degree AV block with associated symptomatic bradycardia regardless of type or site of block Second- or third-degree AV block during exercise in the absence of myocardial ischemia
Class IIa
Persistent third-degree AV block with an escape rate >40 beats/min in asymptomatic adult patients without cardiomegaly Asymptomatic second-degree AV block at intra- or infra-His levels found at electrophysiological study First- or second-degree AV block with symptoms similar to those of pacemaker syndrome or hemodynamic compromise Asymptomatic type II second-degree AV block with a narrow QRS. When type II second-degree AV block occurs with a wide QRS, including isolated right bundle-branch block, pacing becomes a class I recommendation
Class IIb
Neuromuscular diseases such as myotonic muscular dystrophy, Erb dystrophy (limb-girdle muscular dystrophy), and peroneal muscular atrophy with any degree of AV block (including first-degree AV block), with or without symptoms, because there may be unpredictable progression of AV conduction disease AV block in the setting of drug use and/or drug toxicity when the block is expected to recur even after the drug is withdrawn
Class III
Asymptomatic first-degree AV block Asymptomatic type I second-degree AV block at the AVN level or that which is not known to be intra- or infra-Hisian AV block that is expected to resolve and is unlikely to recur (e.g., drug toxicity, Lyme disease, or transient increases in vagal tone, or during hypoxia in sleep apnea syndrome in the absence of symptoms)

AV = atrioventricular; AVN = atrioventricular node; LV = left ventricle.

From Epstein AE, DiMarco JP, Ellenbogen KA, et al: ACC/AHA/HRS 2008 Guidelines for Device-Based Therapy of Cardiac Rhythm Abnormalities: a report of the American College of Cardiology/American Heart Association Task Force on Practice Guidelines (Writing Committee to Revise the ACC/AHA/NASPE 2002 Guideline Update for Implantation of Cardiac Pacemakers and Antiarrhythmia Devices): developed in collaboration with the American Association for Thoracic Surgery and Society of Thoracic Surgeons. Circulation 2008;117:e350-408.

onds) and symptoms similar to pacemaker syndrome, and in those with left ventricular (LV) dysfunction and heart failure symptoms in whom a shorter AV interval results in hemodynamic improvement, presumably by decreasing LA filling pressure. The latter recommendation, however, is now questionable because a conventional DDD(R) pacemaker with an optimized AV delay would have to pace the ventricle almost 100% of the time. The benefit of pacing with optimized AV synchrony (with a shorter AV delay) should be weighed against the impairment of LV function produced by RV pacing with resultant LV dyssynchrony. However, such a determination can be difficult or impossible.[25]

Temporary pacing is sometimes required in patients with acute MI (more often in anterior than inferior wall MI). Patients with asymptomatic first-degree or type 1 second-degree AV block do not require pacing. However, patients with type 2 second-degree or complete AV block should be temporarily paced, even if asymptomatic. In the setting of MI, the criteria for permanent pacing depends less on the presence of symptoms. If type 2 second-degree or complete AV block persists once past the periinfarct period, permanent pacing is indicated. Even if the type 2 or third-degree AV block was transient but associated with BBB that persists following resolution of the AV block, permanent pacing of the post MI patient improves long-term survival.[29]

Most patients with AV block require dual-chamber pacemakers to maintain AV synchrony, prevent development of pacemaker syndrome, and, possibly, prevent subsequent development of AF. In patients with normal sinus node function and AV block, VDD pacing using a single lead with a series of electrodes for atrial sensing and ventricular pacing and sensing is appropriate. In patients with chronic AF and bradycardia, rate-responsive single-chamber ventricular pacing (VVIR) is adequate.

REFERENCES

1. Rubart M, Zipes DP: Genesis of cardiac arrhythmias: Electrophysiological considerations. *In* Zipes DP, Libby P, Bonow R, Braunwald E (eds): Braunwald's Heart Disease: A Textbook of Cardiovascular Medicine, 7th ed. Philadelphia, WB Saunders, 2004, pp 653-688.
2. Cosio FG, Anderson RH, Kuck KH, et al: Living anatomy of the atrioventricular junctions. A guide to electrophysiologic mapping. A Consensus Statement from the Cardiac Nomenclature Study Group, Working Group of Arrhythmias, European Society of Cardiology, and the Task Force on Cardiac Nomenclature from NASPE. Circulation 1999;100:e31.
3. Lockwood D, Otomo K, Wang Z, et al: Electrophysiologic characteristics of atrioventricular nodal reentrant tachycardia: Implication for the reentrant circuits. *In* Zipes DP, Jalife J (eds): Cardiac Electrophysiology: From Cell to Bedside, 4th ed. Philadelphia, WB Saunders, 2004, pp 537-557.
4. Valderrabano M: Atypical atrioventricular nodal reentry with eccentric atrial activation. Is the right target on the left? Heart Rhythm 2007;4:433.
5. Anderson RH, Ho SY: The anatomy of the atrioventricular node (http://hrsonline.org/Education/SelfStudy/Articles/anderson_ho1.cfm).
6. Wu J, Olgin J, Miller J, Zipes DP: Mechanisms for atrioventricular nodal reentry and ventricular tachycardia determined from optical mapping of isolated perfused preparations. *In* Zipes DP, Haissaguerre M (eds): Catheter Ablation of Arrhythmias, 2nd ed. Armonk, NY, Futura, 2002, pp 1-29.
7. Luc PJ: Common form of atrioventricular nodal reentrant tachycardia: Do we really know the circuit we try to ablate? Heart Rhythm 2007;4:711.
8. Mazgalev T: AV nodal physiology (http://hrsonline.org/Education/SelfStudy/Articles/mazgalev.cfm).
9. Shryock J, Belardinelli L: Pharmacology of the AV node (http://hrsonline.org/Education/SelfStudy/Articles/shrbel.cfm).
10. Schwartzman D: Atrioventricular block and atrioventricular dissociation. *In* Zipes DP, Jalife J (eds): Cardiac Electrophysiology: From Cell to Bedside, 4th ed. Philadelphia, WB Saunders, 2004, pp 485-489.
11. Friedman DM, Rupel A, Buyon JP: Epidemiology, etiology, detection, and treatment of autoantibody-associated congenital heart block in neonatal lupus. Curr Rheumatol Rep 2007;9:101.
12. Jayaprasad N, Johnson F, Venugopal K: Congenital complete heart block and maternal connective tissue disease. Int J Cardiol 2006;112:153.
13. Walsh EP: Interventional electrophysiology in patients with congenital heart disease. Circulation 2007;115:3224.
14. Wolbrette DL, Naccarelli GV: Bradycardias: Sinus nodal dysfunction and atrioventricular conduction disturbances. *In* Topol E (ed): Textbook of Cardiovascular Medicine, 2nd ed. Philadelphia, Lippincott Williams & Wilkins, 2002, pp 1385-1402.
15. Wellens HJJ: Atrioventricular nodal and subnodal ventricular disturbances. *In* Willerson J, Cohn J, Wellens H Jr, Holmes D (eds): Cardiovascular Medicine. New York, Springer, 2007, pp 1991-1998.
16. Olgin JE, Zipes DP: Specific Arrhythmias: Diagnosis and Treatment. *In* Zipes DP, Libby P, Bonow R, Braunwald E (eds): Braunwald's Heart Disease: A Textbook of Cardiovascular Medicine, 7th ed. Philadelphia, WB Saunders, 2004, pp 803-864.
17. Sovari AA, Bodine CK, Farokhi F: Cardiovascular manifestations of myotonic dystrophy-1. Cardiol Rev 2007;15:191.

18. Gross GJ, Chiu CC, Hamilton RM, et al: Natural history of postoperative heart block in congenital heart disease: Implications for pacing intervention. Heart Rhythm 2006;3:601.
19. Tucker EM, Pyles LA, Bass JL, Moller JH: Permanent pacemaker for atrioventricular conduction block after operative repair of perimembranous ventricular septal defect. J Am Coll Cardiol 2007;50:1196.
20. Liberman L, Pass RH, Hordof AJ, Spotnitz HM: Late onset of heart block after open heart surgery for congenital heart disease. Pediatr Cardiol 2008;29:56.
21. Topilski I, Rogowski O, Glick A, et al: Catheter-induced mechanical trauma to fast and slow pathways during radiofrequency ablation of atrioventricular nodal reentry tachycardia: Incidence, predictors, and clinical implications. Pacing Clin Electrophysiol 2007;30:1233.
22. Shirayama T, Hadase M, Sakamoto T, et al: Swallowing syncope: Complex mechanisms of the reflex. Intern Med 2002;41:207.
23. Stein R, Medeiros CM, Rosito GA, et al: Intrinsic sinus and atrioventricular node electrophysiologic adaptations in endurance athletes. J Am Coll Cardiol 2002;39: 1033.
24. Barold SS, Hayes DL: Second-degree atrioventricular block: A reappraisal. Mayo Clin Proc 2001;76:44.
25. Barold SS, Ilercil A, Leonelli F, Herweg B: First-degree atrioventricular block. Clinical manifestations, indications for pacing, pacemaker management and consequences during cardiac resynchronization. J Interv Card Electrophysiol 2006;17:139.
26. Josephson ME: Atrioventricular conduction. *In* Josephson ME (ed): Clinical Cardiac Electrophysiology: Techniques and Interpretations, 3rd ed. Philadelphia, Lippincott, Williams & Wilkins, 2002, pp 92-109.
27. Fisch C, Knoebel SB: Atrioventricular and ventriculoatrial conduction and blocks, gap, and overdrive suppression. *In* Fisch C, Knoebel SB (eds): Electrocardiography of Clinical Arrhythmias. Armonk, NY, Futura, 2000, pp 315-344.
28. Fisch C, Knoebel SB. Atrioventricular conduction abnormalities. *In* Fisch C, Knoebel SB (eds): Electrocardiography of Clinical Arrhythmias. Armonk, NY, Futura, 2000, pp 129-149.
29. Gregoratos G, Abrams J, Epstein AE, et al: ACC/AHA/NASPE 2002 Guideline Update for Implantation of Cardiac Pacemakers and Antiarrhythmia Devices—summary article: A report of the American College of Cardiology/American Heart Association Task Force on Practice Guidelines (ACC/AHA/NASPE Committee to Update the 1998 Pacemaker Guidelines). J Am Coll Cardiol 2002;40:1703.

CHAPTER 7

Intraventricular Conduction Abnormalities

GENERAL CONSIDERATIONS

Transient Bundle Branch Block

The term *aberration* is used to describe transient bundle branch block (BBB) and does not include QRS abnormalities caused by preexisting BBB, Wolff-Parkinson-White (WPW) conduction, or the effect of drugs. Transient BBB can have several mechanisms, including phase 3 block, phase 4 block, and concealed conduction. Those mechanisms of aberration can occur anywhere in the His-Purkinje system (HPS) and, unlike chronic BBB, the site of block during aberration can shift. Right bundle branch block (RBBB) is the most common pattern of aberration, occurring in 80% of patients with aberration, and in up to 100% of aberration in normal hearts.[1-7]

Phase 3 Block

Conduction velocity depends, in part, on the rate of rise of phase 0 of the action potential (dV/dt) and the height to which it rises (V_{max}). These factors in turn depend on the membrane potential at the time of stimulation. The more negative the membrane potential, the more fast sodium channels are available for activation, the greater the influx of Na^+ into the cell during phase 0, and the greater the conduction velocity. Therefore, when stimulation occurs during phase 3, before full recovery and at less negative potentials of the cell membrane, a portion of the sodium channels will still be refractory and unavailable for activation. Consequently, the Na^+ current and phase 0 of the next action potential will be reduced, and conduction will then be slower.[5,8-10]

Phase 3 block, also called tachycardia-dependent block, occurs when an impulse arrives at tissues that are still refractory caused by incomplete repolarization. Manifestations of phase 3 block include BBB and fascicular block, as well as complete atrioventricular (AV) block.[2,11]

Functional or physiological phase 3 aberration can occur in normal fibers if the impulse is sufficiently premature to encroach on the physiological refractory period of the preceding beat, when the membrane potential is still reduced. This is commonly seen with very early premature atrial complexes (PACs) that conduct aberrantly. Phase 3 aberration can also occur pathologically if electrical systole and/or the refractory period are abnormally prolonged (with refractoriness extending beyond the action potential duration or the QT interval) and the involved fascicle is stimulated at a relatively rapid rate.[2,11] Transient left bundle branch block (LBBB) is less common than RBBB (25% of phase 3 aberration is of the LBBB type). The block usually occurs in the very proximal portion of the bundle branch.[5,9,10]

Phase 3 block constitutes the physiological explanation of several phenomena, including aberration caused by premature excitation, Ashman's phenomenon, and acceleration-dependent aberration.

Aberration Caused by Premature Excitation. Premature excitation can cause aberration (BBB) by encroaching on the refractory period of the bundle branch prior to full recovery of the action potential, namely during the so-called voltage-dependent refractoriness (see Fig. 2-29).[11] In normal hearts, this type of aberration is almost always in the form of RBBB, whereas such aberration in the abnormal heart can be that of RBBB or LBBB.

The left bundle (LB) effective refractory period (ERP) is shorter than that of the right bundle (RB) at normal heart rates. At faster heart rates, the ERP of both bundle branches shortens; however, at faster rates, the RB ERP shortens to a greater degree than LB ERP, so that the duration of the refractory periods of the two bundles cross over, and the LB ERP becomes longer than that of the RB. This explains the tendency of aberration to be in the form of RBBB when premature excitation occurs during normal heart rates, and in the form of LBBB when it occurs during fast heart rates.[1,2,5,8-10,12]

Ashman's Phenomenon. Ashman's phenomenon refers to aberration occurring when a short cycle follows a long one (long-short cycle sequence) (Fig. 7-1).[11,13] Aberrancy is caused by the physiological changes of the conduction system refractory periods associated with the R-R interval. Normally, the refractory period of the HPS lengthens as the heart rate slows and shortens as the heart rate increases, even when heart rate changes are abrupt. Thus,

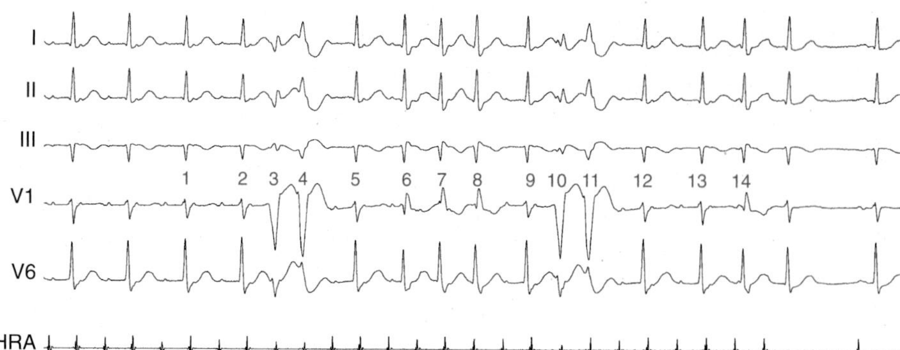

FIGURE 7–1 Atrial tachycardia (AT) with variable atrioventricular (AV) conduction and intermittent aberrancy. **Left,** AT with 2 : 1 AV conduction and normal QRS morphology is observed. Once 1 : 1 AV conduction occurs (QRS 3), left bundle branch block (LBBB) aberration develops (caused by long-short cycle sequence, phase 3 block, Ashman's phenomenon). Phase 3 block develops during QRS 6 but this time it manifests as a right bundle branch block (RBBB) pattern. This is because activation during QRS 4 propagated down the RB and across the septum, activating the LB after some delay (concealed transseptal conduction), so that the LB-LB interval (following QRS 4) and the LB effective refractory period (ERP) became shorter, whereas the RB-RB interval (following QRS 4) was longer and, consequently, the RB ERP was still prolonged following QRS 5, setting the stage for a long-short cycle sequence and RBBB aberration. This scenario is repeated during the following two cycles, but this time the LB-LB interval (following QRS 8 and 9) exhibits long-short cycle sequence and underlies LBBB aberration. Ashman's phenomenon underlies RBBB aberration during QRS 14. Aberration during QRS is secondary to either concealed transseptal conduction or rate-dependent BBB. However, because contralateral BBB was observed during QRS 4 and 11 versus QRS 8 (although those QRSs occurred following a similar cycle length), concealed transseptal conduction is more likely to be the mechanism of aberration.

aberrant conduction can result when a short cycle follows
a long R-R interval. In this scenario, the QRS complex that
7 ends the long pause will be conducted normally but creates
a prolonged ERP of the bundle branches. If the next QRS complex occurs after a short coupling interval, it may be conducted aberrantly, because one of the bundles is still refractory as a result of a lengthening of the refractory period (phase 3 block; see Fig. 7-1).[5-7]

RBBB aberration is more common than LBBB in this setting because the RB has a longer ERP than the LB. Because of the irregularity of the ventricular response during atrial fibrillation (AF), the long-short cycle sequence occurs commonly, and Ashman's phenomenon is seen frequently during AF.

The aberrancy can be present for one beat and have a morphology resembling a premature ventricular complex (PVC), or can involve several sequential complexes, suggesting ventricular tachycardia (VT). In the case of aberrancy during AF, Ashman's phenomenon (long-short cycle sequence) may not be helpful in differentiating aberration from ventricular ectopy. Although a long cycle (pause) sets the stage for Ashman's phenomenon, it also tends to precipitate ventricular ectopy. Furthermore, concealed conduction occurs frequently during AF and, therefore, it is never possible to know from the surface ECG exactly when a bundle branch is activated. Thus, if an aberrant beat does end a long-short cycle sequence during AF, it can be because of refractoriness of a bundle branch secondary to concealed conduction into it rather than because of changes in the length of the ventricular cycle.[8-10,12]

Nevertheless, there are several features of ventricular ectopy that may help distinguish a PVC from an aberrantly conducted or Ashman's beat in the presence of AF. PVCs are usually followed by a longer R-R cycle, indicating the occurrence of a compensatory pause, the result of retrograde conduction into the atrioventricular node (AVN) and anterograde block of the impulse originating in the atrium. A ventricular origin is also likely when there is a fixed coupling cycle between the normal and aberrated QRS complexes. The presence of long and identical R-R cycles after the aberrated beats and the absence of a long-short cycle sequence associated with the wide or aberrated QRS complex also suggest ventricular ectopy. Additionally, the absence of aberrancy, despite the presence of R-R CL combinations that are longer and shorter than those associated with the wide QRS complex, suggests ventricular ectopy. QRS morphology inconsistent with LBBB or RBBB aberrancy argues against aberration (Fig. 7-2).[5,8-10,12]

Aberration caused by Ashman's phenomenon can persist for a number of cycles. The persistence of aberration can reflect a time-dependent adjustment of refractoriness of the bundle branch to an abrupt change in CL, or it can be the result of concealed transseptal activation (see later).

Aberration Caused by Heart Rate Acceleration. As the heart rate accelerates, the HPS refractory period shortens; normal conduction tends to be preserved because of this response. Conversely, the refractory period lengthens as the heart rate slows. Acceleration-dependent BBB is a result of failure of the action potential of the bundle branches to shorten or, in fact, paradoxically, it lengthens, in response to acceleration of the heart rate (Fig. 7-3).[2,11] The ERP of the RB normally shortens to a greater degree than that of the LB at faster heart rates, explaining the more frequent RBBB aberration at longer cycle lengths (CLs) than at shorter CLs.[3,8-10]

This form of aberration is a marker of some type of cardiac abnormality when it appears at relatively slow heart rate (frequently less than 70 beats/min), displays LBBB, appears after a number of cycles of accelerated but regular rate, and/or appears with gradual rather than abrupt acceleration of the heart rate and frequently at CL shortening less than 5 millliseconds. Because of the small changes in duration of the CL that may initiate aberration (critical cycle), recognition of acceleration-dependent aberration may require a long record to document the gradual, and at times minimal, shortening of the R-R interval.[8-10]

With increasing heart rate or persistence of fast heart rate, acceleration-dependent aberration can occasionally disappear. The normalization of a previously aberrant QRS complex can be explained by a greater shortening of the ERP of the bundle branches than that of the AVN and/or a time-dependent gradual shortening of the refractory period of the

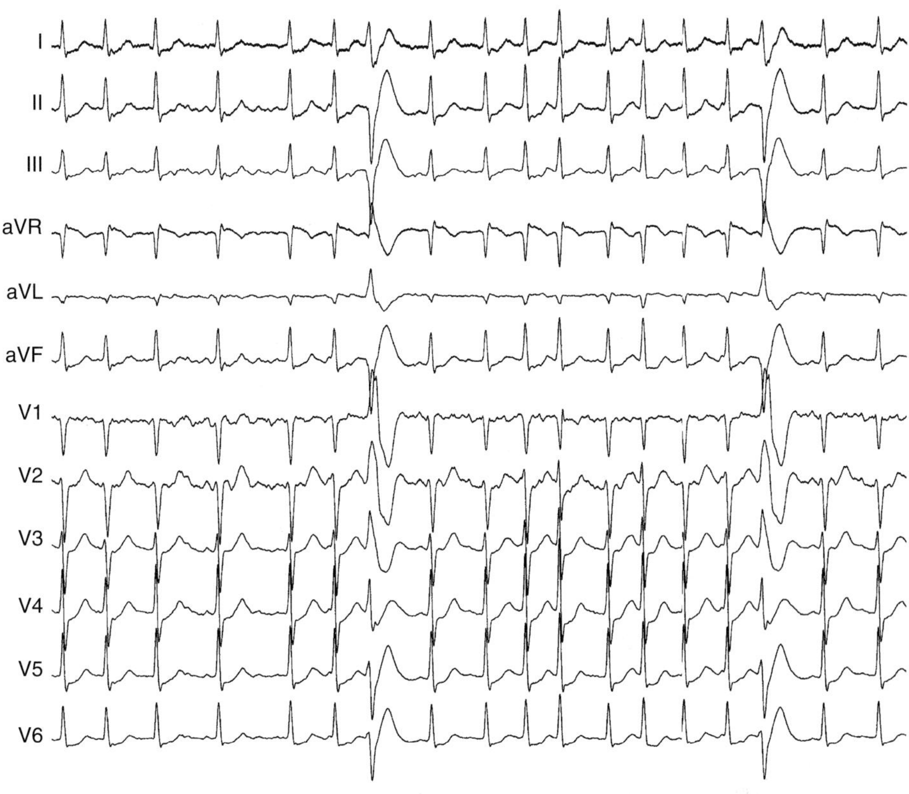

FIGURE 7–2 Premature ventricular complexes (PVCs) during atrial fibrillation (AF). Several features suggest that the wide QRS complexes are caused by ventricular ectopy rather than aberration. QRS morphology is inconsistent with LBBB or RBBB aberrancy. Additionally, there is a fixed coupling cycle between the normal and aberrated QRS complex. The absence of a long-short cycle sequence associated with the wide QRS complex and the absence of aberrancy despite the presence of R-R cycle length combinations that are longer and shorter than those associated with the wide QRS complex also suggest ventricular ectopy.

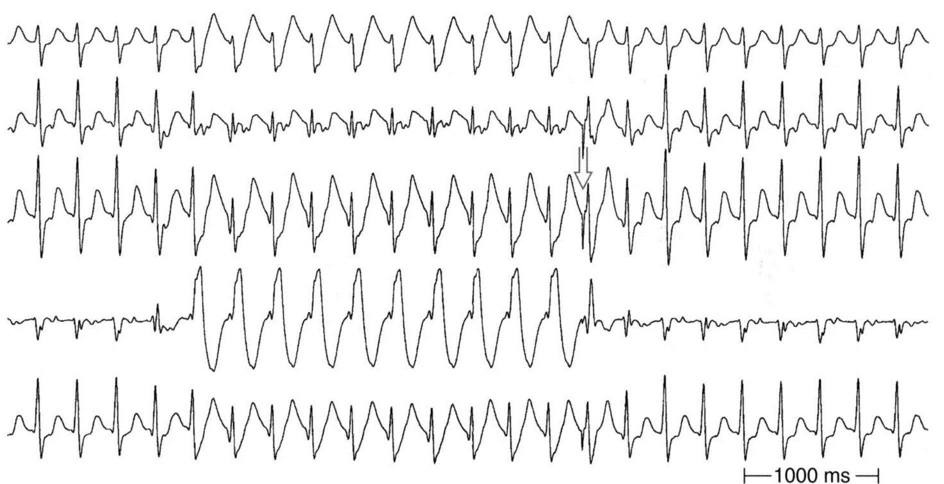

FIGURE 7–3 Supraventricular tachycardia (SVT) with tachycardia-dependent (phase 3) right bundle branch block. Delivery of a late ventricular extrastimulus (arrow) during the SVT preexcites the right bundle branch (and either peels back or shortens its refractoriness) and restores normal conduction.

affected bundle branch (a phenomenon occasionally referred to as restitution).[5]

During slowing of the heart rate, intraventricular conduction often fails to normalize at the critical CL and aberration persists at cycles longer than the critical cycle that initiated the aberration. Once acceleration-dependent BBB is established, the actual cycle for the blocked bundle does not begin until approximately halfway through the QRS complex because of concealed transseptal conduction (see later); thus, it is necessary for the heart rate to slow down more than would be expected to reestablish normal conduction.[8-10]

Phase 4 Block

Phase 4 block occurs when conduction of an impulse is blocked in tissues well after their normal refractory periods have ended.[2,11] Phase 4 block is governed by the same physiological principles as those for phase 3 block. Membrane responsiveness is determined by the relationship of the membrane potential at excitation to the maximum height of phase 0. The availability of the sodium channels is reduced at less negative membrane potentials, and activation at a reduced membrane potential is likely to cause aberration or block.[5]

The cause of membrane depolarization (i.e., reduction of membrane potential) in the case of phase 4 block, however, is different from that in phase 3 block. Enhanced phase 4 depolarization within the bundle branches can be caused by enhanced automaticity and/or partial depolarization of injured myocardial tissue. In such a case, the maximum diastolic potential immediately follows repolarization, from which point the membrane potential is steadily reduced (by the pacemaker current), which in turn results in inactivation of some sodium channels. Thus, an action potential initiated early in the cycle (immediately after repolarization) would have a steeper and higher phase 0 and consequently better conduction than would an action potential initiated later in the cycle, when the membrane potential at the time of the stimulus can be reduced, resulting in reduction in the velocity and height of phase 0 and slower conduction.[8-10,12]

Phase 4 aberration is one explanation for the development of aberration at the end of a long cycle. As a result of a gradual spontaneous depolarization made possible by a prolonged cycle, the cell is activated from a less negative potential, resulting in impaired conduction. This type of aberration is sometimes referred to as bradycardia-dependent BBB.[5]

Phase 4 aberration would be expected in the setting of bradycardia or enhanced normal automaticity. However, despite the fact that bradycardia is common and cells with phase 4 depolarization are abundant, phase 4 block is not commonly seen; most reported cases are associated with structural heart disease. One explanation for this phenomenon is that in normal fibers, conduction is well maintained at membrane potentials more negative than −70 to −75 mV. Significant conduction disturbances are first manifested when the membrane potential is less negative than −70 mV at the time of stimulation; local block appears at −65 to −60 mV. Because the threshold potential for normal His-Purkinje fibers is −70 mV, spontaneous firing occurs before the membrane can actually be reduced to the potential necessary for conduction impairment or block. Phase 4 block is therefore pathological when it does occur, and it requires one or more of the following: (1) the presence of slow diastolic depolarization, which needs to be enhanced; (2) a decrease in excitability (a shift in threshold potential toward
7 zero) so that, in the presence of significant bradycardia, sufficient time elapses before the impulse arrives, enabling the bundle branch fibers to reach a potential at which conduction is impaired; and (3) a deterioration in membrane responsiveness so that significant conduction impairment develops at −75 mV instead of −65 mV; this occurrence would also negate the necessity for such a long cycle before conduction falters.[8-10,12]

Bradycardia-dependent or phase 4 block almost always manifests a LBBB pattern, likely because the LV conduction system is more susceptible to ischemic damage and has a higher rate of spontaneous phase 4 depolarization than the right ventricle (RV).[2]

Both tachycardia-dependent and bradycardia-dependent BBB can be seen in the same patient with an intermediate range of CLs associated with normal conduction. The prognosis of rate-dependent BBB largely depends on the presence and severity of the underlying heart disease. Its clinical implications are not clear, and it usually occurs in diseased tissue and in the setting of myocardial infarction (MI), especially inferior wall MI.[5]

Aberration Caused by Concealed Transseptal Conduction

Concealed transseptal conduction is the underlying mechanism of aberration occurring in several situations, including perpetuation of aberrant conduction during tachyarrhythmias, unexpected persistence of acceleration-dependent aberration, and alternation of aberration during atrial bigeminal rhythm.[8-12,14,15]

Perpetuation of Aberrant Conduction During Tachyarrhythmias. During a supraventricular tachycardia (SVT) with normal ventricular activation, a PVC originating from the LV can activate the LB early, conduct transseptally, and then activate the RB retrogradely. Consequently, while the LB ERP expires in time for the next SVT impulse, the RB remains refractory because its actual cycle began later than the LB. Therefore, the next SVT impulse traveling down the His bundle (HB) encounters an excitable LB and a refractory RB; thus, it propagates to the LV over the LB (with an RBBB pattern, phase 3 aberration). Conduction subsequently propagates from the LV across the septum to the RV. By this time, the distal RB has recovered, allowing for retrograde penetration of the RB by the SVT impulse propagating transseptally, thereby rendering the RB refractory to each subsequent SVT impulse. This scenario is repeated and the RBBB pattern continues until another, well-timed PVC preexcites the RB (and either peels back or shortens its refractoriness) so that the next impulse from above finds the RB fully recovered (see Fig. 7-3).[3,14,15]

Unexpected Persistence of Acceleration-Dependent Aberration. Acceleration-dependent BBB develops at a critical rate faster than the rate at which it disappears. This paradox is most commonly ascribed to concealed conduction from the contralateral conducting bundle branch across the septum with delayed activation of the blocked bundle. Such concealed transseptal activation results in a bundle branch–to–bundle branch interval shorter than the manifest R-R cycle, because the actual cycle for the blocked bundle does not begin until approximately halfway through the QRS complex, because it takes 60 to 100 milliseconds for the impulse to propagate down the RB and transseptally reach the blocked LB. Consequently, for normal conduction to resume, the cycle during deceleration (R-R interval) must be longer than the critical cycle during acceleration by at least 60 to 100 milliseconds.[8-10,12,14,15]

However, unexpected delay of normalization of conduction cannot always be explained by concealed conduction. Sometimes, conduction normalizes with slowing of the heart rate only to recur at cycles that are still longer than the critical cycle. Such a sequence excludes transseptal concealment as the mechanism of recurrence of the aberration. Similarly, when the discrepancy between the critical cycle and the cycle at which normalization finally occurs is longer than the expected transseptal activation time (approximately 60 milliseconds in the normal heart and 100 milliseconds in the diseased states), transseptal concealment alone cannot explain the delay. Fatigue and overdrive suppression have been suggested as possible mechanisms of the delay of normalization of conduction.[8-10]

Alternation of Aberration During Atrial Bigeminal Rhythm. A bigeminal rhythm can be caused by atrial bigeminy, 3:2 AV block, or atrial flutter (AFL) with alternating 2:1 and 4:1 AV conduction. The alternation can be between a normal QRS complex and BBB or between RBBB and LBBB.

When alternation occurs between a normal QRS complex and RBBB during atrial bigeminy, the ERP of both RB and LB starts simultaneously following the normally conducted PAC, and the ERP of both branches is relatively short because of the preceding short cycle. After the pause, the sinus beat conducts normally and the ERP of both bundle branches starts simultaneously but will be relatively long because of the preceding long cycle. However, because the RB ERP is relatively longer than that of the LB, the next PAC encroaches on the RB refractoriness and conducts with an RBBB pattern (phase 3 block). Subsequently, that PAC is conducted down the LB and across the septum, activating the RB after some delay (concealed transseptal conduction), so that the RB-RB interval (during the following pause) and the RB ERP will become shorter. As a result, by the time the next PAC reaches the RB, the RB is fully recovered because of its abbreviated ERP (reflecting the shorter preceding RB-RB interval, which is shorter than the manifest R-R interval during the preceding pause), and normal conduction occurs (see Fig. 7-1).[14,15]

The same phenomenon (concealed transseptal conduction) explains alternating RBBB and LBBB. In the presence of RBBB, transseptal concealed conduction from the LB to the RB shortens the RB-to-RB interval relative to the now longer LB-to-LB interval. As a result, the ERP of the LB is longer and conduction in the LB fails. In the presence of a refractory LB, conduction proceeds along the RB. The delayed transseptal activation of the LB shortens the LB-to-LB interval. The ERP of the RB is now relatively longer, because RB conduction is blocked.[8-10,12]

Chronic Bundle Branch Block

Anatomical Considerations

Normal ventricular activation requires the synchronized participation of the distal components of the specialized conduction system, that is, the main bundle branches and their ramification. An intraventricular conduction defect (IVCD) is the result of abnormal activation of the ventricles caused by conduction delay or block in one or more parts of the specialized conduction system. Abnormalities of local myocardial activation can further alter the specific pattern of activation in that ventricle.[5]

Traditionally, three major fascicles are considered to be operative in normal persons: the RB, the left anterior fascicle (LAF), and the left posterior fascicle (LPF) branches of the LB. An estimated 65% of individuals have a third fascicle of the LB, the left median fascicle (LMF). The HB divides at the junction of the fibrous and muscular boundaries of the intraventricular septum into the RB and LB. The RB is an anatomically compact unit that travels as the extension of the HB after the origin of the LB. The LB and its divisions are, unlike the RB, diffuse structures that fan out just beyond their origin. The LAF represents the superior (anterior) division of the LB, the LPF represents the inferior (posterior) division of the LB, and the LMF represents the septal (median) division of the LB.[5]

The terminal Purkinje fibers connect the ends of the bundle branches to the ventricular myocardium. The Purkinje fibers form interweaving networks on the endocardial surface of both ventricles and penetrate only the inner third of the endocardium, and they tend to be less concentrated at the base of the ventricle and at the papillary muscle tips. The Purkinje fibers facilitate an almost simultaneous propagation of the cardiac impulse to the entire right and left ventricular endocardium.[5]

Characteristics of the Right Bundle. The RB is a long, thin, discrete, and vulnerable structure that consists of fast response Purkinje fibers. The RB courses down the right side of interventricular septum near the endocardium in its upper third, deeper in the muscular portion of the septum in the middle third, and then again near the endocardium in its lower third. The RB does not divide throughout most of its course, and begins to ramify as it approaches the base of the right anterior papillary muscle, with fascicles going to the septal and free walls of the RV.

The RB consists of a bundle of Purkinje cells covered by a dense sheath of connective tissue. The Purkinje cells are specialized to conduct rapidly, at 1 to 3 m/sec, because phase 0 of the action potential is dependent on the rapid inward Na^+ current. The RB is vulnerable to stretch and trauma for two thirds of its course when it is near the subendocardial surface.

Chronic RBBB pattern can result from three levels of conduction delay in the RV—proximal, distal, or terminal.[2] Proximal RBBB is the most common site of conduction delay. Distal RBBB occurs at the level of the moderator band, and it is an unusual site of conduction delay unless there has been transection of the moderator band during surgery. Terminal RBBB involves the distal conduction system of the RB or, more likely, the ventricular muscle itself, and it can be produced by ventriculotomy or transatrial resection of parietal bands in repair of tetralogy of Fallot.

In addition, RBBB can be induced by events in the HB, because certain fibers of the HB are organized longitudinally and predestined to activate only one fascicle or bundle branch. Disease in these areas can result in activation that is asynchronous from that in the rest of the infranodal conducting system, possibly resulting in a bundle branch or fascicular block.

Characteristics of the Left Bundle and Its Fascicles. The main LB penetrates the membranous portion of the interventricular septum under the aortic ring and then divides into several fairly discrete branches. The components of the LB are the predivisional segment, the LAF, the LPF, and the LMF.[2] The LAF crosses the left ventricular outflow tract (LVOT) and terminates in the Purkinje system of the anterolateral wall of the LV. The LPF appears as an extension of the main LB and is large in its initial course. It then fans out extensively posteriorly toward the papillary muscle and inferoposteriorly to the free wall of the LV. The LMF runs to the interventricular septum, and it arises in most cases from the LPF, less frequently from the LAF or from both, and in a few cases has an independent origin from the central part of the main LB at the site of its bifurcation.[16]

The clinical presentation of conduction disturbances in order of decreasing incidence is LAF block, RBBB, LBBB, and lastly LPF block. This rank depends not only on the intrinsic, anatomic, and genetically determined differences among branches and fascicles but also on the manner in which the intraventricular conduction system is exposed to the various pathological processes of the surrounding cardiac structures. The LAF can be injured by diseases that involve primarily the LVOT, the anterior half of the ventricular septum, and the anterolateral LV wall. In fact, isolated LAF block is the most common type of intraventricular conduction defect seen in acute anterior MI. Other pathologies that can also cause LAF block are hypertension, cardiomyopathies, aortic valve disease, Lev and Lenègre diseases, spontaneous and surgical closure of a ventricular septal defect, and other surgical procedures.[16-19]

In contrast, the LPF is the least vulnerable segment of the whole system because it is short and wide and is located in the inflow tract of the LV, which is a less turbulent region than the outflow tract. Additionally, the LPF has a dual blood supply, from the anterior and posterior descending coronary arteries, and it is not related to structures that are so potentially dangerous.[16]

The main LB and its fascicles consist of Purkinje fibers that conduct rapidly at 1 to 3 m/sec, because phase 0 is dependent on the rapid inward sodium current, resulting in almost simultaneous depolarization of the terminal HPS and the adjacent ventricular myocardium. The location of conduction delay in LBBB can be proximal (particularly in diffuse myocardial disease), distal, or a combination of both.

Site of Block

Interest in the site of block stems from the fact that bifascicular block (especially RBBB and LAF block) is the most common ECG pattern preceding the development of AV block. Determining the site of block, therefore, can help predict the risk of AV block.

Despite ECG anatomic correlates, the site of block producing BBB patterns is not certain in all cases. Data suggest that fibers to the RV and LV are already predestined within the HB and that lesions in the HB can produce characteristic BBB patterns. Longitudinal dissociation with asynchronous conduction in the HB can give rise to abnormal patterns of ventricular activation; hence, the conduction problem may not necessarily lie in the individual bundle branch. Moreover, it is not uncommon for intra-Hisian disease to be accompanied with BBB (especially LBBB).[2] Pacing distal to the site of block can normalize the QRS. Furthermore, the problem may not be actual block, because conduction *delay* within the bundle in the range of 10 milliseconds can give rise to an ECG pattern of BBB.

Clinical Relevance

The prognosis of BBB is related largely to the type and severity of the underlying heart disease and to the possible presence of other conduction disturbances. BBB in the absence of apparent structural heart disease and not associated with block in the other fascicles is usually benign. Bifascicular block (especially RBBB and LAF block) is the most common ECG pattern preceding complete heart block in adults. Other forms of IVCD precede the bulk of the remaining cases of complete intra- and infra-Hisian AV block. The incidence of progression to complete AV block is approximately 2% in asymptomatic patients with an IVCD, and approximately 6% in patients with an IVCD and neurological symptoms (such as syncope).[20,21]

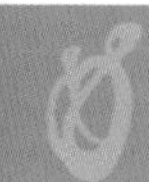

Patients with BBB have an unusually high incidence of cardiac disease and sudden cardiac death. The highest incidence of sudden cardiac death is among patients with LBBB and cardiac disease.[20-23] Most sudden cardiac deaths are caused by VT–ventricular fibrilation (VF), do not seem to be related to AV block, and are not prevented by pacemakers (although pacing can potentially relieve symptoms such as syncope). Complete electrophysiologial (EP) testing and ventricular stimulation are, therefore, necessary in patients with syncope and BBB because VT can be found in 30% to 50%. Although the poor prognosis associated with BBB is related to myocardial dysfunction, heart failure, and VF rather than heart block, symptoms such as syncope are often related to heart block.[24-26]

RBBB is a common finding in the general population. In patients without evidence of structural heart disease, RBBB has no prognostic significance. However, new-onset RBBB does predict a higher rate of coronary artery disease, heart failure, and cardiovascular mortality. When cardiac disease is present, the coexistence of RBBB suggests advanced disease.[18,27]

Isolated LAF block does not imply by itself a risk factor of cardiac morbidity or mortality. In a healthy population, it can be regarded as an incidental ECG finding.[16,18]

LPF block is a rare finding, and rather nonspecific for cardiac disease. LPF block is almost invariably associated with RBBB, in that LPF block and RBBB share cause, pathogenesis, and prognosis. LPF block plus RBBB in acute MI is associated with a high mortality rate (80% to 87%) during the first weeks after the coronary event. Similarly, the risk of progression toward complete AV block (a form of trifascicular block) is also considerable (42%), and approximately 75% of these patients die from pump failure.[16,18]

ELECTROCARDIOGRAPHIC FEATURES

Bundle Branch Block

The ECG criteria of different types fascicular and bundle branch block are listed in Table 7-1. The ECG pattern of BBB can represent complete block or conduction delay (relative to the other fascicles) producing asynchronous ventricular activation without necessarily implying complete failure of conduction in the diseased fascicle. Therefore, an ECG pattern of complete BBB can have varying degrees or alternate with contralateral complete BBB, phenomena explained by a delay rather than complete block as the underlying pathophysiology of the ECG pattern.[2,21,28]

TABLE 7–1 ECG Criteria for Fascicular and Bundle Branch Block

Complete RBBB
QRS duration ≥ 120 msec Broad, notched secondary R waves (rsr′, rsR′, or rSR′ patterns) in right precordial leads (V_1 and V_2) Wide, deep S waves (qRS pattern) in left precordial leads (V_5 and V_6) Delayed intrinsicoid deflection (>50 msec) in right precordial leads
Complete LBBB
QRS duration ≥ 120 msec Broad, notched, monophasic R waves in V_5 and V_6, and usually in leads I and aVL Small or absent initial r waves in V_1 and V_2, followed by deep S waves (rS or QS patterns) Absent septal q waves in left-sided leads (leads I, V_5, and V_6) Delayed intrinsicoid deflection (>60 msec) in V_5 and V_6 ST segment and T wave directed opposite to the predominant deflection of the QRS complex
LAF Block
Frontal plane mean QRS axis of −45 to −90 degrees rS patterns in leads II, III, and aVF (the S wave in lead III is deeper than lead II) qR pattern in aVL Delayed intrinsicoid deflection in aVL QRS duration <120 msec
LPF Block
Frontal plane of mean QRS axis ≥100 degrees rS pattern in leads I and aVL , and qR patterns in leads II, III, and aVF (S1-Q3 pattern) QRS duration <110 msec Exclusion of other factors causing right axis deviation (right ventricular overload patterns, lateral MI) Delayed intrinsicoid deflection in aVF

LAF = left anterior fascicle; LBBB = left bundle branch block; LPF = left posterior fascicle; MI = myocardial infarction; RBBB = right bundle branch block.

BBB leads to prolongation of the QRS duration and sometimes to alterations in the QRS vector. The degree of prolongation of the QRS duration depends on the severity of the impairment. With complete BBB, the QRS is 120 milliseconds or longer in duration; with incomplete BBB, the QRS duration is 100 to 120 milliseconds. The QRS vector in BBB is generally oriented in the direction of the myocardial region in which depolarization is delayed.

BBB is characteristically associated with secondary repolarization (ST-T) abnormalities. The T wave is typically opposite in polarity to the last deflection of the QRS, a discordance that is caused by the altered sequence of repolarization that occurs secondary to altered depolarization.

Right Bundle Branch Block

Development of RBBB alters the activation sequence of the RV but not the LV. Thus, changes in the morphological features of local electrograms can be recorded only in the RV. Because the LB is not affected, the initial septal activation (the initial 30 milliseconds of the QRS complex), which depends on the LB, remains normal, occurring from left to right, and results in septal q waves in leads I, aVL, and V_6 and r waves in leads V_1, V_2, and aVR.[18,27] Thus, the Q wave of a prior MI remains unchanged.

Septal activation is followed by LV activation (within the subsequent 40 to 60 milliseconds), occurring over the LB in a leftward and posterior vector, resulting in R waves in leads I, aVL, and V_6 as well as an s (or S) waves in V_1 and V_2. This appearance is usually similar to that in normal subjects. The asynchronous depolarization caused by RBBB is primarily manifested in the later portion of the QRS, at 80 milliseconds and beyond. During this time, RV activation spreads slowly by conduction through working muscle fibers rather than the specialized conduction system, and occurs predominantly after activation of the LV has been completed. The forces generated by the late, unopposed RV free wall activation result in a terminal rightward and anterior positivity, manifesting as S waves in the left-right leads (I, aVL, and V_6) and a second positive deflection that can be small (r′) or large (R′) in the anterior-posterior leads (V_1 and V_2; Fig. 7-4).[2,18,27]

The QRS axis is unaffected by RBBB; left or right axis deviation can indicate concurrent LAF or LPF block, respectively (see Fig. 7-4).

RBBB also results in an abnormality of ventricular repolarization of the RV myocardium. Thus, there are often secondary ST segment and T wave changes present in the right precordial leads. The ST segment change is usually small but, when present, is discordant (i.e., has an axis in the opposite direction) to the terminal mean QRS spatial vector. The T wave also tends to be discordant to the terminal conduction disturbance, resulting in inverted T waves in the right precordial leads (where there is a terminal R′ wave) and upright T waves in the left precordial leads (where there is a terminal S wave).

Atypical Right Bundle Branch Block. Some patients have an atypical RBBB pattern caused by anterior displacement of the usually posterior midtemporal forces. This change is characterized by attenuation or loss of posterior deflections in the anterior-posterior leads, resulting in an rsR′, qR, or M-shaped QRS pattern in V_1. There are three mechanisms that can account for this pattern—normal variant; a gain of midtemporal anterior forces caused by RV enlargement or by concurrent LAF block; and a loss of posterior forces caused by a posterior wall MI.

Incomplete Right Bundle Branch Block. An incomplete RBBB can result from lesser degrees of conduction delay in the RB. RBBB is arbitrarily said to be complete when the QRS duration is over 120 milliseconds and incomplete when it is between 100 and 120 milliseconds (see Fig. 7-4). An RBBB pattern with a QRS duration shorter than 100 milliseconds can be a normal variant, presumably reflecting a slight delay in the terminal posterobasal forces in some individuals.[18]

Left Bundle Branch Block

The normal sequence of ventricular activation is altered dramatically in LBBB. Complete LBBB results in delayed and abnormal activation and diffuse slowing of conduction throughout the LV. Activation of the LV originates from the RB in a right to left direction, in contrast to the normal situation in which the first part of the LV myocardium to be activated is the septum via a small septal branch of the LB, with subsequent impulse spread in a left to right direction.[18]

LBBB results in reversal of the direction of the initial septal activation sequence (within the initial 30 milliseconds of the QRS complex), with the activation traveling from right to left and from apex to base and to the RV apex and free ventricular wall. However, the septum is a larger structure than the RV free wall; thus, septal activation predominates. The resultant vector is to the left and usually anterior, resulting in loss of the normal small q waves and initiation of a wide, slurred R wave in leads I, aVL, and V_6. In addition, an rS or QS pattern is seen in V1 (Fig. 7-5). Pseudonormalization of septal depolarization in LBBB (i.e., the reappearance of a q wave in leads I and V_6) can reflect damage (infarct) to the septum.[18] Thus, the Q wave of a prior MI becomes lost, and new Q waves can emerge.

Following septal activation, LV activation (starting as late as 30 to 50 milliseconds into the QRS) spreads slowly by conduction through working muscle fibers rather than the specialized conduction system, with spatial vectors oriented to the left and posteriorly because the LV is a leftward and posterior structure. The spatial vector that appears at 80 milliseconds represents the mass of LV myocardial depolarization, resulting in a signal of large amplitude. The amplitude of this signal is further increased because of the lack the opposing RV forces because the RV has already been depolarized and because the thick posterobasal portion of the LV is activated before the thinner anterolateral wall. The terminal activation vector results from depolarization of the anterolateral LV wall, producing a small vector that is also directed to the left and posteriorly.[2,18,26]

The altered activation sequence also changes the sequence of repolarization. Both the ST segment and T wave vectors are discordant from the QRS complex.

Incomplete Left Bundle Branch Block. Incomplete LBBB can result from lesser degrees of conduction delay in the LB. Although LV activation begins abnormally on the right side of the septum (as in complete LBBB), much of the subsequent LV activation occurs via the normal conduction

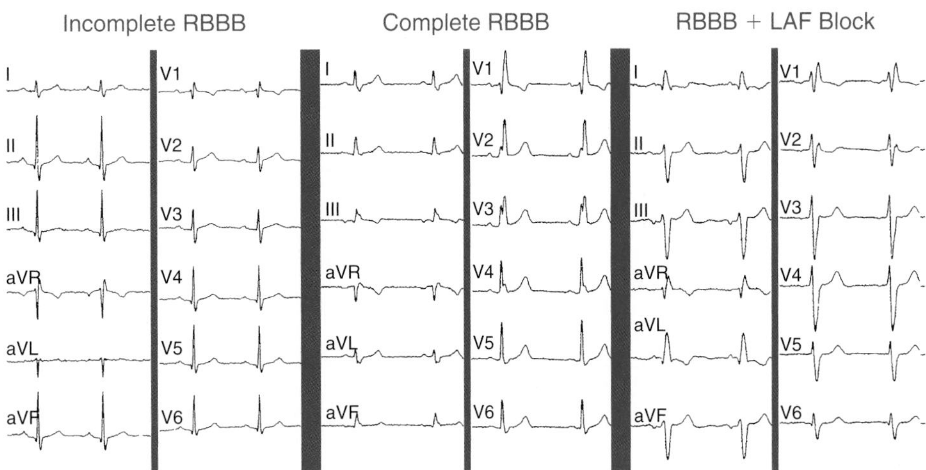

FIGURE 7–4 Surface ECG of incomplete and complete right bundle branch block (RBBB). LAF = left anterior fascicle.

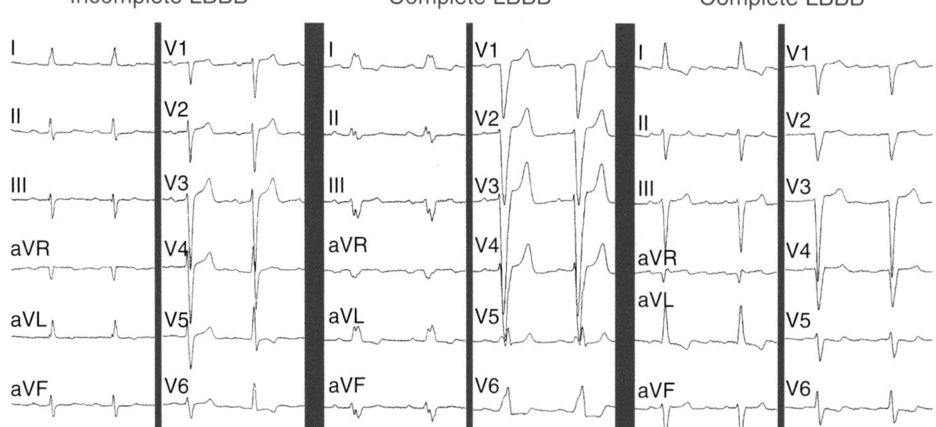

FIGURE 7–5 Surface ECG of incomplete and complete left bundle branch block (LBBB).

system. Incomplete LBBB is characterized by the following: (1) QRS duration of 100 to 120 milliseconds; (2) diminutive or absent q in I and V_6 that is frequently replaced by a slurred initial upstroke (pseudo–delta wave); (3) QRS morphology reminiscent of complete LBBB; and (4) delayed intrinsicoid deflection (time from beginning of QRS to its maximal amplitude in V_6 is more than 60 milliseconds; see Fig. 7-5). This entity can bear an ECG resemblance to WPW ECG pattern secondary to the delayed upstroke of the R wave, although the PR interval is usually short in WPW, whereas it should be normal in cases of incomplete LBBB.

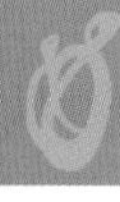

Fascicular Block

Hemiblocks in the LB system affect the LAF, LPF, or LMF. Fascicular block generally does not substantially prolong QRS duration, but only alters the sequence of LV activation. The primary ECG change is a shift in the frontal plane QRS axis, because the conduction disturbance primarily involves the early phases of activation. The QRS duration is usually less than 100 milliseconds (unless complicated by BBB or hypertrophy), although some allow a QRS duration up to 120 milliseconds, or 20 milliseconds above the previous baseline.[16,17,19]

Left Anterior Fascicular Block

The LAF normally initiates activation in the upper part of the septum, the anterolateral LV free wall, and the left anterior papillary muscle. Delayed activation of these regions secondary to damage to the LAF causes unopposed activation wavefronts via by the LPF and LMF early during the QRS complex and unopposed anterosuperior forces late during ventricular activation. The net effect is that the first 20 milliseconds of the QRS vector depicts an inferior and rightward shift in the frontal plane, whereas the main QRS forces are shifted superiorly and to the left. All these changes occur with a QRS that widens no more than 20 milliseconds in pure and uncomplicated LAF block.[16]

The initial activation vector is normal in time, but has an abnormal direction. Rather than proceeding superiorly and to the left, the vector points inferiorly and to the right (55%) or left (45%). If the initial direction is to the right and inferiorly, there will be a small positive deflection, an r wave, in the inferior leads (II, III, and aVF) and a small q wave in leads I, aVL, V_5, and V_6. If the initial direction is to the left and sufficiently inferior, the initial forces can result in small sharp q waves that simulate an old anteroseptal infarction in leads V_2 and V_3 when the electrodes are placed at the normal level and, in almost all cases, when placed in a higher position.[16]

During the midportion of the QRS, the main forces of LV activation are oriented superiorly and to the left, with a wide open counterclockwise rotated loop in the frontal plane caused by delayed depolarization of the areas normally activated by the LAF. As a result, the mean electrical axis is extremely leftward (more than −45 or −60 degrees). The net effect of the late left and superior forces include S waves in the inferior leads, resulting in an rS pattern in leads II, III, and aVF and R waves in the leftward leads, resulting in a qR or R (depending on the initial right or left orientation) pattern in leads I, aVL, V_5, and V_6. Because of the left axis deviation, the QRS complex in aVR and aVL ends in an R wave. Deeper S waves are recorded in leads V_5 and V_6 as a result of the superiorly directed forces (caused by the delayed activation of the high lateral wall, which is normally activated by the LAF). Accordingly, S waves tend to disappear in leads when the electrodes are placed at the normal level and are deeper when the electrodes are placed below the normal level.[16,17,19]

The ECG pattern of LAF block can simulate LV hypertrophy in limb leads I and aVL and, conversely, it can conceal signs of LV hypertrophy in the left precordial leads; it can also hide signs of inferior ischemia.

Left Posterior Fascicular Block

The early unopposed activation of the anterosuperior LV by the normally conducting LAF and LMF causes the initial forces to be oriented superiorly and to the left, producing initial small r waves in leads I, aVL, V_1, and V_6 and small q waves in leads II, III, and aVF. However, the late unopposed forces from the inferoposterior free wall are directed to the right, posteriorly and inferiorly because of delayed depolarization of the areas normally activated by the LPF. This is responsible for the characteristic rightward axis of +120 to +180 degrees. As a result, there is a qR morphology in leads II, III, and aVF and an rS morphology in leads I and aVL. In the frontal plane, the main and terminal forces of the QRS loop are oriented inferiorly and to the right (about +100 degrees) with a wide-open clockwise-rotated loop. In fact, the ECG pattern of LPF block is the exact mirror picture of LAF block in the standard and unipolar leads. LPF block is almost always associated with RBBB. Isolated LPF block is extremely rare, and a firm diagnosis requires that other causes of right axis deviation have been excluded.[16]

Left Median Fascicular Block

The ECG pattern seen with LMF block is probably determined by the differences in the sites of insertion of the median, anterior, and posterior fascicles. Functional block in the LMF can lead to the apparent loss of anterior forces, resulting in the transient development of q waves in leads V_1 and V_2, which normally have a positive initial deflection caused by septal depolarization. These changes are similar to those that occur in septal MI. On the other hand, prominent R waves are seen in the right precordial leads when LMF block leads to a gain of anterior forces. These changes are similar to those caused by true posterior MI. The prominence of the R waves may be increased when LMF block occurs in association with RBBB.

Other Types

Nonspecific Intraventricular Conduction Defect

A nonspecific IVCD is the result of diffuse slowing of impulse conduction involving the entire HPS, resulting in a generalized and uniform delay in activation of the ventricular myocardium. A nonspecific IVCD is diagnosed in the presence of a QRS duration longer than 120 milliseconds and a QRS morphology that does not resemble either LBBB or RBBB, and may even resemble the normal QRS complex. Nonspecific IVCDs can be classified as LV or RV IVCD, depending on the site of delayed intrinsicoid deflection and the direction of the terminal forces.

Bifascicular Blocks

Bifascicular block refers to different combinations of fascicular and bundle branch blocks. Examples of bifascicular block include RBBB with LAF block (most common; see Fig. 7-4), RBBB with LPF block, and LAF block plus LPF block (which manifests as LBBB).

Trifascicular Blocks

Trifascicular block involves conduction delay in the RB and either the main LB or both the LAF and LPF. The resulting ECG pattern will depend on the relative degree of conduction delay in the affected fascicles. Ventricular activation starts at the insertion site of the fastest conducting fascicle, with subsequent spread of activation from that site to the remainder of the ventricles. ECG documentation of trifascicular block during 1:1 AV conduction is rare. ECG manifestations of trifascicular block include the following: (1) complete AV block with a slow ventricular escape rhythm with a wide, bizarre QRS; (2) alternating RBBB and LBBB; and (3) fixed RBBB with alternating LAF and LPF block.

The combination of bifascicular block (RBBB + LAF block, RBBB + LPF block, or LBBB) with first-degree AV block on the surface ECG cannot be considered as trifascicular block because the site of AV block can be in the AVN or HPS, and such a pattern can reflect slow conduction in the AVN with concomitant bifascicular block. In such circumstances, the PR interval on the ECG does not appear to be helpful in selecting those individuals with a prolonged His bundle–ventricular (HV) interval because a normal PR interval can easily conceal a significantly prolonged HV interval and a prolonged PR interval can be caused by a prolonged atrial–His bundle (AH) interval. However, two criteria can be of value: (1) a short PR interval (less than 160 milliseconds) makes a markedly prolonged HV interval (i.e., more than 100 milliseconds) unlikely, and (2) a markedly prolonged PR interval (more than 300 milliseconds) almost always indicates that at least some of the abnormality, if not all, is caused by AVN conduction.

Alternating Bundle Branch Block

Alternating RBBB and LBBB is manifested by QRS complexes with LBBB morphology coexisting with complexes with RBBB morphology (Fig. 7-6). Often, every other complex is a right or left BBB. Spontaneous alternating BBB, especially when associated with a change in the PR interval, represents the most common ominous sign for progression to AV block. Beat-to-beat alternation is the most ominous, whereas a change in BBB noted on different days is less ominous.

This phenomenon implies instability of the HPS and a disease process involving the HB or bundle branches. In most patients with diffuse HPS disease, delay or block in one of the bundle branches consistently predominates, and alternating BBB is uncommon. The HV interval in alternating BBB is almost universally prolonged, and typically varies with the change in BBB. This group has the highest incidence of HV interval exceeding 100 milliseconds.[2]

Alternating BBB is infrequent, and therefore insensitive, but is associated with the most predictable progression to complete AV block (70% develop high-grade AV block within weeks of diagnosis). As a rule, AV conduction delay or block can be assumed to be caused by BBB only in the presence of an alternating or intermittent RBBB and LBBB with a changing PR interval. Not infrequently, the bilateral BBB is caused by acceleration-dependent aberration.

Intermittent Bundle Branch Block

Intermittent BBB, either right or left, is diagnosed on the surface ECG when there are occasional QRS complexes with

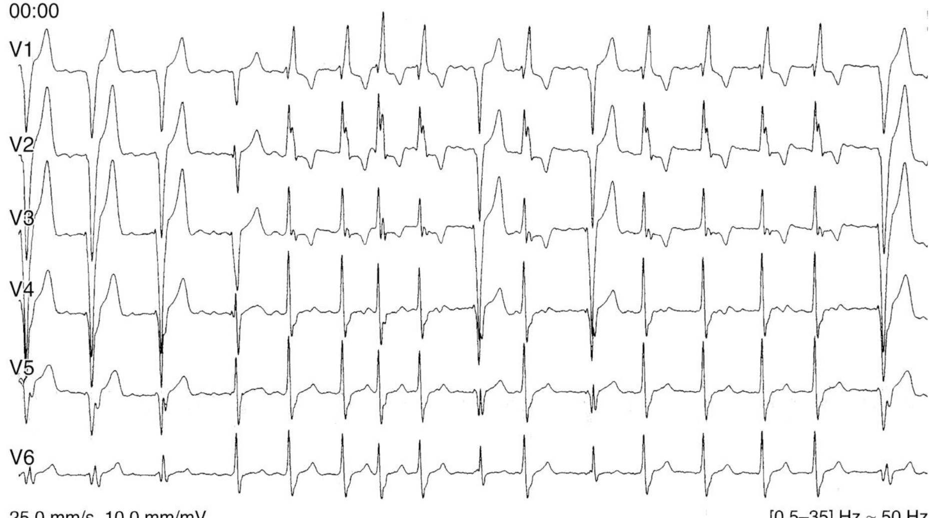

FIGURE 7–6 Alternating bundle branch block—surface ECG precordial leads during atrial fibrillation. QRS complexes with left bundle branch block configuration are observed mostly at long cycle lengths, and complexes with right bundle branch block configuration are observed mostly at shorter cycle lengths.

RBBB or LBBB morphology, interspersed with QRS complexes that have a normal morphology. Most often the intermittent BBB is rate-related; thus, the R-R intervals of the QRS complexes manifesting the BBB are shorter when compared with the intervals of the normal QRS complexes. In other cases, there is no rate-related change in the QRS intervals, but the occurrence of the BBB is a random or sporadic event.

ELECTROPHYSIOLOGICAL TESTING

Baseline Intervals

His Bundle–Ventricular Interval

The use of multipolar catheters to record distal, mid, and proximal HB potentials can help localize the site of conduction delay or block within the HB. The value of prolonged HV interval in predicting the risk of AV block is controversial. Studies have shown that an HV interval longer than 70 milliseconds predicts a higher risk of AV block (especially in symptomatic patients). The risk of AV block, however, even in the high-risk group, only approaches at most 6% per year. An HV interval exceeding 100 milliseconds identifies a group of patients at a very high risk of AV block (25% over 22 months).[2]

In the presence of RBBB with or without additional fascicular block, the HV interval should be normal as long as conduction is unimpaired in the remaining fascicle (Fig. 7-7). However, 50% of patients with RBBB plus LAF block and 75% of those with LBBB have prolonged HV interval;
7 thus, a prolonged HV interval, by itself, is nonspecific as a predictor of AV block.

In the presence of LBBB, and in the absence of a change in the HB–RB and HB–RV intervals, the HV interval might slightly prolong, because the earliest site of depolarization on the left side of the septum via the LB precedes activation of the RB by 5 to 15 milliseconds. Therefore, an HV interval of up to 60 milliseconds in the presence of LBBB should be considered normal and does not by itself indicate associated RB or HB disease (Fig. 7-8).[2]

Catheter manipulation in the LV or RV can inadvertently produce prolongation of the HV interval and varying degrees of AV block and/or BBB, which is usually temporary (see Figs. 7-7 and 7-8). Complete heart block can occur during right-sided heart catheterization in a patient with preexisting LBBB or during LV catheterization (LV angiography or ablation procedures) in a patient with preexisting RBBB.

Localization of the Site of Block in Right Bundle Branch Block

As noted, chronic RBBB pattern can result from three levels of conduction delay in the RV—proximal RBBB, distal RBBB at the level of the moderator band, and terminal RBBB involving the distal conduction system of the RB or, more likely, the muscle itself.

With proximal RBBB, loss of RB potential occurs where it is typically recorded. Activation at these RV septal sites is via transseptal spread following LV activation. The transseptal activation begins at the apex and then sequentially activates the mid-anterior wall and base of the RV. The mid and apical septum is activated at least 30 milliseconds after the onset of the QRS.

With distal RBBB, activation of the HB and proximal RB is normal. RB potentials persist at the base of the moderator band and are absent at the midanterior wall (where the moderator band normally inserts). The apical and midseptum are normally activated, but activation of the free wall at the level of the moderator band is delayed, as is the subsequent activation of the RVOT and the remaining RV.

With terminal RBBB, activation along the HB and RB remains normal up the Purkinje-myocardium junction. Activation of the midanterior wall also remains normal, and only the RVOT shows delayed activation.

Measurement of activation times at different areas of the RV has been used to assess conduction properties of the RB indirectly. In the presence of RBBB, measuring the HV interval, HB–proximal RB, V-RV apex time (from onset of the surface QRS to RV apical local activation), and V-RVOT may help localize the site of block (Fig. 7-9). A normal HV interval and V-RV apex less than 30 milliseconds in the presence of RBBB suggest terminal RBBB. On the other hand, a normal HV interval and V-RV apex less than 30 milliseconds, with delayed activation in the anterior wall (V-RVOT), suggest distal RBBB. A V-RV apex more than 30 milliseconds is consistent with proximal RBBB.

Localization of the Site of Block in Left Bundle Branch Block

Measurement of activation times at different areas of the LV to assess conduction properties of the LB, LAF, and LPF indirectly has many limitations; it is not as feasible as that used for evaluation of the RB, mainly because the LB does not divide into two discrete fascicles, but it rapidly fans out

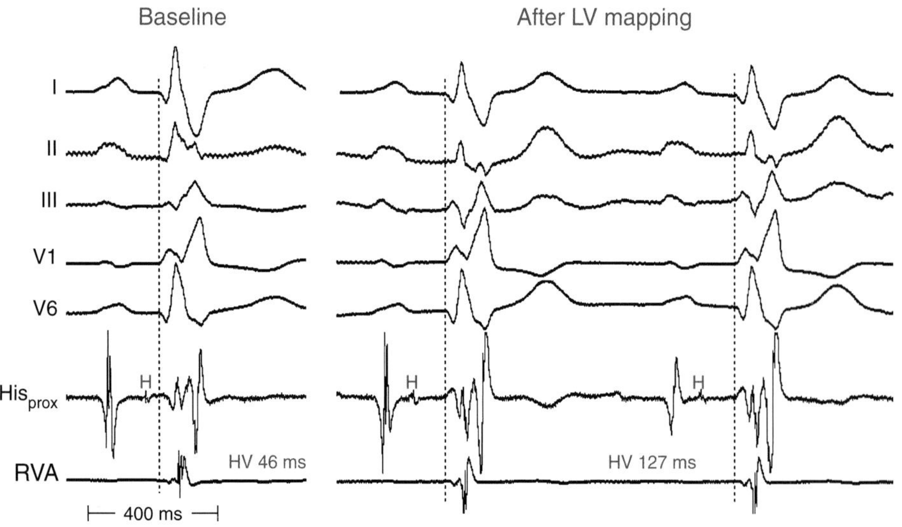

FIGURE 7–7 Catheter-induced His bundle–ventricular interval (HV) prolongation. Right bundle branch block with a normal HV is present at baseline (at left). Prolongation of the HV interval is observed after introducing mapping catheter into the left ventricle (LV), which traumatized a portion of the His-Purkinje system. The QRS is also slightly different than baseline.

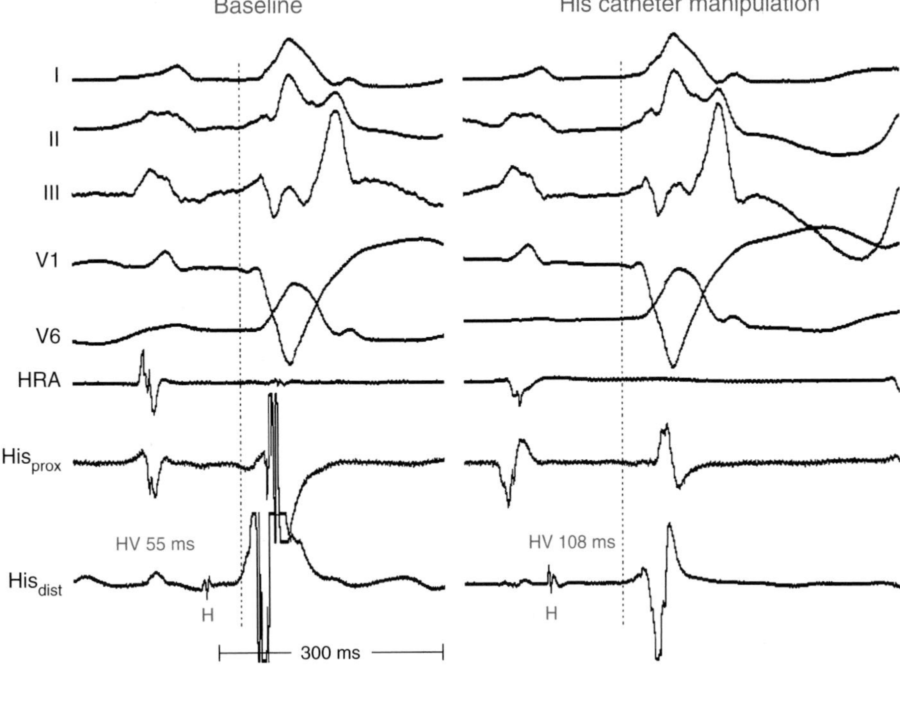

FIGURE 7–8 Catheter-induced His bundle–ventricular (HV) interval prolongation. Left bundle branch block (LBBB) and HV interval at the upper limit of normal are observed at baseline (at left). Manipulation of the His bundle recording catheter results in prolongation of the HV interval. This is not an artifact of the location of His recording, because the PR interval is also prolonged. There is no change in the QRS complex (LBBB pattern), suggesting trauma to the right bundle (RB) or His fibers destined to the RB.

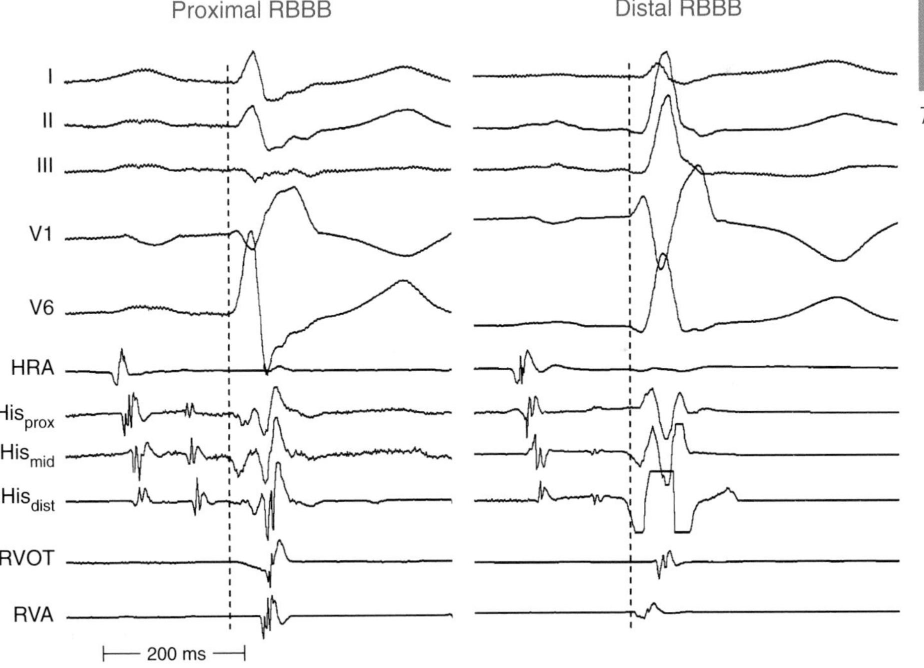

FIGURE 7–9 Localization of the site of block in right bundle branch block (RBBB). Two complexes from different patients are shown, with proximal (left panel) and distal (right panel) RBBB, distinguished by the interval from QRS onset to right ventricle apical (RVA) recording.

over the entire LV. Therefore, for practical reasons, clinical evaluation has primarily focused on the surface ECG pattern and the HV interval.

In chronic LBBB, RV activation occurs relatively earlier in the QRS. A discrete LV breakthrough site is absent, in contrast to normal, in which two or three breakthrough sites may be seen. Moreover, transseptal conduction is slow. In LBBB with normal axis, the latest LV site activated is the AV sulcus (as it is with normal conduction).

The only common observation in patients with LBBB is a delay in transseptal activation. The pattern in which the LV is activated initially (i.e., the site of breakthrough), as well as the remainder of the LV endocardium and transmural activation, depends critically on the nature of the underlying heart disease; the bizarreness of the QRS width and morphology is more a reflection of the underlying LV disease than of the primary conduction disturbance.[2] Patients with normal hearts and those with cardiomyopathy appear to have an intact distal conducting system and, hence, early engagement and rapid spread throughout the rest of the intramural myocardium. In patients with large infarcts, the bulk of their distal specialized conducting system has been destroyed; consequently, endocardial activation occurs via muscle-to-muscle conduction, and thus is much slower.

Diagnostic Maneuvers

Atrial Extrastimulation. Atrial premature stimulation helps determine the ERP of HPS. Normally, the HPS ERP is 450 milliseconds or less and it decreases with decreasing pacing CL. Because the basal AVN functional refractory period usually exceeds the HPS ERP, it can be difficult to evaluate the HPS ERP. Atropine can be useful in measuring the HPS ERP, because it decreases AVN refractoriness but has no effect on the HPS, allowing impulses to reach the HPS earlier.[2]

A grossly prolonged HPS ERP or a paradoxical increase in the HPS ERP in response to shortening of the pacing drive CL indicates an abnormal HPS and predicts a higher risk for progression to AV block.

Atrial Pacing. During incremental-rate atrial pacing, normal shortening of the HPS refractoriness at decreased pacing CLs facilitates 1:1 AV conduction. On the other hand, the development of second or third degree AV block within the HPS (in the absence of changing AH) at pacing CLs more than 400 milliseconds is abnormal and suggests a high risk (50%) for progression to high-grade AV block (Fig. 7-10).

His Bundle Pacing. Normalization of the QRS during HB pacing is suggestive of HB disease proximal to the pacing site (Fig. 7-11).

Ventricular Pacing. Assessment of retrograde VH (or VA) conduction is not useful as an indicator of anterograde HPS reserve. Anterograde RBBB is usually proximal, whereas during RV stimulation, block usually occurs at the gate, which is at the distal HPS–myocardial junction. Bidirectional RBBB is characterized by His activation following local ventricular activation in the HB recording, caused by propagation from the RV pacing site across the interventricular septum to the LB and then to the HB, rather than the more direct route retrogradely up the RB (Fig. 7-12).

Procainamide Challenge. The administration of drugs known to impair the HPS (e.g., procainamide) can unmask

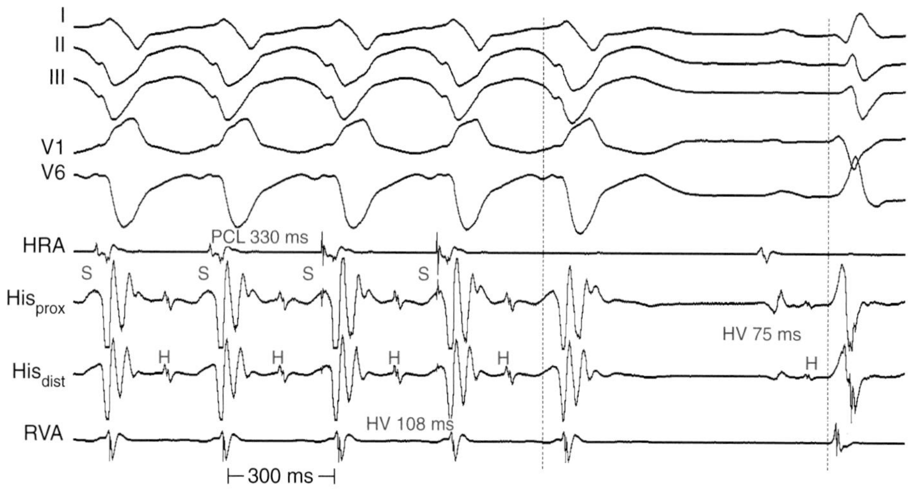

FIGURE 7–10 His-Purkinje system (HPS) disease. The PR interval is borderline (210 milliseconds) and the His bundle–ventricular interval (HV; 75 milliseconds) is prolonged during NSR (at right). Atrial pacing at a cycle length of 330 milliseconds results in stressing the HPS and further prolongation of the HV interval (108 milliseconds). Right bundle branch block also develops during atrial pacing, suggesting slow conduction over the left bundle. PCL = pacing cycle length.

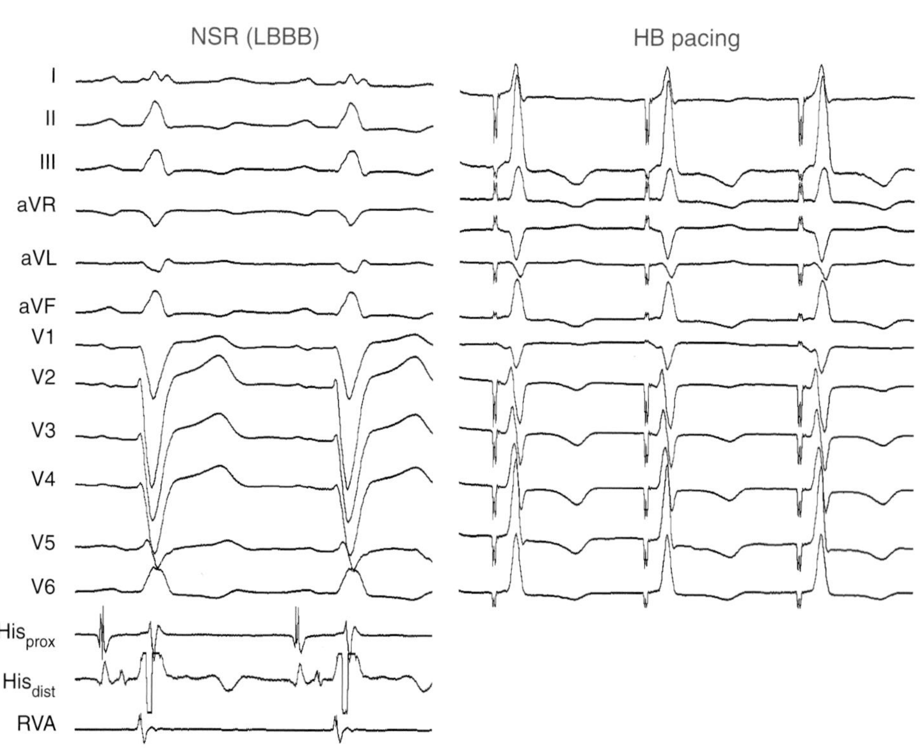

FIGURE 7–11 Left bundle branch block (LBBB) secondary to intra-Hisian disease. **Left panel,** ECG leads and intracardiac recordings in a patient with complete LBBB. **Right panel,** Pacing from the His bundle (HB) pacing normalizes the QRS complex, suggesting that the LBBB is caused by HB disease proximal to the pacing site. NSR = normal sinus rhythm.

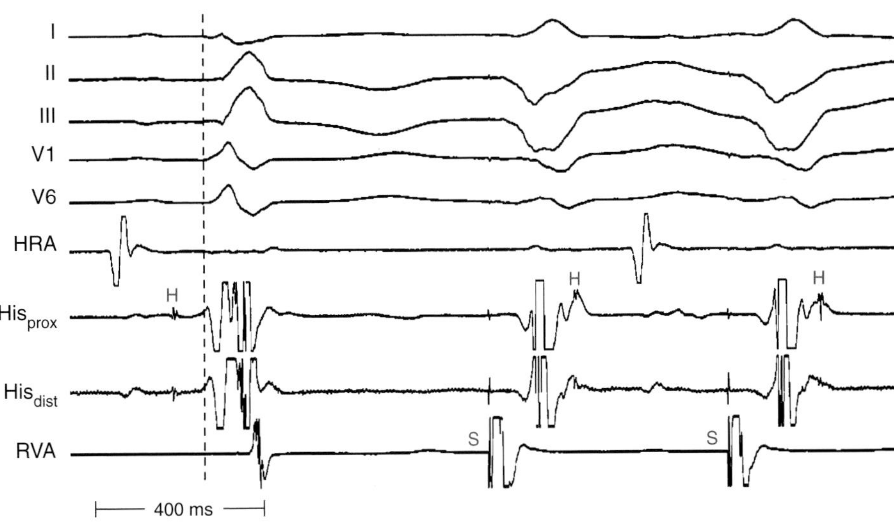

FIGURE 7–12 Bidirectional right bundle branch block (RBBB). The sinus complex at left has proximal RBBB, indicated by a very prolonged ventricular–right ventricular apical (V-RVA) time (more than 100 milliseconds). RV pacing with the next two complexes show His activation following local ventricular activation in the His bundle (HB) recording, caused by propagation from the RV pacing site across the interventricular septum to the left bundle and then to the HB, rather than the more direct route retrogradely up the right bundle. This is consistent with both anterograde and retrograde proximal RBBB.

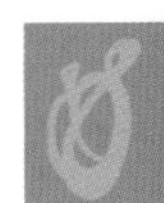

TABLE 7–2 Guidelines for Permanent Pacing in Chronic Bifascicular and Trifascicular Block

Class I
Intermittent third-degree atrioventricular (AV) block Type 2 second-degree AV block Alternating bundle-branch block
Class IIa
Syncope, when other likely causes have been excluded Incidental finding at EP study of HV interval ≥100 msec Pacing-induced block below the bundle of His that is not physiological
Class IIb
Neuromuscular diseases
Class III
Fascicular block without AV block or symptoms Fascicular block with first-degree AV block without symptoms

EP = electrophysiological; HV = His bundle-ventricular.

TABLE 7–3 Role of Electrophysiological (EP) Testing in Patients with Bundle Branch Block

EP Indicators of HPS Disease
HV interval >55 msec Infra-Hisian block at atrial pacing CL ≥ 400 msec HPS ERP ≥ 450 msec HPS ERPs inversely related to pacing CLs Abnormal response to procainamide—prolongation of the HV interval by 100% or to >100 msec, or second- or third-degree infra-Hisian AV block
EP Indicators of High Risk for AV Block in Patients with IVCD
HV interval >100 ms. Infra-Hisian AV block or HV interval prolongation at atrial pacing CL > 400 msec HPS-ERPs inversely related to pacing CLs Infra-Hisian AV block or doubling of the HV interval following procainamide in patients with neurological symptoms compatible with bradyarrhythmia
Recommendations of Pacing in Patients with IVCD
LBBB, RBBB, IVCD, RBBB + LAF block, or RBBB + LPF block associated with the following: HV interval > 100 msec or HV interval = 60-99 msec in presence of unexplained syncope or presyncope Infra-Hisian block at atrial pacing CL ≥ 400 msec (regardless of HV interval or presence of symptoms) Alternating BBB (regardless of HV interval or presence of symptoms)

AV = atrioventricular; BBB = bundle branch block; CL = cycle length; ERP = effective refractory period; HPS = His-Purkinje system; HV = His bundle-ventricular; IVCD = intraventricular conduction defect; LAF = left anterior fascicle; LBBB = left bundle branch block; LPF = left posterior fascicle; RBBB = right bundle branch block.

extraordinary sensitivity to the usual therapeutic doses of the drug, which can itself indicate poor HPS reserve. In normal persons and in most patients with a moderately increased HV interval (55 to 80 milliseconds), procainamide typically produces a 10% to 20% increase in the HV interval.

Abnormal HV interval responses to procainamide representing evidence of a higher risk for infra-Hisian AV block include: (1) doubling of the HV interval, (2) prolongation of the HV interval to more than 100 milliseconds, and/or (3) second- or third-degree infra-Hisian block.

Role of Electrophysiological Testing

The guidelines for pacing in chronic BBB are listed in Table 7-2. EP testing is used to obtain information that could predict which patients are at risk for syncope, AV block, or sudden cardiac death (Table 7-3).[2,29] Complete EP testing with programmed atrial and ventricular stimulation are necessary in patients with syncope and BBB because VT can be induced in 30% to 50% of such patients. Pacemaker therapy clearly can help prevent syncope in those patients in whom that event most likely was caused by transient bradyarrhythmia, but has not been shown to prevent sudden cardiac death or reduce cardiac mortality.[2,29]

REFERENCES

1. Chilson DA, Zipes DP, Heger JJ, et al: Functional bundle branch block: discordant response of right and left bundle branches to changes in heart rate. Am J Cardiol 1984;54:313.
2. Josephson ME: Intraventricular conduction disturbances. *In* Josephson ME (ed): Clinical Cardiac Electrophysiology, 3rd ed. Philadelphia, Lippincott Williams & Wilkins, 2004, pp 110-139.
3. Eckardt L, Breithardt G, Kirchhof P: Approach to wide complex tachycardias in patients without structural heart disease. Heart 2006;92:704.
4. Pavri BB, Kocovic DZ, Hanna M: Long-short RR intervals and the right bundle branch. J Cardiovasc Electrophysiol 1999;10:121.
5. Rubart M, Zipes DP: Genesis of cardiac arrhythmias: Electrophysiological considerations. *In* Zipes DP, Libby P, Bonow R, Braunwald E (eds): Braunwald's Heart Disease: A Textbook of Cardiovascular Medicine, 7th ed. Philadelphia, WB Saunders, 2004, pp 653-688.

6. Smith DC: Ashman's phenomenon—a source of nonsustained wide complex tachycardia. J Emerg Med 1993;11:98.
7. Suyama AC, Sunagawa K, Sugimachi M, et al: Differentiation between aberrant ventricular conduction and ventricular ectopy in atrial fibrillation using RR interval scattergram. Circulation 1993;88(Pt 1):2307.
8. Josephson ME: Miscellaneous phenomena related to atrioventricular conduction. *In* Josephson ME (ed): Clinical Cardiac Electrophysiology, 3rd ed. Philadelphia, Lippincott, Williams & Wilkins, 2004, pp 140-154.
9. Kilborn MF, McGuire MA: Electrocardiographic manifestations of supernormal conduction, concealed conduction, and exit block. *In* Zipes DP, Jalife J (eds): Cardiac Electrophysiology: From Cell to Bedside, 4th ed. Philadelphia, WB Saunders, 2004, pp 733-738.
10. Wellens HJJ, Boss DL, Farre J, Brugada P: Functional bundle branch block during supraventricular tachycardia in man: Observations on mechanisms and their incidence. *In* Zipes DP, Jalife J (eds): Cardiac Electrophysiology and Arrhythmias. New York, Crane & Stratton,1995, pp 435-441.
11. Fisch C, Knoebel SB: Wolff-Parkinson-White syndrome. *In* Fisch C, Knoebel SB (eds): Electrocardiography of Clinical Arrhythmias. Armonk, NY, Futura, 2000, pp 293-314.
12. Fisch C, Knoebel SB: Atrioventricular and ventriculoatrial conduction and blocks, gap, and overdrive suppression. *In* Fisher EA, Knoebel SB (eds): Electrocardiography of Clinical Arrhythmias. Armonk, NY, Futura, 2000, pp 315-344.
13. Gouaux JL, Ashman R: Auricular fibrillation with aberration simulating ventricular paroxysmal tachycardia. Am Heart J 1947;34:366.
14. Fisch C, Zipes DP, McHenry P: Electrocardiographic manifestations of concealed junctional ectopic impulses. Circulation 1976;53:217.
15. Fisch C, Knoebel SB: Concealed conduction. *In* Fisch C, Knoebel SB (eds): Electrocardiography of Clinical Arrhythmias. Armonk, NY, Futura, 2000, pp 153-172.
16. Elizari MV, Acunzo RS, Ferreiro M: Hemiblocks revisited. Circulation 2007;115:1154.
17. Biagini E, Elhendy A, Schinkel AF, et al: Prognostic significance of left anterior hemiblock in patients with suspected coronary artery disease. J Am Coll Cardiol 2005;46:858.
18. Harrigan RA, Pollack ML, Chan TC: Electrocardiographic manifestations: Bundle branch blocks and fascicular blocks. J Emerg Med 2003;25:67.
19. MacAlpin RN: In search of left septal fascicular block. Am Heart J 2002;144:948.
20. Imanishi R, Seto S, Ichimaru S, et al: Prognostic significance of incident complete left bundle branch block observed over a 40-year period. Am J Cardiol 2006;98:644.
21. McCullough PA, Hassan SA, Pallekonda V, et al: Bundle branch block patterns, age, renal dysfunction, and heart failure mortality. Int J Cardiol 2005;102:303.
22. Baldasseroni S, Opasich C, Gorini M, et al: Left bundle-branch block is associated with increased 1-year sudden and total mortality rate in 5517 outpatients with congestive heart failure: A report from the Italian network on congestive heart failure. Am Heart J 2002;143:398.
23. Auricchio A, Fantoni C, Regoli F, et al: Characterization of left ventricular activation in patients with heart failure and left bundle-branch block. Circulation 2004;109:1133.
24. Stenestrand U, Tabrizi F, Lindback J, et al: Comorbidity and myocardial dysfunction are the main explanations for the higher 1-year mortality in acute myocardial infarction with left bundle-branch block. Circulation 2004;110:1896.
25. Wong CK, Stewart RA, Gao W, et al: Prognostic differences between different types of bundle branch block during the early phase of acute myocardial infarction: Insights from the Hirulog and Early Reperfusion or Occlusion (HERO)-2 trial. Eur Heart J 2006;27:21.
26. Francia P, Balla C, Paneni F, Volpe M: Left bundle-branch block—pathophysiology, prognosis, and clinical management. Clin Cardiol 2007;30:110.
27. Agarwal AK, Venugopalan P: Right bundle branch block: Varying electrocardiographic patterns. Aetiological correlation, mechanisms and electrophysiology. Int J Cardiol 1999;71:33.
28. Rogers RL, Mitarai M, Mattu A: Intraventricular conduction abnormalities. Emerg Med Clin North Am 2006;24:41.
29. Englund A, Bergfeldt L, Rehnqvist N, et al: Diagnostic value of programmed ventricular stimulation in patients with bifascicular block: A prospective study of patients with and without syncope. J Am Coll Cardiol 1995;26:1508.

CHAPTER 8

Focal Atrial Tachycardia

CLASSIFICATION OF ATRIAL TACHYCARDIAS

Previous classifications of regular atrial tachycardias (ATs) had been based exclusively on the surface electrocardiogram (ECG). AT is defined as a regular atrial rhythm at a constant rate more than 100 beats/min originating outside the sinus node region. The mechanism can be caused by focal pacemaker activity (automaticity or triggered activity) or reentry (micro- or macroreentry). Atrial flutter (AFL) refers to a pattern of regular tachycardia with a rate of 240 beats/min or more (tachycardia cycle length [CL] 250 milliseconds or less) lacking an isoelectric baseline between deflections. According to this ECG classification, differentiation between AFL and AT depends on a rate cutoff around 240 to 250 beats/min and the presence of an isoelectric baseline between atrial deflections in AT, but not in AFL. Atypical AFL is only a descriptive term for an AT with an ECG pattern of continuous undulation of the atrial complex, different from typical clockwise or counterclockwise isthmus-dependent AFL, at an atrial rate of 240 beats/min or more.

This ECG classification, however, has several major limitations. Neither rate nor lack of isoelectric baseline is specific for any tachycardia mechanism. Rapid AT in a diseased atrium can mimic AFL and, on the other hand, true AFL may show distinct isoelectric intervals between flutter waves. This dilemma is not solvable in terms of analyses of routine ECGs. Moreover, AT mechanisms, defined by electrophysiological (EP) studies and radiofrequency (RF) catheter ablation, do not correlate with ECG patterns as defined currently.

Therefore, the ECG classification is obsolete for this purpose, and a mechanistic classification of ATs has been proposed (Table 8-1).[1,2] If the mechanism of AT or AFL can be elucidated, either through conventional mapping and entrainment, or with special multipoint mapping techniques, description of the mechanism should be stated. However, even when using this classification, there are other tachycardias described in the literature that cannot be well classified because of inadequate understanding of their mechanism(s), including "type II" AFL, inappropriate sinus tachycardia, and fibrillatory conduction from focal source.

This chapter will discuss focal AT; typical and atypical AFL and macroreentrant AT will be discussed in subsequent chapters.

PATHOPHYSIOLOGY

Focal AT is characterized by atrial activation starting rhythmically at a small area (focus) from where it spreads out centrifugally.[1] "Focal" implies that the site of origin cannot be mapped spatially beyond a single point or a few adjacent points with the resolution of a standard 4-mm tip catheter. In contrast, macroreentrant AT is defined by activation that can be recorded over the entire tachycardia CL around a large central obstacle, which is generally several centimeters in diameter.[1] Relatively small reentry circuits may resemble focal AT, especially if a limited number of endocardial recordings are collected.

Focal AT CL is usually more than 250 milliseconds; however, it can be as short as 200 milliseconds. Over a prolonged period of observation (minutes to hours), AT CL can exhibit important variations.

Most focal ATs (83%) arise from the right atrium (RA), about two thirds of which are distributed along the long axis of the crista terminalis (cristal tachycardias) from the sinus node to the coronary sinus (CS) and atrioventricular (AV) junction (called the line of fire), with an apparent gradation in frequency from superior to inferior.[3,4] This particular anatomical distribution of ATs may be related to the marked anisotropy characterizing the region of the crista terminalis. Such anisotropy, which is related to the poor transverse cell-to-cell coupling, favors the development of microreentry by creating regions of slow conduction. Fractionated electrograms often seen at a successful AT ablation site may be markers of the requisite nonuniformly anisotropic substrate. In addition, the normal sinus pacemaker complex is distributed along the long axis of the crista terminalis. The presence of automatic tissue, together with relative cellular uncoupling, may be a requirement

TABLE 8–1	Classification of Atrial Tachycardias	
Focal Atrial Tachycardia	· Automatic atrial tachycardia · Triggered-activity atrial tachycardia · Microreentrant atrial tachycardia	
Macroreentrant Atrial Tachycardia or Atrial Flutter	***Cavotricuspid isthmus-dependent atrial flutters***	· Clockwise and counterclockwise typical atrial flutter · Double-loop reentry · Lower-loop reentry · Intra-isthmus reentry
	Noncavotricuspid isthmus-dependent right atrial flutters	· Upper-loop reentry · Lesional or scar-related right atrial macroreentry
	Left atrial flutters	· Perimitral macroreentry · Pulmonary vein/scar macroreentry · Left septal macroreentry · Postsurgical/ablation macroreentry

for abnormal automaticity such that a normal atrium is prevented from electrotonically inhibiting abnormal phase 4 depolarization. The presence of structural heart disease increases the probability of RA location of the AT, but from sites outside the crista terminalis. Other sites of AT clustering include pulmonary vein (PV) ostia,[5] coronary sinus ostium (CS os),[4,6-9] mitral and tricuspid annuli,[3,5,10,11] bases of RA and left atrial (LA) appendages, para-Hisian region, and atrial septum. Recent experience gained during catheter ablation of atrial fibrillation (AF) has indicated that focal ATs also can arise in the vein of Marshall,[12] superior vena cava (SVC),[13,14] or inferior vena cava (IVC).[15] The distribution of AT foci may differ, depending on the patient population.

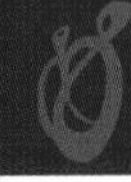
8

Available information suggests that focal activity can be caused by automaticity, triggered activity, or microreentry. There is some overlap based on the pharmacological characterization of these different AT mechanisms. Delineating the mechanism of focal AT, however, can be difficult, and means of distinguishing focal AT mechanism are fraught with exceptions.[16] The major limiting factor in the analysis of mechanisms is the absence of a gold standard for determining the tachycardia mechanism, so these remain largely descriptive. In addition, there is a significant overlap in the electrophysiological characteristics of tachycardias with differing mechanisms.[17] It is especially difficult to discriminate definitively between triggered activity and microreentry as a mechanism of focal AT; therefore, some have classified focal AT as automatic or nonautomatic.[1] Furthermore, it is not clear that making such mechanistic distinctions between various types of focal AT carries any clinical significance, although it is possible that such information could be useful in guiding drug therapy. In contrast, determination of likely focal versus macroreentrant mechanism is critical for planning mapping and ablation strategy.

"Incessant" is applied to an AT that is present for at least 50% of the time that a patient is monitored.[18] Incessant AT frequently is automatic, but can also be secondary to reentry or triggered activity.

Other forms of AT in which EP testing and catheter ablation are not indicated are beyond the scope of this chapter and are discussed briefly. Multifocal AT is usually caused by enhanced automaticity and is characterized by varying morphology of the P waves and the PR interval. This finding suggests that the pacemaker arises in different atrial locations, but a single focus with different exit pathways or abnormalities in intraatrial conduction can produce identical electrocardiographic manifestations. Synonyms include chaotic atrial tachycardia, multifocal atrial rhythm, and wandering atrial pacemaker. Nonparoxysmal AT typically occurs in patients with significant heart disease and/or digitalis toxicity. The latter may be caused by triggered activity. Repetitive automatic AT, also called repetitive focal AT, is thought to be caused in most cases by enhanced automaticity, frequently occurring in patients with structural heart disease, and is often related to some acute event, such as a myocardial infarction, pulmonary decompensation, infection, alcohol excess, hypokalemia, hypoxia, stimulants, cocaine, and theophylline.

Early studies of sinus node function described the response to a single atrial extrastimulus (AES). The curve produced by plotting return cycles against the coupling interval could be divided into several phases, including compensatory pause, reset, interpolation, and reentry. Sinus node reentrant tachycardia was described on the basis of these findings as a tachycardia that could be induced and terminated by programmed electrical stimulation with a P wave morphology identical or similar to sinus P waves and tachycardia CLs of 350 to 550 milliseconds (see Fig. 12-3).[19] There have been some reports of endocardial ablation of sinus node reentrant tachycardias identified by these criteria. However, the precise identification of sinus node reentrant tachycardia remains elusive. The mechanism of focal AT can be reentrant, the CL of such ATs completely overlaps that described for sinus node reentrant tachycardia, and the location of AT foci is often along the crista terminalis, very close to the supposed location of the sinus node. An added problem is that the origin of the sinus activation can be variable, according to epicardial mapping studies. Furthermore, endocardial origin of sinus activation during normal sinus rhythm (NSR) has not been systematically studied in humans, and specific criteria do not exist to pinpoint a specific sinus node area. Finally, reentry strictly limited to the sinus node area has never been demonstrated, and has even been questioned.[19]

CLINICAL CONSIDERATIONS

Epidemiology

Nonsustained AT is frequently found on Holter recordings and is seldom associated with symptoms. Sustained focal ATs are relatively infrequent; they are diagnosed in about 5% to 15% of patients referred for catheter ablation of supraventricular tachycardia (SVT).[20] However, ATs comprise a progressively greater proportion of paroxysmal SVTs with increasing age, accounting for 23% in patients older than 70 years. Age-related changes in the atrial EP substrate (including cellular coupling and autonomic influences) may contribute to the increased incidence of AT in older individuals.[20] In adults, focal AT can occur in the absence of cardiac disease, but it is often associated with underlying cardiac abnormalities. Not infrequently, two or more foci of AT can be found in the same patient.[21]

Clinical Presentation

Focal ATs can present as paroxysmal or incessant tachycardias. When paroxysmal, it presents with the clinical syndrome of paroxysmal SVT. Symptoms, however, may be more severe or associated with cardiac decompensation caused by the more likelihood of the presence of structural heart disease in this group of patients. Incessant AT can result in tachycardia-induced cardiomyopathy and present with symptoms of congestive heart failure. AT can also manifest as a frequently repetitive tachycardia, with frequent episodes of AT interrupted by short periods of NSR. The repetitive type may be tolerated well for years, causing symptoms only in cases of fast heart rates during phases of tachycardia and infrequently inducing dilated cardiomyopathy.

Initial Evaluation

History, physical examination, 12-lead ECG, and echocardiography constitute an appropriate initial evaluation. Differentiation of paroxysmal AT from other mechanisms of SVT can be challenging and may require invasive EP testing. However, diagnosis of the incessant and frequently repetitive forms of AT usually can be readily made based on P wave morphology and the frequent presence of AV block during the tachycardia on ECG recordings. An ECG pattern of AT with discrete P waves and isoelectric baselines is suggestive of a focal mechanism of the AT, but does not rule out macroreentrant AT, especially if complex structural heart disease is present and/or there has been surgery for congenital heart disease. The diagnosis of focal AT can be established with certainty only by an EP study. ATs often occur in older patients and in the context of structural heart disease; therefore, coronary artery disease and left ventricular (LV) dysfunction should be excluded.

Principles of Management

Acute Management

On rare occasions, ATs can be terminated with vagal maneuvers. Conversely, a significant proportion of ATs will terminate with administration of adenosine. Adenosine-sensitive ATs are usually focal in origin. Persistence of the tachycardia with AV block is also a common response to adenosine. In addition, ATs responsive to intravenous verapamil or beta blockers have been reported. It is conceivable that the mechanism of AT in these patients relates to microreentry, involving tissue with slow conduction, or to triggered activity. Class IA or IC drugs can suppress automaticity or prolong action potential duration and hence can be effective for some patients with AT.

For patients with automatic AT, atrial pacing (or adenosine) can result in transient slowing but no tachycardia termination. Similarly, DC cardioversion seldom terminates automatic ATs, but DC cardioversion may be successful for those in whom the tachycardia mechanism is microreentry or triggered activity. An attempt at DC cardioversion should, therefore, be considered for symptomatic patients with drug-resistant arrhythmia.

The usual acute therapy for AT consists of intravenous beta blockers or calcium channel blockers for either termination, which is rare, or to achieve rate control through AV block, which is often difficult to achieve.[18] Direct suppression of the tachycardia focus may be achieved by the use of intravenous class IA and IC or class III agents. Intravenous class IA or IC agents may be taken by patients without cardiac failure, whereas intravenous amiodarone is preferred for those with poor LV function.[18]

Chronic Management

As with other forms of SVT, AT is usually benign and associated with only mild to moderate symptoms. Thus, most patients with AT are treated initially with medical therapy. Patient preference and refractoriness to pharmacological therapy are reasonable indications for catheter ablation.[18]

The efficacy of antiarrhythmic drugs is poorly defined because the clinical definition of focal ATs is often not rigorous. No large studies have been conducted to assess the effect of pharmacological treatment in patients with focal ATs, but both paroxysmal and, especially, incessant ATs are reported to be difficult to treat medically. Available data support a recommendation for initial therapy with calcium channel blockers or beta blockers because these agents may prove to be effective and have minimal side effects. If these drugs are unsuccessful, then class IA, class IC (flecainide and propafenone) in combination with an atrioventricular node (AVN) blocking agent, or class III agents (sotalol and amiodarone) may be tried; however, the potential benefit should be balanced by the potential risks of proarrhythmia and toxicity. Because ATs often occur in older patients and in the context of structural heart disease, class IC agents should be used only after coronary artery disease is excluded.[18]

For patients with drug-refractory AT or incessant AT, especially when tachycardia-induced cardiomyopathy has developed, the best therapy appears to be catheter ablation of the AT focus. In case reports and small series, patients with atrial tachycardia-induced cardiomyopathy frequently have complete resolution of LV dysfunction with successful RF catheter ablation of the atrial focus.[18] Regardless of whether the arrhythmia is caused by abnormal automaticity, triggered activity, or microreentry, focal AT is ablated by targeting the site of origin of the AT. Catheter ablation for focal AT carries an 86% success rate, with a recurrence rate of 8%. The incidence of significant complications is low (1% to 2%) in experienced centers.

ELECTROCARDIOGRAPHIC FEATURES

P Wave Morphology

During AT, typically there are discrete P waves at rates of 130 to 240 beats/min, but possibly as low as 100 beats/min or as high as 300 beats/min. Antiarrhythmic drugs can slow the tachycardia rate without abolishing the AT. Classically, there is a clearly defined isoelectric baseline between the P waves in all leads. However, in the presence of rapid rates, intraatrial conduction disturbances, or both, the P waves can be broad, and there may be no isoelectric baseline. In these cases, the ECG will show an AFL pattern (continuous undulation without isoelectric baseline; Fig. 8-1).[1] Nevertheless, a recent report has demonstrated a high sensitivity (90%) and specificity (90%) of *quantitative* ECG indexes of shorter atrial activation and longer diastolic intervals in distinguishing focal from macroreentrant AT. This approach was effective in cases with and without 1:1 AV conduction and when the P or flutter waves overlay T waves.[22]

P wave morphology depends on the location of the atrial focus, and it can be used to localize the site of origin of the AT approximately. However, the P wave can be partially masked by the preceding ST segment and/or T wave. Vagal maneuvers and adenosine infusion to provide transient AV block can be used to obtain a clear view of the P wave, assuming that the tachycardia does not terminate and responds with AV block. The compensatory pause following a premature ventricular complex (PVC) during the AT can also be used to delineate P wave morphology. It has been suggested that the multilead body surface potential recording can be used to help localize the site of origin of the tachycardia.

Focal automatic ATs start with a P wave identical to the P wave during the arrhythmia and the rate generally increases gradually (warms up) over the first few seconds. In comparison, intraatrial reentry or triggered-activity AT is usually initiated by a P wave from a premature atrial complex (PAC) that generally differs in morphology from the P wave during the established arrhythmia.

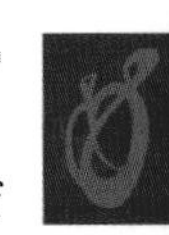

Focal atrial tachycardia

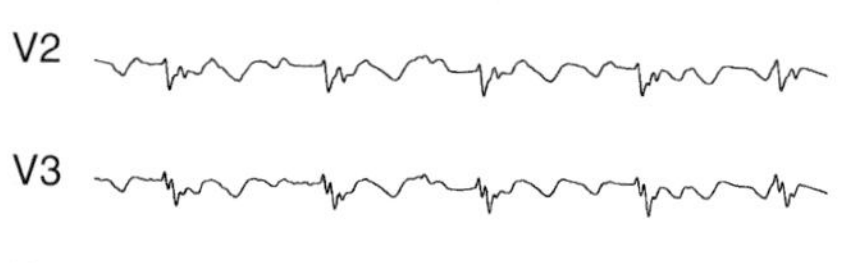

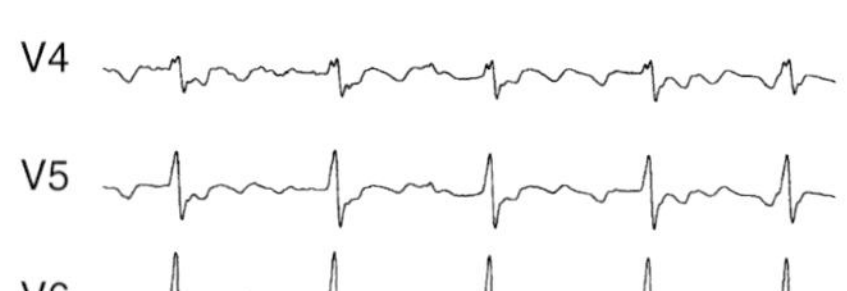

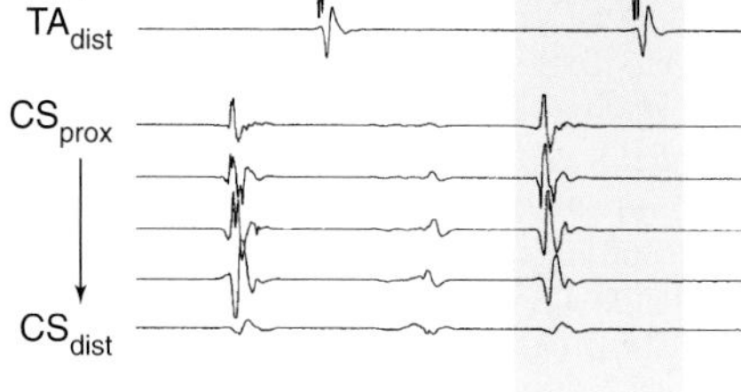

Macroreentrant atrial tachycardia

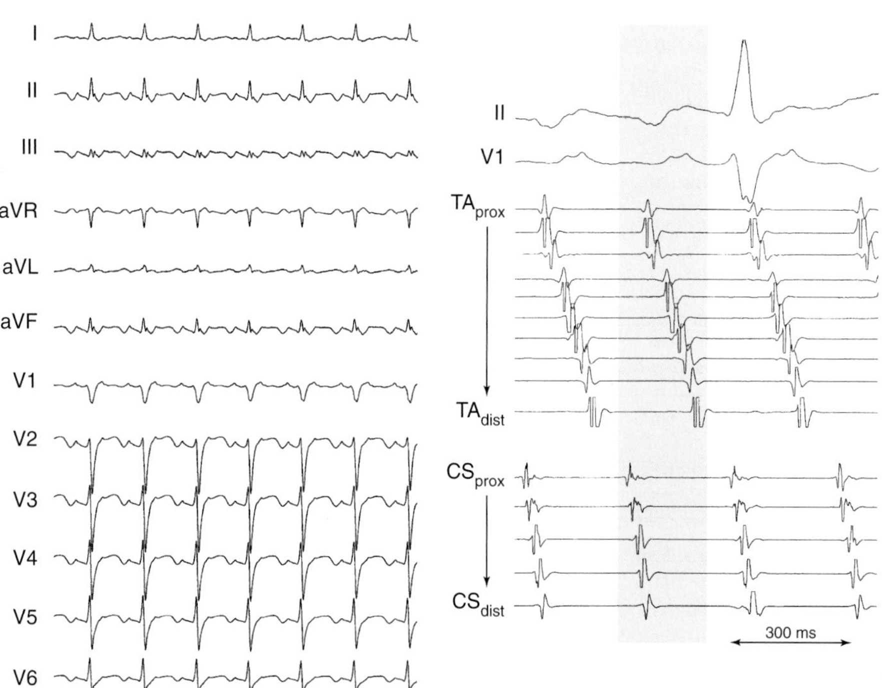

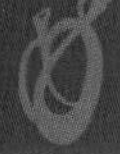

FIGURE 8–1 Comparison of focal and macroreentrant atrial tachycardia (AT). **Upper panel,** Surface ECG and endocardial activation sequence of focal AT originating from inferior aspect of the mitral annulus with 2:1 atrioventricular (AV) conduction. **Lower panel,** Endocardial activation macroreentrant AT around the tricuspid annulus (counterclockwise, typical atrial flutter) with 2:1 AV conduction. As illustrated in this case, discrimination between focal and macroreentry as the mechanism of AT based on the presence of distinct isoelectric intervals between the tachycardia P waves can be challenging caused by superimposition of the QRS and ST-T waves. Endocardial activation (shaded area), however, clearly demonstrates that biatrial activation from all electrodes of the Halo catheter (around the tricuspid annulus, TA) and the coronary sinus (CS) catheter occupies only a small fraction (less than 50%) of the tachycardia cycle length (CL) during focal AT with significant portions of the tachycardia CL without recorded activity. In contrast, biatrial activation occupies most (~90%) of the tachycardia CL during macroreentrant AT.

QRS Morphology

QRS morphology during AT is usually the same as during NSR. However, functional aberration can occur at rapid atrial rates.

P/QRS Relationship

The atrial to ventricular relationship is usually 1:1 during ATs, but Wenckebach or 2:1 AV block can occur at rapid rates, in the presence of AVN disease, or in the presence of drugs that slow AVN conduction. The presence of AV block during an SVT strongly suggests AT, excludes atrioventricular reentrant tachycardia (AVRT), and renders atrioventricular nodal reentrant tachycardia (AVNRT) unlikely.

ATs usually have a long RP interval, but the RP interval can also be short, depending on the degree of AV conduction delay (i.e., PR interval prolongation) during the tachycardia.

Localization of the Atrial Tachycardia Site of Origin Using P Wave Morphology

General Observations Relating P Wave Morphology to Site of Origin of Atrial Tachycardia

P wave morphology provides a useful guide to the localization of focal AT. ECG lead V_1 is the most useful in identifying the likely anatomical site of origin for focal AT. Lead V_1 is located to the right and anteriorly in relation to the atria, which should be considered as right anterior and left posterior. Thus, for example, tachycardias originating from the tricuspid annulus have negative P waves in lead V_1 because of the anterior and rightward location of this structure (i.e., activation travels *away* from lead V_1). The P wave in lead V1 is universally positive for tachycardias originating from the PVs because of the posterior location of these structures (i.e., the impulse travels *toward* lead V_1).[23-25]

In a recent report, a negative or biphasic (positive, then negative) P wave in lead V_1 was associated with a 100% specificity and positive predictive value for a tachycardia arising from the RA. A positive or biphasic (negative, then positive) P wave in lead V_1 was associated with a 100% sensitivity and negative predictive value for tachycardia originating in the LA.[25]

The predictive value of P wave morphology for localizing the atrium of origin is more limited when the tachycardia foci arise from the interatrial septum. Those ATs are associated with variable P wave morphology, with considerable overlap for tachycardias located on the left and right side of the septum. Nevertheless, P waves during ATs arising near the septum are generally narrower than those arising in the RA or LA free wall.

P waves identical to the sinus P wave are suggestive of sinus node reentrant tachycardia or perinodal AT. Negative P waves in the anterior precordial leads suggest an anterior RA or LA free wall location. Negative P waves in the inferior leads suggest a low (inferior) atrial origin.

Several algorithms have been proposed for ECG localization of focal AT using P wave morphology. Figure 8-2 summarizes some of those algorithms.[25,26]

Right Atrial Tachycardias

Cristal ATs (ATs arising from the crista terminalis) are characterized by right-to-left activation sequence resulting in P waves that are positive and broad in leads I and II, positive in lead aVL, and biphasic in lead V_1 (Fig. 8-3). A negative P wave in lead aVR identifies cristal ATs with 100% sensitivity and 93% specificity. High, mid, or low cristal locations can be identified by P wave polarity in the inferior leads.

In anteroseptal ATs (originating above the membranous septum), the P wave is biphasic or negative in lead V_1 and positive in the inferior leads. The P wave during AT is approximately 20 milliseconds narrower than the sinus P wave. Those ATs can mimic slow-fast AVNRT or orthodromic AVRT with superoparaseptal bypass tracts (BTs).[27] Midseptal ATs (originating below the membranous septum and above the CS os) are associated with P waves that are biphasic or negative in lead V_1 and negative in the inferior leads. Those ATs can mimic fast-intermediate AVNRT or orthodromic AVRT with midseptal BTs.[27] With posteroseptal ATs (originating below and around the CS os), the P wave is positive in lead V_1, negative in the inferior leads, and positive in leads aVL and aVR. Those ATs can mimic fast-slow AVNRT or orthodromic AVRT using a posteroseptal BT.[27]

For tricuspid annular ATs, the nonseptal sites demonstrate negative P waves in lead V_1, whereas anteroinferior sites tend to have inverted P waves across the precordial leads, and superior sites closer to the septum show transition from negative in lead V_1 through biphasic to upright in the lateral precordial leads. P wave polarity in the inferior leads differentiate inferior from superior tricuspid annular locations.[3]

Left Atrial Tachycardias

ATs arising from the PVs are characterized by entirely positive P waves in lead V_1 in 100% of cases, isoelectric or negative in lead aVL in 86%, and negative in lead aVR in 96%. Lead aVL can be biphasic or positive in right-sided PV ATs.[26,28,29] Left PV ATs have several characteristics (as compared with right PV ATs): positive notching in the P waves

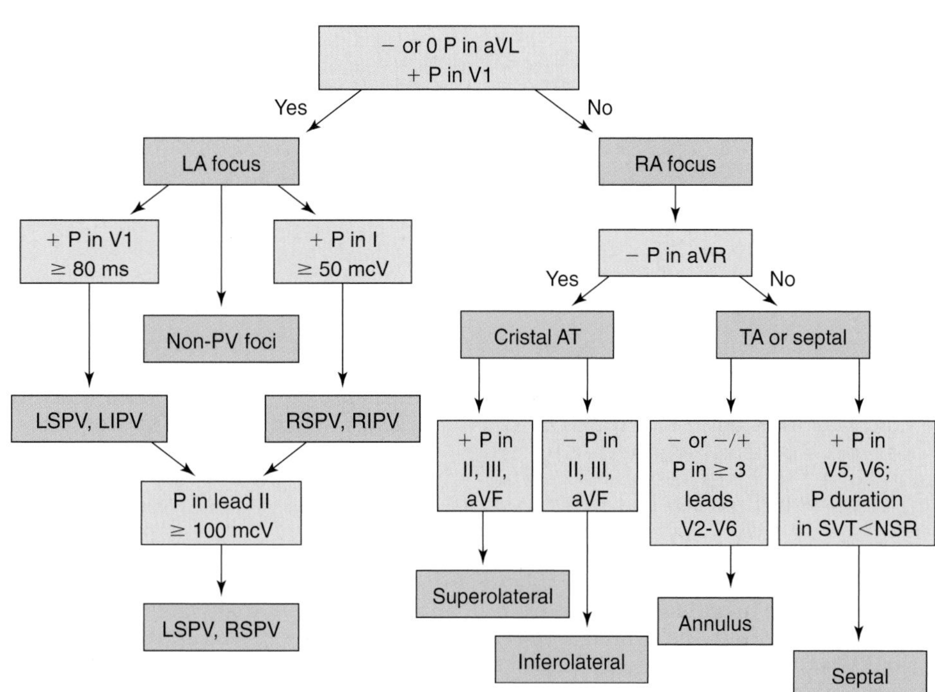

FIGURE 8–2 Algorithm for localization of AT origin based on P wave morphology on the surface ECG. +P = positive P wave; −P = negative P wave; 0 = isoelectric P wave; −/+ = biphasic P wave; LSPV = left superior pulmonary vein; LIPV = left inferior pulmonary vein; RSPV = right superior pulmonary vein; RIPV = right inferior pulmonary vein; SR, sinus rhythm. (From Ellenbogen KA, Wood MA: Atrial tachycardia. *In* Zipes DP, Jalife J [eds]: Cardiac Electrophysiology: From Cell to Bedside, 4th ed. Philadelphia, WB Saunders, 2004, pp 500-511.)

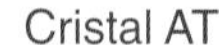

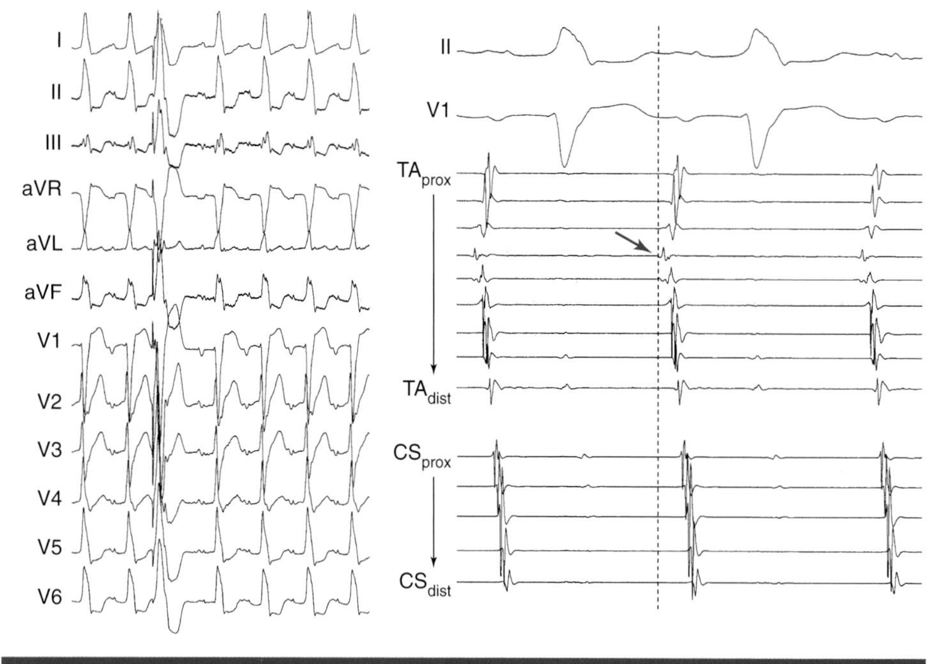

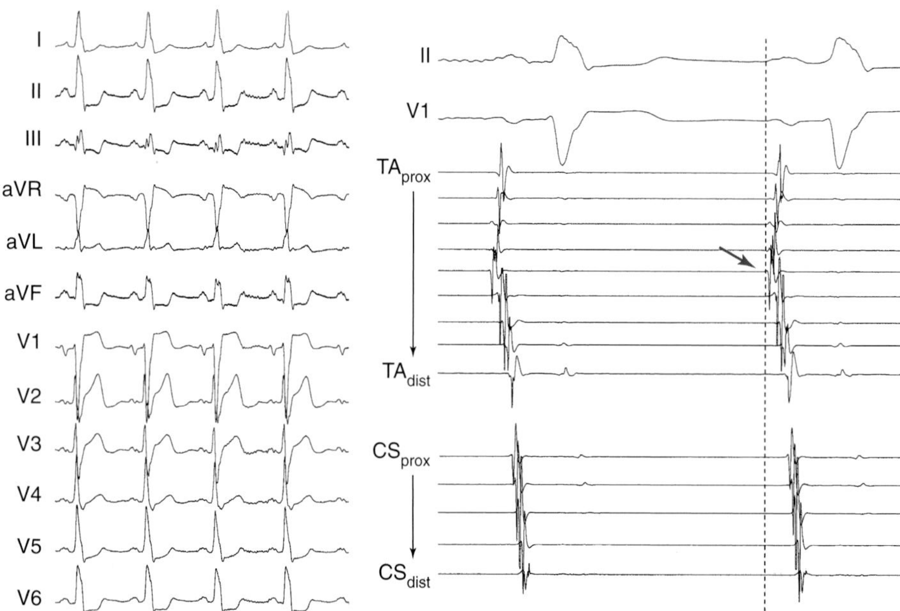

FIGURE 8–3 Comparison of P wave morphology and endocardial atrial activation sequence between focal atrial tachycardia (AT) originating from the crista terminalis **(upper panel)** and normal sinus rhythm (NSR; **lower panel**) in the same patient. A Halo catheter is positioned around the tricuspid annulus (TA).

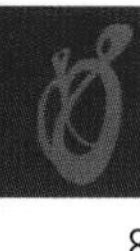

8

in two or more surface leads, an isoelectric or negative P wave in lead I, P wave amplitude in lead III/II ratio > 0.8, and broad P waves in lead V_1. ATs arising from the superior PVs have larger amplitude P waves in the inferior leads than those in ATs arising from the inferior PVs. However, P wave morphology generally is of greater accuracy in distinguishing right-sided from left-sided PVs in contrast to superior from inferior PVs. Despite prior posterior LA ablation, the surface ECG morphology of ATs originating from the PV ostia in patients with prior AF ablation procedures are similar to those in patients without prior ablation. However, ATs originating from the bottom of the right or left PVs after prior PV isolation can have a significant negative component or can be completely negative in the inferior leads. This may be related to prior ablation in the superoposterior LA or to a more inferior origin of the tachycardia after prior ablation outside the PV ostium.[30]

ATs arising from the right superior PV are associated with P waves that are narrow, positive in the inferior leads, of equal amplitude in leads II and III, biphasic or slightly positive in lead V_1, and isoelectric in lead I (Fig. 8-4). The right superior PV is a common site of origin for LA ATs. It is only a few centimeters from the sinus node, and activation rapidly crosses the septum via Bachmann's bundle to activate the RA in a fashion similar to NSR, explaining the similarities in P wave morphology. However, whereas the P wave is biphasic in lead V_1 during NSR, it is positive in that lead during right superior PV AT (Fig. 8-5).[28]

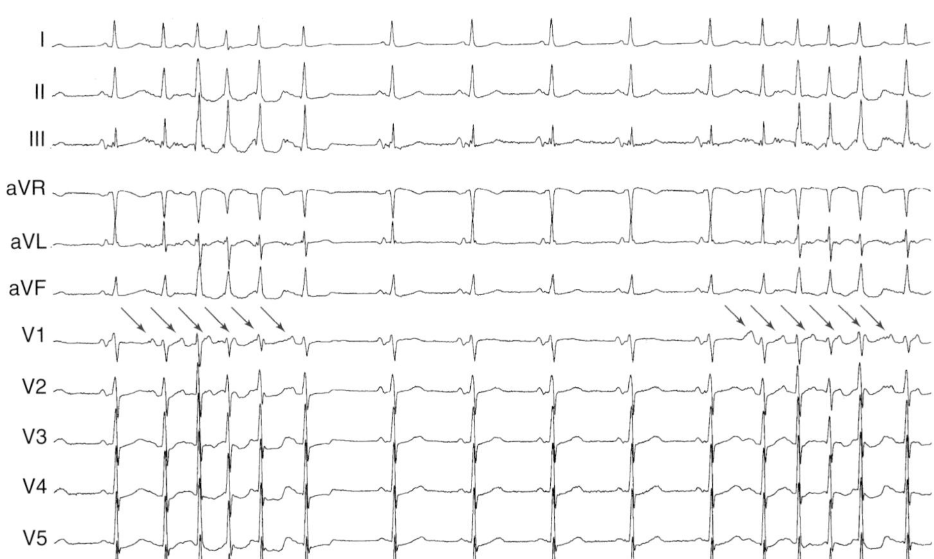

FIGURE 8–4 Surface ECG of repetitive nonsustained atrial tachycardia (AT) originating from the right superior pulmonary vein (PV). Note that the first P wave of the tachycardia is similar in morphology to the subsequent ones, consistent with abnormal automaticity mechanism of the AT. Also, note the similarities between the AT and sinus P waves. However, in lead V_1, the tachycardia P wave is positive, whereas the sinus P wave is biphasic.

With LA appendage ATs, the P wave is positive in the inferior leads (more positive in lead III than in II), positive in lead V_1, and negative in leads I and aVL.

Mitral annular ATs typically cluster at the superior aspect of the mitral annulus in close proximity to the aortomitral continuity. ATs originating in this circumscribed area are characterized by P waves with an initial narrow negative deflection in lead V_1 followed by a positive deflection. The positivity of the P wave becomes progressively less from V_1 through V_6. The P wave is negative in leads I and aVL, and isoelectric or slightly positive in the inferior leads.[10]

ATs arising from the CS musculature typically demonstrate positive P waves in leads V_1, aVL, and aVR and negative P waves in the inferior leads.[4]

ELECTROPHYSIOLOGICAL TESTING

Baseline Observations During Normal Sinus Rhythm

Preexcitation can be present and suggests orthodromic AVRT but does not exclude AT. Also, the presence of dual AVN physiology suggests AVNRT but does not exclude AT. On the other hand, broad sinus P wave and intraatrial conduction delay suggest macroreentrant AT.

Induction of Tachycardia

Frequently, AT foci can become inactive in the EP laboratory environment because of sedative medications, changes in autonomic tone that can be caused by prolonged supine position, patient anxiety, deviation from normal diet, or other changes in daily activities that can have an impact on the circadian variation of AT activity. Thus, in preparation for an AT ablation procedure, several measures should be undertaken. Antiarrhythmic drugs should be discontinued for at least five half-lives before the EP study. Sedation should be minimized throughout the procedure. It may be an appropriate policy to monitor the patient in the EP laboratory initially without sedation. If no spontaneous tachycardia is induced, isoproterenol is administered. If no AT can be induced, a single quadripolar catheter is placed in the RA, and programmed electrical stimulation is performed. If AT remains quiescent, the procedure is aborted and retried at a future date. If AT is inducible at any step, the full EP catheter arrangement and EP study are undertaken (Table 8-2).[16,19,24]

TABLE 8–2 Programmed Electrical Stimulation Protocol for Electrophysiological Testing of Atrial Tachycardia

- Atrial burst pacing from the RA and CS (down to a pacing CL at which 2 : 1 atrial capture occurs)
- Single and double AES at multiple CLs (600-400 msec) from the RA and CS (down to atrial ERP)
- Ventricular burst pacing from the RV apex (down to VA Wenckebach CL)
- Single and double VES at multiple CLs (600-400 msec) from the RV apex (down to ventricular ERP)

AES = atrial extrastimulation; CL = cycle length; CS = coronary sinus; ERP = effective refractory period; RA = right atrium; RV = right ventricle; VA = ventricular-atrial; VES = ventricular extrastimulation.

Initiation by Atrial Extrastimulation or Atrial Pacing

Microreentrant Atrial Tachycardia. Microreentrant AT is usually easy to initiate with a wide range of AES coupling intervals (A_1-A_2 intervals). The initiating AES coupling interval and the interval between the initiating AES and first beat of AT are inversely related.

The first tachycardia P wave is different from subsequent P waves; the first P wave is usually a PAC or AES that is necessary to start the AT (Fig. 8-6). In addition, no delay in AH or PR interval is required for initiation, although it can occur. AV block can also occur at initiation.[19]

Triggered-Activity Atrial Tachycardia. Triggered ATs can be initiated by AES or (more commonly) atrial pacing. Initiation frequently requires catecholamines (isoproterenol). There is usually a direct relationship between the coupling interval or pacing CL initiating the AT and the interval to the onset of the AT and the early CL of the AT.

The first tachycardia P wave is different from subsequent P waves (the first P wave is usually a PAC or AES that is necessary to start the AT). No delay in the AH interval is required for initiation, although it can occur.

Automatic Atrial Tachycardia. Automatic ATs cannot be reproducibly initiated by AES or atrial pacing. The first

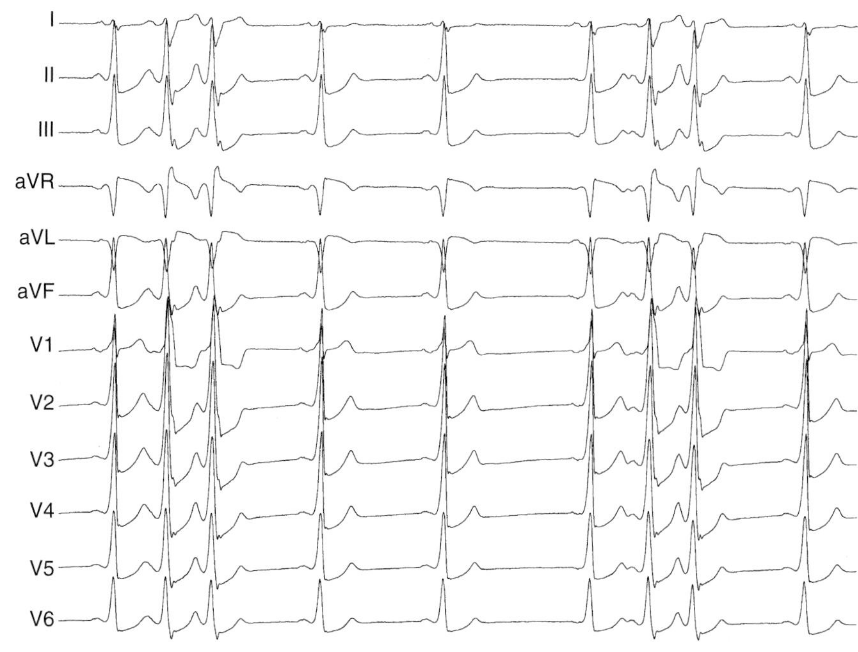

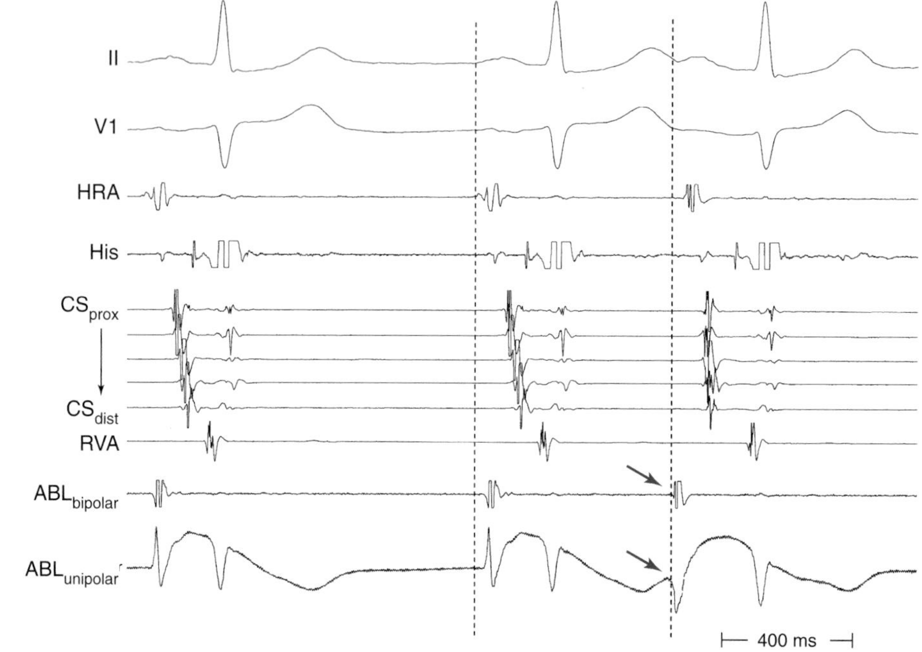

FIGURE 8–5 Premature atrial complexes (PACs) originating from the right superior pulmonary vein (PV). **Upper panel,** 12-lead surface ECG illustrating atrial couplets during normal sinus rhythm (NSR). Note the similarities in P wave morphology during PACs versus NSR. **Lower panel,** Intracardiac recordings from the same patient. Detailed mapping localized the origin of the PACs to the ostium of the right superior PV (as illustrated by bipolar and unipolar recordings from the ablation catheter [ABL]). Note the concordance of timing of the bipolar and unipolar recordings and the QS unipolar electrogram morphology (blue arrows), suggesting the site of origin of activation and a good ablation site.

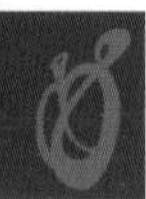

8

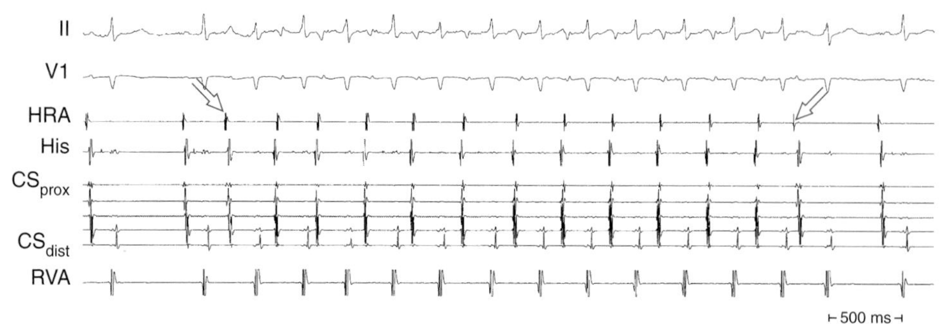

FIGURE 8–6 Spontaneous initiation and termination of a midseptal focal atrial tachycardia (AT; arrows). The tachycardia is initiated and terminated by a premature atrial complex of different morphology from that of the AT, suggesting a nonautomatic mechanism. Note the narrow P wave during AT, consistent with a septal origin.

tachycardia P wave occurs late in the cardiac cycle and is therefore not associated with atrial or AVN conduction delay.

The first tachycardia P wave and subsequent P waves are identical; the AT does not require a PAC to start (see Fig. 8-4). The tachycardia CL tends to progressively shorten (warm up) for several beats until its ultimate rate is achieved. As with other types of AT, no delay in the AH interval is required for initiation, although it can occur.

Initiation by Ventricular Extrastimulation or Ventricular Pacing

It is uncommon to initiate AT with ventricular extrastimulation (VES) or ventricular pacing because decremental retrograde conduction over the AVN prevents adequate prematurity of atrial activation. However, in the presence of an AV BT, fast retrograde atrial activation mediates adequate prematurity of the conducted ventricular stimulus to the atrium, and AT may be induced.[19]

Tachycardia Features

Atrial Activation Sequence

P wave morphology and atrial activation sequence depend on the site of origin of the AT. Intracardiac mapping shows significant portions of the tachycardia CL without recorded atrial activity, and atrial activation time is markedly less than the tachycardia CL (see Fig. 8-1).[19]

Atrial-Ventricular Relationship

The atrial–His bundle (AH) and PR intervals during AT are appropriate for the AT rate and are usually longer than those during NSR. The faster the AT rate, the longer the AH and PR intervals. Thus the PR interval may be shorter, longer, or equal to the RP interval. The PR interval may also be equal to the RR and the P wave may fall inside the preceding QRS, mimicking typical AVNRT.[19]

AV block may be observed during AT because neither the AVN nor the ventricle are part of the AT circuit. Most incessant SVTs with AV block are probably automatic ATs.

Oscillation in the Tachycardia Cycle Length

Analysis of tachycardia CL variability can provide useful diagnostic information for discrimination between the different types of SVT, even when episodes of SVT are nonsustained. SVT CL variability 15 milliseconds or more in magnitude occurs commonly in paroxysmal SVTs. CL variability in AT is a result of changes in the CL of the AT or changes in AVN conduction. Therefore, when there is CL variability in the atrium and ventricle, changes in the atrial CL are expected to precede and predict the changes in the ventricular CL. However, ventricular CL variability can be caused by changes in AV conduction instead of changes in the CL of the AT, in which case ventricular CL variability is not predicted by a prior change in atrial CL during the AT. Because there is no VA conduction during AT, ventricular CL variability by itself is not expected to result in atrial CL variability during AT.[31] Additionally, spontaneous changes in the PR and RP intervals with fixed A-A interval favor AT over other types of SVT (Fig. 8-7).

In contrast to AT, typical AVNRT and orthodromic AVRT generally have CL variability caused by changes in anterograde AVN conduction. Because retrograde conduction through a fast AVN pathway or a BT generally is much less variable than anterograde conduction through the AVN, the changes in ventricular CL that result from variability in anterograde AVN conduction are expected to precede the subsequent changes in atrial CL.[31]

Effects of Bundle Branch Block

Bundle branch block (BBB) may occur during AT but does not affect the tachycardia CL because the ventricles are not part of the AT circuit.[19]

Termination and Response to Physiological and Pharmacological Maneuvers

With spontaneous termination, ATs terminate with a QRS complex following the last P wave of the tachycardia. Most ATs (50% to 80%) are terminated by adenosine; therefore, termination of SVT in response to adenosine is not helpful in differentiating AT from other SVTs.[19,32] Usually (80%), termination of AT in response to adenosine occurs prior to the onset of AV block (i.e., termination occurs with a tachycardia P wave followed by a QRS). Reproducible termination with a P wave not followed by a QRS indicates other types of SVT, because it occurs in AT only if adenosine terminates the AT at the same moment it causes AV block, which is a rare event. In the atrium, adenosine produces antiadrenergic effects (presumably responsible for terminating triggered activity) and increases acetylcholine- or adenosine-activated K^+ current ($I_{K(Ach,Ado)}$), resulting in shortening of the action potential duration and reduction of the resting membrane potential, which may be responsible for terminating atrial microreentry. Adenosine may help identify automatic ATs, which are generally transiently slowed but not terminated, with gradual resumption of the AT rate.[1]

Microreentrant Atrial Tachycardia. Carotid sinus massage, vagal maneuvers, and adenosine reproducibly slow or terminate sinus node reentrant tachycardia and 25% of microreentrant ATs (especially those with long tachycardia CL and those arising in the RA). Spontaneous termination of AT is usually accompanied by progressive

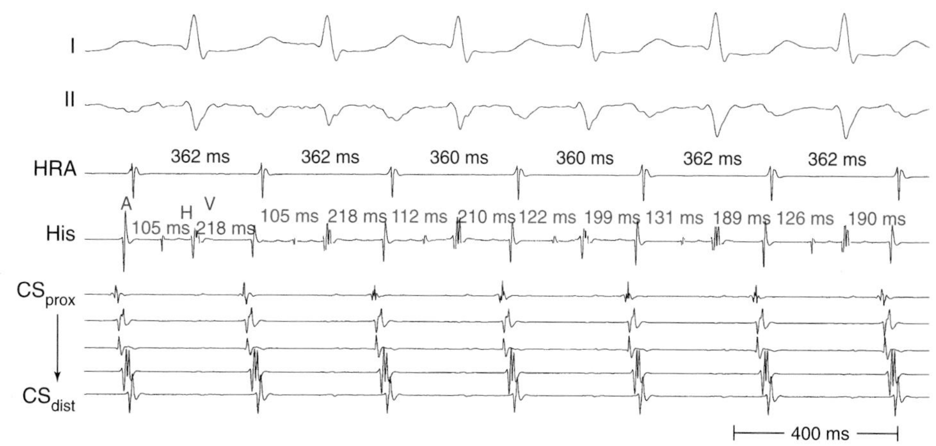

FIGURE 8–7 Supraventricular tachycardia (SVT) with concentric atrial activation sequence. Note the constant atrial cycle length (numbers in black) but variable atrial–His bundle (AH) interval (numbers in red) and ventricular-atrial (VA) interval (numbers in blue). This observation favors atrial tachycardia (originating from the posteroseptal region) as the mechanism of the tachycardia over other types of SVT.

prolongation of the A-A interval, with or without changes in AV conduction.[1]

Triggered-Activity Atrial Tachycardia. Carotid sinus massage, vagal maneuvers, adenosine, verapamil, beta blockers, and sodium channel blockers usually can terminate triggered-activity AT.

Automatic Atrial Tachycardia. Carotid sinus massage can cause AV block but generally does not terminate the AT. Adenosine can slow but not terminate the AT. Only beta blockers have been useful in termination of paroxysmal (but not incessant) automatic AT. Termination of automatic AT is usually preceded by a cool-down phenomenon of the AT rate.[1]

Diagnostic Maneuvers During Tachycardia

Atrial Extrastimulation and Atrial Pacing During Supraventricular Tachycardia

Microreentrant Atrial Tachycardia. AES can reset microreentrant AT with a resetting response classic for reentry (increasing or mixed response). Atrial pacing can entrain microreentrant AT. However, because the microreentrant circuit is very small, only orthodromic capture is usually observed. In addition, constant fusion (at a fixed pacing CL) or progressive fusion (at progressively shorter pacing CLs), as demonstrated by intermediate P wave morphologies on the surface ECG, cannot be demonstrated in case of microreentrant AT. Similarly, collision of activation wavefronts and/or partial activation change during entrainment cannot be demonstrated with multiple endocardial recordings. During entrainment of microreentrant AT, the return CL and post-pacing interval (PPI) will be fixed regardless of the number of beats in the pacing train. AES and atrial pacing can almost always terminate microreentrant AT (especially sinus node reentrant tachycardia).[19]

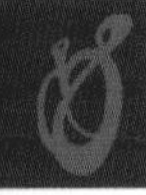
8

Triggered-Activity Atrial Tachycardia. AES can reset triggered-activity AT (with a decreasing resetting response). However, triggered-activity AT cannot be entrained by atrial pacing. Following the delivery of an AES or atrial overdrive pacing during triggered-activity AT, the return CL tends to shorten with shortening of the AES coupling interval or pacing CL. AES and, more effectively, atrial pacing can usually terminate triggered-activity AT.[19]

Automatic Atrial Tachycardia. Response of automatic AT to AES is similar to that of the sinus node. A late-coupled AES collides with the tachycardia impulse already exiting the AT focus (zone of collision), resulting in fusion of atrial activation (fusion between the paced and the tachycardia wavefronts) or paced-only atrial activation sequence, and will not affect the timing of the next AT complex (producing a fully compensatory pause). An earlier coupled AES enters the AT focus before the time of the next tachycardia wavefront, and therefore resets the AT focus (zone of reset), with a return CL that is not fully compensatory. The return cycle usually remains constant over widening coupling intervals during the zone of reset. A very early coupled AES encounters a refractory AT focus (following the last tachycardia complex) and would not be able to enter or reset the AT focus. Therefore, the next AT complex will be on time because the atrium is already fully recovered following that early AES (zone of interpolation).

Automatic AT cannot be entrained by atrial pacing. Rapid atrial pacing results in overdrive suppression of the AT rate, with the return CL following the pacing train prolonging with increasing the duration of pacing. The AT resumes after cessation of atrial pacing but at a slower rate and gradually speeds up (warms up) to return back to prepacing tachycardia CL. Occasionally, overdrive pacing produces no effect at all on automatic AT.[19]

Differential Site Atrial Pacing: Overdrive pacing during the SVT is performed from different atrial sites (high RA and proximal CS) at the same pacing CL, and the maximal difference in the post-pacing VA intervals (the interval from last captured ventricular electrogram to the earliest atrial electrogram of the initial beat after pacing) among the different pacing sites is calculated (ΔVA interval). In one report, a ΔVA interval more than 14 milliseconds was diagnostic of AT, whereas a ΔVA interval less than 14 milliseconds favors AVNRT or orthodromic AVRT over AT (with the sensitivity, specificity, and positive and negative predictive values all equal to 100%).

In orthodromic AVRT and AVNRT, the initial atrial activation following cessation of atrial pacing is linked to the last captured ventricular activation and, therefore, cannot be dissociated from the ventricular activation. In contrast, in AT, the first atrial return cycle following cessation of pacing is dependent on the distance between the AT origin and pacing site, atrial conduction properties, and mode of the resetting response of the AT, and is not related to the preceding ventricular activation. Hence, the post-pacing VA intervals vary among the pacing sites and the ΔVA interval display not zero, but a certain value.

Ventricular Extrastimulation and Ventricular Pacing During Supraventricular Tachycardia

It is uncommon for VES or ventricular pacing to affect an AT unless rapid 1:1 VA conduction is present (especially in the presence of an AV-BT) and the tachycardia CL is relatively long. Cessation of overdrive ventricular pacing during AT (with 1:1 VA conduction without terminating the tachycardia) results in an A-A-V pattern, which is suggestive of AT as the mechanism of the SVT and practically excludes AVNRT and orthodromic AVRT, whereas an A-V pattern is consistent with AVNRT or orthodromic AVRT and makes AT less likely.[19]

Concept of A-V Versus A-A-V Response After Ventricular Pacing During Supraventricular Tachycardia

Technique. During SVT, ventricular pacing is initiated at a pacing CL 10 to 60 milliseconds shorter than the tachycardia CL until 1:1 VA conduction occurs, at which point pacing is discontinued. If pacing results in termination of the tachycardia, SVT is reinduced and the maneuver is repeated. If ventricular pacing does not terminate the tachycardia and the presence of stable 1:1 VA conduction is verified, the electrogram sequence immediately after the last ventricular paced complex is categorized as atrial-ventricular (A-V) or atrial-atrial-ventricular (A-A-V) (Fig. 8-8).

Interpretation. During AVNRT or orthodromic AVRT, when the ventricle is paced at a CL shorter than the tachycardia CL and all electrograms are advanced to the pacing rate without terminating the tachycardia (i.e., entrainment of the tachycardia is achieved), VA conduction occurs through the retrograde limb of the circuit. Therefore, after the last paced ventricular complex, the anterograde limb of the tachycardia circuit is not refractory, and the last entrained retrograde atrial complex can conduct to the ventricle. This results in an A-V response following cessation of pacing. However, when the ventricle is paced during AT and 1:1 VA conduction is produced, retrograde conduction occurs through the AVN. In this case, the last retrograde atrial complex resulting from ventricular pacing is unable to conduct to the ventricle because the AVN is refractory to anterograde conduction, and the result is an A-A-V response.

Pitfalls. This pacing maneuver would not be useful when 1:1 VA conduction during ventricular pacing is absent. Thus, when determining the response after ventricular pacing during SVT, the presence of 1:1 VA conduction

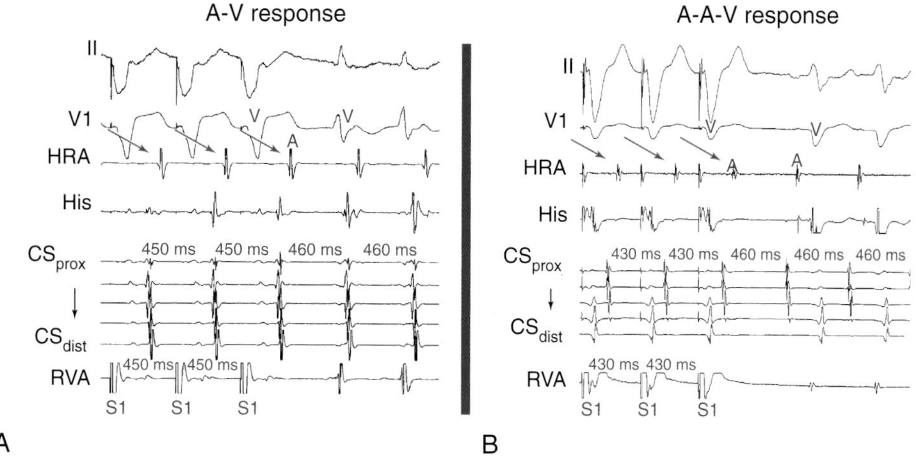

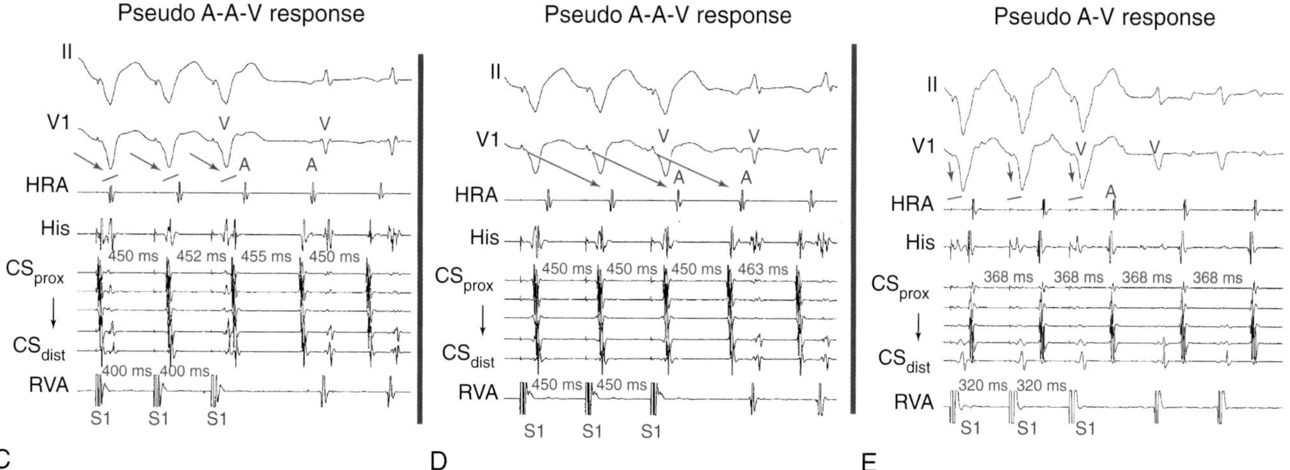

FIGURE 8–8 A-V versus A-A-V response after ventricular pacing during supraventricular tachycardia (SVT). Overdrive ventricular pacing is performed during five SVTs with concentric atrial activation sequence. Red arrows track ventricular-atrial (VA) conduction during ventricular pacing. Numbers indicate ventricular pacing cycle lengths (CLs) and atrial CLs during and after pacing. **A,** A-V response is observed following cessation of pacing during typical atrioventricular nodal reentrant tachycardia (AVNRT), which is inconsistent with atrial tachycardia (AT). **B,** A-A-V response is observed, consistent with AT originating in the posteroseptal region. **C,** Pseudo–A-A-V response is observed during atypical AVNRT secondary to VA dissociation (i.e., absence of VA conduction) during ventricular pacing. **D,** Pseudo–A-A-V response is observed during atypical AVNRT despite the presence of 1 : 1 VA conduction during ventricular pacing. Retrograde conduction during ventricular pacing, however, occurs through the slow atrioventricular node (AVN) pathway with a long VA interval (red arrows) that is longer than the pacing CL; hence, the last ventricular paced impulse will be followed first by the P wave conducted slowly from the previous paced QRS, and then by the P wave resulting from the last paced QRS, mimicking an A-A-V response. This is verified by observing that the last retrograde atrial complex characteristically occurs at an A-A interval equal to the ventricular pacing CL, whereas the first tachycardia atrial complex usually occurs at a different return CL. **E,** Pseudo–A-V response is observed during focal AT secondary to VA dissociation (i.e., absence of VA conduction) during ventricular pacing.

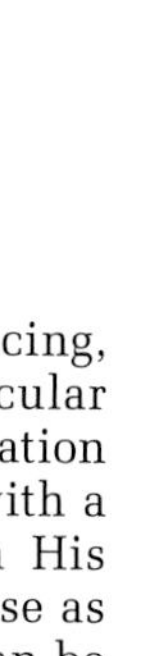

must be confirmed. Isorhythmic VA dissociation can mimic 1 : 1 VA conduction, especially when the pacing train is not long enough or the pacing CL is too slow (see Fig. 8-8).

A pseudo–A-A-V response can occur during atypical AVNRT. Because retrograde conduction during ventricular pacing occurs through the slow pathway, the VA interval is long and can be longer than the pacing CL (V-V interval), so that the last paced QRS is followed first by the atrial complex resulting from slow VA conduction of the preceding paced QRS, and then by the atrial complex resulting from the last paced QRS. Careful examination of the last atrial electrogram that resulted from VA conduction during ventricular pacing will avoid this potential pitfall; the last retrograde atrial complex characteristically occurs at an A-A interval equal to the ventricular pacing CL, whereas the first tachycardia atrial complex usually occurs at a different return CL. A pseudo–A-A-V response may also occur when 1 : 1 VA conduction is absent during overdrive ventricular pacing, during typical AVNRT with long His bundle–ventricular (HV) or short HA intervals during which atrial activation may precede ventricular activation, and in patients with a bystander BT. Replacing ventricular activation with His bundle (HB) activation (i.e., characterizing the response as A-A-H or A-H instead of A-A-V or A-V, respectively) can be more accurate and can help eliminate the pseudo–A-A-V response in patients with AVNRT and long HV intervals, short HA intervals, or both.[33]

On the other hand, a pseudo–A-V response can occur with automatic AT when the maneuver is performed during isoproterenol infusion. Ventricular pacing with 1 : 1 VA conduction can result in overdrive suppression of the atrial focus and isoproterenol may cause an increase in junctional automaticity, so that an apparent A-V response occurs. Therefore, when performed during an isoproterenol infusion, it is important to determine that the response after cessation of ventricular pacing is reproducible.[34]

A pseudo–A-V response can theoretically occur when AT coexists with retrograde dual AVN pathways or bystander BT. In such cases, the last retrograde atrial complex would have an alternative route for anterograde conduction to the ventricle, other than the one used for retrograde VA conduction during ventricular pacing, resulting in an A-V response. However, clinical occurrence of these theoretical scenarios has not been observed, probably because of retrograde penetration of both AVN pathways or of the AVN and the BT during ventricular pacing, so that both pathways are refractory to anterograde conduction on cessation of pacing.[34]

Exclusion of Other Arrhythmia Mechanisms

Focal AT should be differentiated from other SVTs, including AVNRT, orthodromic AVRT, and macroreentrant AT. Programmed electrical stimulation is usually adequate in excluding AVNRT and AVRT as the mechanism of SVT (Tables 8-3 and 8-4).[19,27] Macroreentry, however, can be more difficult to exclude, and electroanatomical mapping is of value in some cases (Table 8-5).

MAPPING

Activation Mapping

Activation mapping entails localizing the site of earliest presystolic activity to the onset of the P wave during AT. Endocardial activation mapping can trace the origin of activation to a specific area, from where it spreads to both atria. Spread of activation from the focus or origin may not be uniformly radial; anatomical or functional pathways and barriers can influence conduction.

There is generally an electrically silent period in the atrial CL reflected by an isoelectric line between atrial deflections on the surface ECG. Intracardiac mapping typically shows significant portions of the tachycardia CL without recorded activity, even when recording from the entire RA, LA, and/or CS (see Fig. 8-1). However, in

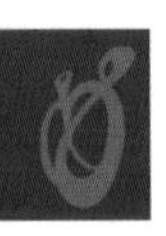

8

TABLE 8–3 Exclusion of Atrioventricular Nodal Reentrant Tachycardia (AVNRT)

Parameter	Features
Atrial activation sequence	Eccentric atrial activation sequence generally excludes AVNRT (except in the case of left variant of AVNRT).
AV block	Spontaneous or induced AV block with continuation of the tachycardia is uncommon in AVNRT.
Spontaneous oscillations of the tachycardia CL	Spontaneous changes in PR and RP intervals with fixed A-A interval excludes AVNRT.
Entrainment of the SVT by ventricular pacing	If overdrive pacing entrains the SVT with an atrial activation sequence different from that during the SVT, AVNRT is unlikely. The presence of an A-A-V electrogram sequence following cessation of overdrive ventricular pacing practically excludes AVNRT.
Entrainment of SVT by atrial pacing	ΔAH ($AH_{atrial\ pacing} - AH_{SVT}$) < 20 msec excludes AVNRT. If entrainment cannot be achieved or overdrive suppression is demonstrated, AVNRT is excluded.
Atrial pacing during NSR at the tachycardia CL	ΔAH ($AH_{atrial\ pacing} - AH_{SVT}$) < 20 msec excludes AVNRT.

AH = atrial-His bundle interval; AV = atrioventricular; CL = cycle length; NSR = normal sinus rhythm; SVT = supraventricular tachycardia.

TABLE 8–4 Exclusion of Orthodromic Atrioventricular Reentrant Tachycardia (AVRT)

Parameter	Features
Atrial activation sequence	Initial atrial activation site away from the AV groove excludes orthodromic AVRT.
VA interval	VA interval <70 msec or V-high RA interval <95 msec during SVT excludes orthodromic AVRT.
AV block	Spontaneous or induced AV block with continuation of the SVT excludes orthodromic AVRT.
Spontaneous oscillations of the tachycardia CL	Spontaneous changes in PR and RP intervals with fixed A-A interval excludes orthodromic AVRT.
VES delivered during the SVT	Failure to reset (advance or delay) atrial activation with early VES on multiple occasions and at different VES coupling intervals, despite advancement of the local ventricular activation at all sites (including the site of the suspected BT) by >30 msec, orthodromic AVRT and presence of AV BT are excluded.
Entrainment of the SVT by ventricular pacing	If overdrive pacing entrains the SVT with an atrial activation sequence different from that during the SVT, orthodromic AVRT is unlikely. The presence of an A-A-V electrogram sequence following cessation of overdrive ventricular pacing practically excludes orthodromic AVRT.
Entrainment of SVT by atrial pacing	If entrainment cannot be achieved or overdrive suppression is demonstrated, orthodromic AVRT is excluded. If the VA interval of the return cycle after cessation of atrial pacing is variable, orthodromic AVRT is excluded.
Ventricular pacing during NSR at the tachycardia CL	If VA block is present, orthodromic AVRT is excluded.

AV = atrioventricular; BT = bypass tract; CL = cycle length; NSR = normal sinus rhythm; RA = right atrium; SVT = supraventricular tachycardia; VA = ventricular-atrial; VES = ventricular extrastimulation.

TABLE 8–5 Exclusion of Macroreentrant Atrial Tachycardia (AT)

Parameter	Features
ECG	Focal AT usually has clearly defined isoelectric baseline between P waves in all leads. Macroreentrant AT usually lacks an isoelectric baseline between deflections.
Atrial activation sequence	Focal AT is characterized by atrial activation starting rhythmically at a small area (focus) and intracardiac mapping shows significant portions of the CL without recorded atrial activity. Macroreentrant AT endocardial recordings typically show activation spanning the whole tachycardia CL.
Programmed electrical stimulation	Focal AT is defined on the basis of dissociation of almost the entire atria from the tachycardia with AES. Macroreentrant AT circuit usually incorporates large portions of the RA or LA, which would be identified with resetting and entrainment mapping.
Entrainment mapping	Focal AT cannot be entrained, except for microreentrant AT, and in this case, because the microreentrant circuit is very small, only orthodromic capture is usually observed. In addition, constant or progressive fusion, as demonstrated by intermediate P wave morphologies on the ECG, cannot be demonstrated. Macroreentrant AT is defined by demonstration of concealed or manifest entrainment of the tachycardia with atrial pacing.
Electroanatomical 3-D mapping	Focal AT is suggested by electroanatomical maps demonstrating radial spreading of activation, from the earliest local activation site in all directions. Macroreentrant AT is suggested by electroanatomical maps demonstrating continuous progression of colors around the RA with close proximity of earliest and latest local activation.
Response to adenosine	Focal AT usually responds to adenosine by slowing or termination. Macroreentrant AT usually is not influenced by adenosine, and may actually accelerate (when the tachycardia CL is refractoriness-dependent) secondary to shortening of atrial refractoriness by adenosine.

AES = atrial extrastimulation; CL = cycle length; LA = left atrium; RA = right atrium.

the presence of complex intraatrial conduction disturbances, intraatrial activation may extend over a large proportion of the tachycardia CL, and conduction spread may follow circular patterns suggestive of macroreentrant activation.[16,19,24,35]

Determining the onset of the P wave is important in activation mapping but may be impossible if the preceding T wave or QRS is superimposed. Thus, the P wave during AT should be assessed using multiple surface ECG leads and choosing the one with the earliest P onset. To facilitate visualization of the P wave, a VES (or a train of ventricular pacing) is delivered to advance ventricular activation and repolarization to permit careful distinction of the P wave onset. After determining P wave onset, a surrogate marker that is easier to track during mapping, such as a high RA or CS electrogram indexed to P wave onset where it is clearly seen, may be used, rather than the P wave onset.

A single roving catheter is used to find the site with the earliest atrial electrogram using unipolar and bipolar recordings. Small movements of the catheter tip in the general target region are undertaken under the guidance of fluoroscopy until the site with the earliest possible atrial activation relative to the P wave is identified.[16,19,24,35] Activation times are generally measured from the onset or the first rapid deflection of the atrial bipolar electrogram to the onset of the P wave or (preferably) surrogate marker during AT. Using the onset of local electrogram is preferable, because it is easier to determine reproducibly when measuring heavily fractionated, low-amplitude atrial electrograms. The distal pole of the mapping catheter should be used for mapping for the earliest atrial activation site, because it is the pole through which RF energy is delivered.

An alternative method of activation mapping is to use two roving catheters. These catheters are each moved in tandem so that the earliest electrogram is recorded. Once the mapping catheter is placed at the site of early presystolic activity, a second catheter can then be manipulated around the reference mapping catheter to find even earlier sites of activation. Then, this catheter is left at those sites, and the first catheter is moved to look for another early site of activation. This is repeated until the earliest definable site is established. This dancing catheter technique is useful in the RA, but cannot be easily applied in the LA, where the CS catheter can serve as an excellent reference catheter, especially in cases of LA ATs arising close to the mitral annulus.

Unipolar recordings from the distal ablation electrode are used to supplement conventional bipolar activation mapping. Unipolar signals can be filtered or unfiltered, but unfiltered signals offer more directional information. Unipolar recordings will be helpful by showing negative (QS) patterns with sharp initial deflections at the location of the focus (see Fig. 8-5). Timing of the unipolar electrograms can help ensure that the tip electrode, which is the ablation electrode, is responsible for the early component of the bipolar electrograms. The site of origin of the AT is defined as the site with the earliest bipolar recording in which the distal tip shows the earliest intrinsic deflection and QS unipolar electrogram configuration (see Fig. 8-5).

Low-amplitude early signals followed by a sharper discrete signal may represent an early component of a fragmented electrogram or a far-field signal associated with a second discrete local signal. This is most likely to happen in the superior posterior RA, where it can actually represent electrical activity generated from the right superior PV. In this situation, the unipolar electrogram will demonstrate sharp negative deflection timing with the later, high-frequency potential on the bipolar electrogram.

Transient catheter-induced interruption of AT by pressure of the catheter may suggest an appropriate site for ablation. This sign is more useful when it is a reproducible phenomenon. Often, however, the tachycardia terminates as the catheter is passing the area, and where the catheter comes to rest may not be the same site as where transient AT termination occurred.

Special attention should be given to ATs mapped to the midseptum and the right anteroseptal region. For ATs mapped to the midseptum, especially if presystolic activity is not particularly early (i.e., less than 30 milliseconds presystolic), the electrogram is not fractionated, and multiple sites have similar activation times, exclusion of LA ATs using transseptal access to the LA is required (Fig. 8-9). For

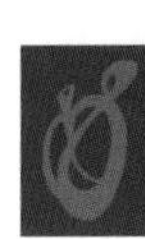

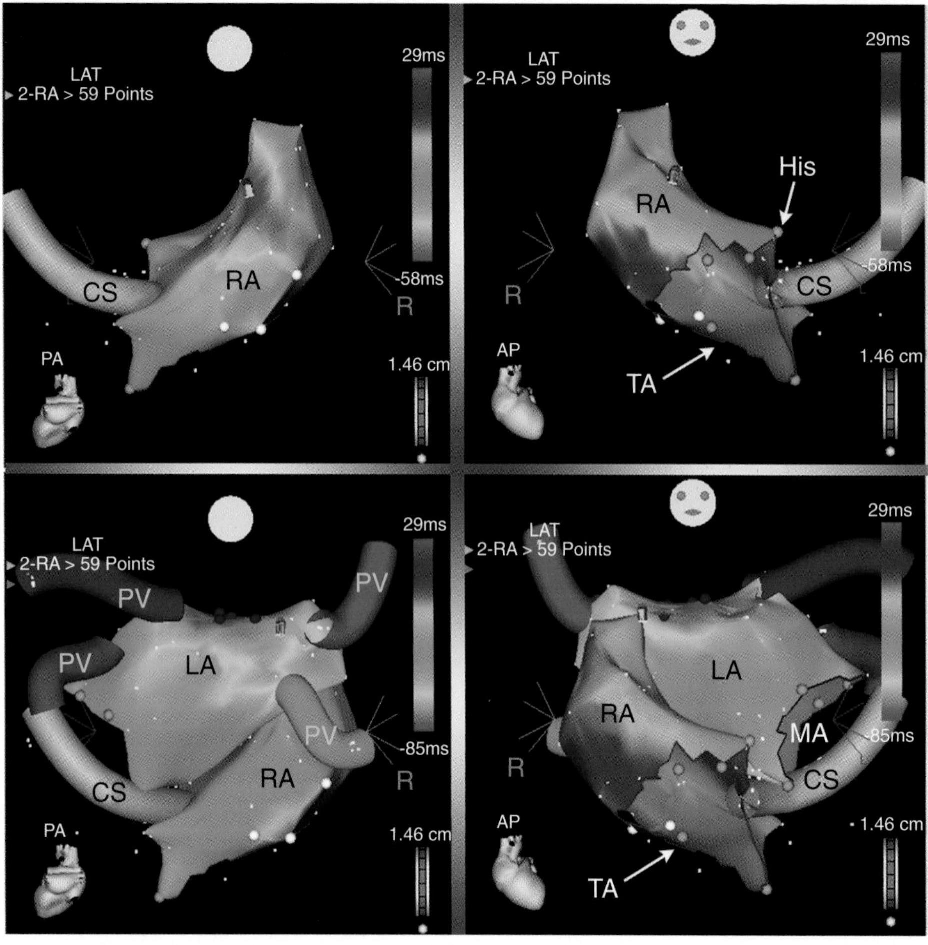

FIGURE 8–9 3-D electroanatomical (CARTO) activation map of focal atrial tachycardia (AT) originating from the left atrial (LA) roof. **Upper panel,** Posteroanterior (PA) and anteroposterior (AP) projections of the CARTO activation map of the right atrium (RA). **Lower panels,** PA and AP projections of the CARTO activation map of both the RA and LA. When mapping is limited to the RA (upper panels), the site of earliest atrial activation was localized to the interatrial septum, with local activation preceding the reference electrogram by 58 milliseconds. When activation mapping is extended to the LA (lower panels), a site with earlier local activation (preceding the reference electrogram by 85 milliseconds) was localized to the LA roof. Radiofrequency ablation (red dots) at that site eliminated the tachycardia. MA = mitral annulus; PV = pulmonary vein; TA = tricuspid annulus.

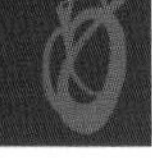

ATs arising from the PVs, CS activation times may not clearly indicate an LA site of origin. For ATs mapped to the right anteroseptal region (HB region), great care must be given to the anteromedial LA septum and LA free wall, because sites in these regions break through early to the right anteroseptal region, where ablation is not only unsuccessful but also can result in AV block.

Pace Mapping

When atrial activation originates from a point-like source, such as during focal AT or during pacing from an electrode catheter, the resultant P wave recorded on the surface ECG is determined by the sequence of atrial activation, which is determined to a large extent by the initial site of myocardial depolarization. Additionally, analysis of specific P wave configurations in multiple leads allows estimation of the pacing site location to within several square centimeters. Therefore, comparing the paced P wave configuration with that of AT is particularly useful for locating a small arrhythmia focus in a structurally normal heart.[5,16,19]

Pace mapping involves pacing from the distal tip of the mapping-ablation catheter at sites of interest. Initially, the exact morphology of the tachycardia complex should be determined and used as a template for pace mapping. Pace mapping during the tachycardia (at a pacing CL 20 to 40 milliseconds shorter than the tachycardia CL) is preferable whenever possible, because it facilitates rapid comparison of tachycardia and paced complexes at the end of pacing train. If sustained tachycardia cannot be induced, mapping is performed during spontaneous nonsustained runs or ectopic beats. Although it is preferable to match the pacing CL and coupling intervals of atrial extrastimuli to those of spontaneous ectopy, some reports have suggested that it is not mandatory to stimulate exactly at the same tachycardia CL to reproduce a similar atrial activation sequence and P wave morphology. Pace mapping is preferably performed with unipolar stimuli (10 mA, 2 milliseconds) from the distal electrode of the mapping catheter (cathode) and an electrode in the IVC (anode), or with closely spaced bipolar pacing at twice the diastolic threshold, so as to eliminate far-field stimulation effects.[16]

The greater the degree of concordance between the morphology during pacing and tachycardia, the closer the catheter is to the site of origin of the tachycardia. Pace maps with identical or near-identical matches of the tachycardia morphology in all 12 surface ECG leads are indicative of the site of origin of the tachycardia (Fig. 8-10).

Pace mapping is used as an adjunct to other methods of mapping to corroborate putative ablation sites. It can be of great help, especially when the AT is difficult to induce. Although there are some limitations to this technique, many studies have demonstrated efficacy using pace mapping to choose ablation target sites; concordance of P wave morphology during pace mapping and AT has a sensitivity of 86% and specificity of 37%. However, difficulties in precisely comparing P wave morphologies and intracardiac activation sequences limit the applicability of pace mapping. Moreover, the spatial resolution of atrial pace mapping is approximately 2 cm, which is too imprecise.

Electroanatomical Mapping

Mapping Technique. Electromagnetic 3-D mapping (CARTO, NavX), uses a single mapping catheter attached to a system that can precisely localize the catheter tip in 3-D

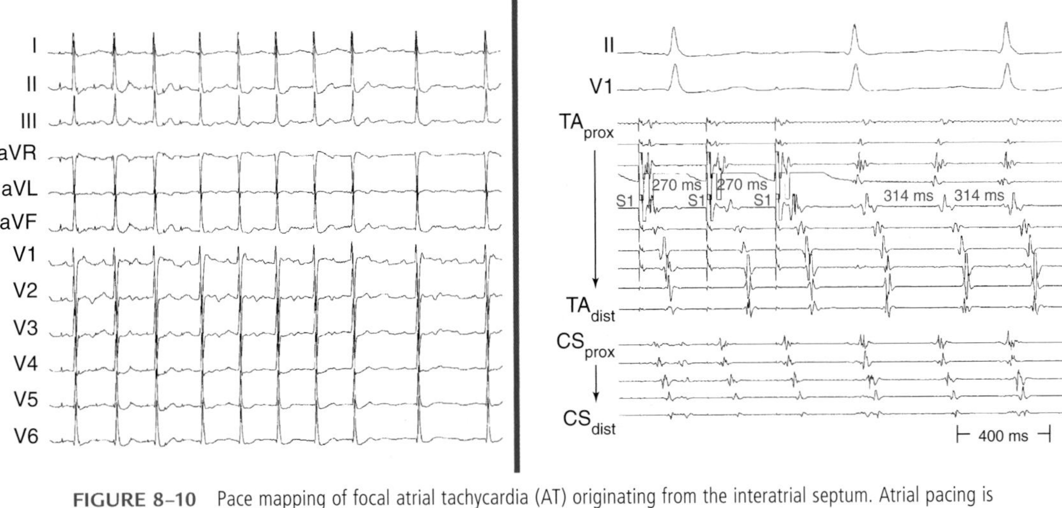

FIGURE 8–10 Pace mapping of focal atrial tachycardia (AT) originating from the interatrial septum. Atrial pacing is performed during the tachycardia at a cycle length (CL) of 270 milliseconds from the site of earliest activation (recorded by the Halo catheter positioned around the tricuspid annulus [TA]). Concordance between paced and tachycardia P wave morphology on the surface ECG (left panel) as well as endocardial atrial activation sequence (right panel) suggests proximity of the pacing site to the AT focus.

space and store activation time on a 3-D anatomical reconstruction.[5,36,37] Initially, selection of the reference electrogram, positioning of the anatomical reference, and determination of the window of interest are undertaken. The reference catheter is usually placed in the CS (because of its stability) using an electrode recording a prominent atrial electrogram, and ensuring that the ventricular electrogram is not the one picked up by the system.

A 4-mm tip mapping-ablation catheter is initially positioned, using fluoroscopy, at known anatomical points that serve as landmarks for the electroanatomical map. Anatomic and EP landmarks (IVC, SVC, CS, HB, and tricuspid annulus for RA mapping, and the mitral annulus and PVs for LA mapping) are tagged. The catheter is then advanced slowly around the chamber walls to sample sequential points along the endocardium, sequentially acquiring the location of its tip together with the local electrogram (see Fig. 8-9).

Activation mapping is performed to define atrial activation sequence. A reasonable number of points homogenously distributed in the RA or LA have to be recorded (approximately 80 to 100 points). The local activation time at each site is determined from the intracardiac bipolar electrogram and is measured in relation to the fixed intracardiac electrogram obtained from the CS (reference) catheter. Points are added to the map only if stability criteria in space and local activation time requirements are met. The end-diastolic location stability criterion is less than 2 mm and the local activation time stability criterion is less than 2 milliseconds. The activation map may also be used to catalogue sites at which pacing maneuvers are performed during assessment of the tachycardia.

Activation maps display the local activation time by a color-coded overlay on the reconstructed 3-D geometry. The selected points of local activation time are color-coded (red for the earliest electrical activation areas; orange, yellow, green, blue, and purple for progressively delayed activation areas). The electroanatomical maps of focal ATs demonstrate radial spreading of activation, from the earliest local activation site (red) in all directions (a well-defined early activation site surrounded by later activation sites); in these cases, activation time—a total range of activation times—is usually markedly shorter than the tachycardia CL (see Fig. 8-9). Conversely, a continuous progression of colors (from red to purple), with close proximity of earliest and latest local activation ("red meeting purple"), suggests the presence of a macroreentrant tachycardia. In these cases, activation time is in a similar range to tachycardia CL (see Fig. 9-6).

A stepwise strategy for mapping of RA and LA focal ATs has been described in a study using CARTO to avoid time-consuming whole-chamber maps.[36] Using this approach, mapping is started with the acquisition of four or five anatomically defined sites at the superior and septal part of the tricuspid annulus, and the mapping procedure is strategically continued according to this initial activation sequence. If the initial four-point activation map shows the earliest atrial activation to be at the superior aspect of the tricuspid annulus, mapping is continued toward the free wall of the RA, including the crista terminalis. In cases in which earliest atrial activation within the four-point area is found at the septal aspect of the tricuspid annulus, the map is expanded to the triangle of Koch and the paraseptal space. This strategy was found to differentiate reliably between ATs arising from the free wall of the RA, including crista terminalis and RA appendage, from those arising from the triangle of Koch and paraseptal space, as well as from left-sided ATs. Once the general area of interest is identified, high-density mapping of this area is undertaken together with conventional electrographic analysis (see earlier) to identify the site of the earliest activation within this target area. If the unipolar electrogram of the point of earliest activation at the RA septum or at the high posterior wall still shows a significant R wave, or RF ablation at that site is unsuccessful, a left-sided AT origin is assumed and the procedure is extended to the LA for dual-chamber maps.

Advantages of Electroanatomical (CARTO) Mapping System. The CARTO system provides a highly accurate geometric rendering of a cardiac chamber with a straightforward geometric display that has the capability to determine the 3-D location and orientation of the ablation catheter accurately.

The capability of the CARTO mapping system to associate relevant EP information with the appropriate spatial location in the heart and the ability to study activation patterns (with high spatial resolution [less than 1 mm]) during tachycardia in relation to normal anatomical structures and areas of scar significantly facilitate the mapping and ablation procedure. It allows for defining the mechanism(s) underlying the arrhythmia, rapid distinction between a

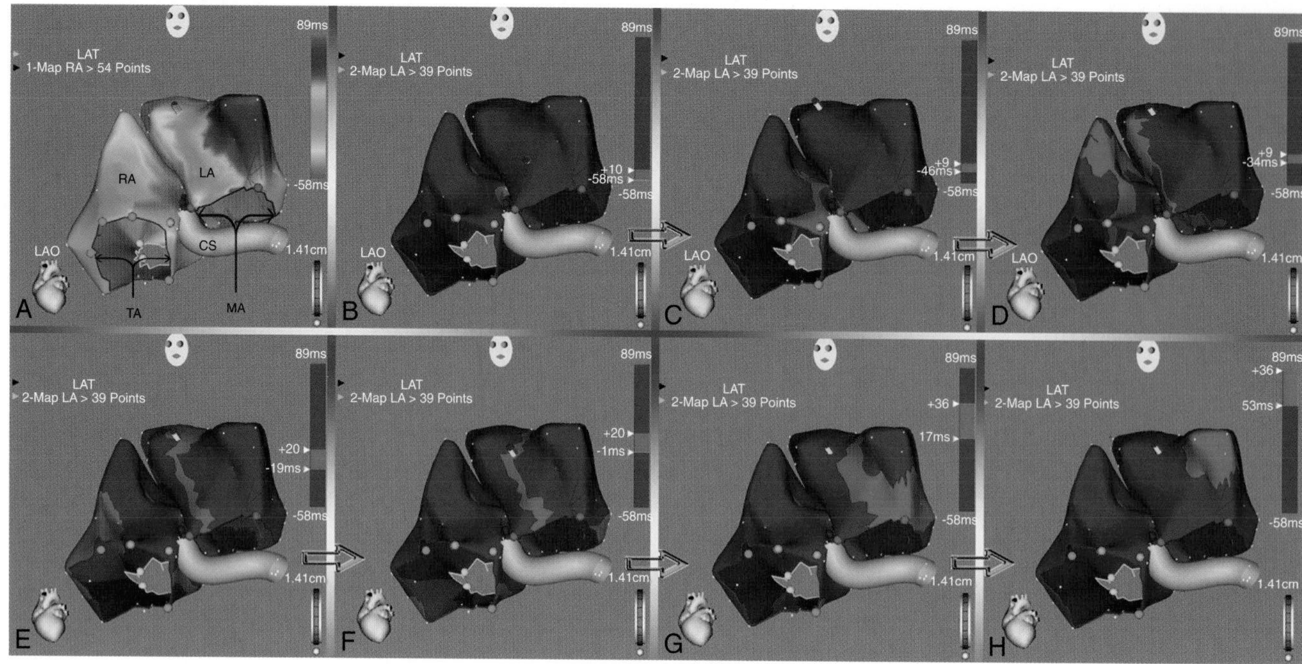

FIGURE 8–11 **A,** 3-D electroanatomical (CARTO) biatrial activation map in the left anterior oblique view constructed during focal atrial tachycardia (AT) originating posterosuperior to the coronary sinus (CS) ostium. During tachycardia, the activation wavefront propagates from the earliest local activation site (red) in all directions, **B to H,** Biatrial propagation map during the focal AT. MA = mitral annulus; TA = tricuspid annulus.

focal origin and macroreentrant tachycardia, and rapid visualization of the activation wavefront (propagation maps; Fig. 8-11), facilitating the identification of appropriate sites for entrainment mapping and pace mapping.

CARTO provides the capability to create and tag several potential points of interest during the mapping process (e.g., double potentials and sites with good pace maps) and return to them with great precision, which provides significant advantages over conventional techniques. The catheter can anatomically and accurately revisit a critically important recording site identified previously during the study, even if the tachycardia is no longer present or inducible and map-guided catheter navigation is no longer possible. This accurate repositioning can allow pace mapping from or further application of RF energy current to critically important sites that otherwise cannot be performed with a high degree of accuracy and reproducibility. Additionally, fluoroscopy time can be reduced via electromagnetic catheter navigation, and the catheter can be accurately guided to positions removed from fluoroscopic markers (see Fig. 8-9).

Limitations of Electroanatomical Mapping System. The sequential data acquisition required for creation of the electroanatomical map remains time-consuming, because the process requires tagging many points, depending on the spatial details needed to analyze a given arrhythmia. Furthermore, because the acquired data are not coherent in time, multiple beats are required and stable, sustained, or frequently repetitive arrhythmia is usually needed for creation of the activation map. Single PACs or nonsustained AT can be mapped, although at the expense of an appreciable amount of time.

Variation of the tachycardia CL of more than 10% may prevent complete understanding of the circuit, and decreases the confidence in the CARTO map. Additionally, the patient or intracardiac reference catheter may move, thus necessitating remapping. Another limitation of the CARTO system is the requirement of a special Biosense Webster mapping catheter; no other catheter types can be used with this system, and bidirectional steerable catheters are not available.

Mapping Nonsustained Focal Atrial Tachycardia

Several alternative mapping modalities can be used when AT is short-lived or cannot be reproducibly initiated, including simultaneous multisite data acquisition systems (noncontact mapping system, basket catheter, or localized high-density mapping). Moreover, the electroanatomical mapping and pace mapping techniques discussed can be used in these situations.

EnSite Noncontact Mapping System

The EnSite 3000 noncontact mapping system (Endocardial Solutions, St. Paul, Minn) consists of a noncontact catheter with a multielectrode array surrounding a 7.5-mL balloon mounted at the distal end. Raw data detected by the multielectrode are transferred to a silicon graphics workstation via a digitalized amplifier system. The multielectrode array is used to construct a 3-D computer model of the virtual endocardium. The system is able to reconstruct more than 3000 unipolar electrograms simultaneously and superimpose them onto the virtual endocardium, producing isopotential maps with a color range representing voltage amplitude. Electrical potentials at the endocardial surface some distance away are calculated. Sites of early endocardial activity, which are likely adjacent to the origin of the AT, are usually identifiable. Noncontact mapping can rapidly identify AT foci and thus delineate starting points for conventional mapping.[38-41]

The biggest advantage of noncontact endocardial mapping is its ability to recreate the endocardial activation sequence from simultaneously acquired multiple data points over a few (theoretically one) tachycardia beats, without requiring sequential point-to-point acquisitions. Therefore, it can be of great value in mapping nonsustained arrhythmias, PACs, irregular ATs, and rhythms that are not hemodynamically stable.[38-41]

Technique of Noncontact Mapping. The EnSite 3000 system requires placing a 9 Fr multielectrode array and a 7 Fr conventional (roving) deflectable mapping-ablation catheter in the cardiac chamber of interest. The balloon catheter is advanced over a 0.035-inch guidewire under fluoroscopy guidance and positioned in the atrium and deployed. The balloon is positioned in the center of the atrium and does not come in contact with the atrial walls being mapped. Activated clotting time (ACT) is kept at 250 to 300 seconds for right-sided and 300 to 400 seconds for left-sided mapping. The mapping-ablation catheter is positioned in the atrium and used to collect geometry information. The mapping catheter is initially moved to known anatomical locations (IVC, SVC, CS, HB, and tricuspid annulus for RA mapping, and mitral annulus and PVs for LA mapping), which are tagged. A detailed geometry of the chamber is then reconstructed by moving the mapping catheter around the atrium.

Unlike the CARTO mapping system, the noncontact system allows for the patient to be in NSR or tachycardia during creation of the geometry. Using this information, the computer creates a model of the atrium. After the chamber geometry is determined, mapping of the arrhythmia can begin. The data acquisition process is performed automatically by the system, and all data for the entire chamber are acquired simultaneously. Following this, the segment must be analyzed by the operator to find the early activation of the AT. The locator technology that was used to collect the geometry information can then be used to guide an ablation catheter to the proper location in the heart.

Limitations of Noncontact Mapping. Very low amplitude signals may not be detected, particularly if the distance between the center of the balloon catheter and endocardial surface exceeds 40 mm, limiting the accurate identification of diastolic signals. Furthermore, a second catheter is still required for additional mapping and for ablation. Aggressive anticoagulation is required using this mapping modality, and special attention and care are necessary during placement of the large balloon electrode in a nondilated atrium.

Multielectrode (Basket) Catheter Mapping

The basket catheter consists of an open-lumen catheter shaft with a collapsible, basket-shaped, distal end. The catheter is composed of 64 electrodes mounted on eight flexible, self-expanding, equidistant metallic splines (each spline carrying eight ring electrodes). The electrodes are equally spaced 4 or 5 mm apart, depending on the size of the basket catheter used (with diameters of 48 or 60 mm, respectively). Each spline is identified by a letter (from A to H) and each electrode by a number (from 1 to 8, with electrode 1 having the distal position on the splines). The basket catheter is constructed of a superelastic material to allow passive deployment of the array catheter and optimization of endocardial contact.[42,43]

Technique of Basket Catheter Mapping. The size of the atrium is initially evaluated (usually with echocardiography) to help select the appropriate size of the basket catheter. The collapsed basket catheter is advanced under fluoroscopy guidance through an 11 Fr long sheath into the RA or LA; the catheter is then expanded (Fig. 8-12). Electric-anatomical relations are determined by fluoroscopically identifiable markers (spline A has one marker and spline B has two markers located near the shaft of the basket cathe-

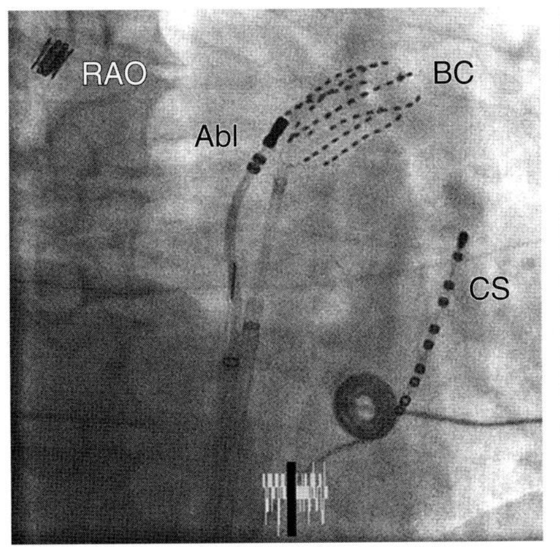

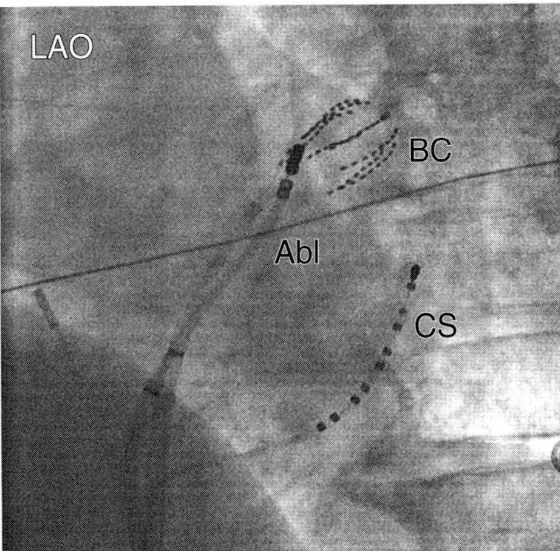

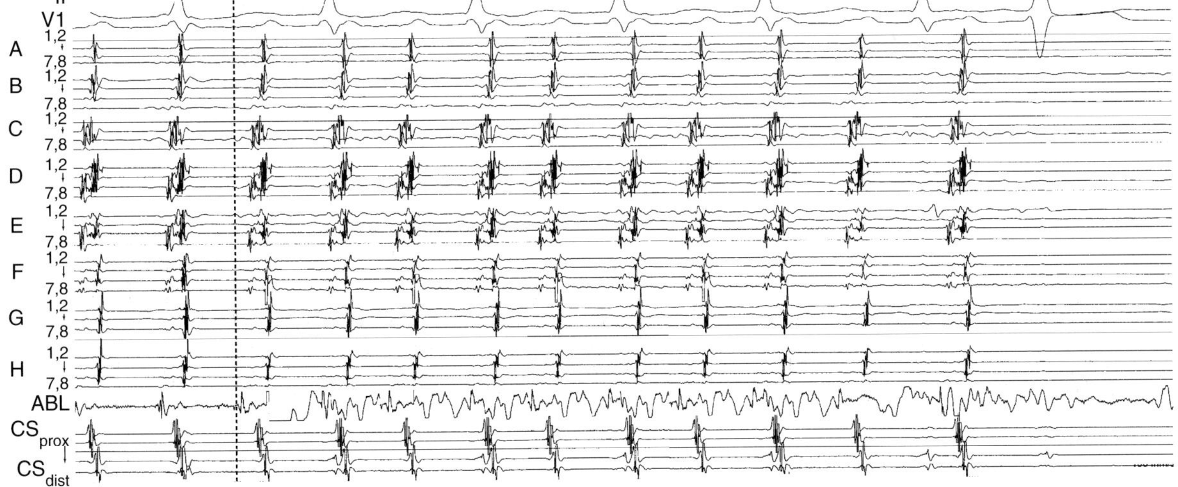

FIGURE 8–12 Basket catheter (BC) mapping of atrial tachycardia (AT) . **Upper panels,** Fluoroscopic views (right anterior oblique, 30 degrees; left anterior oblique, 60 degrees) of the basket catheter positioned at the ostium of the left superior pulmonary vein (PV). **Lower panel,** Basket catheter bipolar electrograms (1-2, 3-4, 5-6, 7-8) from the eight splines (A to H) are displayed. The earliest atrial activation during AT is recorded by the proximal electrodes of the E spline of the basket catheter. Detailed mapping obtained by the ablation catheter (Abl) recorded an even earlier activation (dashed line) at a site in the left atrial roof just outside the PV ostium. Radiofrequency energy delivery at that site resulted in termination of the tachycardia within a few seconds. CS = coronary sinus.

ter). Additionally, the electrical signals recorded from certain electrodes (e.g., annular or HB electrograms) can help identify the location of those particular splines.[42,43]

From the 64 electrodes, 64 unipolar signals and 32 to 56 bipolar signals can be recorded (by combining 1-2, 3-4, 5-6, 7-8 or 1-2, 2-3 until 7-8 electrodes are on each spline). Color-coded activation maps are reconstructed. The concepts of activation mapping discussed earlier are then used to determine the site of origin of the tachycardia. The capacity of pacing from the majority of basket electrodes allows the evaluation of activation patterns, pace mapping, and entrainment mapping. The electrograms recorded from the basket catheter can be used to monitor changes in the activation sequence in real time and thereby indicate the effects of ablation as lesions are created.

After basket catheter deployment, the conventional catheters are introduced and positioned in standard positions. The ablation catheter is placed in the region of earliest activity, and is used for more detailed mapping of the site of origin of the AT (see Fig. 8-12). The Astronomer navigation system permits precise and reproducible guidance of the ablation catheter tip electrode to targets identified by the basket catheter.

Limitations of Basket Approaches. The electrode array does not expand to provide adequate contact with the entire atrium. In addition, the system does not permit immediate correlation of activation times to precise anatomical sites. Furthermore, a second catheter is still required for additional mapping and for ablation.[42,43]

Localized High-Density Mapping Catheter

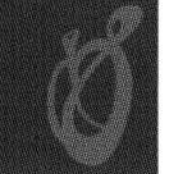

A recent study has evaluated a new mapping approach for AT using a novel high-density multielectrode mapping catheter (PentaRay, Biosense Webster, Diamond Bar, Calif).[44] This 7 Fr steerable catheter (180 degrees of unidirectional
8 flexion) has 20 electrodes distributed over five soft radiating spines (1-mm electrodes separated by 4-4-4 or 2-6-2 mm interelectrode spacing), allowing splaying of the catheter to cover a surface diameter of 3.5 cm. The spines have been nominated with alphabetical nomenclature (A to E), with spines A and B being recognized by radiopaque markers (see Fig. 3-26).

Localization of the atrial focus can be performed during tachycardia or atrial ectopy. Guided by the ECG appearance and previous mapping information, the catheter is sequentially applied to the endocardial surface in various atrial regions to allow rapid activation mapping. Mapping is performed to identify the earliest endocardial activity relative to the P wave and/or to a fixed catheter positioned within the CS. By identifying the earliest site of activation around the circumference of the high-density catheter, vector mapping is performed, moving the catheter and applying it to the endocardium in the direction of earliest activation (outer bipoles) to identify the tachycardia origin and bracket activation—that is, demonstrating later activation in all surrounding regions. Ablation is performed at the site of earliest endocardial activation relative to the P wave when tachycardia is bracketed.

The high-density mapping catheter may offer several potential advantages. Whereas basket catheter mapping has the ability to perform rapid simultaneous contact mapping of the chamber and provides a global density of mapping, its localized resolution is limited. In contrast, this new mapping modality allows splaying of the spines against the endocardial surface to achieve high-density contact mapping to localize and characterize the origin of focal ATs accurately. Additionally, the ability to position multiple electrodes in a circumscribed part of the endocardium is particularly advantageous for use within the LA and for mapping complex focal AT.

ABLATION

Target of Ablation

The site of origin (or focus) of focal AT is the target of ablation.[24,35] Bipolar electrograms at the site of successful ablation are typically fractionated and demonstrate moderate to marked presystolic timing. Average presystolic intervals at sites of successful ablation are generally more than 30 milliseconds (and not mid-diastolic, as in the case of macroreentrant AT). However, the key to successful mapping is finding the earliest site, because there is great variability in the presystolic interval that will be obtained at successful ablation sites (10 to 80 milliseconds). QS unipolar electrogram morphology is highly predictive of the successful ablation site and supplement findings of bipolar mapping. Timing of the earliest bipolar and unipolar electrogram should be in agreement (see Fig. 8-5).

Ablation Technique

RF energy power should be adjusted to achieve a tip temperature of 55° to 65°C.[24,35] The response of the AT focus to a successful RF application should be rapid, typically within a few seconds of RF energy delivery. The most common response to successful ablations is abrupt termination. However, in some patients, transient acceleration precedes termination; in others, gradual slowing precedes termination. If the tachycardia is not affected within 10 to 20 seconds, RF energy application is terminated and the catheter is repositioned slightly for a repeat attempt. Prolonged RF applications beyond 10 to 20 seconds without accompanying changes in AT rate are usually nonproductive.

If the AT terminates or changes rate noticeably during the 10- second application, the RF application is continued for 30 to 60 seconds. However, in some patients, applications that may be just slightly off target can cause acceleration of the AT without terminating it. In these cases, the tachycardia rate usually remains accelerated as long as the RF application is in progress, and it returns immediately to baseline rate when the RF delivery is discontinued. If adequate catheter tip temperature is achieved and good contact is ensured, which might be indicated by observing ST elevation on the unipolar recording, this probably suggests that the catheter is close to, but not exactly at, the proper target area. Continued RF application at a site that produces only acceleration (but not termination) after 15 seconds invites the possibility of transient injury to the AT focus, which impedes further ablation and may result in later AT recurrence.

Ablation of focal ATs near the AVN or HB (in the triangle of Koch) requires special precautions.[27] Titrated RF energy output should be used, starting with 5 W and increasing by 5 W every 10 seconds of energy application, up to a maximum of 40 W. Additionally, it is preferable to deliver RF energy during AT; if AT terminates during RF delivery, the RF application is continued at the same power output for 30 seconds and then repeated for 30 seconds or more. If the AT does not terminate with an RF output of 40 W for 30 seconds, then another site should be sought. If accelerated junctional rhythm develops after AT termination, overdrive atrial pacing should be performed to monitor AV conduction, or RF application should be stopped and other sites sought. To reduce the risk of AV block, RF delivery should be immediately discontinued when (1) impedance rises suddenly (more than 10 Ω), (2) the PR interval (during NSR or atrial pacing) prolongs, (3) AV block develops, (4) retrograde conduction block is observed during junctional ectopy, or (5) fast junctional tachycardia (tachycardia CL less than 350 milliseconds) occurs, which may herald imminent heart block.

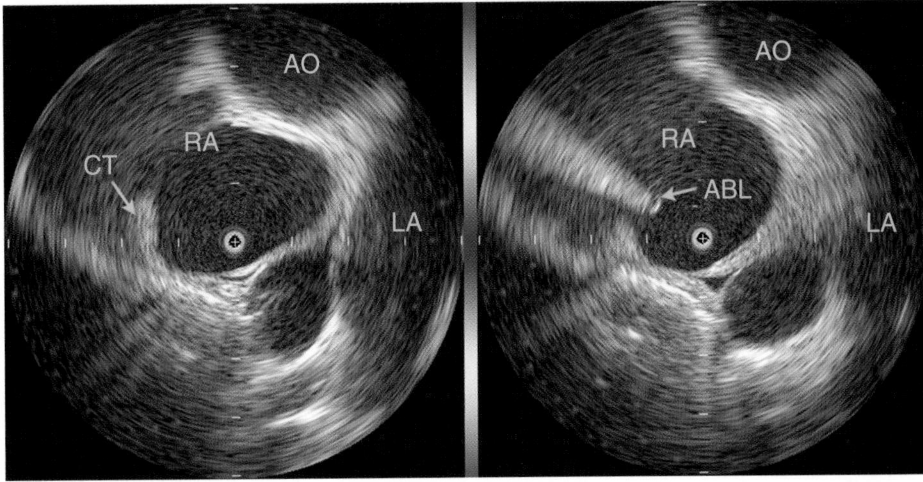

FIGURE 8–13 Intracardiac echocardiographic view of the high crista terminalis (CT) showing the anatomical structures and location of the ablation catheter (ABL) at the site of radiofrequency application (left panel). The ablation catheter is located on the high lateral CT. AO = aorta; LA = left atrium; RA = right atrium.

Use of Intracardiac Echocardiography to Guide Mapping and Ablation

Intracardiac echocardiography (ICE) can be useful to provide focused real-time images of the endocardial surfaces critical for positioning of catheters, establish catheter tip–tissue contact, and monitor energy delivery in the beating heart. In particular, ICE has been used in cristal ATs to assist in accurate positioning of a multipolar catheter along the crista terminalis. In view of the variability in the anatomical course of the crista terminalis, ICE may become necessary for accurate positioning of the multipolar mapping catheter and guiding precise mapping along this structure with the mapping-ablation catheter (Fig. 8-13).

ICE can also help demonstrate the close anatomical relation between the superior crista terminalis and right upper PV and facilitate careful and subtle mapping to determine whether a tachycardia is high cristal or in the right upper PV. This is important when making a decision as to whether it is necessary to proceed with a transseptal puncture, in which case ICE can also be helpful. Echocardiographic lesion characteristics defined by ICE can provide a guide for directing additional RF lesions. The effective RF lesion has an increased and/or changed echodensity completely extending to the epicardium, with the development of a trivial linear low-echodensity or echo-free interstitial space, which suggests a transmural RF lesion.

Endpoints of Ablation

Termination of Atrial Tachycardia During Radiofrequency Delivery. Sudden termination of an incessant AT during RF application suggests a successful ablation. However, reliance on AT termination during RF application as the sole criterion of a successful ablation may be misleading because AT may terminate spontaneously or in response to PACs induced by the RF application, and may not be a result of ablation of the AT focus. Furthermore, the sudden termination of the AT can be associated with catheter dislodgment from the critical site to another site, making it difficult to deliver additional lesions at the critical site.

Lack of Atrial Tachycardia Inducibility. To use this criterion as a reliable endpoint, careful assessment of inducibility should be performed prior to ablation; the feasibility and best method of reproducible induction of the AT should be documented at baseline before ablation. In the setting of easy inducibility prior to ablation, one may consider the lack of inducibility as an indicator of successful ablation. Noninducibility of the arrhythmia is inapplicable if the original arrhythmia is noninducible at baseline or was inadvertently terminated mechanically. Inducibility should be reassessed 30 minutes after the last successful RF application.

Outcome

Acute success rate is variable (range, 69% to 100%; mean, 91%). Complication rates range from 0% to 8% (mean, 3%). Recurrence rates range from 0% to 25% (mean, 9%). The mechanism of AT influences outcome.

Phrenic nerve injury can occur during ablation of ATs in the right or left free wall, SVC, right superior PV, or left PVs. The ability to pace the phrenic nerve should suggest attempting to find a slightly different site or, if this is not possible, applying RF energy at low power and/or for short duration. Even when the phrenic nerve cannot be paced, intermittent fluoroscopic visualization of the ipsilateral diaphragm movement should be performed during RF application at high-risk sites, and RF delivery should be terminated if diaphragmatic excursion decreases.

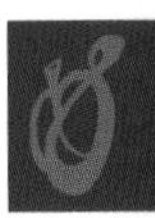

Sinus node dysfunction can develop during ablation of ATs originating near the sinus node. The risk is usually low, except in older patients or in those with preexisting sinus node dysfunction.

AV block can also complicate ablation of ATs originating in the anteroseptal region. When HB potential is detectable at the ablation catheter location, titrated RF energy output and RF application for short duration should be used, coupled with overdrive atrial pacing to monitor AV conduction in case accelerated junctional rhythm occurs. Moreover, detailed mapping in the right and left anteroseptal regions is required, because ATs arising along the anterior and anteroseptal LA will frequently have earliest RA activation at the HB region, with a normal activation pattern along the posterior LA, as recorded by the CS electrodes.

REFERENCES

1. Saoudi N, Cosio F, Waldo A, et al: Classification of atrial flutter and regular atrial tachycardia according to electrophysiologic mechanism and anatomic bases: A statement from a joint expert group from the Working Group of Arrhythmias of the European Society of Cardiology and the North American Society of Pacing and Electrophysiology. J Cardiovasc Electrophysiol 2001;12:852.
2. Scheinman MM, Yang Y, Chen J: Atrial flutter: Part II: Nomenclature. Pacing Clin Electrophysiol 2004;27:504.
3. Morton JB, Sanders P, Das A, et al: Focal atrial tachycardia arising from the tricuspid annulus: electrophysiologic and electrocardiographic characteristics. J Cardiovasc Electrophysiol 2001;12:653.
4. Badhwar N, Kalman JM, Sparks PB, et al: Atrial tachycardia arising from the coronary sinus musculature: Electrophysiological characteristics and long-term outcomes of radiofrequency ablation. J Am Coll Cardiol 2005;46:1921.

5. Hoffmann E, Reithmann C, Nimmermann P, et al: Clinical experience with electroanatomic mapping of ectopic atrial tachycardia. Pacing Clin Electrophysiol 2002;25:49.
6. Tritto M, Zardini M, De PR, Salerno-Uriarte JA: Iterative atrial tachycardia originating from the coronary sinus musculature. J Cardiovasc Electrophysiol 2001;12:1187.
7. Volkmer M, Antz M, Hebe J, Kuck KH: Focal atrial tachycardia originating from the musculature of the coronary sinus. J Cardiovasc Electrophysiol 2002;13:68.
8. Pavin D, Boulmier D, Daubert JC, Mabo P: Permanent left atrial tachycardia: radiofrequency catheter ablation through the coronary sinus. J Cardiovasc Electrophysiol 2002;13:395.
9. Navarrete AJ, Arora R, Hubbard JE, Miller JM: Magnetic electroanatomic mapping of an atrial tachycardia requiring ablation within the coronary sinus. J Cardiovasc Electrophysiol 2003;14:1361.
10. Kistler PM, Sanders P, Hussin A, et al: Focal atrial tachycardia arising from the mitral annulus: electrocardiographic and electrophysiologic characterization. J Am Coll Cardiol 2003;41:2212.
11. Matsuoka K, Kasai A, Fujii E, et al: Electrophysiological features of atrial tachycardia arising from the atrioventricular annulus. Pacing Clin Electrophysiol 2002;25(Pt 1):440.
12. Hwang C, Wu TJ, Doshi RN, et al: Vein of Marshall cannulation for the analysis of electrical activity in patients with focal atrial fibrillation. Circulation 2000;101:1503.
13. Tsai CF, Tai CT, Hsieh MH, et al: Initiation of atrial fibrillation by ectopic beats originating from the superior vena cava: electrophysiological characteristics and results of radiofrequency ablation. Circulation 2000;102:67.
14. Dong J, Schreieck J, Ndrepepa G, Schmitt C: Ectopic tachycardia originating from the superior vena cava. J Cardiovasc Electrophysiol 2002;13:620.
15. Scavee C, Jais P, Weerasooriya R, Haissaguerre M: The inferior vena cava: An exceptional source of atrial fibrillation. J Cardiovasc Electrophysiol 2003 June;14(6):659-662.
16. Wharton M, Shenasa H, Barold H, et al: Ablation of atrial tachycardia in adults. *In* Huang SKS, Wilber DJ (eds): Radiofrequency Catheter Ablation of Cardiac Arrhythmias: Basic Concepts and Clinical Applications, 2nd ed. Armonk, NY, Futura, 2000, pp 139-164.
17. Roberts-Thomson KC, Kistler PM, Kalman JM: Focal atrial tachycardia I: Clinical features, diagnosis, mechanisms, and anatomic location. Pacing Clin Electrophysiol 2006;29:643.
18. Blomström-Lundqvist C, Scheinman MM, et al: American College of Cardiology; American Heart Association Task Force on Practice Guidelines; European Society of Cardiology Committee for Practice Guidelines. Writing Committee to Develop Guidelines for the Management of Patients With Supraventricular Arrhythmias: ACC/AHA/ESC guidelines for the management of patients with supraventricular arrhythmias—executive summary: A report of the American College of Cardiology/American Heart Association Task Force on Practice Guidelines and the European Society of Cardiology Committee for Practice Guidelines. Circulation 2003;108:1871.

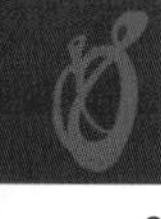

8

19. Josephson ME: Supraventricular tachycardias. *In* Josephson ME (ed): Clinical Cardiac Electrophysiology, 3rd ed. Philadelphia, Lippincott Williams & Wilkins, 2002, pp 168-271.
20. Porter MJ, Morton JB, Denman R, et al: Influence of age and gender on the mechanism of supraventricular tachycardia. Heart Rhythm 2004;1:393.
21. Hillock RJ, Kalman JM, Roberts-Thomson KC, et al: Multiple focal atrial tachycardias in a healthy adult population: Characterization and description of successful radiofrequency ablation. Heart Rhythm 2007;4:435.
22. Brown JP, Krummen DE, Feld GK, Narayan SM: Using electrocardiographic activation time and diastolic intervals to separate focal from macro-re-entrant atrial tachycardias. J Am Coll Cardiol 2007;49:1965.
23. Ellenbogen KA, Wood MA: Atrial tachycardia. *In* Zipes DP, Jalife J (eds): Cardiac Electrophysiology: From Cell to Bedside, 4th ed. Philadelphia, WB Saunders, 2004, pp 500-511.
24. Hsieh MH, Chen SA: Catheter ablation of focal atrial tachycardia. *In* Zipes DP, Haissaguerre M (eds): Catheter Ablation of Arrhythmias. Armonk, NY, Futura, 2002, pp 185-204.
25. Kistler PM, Roberts-Thomson KC, Haqqani HM, et al: P-wave morphology in focal atrial tachycardia: development of an algorithm to predict the anatomic site of origin. J Am Coll Cardiol 2006;48:1010.
26. Yamane T, Shah DC, Peng JT, et al: Morphological characteristics of P waves during selective pulmonary vein pacing. J Am Coll Cardiol 2001;38:1505.
27. Lai LP, Lin JL, Huang S: Ablation of atrial tachycardia within the triangle of Koch. *In* Huang SKS, Wilber DJ (eds): Radiofrequency Catheter Ablation of Cardiac Arrhythmias: Basic Concepts and Clinical Applications, 2nd ed. Armonk, Futura, 2000, pp 175-184.
28. Kistler PM, Sanders P, Fynn SP, et al: Electrophysiological and electrocardiographic characteristics of focal atrial tachycardia originating from the pulmonary veins: acute and long-term outcomes of radiofrequency ablation. Circulation 2003;108:1968.
29. Anguera I, Brugada J, Roba M, et al: Outcomes after radiofrequency catheter ablation of atrial tachycardia. Am J Cardiol 2001;87:886.
30. Gerstenfeld EP, Dixit S, Bala R, et al: Surface electrocardiogram characteristics of atrial tachycardias occurring after pulmonary vein isolation. Heart Rhythm 2007;4:1136.
31. Crawford TC, Mukerji S, Good E, et al: Utility of atrial and ventricular cycle length variability in determining the mechanism of paroxysmal supraventricular tachycardia. J Cardiovasc Electrophysiol 2007;18:698.
32. Iwai S, Markowitz SM, Stein KM, et al: Response to adenosine differentiates focal from macroreentrant atrial tachycardia: Validation using three-dimensional electroanatomic mapping. Circulation 2002;106:2793.
33. Vijayaraman P, Lee BP, Kalahasty G, et al: Reanalysis of the "pseudo A-A-V" response to ventricular entrainment of supraventricular tachycardia: Importance of His-bundle timing. J Cardiovasc Electrophysiol 2006;17:25.
34. Maruyama M, Kobayashi Y, Miyauchi Y, et al: The VA relationship after differential atrial overdrive pacing: A novel tool for the diagnosis of atrial tachycardia in the electrophysiologic laboratory. J Cardiovasc Electrophysiol 2007;18:1127.
35. Josephson ME: Catheter and surgical ablation in the therapy of arrhythmias. *In* Josephson ME (ed): Clinical Cardiac Electrophysiology, 3rd ed. Philadelphia, Lippincott Williams & Wilkins. 2002, pp 710-836.
36. Wetzel U, Hindricks G, Schirdewahn P, et al: A stepwise mapping approach for localization and ablation of ectopic right, left, and septal atrial foci using electroanatomic mapping. Eur Heart J 2002;23:1387.
37. Khongphatthanayothin A, Kosar E, Nademanee K: Nonfluoroscopic three-dimensional mapping for arrhythmia ablation: tool or toy? J Cardiovasc Electrophysiol 2000;11:239.
38. Seidl K, Schwacke H, Rameken M, et al: Noncontact mapping of ectopic atrial tachycardias: different characteristics of isopotential maps and unipolar electrogram. Pacing Clin Electrophysiol 2003;26(Pt 1):16.
39. Schmitt H, Weber S, Schwab JO, et al: Diagnosis and ablation of focal right atrial tachycardia using a new high-resolution, non-contact mapping system. Am J Cardiol 2001;87:1017.
40. Paul T, Windhagen-Mahnert B, Kriebel T, et al: Atrial reentrant tachycardia after surgery for congenital heart disease: Endocardial mapping and radiofrequency catheter ablation using a novel, noncontact mapping system. Circulation 2001;103:2266.
41. Higa S, Tai CT, Lin YJ, et al: Focal atrial tachycardia: New insight from noncontact mapping and catheter ablation. Circulation 2004;109:84.
42. Rodriguez E, Callans D, Kantharia B, et al: Basket catheter localization of the origin of atrial tachycardia with atypical morphology after atrial flutter ablation. Pacing Clin Electrophysiol 2000;23:269.
43. Zrenner B, Ndrepepa G, Schneider M, et al: Basket catheter-guided three-dimensional activation patterns construction and ablation of common type atrial flutter. Pacing Clin Electrophysiol 2000;23:1350.
44. Sanders P, Hocini M, Jais P, et al: Characterization of focal atrial tachycardia using high-density mapping. J Am Coll Cardiol 2005;46:2088.

CHAPTER 9

Isthmus-Dependent Atrial Flutter

PATHOPHYSIOLOGY

Right Atrial Anatomy

The right atrial endocardial surface is comprised of many orifices and embryonic remnants, accounting for an irregular complex surface. Orifices of the superior vena cava (SVC) and inferior vena cava (IVC) lie in the superior and inferior aspects of the right atrium (RA), respectively. The tricuspid annulus lies anterior to the body of the RA. The RA endocardium is architecturally divided into the anterolateral trabeculated RA, derived from the true embryonic RA, and the posterior smooth-walled RA, derived from the embryonic sinus venosus. These distinct anatomical regions of the RA are separated by the crista terminalis on the lateral wall and the eustachian ridge in the inferior aspect.

The crista terminalis is formed at the junction between the sinus venosus part of the RA and the "true" RA contributing to the RA appendage and free wall. The crista runs from the high septum, anterior to the orifice of the SVC superiorly, and courses caudally along the posterolateral aspect of the RA. In its inferior extent, it courses anteriorly to the orifice of the IVC. As it reaches the region of the IVC, it is extended by the eustachian valve ridge (the remnant of the embryonic sinus venosus valve), which courses superiorly along the floor of the RA to the coronary sinus ostium (CS os), to join the valve of the CS and form the tendon of Todaro.

The inferior portion of the tricuspid annulus lies a short distance (approximately 1 to 4 cm) anterior to the eustachian ridge, though its course varies among individuals. In some patients, it may bifurcate and may terminate anterior or posterior to the CS os. The CS os lies medial to the orifice of the IVC as the floor of the RA becomes the septum. On the lower third of the interatrial septum lies the fossa ovalis.[1]

Types of Isthmus-Dependent Atrial Flutter

1. Clockwise and Counterclockwise "Typical" Atrial Flutter

Typical atrial flutter (AFL) is a macroreentrant atrial tachycardia (AT) that uses the cavotricuspid isthmus as an essential part of its circuit. The circuit boundaries are the tricuspid annulus, crista terminalis, IVC, eustachian ridge, CS os, and probably the fossa ovalis. These barriers (lines of conduction block) can be functional or anatomical, and are necessary to provide adequate path length for the flutter reentry circuit. The tricuspid annulus forms the anterior border of the flutter circuit, whereas the posterior border occurs at a variable distance from this anterior border; it is narrowest in the region of the eustachian ridge and widest in the anterior part of the RA.[1-3]

The cavotricuspid isthmus runs in an anterolateral to posteromedial direction, from the low anterior RA to the low septal RA (see Fig. 13-1). Its width and muscle thickness are variable, from a few millimeters to more than 3 cm in width and more than 1 cm in depth.[4] Its posterior rim is made of the IVC orifice and the eustachian ridge that extends toward the CS os. The cavotricuspid isthmus provides the protected zone of slow conduction necessary for the flutter reentry circuit. Conduction velocity in the isthmus during pacing in sinus rhythm is slower in patients with typical AFL compared with those without any history of AFL. The mechanism of the slower conduction velocity in the cavotricuspid isthmus, relative to the interatrial septum and RA free wall, is uncertain but can be related to the anisotropic fiber orientation. With aging or atrial dilation, intercellular fibrosis can change the density of gap junctions and produce nonuniform anisotropic conduction through the trabeculations of the cavotricuspid isthmus. Additionally, the isthmus and RA in patients with typical AFL are significantly larger than those in a control population.[3]

Typical AFL is of two types, counterclockwise and clockwise.[2] In counterclockwise AFL, activation proceeds caudocephalic up the septal side of the tricuspid annulus toward the crista terminalis and moves cephalocaudal along the lateral wall of the RA to reach the lateral tricuspid annulus, after which it propagates through the isthmus defined by the IVC, CS, and tricuspid annulus (counterclockwise as viewed in the left anterior oblique [LAO] view from the ventricular side of the tricuspid annulus). The circuit is entirely in the RA. Left atrial activation occurs as a bystander and follows transseptal conduction across the inferior CS-left atrium (LA) connection, Bachmann's bundle, and/or fossa ovalis. In clockwise (reverse typical) AFL, activation propagates in the opposite direction (Fig. 9-1).[1,3]

Clockwise AFL is observed in only 10% of clinical cases, despite the fact that it is easily inducible in the electrophysiology (EP) laboratory with programmed electrical stimulation. Clockwise AFL can be induced in the EP laboratory in about 50% of patients who clinically present with only counterclockwise AFL. The 9:1 clinical predominance of counterclockwise AFL can be related to the localization of an area with a low safety factor for conduction in the cavotricuspid isthmus, close to the atrial septum. Furthermore, counterclockwise AFL is more likely to be induced with rapid atrial pacing from the CS os and, conversely, clockwise AFL is more likely to be induced with pacing from the low lateral RA pacing. These observations may be related to the anisotropic properties of the cavotricuspid isthmus and the development of rate-dependent conduction delays and unidirectional block necessary for tachycardia induction, which may be affected by the site of stimulation.[1,3]

2. Double-Wave Reentry

A typical AFL circuit with a large excitable gap may allow a second excitation wave to be introduced into the flutter circuit by a critically timed atrial extrastimulus (AES), so that two wavefronts occupy the same circuit simultaneously. This type of AFL is designated as double-wave reentry.[5]

Double-wave reentry is manifest by acceleration of the tachycardia rate but with identical surface and intracardiac electrogram morphology. It can be recognized by the simultaneous activation of the superior and inferior regions of the tricuspid annulus, with all activation being sequential. This rhythm rarely lasts for more than a few beats, and can serve as a trigger for atrial fibrillation (AF). Because the cavotricuspid isthmus is still a necessary part of the circuit, double-wave reentry is amenable to cavotricuspid isthmus ablation.[1,3,5]

3. Lower Loop Reentry

Lower loop reentry is a form of isthmus-dependent AFL with a reentrant circuit around the IVC; therefore, it is confined to the lower part of the RA. It often coexists with typical counterclockwise or clockwise AFL and involves posterior breakthrough(s) across the crista terminalis. Lower loop reentry can rotate around the IVC in a counterclockwise (i.e., the impulse within the cavotricuspid isthmus travels from the septum to the lateral wall) or clockwise fashion. A breakdown in the inferoposterior boundaries of the cavotricuspid isthmus produced by the eustachian ridge and lower crista terminalis causes the circuit to revolve around the IVC (instead of around the tricuspid annulus), across the eustachian ridge, and through the crista terminalis, conducting slowly because of transverse activation through that structure. Alternatively, the circuit can exit at the apex of Koch's triangle and come behind the eustachian ridge to break through across the crista terminalis behind the IVC and then return to the cavotricuspid isthmus.[1,3,6-8]

This arrhythmia is usually transient and terminates by itself or converts spontaneously into AFL or AF. Because

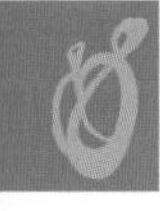

9

Counterclockwise typical AFL

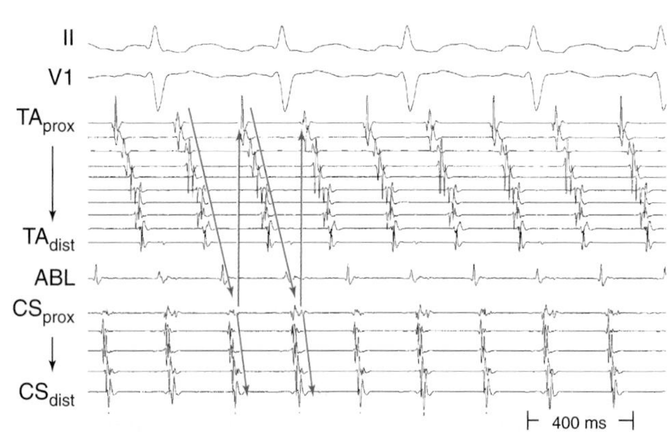

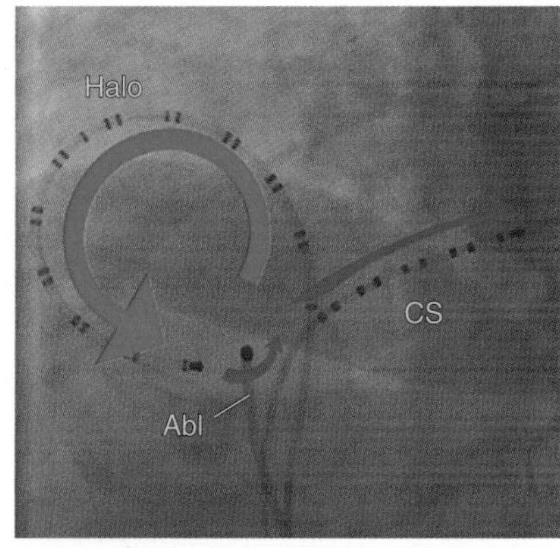

Clockwise typical AFL

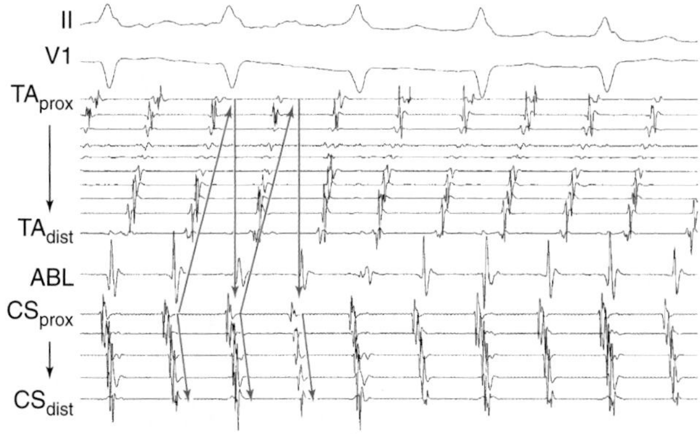

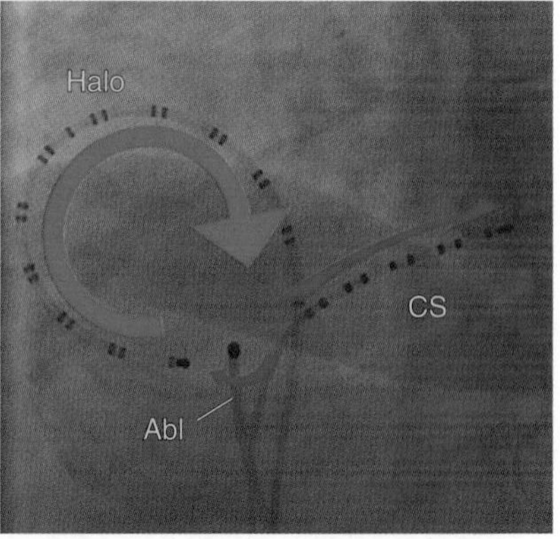

FIGURE 9–1 Endocardial activation during counterclockwise (upper panel) and clockwise (lower panel) typical atrial flutter (AFL) in the same patient. Catheter position and wavefront activation during the tachycardia are illustrated in a left anterior oblique (LAO) fluoroscopic view (right side). The ablation catheter (Abl) is positioned at the cavotricuspid isthmus, and the Halo catheter is positioned around the tricuspid annulus, with the distal end at the lateral aspect of the cavotricuspid isthmus.

the cavotricuspid isthmus is still a necessary part of the circuit, lower loop reentry is amenable to cavotricuspid isthmus ablation, as is true for patients with typical AFL.[6-8]

4. *Intraisthmus Reentry*

Intraisthmus reentry is a recently reported reentrant circuit within the region bounded by the medial cavotricuspid isthmus and CS os. In this form of isthmus-dependent AFL, entrainment pacing from the lateral cavotricuspid isthmus shows a post-pacing interval (PPI) longer than the tachycardia cycle length (CL), indicating that the lateral cavotricuspid isthmus is not part of the reentrant circuit; on the other hand, pacing from the region of medial cavotricuspid isthmus or CS os shows concealed entrainment with PPI equal to the tachycardia CL. Fractionated or double potentials usually can be recorded in this area and can be entrained. Although the anatomical basis of this arrhythmia remains unknown, a linear lesion across the medial, not lateral, cavotricuspid isthmus can cure the tachycardia.[6,9,10]

CLINICAL CONSIDERATIONS

Epidemiology

Paroxysmal AFL can occur in patients with no apparent structural heart disease, whereas chronic AFL is usually associated with underlying heart disease, such as valvular or ischemic heart disease or cardiomyopathy. In approximately 60% of patients, AFL occurs as part of an acute disease process, such as exacerbation of pulmonary disease, following cardiac or pulmonary surgery, or during acute myocardial infarction. AFL accounts for approximately 15% of supraventricular arrhythmias, and frequently coexists with or precedes AF.

Clinical Presentation

Patients with AFL may present with a spectrum of symptoms ranging from palpitations, lightheadedness, fatigue, or dyspnea to acute pulmonary edema or acute coronary syndrome. The severity of symptoms usually depends on ventricular rate during the AFL, presence of structural heart disease, and baseline LV function. AFL occurs in approximately 25% to 35% of patients with AF and may be associated with more intense symptoms because of more rapid ventricular rates.

Initial Evaluation

ECG diagnosis of typical AFL is frequently accurate, but can occasionally be misleading (see later). Cardiac evaluation with echocardiography is required to evaluate for structural heart disease. Other tests may be required to evaluate for potential substrates and/or triggers of AFL.

Principles of Management

Acute Management

Acute therapy for patients with AFL depends on the clinical presentation and may include cardioversion and the use of atrioventricular nodal (AVN) blockers to slow the ventricular rate during the AFL. Cardioversion (electrical or chemical) is commonly the initial treatment of choice. Electrical cardioversion is almost always successful in terminating AFL, and often requires relatively low energies (less than 50 J). Chemical cardioversion can be achieved with intravenous ibutilide in 38% to 76% of cases, which is more effective than intravenous amiodarone, sotalol, and class IC agents. Overdrive atrial pacing (via a catheter in the esophagus or the RA) can effectively terminate typical AFL, but can also induce conversion of AFL into AF. Anticoagulation in the pericardioversion period should be considered and is guided by the duration of the AFL and the patient's stroke risk factors, using the same criteria as for AF.[11]

Rate control is typically achieved with oral or intravenous AVN blockers such as verapamil, diltiazem, beta blockers, and digoxin. Rate control tends to be more difficult to achieve during AFL than AF because of the slower atrial rate.

Chronic Management

When AFL occurs as part of an acute disease process, chronic therapy of the arrhythmia is usually not required after sinus rhythm is restored and the patient survives the underlying disease process. Long-term success rate of antiarrhythmic drugs to prevent AFL recurrence appears to be limited, and complete suppression of AFL can be difficult to achieve. Therefore, catheter ablation of the cavotricuspid isthmus is the treatment of choice for typical AFL, whether paroxysmal or persistent, and long-term drug therapy is rarely indicated and should be reserved for unusual circumstances.[1]

Several antiarrhythmic drugs have demonstrated efficacy in suppression of AFL, including class IA (quinidine, procainamide, and disopyramide), class IC (flecainide and propafenone), and class III (sotalol, amiodarone, and dofetilide) agents. In the absence of structural heart disease, class IC agents are the drugs of choice. The use of antiarrhythmic agents should be instituted in conjunction with AVN blockers to avoid the risk of rapid ventricular rates secondary to the vagolytic effects of class I drugs and slowing of the flutter rate.[11]

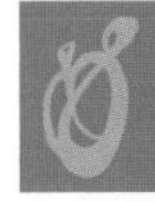

Ablation of the atrioventricular (AV) junction and pacemaker implantation may be indicated for patients who failed curative ablation of the AFL, antiarrhythmic therapy, and rate control strategies. Stroke prevention is recommended and is usually achieved with aspirin or warfarin, depending on the patient's stroke risk factors, using the same criteria as for AF.

ELECTROCARDIOGRAPHIC FEATURES

Typical Atrial Flutter

P Waves. Flutter waves appear as atrial complexes of constant morphology, polarity, and CL. Typically, flutter waves are most prominent in the inferior leads (II, III, aVF) and V_1. In the inferior leads, they appear as a picket fence (sawtooth) because the leads are primarily negative. This consists of a downsloping segment, followed by a sharper negative deflection, and then a sharp positive deflection, with a positive overshoot leading to the next downsloping plateau. The relative size of each component can vary markedly.[1]

Counterclockwise AFL (Fig. 9-2) can be characterized by pure negative deflections in the inferior leads, negative and then positive deflections that are equal in size, or a small negative and then a larger positive deflection. Those three varieties coexist with tall positive, small positive, or biphasic P waves in V_1, respectively. The degree of positivity in the inferior leads appears to be related to the coexistence of heart disease and LA enlargement. Counterclockwise AFL will always have a negative deflection preceding the positive deflection in the inferior leads. Leads I and aVL characteristically show low-voltage deflections. Clockwise AFL

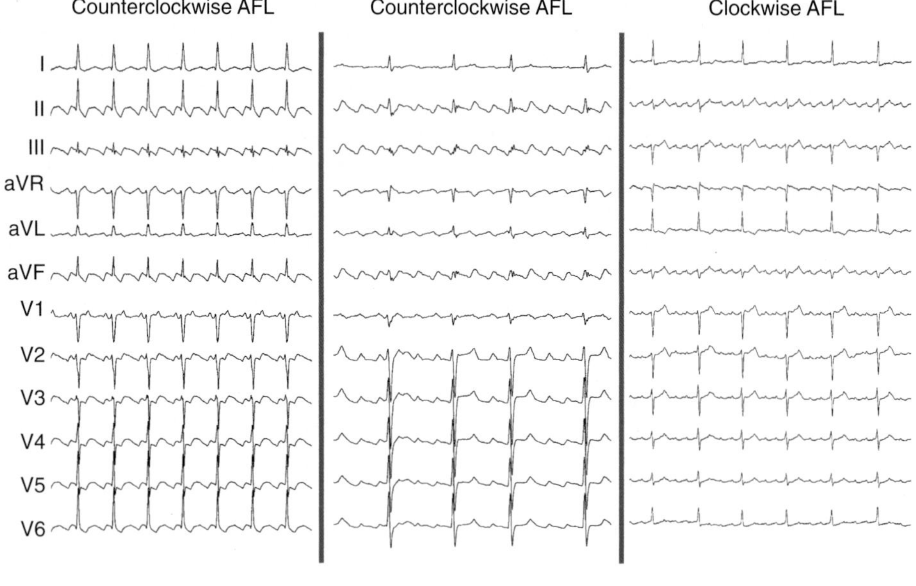

FIGURE 9–2 Surface ECG of counterclockwise typical atrial flutter (AFL) with 2:1 atrioventricular (AV) conduction (left), counterclockwise typical AFL with variable AV conduction (middle), and clockwise typical AFL with 4:1 AV conduction (right).

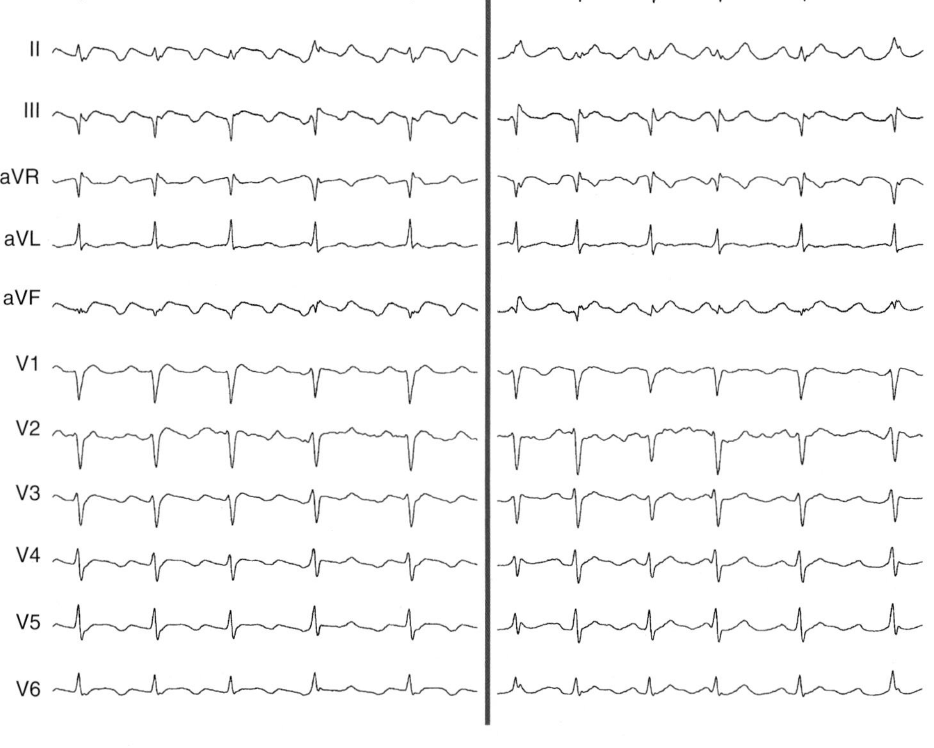

FIGURE 9–3 Surface 12-lead ECGs during counterclockwise (left) and clockwise (right) typical atrial flutter (AFL) in a patient on flecainide therapy. Note the slow flutter cycle length (approximately 350 milliseconds) secondary to the effects of flecainide.

generally has broad positive deflections in the inferior leads and wide negative deflections in V_1 (see Fig. 9-2).[1]

Typical AFL usually has a CL between 190 and 250 milliseconds (flutter rate of 240 to 340 beats/min), with 2% or less cycle-to-cycle variation. However, AFL may be slower in patients receiving antiarrhythmic agents (Fig. 9-3). It is not uncommon for clockwise and counterclockwise AFLs to be seen in the same patient and often have similar rates, although clockwise AFL can have a slower rate.

If the ventricular response is half the atrial rate, it can be difficult to identify the flutter waves because they can be superimposed on the QRS or T waves (see Fig. 9-2). Close inspection of the QRS and T waves, and comparing them with those in normal sinus rhythm (NSR), can help identify buried flutter waves. Furthermore, vagal maneuvers and AVN blockers can slow AV conduction and unmask the flutter waves.

Atrioventricular Conduction. Most commonly, 2:1 AV conduction is present during AFL. Variable AV conduction and/or larger multiples (e.g., 4:1 or 6:1) are not uncommon. Variable AV block is the result of multilevel block; for example, proximal 2:1 AV block and more distal 3:2 Wenckebach block result in 5:2 AV Wenckebach block. It is likely that the proximal 2:1 block occurs in the upper part of the AVN, whereas Wenckebach block occurs in the lower part of the AVN. Distal Wenckebach behavior in the His bundle (HB) would result in a similar AV conduction pattern but is unlikely to occur. In most cases, the nonconducted flutter beats block in the AVN; however, infranodal AV block can occur, especially in the presence of prolonged His-

Purkinje system (HPS) refractoriness caused by class I antiarrhythmic agents or during Wenckebach cycles in the AVN, which leads to long-short cycle activation of the HPS.[12]

Slowing the atrial rate during AFL by antiarrhythmic agents can result in a paradoxical increase in the ventricular rate caused by better AVN conduction of the slower flutter beats. Rapid 1:1 AV conduction is most commonly seen in patients with Wolff-Parkinson-White (WPW) syndrome (Fig. 9-4), but may also be present in cases of enhanced AVN conduction secondary to high sympathetic tone (e.g., exercise, sympathomimetic drugs).[1]

QRS Morphology. The QRS complex during AFL is often identical to that during NSR. However, flutter beats can be aberrantly conducted because of functional bundle branch block (BBB), most frequently right bundle branch block (RBBB). Even with normal ventricular conduction, the QRS complex may be slightly distorted by temporal superimposition of flutter waves on the QRS complex. Thus, the QRS complex can appear to acquire a new or larger R, S, or Q wave.[1]

Atypical Isthmus-Dependent Atrial Flutter

Double-Wave Reentry. P wave morphology on all surface ECG leads during double-wave reentry is identical to that during typical AFL, but at a faster rate.[5]

Lower Loop Reentry. The surface morphology of lower loop reentry is highly variable and can be similar to that of counterclockwise or clockwise AFL, but lower loop reentry associated with higher cristal breaks can produce unusual ECG patterns. Sometimes, the changes are manifested by decreased amplitude of the late positive waves in the inferior leads, probably as a result of wavefront collision over the lateral RA wall.[8]

ELECTROPHYSIOLOGICAL TESTING

Induction of Tachycardia

Typically, a decapolar catheter (positioned into the CS with the proximal electrodes bracketing the CS os) and a multipolar (20-pole) Halo catheter (positioned at the tricuspid annulus) are used to map AFL. The distal tip of the Halo catheter is positioned at 6 to 7 o'clock in LAO view, so that the distal electrodes will record the middle and lateral aspects of the cavotricuspid isthmus, the middle electrodes will record the anterolateral RA, and the proximal electrodes may record the RA septum (depending on the catheter used). Instead of the Halo and CS catheters described, some laboratories use a single duodecapolar catheter around the tricuspid annulus, while extending the catheter tip

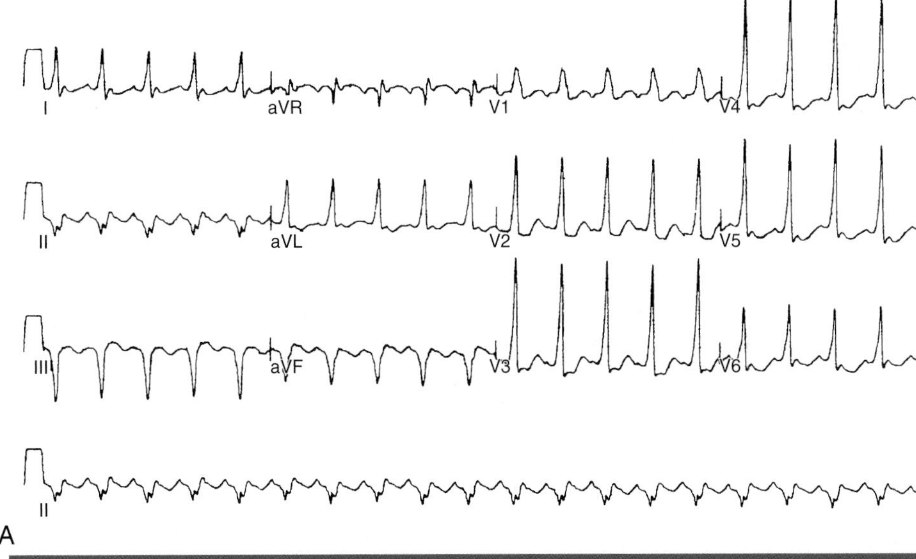

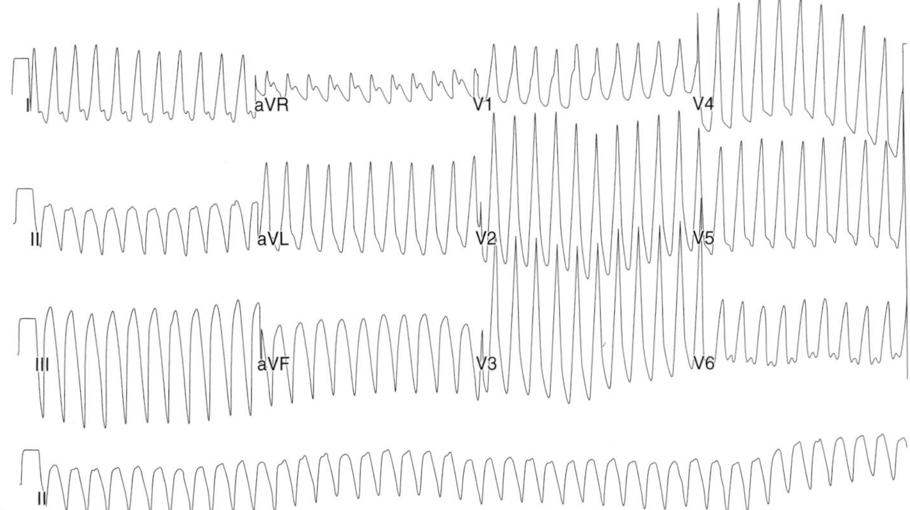

FIGURE 9–4 Surface 12-lead ECGs during clockwise typical atrial flutter (AFL) in a patient with a left posteroseptal bypass tract (BT). **A,** 2:1 atrioventricular (AV) conduction with QRS fusion (secondary to conduction over both the BT and atrioventricular node). **B,** 1:1 AV conduction with fully preexcited QRS morphology.

inside the CS. Such a catheter would straddle the cavotricuspid isthmus and provide recording and pacing from the medial and lateral aspects of the isthmus.

Programmed electrical stimulation protocol typically involves atrial burst pacing from the high RA and CS (down to the pacing CL at which 2:1 atrial capture occurs) and single and double AESs (down to the atrial effective refractory period [ERP]) at multiple CLs (600 to 200 milliseconds) from the high RA and CS. Administration of an isoproterenol infusion (0.5 to 4 µg/min) may be required to facilitate tachycardia induction.

AFL can be induced readily with programmed electrical stimulation in most patients with a clinical history of AFL. Reproducible initiation of counterclockwise AFL is possible in more than 95% of patients.[13] Rapid atrial pacing is more likely to induce AFL than a single AES, but as likely as introducing two AESs. On the other hand, the frequency of single or double AESs initiating AFL is low in patients without a history of AFL (less than 10%). Counterclockwise AFL is more likely to be induced by stimulation from the CS os and, conversely, clockwise AFL is more likely to be induced with low lateral RA pacing. The faster the pacing rate and the shorter the AES coupling intervals, the more likely that AF is induced, which is usually self-terminating but can be sustained in less than 10% of patients. The significance of induction of AF in these patients is uncertain.

Tachycardia Features

The RA activation sequence during counterclockwise AFL occurs sequentially down the lateral RA wall and adjacent to the crista terminalis, across the cavotricuspid isthmus (with some delay because of slow conduction across the isthmus), past the CS os, up the atrial septum, over the roof of the RA, and back to the lateral free wall of the RA (in a proximal-to-distal direction along the Halo electrodes; see Fig. 9-1). This sequence is reversed during clockwise AFL (see Fig. 9-1).

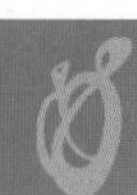

This sequence of atrial activation is different from that of NSR or focal AT originating from the upper RA or LA, in which the activation wavefront propagates from the upper RA (middle or proximal Halo electrodes) down both the RA septum and lateral wall in a craniocaudal direction, toward the distal and proximal most Halo electrodes.

Occasionally, P wave morphology on the surface ECG resembles typical AFL, but intracardiac recordings show that parts of the atria (commonly the LA) have disorganized atrial activity. Such rhythms behave more like AF than AFL, but may be converted to true typical AFL with class I antiarrhythmic drugs or amiodarone.[13]

During AFL, double potentials are seen on the crista terminalis and along the eustachian ridge, indicating lines of block (fixed or functional) along those structures.

Diagnostic Maneuvers During Tachycardia

Goals of Programmed Stimulation During Atrial Flutter

The goals of EP testing in AFL are (1) to confirm that the tachycardia is a macroreentrant circuit (as demonstrated by resetting and entrainment maneuvers), and (2) to confirm that the cavotricuspid isthmus is an integral part of the reentrant circuit (as demonstrated by entrainment maneuvers).

Atrial Extrastimulation During Atrial Flutter. An AES from the high RA or CS or along the Halo catheter are introduced at a coupling CL 10 milliseconds shorter than the flutter CL, with progressive shortening of the coupling CL by 10 to 30 milliseconds.

An AES commonly results in resetting of the AFL circuit.[13] The closer the site of atrial stimulation, the easier the resetting of the AFL circuit at longer coupling intervals. AFL has a resetting response pattern typical of reentrant circuits with fully excitable gaps—flat (for approximately 15% to 30% of the tachycardia CL, equal to approximately 30 to 63 milliseconds in the absence of drugs, and up to 100 milliseconds with class I antiarrhythmic agents) and then an upward return CL with progressively shorter coupling intervals. The ability to capture the atrium without affecting (resetting) the AFL circuit timing indicates that the pacing site is outside the AFL circuit (e.g., RA appendage or distal CS).

It is usually difficult for a single AES to terminate AFL because AFL has a sizable fully excitable gap (15% to 30% of the tachycardia CL), which makes it difficult for a single AES to penetrate the AFL circuit with adequate prematurity to terminate the AFL without intervening atrial refractoriness and intraatrial conduction delays. An AES delivered in the region of the cavotricuspid isthmus will have the greatest chance of terminating AFL because it can capture the isthmus tissue with a very short coupling interval (down to the ERP of this critical site) because of lack of intervening tissue between the stimulation site and isthmus. Termination of AFL always occurs because of conduction block in the isthmus.

Atrial Pacing During Atrial Flutter. Burst pacing from the high RA or CS or along the Halo catheter is started at a CL 10 to 20 milliseconds shorter than the flutter CL, and then progressively shortening the pacing CL by 10 to 20 milliseconds.

Entrainment can usually be demonstrated with atrial pacing at CL 10-30 milliseconds shorter than the tachycardia CL. Occurrence of entrainment should first be confirmed before interpretation of the PPI. Entrainment is used to estimate qualitatively how far the reentrant circuit is from the pacing site (Table 9-1; Fig. 9-5).

More rapid atrial burst pacing (pacing CL 20 to 50 milliseconds shorter than the AFL CL) results in termination of AFL in most cases.[13] Termination of AFL during rapid pacing can be indicated by a sudden change of P wave morphology on the surface ECG and by a change of atrial activation sequence in the HB and CS os recordings. This is seen particularly with high RA pacing during counterclockwise AFL, whereby on termination of AFL, the negative flutter waves in the inferior leads change suddenly into upright P waves, reflecting a change in the atrial activation sequence to one of high RA pacing (i.e., simultaneous RA lateral and septal activation in a craniocaudal direction).[2] However, if the pacing site is distant from the AFL circuit (e.g., distal CS), a large mass of the atrial tissue can be captured by the pacing stimulus, producing a marked change in P wave morphology (i.e., manifest fusion) without terminating the AFL.

Failure to terminate AFL with rapid pacing can be caused by the following: (1) a short period of pacing or pacing at a relatively long CL—the closer the pacing CL to the tachycardia CL, the longer the pacing duration needed to terminate the tachycardia; (2) a pacing site distant from the AFL circuit, with the intervening atrial tissue preventing penetration of the AFL circuit; and/or (3) an apparent AFL on the ECG may actually be AF with streaming of the RA activation wavefront or may be a focal nonreentrant AT.[2,13]

Rapid atrial burst pacing may convert AFL into AF. This is less likely with a slower pacing CL or pacing from sites within the AFL circuit.[2] Atrial pacing can also accelerate AFL into one of two different tachycardias, double-wave reentry or lower loop reentry.[13] Double-wave reentry is manifest by acceleration of the tachycardia rate but with identical surface and intracardiac electrogram morphology. It can be recognized by having simultaneous activation of the superior and inferior regions of the tricuspid annulus, with all activation being sequential. This rhythm rarely lasts for more than a few beats, and may serve as a trigger for AF. Lower loop reentry is usually transient and stops by itself or terminates into typical AFL or AF.

Electroanatomical Mapping

High-density three-dimensional (3-D) electroanatomical maps during AFL can be useful in delineating the specific features of the AFL circuit and global RA activation during AFL. The activation map typically demonstrates a continuous progression of colors (from red to purple) around the tricuspid annulus with close proximity of earliest and latest local activation (red meeting purple), consistent with macroreentry (Fig. 9-6). The activation wavefront exits the cavotricuspid isthmus as a broad wavefront, spreading

TABLE 9–1 Entrainment Mapping of Typical Atrial Flutter (AFL)

Pacing from sites *outside* the AFL circuit (e.g., from RA appendage or mid or distal CS) results in: Manifest atrial fusion on the surface ECG and/or intracardiac recordings (fixed fusion at a single pacing CL, and progressive fusion on progressively shorter pacing CLs). During entrainment, any difference in atrial activation sequence compared with that during tachycardia (as determined by analysis of all available surface ECG and intracardiac recordings) is considered to represent manifest fusion. PPI—tachycardia CL > 30 msec: the interval between the stimulus artifact to the onset of the flutter wave on the surface ECG is longer than the interval between the local electrogram on the pacing site to the onset of flutter wave on the surface ECG.
Pacing from sites inside the AFL circuit (e.g., from CS os or Halo) results in: Manifest atrial fusion on surface ECG and/or intracardiac recordings (fixed fusion at a single pacing CL, and progressive fusion on progressively shorter pacing CL). PPI—tachycardia CL < 30 msec: the interval between the stimulus artifact to the onset of the flutter wave on the surface ECG is equal to the interval between the local electrogram on the pacing site to the onset of the flutter wave on the surface ECG.
Pacing from a protected isthmus inside the circuit (cavotricuspid isthmus) results in: Concealed atrial fusion (i.e., paced atrial waveform on the surface ECG and intracardiac recordings are identical to the AFL waveform). PPI—tachycardia CL < 30 msec: the interval between the stimulus artifact to the onset of the flutter wave on the surface ECG is equal to the interval between the local electrogram on the pacing site to the onset of the flutter wave on the surface ECG.

CL = cycle length; CS = coronary sinus; CS os = coronary sinus ostium; PPI = post-pacing interval; RA = right atrium.

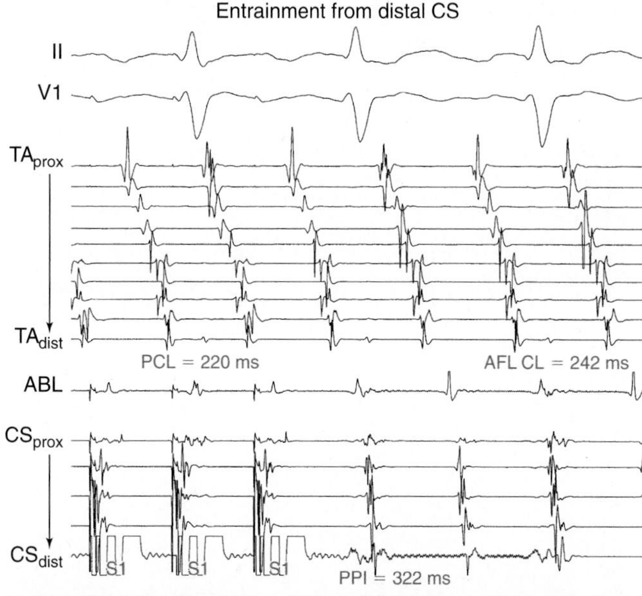

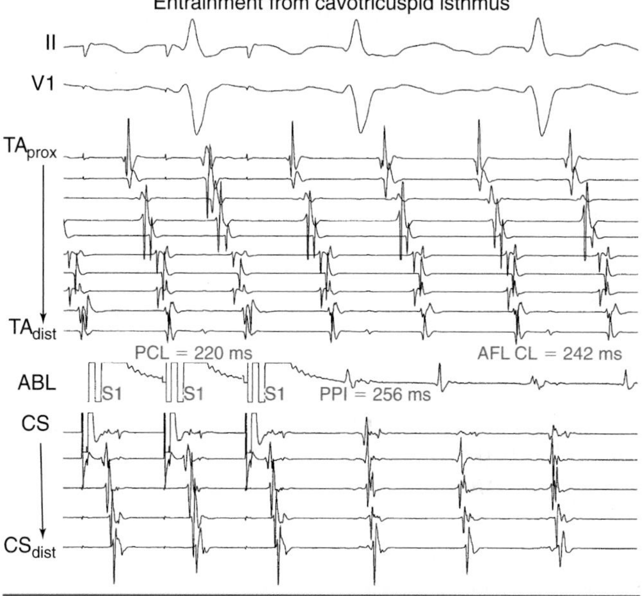

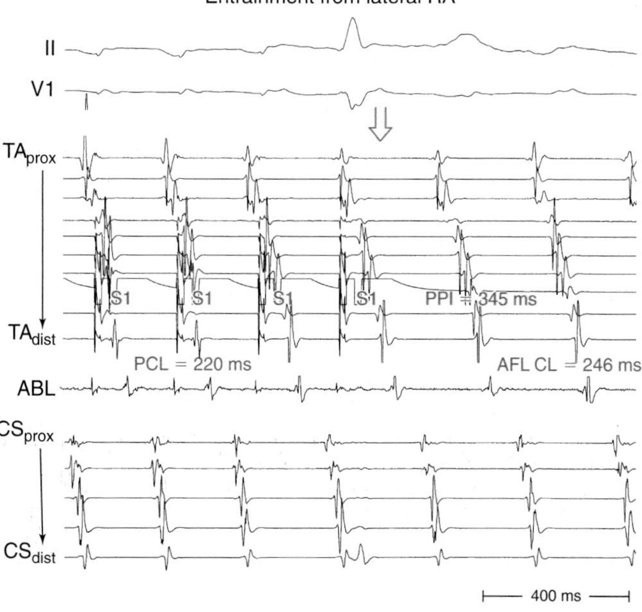

FIGURE 9–5 Entrainment of counterclockwise typical atrial flutter (AFL). **Upper panel,** Entrainment from the distal coronary sinus (CS) results in manifest atrial fusion and a long post-pacing interval (PPI; PPI – AFL cycle length [CL] = 80 milliseconds), because the distal CS is far from the reentrant circuit. **Middle panel,** Entrainment from ablation catheter positioned at the cavotricuspid isthmus results in concealed atrial fusion with a short PPI (PPI – AFL CL = 14 milliseconds), indicating that the cavotricuspid isthmus is part of the reentrant circuit. **Lower panel,** Entrainment from the lateral RA wall is attempted; however, the last paced stimulus fails to capture the atrium (open arrow); therefore, calculation of the PPI in this case is invalid and produces erroneous results. PCL = pacing cycle length.

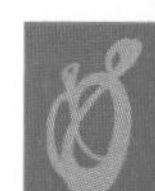

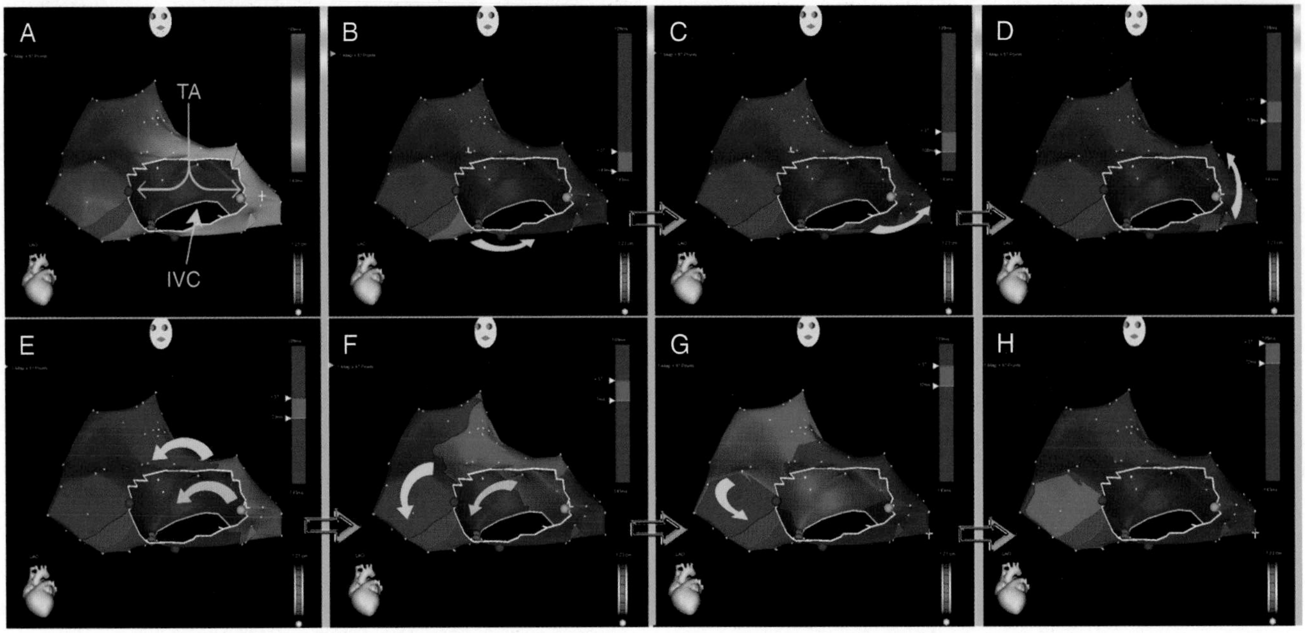

FIGURE 9–6 **A,** 3-D electroanatomical (CARTO) activation map of the right atrium (RA) in the left anterior oblique (LAO) view constructed during counterclockwise typical atrial flutter (AFL). During tachycardia, the depolarization wavefront travels counterclockwise around the tricuspid annulus (TA), as indicated by a continuous progression of colors (from red to purple) with close proximity of earliest and latest local activation (red meeting purple). **B to H,** Propagation map of the RA during counterclockwise typical AFL.

anterosuperiorly around the tricuspid annulus and posterosuperiorly (see Fig. 9-6). Lateral spread of the posterior wavefront is blocked along the vertical line in the posterolateral RA, a region marked by double potentials that coincides with the crista terminalis. The posterior wavefront proceeds cranially around the SVC to merge with the activation wavefront circulating around the tricuspid annulus. The anterolateral wall of the RA is the last to activate as the wavefront reenters the lateral aspect cavotricuspid isthmus.[14]

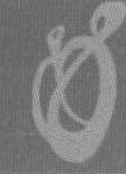

9

3-D electroanatomical maps can also provide information about the voltage characteristics of the tissues involved in the cavotricuspid isthmus. The lower the voltage, the easier it is to achieve block in the tissue. Thus, 3-D electroanatomical mapping may help choose a path in the cavotricuspid isthmus that is easier to ablate, which may not necessarily be the shortest path across the isthmus.[14]

Noncontact Mapping

Typical AFL is usually readily treated using standard ablation techniques. However, noncontact mapping can be used to confirm the anatomical location of the flutter circuit, reduce fluoroscopy time, and confirm isthmus block. Noncontact mapping has also been used to identify and guide RF ablation of the site of residual conduction following incomplete linear ablation lesions at the isthmus. Because of its ability to record from multiple sites simultaneously, noncontact mapping can rapidly identify gaps in linear lesions. This is accomplished by analysis of one or more paced complexes originating adjacent to the line being assessed. This capability can be particularly helpful in patients who have recurrent AFL following a previous ablation.[15-17] Because any number of maps can be superimposed on the initial geometry, bidirectional block at the ablation site can be rapidly identified during pacing following ablation. Tagging ablation areas during delivery of each RF impulse and a constantly visible ablation line offer another advantage—they ensure that no area is overlooked or ablated repeatedly.

ABLATION

Target of Ablation

The cavotricuspid isthmus, which represents the central portion of the inferior RA isthmus, is the ideal target of AFL ablation because it is accessible, relatively narrow, short, and safe to ablate, and essential for the AFL circuit (and not because it is the diseased area or causing the AFL).[18] The central part of the isthmus (the 6 o'clock region in a fluoroscopic LAO view) appears to be the optimal target site because it is the shortest (19 ± 4 mm; range, 13 to 26 mm). It is also there that the thinner isthmus is less likely to resist RF ablation, because it is composed of fibrofatty tissue. Another advantage of the central isthmus is the increased distance from the paraseptal isthmus, which contains, in 10% of cases, extensions of the AVN or AV nodal artery, and also the increased distance from the inferolateral isthmus, where the right coronary artery is in close proximity to the endocardium (less than 4 mm).[19]

Alternatively, the tricuspid annulus–CS or IVC-CS isthmuses may be targeted (Fig. 9-7); however, for this approach to be successful, ablation within the CS is probably necessary. Such approaches are less successful in curing AFL.[13] As noted, the paraseptal isthmus (tricuspid annulus–CS isthmus) has the thickest wall, compared with other parts of the inferior RA isthmus, although there is significant interindividual variability, is close to the arterial branch supplying the AVN and, in some cases, can contain the inferior extensions of the AVN. The inferolateral isthmus is the longest and is in closest proximity to the right coronary artery.[19]

Ablation Technique

Catheter Positioning

A steerable ablation catheter with a distal ablation electrode of 4 or 8 mm is generally used.[20-23] The catheter's curve size and shape can affect the ability to position the catheter on the isthmus, and the use of preshaped guiding sheaths (e.g., SR0, SL1, or ramp sheath; Daig, Minnetonka, Minn) can help stabilize the catheter position and prevent the catheter from sliding off the cavotricuspid isthmus and in and out of the right ventricle (RV).

The cavotricuspid isthmus can be localized electroanatomically. The ablation catheter is advanced to the RV under fluoroscopy (right anterior oblique [RAO] view); the tip is deflected to achieve contact with RV inferior wall and withdrawn progressively until the electrogram shows small atrial and large ventricular electrograms. The distal tip of the ablation catheter is then adjusted under fluoroscopy on the cavotricuspid isthmus in the LAO view until it is midway between the atrial septum and RA lateral wall (pointing toward 6 o'clock in a 45-degree LAO view; Fig. 9-8).

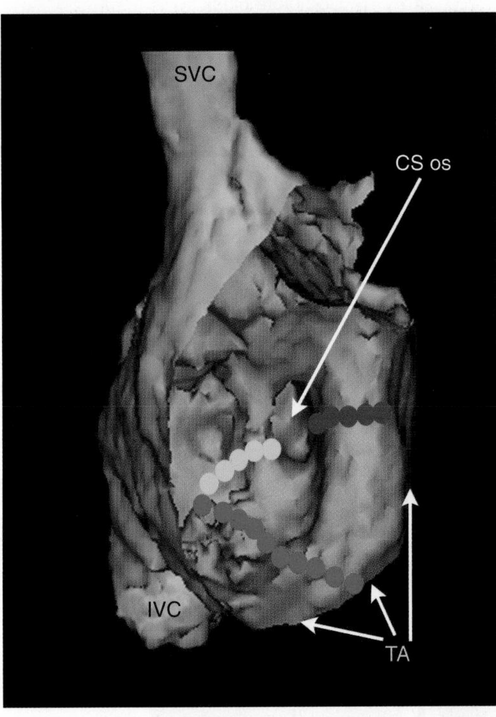

FIGURE 9-7 Computed tomography scan of the right atrium (RA; cardioscopic view) illustrating the typical location for linear ablation of the cavotricuspid isthmus (red dots), the tricuspid valve–coronary sinus (CS) isthmus (blue dots), and the CS–inferior vena cava (IVC) isthmus (yellow dots).

The ratio of the atrial and ventricular electrogram amplitude can help localize the position of the ablation catheter; the A/V ratio is typically 1:4 or less at the tricuspid annulus, 1:2 to 1:1 at the isthmus, and 2:1 to 4:1 near the IVC. The location of the catheter at the cavotricuspid isthmus can also be confirmed by demonstrating entrainment with concealed fusion during AFL.

Radiofrequency Ablation

After positioning of the ablation catheter on or near the tricuspid annulus, it is either gradually withdrawn toward the IVC during a continuous energy application (50 to 70 W, 60 to 120 seconds, targeting a temperature of 55° to 60°C), or in a stepwise manner with sequentially interrupted point by point application of radiofrequency (RF) energy (50 to 70 W, 30 to 60 seconds, targeting a temperature of 55° to 60°C). The first RF lesion is initiated from the tricuspid annulus edge with large ventricular and small atrial electrograms and the last lesion is completed at the IVC edge. It is important that linear lesions span completely from the tricuspid annulus to the IVC (Fig. 9-9). After each RF application, the electrogram will lose voltage and m ay become fragmented; the catheter is then withdrawn (2 to 4 mm at a time) toward the IVC until a new area of sharp atrial electrogram is reached, and the next RF application is delivered. This is repeated until the lack of atrial electrograms indicates that the catheter has reached the IVC. Before each RF application, the position of the ablation catheter is confirmed fluoroscopically, as described, or by using a 3-D mapping-navigation system.

During delivery of RF applications, AFL can terminate or its CL can increase transiently or permanently, and a gradual delay in activation of the low lateral RA wall can occur. This indicates that the ablation lesions have affected the circuit and should lead to continuation of RF delivery or extension of the lesion to ensure the achievement of complete conduction block across the isthmus.

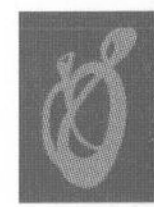

Ablation of the cavotricuspid isthmus may require more than one pass of RF delivery across the isthmus. It may be necessary to rotate the ablation catheter away from the initial line of energy application, medially or laterally in the isthmus, to create new or additional lines of block. At the time of the second pass-over, the ablation line isthmus electrograms will be fragmented, of low voltage, and often double.

A complete line of block is identified by a continuous corridor of double potentials separated by an isoelectric interval (Fig. 9-10). Further ablation is usually not needed

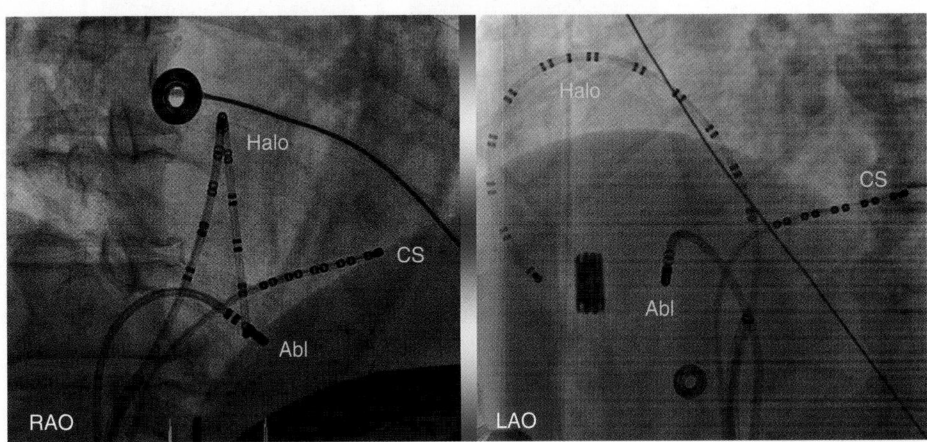

FIGURE 9-8 Fluoroscopic views (right anterior oblique [RAO] and left anterior oblique [LAO]) illustrating catheter location during ablation (Abl) of the cavotricuspid isthmus. CS = coronary sinus.

FIGURE 9–9 Ablation of the cavotricuspid isthmus guided by CARTO. The left anterior oblique (LAO) and inferior views of the reconstructed right atrium (RA) geometry are shown. Linear ablation (red dots) is performed across the cavotricuspid isthmus between the tricuspid annulus (TA) and inferior vena cava (IVC). CS = coronary sinus.

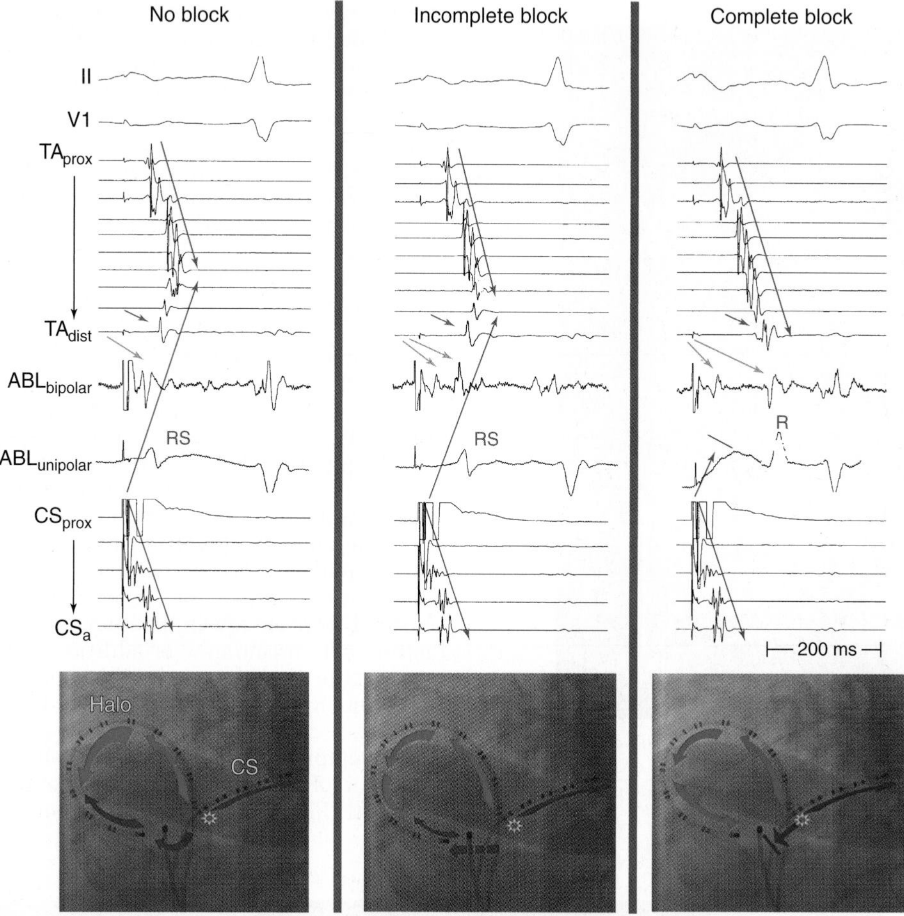

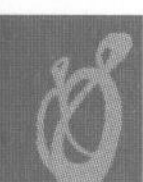

FIGURE 9–10 The use of coronary sinus (CS) pacing to verify the presence of clockwise cavotricuspid isthmus block. **Upper panels,** Intracardiac recordings from the right atrium (RA), CS, and cavotricuspid isthmus. **Lower panels,** Left anterior oblique fluoroscopic view illustrating position of the ablation catheter (Abl) at the cavotricuspid isthmus, and the Halo catheter around the tricuspid annulus (TA), with the distal end at the lateral end of the cavotricuspid isthmus. When isthmus conduction is intact (left panel), pacing from the coronary sinus ostium results in the collision of activation wavefronts in the lateral RA wall (red and blue arrows). **Middle panel,** The collision point moves toward the low lateral RA wall when incomplete block is present. **Right panel,** Complete clockwise isthmus block is indicated by the observation of a purely descending wavefront at the lateral wall down to the cavotricuspid isthmus (proximal-to-distal Halo sequence). Bipolar electrogram recording from the cavotricuspid isthmus initially shows a single atrial potential (left panel, orange arrow). With partial isthmus ablation, the atrial electrogram splits into two closely adjacent potentials (middle panel, orange arrows). Complete isthmus block is indicated by the observation of double potentials separated by an isoelectric interval (right panel, orange arrows). Additionally, bipolar electrogram polarity reversal is observed in the distal Halo and the distal ablation electrodes recordings when complete block is achieved, indicating reversal of the direction of the activation wavefront lateral to the line of block (green and orange arrows). Positive (R wave) morphology of the unipolar recording lateral to the line of block also indicates complete isthmus block (in contrast to biphasic [RS] electrogram morphology when intact conduction or only incomplete block is present).

at sites that exhibit double potentials, because this finding generally indicates that local conduction block is already present. Gaps in the ablation line (i.e., sites of persistent conduction) are characterized by single- or triple-fractionated potentials centered on or occupying the isoelectric interval of the adjacent double potential (see Fig. 9-10). These gaps should be ablated until complete isthmus block is achieved. In 15% to 20% of cases, it can be extremely difficult to produce isthmus block, which can be secondary to one or more of the following: (1) a very prominent eustachian ridge; (2) a thick isthmus, preventing transmural ablation; and (3) local edema, clot, and/or superficial damage forming a barrier for deeper penetration of subsequent RF applications.[18]

Advances in catheter design have enhanced the ability to create complete lines of block in the cavotricuspid isthmus. Because of the pouches, recesses, ridges, and trabeculations that can occur in the isthmus, it often is advantageous to create lesions that are larger than those created with conventional 4-mm–tip ablation catheters. RF ablation catheters that have an 8-mm distal electrode allow the creation of larger lesions in high- and low-flow regions. These catheters may facilitate AFL ablation by achieving a high success rate with a smaller number of RF lesions, shorter procedure, and less fluoroscopy exposure.

Cooled- or irrigated-tip catheters also allow the creation of larger lesions in high- and low-flow regions. Several studies have demonstrated that complete cavotricuspid isthmus block is more reliably achieved with a cooled- or irrigated-tip catheter than with a conventional ablation catheter. RF ablation with a cooled RF catheter is as safe as standard RF ablation, and it facilitates the creation of cavotricuspid isthmus line of block more rapidly, with fewer RF applications.[22,24-27]

Maximum Voltage-Guided Technique

The maximum voltage-guided technique is based on the hypothesis that discrete muscle bundles in the cavotricuspid isthmus participate in the flutter circuit. Large atrial electrogram voltages identify the location of these muscle bundles along the isthmus and are selectively targeted for ablation. This technique has demonstrated significantly reduced ablation times compared with a purely anatomical approach.[28-30]

Using this technique, the cavotricuspid isthmus is mapped in the 6 o'clock position (as viewed in a 30-degree LAO projection) and bipolar atrial electrograms (during AFL or, preferably, during NSR or CS pacing) are measured peak to peak during a continuous pullback along the isthmus. The site of maximum voltage is noted and used as a marker for a presumed muscle bundle. The ablation catheter is positioned at this site, regardless of the location along the line, and RF ablation is performed for 40 to 60 seconds until an amplitude reduction of 50% or more is achieved. If the ablation lesion does not result in bidirectional isthmus block, the line is remapped and the next largest atrial electrogram is sequentially targeted for ablation. This is repeated until bidirectional isthmus block is achieved. This technique therefore targets the signals with highest amplitude along the cavotricuspid isthmus and does not necessitate a contiguous line of ablation.[29,30]

Cryoablation

Complete cavotricuspid isthmus block can also be achieved by cryothermal ablation. Although there is no reason to believe that cryothermal ablation will be more effective than RF ablation of the cavotricuspid isthmus, cryothermal ablation has the advantage of being less painful. Short-term and long-term success rates are comparable to those for RF ablation.[31] However, compared with RF ablation, cryoablation is associated with significantly longer procedure times. This is driven mainly by differences in ablation duration, which can be attributed to the longer duration of each cryoablation (4 minutes) compared with RF ablation (up to 60 seconds).[32]

Role of 3-D Electroanatomical Mapping-Navigation Systems

Electroanatomical mapping systems (CARTO or NavX) can provide precise spatial localization and tracking of the ablation catheter along the cavotricuspid isthmus, which potentially helps shorten radiation exposure and procedure time. Electroanatomical mapping can also provide anatomical localization of serial RF applications. The main advantage of using this mapping system for AFL is the visibility of an ablation line as the procedure is carried out so that no area is left out or repeatedly ablated. Therefore, it facilitates the creation of ablation lines devoid of gaps across the entire isthmus (see Fig. 9-9).[14,33]

Such systems also provide information about the voltage characteristics of the tissues involved in the cavotricuspid isthmus. After taking the usual anatomical landmarks, detailed cavotricuspid isthmus mapping is performed by withdrawing the catheter at 2- to 3-mm intervals and taking several points along the line. Voltage, activation, and propagation maps are then created to look for any high-voltage areas that are better avoided in first-time ablations. Bipolar electrograms recorded from the mapping catheter are filtered at 30 to 400 Hz. Areas showing voltages of less than 1 mV are considered to represent scar tissue. The lower the voltage, the easier it is to achieve block in the tissue. Thus, it may help choose a path in the isthmus that is easier to ablate, which may not necessarily be the shortest path across the cavotricuspid isthmus.[14]

Electroanatomical mapping can also help delineation of cavotricuspid isthmus geometry. As the catheter is dragged across the isthmus, each point is acquired and tagged. The isthmus region forms a relatively flat rectangular surface in a caudal projection, and a side-on view is provided by the RAO projection. The ablation line can be planned by a trial run. Typically, the most anterior and posterior points in the cavotricuspid isthmus are tagged; during RF application, the line is placed to connect the tags. Each tag is approximately 4 mm in diameter, permitting visual estimation of the density of applications needed to produce a linear lesion during the drag. This helps avoid redundant lesion application and can identify potential gaps in the ablation line.[14,33]

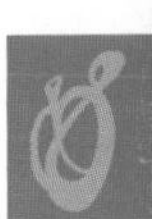

In patients with recurrent AFL following previous ablation attempts, electroanatomical mapping is particularly helpful. A detailed map of the isthmus is constructed. Because the system records the activation time and electrogram amplitude from each point selected, a voltage map that reveals the unablated area can be prepared. This helps localize high-voltage and breakthrough sites, because these sites should be targeted under these circumstances. The RF energy can then be delivered to these sites with more precision.[14]

Verification of cavotricuspid isthmus conduction block following ablation can also be carried out using electroanatomical mapping systems. The activation wavefront during AFL halts at the previously completed line but continues through the breakthrough site (see later).

Endpoints of Ablation

Ablation can be performed during AFL or CS pacing.[34] If ablation is carried out during AFL, the first endpoint is to terminate AFL during RF energy delivery. If AFL is terminated, programmed electrical stimulation and burst atrial pacing should be performed immediately to determine whether AFL is still reinducible. If AFL is not terminated or is reinducible, ablation should be repeated. If AFL is terminated and is not reinducible, pacing maneuvers should be performed to determine whether there is bidirectional block in the cavotricuspid isthmus. Termination of AFL during RF delivery is often not associated with complete bidirectional cavotricuspid isthmus block, and should not be considered a reliable ablation endpoint by itself. Once complete bidirectional isthmus block has been achieved, reconfirmation should be repeated 30 minutes after the last RF application.[1,3]

If ablation is performed during NSR, it is usually performed during CS pacing to help monitor the activation sequence in the lateral RA wall. During ablation of the cavotricuspid isthmus, gradual delay in activation of the low lateral RA can be observed prior to achieving complete bidirectional isthmus block.

Confirmation of Bidirectional Cavotricuspid Isthmus Block

1. Atrial Activation Sequence During Atrial Pacing. Complete bidirectional isthmus block is demonstrated by pacing from the CS and RA lateral wall and observing that sequential atrial activation terminates at the ablation line, on the contralateral side from the pacing site. Atrial pacing at a CL of approximately 600 milliseconds is performed from the CS os and then from the low lateral RA.

During CS os pacing, the baseline RA activation sequence (with intact clockwise cavotricuspid isthmus conduction) is characterized by two RA wavefronts of impulse propagation. One wavefront propagates from the CS pacing site in a clockwise direction through the cavotricuspid isthmus to the low lateral RA. The other wavefront from the CS os ascends up the atrial septum to the high RA in a counterclockwise direction, with resulting collision of wavefronts at the upper part of the lateral RA (the exact location of wavefront collision depends on the relative conduction velocities of the RA and the cavotricuspid isthmus) and generating an atrial activation sequence with a chevron pattern (see Fig. 9-10). Clockwise isthmus block is indicated by the observation of a purely descending wavefront at the lateral wall down to the cavotricuspid isthmus (proximal to distal Halo sequence) when pacing from the CS os (i.e., pacing of the septal side of the ablation line). This block is associated with a marked prolongation of the cavotricuspid isthmus conduction duration (i.e., the interval from the CS os to the low lateral RA; see Fig. 9-10). Incomplete clockwise isthmus block is said to occur when a descending wavefront at the lateral RA wall still allows the lateral part of the cavotricuspid isthmus to be activated from the CS os in a clockwise direction across the cavotricuspid isthmus but at a slower conduction velocity, resulting in displacement of collision of the clockwise and counterclockwise wavefronts to the lower part of lateral RA. The distal bipole of the Halo catheter (Halo 1,2) at the lateral part of the cavotricuspid isthmus is activated slightly before or at the same time as bipole Halo 3,4, situated more laterally (see Fig. 9-10).[1,3]

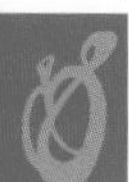

9

It is important to recognize that monitoring only the atrial activation sequence of the RA lateral wall recorded by the Halo catheter during CS pacing can lead to diagnostic errors in a large percentage of patients. This is because of the inability to detect residual isthmus conduction slow enough to allow the wavefront propagating in an opposite direction to reach the ablation line earlier than the trans-isthmus conduction. Theoretically, slow but persistent isthmus conduction that can be confined within the ablation line or part of the isthmus distant from an area mapped by the multipolar catheter can therefore be misdiagnosed, no matter how close the distal tip of the Halo catheter is placed to the ablation line, or even if the Halo catheter is positioned across the ablation line.[1,3]

During low lateral RA pacing, the baseline RA activation sequence (with intact counterclockwise cavotricuspid isthmus conduction) exhibits two ascending wavefronts (septal and lateral) leading to impulse collision at the high lateral wall; the caudocranial activation of the RA septum following counterclockwise propagation of the paced wavefront through the cavotricuspid isthmus results in atrial activation in the CS os electrode preceding that in the HB electrode (Fig. 9-11). Furthermore, intact conduction through the cavotricuspid isthmus permits the paced wavefront to proceed rapidly to activate the LA from below (and CS activation spreads from proximal CS to distal CS), giving rise to an inverted P wave in the inferior leads.[35] Counterclockwise isthmus block is indicated by the observation of a

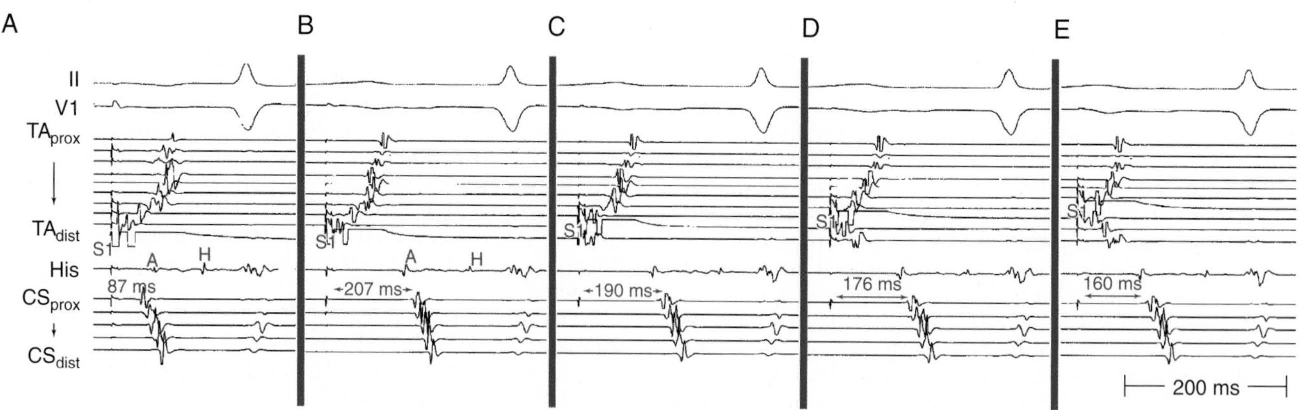

FIGURE 9–11 The use of differential pacing from the lateral right atrial (RA) wall to verify the presence of counterclockwise cavotricuspid isthmus block. **A,** Pacing from the lateral aspect of the isthmus (Halo 1,2) before isthmus ablation. **B** to **E,** Pacing from different lateral RA sites along the Halo catheter after isthmus ablation (**B,** pacing from Halo 3,4; **C,** pacing from Halo 5,6; **D,** pacing from Halo 7,8; **E,** pacing from Halo 9,10). When isthmus conduction is intact, coronary sinus ostium (CS os) activation occurs via a counterclockwise wavefront across the isthmus and, because the CS os is anatomically closer to the pacing site than the His bundle (HB), atrial activation in the CS os electrode precedes that in the HB electrode. In the presence of counterclockwise isthmus block, CS os activation occurs via the wavefront propagating in a clockwise direction up the RA lateral wall, over the RA roof, and then down the septum. Consequently, CS os activation (as measured by the stimulus–to–local electrogram interval) occurs progressively earlier during pacing from more cephalic sites along the lateral RA wall (**B** to **E**). Additionally, activation of the CS os occurs after the high RA and the HB region.

single ascending wavefront at the lateral wall (distal-to-proximal Halo sequence) followed by a completely descending wavefront at the septum to reach the CS os. Therefore, compared with baseline, a counterclockwise isthmus block is associated with inversion of the direction of the septal activation from ascending to descending. Furthermore, the CS os electrogram is activated after the high RA and the HB region (see Fig. 9-11). Additionally, counterclockwise conduction block in the cavotricuspid isthmus forces the wavefront to activate the LA from above via Bachmann's bundle—and CS activation spreads from the distal to proximal CS—giving rise to a different P wave morphology, with the terminal portion positive in the inferior leads.[1,3,35]

2. Transisthmus Conduction Interval. Transisthmus conduction interval is measured during CS os or low lateral RA pacing; it is equal to the interval from the stimulus artifact from one side of the isthmus to the atrial electrogram on the contralateral side. Prolongation of this interval by more than 50% (and/or to an absolute value of 150 milliseconds or more) indicates isthmus block (see Fig. 9-10).[36] This criterion has sensitivity and negative predictive values of 100%. However, the specificity and positive predictive values are less than 90%.

3. Double Potentials. Double potentials, separated by an isoelectric interval of 30 milliseconds or longer, straddle a line of block. Double potentials along the ablation line across the cavotricuspid isthmus are generally considered the gold standard for determining complete bidirectional block (see Fig. 9-10).[37] When there is a gap in a line of block, the isoelectric period between the double potentials shortens the closer the electrograms are to the gap. At the gap, in the line of block, double potentials are no longer present, and the electrogram is typically long and fractionated but can also be discrete. When the interval between the double potentials is more than 110 milliseconds, isthmus block is present. When that interval is less than 90 milliseconds, complete bidirectional block is absent. This technique is probably more difficult to perform than the classic activation mapping technique, mainly because of the ambiguity of electrogram interpretation along the ablation line, especially after extensive ablation attempts.[37]

4. Unipolar Electrogram Configuration. The morphology of the unfiltered unipolar recording indicates the direction of wavefront propagation. Positive deflections (R waves) are generated by propagation toward the recording electrode; negative deflections (QS complexes) are generated by propagation away from the electrode. During proximal CS pacing, the unfiltered unipolar signals recorded from the cavotricuspid isthmus typically demonstrate an RS configuration as the paced impulse propagates clockwise across the isthmus. Also, because atrial depolarization along the cavotricuspid isthmus occurs sequentially in the clockwise direction, the polarity of the initial depolarization is the same from each pair of recording electrodes using unfiltered unipolar recording on the cavotricuspid isthmus. When complete clockwise isthmus block is achieved, depolarization of the electrode just medial to the line of block retains its original polarity, but its morphology changes to a single positive deflection (monophasic R wave) because the recording site becomes a dead end for impulse conduction. On the other hand, atrial tissue lateral to the line of block is depolarized from the counterclockwise direction, which is opposite to the original direction of depolarization and, accordingly, the polarity of the atrial electrograms on the cavotricuspid isthmus lateral to the line of block reverses (see Fig. 9-10).[38,39] The same maneuver can be performed with pacing from the low lateral RA to evaluate counterclockwise isthmus block.

Some studies have suggested that bipolar electrogram morphology could also be used for this purpose, although it is important to emphasize that bipolar recordings predominantly reflect local activation time. Signal subtraction used to create a bipolar signal largely eliminates morphology information at either electrode. Bipolar electrogram polarity reversal, however, may indicate a reversed wavefront direction that has been used in addition to the activation sequence for verifying bidirectional cavotricuspid isthmus block (see Fig. 9-10).[40]

5. Differential Pacing. During unidirectional activation of the cavotricuspid isthmus (e.g., low lateral RA pacing), the double electrograms recorded along the ablation line reflect activation in its immediate vicinity. The initial component reflects activation at the ipsilateral border, and the terminal component reflects that at the contralateral border. Pacing from another site farther away from the ablation line (e.g., midlateral RA), would obviously delay the stimulus to initial component timing, whereas the response of the terminal component would depend on the presence or absence of conduction through the ablation line.[41] If the two components of the electrogram represent slow conduction across the isthmus ablation line, the terminal component would be delayed similar to that of the initial component because both components are activated by the same wavefront penetrating through the ablation line. In contrast, when complete cavotricuspid isthmus block is achieved, the two components represent two opposing activation wavefronts; the second component will be advanced because it is activated by the wavefront going around, instead of through, the ablation line since the length of the detour is shortened by withdrawal of the pacing site.

Using the same principle, the local activation time at the CS os electrode during fixed rate pacing performed from the low lateral and midlateral RA can be used for evaluation of counterclockwise cavotricuspid isthmus block. Normally (with intact isthmus conduction), CS os activation occurs via propagation of the paced wavefront across the isthmus in a counterclockwise direction. Therefore, CS os activation occurs earlier during pacing from the low lateral compared with the midlateral RA, because the low lateral RA is anatomically closer to the CS os. In contrast, when counterclockwise isthmus block is present, CS os activation occurs via the wavefront propagating in a clockwise direction up the RA lateral wall, over the RA roof, and then down the septum (see Fig. 9-11). Consequently, CS os activation occurs earlier during pacing from the midlateral compared with the low lateral RA because the length of the detour is shortened by pacing from the midlateral RA.

6. Rate-Dependent Isthmus Block. Incomplete cavotricuspid isthmus block can mimic the activation pattern related to complete block, producing intraatrial conduction delay at the low lateral RA. Residual isthmus conduction is usually decremental and is worsened at faster pacing rates. Rate-dependent isthmus block (during CS os or low lateral RA pacing) is associated with a change of the direction of impulse propagation and an increase of conduction time when the pacing rate is increased.

This maneuver helps distinguish isthmus block from long local conduction delay across the isthmus. With incomplete isthmus block, activation of the low lateral RA during CS os pacing can be delayed, but can still occur via the cavotricuspid isthmus at the same time or just earlier than the wavefront coming to the low lateral RA from the counterclockwise direction. Increasing the pacing rate results in decremental conduction across the now diseased isthmus, causing further delay in activation of the low lateral RA. In contrast, when complete isthmus block is present, the lateral RA is activated in a counterclockwise direction across the atrial septum and RA roof. Because these atrial regions conduct nondecrementally, pacing at faster rates should not change the timing of low lateral RA activation significantly,

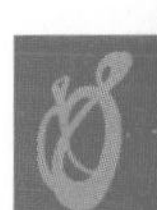

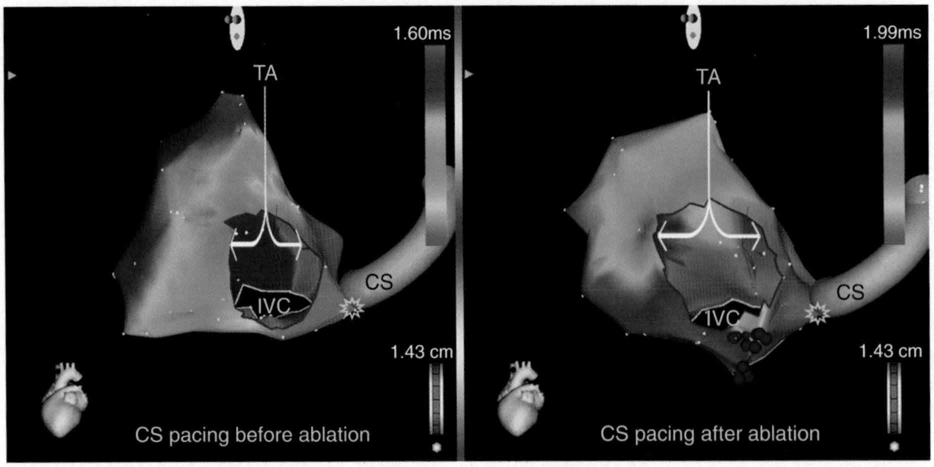

FIGURE 9–12 CARTO activation map of coronary sinus (CS) pacing before (left) and after (right) cavotricuspid isthmus ablation. During CS ostium pacing (yellow star), complete isthmus block in the clockwise direction is indicated by the absence of activation proceeding through the ablation line (red dots); activation of the entire tricuspid annulus (TA) remains counterclockwise, except for the small portion that is situated between the pacing site and the line of block. IVC = inferior vena cava.

as long as the pacing CL is longer than atrial refractoriness. The same maneuver can be performed with pacing from the low lateral RA to evaluate counterclockwise isthmus block.

7. 3-D Electroanatomical Mapping. Electroanatomical 3-D activation mapping can be used to verify isthmus block. When clockwise block in the isthmus is achieved, proximal CS pacing results in an activation wavefront propagating in a counterclockwise fashion, with the latest activation in the cavotricuspid isthmus immediately lateral to the ablation line (Fig. 9-12). When conduction across the cavotricuspid isthmus is still intact, CS pacing produces an activation wavefront that propagates rapidly through the cavotricuspid isthmus, with the anterolateral RA wall being activated last. Similar maps can be generated during low lateral RA pacing to confirm counterclockwise block in the cavotricuspid isthmus. CARTO maps can also be evaluated for the presence of gaps in the ablation lines, indicated by the early breakthroughs from the ablation line. However, following isthmus ablation, the local electrograms at the ablation line can be complex—with double, triple, or fragmented potentials, and unclear local activation time—and electroanatomical activation mapping can be challenging.

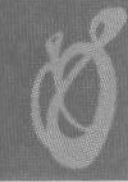

Outcome

With the availability of precise catheter locator systems, more effective ablation tools, and accurate endpoints for ablation, the inability to create complete cavotricuspid isthmus block and to eliminate recurrences of isthmus-dependent AFL successfully is unusual in contemporary practice. Acute success rate of ablation of typical AFL approaches 99%.[42] A repeat ablation procedure is performed in 5% to 15% of patients and the long-term success rate in preventing recurrent AFL is 97%.[42] For patients in whom typical AFL recurs after ablation, conduction through the cavotricuspid isthmus is usually elicited. Presumably, such recurrences reflect failure to achieve bidirectional isthmus block at the initial procedure, incorrect initial assessment of bidirectional block, or resumption of conduction across an initially blocked isthmus. Following AFL ablation, AF can develop in approximately 20% to 30% (with short-term follow-up, approximately 1 year) and in up to 82% (with long-term follow-up, approximately 4 years) of patients with or without prior history of AF.[1,3,43]

Serious complications associated with AFL ablation are rare (0.4%) and include AV block (most common, 0.2%), cardiac tamponade, groin hematoma, transient inferior ST segment elevation or acute occlusion of the right coronary artery,[44] thromboembolic complications, and ventricular tahycardia.[42,45]

REFERENCES

1. Waldo AL: Atrial flutter: Mechanisms, clinical features, and management. *In* Zipes DP, Jalife J (eds): Cardiac Electrophysiology: From Cell to Bedside, 4th ed. Philadelphia, WB Saunders, 2004, pp 490-499.
2. Waldo AL: Atrial flutter. From mechanism to treatment. *In* Camm AJ (ed): Clinical Approaches to Tachyarrhythmias. Armonk, NY, Futura, 2001, pp 1-56.
3. Feld G, Srivatsa U, Hoppe B: Ablation of isthmus-dependent atrial flutters. *In* Huang SKS, Wood M (eds): Catheter Ablation of Cardiac Arrhythmias. Philadelphia, WB Saunders, 2006, pp 195-218.
4. Waki K, Saito T, Becker AE: Right atrial flutter isthmus revisited: Normal anatomy favors nonuniform anisotropic conduction. J Cardiovasc Electrophysiol 2000; 11:90.
5. Yang Y, Mangat I, Glatter KA, et al: Mechanism of conversion of atypical right atrial flutter to atrial fibrillation. Am J Cardiol 2003;91:46.
6. Yang Y, Cheng J, Bochoeyer A, et al: Atypical right atrial flutter patterns. Circulation 2001;103:3092.
7. Zhang S, Younis G, Hariharan R, et al: Lower loop reentry as a mechanism of clockwise right atrial flutter. Circulation 2004;109:1630.
8. Bochoeyer A, Yang Y, Cheng J, et al: Surface electrocardiographic characteristics of right and left atrial flutter. Circulation 2003;108:60.
9. Yang Y, Varma N, Keung EC, Scheinman MM: Reentry within the cavotricuspid isthmus: An isthmus dependent circuit. Pacing Clin Electrophysiol 2005 August; 28(8):808-818.
10. Yang Y, Varma N, Keung EC: Surface ECG characteristics of Intraisthmus reentry. Pacing Clin Electrophysiol 2003;26:1032.
11. Blomström-Lundqvist C, Scheinman MM, Aliot EM, et al. American College of Cardiology; American Heart Association Task Force on Practice Guidelines; European Society of Cardiology Committee for Practice Guidelines. Writing Committee to Develop Guidelines for the Management of Patients With Supraventricular Arrhythmias: ACC/AHA/ESC guidlines for the managementof patients with supraventricular arrhythmias: executive summary: A report of the Amerian College of Cardiology/American Heart Association Task Force on Practice Guidelines and the European Society of Cardiology Committee for Practice Guidelines. Circulation 2003;108:1871.
12. Duytschaever M, Dierickx C, Tavernier R: Variable atrioventricular block during atrial flutter: What is the mechanism? J Cardiovasc Electrophysiol 2002;13:950.
13. Josephson ME: Atrial flutter and fibrillation. *In* Josephson ME (ed): Clinical Cardiac Electrophysiology. Philadelphia, Lippincott, Williams & Wilkins, 2002, pp 272-321.
14. Kottkamp H, Hugl B, Krauss B, et al: Electromagnetic versus fluoroscopic mapping of the inferior isthmus for ablation of typical atrial flutter: A prospective randomized study. Circulation 2000;102:2082.
15. Friedman PA: Novel mapping techniques for cardiac electrophysiology. Heart 2002;87:575.
16. Schneider MA, Ndrepepa G, Zrenner B, et al: Noncontact mapping-guided ablation of atrial flutter and enhanced-density mapping of the inferior vena caval–tricuspid annulus isthmus. Pacing Clin Electrophysiol 2001;24:1755.
17. Betts TR, Roberts PR, Allen SA, et al: Electrophysiological mapping and ablation of intra-atrial reentry tachycardia after Fontan surgery with the use of a noncontact mapping system. Circulation 2000;102:419.
18. Cosio FG, Pastor A, Nunez A, Goicolea A: Catheter ablation of typical atrial flutter. *In* Zipes DP, Haissaguerre M (eds): Catheter Ablation of Arrhythmias. Armonk, Futura, 2002, pp 131-152.
19. Nakao M, Saoudi N: More on isthmus anatomy for safety and efficacy. J Cardiovasc Electrophysiol 2005;16:409.

20. Kasai A, Anselme F, Teo WS, et al: Comparison of effectiveness of an 8-mm versus a 4-mm tip electrode catheter for radiofrequency ablation of typical atrial flutter. Am J Cardiol 2000;86:1029.
21. Rodriguez LM, Nabar A, Timmermans C, Wellens HJ: Comparison of results of an 8-mm split-tip versus a 4-mm tip ablation catheter to perform radiofrequency ablation of type I atrial flutter. Am J Cardiol 2000;85:109.
22. Marrouche NF, Schweikert R, Saliba W, et al: Use of different catheter ablation technologies for treatment of typical atrial flutter: Acute results and long-term follow-up. Pacing Clin Electrophysiol 2003;26:743.
23. Ventura R, Willems S, Weiss C, et al: Large tip electrodes for successful elimination of atrial flutter resistant to conventional catheter ablation. J Interv Card Electrophysiol 2003;8:149.
24. Jais P, Shah DC, Haissaguerre M, et al: Prospective randomized comparison of irrigated-tip versus conventional-tip catheters for ablation of common flutter. Circulation 2000;22;101:772.
25. Jais P, Hocini M, Gillet T, et al: Effectiveness of irrigated tip catheter ablation of common atrial flutter. Am J Cardiol 2001;88:433.
26. Atiga WL, Worley SJ, Hummel J, et al: Prospective randomized comparison of cooled radiofrequency versus standard radiofrequency energy for ablation of typical atrial flutter. Pacing Clin Electrophysiol 2002;25:1172.
27. Schreieck J, Zrenner B, Kumpmann J, et al: Prospective randomized comparison of closed cooled-tip versus 8-mm-tip catheters for radiofrequency ablation of typical atrial flutter. J Cardiovasc Electrophysiol 2002;13:980.
28. Ozaydin M, Tada H, Chugh A, et al: Atrial electrogram amplitude and efficacy of cavotricuspid isthmus ablation for atrial flutter. Pacing Clin Electrophysiol 2003;26:1859.
29. Redfearn DP, Skanes AC, Gula LJ, et al: Cavotricuspid isthmus conduction is dependent on underlying anatomical bundle architecture: Observations using a maximum voltage-guided ablation technique. J Cardiovasc Electrophysiol 2006;17:832.
30. Subbiah RN, Gula LJ, Krahn AD, et al: Rapid ablation for atrial flutter by targeting maximum voltage—factors associated with short ablation times. J Cardiovasc Electrophysiol 2007;18:612.
31. Timmermans C, Ayers GM, Crijns HJ, Rodriguez LM: Randomized study comparing radiofrequency ablation with cryoablation for the treatment of atrial flutter with emphasis on pain perception. Circulation 2003;107:1250.
32. Collins NJ, Barlow M, Varghese P, Leitch J: Cryoablation versus radiofrequency ablation in the treatment of atrial flutter trial (CRAAFT). J Interv Card Electrophysiol 2006;16:1.
33. Ventura R, Rostock T, Klemm HU, et al: Catheter ablation of common-type atrial flutter guided by three-dimensional right atrial geometry reconstruction and catheter tracking using cutaneous patches: A randomized prospective study. J Cardiovasc Electrophysiol 2004;15:1157.
34. Tada H, Oral H, Ozaydin M, et al: Randomized comparison of anatomical and electrogram mapping approaches to ablation of typical atrial flutter. J Cardiovasc Electrophysiol 2002;13:662.
35. Shah DC, Takahashi A, Jais P, et al: Tracking dynamic conduction recovery across the cavotricuspid isthmus. J Am Coll Cardiol 2000;35:1478.
36. Oral H, Sticherling C, Tada H, et al: Role of transisthmus conduction intervals in predicting bidirectional block after ablation of typical atrial flutter. J Cardiovasc Electrophysiol 2001;12:169.
37. Anselme F, Savoure A, Cribier A, Saoudi N: Catheter ablation of typical atrial flutter: A randomized comparison of two methods for determining complete bidirectional isthmus block. Circulation 2001;103:1434.
38. Villacastin J, Almendral J, Arenal A, et al: Usefulness of unipolar electrograms to detect isthmus block after radiofrequency ablation of typical atrial flutter. Circulation 2000;102:3080.
39. Tada H, Oral H, Sticherling C, et al: Electrogram polarity and cavotricuspid isthmus block during ablation of typical atrial flutter. J Cardiovasc Electrophysiol 2001;12: 393.
40. Andronache M, de CC, Miljoen H, et al: Correlation between electrogram morphology and standard criteria to validate bidirectional cavotricuspid block in common atrial flutter ablation. Europace 2003;5:335.
41. Haissaguerre M, Jais P, Shah DC, et al: Electrophysiological end point for catheter ablation of atrial fibrillation initiated from multiple pulmonary venous foci. Circulation 2000;101:1409.
42. Morady F: Catheter ablation of supraventricular arrhythmias: state of the art. J Cardiovasc Electrophysiol 2004;15:124.
43. Ellis K, Wazni O, Marrouche N, et al: Incidence of atrial fibrillation post-cavotricuspid isthmus ablation in patients with typical atrial flutter: Left-atrial size as an independent predictor of atrial fibrillation recurrence. J Cardiovasc Electrophysiol 2007;18:799.
44. Ouali S, Anselme F, Savoure A, Cribier A: Acute coronary occlusion during radiofrequency catheter ablation of typical atrial flutter. J Cardiovasc Electrophysiol 2002;13:1047.
45. Ramanna H, Derksen R, Elvan A, et al: Ventricular tachycardia as a complication of atrial flutter ablation. J Cardiovasc Electrophysiol 2000;11:472.

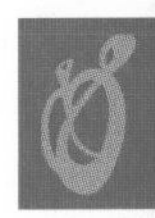

CHAPTER 10

Atypical (Non–Isthmus-Dependent) Atrial Flutter

PATHOPHYSIOLOGY

The term *typical atrial flutter* (AFL) is reserved for an atrial macroreentrant arrhythmia rotating clockwise or counterclockwise around the tricuspid annulus and using the cavotricuspid isthmus as an essential part of the reentrant circuit. Any other atrial *macroreentrant* tachycardia, regardless of the atrial cycle length (CL), is classified as atypical AFL.

The mechanism of macroreentrant atrial tachycardia (AT) is reentrant activation around a large central obstacle, generally several centimeters in diameter, at least in one of its dimensions. The central obstacle can consist of normal or abnormal structures. Additionally, the obstacle can be fixed, functional, or a combination of both. There is no single point of origin of activation, and atrial tissues outside the circuit are activated from various parts of the circuit.

A description of macroreentrant AT mechanisms must be made in relation to atrial anatomy, including a detailed description of the obstacles or boundaries of the circuit and the critical isthmuses that may be targets for therapeutic action. Typically, chronic or long-lasting ATs are macroreentrant. Focal ATs are more frequently responsible for irregular ATs with frequent spontaneous interruption and reinitiation than those observed with macroreentry.

Right Atrial Non–Isthmus-Dependent Flutter

1. Lesional Right Atrial Macroreentrant Tachycardia. In this macroreentrant AT, the central obstacle of the circuit is an atriotomy scar, a septal prosthetic patch, a suture line, or a line of fixed block secondary to radiofrequency (RF) ablation. Other obstacles can also include anatomical structures located in the vicinity of the scar (superior vena cava [SVC], inferior vena cava [IVC]). Rarely, such ATs are associated with areas of electrical silence suggesting atrial scarring in patients who have not undergone prior atrial surgery. These patients have a characteristic posterolateral and lateral distribution of right atrial (RA) scarring and frequently have more than one tachycardia mechanism.[1-4] Low-voltage electrograms characterizing areas of scar and double potentials characterizing a line of block can be observed during both normal sinus rhythm (NSR) and AT.[1,3,5-10]

For macroreentrant ATs in adults with repaired congenital heart disease, three RA circuits are generally identified: lateral wall circuits with reentry around or related to the lateral atriotomy scar; septal circuits with reentry around an atrial septal patch; and typical AFL circuits using the cavotricuspid isthmus. Left atrial (LA) macroreentrant circuits are infrequent in this group of patients.[11] Very complex and/or multiple reentry circuits can be seen after placement of an intraatrial baffle (Mustard, Senning) in a very dilated RA after a Fontan procedure, after maze surgery, and after RF catheter ablation of atrial fibrillation (AF).[8]

The best characterization of macroreentrant AT caused by atriotomy is from activation around an incision scar in the lateral RA wall, with a main superoinferior axis (Fig. 10-1). This is a common problem in patients who have undergone surgery for congenital or valvular heart disease. Typically, the reentry circuit is located in the lateral RA wall and the central obstacle not only includes the scar, but functional block can magnify this obstacle to include the SVC.[7,9] The anterior RA wall is commonly activated superoinferiorly (descending), as in typical AFL. However, the septal wall frequently lacks a clear-cut inferosuperior (ascending) activation pattern. Participation of the anterior RA wall in the circuit can be confirmed with entrainment mapping, when the post-pacing interval (PPI) is equal to the tachycardia CL. A line of double potentials is recorded in the lateral RA, extending superoinferiorly. Double potential separation can be more marked and demonstrate a voltage lower than in typical AFL. Narrow passages (isthmuses) in the circuit can be found between the SVC and superior end of the atriotomy scar, IVC and inferior end of the atriotomy, atriotomy scar and tricuspid annulus, or even within the scar itself (Fig. 10-2). These isthmuses can be areas of slow conduction. Stable pacing of the critical isthmus can be difficult or impossible in RA atriotomy tachycardia because of tachy-

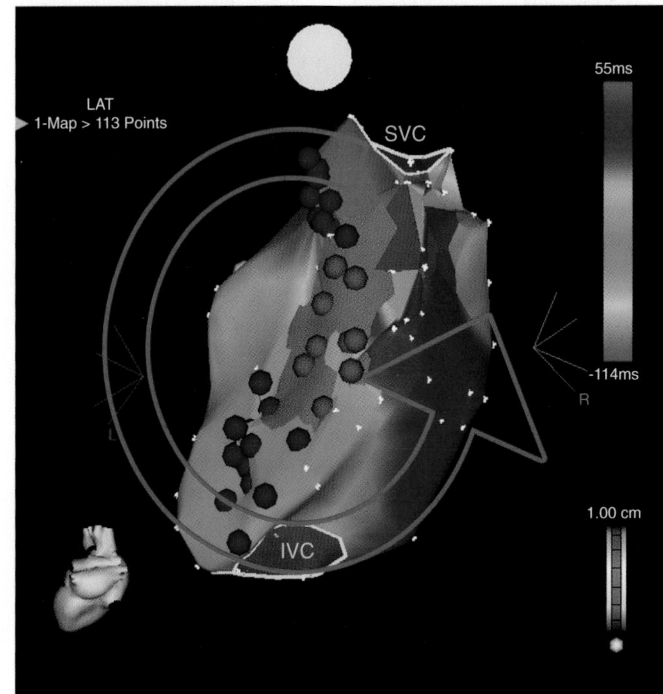

FIGURE 10–1 3-D electroanatomical (CARTO) activation map of macroreentrant atrial tachycardia (AT) in a patient with previous surgical repair of atrial septal defect. Gray areas in the posterolateral right atrium represent areas of unexcitable scar related to previous atriotomy, characterized by very low-voltage electrograms. During tachycardia, the activation wavefront travels in a macroreentrant circuit around the atriotomy scar. Ablation lines (red dots) connecting the atriotomy scar to the inferior vena cava (IVC) and superior vena cava (SVC) successfully eliminated the tachycardia.

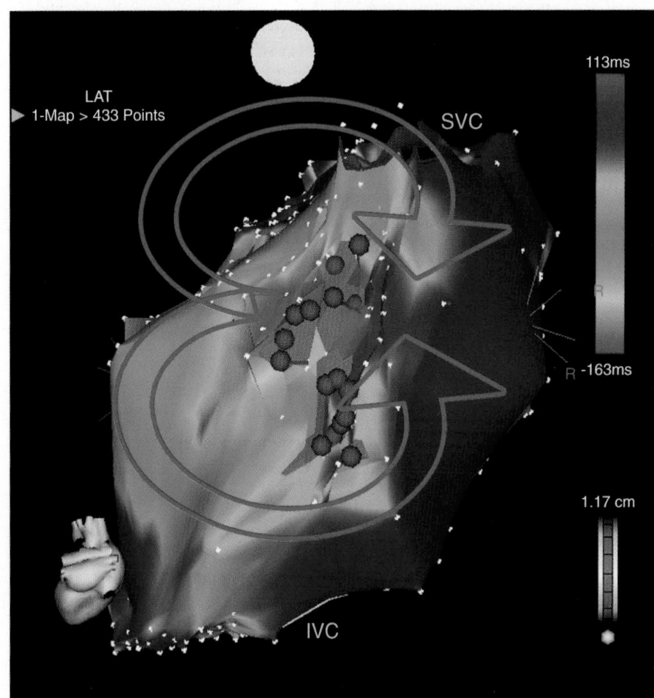

FIGURE 10–2 3-D electroanatomical (CARTO) activation map of macroreentrant atrial tachycardia (AT) in a patient with previous surgical repair of atrial septal defect. Gray areas in the posterolateral right atrium (RA) represent areas of unexcitable scar related to previous atriotomy, characterized by very low-voltage electrograms. During tachycardia, the activation wavefront travels from the midposterior RA superiorly and inferiorly, and both counterclockwise and clockwise wavefronts return to the region proximal to the exit site (purple) to complete the circuit by propagating through a narrow isthmus bounded by two areas of unexcitable scar (figure-of-8 reentry). Radiofrequency ablation targeting the gap in the atriotomy scar successfully eliminated the tachycardia. IVC = inferior vena cava; SVC = superior vena cava.

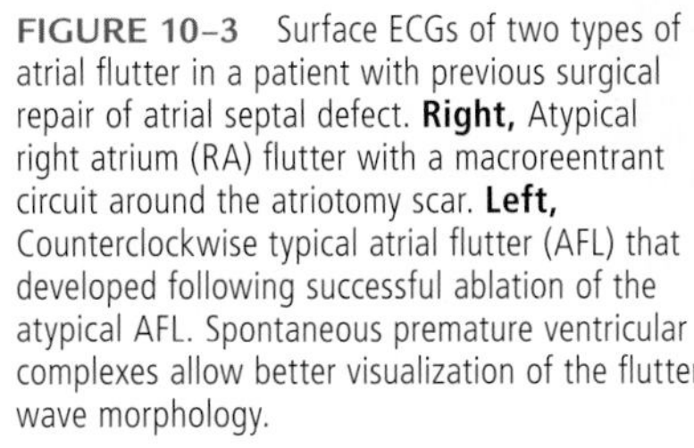

FIGURE 10–3 Surface ECGs of two types of atrial flutter in a patient with previous surgical repair of atrial septal defect. **Right,** Atypical right atrium (RA) flutter with a macroreentrant circuit around the atriotomy scar. **Left,** Counterclockwise typical atrial flutter (AFL) that developed following successful ablation of the atypical AFL. Spontaneous premature ventricular complexes allow better visualization of the flutter wave morphology.

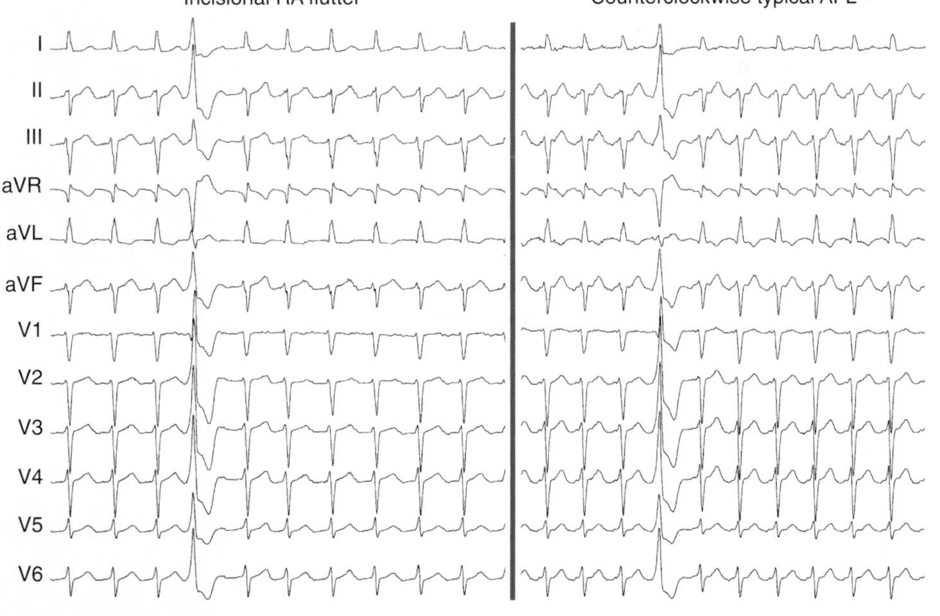

cardia interruption. Isthmus participation in the circuit is often proven by tachycardia interruption with catheter pressure, and by tachycardia interruption and noninducibility after RF application in the area. A single, wide, fractionated electrogram can be recorded from the lower pivot point of the circuit in the low lateral RA, close to the IVC, and perhaps also from other isthmuses of the circuit. The line of double potentials or fractionated, low-voltage electrograms can also often be recorded in NSR allowing tentative localization of the scar and the associated anatomical isthmuses.[1,3,5-10]

Typical AFL is also often associated with RA atriotomy tachycardia. In fact, the most common macroreentrant AT in these patients is typical isthmus-dependent AFL (Fig. 10-3). Not uncommonly, ablation of one tachycardia will unmask the other, and ablation of both circuits will be necessary for clinical success. Detection of this change requires careful attention to the atrial activation sequence and ECG pattern after each RF application. The recording of multiple simultaneous electrograms, as continuous endocardial references, will facilitate detection of these activation changes.[11-13] Moreover, the cavotricuspid isthmus was found to be part of the reentrant circuit in approximately 70% of patients with postoperative intraatrial reentrant tachycardia and, in one report, ablation of this isthmus alone resulted in elimination of the tachycardia in 27% of these patients.[9,13]

2. Upper Loop Reentry. This type of atypical AFL involves the upper portion of the RA, with transverse conduction over the crista terminalis and wavefront collision occurring at a lower part of the RA or within the cavotricuspid isthmus. When upper loop reentry was first reported, it was thought to be a reentrant circuit using the channel between the SVC, fossa ovalis, and crista terminalis. Noncontact mapping techniques have shown that this form of AFL is a macroreentrant tachycardia in the RA, with the crista terminalis as its functional central obstacle. The impulse rotating in the circuit can be in a counterclockwise or clockwise direction. The cavotricuspid isthmus is not an intrinsic part of the reentrant circuit.[1,14]

Upper loop reentry can occur in conjunction with typical clockwise and/or counterclockwise AFL, as well as lower loop reentry (when two of these circuits coexist at the same time, they create the so-called *dual loop reentry*). Upper loop reentry can be abolished by linear ablation of the gap in the crista terminalis.[1,14]

Left Atrial Macroreentrant Tachycardia

LA flutter circuits are frequently related to or coexist with AF. Cardiac surgery involving the LA or atrial septum can produce different LA flutter circuits, but LA circuits also can be found in patients without a history of atriotomy. Electroanatomical maps in these patients often show low voltage or areas of scar in the LA, which act as a central obstacle or barrier in the circuit.

1. Mitral Annulus (Perimitral) Atrial Flutter. This circuit involves reentry around the mitral annulus in a counterclockwise or clockwise fashion (Fig. 10-4). This arrhythmia is more common in patients with structural heart disease; however, it has been described in patients without obvious structural heart disease but, in these patients, electroanatomical voltage mapping often shows scar or low-voltage area(s) on the posterior wall of the LA as a posterior boundary of this circuit.[4,10,15,16] Perimitral AFL is the most common macroreentrant AT in patients with prior LA ablation procedures for AF.[17]

2. Circuits Involving the Pulmonary Vein(s) with or Without Left Atrial Scar. Various reentrant circuits involve the pulmonary veins (PVs), especially in patients with AF or mitral valve disease and those with prior catheter ablation of AF (especially with linear LA ablation lesions), including reentrant circuits around two or more PVs (it is unusual for a circuit to involve one PV) and posterior scar or low-voltage area(s).[4,6,10,15-18]

3. Left Septal Circuits. These circuits involve the fossa ovalis, which acts as a central obstacle for the reen-

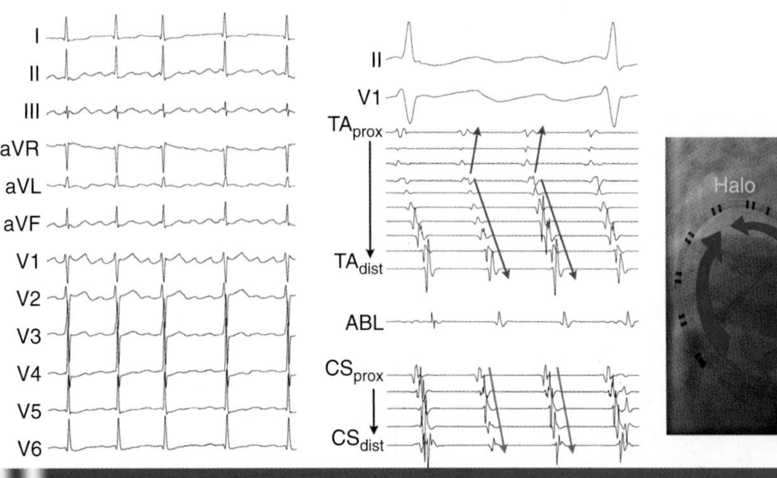

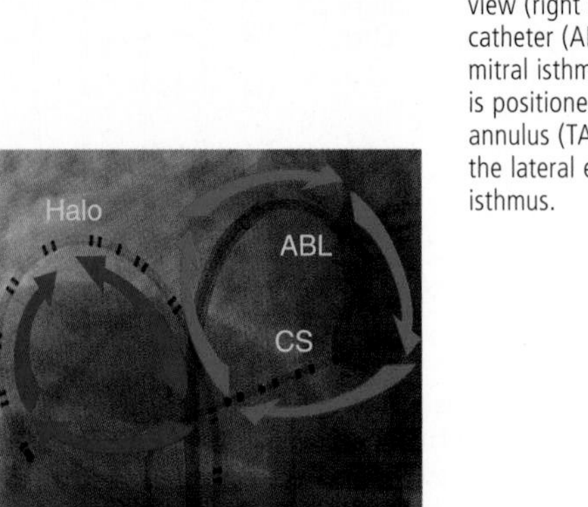

FIGURE 10–4 Surface ECGs and intracardiac recordings during clockwise (lower panel) and counterclockwise (upper panel) perimitral atrial flutter (AFL). Catheter position and wavefront activation during the tachycardia are illustrated in a left anterior oblique fluoroscopic view (right side). The ablation catheter (ABL) is positioned at the mitral isthmus, and the Halo catheter is positioned around the tricuspid annulus (TA), with the distal end at the lateral end of the cavotricuspid isthmus.

trant circuit. The right PVs serve as its posterior boundary whereas the mitral annulus serves as its anterior boundary. In patients with a history of surgery for atrial septal defects, scars or the patch on the septum can serve as the anatomical substrate of left septal circuits.[16,19]

4. Post–Maze Procedure Atrial Flutter. Atrial tachyarrhythmias have been observed in more than 10% of patients following the maze procedure for AF. The most common mechanism of AFL following surgical maze is LA macroreentry, typically involving posterior or anterior circuits stabilized by zones of block created by surgical ablation or LA appendage amputation. Perimitral reentry is infrequent.

CLINICAL CONSIDERATIONS

Epidemiology

Atypical AFL comprises a heterogeneous group of right or left atrial macroreentrant circuits related to different anatomical and electrophysiological (EP) substrates. Such ATs are frequently associated with structural heart disease, congenital cardiac defects, previous cardiac surgeries, and/or surgical or catheter ablation procedures for AF. Often, these arrhythmias coexist with AF. However, macroreentrant AT occasionally occurs in a patient with no apparent structural heart disease.

Surgical incisions in the RA for repair of atrial septal defects are probably the most common cause of lesion-related reentry in adults. Macroreentrant AT is also especially common after the Fontan procedure (5% to 20% perioperatively, 16% to 50% late) and Mustard or Senning atrial switch procedures (15% to 48%), and increases in prevalence over time. ATs also occur commonly (12% to 34%) during late follow-up after tetralogy of Fallot repair. It should be recognized, however, that typical AFL is more common than non–isthmus-dependent AFL even in this population and typical and atypical flutter circuits often coexist in a single patient.[20]

Macroreentrant AT is the most common mechanism for symptomatic tachycardia in the adult congenital heart disease population.[20] Usually, macroreentrant AT appears many years after operations that involved an atriotomy or other surgical manipulation of RA tissue. It can follow simple procedures, such as closure of an atrial septal defect (occasionally), but the incidence is highest among patients with advanced dilation, thickening, and scarring of their RA. Other risk factors for macroreentrant AT include concomitant sinus node dysfunction and older age at time of heart surgery. Hence, macroreentrant AT is especially problematic for older patients who have undergone the Mustard, Senning, or older style Fontan operations, in which extensive suture lines and long-term hemodynamic stress result in markedly abnormal atrial myocardium.[20]

Clinical Presentation

Macroreentrant ATs are typically chronic or long-lasting and, similar to AF and typical AFL, patients can present with symptoms related to rapid ventricular response, tachycardia-induced cardiomyopathy, or deterioration of preexisting cardiac disease.

Generally, in the adult congenital heart disease population, macroreentrant ATs tend to be slower than typical AFL, with atrial rates in the range of 150 to 250/min. In the setting of a healthy atrioventricular node (AVN), such rates will frequently conduct in a rapid 1:1 A:V pattern that can result in hypotension, syncope, or possibly circulatory collapse in patients with limited myocardial reserve. Even if the ventricular response rate is safely titrated, sustained macroreentrant AT can cause debilitating symptoms in some patients because of loss of atrioventricular (AV) synchrony and can contribute to thromboembolic complications when the duration is protracted.[20]

Initial Evaluation

Outside typical AFL, the clinician is faced with a wide spectrum of ATs in which therapy and prognosis cannot be defined with routine noninvasive testing, and definitive diagnosis typically requires intracardiac mapping. ECG alone is frequently inadequate to distinguish atypical AFL from focal AT or typical AFL. Detailed cardiac evaluation of cardiac function and anatomy is typically required, especially in patients with congenital heart disease and those with previous cardiac procedures (surgical or catheter-based). Additionally, detailed knowledge of the congenital anomaly and previous surgical or ablative procedures is very important.

Principles of Management

Medical management of atypical AFL is practically similar to that for AF. Antiarrhythmic drugs (class IA, IC, and III) have been first-line therapy. Chronic anticoagulation for stroke prevention is typically recommended. Rate control versus rhythm control strategies are evaluated depending on several factors, including severity of symptoms, response to rate-controlling medications, cardiac function, and associated noncardiac diseases.

Ablation of atypical AFL can be effective, but the number of patients studied is small and the efficacy and adverse effects of ablation are not yet well defined. Ablation of non–isthmus-dependent AFL can also be substantially more difficult than for typical AFL. These arrhythmias can have complex reentrant circuits that demand a thorough knowledge of atrial anatomy and a great deal of experience to correlate activation patterns with anatomical landmarks. When this type of AFL is suspected, such as in patients with congenital heart disease who have had surgery, referral to an experienced center should be considered. Therefore, ablation is typically reserved for symptomatic patients not responding to, or intolerant of, antiarrhythmic medications. Therapeutic decisions are made case by case. Further advances in our understanding of arrhythmia substrate and the technology to visualize and modify it will improve the outcomes of ablative therapy and expand its role in the management of these arrhythmias.

Catheter ablation of the AV junction and pacemaker insertion should be considered if catheter ablative cure is not possible and the patient has a rapid ventricular response not responding to drug therapy.

ELECTROCARDIOGRAPHIC FEATURES

Incisional Right Atrial Macroreentrant Tachycardia. In a patient with a previous atriotomy, any ECG pattern can result from incisional macroreentrant AT (see Fig. 10-3). The morphology of the atrial complex on the surface ECG can range from that similar to typical AFL to that characteristic of focal AT.[16,21-25]

Often, more than one AT mechanism can be demonstrated and related to more than one ECG pattern. The surface ECG manifestations can vary depending on the location of the scar(s) and low-voltage area(s) and how the wavefronts exit the circuits.

Upper Loop Reentry. The surface ECG of upper loop reentry closely mimics that of clockwise isthmus-dependent AFL.[1,14,25]

Left Atrial Macroreentrant Tachycardia. The ECG morphology of LA flutter caused by the different reentrant circuits is variable. LA flutters can result in ECG patterns of focal AT (discrete P waves and isoelectric baseline), typical AFL, or atypical AFL.[10,15,16,24-27]

Perimitral Atrial Flutter. Most of these tachycardias show prominent forces in leads V_1 and V_2, with diminished amplitude in the inferior leads (see Fig. 10-4). It has been suggested that a posterior LA scar allows for domination by anterior LA forces. This constellation of findings might mimic counterclockwise or clockwise isthmus-dependent AFL, but the decreased amplitude of frontal plane forces suggests an LA circuit. In patients with prior PV isolation procedures, the surface ECG morphology for counterclockwise perimitral AFL can be different from that in patients without prior ablation, possibly related to varying degrees of prior LA ablation or scar. In these patients, counterclockwise perimitral AFL demonstrates positive flutter waves in the inferior and precordial leads and a significant negative component in leads I and aVL.[28] Furthermore, counterclockwise perimitral AFL in these patients can have a morphology similar to that of left PV ATs; however, counterclockwise perimitral AFL is suggested by a more negative component in lead I, initial negative component in lead V_2, and lack of any isoelectric interval between flutter waves. Clockwise perimitral AFL has the converse limb lead morphology to that of counterclockwise perimitral AFL and an initial negative component in the lateral precordial leads. The positive flutter wave in leads I and aVL differentiates clockwise perimitral AFL from counterclockwise isthmus-dependent atrial flutter and left PV AT.[28]

Pulmonary Vein Circuits. Because these circuits are related to low-voltage or scar area(s), the surface ECG usually shows low-amplitude or flat flutter waves. These tachycardias have the most variable surface ECG patterns.

Left Septal Circuits. Because the reentry circuit is on the septum, the surface ECG shows prominent, usually positive, flutter waves only in lead V_1 or V_2, and almost flat waves in most other leads (Fig. 10-5). This pattern can be caused by a septal circuit with anterior-posterior forces projecting in lead V_1 and the cancellation of caudocranial forces. This pattern was 100% sensitive for a LA septal circuit, but the specificity of this pattern for any LA AFL was only 64%.

ELECTROPHYSIOLOGICAL TESTING

Induction of Tachycardia

The programmed electrical stimulation protocol should include atrial burst pacing from the high RA and coronary sinus (CS)—down to a pacing CL at which 2:1 atrial capture occurs—and atrial extrastimulation (AES), single and double, at multiple CLs (600 to 300 milliseconds) from the high RA and CS (down to the atrial effective refractory period [ERP]). Isoproterenol infusion (0.5 to 4 µg/min) is administered as needed to facilitate tachycardia induction. Goals of EP testing in patients with macroreentrant AT are listed in Table 10-1.

Diagnostic Maneuvers During Tachycardia

Atrial Extrastimulation

Once the diagnosis of macroreentry is confirmed, AES is not necessary, but may be performed during the tachycardia to

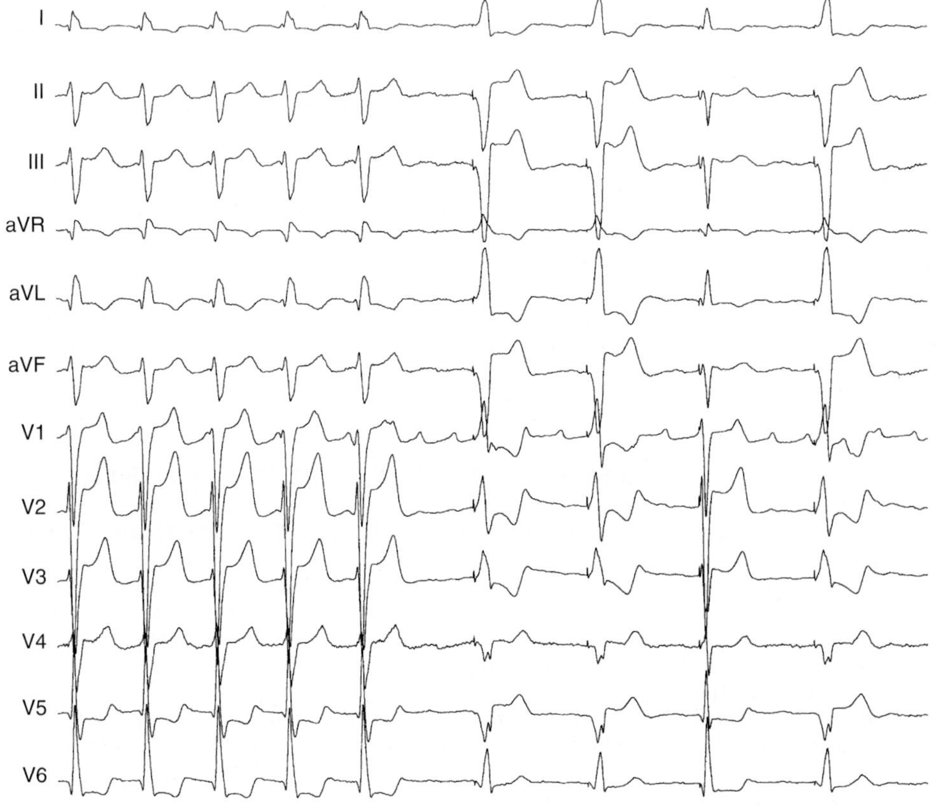

FIGURE 10–5 Surface ECG of left septal atrial flutter (AFL) in a patient with tachycardia-bradycardia syndrome and permanent pacemaker implantation. The flutter waves are masked by the QRS and T waves during 2:1 atrioventricular (AV) conduction. Administration of adenosine results in AV block and reveals flutter wave morphology. Note the prominent positive flutter waves only in lead V_1 and almost flat waves in most of the other leads.

TABLE 10–1	Goals of Programmed Stimulation During Macroreentrant Atrial Tachycardia (AT)
1. To confirm that the tachycardia is AT	
2. To confirm that the AT is a macroreentrant circuit · Atrial activation spanning the tachycardia cycle length (CL) · Resetting response consistent with reentry · Entrainment mapping consistent with reentry	
3. To exclude cavotricuspid isthmus-dependent atrial flutter · Entrainment mapping at the cavotricuspid isthmus	
4. Localization of the circuit in the right atrium (RA) versus left atrium (LA) · ECG morphology of the atrial complex · Isolated variation of RA CL · RA activation time < 50% of tachycardia CL · Entrainment pacing from different RA sites	
5. To define the tachycardia circuit · Entrainment mapping	
6. To define the critical isthmus in the tachycardia circuit · Entrainment mapping	

study the resetting response. Macroreentrant tachycardia will have an increasing or mixed (flat, then increasing) resetting response.

Atrial Pacing

Entrainment Mapping. Entrainment mapping provides information about sites of the RA or LA that are part of the reentrant circuit, those that are outside the circuit, and the critical isthmus in the macroreentrant circuit (Fig. 10-6). Pacing is performed from the cavotricuspid isthmus, high RA, and midlateral RA, but not on the septum, to avoid the possibility of capturing the LA, which could be confusing in distinguishing RA from LA flutters.[4,15,25,29-33]

Analysis of Entrainment. Entrainment can usually be demonstrated with pacing from different atrial sites at a CL approximately 10 to 30 milliseconds shorter than the tachycardia CL. Occurrence of entrainment should first be confirmed before interpretation of the PPI. Achievement of entrainment of the AT establishes a reentrant mechanism of the tachycardia, and excludes triggered activity and abnormal automaticity as potential mechanisms. Entrainment can also be used to estimate qualitatively how far the reentrant circuit is from the pacing site (Table 10-2).

Limitation of Entrainment Mapping. Entrainment techniques can be difficult in patients with incisional AT caused by low-amplitude or absent atrial potentials in the area of surgical incisions. Fusion is difficult to assess on the surface ECG, because the pacing artifact and/or QRS complex frequently obscure the surface P waves, which often have low amplitude in these patients.

Furthermore, methodological problems can affect the validity of the PPI. Decremental conduction during pacing increases the PPI, causing false-negative assessment at some reentry circuit sites. The occasional presence of far-field potentials can also impair the accuracy of entrainment mapping. Additionally, it is difficult to identify exact catheter positions in relation to anatomical barriers, because visualization of these barriers is not possible fluoroscopically. Spontaneous changes in the tachycardia CL in some macroreentrant ATs can also make interpretation of the PPI impossible. Combining entrainment mapping with electroanatomical mapping can reduce the difficulties created by some of these limitations.

Finally, reconstruction of the complete circuit can be extremely difficult to achieve and the risk of transformation of the clinical tachycardia to another morphology or to

TABLE 10–2	Entrainment Mapping of Macroreentrant Atrial Tachycardia (AT)
Pacing from sites *outside* the AT circuit results in manifest entrainment: 1. Manifest atrial fusion on surface ECG and intracardiac recordings (fixed fusion at a single pacing cycle length [PCL], and progressive fusion on progressively shorter PCLs). Any change in atrial activation sequence, compared with baseline tachycardia and that of pure pacing, as determined by analysis of all available surface and intracardiac ECG recordings, is considered to represent manifest fusion. 2. PPI – AT CL > 30 msec 3. The interval between the stimulus artifact to the onset of P wave on surface ECG is longer than the interval between the local electrogram on the pacing site to the onset of the P wave on the surface ECG.	
Pacing from sites *inside* the AT circuit results in manifest entrainment: 1. Manifest atrial fusion on the surface ECG and intracardiac recordings (fixed fusion at a single PCL, and progressive fusion on progressively shorter PCLs) 2. PPI – AT CL < 30 msec 3. The interval between the stimulus artifact to the onset of P wave on surface ECG equals the interval between the local electrogram on the pacing site to the onset of P wave on surface ECG.	
Pacing from *a protected isthmus* inside the circuit results in concealed entrainment: 1. Concealed atrial fusion (i.e., paced atrial waveform on the surface ECG and intracardiac recordings is identical to the tachycardia waveform) 2. PPI – AT CL < 30 msec 3. The interval between the stimulus artifact to the onset of P wave on surface ECG equals the interval between the local electrogram on the pacing site to the onset of the P wave on the surface ECG.	

PPI = post-pacing interval.

AF is high. Therefore, it is advisable to begin with electroanatomical (e.g., CARTO) mapping, while pacing maneuvers are used sparingly, just to confirm the participation of precise areas in the reentry circuit and to improve understanding of the tachycardia further.

MAPPING

Because the reentrant circuit can involve any of multiple barriers, the usual anatomically guided ablation, as is performed for typical isthmus-dependent AFL, is not possible. Mapping is required to determine the precise circuit and define its vulnerable segment (critical isthmus) to provide a specifically tailored ablation solution.[10,21,25,33] Goals of mapping of macroreentrant circuits include localization of the tachycardia circuit (RA versus LA), identification of possible lines of block, identification of an isthmus of tissue bounded between two long barriers, and determination of whether the line of block is a critical part of the circuit.

Detailed knowledge of the congenital anomaly and the surgical procedure, if present, is important in the interpretation of the results of mapping, how to access the RA, the feasibility of the transseptal puncture, and whether fluoroscopy is helpful in localizing the catheters or whether transesophageal echocardiography is needed.[10,21,25,33,34]

Localization of the Reentrant Circuit Chamber (Right Atrium Versus Left Atrium)

Patient History. A history of prior surgery or ablation within a particular atrial chamber should focus the inten-

Entrainment from distal CS

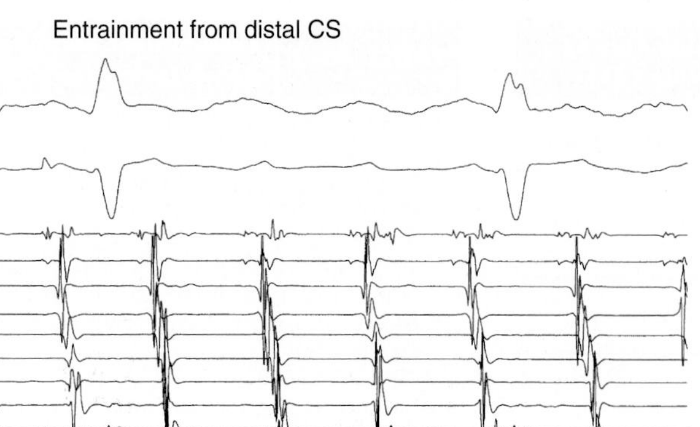

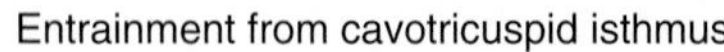

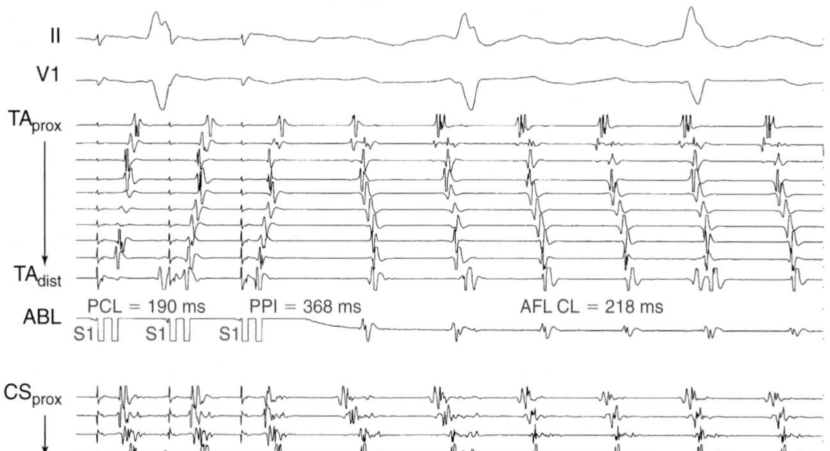

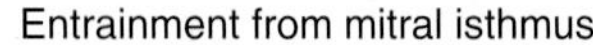

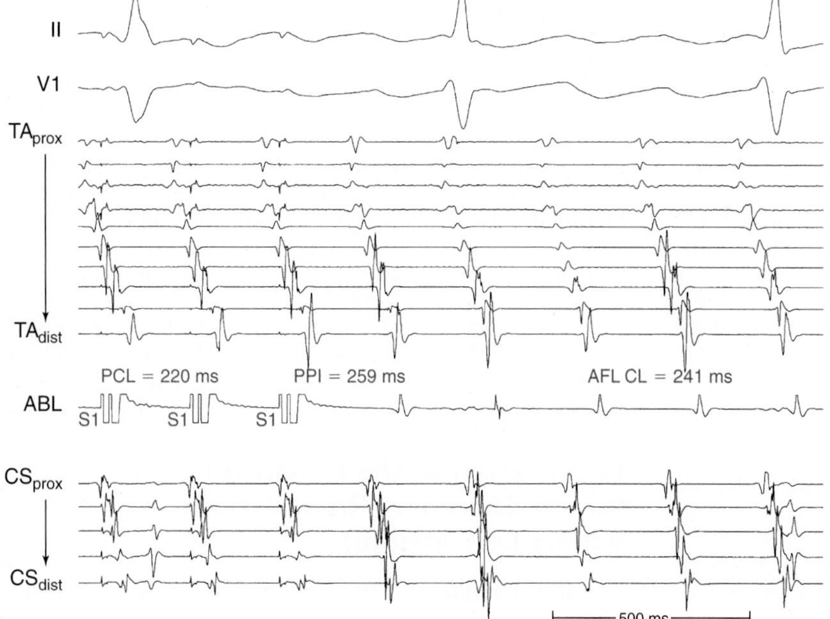

FIGURE 10–6 Entrainment of counterclockwise perimitral atrial flutter (AFL). **Upper panel,** Entrainment from the distal coronary sinus (CS) results in intracardiac atrial fusion (as demonstrated in CS activation sequence) and a short post-pacing interval (PPI)—PPI – AFL CL = 14 msec—because the distal CS is close to the reentrant circuit. **Middle panel,** Entrainment from ablation catheter positioned at the cavotricuspid isthmus results in manifest atrial fusion with a long PPI—PPI – AFL CL = 150 msec—suggesting that the cavotricuspid isthmus is not part of the reentrant circuit. **Lower panel,** Entrainment from ablation catheter positioned at the mitral isthmus, concealed atrial fusion, and a short PPI—PPI – AFL CL = 18 msec—suggesting that the mitral isthmus is the critical isthmus of the reentrant circuit. CL = cycle length; PCL = pacing CL.

sity of the search for the arrhythmia substrate in that chamber. Such macroreentrant arrhythmias can occur in isolation or involve anatomical structures to create dual- or multiple-loop or circuit reentry.

In the setting of previous cardiac surgery, a right-sided location of the arrhythmia is more likely and is often seen years later in patients who have had a right lateral atriotomy and underwent surgical closure of an atrial or ventricular septal defect or valve repair. These arrhythmias can also be seen in more complex surgical correction of congenital heart disease, such as the Mustard or Senning correction for transposition of the great vessels, and also after tricuspid valve surgery.

Left-sided flutters are more likely in the presence of left heart disease, such as hypertrophic cardiomyopathy or mitral valve disease and following catheter or surgical ablation of AF. In these patients, spontaneous conduction abnormalities and areas of electrical silence forming the substrate for arrhythmia have been recently observed.

Electrocardiographic Findings. In the absence of previous cardiac surgery and/or catheter ablation (particularly involving linear lesions in the LA), a completely negative flutter wave in lead V_1 (particularly if it involves all the anterior chest leads) is more frequently associated with RA free wall circuits. Conversely, in the absence of counterclockwise isthmus-dependent AFL, positive (or biphasic positive-negative) flutter waves in lead V_1 are more frequently associated with LA circuits. LA circuits have also been reported to generate low-amplitude flutter waves frequently, with some of them having visible waves only in lead V_1.

Isolated Variation of the Right Atrial Cycle Length. Large spontaneous variations (30 to 125 milliseconds) or even 2:1 conduction in the RA CL with concomitant variations less than 20 milliseconds in CS recordings suggest an LA origin of the macroreentrant circuit (Fig. 10-7).[10]

Exclusion of Cavotricuspid Isthmus Dependence. - Exclusion of cavotricuspid isthmus as part of the reentrant circuit is an important initial step and can be established by the following: (1) demonstration of bidirectional activation of the cavotricuspid isthmus during AT, resulting in collision or fusion within the isthmus by activation from opposing directions (the low lateral RA and CS; see Fig. 10-4); (2) recording of double potentials separated by an isoelectric and constant interval throughout the full extent of the cavotricuspid isthmus during tachycardia; and/or (3) entrainment mapping from the cavotricuspid isthmus demonstrating manifest atrial fusion with a long PPI (see Fig. 10-6).

Activation Mapping

Right Atrial Activation Time. Activation from evenly distributed 10 sites in the RA, including three or four points at the tricuspid annulus, is recorded, and local activation time at each of these sites is measured relative to a reference intracardiac electrogram (e.g., the CS). If less than 50% of the tachycardia CL is recorded among these 10 points, the arrhythmia is probably not located in the RA. The only exception is the presence of a small reentrant circuit in the RA.[4,10,25,33]

Right Atrial Activation During Left Atrial Flutter. In the absence of LA mapping through transseptal catheterization, long segments of the tachycardia CL may not be covered by recorded electrograms. RA mapping typically shows nonreentrant activation patterns, clearly different from typical clockwise and counterclockwise AFL. Early RA septal activation relative to other parts of the RA can suggest a focal septal origin in some cases when LA recordings are not obtained (see Figs. 10-4 and Fig. 10-7). Local RA conduction disturbances, such as cavotricuspid isthmus block (from prior isthmus ablation), transverse block at the crista terminalis, or both, can result in activation of the anterior and septal RA in opposite directions, mimicking reentrant RA activation of typical AFL. In these cases, entrainment mapping will clarify the location of the reentrant circuit.

Coronary Sinus Activation Sequence. CS activation sequence has frequently been suggested as a useful way to determine the chamber of interest; however, this is not without limitations. Whereas in RA flutter the CS is frequently activated from proximal to distal, this is not always true, particularly with AFL localized to the superior RA. Similarly, although most circuits with distal to proximal activation of the CS are caused by LA flutter, this sequence may also be seen in some cases of RA flutter (see Fig. 10-4). Furthermore, some LA flutter may activate the CS proximally to distally (e.g., counterclockwise perimitral AFL).

Entrainment Mapping. A PPI – AFL CL longer than 40 milliseconds at three or more different points in the RA (including the cavotricuspid isthmus and RA free wall, but excluding the septum and CS) indicates an LA circuit (see Fig. 3-20). When entrainment does not localize the circuit in the LA or RA, a focal or small reentrant arrhythmia should be considered.[4,10,11,15,21,25,29-33]

Identification of Possible Lines of Block (Barriers)

Tachycardia circuit barriers should be identified. For RA flutter, the tricuspid annulus often provides one important barrier. Other naturally fixed barriers (i.e., independent of the precise form of activation and present also in NSR) include the IVC, SVC, and coronary sinus ostium (CS os). For LA flutters, the mitral annulus and PVs often provide important barriers. Acquired barriers include surgical incisions or patches and mute regions devoid of electrical activity (of uncertain cause).[4,10,21,35]

A line of block can be identified by the presence of double potentials, reflecting conduction up one side of the barrier and down the other side, with the bipolar electrogram recording both waves of activation. Significant large areas devoid of electrical activity can be easily recognized as electrical scars, provided that catheter contact is verified. Narrow lines of block can easily be missed unless the conduction delay across them is maximized by the appropriate choice of pacing sites and CLs. Therefore, to avoid overlooking any such scar, it may be necessary to perform mapping during more than one form of activation (e.g., during both proximal CS and low lateral RA pacing).[4,10,21,35]

Identification of the Complete Reentrant Circuit

The complete reentrant circuit may be defined as the spatially shortest route of unidirectional activation encompassing the complete CL of the tachycardia in terms of activation timing, and returning to the site of earliest activation. Endocardial recordings will often show activation during the isoelectric intervals on the surface ECG. The concept of early activation is not applicable to any particular site in the reentrant circuit. Activation can be continuously mapped, and an earlier activation time can always be found for any particular point of the circuit. For illustrative purposes, a particular reference point may be designated as the origin of activation (time 0), but it should be understood that this is always arbitrary.[4,10,21,25,33]

Activation wavefronts that do not fulfill these conditions are bystander wavefronts and are not critical to the arrhythmia circuit. However, incomplete mapping can lead to con-

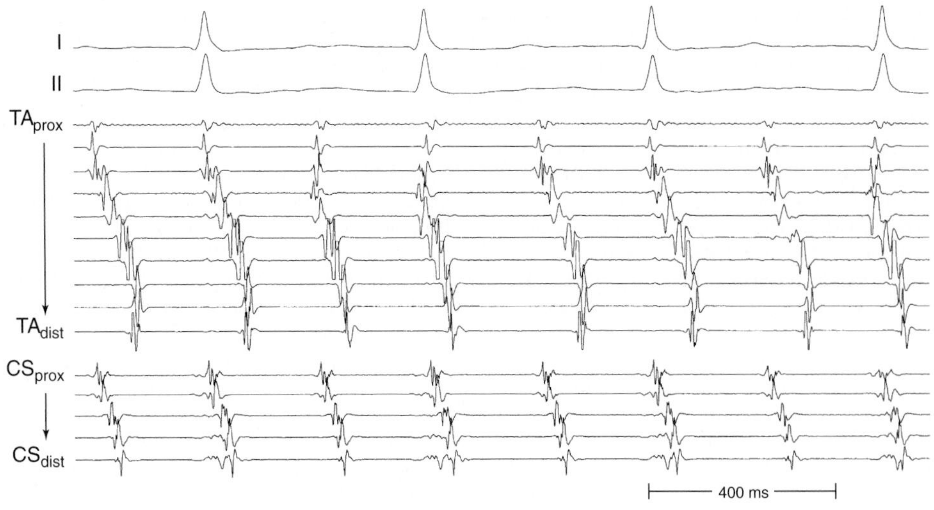

FIGURE 10–7 Surface ECG leads I and II and intracardiac recording during left atrial (LA) flutter. Note the large spontaneous variations in the right atrial cycle length (CL) and activation sequence (as recorded by a Halo catheter around the tricuspid annulus, TA), with a constant LA CL and activation sequence (as recorded by the coronary sinus [CS] catheter).

fusion about the bystander status of a given activation wavefront or loop, with an incomplete loop being mistaken for a complete one. High-density mapping or entrainment mapping can clarify this situation by documenting wavefront collision or a long PPI, respectively.

For LA flutter, identification of the complete reentrant circuit can be challenging. The initial step is activation mapping to determine whether activation of the entire tachycardia CL can be recorded within the LA. In particular, mapping should be carefully carried out around the mitral annulus because this maneuver is easy to perform and identifies a common form of LA flutter, perimitral AFL.

If activation recorded at different atrial locations does not cover most of the tachycardia CL, two possibilities must be considered: focal AT and small, localized reentrant circuits, which require much more detailed activation mapping in order to be identified.

Sometimes, it can be impossible to map the entire circuit, especially in patients with repaired congenital heart disease, caused by the complex suture lines, baffles, or both. Entrainment then becomes an essential tool in these cases to confirm participation of specific areas in the circuit and to try to

locate a suitable isthmus area from which concealed entrainment can be demonstrated. However, fusion can be, and usually is, difficult to analyze on the ECG because of atypical low-voltage atrial complexes on the ECG, and assessment of concealed entrainment can be challenging. Multiple endocardial recordings can help by showing local activation change (surrogate of fusion) during entrainment.[11]

Identification of the Critical Isthmus

Once a scar or fixed barrier is localized, its role for supporting reentry is important in determining whether the isthmuses formed around it need ablation. Identification of whether an isthmus is a critical part of the reentrant circuit can be achieved by activation mapping during sustained stable reentry and entrainment mapping (see earlier).[4,10,21,25,33]

The presence of multiple fixed barriers in the atrium can provide more than one isthmus for reentry. Because wavefront collision can be functional in origin, recurrence may result from a different arrhythmia or transformation of the same arrhythmia, with reentry occurring after ablation and block in only one of the potential circuit isthmuses.

Behavior of the Tachycardia

A change in ECG morphology without a change in the tachycardia CL can be secondary to transformation of a multiple loop tachycardia by interruption of one loop, change in bystander activation sufficient to be visible on the surface ECG (typified by the change in CS and LA activation observed during incomplete ablation of the cavotricuspid isthmus in counterclockwise typical AFL), or activation of the same circuit in the opposite direction.[10,21,36]

Variations in the tachycardia CL can suggest variations in activation pathways resulting from circuit transformation or simply changes in conduction time; the latter is usually manifest as CL alternans. The absence of ECG changes accompanying changes in activation sequences can occur because of an insufficient change in electromotive force, either because of distance from the recording electrodes or because of insufficient electrically active tissue. At all points of time, it is necessary to ensure that the change of activation sequence is not secondary to unintentional movement of the recording catheters. A single-loop tachycardia with a fixed barrier as its core typically remains stable and unchanged during catheter manipulation, and may even be difficult to pace-terminate, although mechanical bump termination rendering the tachycardia noninducible suggests mechanical stimulation close to a restricted and relatively fragile isthmus.

Electroanatomical Mapping

Electroanatomical mapping can help distinguish between a focal origin and macroreentrant tachycardia by providing precise description of the macroreentrant circuit and sequence of atrial activation during the tachycardia and rapid visualization of the activation wavefront. This can contribute to the understanding of the reentrant circuit in relation to native barriers and surgical scars, identification of all slow-conducting pathways and appropriate sites for entrainment mapping, planning of ablation lines, navigation of ablation catheter, and verification of conduction block produced by RF ablation.*

CARTO Mapping Technique. The reference catheter is usually placed in the CS (because of stability) using an electrode recording a prominent atrial electrogram, and ensuring that the ventricular electrogram is not the one picked up by the system. Anatomical and EP landmarks (IVC, SVC, CS, His bundle [HB], and tricuspid annulus for RA mapping, and mitral annulus and PVs for LA mapping) are marked.

Activation mapping is performed to define the atrial activation sequence. A reasonable number of points homoge-

*References 6, 9-11, 15, 18, 21-23, 32, 37, and 38.

nously distributed in the RA and/or LA have to be recorded (80 to 100). Each point is tagged on the 3-D map as follows: The local activation time at each site is determined from the intracardiac bipolar electrogram and is measured in relation to the fixed intracardiac electrogram obtained from the CS (reference) catheter. Points are added to the map only if stability criteria in space and local activation time are met. The end-diastolic location stability criterion is less than 2 mm and the local activation time stability criterion is less than 2 milliseconds. Lines of block (manifest as double potentials) are tagged for easy identification, because they can serve as boundaries for a subsequent design of ablation strategies. Silent areas are defined as an atrial potential amplitude less than 0.05 mV, which is the baseline noise in the Biosense system, and the absence of atrial capture at 20 mA. Such areas and surgically related scars, such as atriotomy scars in the lateral RA or atrial septal defect closure, are tagged as "scar" and therefore appear in gray on the 3-D maps (see Figs. 10-1 and 10-2). The activation map can also be used to catalogue sites at which pacing maneuvers are performed during assessment of the tachycardia.

When two potentials are present, the CARTO system is configured initially to select the potential with the fastest negative slope as the site of activation. At selected double potential sites, entrainment of the tachycardia can help evaluate which potentials are captured by the pacing stimulus. Local activation times are then reviewed, and the apparent far-field signal is excluded from the activation maps.

Activation Map. A continuous progression of colors (e.g., from red to purple) around the RA (or LA), with close proximity of earliest and latest local activation, suggests the presence of an RA (or LA) macroreentrant tachycardia. In these cases, RA (or LA) activation time is in a similar range as the tachycardia CL (Fig. 10-8). Conversely, the electroanatomical maps of focal ATs demonstrate radial spreading of activation, from the earliest local activation site (red) in all directions and, in these cases, atrial activation time is markedly shorter than the tachycardia CL.

Voltage Map. Voltage mapping is performed to define areas of electrical scars, and it serves as boundaries for the subsequent design of ablation strategies. Silent areas are defined as atrial potential amplitude less than 0.05 mV and the absence of atrial capture at 20 mA.

Propagation Map. Propagation of electrical activation superimposed on the 3-D anatomy of the RA or LA is visualized as a propagation map in relation to the anatomical landmarks and barriers. Analysis of the propagation map may allow estimation of the conduction velocity along the reentrant circuit and identification of areas of slow conduction, and thus help locate appropriate sites for entrainment mapping and catheter ablation.

In the propagation map, electrically activated myocardium is colored red and nonactivated myocardium is colored blue. A propagation map of RA (or LA) activation can be superimposed on the anatomical reconstruction of the RA (or LA), allowing visualization of the reentrant circuit of AT in relation to native barriers and surgical scars.

Limitation of the Use of Electroanatomical Mapping. Variation of the tachycardia CL of more than 10% of the tachycardia CL may prevent complete understanding of the circuit, and decreases the confidence in the CARTO map. Similarly, electroanatomical mapping can be difficult or even impossible in patients with nonsustained AT. In these cases, 3-D mapping systems based on a single-beat analysis, such as the multielectrode basket catheter or the noncontact mapping system, may be an alternative to electroanatomical mapping technology. For unstable tachycardia with changes in morphology or CL, flecainide or amiodarone infusion can help stabilize the arrhythmia. If the tachycardia CL is too variable, it has to be considered as AF.

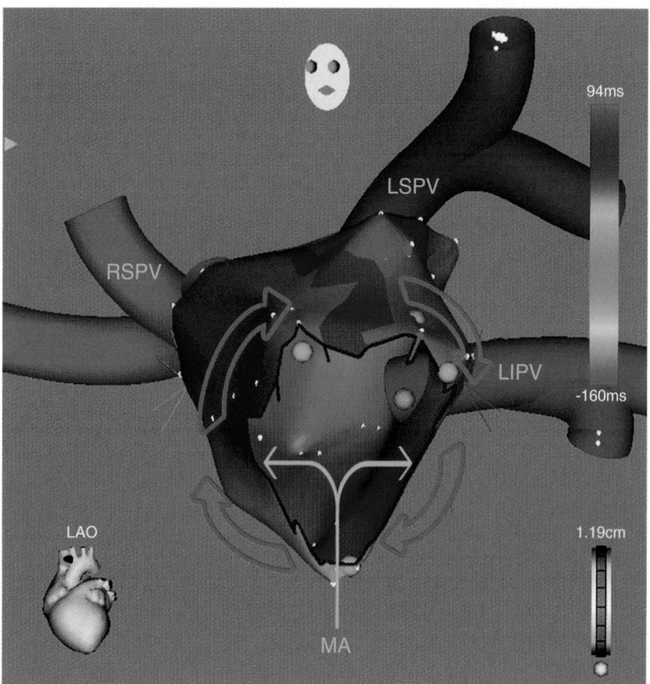

FIGURE 10–8 3-D electroanatomical (CARTO) activation map of the left atrium (LA) in the left anterior oblique (LAO) view constructed during clockwise perimitral atrial flutter. During tachycardia, the activation wavefront travels clockwise around the mitral annulus, as indicated by a continuous progression of colors (from red to purple) with close proximity of earliest and latest local activation (red meeting purple). MA = mitral annulus; LIPV = left inferior pulmonary vein; LSPV = left superior pulmonary vein; RSPV = right superior pulmonary vein.

Noncontact Mapping

When AT is short-lived or cannot be reproducibly initiated, simultaneous multisite data acquisition using the noncontact mapping system (EnSite 3000, Endocardial Solutions, St. Paul, Minn) can help localize the AT origin.[37,39] This system can recreate the endocardial activation sequence from simultaneously acquired multiple data points over a few tachycardia beats, without requiring sequential point-to-point acquisitions.

The EnSite 3000 system requires a 9 Fr multielectrode array and a 7 Fr mapping-ablation catheter. To create a map, the balloon catheter is positioned over a 0.035-inch guidewire under fluoroscopic guidance in the cardiac chamber of interest. The balloon is then deployed, and it can be filled with contrast dye to be visualized fluoroscopically. The balloon is positioned in the center of the atrium and does not come into physical contact with the atrial walls being mapped.

Systemic anticoagulation is critical to avoid thromboembolic complications. Intravenous heparin is usually given to maintain the activated clotting time (ACT) at 250 to 300 seconds and 300 to 350 seconds for right-sided and left-sided mapping, respectively.

A conventional deflectable mapping-ablation catheter is also positioned in the chamber and used to collect geometry information. The mapping catheter is initially moved to known anatomical locations (IVC, SVC, CS, HB, and tricuspid annulus for RA mapping, and mitral annulus and PVs for LA mapping), which are tagged. Subsequently, a detailed geometry of the chamber is reconstructed by moving the mapping catheter around the atrium. Using this information, the computer creates a model, called a convex hull, of the chamber during diastole. Unlike the CARTO mapping system, the noncontact system allows the patient to be in NSR or tachycardia during creation of the geometry.

Once chamber geometry has been delineated, tachycardia is induced and mapping can begin. The data acquisition process is performed automatically by the system, and all data for the entire chamber are acquired simultaneously. Following this, the segment must be analyzed by the operator to find the early activation or vulnerable region of the reentry circuit. The locator technology used to collect the geometry information for the convex hull can then be used to guide an ablation catheter to the proper location in the heart.

The noncontact mapping system is capable of reconstructing and interpolating more than 3000 unipolar electrograms over the endocardium during mapping and, in turn, isopotential or isochronal maps can be reconstructed from these electrograms. Because of the high density of data, color-coded isopotential maps are used to depict graphically regions that are depolarized, and wavefront propagation is displayed as a user-controlled 3-D "movie." The color range represents voltage or timing of onset. In addition, the system can simultaneously display as many as 32 electrograms as waveforms. Unipolar or bipolar electrograms (virtual electrograms) can be selected (at any given interval of the tachycardia cycle) using the mouse from any part of the created geometry and displayed as waveforms as if from point, array, or plaque electrodes. The reconstructed electrograms are subject to the same electrical principles as contact catheter electrograms, because they contain far-field electrical information from the surrounding endocardium as well as the underlying myocardium signal vector, and distance from measurement can affect the contribution to the electrogram. The maps are particularly useful for identifying slowly conducting pathways, such as the critical slow pathways and rapid breakthrough points of macroreentrant AT. The reentry circuit can be fully identifiable, along with other aspects such as the slowing, narrowing, and splitting of activation wavefronts in the isthmus.

Limitations of Noncontact Mapping. Very low-amplitude signals may not be detected, particularly if the distance between the center of the balloon catheter and endocardial surface exceeds 40 mm, limiting the accurate identification of diastolic signals. In addition, the acquired geometry with the current version of software is somewhat distorted, requiring multiple set points to establish the origin and shape of complicated structures clearly, such as the LA appendage or PVs. Otherwise, these structures might be lost in the interpolation between several neighboring points.

A second catheter is still required for more detailed mapping to find the precise site to ablate, and sometimes it is difficult to manipulate an ablation catheter around the outside of the balloon, especially during mapping in the LA. Moreover, aggressive anticoagulation is required when using this system, and special attention and care are necessary during placement of the large balloon electrode in a nondilated atrium.

ABLATION

Target of Ablation

The choice of ablation sites should be among those segments of the reentry circuit that offer the most convenient and safest opportunity for creating conduction block. Among other factors are the isthmus size, anticipated catheter stability, and risk of damage to adjacent structures (e.g., phrenic nerve, sinus node, and AVN).

Ablation is performed by targeting the narrowest identifiable isthmus of conduction accessible within the circuit (allowing the best electrode-tissue contact along the desired line). The ablation line is chosen to transect an area critical for the circuit and, at the same time, connect two anatomical areas of block, an electrically silent area to an anatomical zone of block (e.g., IVC, SVC, tricuspid annulus, PV, or mitral annulus), or two electrically silent areas. In patients with incomplete maps, the ablation is guided by conventional activation and entrainment mapping targeting a critical isthmus and/or a zone of slow conduction shown to be part of the circuit by pacing maneuvers. For example, for lateral RA incisional flutter, ablation is most commonly performed to extend the surgical scar to the closest fixed obstacle (usually the IVC).

When double potentials separated by an isoelectric interval can be traced in a convergent configuration, with a progressively decreasing inter-potential interval, and culminate in a fractionated continuous electrogram, this indicates one end of a line of block and activation through the resulting isthmus or around a pivot point at the end of the line of block.[4,35] If the fractionated low-amplitude electrogram is of longer duration, this suggests a protected corridor of slow conduction, whereas single high-amplitude electrograms suggest a wider and relatively large ablation target. An electrophysiologically defined isthmus may therefore be smaller than the anatomically defined one. EP guidance for determining the target site probably offers greater certitude of RF delivery at a desired location, because the same tip electrode(s) are used for both localization and RF delivery.

Voltage maps can be used to guide the choice of the ablation site; the likelihood of achieving a complete and transmural ablation line is probably greater in low-amplitude areas.

Right Atrial Flutter

Atypical RA flutter is frequently localized to the free wall of the RA, either because of previous atriotomy or spontaneous area of conduction block. In the latter situation, the area with slow conduction is the target of choice. In the setting of previous surgery, the ablation strategy is as follows: (1) to ablate the cavotricuspid isthmus (which is critical to RA flutter in most patients with prior right atriotomy, so it seems reasonable to ablate it in every patient presenting with such a tachycardia);[9,13] (2) to target the slow conduction area; (3) to extend the atriotomy (double potential or scar) to the IVC (see Fig. 10-1); and/or (4) to extend the scar area to the SVC; however, this may lead to injury of the sinus node so, when possible, extending the atriotomy to the IVC is preferable.[21,25,33,40-42]

Rarely, more complex circuits, such as around the right septal patch or as seen in patients with Mustard or Senning repairs, are observed.[8] However, the approach to ablation is the same—the area with slow conduction or scar is extended to an anatomical obstacle.

Left Atrial Flutter

In Setting of Previous Surgery or Spontaneous Regions of Scar. The goal is to localize the area with scar and to extend this line of conduction block to an anatomical obstacle, or to transect the circuit by joining anatomical structures. Although this strategy is achievable in most of the atria, it is advisable to avoid attempting to connect the anterior septal region to the mitral annulus in the region of the low left septum, because the thickness of the tissue prohibits complete lesions in approximately 40% of patients despite the use of irrigated-tip catheters. The exception to this is the presence of a narrow channel; this target is then preferable and usually much easier than longer linear lesions.[10,25,40-42]

Atypical Atrial Flutter Following Ablation of Atrial Fibrillation. These flutters are usually caused by recovered PV conduction or gaps in linear lesion(s) with a circuit propagating through a gap. However, PV isolation can also be associated with circuits around the mitral annulus or around the PVs caused by creation of regions of conduction block within the atrium. As such, detailed mapping of the previously performed ablation lesions is critical to determine whether the ablation lines, PV isolation, or both are complete. In the absence of complete block across the old ablation lines, the gaps must be reablated. In patients for whom the previous AF ablation was limited to PV isolation alone, two atypical circuits are dominant—around the mitral annulus or around PVs.

Left Atrial Flutter in the Absence of Previous Surgery or Atrial Fibrillation Ablation. Spontaneous LA circuits have been observed. The circuits can propagate around spontaneous scars, frequently located in the posterior LA, but also around the mitral annulus or PVs. More recently, LA circuits have been reported to rotate around the fossa ovalis, amenable to RF ablation using a linear lesion connecting the fossa ovalis to the mitral annulus.

Perimitral Atrial Flutter. An ablation lesion connecting the mitral annulus and one other anatomical barrier (usually the left inferior PV; Fig. 10-9) or the posterior scar can eliminate this arrhythmia. Another option is to use an anterior line from the anterior mitral annulus to the ostium of the right inferior PV or to a region of scar through the anterior LA. The latter is technically more challenging.

Atrial Flutter Around the Right Pulmonary Veins. Circuits propagating around the right PVs demonstrate colliding wavefronts along the mitral annulus and a PPI during entrainment that is much longer at the mitral isthmus than at the roof or posterior LA. This arrhythmia is being observed more frequently in the current approach of atrial ablation to isolate the PVs, because the lesions performed to isolate right and left PVs may create a narrow isthmus in the posterior LA that then forms the substrate for AFL. A linear lesion connecting both superior PVs through the roof is the best option. This is best performed along the roof rather than the posterior wall to avoid the potential risk of atrioesophageal fistulas.

Atrial Flutter Around the Left Pulmonary Veins. Circuits around the left PVs seem rare; they can be treated with a linear lesion joining the left inferior PV to the mitral annulus or with a roofline connecting both superior PVs.

Left Septal Circuits. A linear lesion from right PVs to the fossa ovalis or from the mitral annulus to the fossa ovalis usually terminates the tachycardia.

Unmappable Left Atrial Flutters. Atypical LA flutters may show some degree of variation in their CL during mapping, in which case conventional and electroanatomical mapping is less useful. An empirical strategy that commences with ablation at the mitral isthmus and the LA roof is then justified, because such ablation lines interrupt the most dominant circuits in the LA.

Ablation Technique

Once the ablation target is identified, ablation involves placing a series of RF lesions to sever the critical isthmus to connect two anatomical and/or surgical barriers. RF energy can be delivered sequentially point by point to span the targeted isthmus, or by dragging the ablation catheter tip during continuous energy administration. RF energy is maintained for up to 60 to 120 seconds until the bipolar atrial potential recorded from the ablation electrode is decreased by 80% or split into double potentials, indicating local conduction block. Lesion contiguity and continuity depend on ensuring the coalescence of multiple transmural lesions; this is best ensured by documenting the breakdown of the target electrogram (at each site) into double potentials, and continuing RF delivery at this point for 30 to 40 seconds more to ensure a stable lesion. The documentation of electrogram breakdown into double potentials depends on the direction of activation relative to the ablation lesion and its size relative to that of the recording bipole, and is maximized by activation orthogonal to the lesion's largest dimension.

During delivery of RF energy, the tachycardia can terminate or its CL can increase transiently or permanently. This indicates that the lesions have affected the circuit, and should lead to continuation of RF delivery or extension of the lesion to ensure the achievement of complete conduction block across the isthmus.

The coalescence of multiple RF lesions can be facilitated by any 3-D localization system (e.g., CARTO, NavX, RPM). Ablation sites may be tagged to permit visualization of the ablation line on the electroanatomical map. CARTO is also invaluable in localizing the gaps in the scar line through which the impulse can propagate. Focal ablation of these gaps can abolish the tachycardia.

Ablation of the Mitral Isthmus

The mitral isthmus is short (2 to 4 cm), anatomically bounded by the mitral annulus, left inferior PV ostium, and superiorly by the LA appendage (see Fig. 10-9). Mitral isthmus ablation is performed by linear ablation to join the lateral mitral isthmus to the left inferior PV.

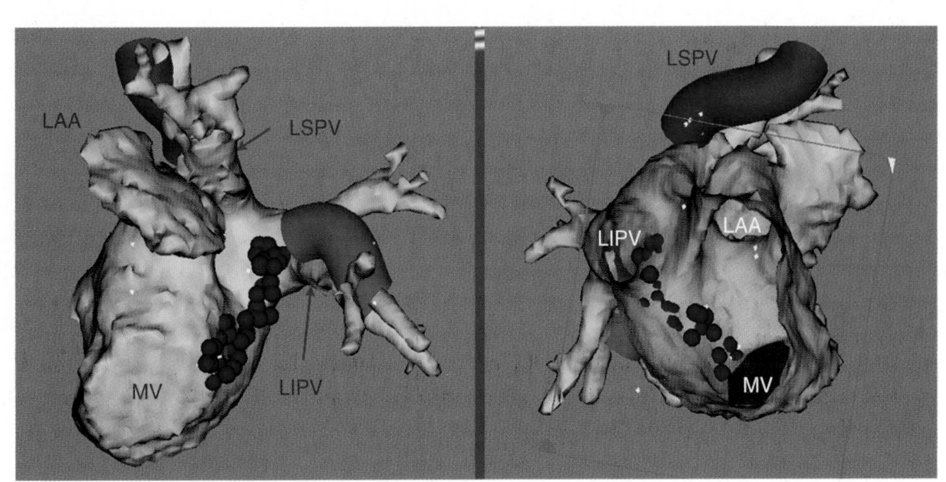

FIGURE 10–9 Integrated computed tomography (CT) and electroanatomical (CARTO) map of the left atrium (LA) acquired during catheter ablation of the mitral isthmus. Left anterior oblique and cardioscopic views of the CT scan are shown. Tubular-appearing structures are pulmonary veins (PVs); small red circles are tagged sites at which RF energy was applied across the isthmus between the annulus of the mitral valve (MV) and left inferior PV (LIPV). LAA = LA appendage; LSPV = left superior PV.

The CS catheter is positioned to bracket the potential linear lesion between its proximal and distal bipoles. The ablation catheter, bent with a 90- to 180-degree curve and introduced through a long sheath to achieve good contact and stability, is first positioned at the ventricular edge of the lateral mitral annulus, where the A:V electrogram shows a 1:1 to 2:1 ratio, to begin ablation. The sheath and catheter are then rotated clockwise to extend the lesion posteriorly, ending at the left inferior PV ostium (Fig. 10-10).[43,44] In general, ablation is commenced at about the 3 or 4 o'clock position on the mitral isthmus and reaches the 2 to 3 o'clock position at the upper end of the line. A more anterior extension to the posterior root of the LA appendage occasionally is required.

RF energy is delivered with the temperature limited to 50°C and power of 40 W, and for 90 to 120 seconds' duration at each site. The stability of the catheter is monitored during RF applications using electrography and intermittent fluoroscopy to exclude inadvertent displacement, which could result in high-energy delivery in the left inferior PV ostium or LA appendage.

When ablation is performed during NSR, the effect of each RF application is assessed on the local electrogram during pacing from the proximal bipole of the CS catheter located immediately septal of the line to maximize conduction delay. Splitting of the local potentials, resulting in an increase in the delay from the pacing artifact, is considered evidence of an effective local lesion. After the initial attempt to create this line, mapping is performed along the line to identify and ablate endocardial gaps, defined as sites showing the shortest delay between the pacing artifact and the local atrial potential, which can be single, narrow double, or fractionated.[43,44]

Persisting epicardial conduction is suspected when the linear lesion results in an endocardial conduction delay recorded on the ablation catheter but not on the adjacent distal bipole of the CS catheter (lateral to the ablation line). The ablation catheter is then withdrawn from the LA and introduced into the CS to map the epicardial side of the isthmus and identify fractionated or early potentials suggestive of an epicardial gap. Ablation within the CS is performed with a target temperature of 50°C and a power of 20 to 30 W (see Fig. 10-10).[43,44]

Endpoints of Ablation

Termination of Atrial Tachycardia During Radiofrequency Energy Application. Sudden termination of an incessant AT during RF application suggests that the lesion has severed a critical isthmus, and that site should be targeted for additional lesions. However, reliance on AT termination during RF application as the sole criterion of a successful ablation is hazardous because such an AT can terminate spontaneously, in which case termination can be misleading. RF application itself can induce PACs that can then terminate AT without eliminating the substrate. Moreover, the sudden termination of AT can be accompanied by catheter displacement from the critical site to another site, making it difficult to deliver additional energy applications at the critical site. Additionally, RF application can cause a transient but not permanent block in the critical isthmus. Such a block can last long enough to terminate the tachycardia, but can resolve after seconds or minutes.[10,21,25,33]

Lack of Atrial Tachycardia Inducibility. To use this criterion as a reliable endpoint, careful assessment of inducibility should be performed prior to ablation and the feasibility and best method of reproducible induction of the AT should be documented at baseline before ablation. In the setting of easy inducibility prior to ablation, one can consider the lack of inducibility as an indicator of successful ablation. Noninducibility of the arrhythmia is inapplicable

10

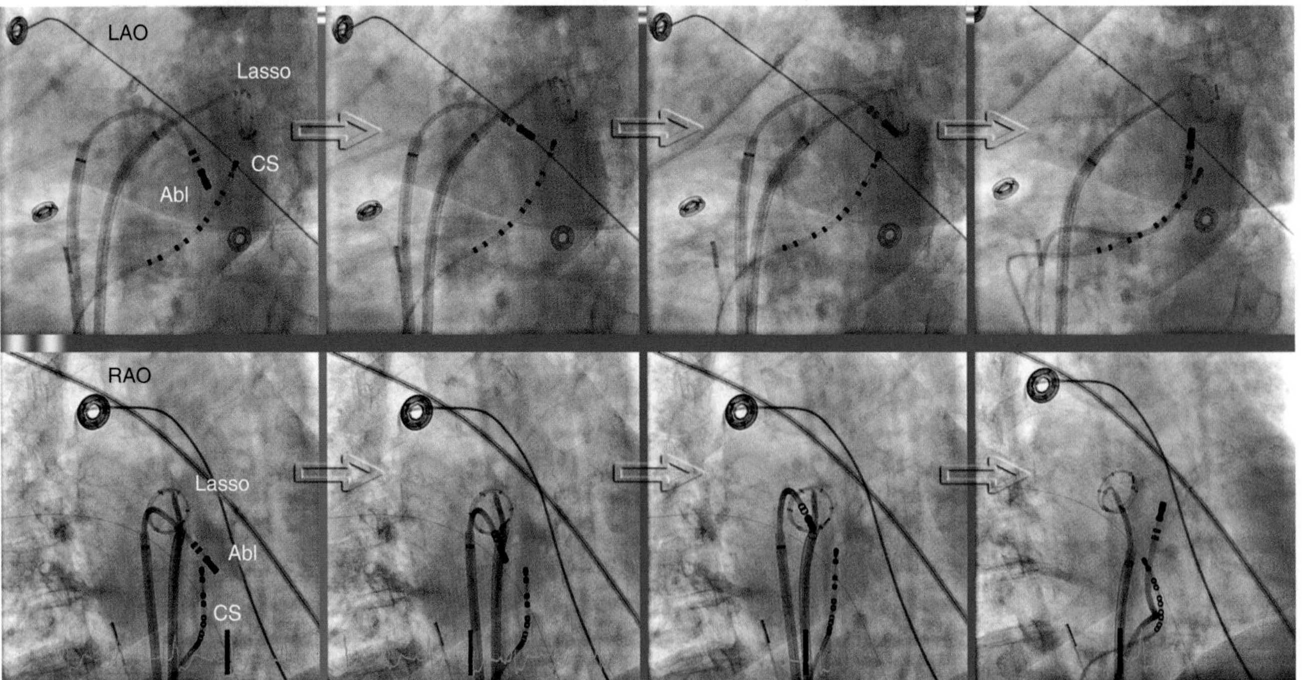

FIGURE 10–10 Right anterior oblique (RAO; upper panels) and left anterior oblique (LAO; lower panels) fluoroscopy views of catheter placement during mitral isthmus ablation. A ring catheter (Lasso) is positioned at the ostium of the left inferior pulmonary vein (PV). Ablation is started with the ablation catheter (Abl) at the ventricular edge of the mitral annulus (left panel). The catheter is then moved gradually to the midisthmus and subsequently to the junction with the ostium of the left inferior PV (middle panels). When the endocardial approach fails, epicardial ablation of the mitral isthmus is attempted via the coronary sinus (CS; right panel).

if the original arrhythmia is either noninducible at baseline or was inadvertently terminated mechanically. Noninducibility may also reflect conduction delay in the critical isthmus, and not stable block, or may be secondary to changes in autonomic tone.[10,21,25,33]

Documentation of a Line of Block. Complete stable conduction block within the reentry path is the most useful and objective endpoint. However, achieving this endpoint can be challenging and is not as feasible as in typical AFL ablation. To confirm complete conduction block following ablation, the mapping catheter is used to retrace the same ablation line (during NSR or atrial pacing), showing the absence of electrograms or a complete line of block demonstrated by parallel double potentials recorded all along the line.[10,21,25,33]

Pacing close to the ablation line (at a site within 30 milliseconds of conduction time to the ablation lesion) and demonstration of marked delay and reversal in the direction of activation on the opposite side of the linear lesion across the isthmus indicates isthmus block, although very slow conduction can be difficult to exclude. For a vertically oriented RA free wall atriotomy, a multielectrode Halo-type catheter can document activation sequences anterior and posterior to the scar, so that when pacing close to the contiguously ablated isthmus, the absence of a wavefront penetrating the scar and isthmus is used to indicate conduction block.

Confirmation of Mitral Isthmus Block. For perimitral AFL, the mitral isthmus is the target of ablation. Mitral isthmus ablation has a well-defined demonstrable procedural endpoint of bidirectional conduction block analogous to cavotricuspid isthmus ablation. Validation of mitral isthmus conduction block is greatly facilitated by its proximity to the CS, allowing pacing and recording on either side of the ablation line to confirm bidirectional block. Differential pacing can also be performed to exclude slow conduction through an incomplete line.[43,44]

Several criteria are used to confirm the presence of bidirectional mitral isthmus block:

1. The presence of widely separated (by 150- to 300-millisecond intervals) local double potentials along the length of the ablation line during CS pacing septal of the ablation line.
2. Mapping the activation detour during pacing from either side of the ablation line. Pacing on the septal side of the line via the CS demonstrates activation toward the line both septally and laterally. Pacing lateral to the line through the ablation catheter placed endocardially demonstrates a proximal-to-distal activation sequence along the CS septal of the line, thus confirming bidirectional conduction block (Fig. 10-11). Such an activation detour can also be determined using 3-D electroanatomical mapping.
3. Differential pacing to distinguish slow conduction across the mitral isthmus from complete block. With the distal bipole of the CS catheter placed just septal to the linear lesion, the pacing site is changed from the distal to the proximal bipole of the CS catheter without moving any of the catheters. The stimulus-to-electrogram timing at a site lateral to the ablation line is measured before and after changing the pacing site. With complete block, the stimulus-to-electrogram interval is shortened after shifting the pacing site from the distal to proximal CS bipole (see Fig. 10-11).[43,44]

Failure of Radiofrequency Ablation. Atrial enlargement can interfere with RF energy delivery secondary to difficulty in achieving stable, firm catheter contact and to the probable high convective heat loss associated with the large chamber volume. In addition, targets for ablation can have low surrounding blood flow; thus, target temperature can be achieved at very low energy outputs because of inadequate cooling of the catheter tip, with consequent limited energy delivery. Furthermore, some surgical repairs are associated with myocardial hypertrophy, making the achievement of a transmural lesion difficult or impossible.[10,21,25,33]

Outcome

Success

Acute success rates are reasonably good (approximately 90%). Recurrence rates of the same or other tachycardias are high, up to 54% of cases requiring repeat ablation in some studies. The long-term success rate is approximately 72%. The highest success rate is in patients with simple defects (e.g., atrial septal defect).[9,10,21,25,33] Block at the mitral isthmus can be achieved in 76% to 92% of patients with 20 ± 10 minutes of endocardial RF application and an additional 5 ± 4 minutes of epicardial RF application from within the CS in 68% of patients.

Despite frequent underlying structural heart disease, the incidence of AF after ablation is relatively low (9% to 21%). This may be related to the presence of silent areas and lines of block (spontaneous and created by RF), which could reduce the electrically active atrial mass below the critical threshold for AF. In the context of flutter propagating through incomplete lines of block delivered for AF ablation, the long-term follow-up is even better, at least in patients for whom complete block is achieved.

Safety of Left Atrial Flutter Ablation

Thromboembolic risk during LA ablation can be reduced by the following: (1) anticoagulation for 4 weeks prior to the procedure; (2) preprocedural transesophageal echocardiography to exclude the presence of atrial clots; (3) perfusion of the LA sheath under pressure to achieve a flow of approximately 2 to 4 mL/min; (4) intravenous heparin administration immediately before or immediately after transseptal puncture and throughout the LA procedure to maintain an activated clotting time between 250 and 350 seconds; and (5) the use of irrigated-tip catheters.[9,10,25]

Free wall perforation can occur during atrial puncture or during the rest of the procedure. The LA appendage is the site of the highest risk of perforation because of the very thin tissue encountered between the pectinate muscles. To prevent perforation caused by steam popping during RF delivery, it is important to limit the delivered power, especially around PVs, posterior LA, and LA dome.

PV stenosis is another potential complication, and using irrigated-tip catheters or limiting RF power to less than 50 W can reduce this risk. Left phrenic palsy is uncommon and is usually associated with RF delivery at the anterior LA and/or base of the LA appendage. Right phrenic nerve injury can be observed during ablation at the anterior aspect of the right PVs.

Safety of Right Atrial Flutter Ablation

Right phrenic nerve injury can be observed during ablation at the anterior aspect of the SVC and lateral RA. Early recognition of phrenic injury, based on cough, hiccup, or reduced diaphragmatic respiratory motion, is critical, because it is usually associated with rapid recovery. Pacing from the ablation catheter at the site without capture of the phrenic nerve is reassuring but its efficacy has never been assessed. In addition, limiting the power delivered to 20 to 25 W and monitoring diaphragmatic movements during ablation further minimize the risk of this complication.[9,21,33]

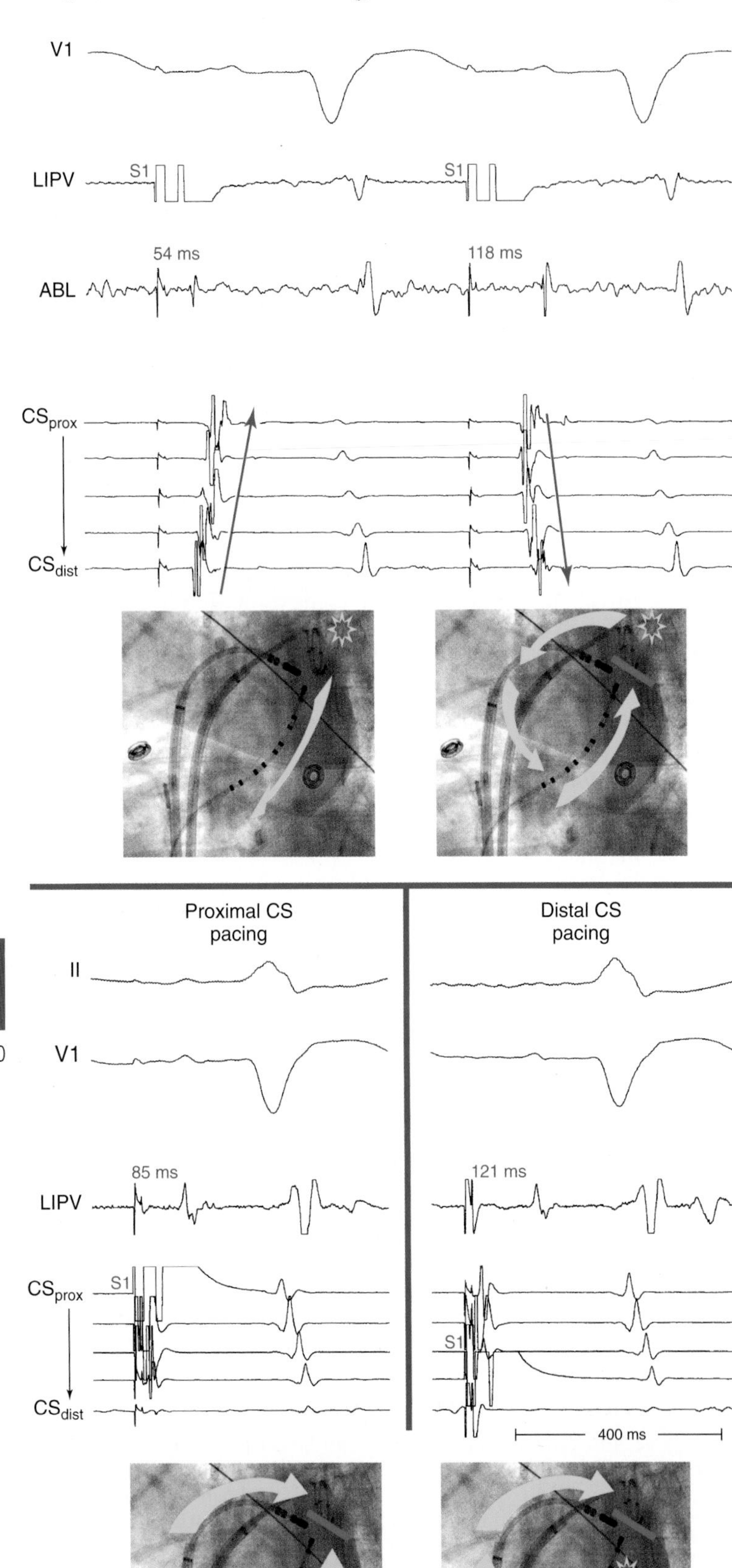

FIGURE 10–11 Verification of bidirectional mitral isthmus block. **Upper panel,** Ablation of the mitral isthmus is performed during pacing lateral to the ablation line (a Lasso catheter positioned at the ostium of the left inferior pulmonary vein [PV], LIPV, is used in this case). With intact isthmus conduction, coronary sinus (CS) activation occurs via the wavefront propagating in the counterclockwise direction; thus, a distal-to-proximal CS activation sequence is observed. When clockwise isthmus block is achieved, CS activation occurs via the wavefront propagating in the clockwise direction; thus, reversal of the CS activation sequence is observed. The ablation catheter (ABL) is positioned at the septal aspect of the line of block. The stimulus-to-electrogram interval recorded by the ablation catheter prolongs suddenly on development of clockwise isthmus block. **Lower panels,** Differential pacing is performed from the proximal and distal CS bipoles (both positioned at the septal aspect of the ablation line) to verify the presence of counterclockwise isthmus block. In the presence of counterclockwise block, activation lateral to the ablation line (as recorded by the Lasso catheter in the LIPV) occurs via the wavefront propagating in a clockwise direction up the left atrial (LA) septal wall and over the LA roof. Consequently, LIPV activation occurs earlier during pacing from the proximal CS (left panel) compared to the distal CS (right panel). A yellow star marks the pacing site.

REFERENCES

1. Yang Y, Cheng J, Bochoeyer A, et al: Atypical right atrial flutter patterns. Circulation 2001;103:3092.
2. Iesaka Y, Takahashi A, Goya M, et al: Nonlinear ablation targeting an isthmus of critically slow conduction detected by high-density electroanatomical al mapping for atypical atrial flutter. Pacing Clin Electrophysiol 2000;23(Pt 2):1911.
3. Kall JG, Rubenstein DS, Kopp DE, et al: Atypical atrial flutter originating in the right atrial free wall. Circulation 2000;101:270.
4. Cosio FG, Martin-Penato A, Pastor A, et al: Atypical flutter: a review. Pacing Clin Electrophysiol 2003;26:2157.
5. Nakagawa H, Shah N, Matsudaira K, et al: Characterization of reentrant circuit in macroreentrant right atrial tachycardia after surgical repair of congenital heart disease: Isolated channels between scars allow "focal" ablation. Circulation 2001;103:699.
6. Markowitz SM, Brodman RF, Stein KM, et al: Lesional tachycardias related to mitral valve surgery. J Am Coll Cardiol 2002;39:1973.
7. Tomita Y, Matsuo K, Sahadevan J, et al: Role of functional block extension in lesion-related atrial flutter. Circulation 2001;103:1025.
8. Triedman JK, Alexander ME, Love BA, et al: Influence of patient factors and ablative technologies on outcomes of radiofrequency ablation of intra-atrial re-entrant tachycardia in patients with congenital heart disease. J Am Coll Cardiol 2002;39:1827.
9. Magnin-Poull I, de CC, Miljoen H, et al: Mechanisms of right atrial tachycardia occurring late after surgical closure of atrial septal defects. J Cardiovasc Electrophysiol 2005;16:681.
10. Jais P, Shah DC, MacLe L, et al: Catheter ablation of atypical left atrial flutter. *In* Zipes DP, Haissaguerre M (eds): Catheter Ablation of Arrhythmias. Armonk, NY, Futura, 2002, pp 169-184.
11. Delacretaz E, Ganz LI, Soejima K, et al: Multi atrial maco-re-entry circuits in adults with repaired congenital heart disease: Entrainment mapping combined with three-dimensional electroanatomical mapping. J Am Coll Cardiol 2001;37:1665.
12. Shah D, Jais P, Takahashi A, et al: Dual loop intra-atrial reentry in humans. Circulation 2000;101:631.
13. Chan DP, Van Hare GF, Mackall JA, et al: Importance of atrial flutter isthmus in postoperative intra-atrial reentrant tachycardia. Circulation 2000;102:1283.
14. Tai CT, Huang JL, Lin YK, et al: Noncontact three-dimensional mapping and ablation of upper loop re-entry originating in the right atrium. J Am Coll Cardiol 2002;40:746.
15. Jais P, Shah DC, Haissaguerre M, et al: Mapping and ablation of left atrial flutters. Circulation 2000;101:2928.
16. Bochoeyer A, Yang Y, Cheng J, et al: Surface electrocardiographic characteristics of right and left atrial flutter. Circulation 2003;108:60.
17. Gerstenfeld EP, Marchlinski FE: Mapping and ablation of left atrial tachycardias occurring after atrial fibrillation ablation. Heart Rhythm 2007;4(Suppl 3):S65.
18. Ouyang F, Ernst S, Vogtmann T, et al: Characterization of reentrant circuits in left atrial macroreentrant tachycardia: Critical isthmus block can prevent atrial tachycardia recurrence. Circulation 2002;105:1934.
19. Marrouche NF, Natale A, Wazni OM, et al: Left septal atrial flutter: Electrophysiology, anatomy, and results of ablation. Circulation 2004;109:2440.
20. Walsh EP, Cecchin F: Arrhythmias in adult patients with congenital heart disease. Circulation 2007;115:534.
21. Shah DC, Jais P, Hocini M, et al: Catheter ablation of atypical right atrial flutter. *In* Zipes DP, Haissaguerre M (eds): Catheter Ablation of Arrhythmias. Armonk, NY, Futura, 2002, pp 153-168.
22. Rodriguez LM, Timmermans C, Nabar A, et al: Biatrial activation in isthmus-dependent atrial flutter. Circulation 2001;104:2545.
23. Ndrepepa G, Zrenner B, Weyerbrock S, et al: Activation patterns in the left atrium during counterclockwise and clockwise atrial flutter. J Cardiovasc Electrophysiol 2001;12:893.
24. Ellenbogen KA, Wood MA: Atrial tachycardia. *In* Zipes DP, Jalife J (eds): Cardiac Electrophysiology: From Cell to Bedside, 4th ed. Philadelphia, PA: Saunders; 2004. pp 683-688.
25. Kall JG, Wilber DJ: Ablation of atypical atrial flutter. *In* Huang SK, Wilber DJ (eds): Radiofrequency Catheter Ablation of Cardiac Arrhythmias: Basic Concepts and Clinical Applications. Armonk, Futura, 2000, pp 233-256.
26. Sehra R, Coppess MA, Altemose GT, et al: Atrial tachycardia masquerading as atrial flutter following ablation of the subeustachian isthmus. J Cardiovasc Electrophysiol 2000;11:582.
27. Ricard P, Imianitoff M, Yaici K, et al: Atypical atrial flutters. Europace 2002;4:229.
28. Gerstenfeld EP, Dixit S, Bala R, et al: Surface electrocardiogram characteristics of atrial tachycardias occurring after pulmonary vein isolation. Heart Rhythm 2007;4:1136.
29. Morton JB, Sanders P, Deen V, et al: Sensitivity and specificity of concealed entrainment for the identification of a critical isthmus in the atrium: relationship to rate, anatomical location and antidromic penetration. J Am Coll Cardiol 2002;39:896.
30. Cantale CP, Garcia-Cosio F, Montero MA, et al: [Electrophysiological and clinical characterization of left atrial macroreentrant tachycardia.] Rev Esp Cardiol 2002;55:45.
31. Hammer PE, Brooks DH, Triedman JK: Estimation of entrainment response using electrograms from remote sites: Validation in animal and computer models of reentrant tachycardia. J Cardiovasc Electrophysiol 2003;14:52.
32. Della Bella P, Fraticelli A, Tondo C: Atypical atrial flutter: Clinical features, electrophysiological characteristics and response to radiofrequency catheter ablation. Europace 2002;4:241.
33. Hare GV. Ablation of reentrant atrial tachycardia associated with structural heart disease. *In* Huang SK, Wilber DJ (eds): Radiofrequency Catheter Ablation of Cardiac Arrhythmias: Basic Concepts and Clinical Applications. Armonk, NY, Futura, 2000, pp 185-208.
34. Perry JC, Boramanand NK, Ing FF: "Transseptal" technique through atrial baffles for 3-dimensional mapping and ablation of atrial tachycardia in patients with d-transposition of the great arteries. J Interv Cardiol Electrophysiol 2003;9:365.
35. Cosio FG, Pastor A, Nunez A, Montero MA: How to map and ablate atrial scar macroreentrant tachycardia of the right atrium. Europace 2000;2:193.
36. Zrenner B, Ndrepepa G, Karch M, et al: Block of the lower interatrial connections: Insight into the sources of electrocardiographic diversities in common type atrial flutter. Pacing Clin Electrophysiol 2000;23:917.
37. Betts TR, Roberts PR, Allen SA, et al: Electrophysiological mapping and ablation of intra-atrial reentry tachycardia after Fontan surgery with the use of a noncontact mapping system. Circulation 2000;102:419.
38. Reithmann C, Hoffmann E, Dorwarth U, et al: Electroanatomical al mapping for visualization of atrial activation in patients with incisional atrial tachycardias. Eur Heart J 2001;22:237.
39. Paul T, Windhagen-Mahnert B, Krebel T: Atrial reentrant tachycardia after surgery for congenital heart disease: Endocardial mapping and radiofrequency catheter ablation using a novel, noncontact mapping system. Circulation 2001;103:2266.
40. Mandapati R, Walsh EP, Triedman JK: Pericaval and periannular intra-atrial reentrant tachycardias in patients with congenital heart disease. J Cardiovasc Electrophysiol 2003;14:119.
41. Kannankeril PJ, Fish FA: Management of intra-atrial reentrant tachycardia. Curr Opin Cardiol 2005;20:89.
42. Morady F: Catheter ablation of supraventricular arrhythmias: State of the art. J Cardiovasc Electrophysiol 2004;15:124.
43. Jais P, Hocini M, Hsu LF, et al: Technique and results of linear ablation at the mitral isthmus. Circulation 2004;110:2996.
44. Fassini G, Riva S, Chiodelli R, et al: Left mitral isthmus ablation associated with PV isolation: Long-term results of a prospective randomized study. J Cardiovasc Electrophysiol 2005;16:1150.

CHAPTER 11

Atrial Fibrillation

PATHOPHYSIOLOGY

Classification of Atrial Fibrillation

Atrial fibrillation (AF) has been described in various ways, such as paroxysmal or chronic, lone, idiopathic, nonvalvular, valvular, or self-terminating. Each of these classifications has implications for the response to therapy, and the lack of a consistent nomenclature has led to difficulties in comparing one study with another.

At the initial detection of AF, it may be difficult to be certain of the subsequent pattern of duration and frequency of recurrences. Thus, a designation of first detected episode of AF is made on the initial diagnosis. When the patient has experienced two or more episodes, AF is classified as recurrent.[1,2] After the termination of an episode of AF, the rhythm can be classified as paroxysmal or persistent. Paroxysmal AF is characterized by self-terminating episodes that generally last less than 7 days. Persistent AF generally lasts longer than 7 days and often requires electrical or pharmacological cardioversion. Permanent AF refers to AF that has failed cardioversion or has been sustained for more than 1 year, or when further attempts to terminate the arrhythmia are deemed futile.

Although useful, this arbitrary classification does not account for all presentations of AF and is not clearly related to any specific pathophysiology or mechanism of arrhythmogenesis. Additionally, the pattern of AF may change in response to treatment. Paroxysmal AF often progresses to longer, non–self-terminating episodes. Moreover, AF initially responsive to pharmacological or electrical cardioversion tends to become resistant and cannot then be converted to normal sinus rhythm (NSR). Additionally, AF that has been persistent may become paroxysmal with antiarrhythmic drug therapy, and AF that had been permanent may be cured or made paroxysmal by surgical or catheter-based ablation. Furthermore, the distinction between persistent and permanent AF is not only a function of the underlying arrhythmia but also the clinical pragmatism of the patient and physician.[3] The severity of symptoms associated with AF, anticoagulation status, and patient preference affect the decision of whether and when cardioversion is attempted, which would then affect the duration of sustained AF, leading to a diagnosis of persistent or permanent AF.

Mechanism of Atrial Fibrillation

Two concepts of the underlying mechanism of AF have received considerable attention—factors that trigger the onset and factors that perpetuate this arrhythmia.[3] In general, patients with frequent, self-terminating episodes of AF are likely to have a predominance of factors that trigger AF, whereas patients with AF that does not terminate spontaneously are more likely to have a predominance of perpetuating factors. Although such a gross generalization has clinical usefulness, there is often considerable overlap of these mechanisms. The typical patient with paroxysmal AF has identifiable ectopic foci initiating the arrhythmia, but these triggers cannot be recorded in all patients. Conversely, occasional patients with persistent or permanent AF may be cured of their arrhythmia by ablation of a single triggering focus, suggesting that perpetual firing of the focus may be the mechanism sustaining this arrhythmia in some cases.

In recent years, advanced mapping technologies, along with studies in animal models, have suggested the potential for complex pathophysiological mechanisms responsible for AF, including the following: (1) continuous aging or degeneration of atrial tissue and the cardiac conduction system; (2) progression of structural heart disease, such as valvular heart disease and cardiomyopathy; (3) myocardial ischemia, local hypoxia, electrolyte derangement, and metabolic disorders (e.g., atherosclerotic heart disease, chronic lung disease, hypokalemia, and hyperthyroidism); (4) inflammation related to pericarditis or myocarditis, with or without cardiac surgery; (5) genetic predisposition; and (6) spontaneous or drug-induced autonomic dysfunction.[2,3]

The electrophysiological (EP) mechanisms responsible for AF may include a rapid focal tachyarrhythmia in the pulmonary veins (PVs) and/or other atrial regions with fibrillatory conduction, multiple reentrant wavelet conduction initiated by premature atrial complexes (PACs) and/or atrial tachyarrhythmias, and/or formation of stable or unstable reentrant circuits of very short cycle lengths (CLs) that generate fibrillatory conduction.[2,3] Additionally, AF can in itself lead to functional and structural changes in the atrial myocardium that favor its maintenance. These remodeling processes are probably precipitated by high rate activity and intracellular calcium overload, followed by activation or enhancement of multiple subcellular mechanisms.[4]

Mechanism of Initiation of Atrial Fibrillation

The factors responsible for the onset of AF include triggers that induce the arrhythmia and the substrate that sustains it. The triggers are diverse yet do not cause AF in the absence of other contributors.[2] There are two different types of arrhythmias that may play a role in generating AF, PACs that initiate AF ("focal triggers") and focal tachycardia that either induces fibrillation in the atria or mimics AF by creating a pattern of rapid and irregular depolarization wavefronts in the atria.[2,5] Studies have suggested that in most cases, AF begins with a rapid focal activity in the PVs and, less commonly, in the superior vena cava (SVC), coronary sinus (CS), or ligament of Marshall.[6]

The mechanism of initiation of AF is not certain in most cases and likely is multifactorial. Triggers propagating into atrial myocardium may initiate multiple reentering wavelets and AF.[2,5] In some patients with paroxysmal AF, impulses initiated by ectopic focal activity propagate into the left atrium (LA) and encounter heterogeneously recovered tissue. If reentry is assumed to be the mechanism of AF, initiation would require an area of conduction block and a wavelength of activation short enough to allow the reentrant circuit in the myocardium.

The triggered AF may be self-sustained, in which case the continued firing of the focus is not required for maintenance of AF and ablation of the focus does not terminate AF, but rather prevents the reinitiation of AF. Conversely, initiation and maintenance of AF may depend on uninterrupted periodic activity of a few discrete reentrant sources localized to the LA (i.e., focal driver), emanating from such sources to propagate through both atria and interact with anatomical or functional obstacles, or both, leading to fragmentation and wavelet formation. Factors such as wavefront curvature, sink-source relationships, and spatial and temporal organization all are relevant to our understanding of the initiation of AF by the interaction of the propagating wavefronts with such anatomical or functional obstacles. Indeed, all these factors, which differ from triggers, may be considered initiators of AF.

AF triggering factors include sympathetic or parasympathetic stimulation, bradycardia, PACs (which are the most common cause; Fig. 11-1), atrial flutter (AFL), supraventricular tachycardias (SVTs; especially those mediated by atrioventricular [AV] bypass tracts [BTs]; Fig. 11-2), and acute

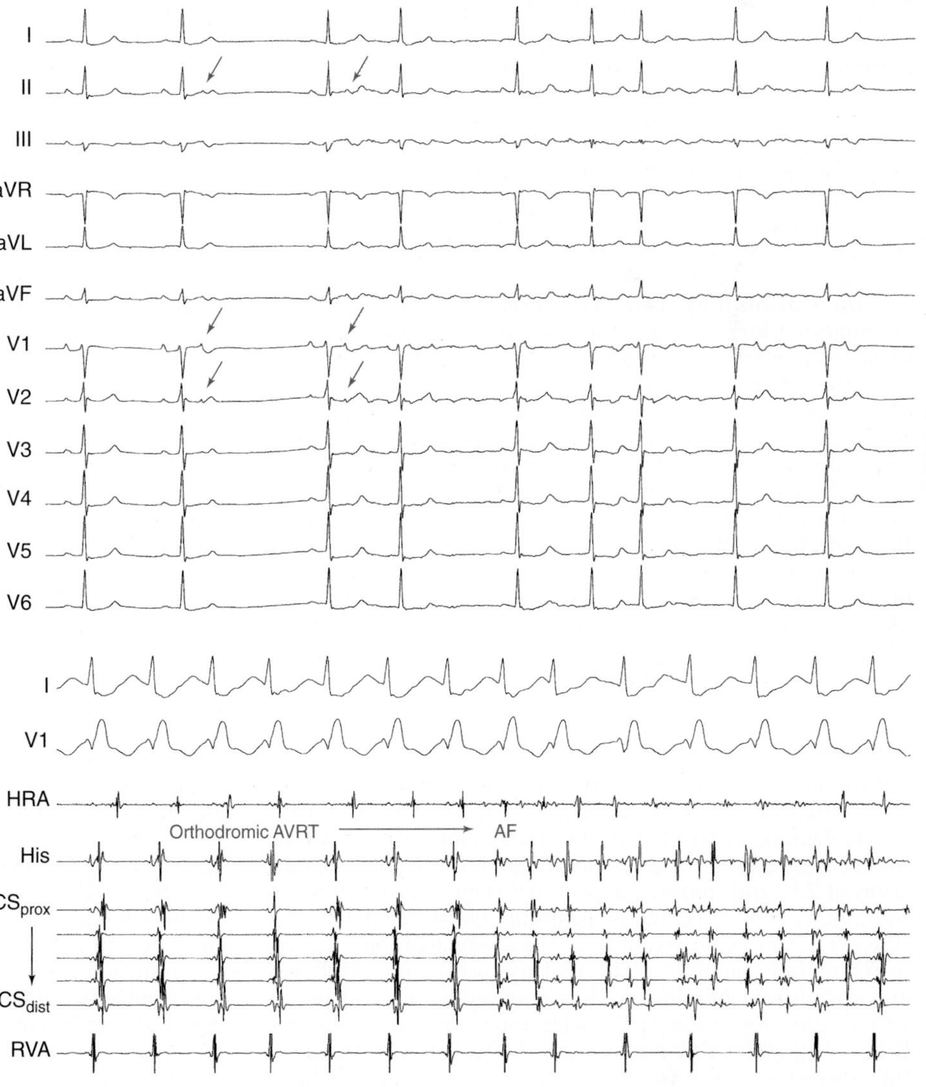

FIGURE 11-1 Atrial fibrillation (AF) induction by premature atrial complexes (PACs) originating from the right superior pulmonary vein (PV). Two monomorphic PACs (arrows) occur at short coupling intervals and are inscribed within the T wave. The second PAC (red arrows) triggers AF.

FIGURE 11–2 Atrial fibrillation (AF) induction by orthodromic atrioventricular reentrant tachycardia (AVRT).

atrial stretch. Identification of these triggers has clinical importance because treatment approaches directed at elimination of the triggers (e.g., radiofrequency [RF] ablation of the initiating PACs or SVT) may be curative.

Pulmonary Vein Triggers. Triggering foci of rapidly firing cells within the sleeves of atrial myocytes extending into the PVs have been clearly shown to be the underlying mechanism of most paroxysmal AF.[5,6] Supporting this idea are clinical studies of impulses generated by single foci propagating from individual PVs or other atrial regions to the remainder of the atria as fibrillatory waves and abolition of AF by RF ablation to isolate the venous foci.[6]

Based on a number of features, the thoracic veins are highly arrhythmogenic. The PV-LA junction has discontinuous myocardial fibers separated by fibrotic tissues and, therefore, is highly anisotropic. Insulated muscle fibers can promote reentrant excitation, automaticity, and triggered activity. These regions likely resemble the juxtaposed islets of atrial myocardium and vascular smooth muscle in the CS and AV valves that, under normal circumstances, manifest synchronous electrical activity but develop delayed afterdepolarizations and triggered activity in response to catecholamine stimulation, rapid atrial pacing, or acute stretch.[7]

Furthermore, the PVs of patients with paroxysmal AF demonstrate abnormal properties of conduction so that there is markedly reduced refractory periods within the PVs, progressive conduction delay within the PV in response to rapid pacing or programmed stimulation, and often conduction block between the PV and LA. Such findings are much more common in patients with paroxysmal AF than in normal subjects.[5,8-11] Rapidly firing foci can often be recorded within the PVs with conduction block to the LA. Administration of catecholamines such as isoproterenol can lead to shortening of the LA refractory period, thereby allowing these foci to propagate to the LA with the induction of spontaneous AF.[9] These discontinuous properties of conduction within the PV may also provide a substrate for reentry within the PV itself, although this remains to be proven.[7]

Non–Pulmonary Vein Triggers. Although over 90% of triggering foci that are mapped during EP studies occur in the PVs in patients with paroxysmal AF, foci within the SVC, the ligament of Marshall, and the musculature of the CS have been identified.[6] Although these latter locations of triggering foci are uncommon in patients with paroxysmal AF, the common factor is that the site of origin is often within a venous structure that connects to the atrium. PACs
11 may originate from the SVC (within 19 mm above the junction with the right atrium [RA]), occurring in 6% of patients in one report. Myocardial sleeves in the CS and small muscle bundles in the ligament of Marshall have also been identified as a source of initiating triggers of AF. Other sites of initiating foci may be recorded in the LA wall or along the crista terminalis in the RA.[7,12]

Mechanism of Maintenance of Atrial Fibrillation

Having been initiated, AF may be brief; however, various factors may act as perpetuators, ensuring the maintenance of AF.[2] One is persistence of the triggers and initiators that induced the AF, acting as an engine that drives the continuation of AF, and maintenance of AF then is dependent on the continued firing of the focus (the so-called focal drivers). However, AF can persist even in the absence of the triggers, in which case persistence of AF may result from electrical and structural remodeling, characterized by atrial dilation and shortening of the atrial refractoriness. This combination, along with other remodeling changes, likely promotes the appearance of multiple reentrant wavelets (a final common pathway for AF) by decreasing the wavelength of reentry, the product of the refractory period and the conduction velocity.

Various EP and structural factors promote the perpetuation of AF. Classic theories have implicated the presence of multiple-circuit reentry, single-circuit reentry, or rapidly discharging atrial focus with fibrillatory conduction.

Multiple-Wavelet Hypothesis. For many years, the most widely held theory on the maintenance of AF was the "multiple-wavelet" hypothesis, which was a key development in our understanding of the mechanism of AF. Moe has noted that, "The grossly irregular wavefront becomes fractionated as it divides about islets or strands of refractory tissue, and each of the daughter wavelets may now be considered as independent offspring. Such a wavelet may accelerate or decelerate as it encounters tissue in a more or less advanced state of recovery." Moe subsequently hypothesized that AF is sustained by multiple randomly wandering wavelets that collided with each other and were extinguished, or divided into daughter wavelets that continually reexcited the atria.[13] Those functional reentrant circuits are therefore unstable; some disappear, whereas others reform. These circuits have variable, but short, cycle lengths, resulting in multiple circuits to which atrial tissue cannot respond in a 1 : 1 fashion. As a result, functional block, slow conduction, and multiple wavefronts develop. It has been suggested that at least four to six independent wavelets are required to maintain AF. These wavelets rarely reenter themselves but can reexcite portions of the myocardium recently activated by another wavefront, a process called random reentry. As a result, there are multiple wavefronts of activation that may collide with each other, extinguishing themselves or creating new wavelets and wavefronts, thereby perpetuating the arrhythmia.

The persistence of multiple-circuit reentry depends on the ability of a tissue to maintain enough simultaneously reentering wavefronts that activity is unlikely to extinguish simultaneously in all parts of the atria. Therefore, the more wavelets present, the more likely it is that the arrhythmia will sustain. The number of wavelets on the heart at any moment depends on the atrial mass, refractory period, conduction velocity, and anatomical obstacles in different portions of the atria. In essence, a large atrial mass with short refractory periods and conduction delay would yield increased wavelets and would present the most favorable situation for AF to be sustained.[2]

Mother Circuit. Studies in isolated human atrial preparations have questioned the randomness of atrial activity and have shown that a single meandering functional reentrant wavefront produces AF.[14] This model suggests the presence of a single source of stable reentrant activity (mother circuit) that serves as a periodic background focus; the presence of anatomical obstacles (scar, orifices) serve to break up the wavefront from the mother circuit into multiple wavelets that spread in various directions.[14] Functional reentry (or anatomical reentry with a functional component), in the form of spiral waves rotating around microreentrant circuits approximately 1 cm in diameter, was suggested to be the most likely cause of AF in this model.[14] In other experiments, it was shown that these dominant rotors that drive AF invariably originate and anchor in the LA, with the RA being activated passively.

Focal Drivers with Fibrillatory Conduction. Although multiple wandering wavelets probably account for most AF, in some cases a single, rapidly firing focus could be identified with EP mapping. Impulses initiated by ectopic focal activity propagate into the atria to encounter heterogeneously recovered tissue. When cardiac impulses are continuously generated at a rapid rate from any source or any mechanism, they will activate the tissue of that cardiac chamber in a 1:1 manner, up to a critical rate. However, when this critical rate is exceeded, so that not all the tissue of that cardiac chamber can respond in a 1:1 fashion (e.g., because the CL of the driver is shorter than the refractory periods of those tissues), fibrillatory conduction will develop. Fibrillatory conduction can be caused by spatially varying refractory periods or to the structural properties of atrial tissue with source-sink mismatches providing spatial gradients in the response.[2] Thus, fibrillatory conduction is characterized by activation of tissues at variable CLs, all longer than the CL of the driver, because of variable conduction block. In that manner, activation is fragmented.[2] This is the mechanism of AF in several animal models in which the driver consists of a stable, abnormally automatic focus of a very short CL, a stable reentrant circuit with a very short CL, or an unstable reentrant circuit with a very short CL. It also appears to be the mechanism of AF in patients in whom activation of the atria at very short CLs originates in one or more PVs. The impulses from the PVs seem to precipitate and maintain AF. Of note, it has also been suggested that fibrillatory conduction caused by a reentrant driver may be the cause of ventricular fibrillation (VF).

Substrate for Atrial Fibrillation

Pathological conditions that predispose to AF, such as heart failure and sinus node dysfunction, have been associated with electrical remodeling of the atria. These conditions are likely associated with increased dispersion in atrial refractoriness and increased and inhomogeneous dispersion of conduction abnormalities, including block, slow conduction, and uncoupling of muscle bundles. Similar phenomena have also been demonstrated in older patients and those with single-chamber ventricular pacemakers, with both groups having a high prevalence of AF. The age-related development of interstitial fibrosis results in decreased conduction velocity and provides the substrate for reentry. However, although such remodeling is important in providing a substrate for AF, its relationship to AF triggers, such as PV ectopy, is less clear. It has been shown that the frequency of atrial ectopy increases with age and hypertension.

It has also been demonstrated that critically timed atrial extrastimuli during chronic AFL could result in degeneration of AFL to AF in an experimental model. This effect was not seen at baseline, prior to any electrical remodeling of the atria. Such work suggests an interaction between triggers and substrate in the genesis of AF. However, the exact nature of this interaction, and specifically the relationship between the frequency of triggers and arrhythmogenic substrate, remains to be elucidated. Moreover, factors determining the point of no return to sinus rhythm are not yet characterized.

Electrophysiological Properties

The normal atrial myocardium consists of so-called fast response tissues that depend on the rapidly activating sodium current for phase 0 of the action potential. As a result, the atrium has several properties that permit the development of very complex patterns of conduction and an extremely rapid atrial rate, as seen in AF—the action potential duration is relatively short, reactivation can occur partially during phase 3 and usually completely within 10 to 50 milliseconds after return to the diastolic potential, the refractory period shortens with increasing rate, and very rapid conduction can occur.

Patients with idiopathic AF appear to have increased dispersion of atrial refractoriness, which correlates with enhanced inducibility of AF and spontaneous episodes. Some patients have site-specific dispersion of atrial refractoriness and intraatrial conduction delays resulting from nonuniform atrial anisotropy. This appears to be a common property of normal atrial tissue, but there are further conduction delays to and within the posterior triangle of Koch in patients with induced AF, which suggests an important role for the low RA in the genesis of AF.

Interstitial Atrial Fibrosis

Interstitial atrial fibrosis predisposes to intraatrial reentry and AF.[3] Fibrosis of the atria may produce inhomogeneity of conduction within the atria, leading to conduction block and intraatrial reentry. When combined with inhomogeneous dispersion of refractoriness within the atria, conduction block is an ideal substrate for reentry. The greater the slowing of conduction velocity in scarred myocardium, the shorter the anatomical circuit that can sustain a reentrant wavelet.

The normal aging process results in anatomical changes likely to yield inhomogeneity in conduction that may create the milieu necessary for the development of reentry. These changes are likely magnified by the presence of certain disease processes, such as coronary artery disease and heart failure. The strong association of sinus node dysfunction and AF (the bradycardia-tachycardia syndrome) also suggests that replacement of atrial myocytes by interstitial fibrosis may play an important part in the pathogenesis of AF in older adults. Furthermore, AF itself seems to produce various alterations of atrial architecture that further contribute to atrial remodeling, mechanical dysfunction, and perpetuation of fibrillation. Long-standing AF results in loss of myofibrils, accumulation of glycogen granules, disruption in cell-to-cell coupling at gap junctions, and organelle aggregates.

Changes in AF characteristics during evolving fibrosis also have a direct impact on why electrical or drug treatment, or both, ultimately fails to achieve conversion to NSR.[3] Fibrotic myocardium exhibits slow conduction, whose low macroscopic propagation velocities are explained by microscopically zigzagging circuits or by the special conduction characteristics of tissues with discontinuous branching architecture. Reentrant circuits can be only a few millimeters in diameter in discontinuously conducting tissue. Thus, atrial regions with advanced fibrosis can be local sources for AF. Such a hypothesis would not preclude the remainder of the atria from showing fibrillatory conduction and/or intact, functional reentrant waves. A highly fibrotic atrial region or regions would explain the refractoriness of AF to therapeutic interventions.[3] In any markedly discontinuous tissue (e.g., discontinuous anisotropy, marked degree of gap junctional uncoupling, branching), the safety factor for propagation is even higher than in normal tissue. Thus, blocking Na^+ current to the same degree as is necessary for the termination of functional reentry may not terminate reentry caused by slow and fractionated conduction in fibrotic scars of remodeled atria.[3] Conduction in discontinuous tissue is mostly structurally determined, which will lead to excitable gaps behind the wavefronts. If a gap is of critical size, the effectiveness of drugs that prolong atrial refractoriness will be limited.[3] Furthermore, scar tissue is likely to exhibit multiple entry and exit points and multiple sites at which unidirectional block occurs. This may lead to activity whose appearance in local extracellular electrograms changes from beat to beat, as well as beat-to-beat CL variability. Although such regions may be expected to respond to defibrillation, AF may resume after extrasystoles or normal sinus beats immediately after conversion, with unidirectional block recurring as a result of the presence of scar.[3] Apoptosis (programmed cell death) is another likely contributor to the structural substrate of AF. Apoptosis normally controls expression of specific cell types, but under pathophysiological conditions, it can occur inappropriately. When this happens in heart, myocytes die and contractile capacity and electrical activity are permanently altered.[3]

Atrial Stretch

The structure of the dilated atria may have important EP effects related to stretch of the atrial myocardium, which may affect automaticity and reentry.[3] Electromechanical feedback refers to changes in the EP properties of the LA induced by dilation and an increase in pressure (caused by volume or pressure overload); this manifests as a decrease in the atrial refractory period and action potential duration in addition to an increase in dispersion of refractoriness, thereby predisposing to AF. Lowering LA pressure may result in prompt reversion of the arrhythmia.[3,4]

The echocardiographic LA volume index and restrictive transmitral Doppler flow pattern are strong predictors for the development of nonvalvular AF. Thus, clinical evidence for diastolic dysfunction strongly supports the concept that myocardial stretch is an important mechanism of AF in older adults.

The effects of changes in stretch are many, even in normal hearts. Regional stretch for less than 30 minutes turns on the immediate early gene program, initiating hypertrophy and altering action potential duration in affected areas. Moreover, acutely altered stress and strain patterns augment the synthesis of angiotensin II, which induces myocyte hypertrophy. By regionally increasing L-type Ca^{2+} current and decreasing the transient outward K^+ current, I_{to}, angiotensin II can contribute to arrhythmogenic electrical dispersion.[3] Altered stretch on atrial myocytes also results in opening of stretch-activated channels, which increases G protein–coupled pathways. This leads to increased protein kinase A and C activity and increased L-type Ca^{2+} current through the cell membrane and release of Ca^{2+} from the sarcoplasmic reticulum, promoting afterdepolarizations and triggered activity.

"Atrial Fibrillation Begets Atrial Fibrillation"

It is well known from clinical practice that AF is a progressive arrhythmia. Eventually, in 14% to 24% of patients with paroxysmal AF, persistent AF will develop, even in the absence of progressive underlying heart disease. Furthermore, conversion of AF to NSR, electrically or pharmacologically, becomes more difficult when the arrhythmia has been present for a longer period. This suggests that the arrhythmia itself results in a cascade of electrical and ana-
11 tomical changes in the atria that may be themselves conducive to the perpetuation of the arrhythmia ("AF begets AF").[4] Recurrent AF may lead to irreversible atrial remodeling and eventually permanent structural changes that account for the progression of paroxysmal to persistent and finally to permanent AF, characterized by the failure of electrical cardioversion and/or pharmacological therapy to restore and maintain NSR.

Changes in atrial electrophysiology that are induced by AF and promote its perpetuation may occur through alteration in ion channel activities with partial depolarization and shortened atrial refractory period (electrical remodeling), which favors the initiation and perpetuation of AF, and modification of cellular calcium handling, which causes contractile dysfunction (contractile remodeling), as well as atrial dilation, with associated structural changes (structural remodeling).

Electrical remodeling results from the high rate of electrical activation. The EP changes typical of atrial myocytes during AF are a decrease in atrial refractory period, decrease in action potential duration, reduction in the amplitude of the action potential plateau, and loss of response of action potential duration to changes in rate (abnormal restitution).[3] Whereas the normal atrial action potential duration shortens in response to pacing at shorter CLs, AF results in loss of this rate dependence of atrial action potential duration, and the atrial refractory period fails to lengthen appropriately at slow rates (e.g., with return to NSR). These changes may explain the increased duration of AF because, according to the multiple-wavelet theory, a short wavelength will result in smaller wavelets, which would increase the maximum number of wavelets, given a certain atrial surface.[2,4] Tachycardia-induced changes in refractoriness are spatially heterogeneous and there is increased variability both within and among various atrial regions, which may promote atrial vulnerability and AF maintenance and provide a substrate for reentry.[2,4]

The mechanism for electrical remodeling and shortening of the atrial refractory period is not entirely clear. Several potential explanations exist, including ion channel remodeling, angiotensin II, and atrial ischemia. Shortening of the atrial refractory period and the atrial action potential may be caused by a net decrease of inward ionic currents (Na^+ or Ca^{2+}), a net increase of outward currents (K^+), or a combination of both. The decrease of L-type Ca^{2+} current seems to be responsible for shortening of the atrial action potential, whereas the decrease of transient outward K^+ current (I_{to}) is considered to result in loss of physiological rate adaptation of the action potential. The reduction in L-type Ca^{2+} current may be explained by a decreased expression of the L-type calcium channel α1c subunit.[3] Verapamil, an L-type calcium antagonist, was shown to prevent electric remodeling and hasten complete recovery without affecting inducibility of AF, whereas intracellular calcium overload, induced by hypercalcemia or digoxin, enhances electrical remodeling. Electrical remodeling can be attenuated by the sarcoplasmic reticulum's release of the calcium antagonist ryanodine, suggesting the importance of increased intracellular calcium to the maladaptation of atrial myocardium during AF.[3] Angiotensin II may also be involved in electrical and atrial myocardial remodeling, and angiotensin II inhibitors may prevent atrial electrical remodeling. Angiotensin-converting enzyme (ACE) inhibitors reduce the incidence of AF in patients with LV dysfunction after myocardial infarction and in patients with chronic ischemic cardiomyopathy. Atrial ischemia is another possible contributor to electrical remodeling and shortening of the atrial refractory period via activation of the sodium-hydrogen exchanger.

Furthermore, chronic, rapid atrial pacing–induced AF results in other changes within the atria, including gap junctional remodeling, cellular remodeling, atrial structural remodeling, and sinus node remodeling. Gap junctional remodeling is manifest as an increase in the expression and distribution of connexin 43 and heterogeneity in the distribution of connexin 40, both of which are intercellular gap junction proteins.[4] Cellular remodeling is caused by the apoptotic death of myocytes with myolysis, which may not be entirely reversible. AF results in marked changes in atrial cellular substructures, including loss of myofibrils, accumulation of glycogen, changes in mitochondrial shape and size, fragmentation of sarcoplasmic reticulum, and dispersion of nuclear chromatin.[4] Sustained fibrillation has also been associated with structural changes, such as myocyte hypertrophy, myocyte death, impaired atrial contractility, and atrial stretch and dilation, which act to reduce conduction velocity.[4,15] In addition to remodeling of the atria, the sinus node may undergo remodeling as well, resulting in sinus node dysfunction and bradyarrhythmias caused by reduced sinus node automaticity or prolonged sinoatrial conduction. The phenomenon of sinus node remodeling may contribute to the episodes of bradycardia seen in the tachycardia-bradycardia syndrome and may reduce sinus rhythm stability and increase the stability of AF.[4]

Structural changes in the atria after remodeling, such as stretch, may also result in increased PV activity. Atrial stretch may lead to increased intraatrial pressure, causing a rise in the rate and spatiotemporal organization of electrical waves originating in the PVs.[16] Rapid atrial pacing has also been shown to reduce atrial refractory period and action potential duration within PV myocytes. These changes imply that electrical and structural remodeling increase the likelihood of ectopic PV automaticity and AF maintenance. Therefore, rather than AF begets AF, one can have a variation on that theme: "PV-induced paroxysmal AF begets PV-induced chronic AF."

Atrial tachycardia–induced remodeling may underlie various clinically important phenomena, such as the tendency of patients with other forms of supraventricular arrhythmias to develop AF, the tendency of AF to recur early after electrical cardioversion, the resistance of longer duration AF to antiarrhythmic medications, and the tendency of paroxysmal AF to become persistent.[2]

If NSR is restored within a reasonable period of time, EP changes and atrial electrical remodeling appear to normalize gradually, atrial size decreases, and restoration of atrial mechanical function occurs.[3] These observations lend support to the idea that the negative downhill spiral in which AF begets AF can be arrested with NSR that perpetuates NSR, and restoration of NSR may forestall progressive remodeling and the increase in duration and frequency of arrhythmic episodes.[3]

Role of Autonomic Nervous System in Atrial Fibrillation

A number of studies have suggested that both divisions of the autonomic nervous system are involved in the initiation, maintenance, and termination of AF, with a predominant role of the parasympathetic system. Basic reports have shown that electrical stimulation of autonomic nerves on the heart itself can facilitate the induction of AF.[17] Increased vagal tone is frequently involved in the onset of AF in patients with structurally normal hearts. Parasympathetic stimulation shortens the atrial refractory period, increases its dispersion, and decreases the wavelength of reentrant circuits that facilitate initiation and perpetuation of AF.[18] Long-term vagal denervation of the atria renders AF less easily inducible in animal experiments, presumably because of increased electrophysiological homogeneity. On the other hand, vagal stimulation results in maintenance of AF, and catheter ablation of the parasympathetic autonomic nerves entering the RA from the SVC prevents vagally induced AF in animal models.

Spatial heterogeneity of refractoriness can also be produced by the heterogeneity of autonomic innervation.[19] It has been well established that vagal innervation of the atria is heterogeneous and vagal stimulation can precipitate AF as a result of heterogeneity of atrial refractoriness. Heterogeneity of sympathetic neural inputs also plays a role in AF. In animal models, sympathetic atrial denervation facilitates sustained AF and AF induced by rapid RA pacing is associated with nerve sprouting and a heterogeneous increase in sympathetic innervation. Enhanced sympathetic activity may promote automaticity, delayed afterdepolarization–related atrial tachycardia (AT), and focal AF. Sympathetic stimulation also shortens atrial refractoriness and may facilitate the induction of AF in patients with structural heart disease, in whom possible heterogeneous sympathetic denervation leads to increased refractoriness heterogeneity.[19]

There is some experimental evidence to suggest that the electrical properties of the PVs can be modulated by changes in autonomic tone.[9] For patients with PV foci, a primary increase in adrenergic tone followed by a marked vagal predominance has been reported just prior to the onset of paroxysmal AF. A similar pattern of autonomic tone has been reported in an unselected group of patients with paroxysmal AF and various cardiac conditions.[18] The initial investigations found that the lowest threshold for inducing AF was at the entrances of the PVs. Moreover, beta blockade blunted this response, whereas atropine abolished AF inducibility.[17] Anatomical studies have revealed that the LA and PVs are innervated by adrenergic and cholinergic nerve fibers. A collection of ganglia was localized on the posterior wall of the LA between the superior PVs. Subsequent studies have found that ganglionated plexi clustered at the PV entrances (within fat pads) could be stimulated without atrial excitation. Now, premature beats induced in the PVs could be converted to AF, with a significantly greater propensity than without ganglionated plexi stimulation. Furthermore, ablation of these ganglionated plexi abolished AF inducibility.

More recent basic and clinical findings may allow targeting autonomic elements at a few specific sites on the heart directly related to arrhythmia formation—namely, the ganglionated plexi located at the atrial entrances or antra of the PVs. This substantially increases the success rate or freedom from AF recurrence compared with the technique of isolating the PVs electrically from the atria.[18]

Role of Pulmonary Veins in Atrial Fibrillation

There is little controversy now that the PVs play a major role in triggering and maintaining AF, as established by animal and human models. First, fibrillatory conduction is likely initiated by rapid discharges from one or several focal sources within the atria. Haissaguerre and colleagues[6] have demonstrated that in most AF patients (94%), the focus is in one of the PVs (see Fig. 11-1). Extra-PV sites may trigger AF, but this occurs in the minority of cases, likely no more than 6% to 10% of patients. AF is also perpetuated by microreentrant circuits, or rotors, that exhibit high-frequency periodic activity from which spiral wavefronts of activation radiate into surrounding atrial tissue. Conduction becomes slower and less organized with increasing distance from the rotors, likely because of atrial structural remodeling, resulting in fibrillatory conduction. Interestingly, the dominant rotors in AF are localized primarily in the junction between the LA and PVs. One study has also demonstrated that the PV-LA region has heterogeneous EP properties capable of sustaining reentry (micro- or macro-). Finally, vagal inputs may be important in triggering and maintaining AF, and many of these inputs are clustered close to the PV-LA junction. Thus, the PVs play a critical role in triggering and maintaining AF.

Pulmonary Vein Anatomy

PVs can have variable anatomy, with most hearts examined found to have four PVs with discrete ostia, but the remainder (approximately 25%) having a common ostium, either on the left or on the right (Fig. 11-3).[5] The PV ostia are ellipsoid with a longer superoinferior dimension, and funnel-shaped ostia are frequently noted in AF patients. The right superior PV is located close to the SVC or RA, and the right inferior PV projects horizontally. The left superior PV is close to the vicinity of the LA appendage, and the left inferior PV courses near the descending aorta. PVs are larger in AF patients, men versus women, and persistent versus par-

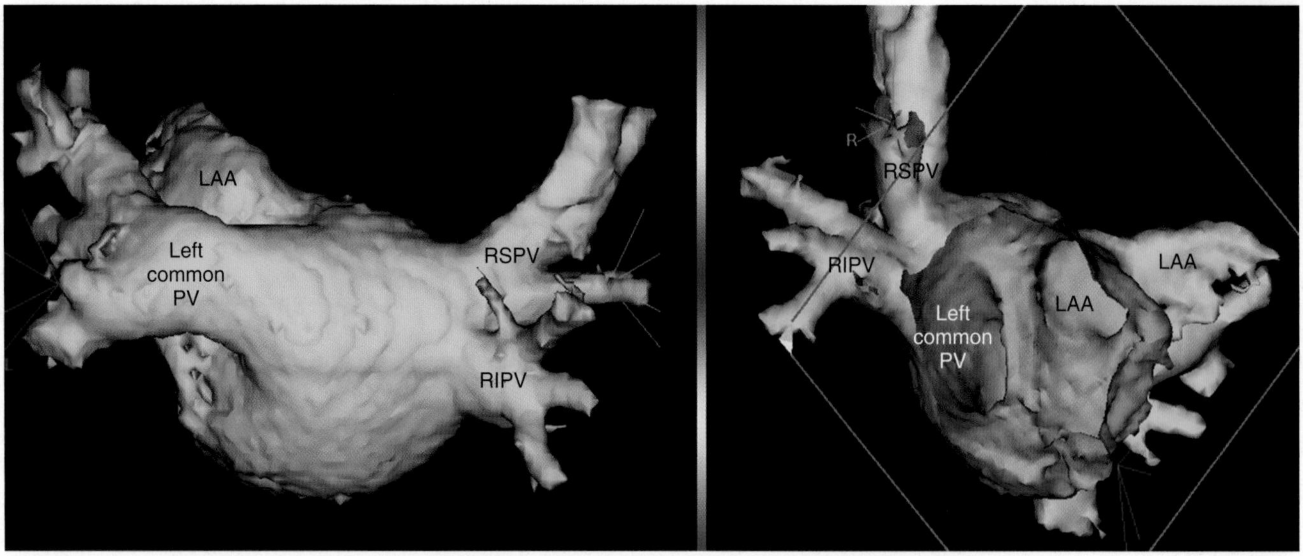

FIGURE 11–3 Cardiac CT angiogram (posteroanterior and cardioscopic views) showing common ostium for left pulmonary vein (PVs). LAA = LA appendage; RIPV = right inferior PV; RSPV = right superior PV.

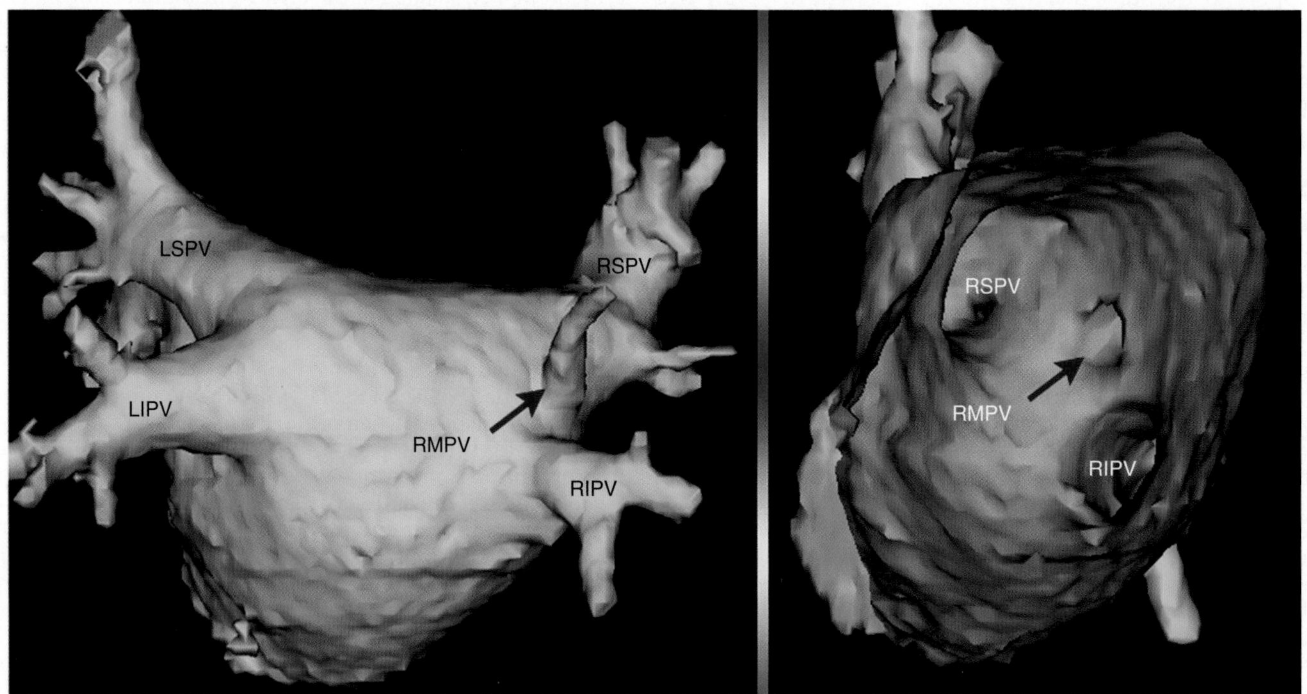

FIGURE 11–4 Cardiac CT angiogram (posteroanterior and cardioscopic views) showing right middle PV (RMPV). LIPV = left inferior PV; LSPV = left superior PV; RIPV = right inferior PV; RSPV = right superior PV.

oxysmal AF. Significant variability of PV morphologies, however, exist, including supernumerary right PVs (in 8% to 29% of patients; Fig. 11-4), multiple ramification and early branching (especially of the right inferior PV), and common ostium of left-sided or, less frequently, right-sided PVs.

The PVs are covered by myocardial sleeves formed by one or more layers of myocardial fibers oriented in a circular, longitudinal, oblique, or spiral direction. These sleeves, continuing from the LA into the PV, vary from 2 to 25 mm in length, with a mean extent of 13 mm. The length of the myocardial sleeves usually has a distinctive distribution; superior PVs have longer and better developed myocardial sleeves than inferior PVs, which may explain why arrhythmogenic foci are found more often in the superior than in inferior PVs.[5,7]

The walls of the PVs are composed of a thin endothelium, a media of smooth muscle, and a thick outer fibrous adventitia. The transition from atrial to venous walls is gradual because the myocardial sleeves from the LA overlap with the smooth muscle of the venous wall. The myocardial sleeves are thickest at the venoatrial junction (mean, 1.1 mm) and then gradually taper distally. Furthermore, the thickness of the sleeves is not uniform, with the inferior walls of the superior veins and the superior walls of the inferior veins having the thicker sleeves. Throughout the PV, and even at the venoatrial junction, there are gaps in the myocardial sleeves mainly composed of fibrous tissue. The arrangement of the myocyte bundles within the sleeves is rather complex. There appears to be a mesh-like arrangement of muscle fascicles made up of circularly oriented bundles (spiraling around the long axis of the vein) that interconnect with bundles that run in a longitudinal orientation (along the long axis of the vein). Such an arrangement, together with the patchy areas of fibrosis seen, may be relevant to the role of the PVs in the initiation of AF.[5]

Electrophysiology of Pulmonary Vein Musculature

The PVs play a role in the initiation and maintenance of AF. However, it is not clear what makes this region so susceptible to the arrhythmia.[5,6,9,20,21] There are, at present, limited data available on the ionic mechanisms that may underlie the arrhythmogenicity of PVs. Detailed mapping studies have suggested that reentry within the PVs is most likely responsible for their arrhythmogenicity, although focal or triggered activity cannot be excluded.

The electrophysiology of the PV, with its distinct area of slow conduction, decremental conduction, nonuniform anisotropy, and heterogeneous repolarization, is a potential substrate for reentry. The heterogeneous fiber orientation in the transition from the LA to the PV sleeve results in unique conduction properties in this area.[5,8-11] It is possible that the complex arrangement of muscle fibers within the myocardial sleeves and the uneven distribution of interspersed connective and adipose tissue account for the greater degree of decremental conduction observed in the myocardial sleeves than in the LA, and for the heterogeneity in conduction properties and refractory periods among the fascicles in the myocardial sleeves. Therefore, the fractionation of PV potentials commonly observed during premature stimulation (which usually indicates local slowing of conduction) is consistent with anisotropic properties that may be attributable to the complex arrangement of muscle fascicles within the myocardial sleeves.[7]

Several studies have suggested that abnormal automaticity or triggered activity, either alone or in combination with the reentrant mechanisms described above, may play a role in the initiation of AF. These studies would suggest that the propensity of PVs to exhibit focal or triggered activity is enhanced by pathological conditions.[5,8] Further work also implicates the posterior LA in the genesis of AF. Recent studies have suggested that the PVs, together with the posterior LA, have an important role in the persistent form of AF. However, the nature of the relationship between this arrhythmogenic region and the pathological conditions that provide a substrate for AF has not been elucidated. Whether the critical region is the posterior LA, the PVs, or both, has been the source of ongoing debate.[9]

There is some experimental evidence to suggest that the electrical properties of the PVs can be modulated by changes in autonomic tone. Anatomical studies have revealed that the LA and PVs are innervated by adrenergic and cholinergic nerve fibers. The role of this innervation has been further highlighted by a clinical study that suggested that the risk of AF recurrence following circumferential PV ablation is further reduced if ablation abolishes all vagal reflexes around the PV ostia.

Pulmonary Vein Tachycardia Versus Pulmonary Vein Fibrillation

In patients with paroxysmal AF originating from the PVs, a wide spectrum of atrial arrhythmias may coexist. Extensive monitoring will frequently document coexisting paroxysms of AT and AF. Furthermore, patients with paroxysmal AF usually have multiple PV foci in multiple veins and many of these foci originate distally in those veins.[22,23]

In patients whose only clinical arrhythmia is PV AT, the clinical course is more comparable to patients with AT from other anatomical locations than to patients with PV AF.[22] Those patients demonstrate a largely focal process, without evidence of a more progressive and diffuse process as observed in the paroxysmal AF population, and there is no tendency to develop further atrial arrhythmias during long-term follow-up. Notably, when patients with PV AT present with recurrence, in almost all cases this is from the original focus.[22,23] In contrast, patients with paroxysmal AF have recurrences from foci in other PVs and from within the body of the LA. Importantly, in most patients with PV AT, the focus is located at the ostium of the vein (or within 1 cm of the designated ostium) rather than from further distally (2 to 4 cm).[22,23] These observations suggest that patients with focal PV AT may represent a different population from those with PV AF. PV AT patients have a discrete and focally curable process in contrast to the more diffuse process involving multiple PVs and the LA seen in AF.

The spontaneous onset of focal AT from the PVs and its lack of inducibility with programmed stimulation suggest that this arrhythmia is more likely to be caused by abnormal automaticity or triggered activity rather than reentry. However, attempts to definitively classify the arrhythmia mechanism of focal AT in the EP laboratory are limited because of the significant overlap in the arrhythmia characteristics (initiation, response to drugs).[22]

CLINICAL CONSIDERATIONS

Epidemiology

AF is the most common clinically significant cardiac arrhythmia, accounting for approximately one third of hospitalizations for cardiac rhythm disturbance. It has been estimated that 2.3 million people in the United States and 4.5 million in the European Union have paroxysmal or persistent AF.

The prevalence of AF is estimated at 0.4% to 1.0% of the general population, increasing with age. AF is uncommon in childhood except after cardiac surgery. It occurs in less than 1% of those younger than 60 years but in more than 6% of those older than 80 years. The age-adjusted prevalence is higher in men. Blacks have less than half the age-adjusted risk of developing AF than whites. The frequency of lone AF was less than 12% of all cases of AF in some series but more than 30% in others.[24]

AF is associated with an increased long-term risk of stroke, heart failure, and all-cause mortality, especially in women. The mortality rate of patients with AF is about double that of patients in NSR and is linked to the severity of underlying heart disease.[24]

The most devastating consequence of AF is stroke as a result of thromboembolism, typically emanating from the LA appendage. Patients with paroxysmal and persistent AF appear to have a risk of stroke similar to that in patients with permanent AF. The rate of ischemic stroke in patients with nonrheumatic AF averages 5% per year, which is two to seven times the rate for people without AF. One of every six strokes occurs in patients with AF. Including transient ischemic attacks and clinically silent strokes detected radiographically, the rate of brain ischemia accompanying nonvalvular AF exceeds 7% per year. In the Framingham Heart Study, patients with rheumatic heart disease and AF had a 17-fold increased risk of stroke compared with age-matched controls, and the attributable risk was five times greater than in those with nonrheumatic AF. The annual risk of stroke attributable to AF increased from 1.5% in Framingham Study participants aged 50 to 59 years to 23.5% for those aged 80 to 89 years.[24]

Clinical Risk Factors Predisposing to Atrial Fibrillation

AF can be related to a transient reversible cause, such as thyrotoxicosis, acute myocardial infarction, acute pericarditis, recent cardiac surgery, acute pulmonary disease, alcohol intake, or electrocution. In these cases, AF is generally eliminated by treatment of the underlying precipitating condition.

AF is the final arrhythmic expression of a diverse family of diseases. AF derives from a complex continuum of predisposing factors that appear to involve disease processes that contribute to the triggering of AF (e.g., sympathetic and parasympathetic nervous systems [neurogenic AF], predisposing arrhythmias, ectopic foci in PVs), increase atrial distention (e.g., valvular heart disease, hypertension, and heart failure), decrease the ratio of atrial myocyte to fibrotic tissue, possibly including an increased rate of apoptotic cell death (e.g., hypertension and ischemic heart disease), disrupt transmyocyte communications (e.g., pericarditis and edema), increase inflammatory mediators (e.g., pericarditis and myocarditis), and/or alter energy and redox states that modulate the function of ion channels and gap junctions.[3]

In the West, about 5% of the population older than 65 years is afflicted with AF.[3] The most frequent causes of acute AF are myocardial infarction (5% to 10% of patients with infarct) and cardiothoracic surgery (up to 40% of patients).[3] The most common clinical settings for permanent AF are hypertension and ischemic heart disease, with the subset of patients having congestive heart failure most likely to experience the arrhythmia. In the developing world, hypertension and rheumatic valvular (usually mitral) and congenital heart diseases are the most commonly related conditions.

Adrenergic and vagotonic forms of paroxysmal AF are uncommon. Nonetheless, patients with lone AF often have attacks against the background of parasympathetic predominance, whereas paroxysms in patients with structural heart disease more usually occur in a sympathetic setting.[3]

In younger patients, approximately 30% to 45% of paroxysmal cases and 20% to 25% of persistent cases of AF occur as lone AF.

Clinical Presentation

AF can be symptomatic or asymptomatic, even in the same patient. Asymptomatic, or silent, AF occurs frequently; in patients with paroxysmal AF, up to 90% of episodes are not
11 recognized by the patient, including some lasting longer than 48 hours. On the other hand, continuous monitoring with a pacemaker with dedicated functions for AF detection and electrogram storage has shown that as many as 40% of patients have episodes of AF-like symptoms in the absence of AF. Up to 21% of patients with newly diagnosed AF are asymptomatic.

Symptoms associated with AF vary with the ventricular rate, underlying functional status, duration of AF, presence and degree of structural heart disease, and individual patient perception. The hemodynamic consequences of AF are related to the loss of atrial mechanical function, irregularity of ventricular response, and fast heart rate. These consequences are magnified in the presence of impaired diastolic ventricular filling, hypertension, mitral stenosis, left ventricular (LV) hypertrophy, and restrictive cardiomyopathy. Irregularity of the cardiac cycle, especially when accompanied by short coupling intervals, and rapid heart rates in AF lead to a reduction in diastolic filling, stroke volume, and cardiac output.[24]

Most patients with AF complain of palpitations, angina, dyspnea, fatigue, or dizziness. Furthermore, AF with a chronically elevated heart rate (≥130 beats/min) can lead to tachycardia-mediated cardiomyopathy. Syncope is an uncommon complication of AF that can occur on conversion in patients with sinus node dysfunction or because of rapid ventricular rates in patients with hypertrophic cardiomyopathy, in patients with valvular aortic stenosis, or in patients with an accessory pathway present. The first presentation of asymptomatic AF may be catastrophic—an embolic complication or exacerbation of heart failure.[24]

Initial Evaluation

The initial evaluation of a patient with suspected or documented AF includes characterizing the pattern of the arrhythmia (e.g., paroxysmal or persistent), determining underlying causes (e.g., heart failure, pulmonary problems, hypertension, or hyperthyroidism), and defining associated cardiac and extracardiac conditions. A careful history will result in a well-planned focused workup that serves as an effective guide to therapy.

The physical examination may suggest AF on the basis of irregular pulse, irregular jugular venous pulsations, and variation in the intensity of the first heart sound. Examination may also disclose associated valvular heart disease, myocardial abnormalities, or heart failure.

Exercise testing is often used to assess the adequacy of rate control with exercise in permanent AF, to reproduce exercise-induced AF, and to evaluate for associated ischemic heart disease, which is not a common cause of AF. Identifying underlying coronary artery disease is particularly important if a class IC antiarrhythmic drug is used. Ambulatory cardiac monitoring may also be required for documentation of AF, its relation to symptoms, and evaluation of the adequacy of heart rate control.[24]

Assessment for hyperthyroidism is indicated for all patients with a first episode of AF, when the ventricular response to AF is difficult to control, or when AF recurs unexpectedly after cardioversion. Serum should be obtained for measurement of thyroid-stimulating hormone (TSH) and free thyroxine (T_4), even if there are no symptoms suggestive of hyperthyroidism, because the risk of AF is increased up to threefold in patients with subclinical hyperthyroidism.

Rarely, EP testing can be required, especially in patients with wide QRS complex tachycardia or a possible predisposing arrhythmia, such as AFL or paroxysmal SVT.

Principles of Management

There are four main issues that must be addressed in the treatment of AF: (1) prevention of systemic embolization, (2) rate control, (3) rhythm control, and (4) choosing between rhythm and rate control. The choice of therapy is influenced by patient preference, associated structural heart disease, severity of symptoms, and whether the AF is recurrent paroxysmal, recurrent persistent, or permanent (chronic). In addition, patient education is critical, given the potential morbidity associated with AF and its treatment.[24]

Prevention of Systemic Embolization

Anticoagulation During the Pericardioversion Period. Based on observational studies, the American College of Cardiology–American Heart Association (ACC/AHA) has strongly recommended that outpatients without a contraindication to warfarin who have been in AF for more than 48 hours should receive 3 to 4 weeks of warfarin prior to and after cardioversion. This approach is also recommended for patients with AF who have valvular disease, evidence of LV dysfunction, recent thromboembolism, or AF of unknown duration.[24]

The rationale for anticoagulation prior to cardioversion is that more than 85% of LA thrombi resolve after 4 weeks of warfarin therapy. Thromboembolic events have been reported in 1% to 7% of patients who did not receive anticoagulation before cardioversion. The recommended target international normalized ratio (INR) is 2.5 (range, 2.0 to 3.0). It has been suggested that it may be prudent to aim for an INR higher than 2.5 before cardioversion to provide the greatest protection against embolic events. Probably more important is to document that the INR has consistently been higher than 2.0 in the weeks before cardioversion.[24]

An alternative approach that eliminates the need for prolonged anticoagulation prior to cardioversion, particularly in low-risk patients who would benefit from earlier cardioversion, is the use of transesophageal echocardiography (TEE)–guided cardioversion. Cardioversion is performed if TEE excludes the presence of intracardiac clots. Anticoagulation after cardioversion, however, is still necessary.

After cardioversion, it is recommended to continue warfarin therapy for at least 4 weeks, with a target INR of 2.5 (range, 2.0 to 3.0). This recommendation only deals with protection from embolic events related to the cardioversion period. Subsequently, the long-term recommendations for patients who have been cardioverted to NSR but are at high risk for thromboembolism are similar to those for patients with chronic AF, even though the patients are in NSR.[24]

A different approach with respect to anticoagulation can be used in low-risk patients (no mitral valve disease, severe LV dysfunction, or history of recent thromboembolism) in whom there is reasonable certainty that AF has been present for less than 48 hours. Such patients have a low risk of clinical thromboembolism if converted early (0.8% in one study), even without screening TEE. The ACC/AHA guidelines do not recommend long-term anticoagulation prior to cardioversion in such patients, but do recommend heparin use at presentation and during the pericardioversion period. The optimal therapy after cardioversion in this group is uncertain. A common practice is to administer aspirin for a first episode of AF that converts spontaneously and warfarin for at least 4 weeks to all other patients. Aspirin should not be considered for patients with AF less than 48 hours' duration if there is associated rheumatic mitral valve disease, severe LV dysfunction, or recent thromboembolism. Such patients should be treated the same as patients with AF of longer duration: 1 month of oral anticoagulation with warfarin or shorter term anticoagulation with screening TEE prior to elective electrical or pharmacological cardioversion, followed by prolonged warfarin therapy after cardioversion.[24]

Long-Term Anticoagulation. Compared with the general population, AF significantly increases the risk of stroke (relative risk, 2.4 in men and 3.0 in women). However, the risk varies markedly among patients. The incidence of stroke is relatively low in patients with AF younger than 65 years who have no risk factors. The prevalence of stroke associated with AF increases strikingly with age and with other risk factors, including diabetes, hypertension, previous stroke, and LV dysfunction.[24]

The stroke risk appears to be equivalent in paroxysmal and chronic AF and, as noted in the AFFIRM and RACE trials, equivalent with a rate control or rhythm control management strategy.[25,26] Furthermore, the reduction in ischemic stroke with oral anticoagulation in patients with paroxysmal AF is probably similar to that in patients with chronic AF. There are at least two reasons for the risk of embolization, even when NSR is present most of the time. First, recurrent episodes of paroxysmal AF are common and asymptomatic in up to 90% of patients; even episodes lasting longer than 48 hours may not be recognized by the patient. Second, some patients have other reasons for embolic risk, such as complex aortic plaque or LV systolic dysfunction.[24]

The choice of therapy (warfarin versus aspirin) varies with the estimated embolic risk. Although a number of risk stratification models are available for patients with chronic AF, the $CHADS_2$ score is currently the best validated and most clinically useful (Table 11-1). Patients with a $CHADS_2$ score of 0 are at low risk of embolization (0.5% per year in the absence of warfarin) and can be managed with aspirin. Patients with a $CHADS_2$ score higher than 3 are at high risk (5.3% to 6.9% per year) and should, in the absence of a contraindication, be treated with warfarin. Patients with a $CHADS_2$ score of 1 or 2 are at intermediate risk of embolization (1.5% to 2.5% per year). In this group, the choice between warfarin therapy and aspirin will depend on many factors, including patient preference.[24,27]

Anticoagulation is beneficial in all age groups, including patients older than 75 years and when given for secondary prevention in patients with nonrheumatic AF who have had a recent stroke. The true efficacy of warfarin is likely to be even higher than suggested by trial results, because many of the strokes in the warfarin-treated groups occurred in patients who were noncompliant at the time of the stroke.[24]

An INR between 2.0 and 3.0 is recommended for most patients with AF who receive warfarin therapy. The risk of stroke doubles when the INR falls to 1.7, and values up to 3.5 do not convey an increased risk of bleeding complications. A higher goal (INR between 2.5 and 3.5) is reasonable for patients at particularly high risk for embolization (e.g., prior thromboembolism, rheumatic heart disease, prosthetic heart valves). A possible exception to the latter recommendation occurs in patients older than 75 years who are at increased risk for major bleeding. A target INR of 1.8 to 2.5 may be a reasonable compromise between toxicity and efficacy for this age group.[24,28]

TABLE 11–1 Stroke Risk in Patients with Nonvalvular Atrial Fibrillation According to $CHADS_2$ Index*

$CHADS_2$ Risk Criteria		Point(s)
Prior stroke or TIA		2
Age > 75 yr		1
Hypertension		1
Diabetes mellitus		1
Heart failure		1
Patients (N = 1733)	**Adjusted Stroke Rate† (5%/yr) (95% CI)**	**$CHADS_2$ Score**
120	1.9 (1.2-3.0)	0
463	2.8 (2.0-3.8)	1
523	4.0 (3.1-5.1)	2
337	5.9 (4.6-7.3)	3
220	8.5 (6.3-11.1)	4
65	12.5 (8.2-17.5)	5
5	18.2 (10.5-27.4)	6

*Not treated with anticoagulation.

†The adjusted stroke rate was derived from multivariate analysis assuming no aspirin usage.

$CHADS_2$ = *c*ardiac failure, *h*ypertension, *a*ge, *d*iabetes, and *s*troke (doubled); CI = confidence interval; TIA = transient ischemic attack.

From Gage BF, Waterman AD, Shannon W, et al: Validation of clinical classification schemes for predicting stroke: Results from the National Registry of Atrial Fibrillation. JAMA 2001;285:2864-2870.

Rate Control

Rate control during AF is important to prevent hemodynamic instability and/or symptoms such as palpitations, heart failure, lightheadedness, and poor exercise capacity and, over the long-term, to prevent tachycardia-mediated cardiomyopathy. Beta blockers (e.g., atenolol or metoprolol), diltiazem, and verapamil are recommended for rate control during rest and exercise; digoxin is not effective during exercise and should be used in patients with heart failure or hypotension, or as a second-line agent. Adequacy of rate control should be assessed at rest and with exertion. Goals include a resting heart rate of 60 to 80 beats/min and 90 to 115 beats/min during exercise, and a 24-hour Holter average heart rate less than 100 beats/min and no heart rate higher than 110% of the age-predicted maximum.[24]

AV junction ablation and permanent pacemaker implantation are highly effective means of improving symptoms in patients with AF who experience symptoms related to a rapid ventricular rate during AF that cannot be adequately controlled with antiarrhythmic or negative chronotropic medications. AV junction ablation is especially useful when an excessive ventricular rate induces a tachycardia-mediated decline in ventricular systolic function, despite appropriate medical therapy.[29]

Rhythm Control

Reversion to Normal Sinus Rhythm. Reasons for restoration and maintenance of sinus rhythm in patients with AF include relief of symptoms, prevention of embolism, and avoidance of cardiomyopathy. When rhythm control is chosen, both electrical and pharmacological cardioversion are appropriate options. The timing of attempted cardioversion is influenced by the duration of AF. In particular, patients with AF longer than 48 hours' duration or unknown duration may have atrial thrombi that can embolize. In such patients, cardioversion should be delayed until the patient has been anticoagulated at appropriate levels for 3 to 4 weeks or TEE has excluded atrial thrombi.[24]

Electrical cardioversion is indicated for patients who are hemodynamically unstable, a setting in which the AF is typically of short duration. In stable patients in whom spontaneous reversion caused by correction of an underlying disease is not likely, electrical or pharmacological cardioversion can be performed. Electrical cardioversion is usually preferred because of greater efficacy and a low risk of proarrhythmia. The overall success rate (at any level of energy) of electrical cardioversion for AF is 75% to 93% and is
11 related inversely to the duration of AF and to LA size.

A number of antiarrhythmic drugs have been found to be more effective than placebo for cardioversion of AF, converting 30% to 60% of patients. Evidence of efficacy from randomized trials has been best established for dofetilide, flecainide, ibutilide, propafenone, amiodarone, and quinidine. The ACC/AHA guidelines have concluded that evidence for benefit from specific antiarrhythmic drugs varies with the duration of AF—dofetilide, flecainide, ibutilide, propafenone or, to a lesser degree, amiodarone (unless the patient has LV dysfunction or heart failure) if less than 7 days' duration; and dofetilide or, to a lesser degree, amiodarone or ibutilide if AF is more prolonged. Rate control with an atrioventricular nodal (AVN) blocker (beta blocker, diltiazem, verapamil or, if the patient has heart failure or hypotension, digoxin) should be attained before instituting a class IA drug because of possible recurrence with AFL and a very rapid ventricular rate.[24]

Maintenance of Normal Sinus Rhythm. Only 20% to 30% of patients who are successfully cardioverted maintain NSR for more than 1 year without chronic antiarrhythmic therapy. This is more likely to occur in patients with AF for less than 1 year, no enlargement of the LA (less than 4.0 cm), and a reversible cause of AF, such as hyperthyroidism, pericarditis, pulmonary embolism, or cardiac surgery. It has been thought that the drugs most likely to maintain NSR suppress triggering ectopic beats and arrhythmias, and affect atrial EP properties to diminish the likelihood of AF. There is, therefore, a strong rationale for prophylactic antiarrhythmic drug therapy in patients who have a moderate to high risk for recurrence, provided that it is effective and that toxic and proarrhythmic effects are low. Prophylactic drug treatment is seldom indicated in patients with a first-detected episode of AF and can also be avoided in patients with infrequent and well-tolerated paroxysmal AF.[24]

Evidence of efficacy from randomized trials is best for amiodarone, propafenone, disopyramide, sotalol, flecainide, dofetilide, and quinidine. The choice, as recommended by the ACC/AHA guidelines, varies with the clinical setting. As examples, flecainide and propafenone are preferred for patients with no or minimal heart disease, whereas amiodarone and dofetilide are preferred for patients with reduced LV ejection fraction or heart failure and sotalol for patients with coronary artery disease. Concurrent administration of an AVN blocker is indicated for patients who have demonstrated a moderate to rapid ventricular response to AF.

In patients with lone AF, a beta blocker may be tried first, but flecainide, propafenone, and sotalol are particularly effective. Amiodarone and dofetilide are recommended as alternative therapy. Quinidine, procainamide, and disopyramide are not favored unless amiodarone fails or is contraindicated. The anticholinergic activity of long-acting disopyramide makes this a relatively attractive choice for patients with a predilection to vagally induced AF. Propafenone is not recommended in vagally mediated AF because its (weak) intrinsic beta-blocking activity may aggravate this type of paroxysmal AF. In patients with adrenergically mediated AF, beta blockers represent first-line treatment, followed by sotalol. In patients with lone AF, amiodarone should be chosen later in the sequence of drug therapy because of its potential toxicity. Overall, when treatment with a single drug fails, combinations of antiarrhythmic drugs may be tried. Useful combinations include a beta blocker, sotalol, or amiodarone, plus a type IC agent.[24] When AF recurrences are infrequent and tolerated, patients experiencing breakthrough arrhythmias might not require a change in antiarrhythmic drug therapy.

Antiarrhythmic therapy should be chosen on the basis of the patient's underlying cardiac condition. Class IC agents are reserved to treat patients without a structural cardiac abnormality, and may be prescribed for outpatients with acute conversion of paroxysmal AF (i.e., the so-called pill in the pocket approach). Class IA and III agents should be avoided by patients with prolongation of the QT interval or LV hypertrophy because of the potential for ventricular arrhythmias. On the one hand, amiodarone, which has a low risk of proarrhythmia (less than 1% per year), causes substantial noncardiac toxic effects and is therefore generally reserved for second-line therapy, except in the treatment of patients with severe cardiomyopathy. On the other hand, it is the most effective antifibrillatory agent; in one trial, 65% of patients treated with amiodarone were free from recurrence after 16 months of therapy, as compared with 37% of those who were treated with propafenone or sotalol.[24]

Rhythm Control Versus Rate Control. In the past, many physicians preferred rhythm to rate control. Reversion of AF and maintenance of NSR restores normal hemodynamics and had been thought to reduce the frequency of embolism. However, two major clinical trials (AFFIRM and RACE) have compared rhythm and rate control and found that embolic events occur with equal frequency, regardless of whether a rate control or rhythm control strategy is pursued, and occur most often after warfarin has been stopped or when the INR is subtherapeutic. Both studies also have shown an almost significant trend toward a lower incidence of the primary endpoint with rate control (hazard ratio, 0.87 for mortality in AFFIRM and 0.73 for a composite endpoint in RACE). There was no difference in the functional status or quality of life. Thus, both rhythm and rate control are acceptable approaches and both require anticoagulation. The trials have provided supportive evidence for the rate control option in most patients.[30-32]

However, it would be incorrect to extrapolate that NSR offers no benefit over AF and that effective treatments to maintain NSR need not be pursued. First, these trials were not comparisons of NSR and AF. They compared a rate control strategy to a rhythm control strategy that attempted to maintain NSR but fell short. The failure of AFFIRM and RACE in showing any difference between rate and rhythm control is not so much a positive statement for rate control but rather a testimony to the ineffectiveness of the rhythm control methods used. Failure of rhythm control to demonstrate superiority over rate control is caused by failure to achieve maintenance of NSR over the long term. Several trials have demonstrated that the success of antiarrhythmic therapy in maintaining NSR is borderline, at best, with increasing failure rates over time. When the data from these trials are analyzed according to the patient's actual rhythm (as opposed to his or her treatment strategy), the benefit of NSR over AF becomes apparent—the presence of NSR is found to be one of the most powerful independent predictors of survival, along with the use of warfarin, even after adjustment for all other relevant clinical variables. Patients in NSR are almost half as likely to die compared with those with AF. This benefit, however, is offset by the use of antiarrhythmic drug therapy, which increases the risk of death.[30-32]

Nonpharmacological Approaches. There are several alternative methods to maintain NSR in patients who are refractory to conventional therapy, including surgery, catheter ablation, atrial defibrillators, and pacemakers. Device-based therapy, however, has demonstrated poor efficacy in treating AF. Burst atrial pacing may effectively convert atrial tachycardia or flutter but fails to terminate or minimize AF. Atrial defibrillators can terminate AF with high acute success rates, but the need for repeated shocks and the resulting patient discomfort often render this option intolerable. Similarly, dual-site atrial pacing has failed to demonstrate any consistent reduction in AF burden or improvement in AF symptoms.

Although surgical ablation of AF is the most effective means of curing this arrhythmia, with the classic maze procedure eliminating AF in more than 90% of patients, the maze procedure is a complex operation and has been applied by relatively few surgeons. Several modifications have been made over time; in addition to the standard cut and sew surgical technique, cryoablation, unipolar or bipolar RF ablation, and microwave ablation have been introduced as alternatives. Most surgical ablation procedures have been performed in conjunction with mitral valve surgery; the combination of mitral valve repair and cure of AF enables patients to avoid lifelong anticoagulation. Developed surgical instrumentation now enables thoracoscopic and keyhole approaches, facilitating the extension of epicardial AF ablation and excision of the LA appendage to patients with isolated AF and no other indication for cardiac surgery.[33]

Currently, the mainstay of nonpharmacological rhythm control is catheter ablation, which has emerged as a curative approach for AF. Catheter ablation of AF can help maintain NSR without the risk associated with long-term antiarrhythmic therapy. Restoration of NSR after catheter ablation for AF significantly improved LV function, exercise capacity, symptoms, and quality of life (usually within the first 3 to 6 months), even in the presence of concurrent heart disease and when ventricular rate control was adequate before ablation. Catheter ablation of AF should be considered after failure of antiarrhythmic medication. In the absence of any large, randomized trial of catheter ablation as a first-line therapy for AF in symptomatic or asymptomatic patients, a history of symptoms, despite therapeutic doses of antiarrhythmic medication (type IA, IC, or III), is widely accepted as the minimum qualifying criterion for catheter ablation. With improved efficacy of ablation techniques, however, the threshold for ablation will continue to fall.[34]

ELECTROCARDIOGRAPHIC AND ELECTROPHYSIOLOGICAL FEATURES

Atrial Activity

AF is characterized by rapid and irregular atrial fibrillatory waves (f waves) and lack of clearly defined P waves, with an undulating baseline that may alternate between recognizable atrial activity and a nearly flat line (Fig. 11-5). Atrial fibrillatory activity is generally best seen in lead V_1 and in the inferior leads. Less often, the f waves are most prominent in leads I and aVL.

The rate of the fibrillatory waves is generally between 350 and 600 beats/min. With up to 600 pulses being generated

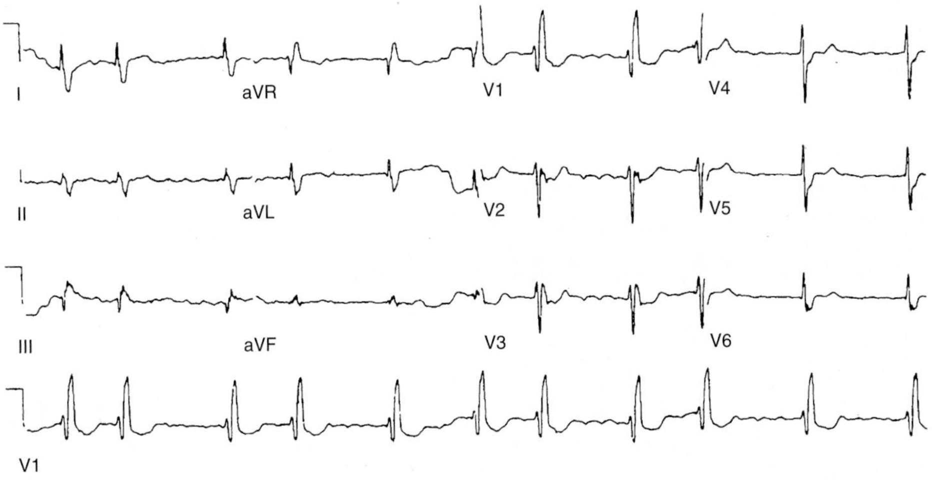

FIGURE 11–5 Surface ECG of AF with chronic right bundle branch block.

every minute, syncytial contraction of the atria is replaced by irregular atrial twitches. Therefore, the fibrillating atria look like bags of worms in that the contractions are very rapid and irregular. The f waves vary in amplitude, morphology, and intervals, reflecting the multiple potential types of atrial activation that may be present at the same time at different locations throughout the atria. The f waves can be fine (amplitude less than 0.5 mm on ECG) or coarse (amplitude more than 0.5 mm). On occasion, the f waves may be inapparent on the standard and precordial leads, which is most likely to occur in permanent AF. It was initially thought that the amplitude of the f waves correlated with increasing atrial size; however, echocardiographic studies have failed to show a correlation among the amplitude of the f waves, the size of the atria, and the type of heart disease. The amplitude, however, may correlate with the duration of AF.

AF should be distinguished from other rhythms in which the R-R intervals are irregularly irregular. These include multifocal atrial tachycardia, wandering atrial pacemaker, multifocal PACs, and AT or AFL with varying AV block. In general, distinct (although often abnormal and possibly variable) P (or flutter) waves are present during these arrhythmias, in contrast to AF. Patients with rheumatic mitral stenosis often demonstrate large-amplitude fibrillatory waves in the anterior precordial leads (V_1 and V_2), which can be confused with AFL. However, careful examination of the fibrillatory waves reveals them to have a varying CL and morphology. The distinction between AF and AFL can also be confusing in patients who demonstrate a transition between these arrhythmias. Thus, AF may organize to AFL or AFL may degenerate to AF. Occasionally, extracardiac artifacts (e.g., 60 cycle/min muscle tremors, as in parkinsonism) can simulate f waves.

Intracardiac recordings demonstrate variability in the atrial electrogram morphology, amplitude, and CL from beat to beat. The different patterns of conduction during AF may be reflected in the morphology of atrial electrograms recorded with mapping during induced AF. Single potentials usually indicate rapid uniform conduction, short double potentials may indicate collision, long double potentials are usually indicative of conduction block, and fragmented potentials and complex fractionated atrial electrograms are markers for pivoting points or slow conduction.

One study attempted to codify AF using RA epicardial electrograms after cardiac surgery. Four distinct types of AF were identified. Type I AF showed atrial electrograms with discrete complexes of variable morphology separated by an isoelectric baseline. The mean atrial rate ranged from 291 to 405 beats/min. Type II AF demonstrated discrete atrial electrograms in the absence of an isoelectric baseline. The mean atrial rate was 383 beats/min. Type III AF was characterized by the absence of discrete atrial complexes or isoelectric intervals. Type IV AF involved the alternation of type III with type I or II electrograms.

Atrioventricular Conduction During Atrial Fibrillation

The ventricular response in AF is typically irregularly irregular, and the ventricular rate depends on multiple factors, including the EP properties of the AVN, rate and organization of atrial inputs to the AVN, level of autonomic tone, effects of medications that act on the AV conduction system, and presence of preexcitation over an AV BT.

The ventricular rate in untreated patients usually ranges from 90 up to 170 beats/min. Ventricular rates that are clearly outside this range suggest some concurrent problem. Ventricular rates below 60 beats/min are seen with AVN disease, and can be associated with the sick sinus syndrome, drugs that affect conduction, and high vagal tone, as can occur in a well-conditioned athlete. The ventricular rate in AF can become rapid (more than 200 beats/min) during exercise, with catecholamine excess (Fig. 11-6), parasympathetic withdrawal, thyrotoxicosis, or preexcitation (Fig. 11-7). The ventricular rate can be very rapid (more than 300 beats/min) in patients with the Wolff-Parkinson-White (WPW) syndrome, with conduction over AV BTs having short anterograde refractory periods.

The compact AVN is located anteriorly in the triangle of Koch. There are two distinct atrial inputs to the AVN, anteriorly via the interatrial septum and posteriorly via the crista terminalis. Experiments in a rabbit AVN preparation have demonstrated that propagation of impulses during AF through the AVN to the His bundle (HB) is critically dependent on the relative timing of activation of septal inputs to the AVN at the crista terminalis and interatrial septum. Other investigators have shown that the ventricular response also depends on atrial input frequency.

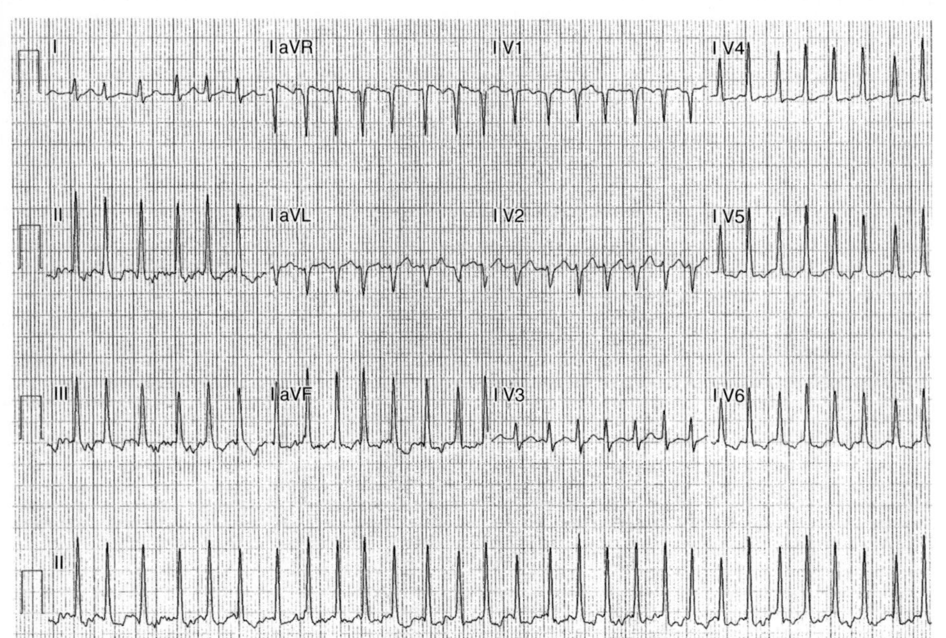

FIGURE 11–6 Surface ECG of atrial fibrillation (AF) with fast ventricular response (207 beats/min) in a patient with septic shock on dopamine infusion.

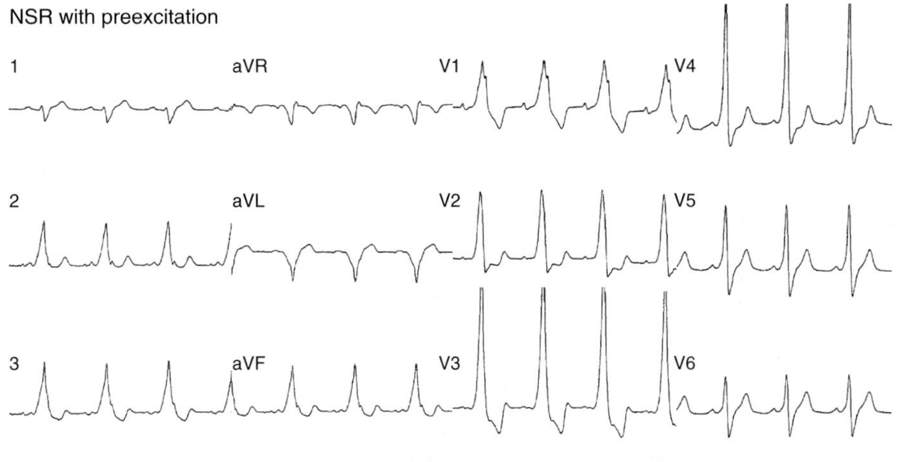

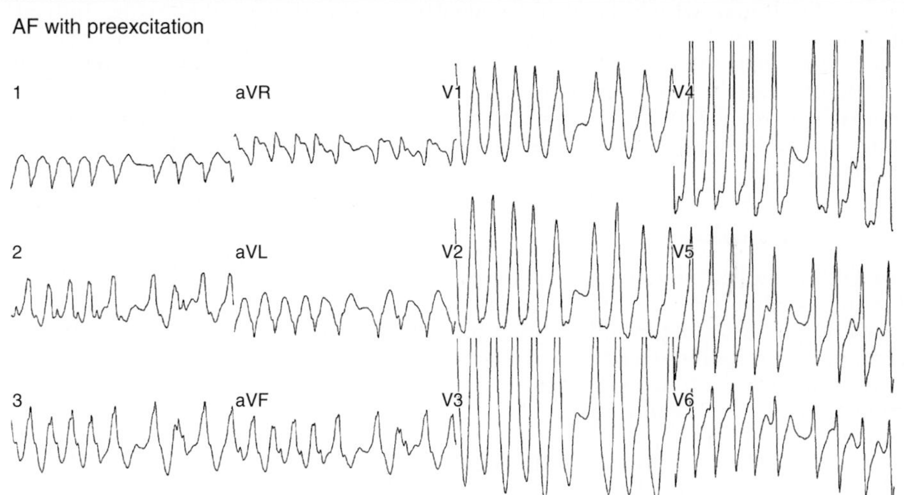

FIGURE 11–7 Preexcited atrial fibrillation (AF). **Upper panel,** ECG showing normal sinus rhythm (NSR) with Wolff-Parkinson-White (WPW) pattern and preexcitation using a left lateral bypass tract (BT). **Lower panel,** ECG showing preexcited AF.

Concealed conduction likely plays the predominant role in determining ventricular response during AF. The constant bombardment of atrial impulses into the AVN creates substantial and varying degrees of concealed conduction, with atrial impulses that enter the AVN but do not conduct to the ventricle, leaving a wake of refractoriness encountered by subsequent impulses. This also accounts for the irregular ventricular response during AF; although the AVN would be expected to conduct whenever it recovers excitability after the last conducted atrial impulse, which would then be at regular intervals, the ventricular response is irregularly irregular because of the varying depth of penetration of the numerous fibrillatory impulses approaching the AVN, leaving it refractory in the face of subsequent atrial impulses.

Alterations of autonomic tone can have profound effects on AVN conduction. Enhanced parasympathetic and sympathetic tone have negative and positive dromotropic effects, respectively, on AVN conduction. An additional factor is the use of AVN blocking agents such as digoxin, calcium channel blockers, or beta blockers. There also may be a circadian rhythm for both AVN refractoriness and concealed conduction, accounting for the circadian variation in ventricular rate.

Preexcitation During Atrial Fibrillation. The presence of a grossly irregular, very rapid ventricular response during AF rarely results from conduction over the AVN and is diagnostic of conduction over an AV BT, with rare exceptions (see Fig. 11-7). At very fast heart rates, there is usually a tendency toward regularization of the R-R intervals; therefore, distinguishing the preexcited AF from VT or preexcited SVT can be difficult. However, careful measurement always discloses definite irregularities. Moreover, very rapid and irregular VTs are usually unstable and quickly degenerate into VF. Thus, when a rapid, irregular wide QRS complex tachycardia is noted in a patient who has a reasonably stable hemodynamic state, preexcited AF is the most likely diagnosis.

The ability to conduct rapidly over an AV BT is determined primarily by the intrinsic conduction and refractory properties of the AV BT. However, as with AVN conduction, factors such as spatial and temporal characteristics of atrial wavefronts during AF, autonomic tone, and concealed conduction influence activation over the AV BT. Very rapid AV conduction during AF can occur in the presence of AV BTs with very short refractoriness, especially when normal conduction through the AVN and His-Purkinje system (HPS) is blocked (such as occurs with AVN blocking drugs) and ventricular activation occurs only via the rapidly conducting BT, which would then eliminate retrograde concealment into the BT. This would result in extremely rapid ventricular rates, possibly more than 300 beats/min, which may occasionally degenerate into VF.

Regular Ventricular Rate During Atrial Fibrillation. Regular ventricular rate during AF indicates associated abnormalities. A regular, slow ventricular rhythm during AF suggests a junctional, subjunctional, or ventricular rhythm, either as an escape mechanism with complete AV block or as an accelerated pacemaker activity with AV dissociation (see Fig. 6-22). Rarely, the R-R interval may be regularly irregular and show group beating with the combination of complete heart block and a lower nodal pacemaker with a Wenckebach type of exit block. Patients with severe underlying heart disease may develop the combination of AF and VT, leading to a rapid, regular, wide QRS complex tachycardia.

Effect of Digitalis Toxicity on Ventricular Response. With increasing degrees of digitalis toxicity, high-grade but not complete AV block during AF initially leads to single junctional, subjunctional, or ventricular escape beats. Higher degrees of AV block result in so few atrial impulses being conducted that the lower pacemaker takes over, leading to an escape junctional, subjunctional, or ventricular rhythm with a regular R-R interval for two or more cycles. Complete AV block is marked by a regular escape rhythm with no conducted beats, which may lead to the erroneous assumption that the patient has converted to NSR. Infrequently, impulses from the lower pacemaker travel alternately down the right and left bundle branches, resulting in a bidirectional tachycardia. This arrhythmia, which is also frequently a reflection of marked digitalis toxicity, may be considered to be ventricular bigeminy. In true bigeminy, however, the ventricular beat in the bigeminal pattern is premature. In comparison, the R-R interval is regular with a bidirectional tachycardia, because all the beats arise from a single pacemaker.

QRS Morphology

The QRS complexes during AF are narrow unless AV conduction is abnormal because of functional (rate-related) aberration, preexisting bundle branch block (BBB; see Fig. 11-5), or preexcitation over an AV BT (see Fig. 11-7).

Aberrant conduction commonly occurs during AF. Aberrancy is caused by the physiological changes of the conduction system refractory periods that are associated with the R-R interval. The refractoriness of the HPS tissue is directly related to the preceding heart rate. Thus, there can be aberrant conduction as the result of a long R-R interval followed by a short cycle. In this scenario, the refractory period of the bundles increases during the long R-R interval (long cycle). The QRS complex that ends the long pause will be conducted normally but is followed by a prolonged refractory period of the bundle branches. If the next QRS complex occurs after a short coupling interval, it can be conducted aberrantly because one of the bundles is still refractory as a result of a lengthening of the refractory period (Ashman's phenomenon). The gross irregularity of ventricular response during AF yields an abundance of R-R cycle lengths; there-

fore, the long-short cycle sequence occurs commonly, and Ashman's phenomenon is seen frequently during AF. Right bundle branch block (RBBB) aberrancy is more common than left bundle branch block (LBBB) aberrancy, probably because the right bundle (RB) has a longer refractory period at slower heart rates. The left anterior fascicle is also frequently involved, often in combination with RBBB. In contrast, functional aberration is uncommon in the HB, the left posterior fascicle, or the main left bundle (LB). Moreover, CLs preceding the pause may also affect the chance for aberrancy after the pause.

The aberrancy caused by Ashman's phenomenon may be present for one beat and have a morphology that resembles a PVC, or may involve several sequential complexes, suggesting a VT. The persistence of aberrancy may reflect a time-dependent adjustment of refractoriness of the bundle branch to an abrupt change in CL, or it may be the result of concealed transseptal activation.

Although functional BBB is common in AF, PVCs are even more frequent, and it is important to differentiate between aberrant ventricular conduction and VT when repetitive wide QRS complexes occur during AF. The presence or absence of a long-short cycle sequence was not found to be helpful in differentiating aberration from ectopy for two reasons. Although a long cycle (pause) sets the stage for Ashman's phenomenon, it also tends to precipitate ventricular ectopy. Moreover, concealed conduction occurs frequently during AF and therefore it is never possible to determine exactly when a bundle branch is activated from the surface ECG. Thus, if an aberrant beat does end a long-short cycle sequence during AF, it may be because of refractoriness of a bundle branch secondary to concealed conduction into it rather than because of changes in the length of the ventricular cycle.

The proper diagnosis of aberrant conduction is a continuing challenge, but can usually be accomplished by careful analysis of the rhythm strip and application of certain criteria. An aberrantly conducted beat caused by BBB generally has the pattern of a classic bundle branch or fascicular block. A PVC is usually followed by a longer R-R cycle, indicating the occurrence of a compensatory pause, the result of retrograde conduction into the AVN and anterograde block of the impulse originating in the atrium. The presence of long R-R cycles after the aberrant beat that have identical CLs also suggests a ventricular origin (see Fig. 7-2). Furthermore, the absence of a long-short cycle sequence associated with the wide or aberrant QRS complex suggests that it is of ventricular origin. Aberrancy is not present if, with inspection of a long ECG rhythm strip, there are R-R cycle length combinations that are longer and shorter than those associated with the wide QRS complex. Also, a ventricular origin is likely if there is a fixed coupling cycle between the normal and aberrated QRS complex.

CATHETER ABLATION OF ATRIAL FIBRILLATION

Evolution of Catheter Ablation of Atrial Fibrillation

Over the past 13 years, catheter ablation for the treatment of AF has evolved from an investigational procedure to one that is now performed on thousands of patients annually in many medical centers worldwide. The growing acceptance of this procedure has been brought about by a steadily increasing number of reports showing the safety and efficacy of catheter ablation of AF targeting the PVs and posterior LA.

Catheter Ablation of Atrial Fibrillation: Substrate Modification

Cox and colleagues developed a series of techniques for the surgical disruption of AF.[35] The final iteration, the maze III procedure, was based on a model of AF in which maintenance of the arrhythmia requires maintenance of a critical number of circulating wavelets of reentry, each of which requires a critical mass of atrial tissue to sustain it.[33] The concept behind the maze III, in which a series of complete incisions are made in the left and right atria, was that by dividing the atria into small enough electrically isolated compartments, reentrant activity was no longer possible and maintenance of AF could be prevented, regardless of the mode of initiation.[33] However, application of the maze III operation has been limited by the morbidity and risk associated with sternotomy-thoracotomy and cardiopulmonary bypass, as well as by limited adoption by cardiothoracic surgeons. With the success of the Cox maze procedure, multiple variations of the procedure have been performed, most of which have involved the use of a smaller lesion set. The LA lesion set was found to be fairly adequate to prevent

AF, whereas RA lesions were required to prevent the development of AFL. Isolation of the PVs and posterior LA was a feature common to all successful iterations of the maze procedure. Therefore, this and other similar compartmentalization procedures have evolved over time and now predominantly involve the LA. In general, all these approaches have lower success rates than the maze III procedure.[36]

The success of surgical linear lesions has led to the development of the catheter-based approach to perform linear ablation. Initial attempts at delivering long lines of RF ablation aimed at mimicking the lines of the surgical maze. Schwartz and associates have reported recreation of the maze III lesion set in a small series of patients using specially designed sheaths and standard RF catheters.[37] Although the efficacy was modest, complication rates were high, and procedure and fluoroscopy times were exceedingly long, this report demonstrated a proof of concept that led others to try to improve the catheter-based approach. Further refinement of the linear catheter ablation technique involved creating a series of ablation lesions using RF catheters to create specific lesion sets in the RA (two lines) and LA (three or four lines). The RA lesion sets consisted of an intercaval line along the interatrial septum and a cavotricuspid isthmus line to prevent AFL. LA lesions were designed to connect the four PVs to each other and to the mitral annulus.[38] As increasing evidence emerged regarding the importance of the LA in the maintenance of AF, ablation targets have become limited to the LA.

In the late 1990s, Pappone and coworkers[39] developed the wide circumferential ablation approach using 3-D electroanatomical mapping. RF ablation was performed circumferentially around ipsilateral PVs, with the endpoint of ablation being the absence or marked reduction (80%) in the amplitude of electrical signals within the encircling lesions (Fig. 11-8). Despite lack of evidence showing that PVs treated in this way are electrically isolated from the LA, this group began reporting results for paroxysmal AF which were just as good as or better than those working with the ostial segmental PV isolation approach (see later). Furthermore, patients with persistent or permanent AF treated with the Pappone approach achieved freedom from AF almost as good as those with paroxysmal AF and far better than reports of patients treated with segmental PV isolation. Further improvements have required a strategy closer to the surgical maze—that is, lines to connect the ipsilateral pairs of the PVs and a line to link the left PV encircling lesion to the mitral annulus, which can be described as the *catheter maze*.[38] Such lines further improved the outcomes of paroxysmal AF and have produced good results for permanent AF ablation as well. It is clear that producing lines with proven transmural conduction block leads to a smaller recurrence of AF; however, achieving this is technically challenging and requires long, arduous procedures. Also, gaps in these lines may promote macroreentrant AT.[38]

More recently, fractionated electrograms and autonomic responses have been used to guide substrate modification for AF ablation (see Fig. 11-8). The ablation of all fractionated electrograms in the RA and LA was based on the hypothesis that these are consistent sites where fibrillating wavefronts turn or split. By ablating these areas, the propagating random wavefronts are progressively restricted until the atria can no longer support AF.[40] Other studies have also provided strong presumptive evidence that hyperactivity of the intrinsic autonomic nervous system constitutes a dysautonomia can lead to a greater propensity for AF, both paroxysmal and sustained forms. Targeting autonomic nerves at a few specific sites on the heart that are directly related to arrhythmia formation may help reduce extensive damage to healthy myocardium while curtailing the ability to induce or maintain AF.[18]

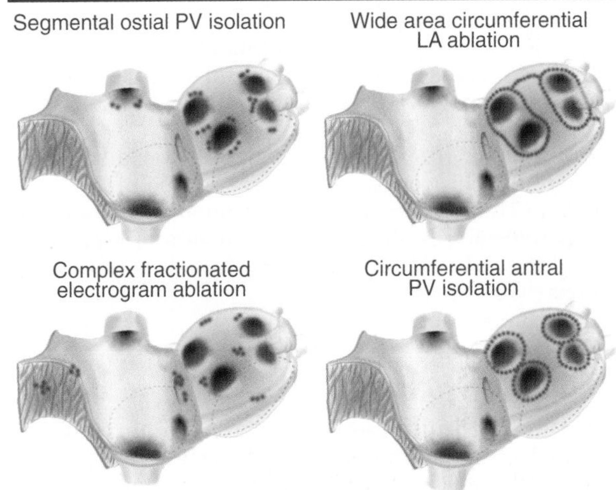

FIGURE 11–8 Catheter ablation of atrial fibrillation (AF). Atrial anatomy is shown at top; both atria are opened and viewed from the front. Various procedures for catheter ablation of AF are shown (red dots are ablation lesions). See text for further discussion. LA = left atrium; PV = pulmonary vein.

Catheter Ablation of Atrial Fibrillation: Elimination of Triggers

Focal Ablation of Triggers. The landmark publication of Haissaguerre and colleagues[6] in 1998 demonstrated that paroxysmal episodes of AF are consistently initiated by spontaneous triggers or atrial extrasystoles. Remarkably, 94% of those triggers originated within the PVs, most within 2 to 4 cm of the ostium.[6] The electrophysiological basis of these focal sources appeared to be the sleeves of LA muscle investing the PVs. One or more veins develop abnormal, paroxysmal, rapid automaticity, triggering AF as a result. Despite extensive research, the pathophysiology of this process remains poorly understood. AF was initiated with a burst of rapid firing from the foci and was abolished with RF ablation at the site of origin.

The initial technique was to identify and ablate the culprit focus within the PV, but this approach was limited by the complication of PV stenosis and the recognition that multiple veins are involved in most patients, which leads to frequent recurrences after a successful procedure. Moreover, it is frequently difficult to elicit PV arrhythmia in the EP laboratory to allow adequate mapping and ablation.[6,12]

Pulmonary Vein Isolation. Recognition of major limitations of focal ablation has led to the development of the PV electrical isolation technique. Recognizing that PV musculature conducts to LA musculature by discrete connections has allowed investigators to target those connections using multipolar catheters shaped into rings or baskets. Ablation is performed with a separate roving catheter at the site of earliest activation sequentially until PV electrical activity disappears or becomes dissociated from LA activity (see Fig. 11-8). Using this strategy, between 20% and 60% of the PV circumference is targeted for ablation.[41,42] PV isolation has the additional advantage of simultaneously treating all triggering foci within the vein, thereby obviating the need to elicit and map those foci individually. For the same reason, investigators were soon led to attempt to isolate as many PVs as possible at the initial ablation session. Comparative case series ultimately demonstrated that empirical isolation of the four PVs led to superior outcomes over isolating fewer veins.

It was subsequently found that by ablating at or just outside the PV ostia, the incidence of PV stenosis could be reduced significantly. Using this approach, RF ablation is performed circumferentially around the antrum of each of the four PVs (see Fig. 11-8). In patients in whom the inferior and superior veins were closely spaced or shared a common ostium, a single large circumferential RF lesion set was performed.[41]

With further research in this area, it was also observed that non-PV foci were an important source of AF in some patients, although percentages vary among different groups. Among the sources identified are the vein of Marshall, the CS, and the SVC, all thoracic veins. Targeting those triggers by electrical isolation of the involved thoracic veins has been attempted in selected patients.[12,43]

Preablation Preparation

Antiarrhythmic Agents. Antiarrhythmic medications are usually stopped more than 5 days (more than 5 half-lives) before the ablation procedure, except for amiodarone, which may be continued or discontinued before or after ablation.

Anticoagulation. Patients with high risk for thromboembolism are anticoagulated with warfarin (INR, 2 to 3) for more than 4 to 6 weeks before the ablation procedure. Warfarin is usually stopped 2 to 5 days before the procedure, and replaced with enoxaparin or intravenous heparin once INR is lower than 2.0. Enoxaparin is stopped 12 to 24 hours and heparin is stopped 4 to 6 hours before ablation (because transseptal catheterization is frequently required). Alternatively, some laboratories have performed these procedures while the patient is on warfarin with therapeutic INR levels. The latter approach can potentially reduce the risk of thromboembolism by avoiding interruption of anticoagulation at any point before and after the procedure, and it may also help avoid some of the vascular complications exacerbated by the combination of warfarin and enoxaparin.[44] However, the concern about this approach is that acute bleeding complications, particularly pericardial tamponade, may be more difficult to control if anticoagulation cannot be immediately reversed in that setting.[45]

Transesophageal Echocardiography. TEE is performed in most patients undergoing AF ablation to screen for LA thrombus. Although it is optional in patients with paroxysmal AF and no structural heart disease, preablation TEE is mandatory in patients who are in AF at the time of the procedure, regardless of the anticoagulation status prior to ablation. The presence of intracardiac thrombus should prompt cancellation of the procedure and mandate 4 to 8 more weeks of anticoagulation, followed by another TEE. Recently, 64-slice computed tomography (CT) scanning has been used to identify LA thrombus, but TEE remains the gold standard.

Pulmonary Vein Imaging. Magnetic resonance (MR) imaging or contrast-enhanced, multislice CT scan of the LA with 3-D reconstruction is performed to define the anatomy of the PVs before the procedure (see Figs. 11-3 and 11-4).

Technical Aspects Common to Different Methods of Ablation

Sedation During Ablation. In most patients, conscious sedation or general anesthesia is used; the choice is determined by the institutional preference and also by assessment of the patient's suitability for conscious sedation. General anesthesia is generally used for patients at risk of airway obstruction, those with history of sleep apnea, and those at increased risk of pulmonary edema. General anesthesia may also be used electively in healthy patients to improve patient tolerance of the procedure.[45]

Left Atrial Access. Mapping and ablation in the LA are performed through a transseptal approach. Search for a patent foramen ovale is initially performed. If one is absent, a transseptal puncture is performed (see detailed discussion in Chap. 2). Generally, one or two transseptal punctures are performed under fluoroscopic (with or without intracardiac echocardiography [ICE]) guidance and one or two long vascular sheaths (SR0, SL1, or Mullins sheath, St. Jude Medical, Minnetonka, Minn) are introduced into the LA. The long sheaths are flushed with heparinized saline at a flow rate of 3 mL/min during the entire procedure.

Anticoagulation. Once vascular access is achieved, intravenous heparin (bolus of 100 U/kg, then infusion of 10 U/kg/hr) is administered. During the initial experience with AF ablation, anticoagulation with heparin was delayed until after LA access had been achieved because of fear of complications with transseptal puncture. Later, it became evident that such a strategy can allow thrombus formation on sheaths, catheters, and in the RA before transseptal puncture, and these thrombi could potentially travel to the LA. More recently, experienced operators have favored complete heparinization after vascular access, and clearly before transseptal puncture, especially when intracardiac echocardiography (ICE) is used to guide transseptal puncture. Even in patients fully anticoagulated with warfarin therapy at the time of ablation, it is still recommended to administer intravenous heparin during the ablation procedure.[44]

The activated clotting time (ACT) should be checked at 10- to 15-minute intervals until therapeutic anticoagulation is achieved and then at 30-minute intervals during the procedure, and the heparin dose is adjusted accordingly. The lower level of anticoagulation should be maintained at an ACT of at least 300 to 350 seconds throughout the period of mapping and ablation in the LA. If significant LA enlargement or spontaneous echo contrast is observed, targeting a higher ACT level (350 to 400 seconds) is probably more appropriate. To reduce the risk of bleeding complications, antiplatelet therapy (especially IIB/IIIA glycoprotein receptor blockers and clopidogrel) should be avoided, if possible.[45]

Identification of the Pulmonary Veins. Initial approaches of focal ablation targeting arrhythmic foci within the PVs were associated with high incidences of PV stenosis. To avoid this serious complication, the ablation procedure has evolved over time to an increasingly proximal ablation, first at the venous ostium or venoatrial junction and most recently proximal to the PV to encompass the antral region. However, the more proximal ablation approaches require correct identification of the ostia and PV-LA junction and, given the marked variation in PV anatomy, assessment of the number of PVs and anatomy of the ostia is essential when planning an ablation strategy. Various imaging techniques have been developed in an attempt to identify the PV ostium more accurately, but exact localization of this structure remains difficult, and the exact definition of the PV ostium varies, depending on the imaging modality used. Ultimately, however, the choice of imaging modality will be dictated by local availability.

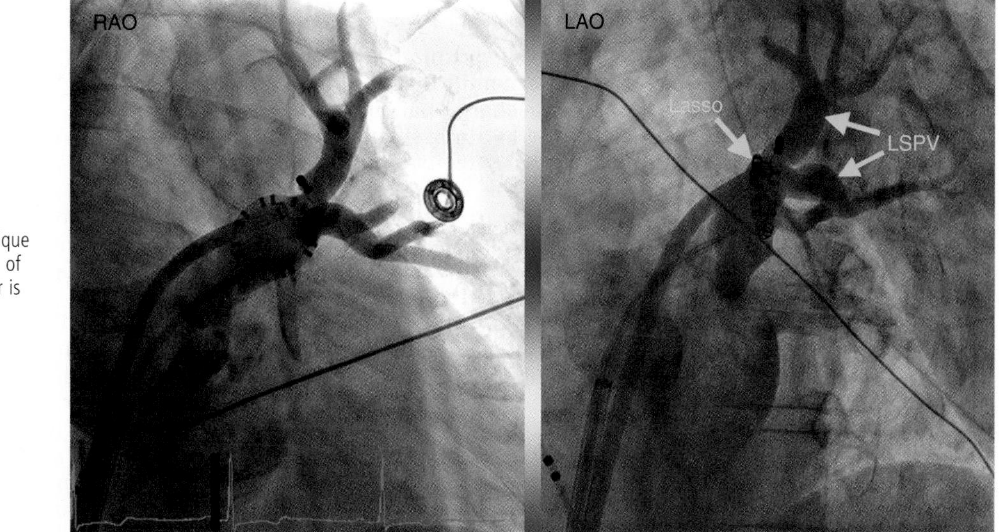

FIGURE 11–9 Pulmonary vein (PV) angiography. Fluoroscopic (right anterior oblique [RAO] and left anterior oblique [LAO]) views of the left superior PV (LSPV). The ring catheter is positioned at the PV ostium.

Fluoroscopy. Entry into the PV is clearly identified as the catheter leaves the cardiac shadow on fluoroscopy and electrical activity disappears. The inferior portion of the PV ostia can be localized by advancing the catheter into the PV with downward deflection of the tip and then dragging back while fluoroscopically monitoring the drop off the ostial edge of the catheter.

Pulmonary Vein Angiography. PV angiography has traditionally been used at the time of catheter ablation to detail PV anatomy. Selective PV angiography is performed using a 5- to 10-mL hand injection of contrast medium through a long sheath (for angiography of right superior, left superior, and left inferior PVs) or NIH catheter (for angiography of right inferior PV; Fig. 11-9). Alternatively, PV angiography is performed by injecting contrast in the left and right pulmonary arteries or the pulmonary trunk; PVs are then assessed during the venous phase of pulmonary arteriography. A third technique used for PV angiography involves contrast injection in the body of the LA or at the roof of the right or left superior PV ostium immediately after administration of an adenosine intravenous bolus to induce AV block; the contrast medium will fill the LA body, PV antrum, and proximal part of the PV during the phase of ventricular asystole. An important limitation of PV angiography is that it images only the tubular portion and does not adequately define the full posterior extension of the PV. Studies of PV anatomy from pathological specimens and 3-D CT scans have shown that the PV is funnel-shaped, with a tube that fans out into a proximal cup that blends into the posterior atrial wall, referred to as the antrum. Furthermore, the PV antrum connects to the LA wall at an oblique angle. The posterior aspect of each PV is more proximal, whereas the anterior segments of the PVs are more distal.

Intracardiac Echocardiography. Phased-array ICE can be used to visualize the antrum and ostium of the PVs (see detailed discussion in Chap. 3). ICE has the advantage of providing real-time imaging of the PVs. In contrast to angiography, ICE can define the proximal edge of the PV antrum (see Fig. 3-42). Important drawbacks of the technique are the need for an additional sheath for placement of the ICE catheter and the expense.

3-D Electroanatomical Mapping. CARTO, NavX, and RPM electroanatomical mapping systems have been used to construct a 3-D shell of the LA and identify the PVs. However, definition of the true PV ostium using these systems alone may be difficult because of variants in 3-D vein morphology.

Combining Electroanatomical Mapping Systems with Contrast-Enhanced, Multislice Cardiac CT or MR. 3-D CT and MR provide critical information regarding the number, location, and size of the PVs, which is needed in planning the ablation and selecting appropriately sized mapping and ablation devices. In addition, preacquired CT and MR scans have the advantage of allowing full integration with 3-D mapping systems and real-time catheter navigation on a 3-D CT or MR image, which offers great potential for accurate identification of PV ostia and ablation targets (see detailed discussion in Chap. 3).

Impedance Mapping. Impedance monitoring can be used to identify the LA-PV junction.[46] With catheter entry into the PV, the impedance usually rises above 140 to 150 Ω. At the PV ostium the impedance typically is more than 4 Ω above the mean LA impedance.

Catheterization of the Pulmonary Veins. In the anteroposterior fluoroscopic view, the PV ostia are situated on both sides of the spine. Clockwise rotation of the catheter inside the LA directs its tip posteriorly and toward the PVs. It is frequently necessary to apply clockwise torque to both the catheter and its long sheath. For catheterization of the left PVs, the catheter should be directed anteroposteriorly in the right anterior oblique (RAO) view and to the left in the left anterior oblique (LAO) view. Care must be taken to avoid advancing the catheter into the LA appendage, in which case the catheter is directed to the right (anteriorly) in the RAO view and not anteroposteriorly. For catheterization of the right PVs, the catheter is rotated further clockwise and is directed to the right in the RAO view and anteroposteriorly in the LAO view. An alternative method for reaching the ostia of the right PVs is to loop the catheter around the lateral, inferior, and then septal LA walls, laying the catheter down along the wall, and dragging the catheter by withdrawing it along the posterior right ostia. Forming a tight loop with maximal deflection of the catheter and using rotational movements can provide greater stability during ablation, particularly at the anterior aspect of the PVs. Counterclockwise rotation of the catheter inside the LA would lead the catheter into the LV. Care must be taken not to get the circular (Lasso) catheter trapped with the mitral valve apparatus. Usually, reversal of the catheter movement (clockwise torque) that resulted in this situation helps correct it.

Postablation Management

Cardiac Monitoring. Patients are generally hospitalized the night after the procedure, with cardiac monitoring, and discharged home the following day. After discharge, patients who report symptoms compatible with an arrhythmia should undergo ambulatory monitoring. Because early recurrences of atrial arrhythmias are common during the first 1 to 3 months following ablation and many of them resolve spontaneously, arrhythmia monitoring to assess the efficacy of the ablation procedure is typically delayed for at least 3 months following catheter ablation. Periodic Holter monitoring to screen asymptomatic occurrences of atrial arrhythmias may be considered. Event monitoring, even in asymptomatic patients, may also help screen for recurrent episodes of AF. The patient is encouraged to activate the event monitor whenever he or she develops symptoms and randomly a few times a day. Patients are also encouraged to take their pulse periodically and monitor for irregularity. Twelve-lead ECGs should be obtained at all follow-up visits.[45]

Anticoagulation. At the conclusion of the ablation procedure, sheath removal requires interruption of anticoagulation to achieve adequate hemostasis. Heparin infusion can be discontinued and the sheaths removed when the ACT is less than 200 seconds. Alternatively, protamine can be administered to reverse heparin effects (1 mg of protamine/100 U heparin received in the previous 2 hours). Warfarin is restarted after the procedure and continued for a minimum of 2 to 3 months. Intravenous heparin (therapeutic loading doses) or subcutaneous enoxaparin (0.5 mg/kg twice daily) is administered 4 to 6 hours after sheath removal and continued until the INR reaches therapeutic levels. In patients undergoing the ablation procedure while fully anticoagulated with warfarin, no heparin or enoxaparin is required following ablation as long as INR levels are maintained in the therapeutic range.[44] Decisions regarding the use of warfarin more than 2 to 3 months following ablation should be based on the patient's risk factors for stroke and not on the presence or absence of AF. Discontinuation of warfarin therapy postablation is generally not recommended in patients who have a $CHADS_2$ score of 2 or higher.[45] Although a recent study has shown that discontinuation of warfarin therapy 3 months after successful catheter ablation may be safe over medium-term follow-up in some subsets of patients, this has never been confirmed by a large prospective randomized trial and therefore remains unproven.[45,47] Even when discontinuation of warfarin therapy is being considered, recurrences of AF should be excluded with confidence. Reliance only on symptoms as an indictor for AF recurrence or ambulatory monitoring can be misleading and can underestimate the incidence of recurrence. With transtelephonic ECGs, the rate of recurrent AF is much higher (28% versus 14% with serial ECG and Holter monitoring in one report). Moreover, a high rate of asymptomatic AF episodes, with some lasting more than 48 hours, has also been noted in patients with paroxysmal AF, even in patients who were significantly symptomatic before the ablation procedure. Therefore, without reliable documentation of the absence of AF recurrences, patients should be anticoagulated according to the guidelines for other patients with AF. The $CHADS_2$ score is recommended for risk stratification to determine which patients require long-term warfarin and which patients can be treated with aspirin. One exception is that patients who would be treated with aspirin receive warfarin anticoagulation for 2 to 3 months after the ablation procedure. In high-risk patients with previous stroke or other indications for anticoagulation, warfarin should be continued indefinitely. Some investigators have also suggested continuation of anticoagulation therapy if significant PV stenosis (more than 50%) is detected.

Pulmonary Vein Imaging. CT or MR imaging to evaluate for evidence of PV stenosis is important in patients with clinical suspicion of PV stenosis. The value of routine follow-up PV imaging to screen for asymptomatic PV stenosis is still unknown, but may be considered during the initial experience of a new AF ablation procedure to confirm quality assurance.[45]

Antiarrhythmic Medications. Continuing antiarrhythmic drug therapy in patients who undergo catheter ablation for AF does not seem to lower the rate of AF recurrences, although it may increase the proportion of patients with asymptomatic AF episodes. Therefore, it seems unnecessary to continue antiarrhythmic drug therapy following ablation with a view to the prevention of arrhythmia recurrences. On the other hand, it may be useful in the management of recurrences soon after the procedure, when they are usually frequent and transient and in patients with long-term recurrences to alleviate symptoms. Continuation of antiarrhythmic treatment may also be considered in the case of incomplete or unsuccessful ablation procedure, such as incomplete isolation of the targeted PVs in patients with a history of persistent or permanent AF (because early recurrences are common but do not necessarily predict failure of the procedure), and in patients with recurrence of AF or AFL during the 24-hour observation period after the procedure. Typically, a class IC agent—sotalol, dofetilide, or amiodarone—is used. In patients discharged on antiarrhythmic drug therapy, such therapy is discontinued after 1 to 3 months if no recurrence of AF is observed. In patients discharged without antiarrhythmic drug therapy who develop recurrent AF, antiarrhythmic drug therapy is initiated unless the patient is satisfied with the extent of symptomatic improvement or elects to undergo a repeat ablation procedure.

FOCAL ABLATION OF PULMONARY VEIN TRIGGERS

Rationale

There are two different types of arrhythmias that may play a role in generating AF, and both may be addressed by focal ablation. One type is a PAC (or runs of PACs) that triggers self-sustained AF (focal triggers). Ablation of a focal trigger will not terminate AF but prevents its reinitiation (see Fig. 11-1).[5] A second type is a focal tachycardia that either induces fibrillation in the atria or mimics AF by creating a pattern of rapid and irregular depolarization wavefronts in the atria. Such tachycardia acts as a focal driver and is necessary for the continuation and maintenance of AF. Ablation of a focal driver results in the termination of AF and prevention of its reinitiation. Focal tachycardias that initiate or mimic AF can be recognized in the EP laboratory because they are frequently associated with exit block between the site of origin of the tachycardia and the rest of the atria (Fig. 11-10).[5,20]

Several observations have provided evidence that the electrical activity that arises in the PVs plays a role in the maintenance of AF. By analyzing surface ECG and 24-hour Holter recordings, studies have shown that most paroxysmal AF episodes are initiated by a single PAC. Although focal sources of AF may be found in the RA, LA, CS, SVC, or vein of Marshall, 94% of foci are located within a PV.[5,6,12,48] It is possible that intermittent bursts of PV tachycardia serve to perpetuate AF in the same fashion as aconitine-induced rapid firing or bursts of rapid atrial pacing (see Fig. 11-10).

There may be a subset of patients with focally induced AF in whom ablation of a single dominant focus can result

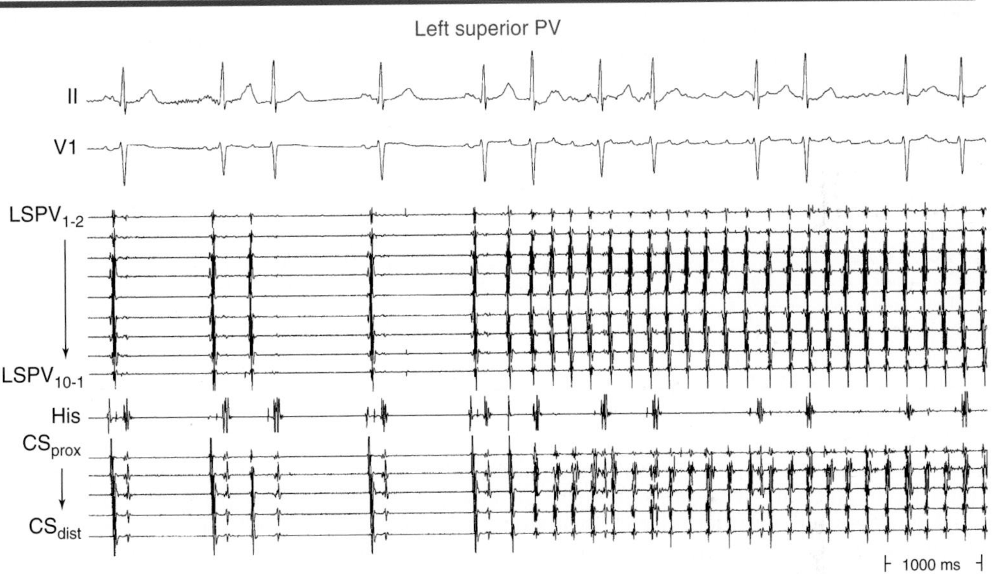

FIGURE 11–10 Atrial fibrillation (AF) initiation from the right superior pulmonary vein (RSPV). **Upper panel,** A burst of nonsustained PV tachycardia followed by a second sustained episode. Note that the local cycle length (CL) in the ring catheter recordings from the RSPV is significantly shorter than atrial CL recorded in the coronary sinus (CS) during AF, indicating that this PV is the source and driver of AF. **Lower panel,** Recording from the left superior PV (LSPV) in the same patient during spontaneous initiation of AF showing LSPV activity having a similar CL as the atrial CL, suggesting that this PV is activated passively.

in cure, without the need for empirical isolation of all PVs. A more limited ablation approach requires shorter procedure and fluoroscopy times and may be safer. These are important considerations in a relatively young patient population.

Identification of Arrhythmogenic Pulmonary Veins

Definition of an Arrhythmogenic Pulmonary Vein. An arrhythmogenic PV is defined by single or multiple ectopy originating from the PV, with or without conduction to the LA. During ectopy from an arrhythmogenic PV, there is a reversal in activation sequence, from the distal PV trunk (source) to the ostium and LA (exit), with the PV potential preceding the LA potential (Figs. 11-11 and 11-12).[6] Conversely, if the explored PV was not the origin of ectopy, it is passively activated, as in NSR, with a proximal-to-distal sequence and a PV potential after or fusing with the LA potential.

Ectopic discharges with a short coupling interval may not be conducted to the LA, producing isolated PV potentials confined within the PV. These can be recognized as a PV potential coincident with or just after the ventricular electrogram and can be distinguished from a potential of ventricular origin by their spontaneous disappearance (intermittent PV potential) or suppression during atrial pacing.[6] Multiple foci in the same PV are defined by the presence of two different sources and exits at opposite locations of the PV perimeter (e.g., roof and bottom).

During an episode of AF, rapid rhythms arising in the PVs (variably referred to as rapid focal activity, repetitive rapid activity, intermittent PV tachycardia, or paroxysmal CL shortening) are common and may play an important role in the maintenance of AF or may be a marker of an arrhythmogenic PV that triggers AF during NSR. The CL of local activity within the arrhythmogenic PV is shorter than that of the atrium. In contrast, the local CL in passively activated PVs is similar to or longer than that of the atrium (see Fig. 11-10).

Provocation of Pulmonary Vein Ectopy. If PV ectopy does not spontaneously develop during EP monitoring or is not sufficiently sustained, one or a combination of several provocative maneuvers can be tried to induce the arrhythmia, including physiological procedures (e.g., Valsalva maneuvers, carotid sinus massage, or deep breathing), pharmacological agents (isoproterenol, 1 to 8 μg/min, and adenosine, rapid IV injection, 12 mg and then 18 mg, up to 20 to 60 mg), and slow-rate atrial pacing (bursts of 3 to 10

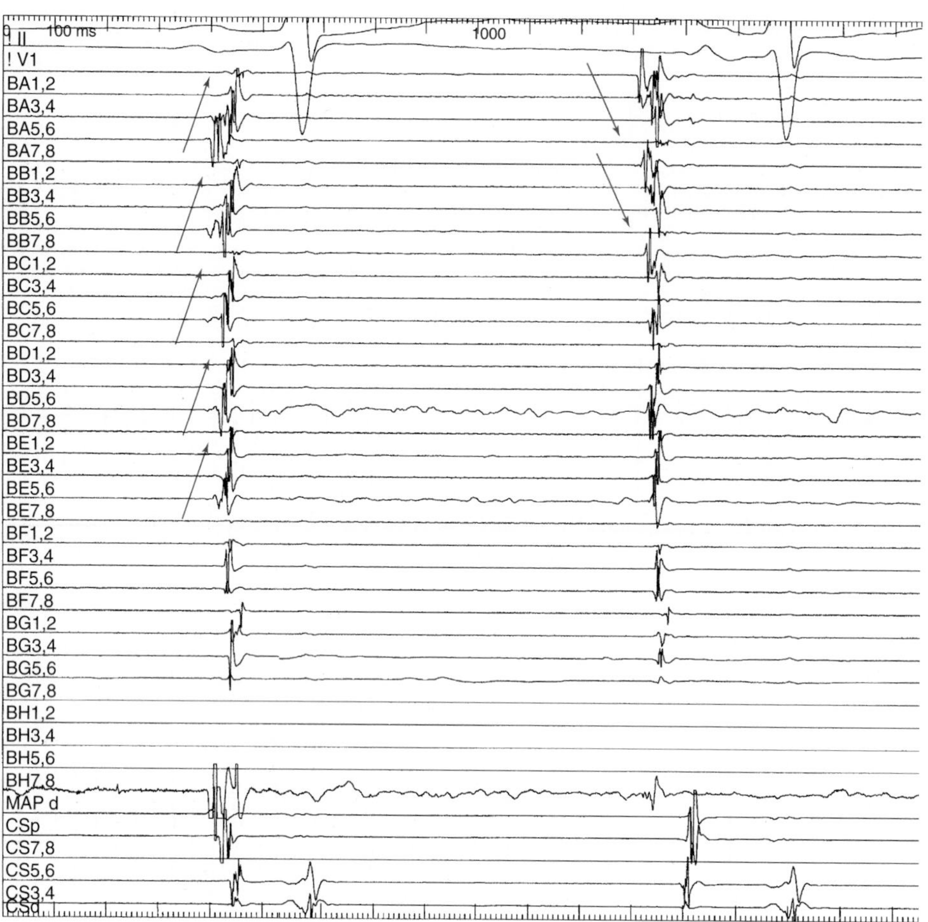

FIGURE 11–11 Mapping of pulmonary vein (PV) ectopy using a basket catheter. The basket catheter is positioned in the left superior PV. Bipolar recordings are obtained from the eight electrodes (1-2, 3-4, 5-6, 7-8) on each of the eight splines (BA through BH) of the basket catheter. **Left,** During normal sinus rhythm (NSR), PV activation propagates from proximal (ostial) to distal, as reflected by earlier activation timing on the proximal basket electrodes than the distal ones (blue arrows). **Right,** In contrast, during a premature atrial complex (PAC) originating from this PV, activation occurs earliest deep in the vein and progressively later toward the ostium and the left atrial (LA) exit, resulting in distal to proximal venous activation on the basket catheter recordings (red arrows). Note that the PV potentials precede the onset of the P wave on the surface ECG during PV ectopy, but occur late after P wave onset during NSR.

stimuli at 100 to 200 beats/min for postpause ectopy).[6] Additionally, in patients who present with AF at the time of ablation, external or internal cardioversion of AF can be attempted, which can reproducibly induce PACs from the same location as spontaneous PACs, and such PACs following cardioversion can reinitiate AF. There is a high degree of correlation between spontaneous and postcardioversion PACs or PACs inducing AF. If AF is not present at baseline,

11

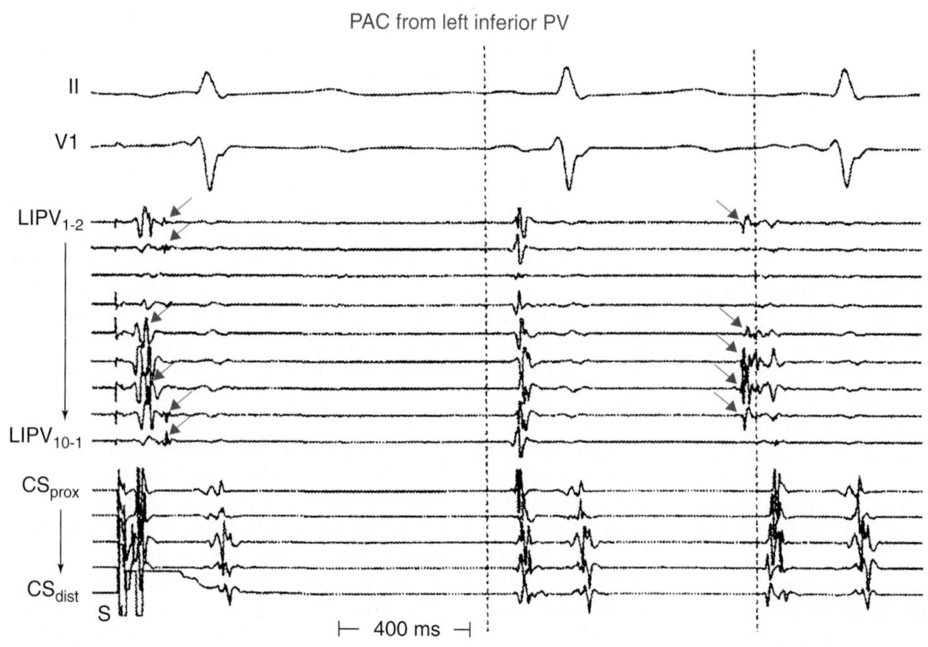

FIGURE 11–12 Mapping pulmonary vein (PV) ectopy using a ring catheter. The ring catheter is positioned at the ostium of the left inferior PV (LIPV). **Left,** During pacing from the distal coronary sinus (CS) (at left), PV potentials (red arrows) follow the left atrium (LA) potentials. During normal sinus rhythm (NSR; middle complex), LA and PV potentials overlap, and they occur in the second half of the P wave. **Right,** During a premature atrial complex (PAC) originating from the LIPV, reversal of the electrogram sequence in the ring catheter recording is observed, with the PV potentials (red arrows) preceding the LA potentials and occurring well before the onset of the P wave on surface ECG (dashed line).

rapid burst atrial pacing to induce AF, followed by electrical cardioversion, may also be attempted to identify early post-cardioversion PV triggers.

Mapping of Pulmonary Vein Ectopy

ECG Localization of Pulmonary Vein Ectopy

ATs arising from the PVs are characterized by entirely positive P waves in lead V_1 in 100% of cases, isoelectric or negative in aVL in 86%, and negative in lead aVR in 96%; lead aVL may be biphasic or positive in right-sided PV ATs (Fig. 11-13).[23]

Left PV ATs have several characteristics (as compared with right PV ATs), including positive notching in the P waves in two or more surface leads, isoelectric or negative P wave in lead I, P wave amplitude in lead III/II ratio >0.8, and broad P waves in lead V_1 (see Fig. 11-13).

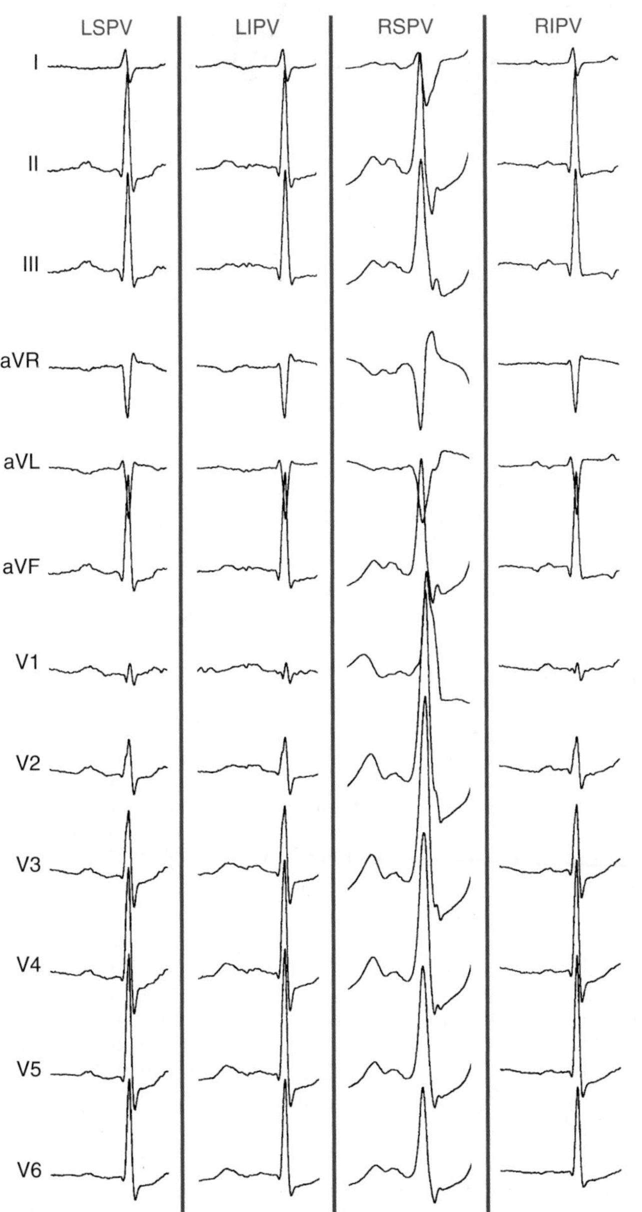

FIGURE 11–13 Surface ECG of spontaneous premature atrial complexes (PACs) originating from the pulmonary veins (PVs). LIPV = left inferior PV; LSPV = left superior PV; RIPV = right inferior PV; RSPV = right superior PV.

ATs arising from superior PVs have larger amplitude P waves in inferior leads than those in ATs arising from inferior PVs (see Fig. 11-13). However, P wave morphology generally is of greater accuracy in distinguishing right-sided from left-sided veins, in contrast to superior from inferior.

During right superior PV ATs, the P waves are narrow, positive in inferior leads, of equal amplitude in leads II and III, biphasic or slightly positive in lead V_1, and isoelectric in lead I (see Fig. 11-13). The right superior PV is a common site of origin for LA ATs. It is only a few centimeters from the sinus node. Activation rapidly crosses the septum via Bachmann's bundle to activate the RA in a fashion similar to NSR, explaining the similarities in P wave morphology. However, whereas the P wave is biphasic in lead V_1 during NSR, it is positive in that lead during right superior PV AT (see Fig. 11-13).[23]

Endocardial Activation Mapping

Initially, the PV of interest is identified based on earliest activation of triggers in the CS and RA catheters. If no sharp bipolar activity is recorded in the RA less than 10 milliseconds before the onset of the ectopic P wave, the ectopic beats are considered to have originated in the LA.[6] Following initial identification, a 4-mm-tip ablation catheter is placed and maneuvered to the appropriate PV.

Activation mapping within the PV is performed during ectopy. It is important to have adequate frequency of PACs from each focus, so as to be able to acquire enough points and identify the earliest activation sequence. Multielectrode mapping catheters, such as the ring catheter (a decapolar catheter with a distal ring configuration) or basket catheter positioned in the PV, can be of value in mapping the source of ectopy. The ectopic focus is localized inside the selected PV according to the earliest atrial activity relative to the reference electrogram or the onset of the ectopic P wave. PV depolarization during ectopy is marked by a spike (an electrogram of sharp onset and short duration) preceding the onset of the ectopic P wave by 106 ± 24 milliseconds (range, 40 to 160 milliseconds; see Figs. 11-11 and 11-12).[6] The spike is typically localized, and its amplitude rapidly decreases, when the catheter tip is turned or moved a few millimeters. Bystander or far-field activity from contiguous branches can be distinguished by temporal delay or lower amplitude. The spike occurs earliest deep in the vein and progressively later toward the ostium and LA exit, resulting in distal-to-proximal venous activation during multipolar recordings (see Fig. 11-11). A second electrographic component with a slow deflection (depolarization rate [dV/dt] < 0.5 mV/msec), reflecting later LA activation, is temporally distinct from the spike inside the vein and then approaches and becomes continuous with the spike at the ostium.

Mechanically induced beats are prevented by avoiding manipulation of the catheters during the recordings. These beats are excluded by comparing the ECG pattern and intracardiac activation sequence with the confirmed spontaneous ectopic beats.[6]

If still insufficient spontaneous or induced ectopy is present, focal mapping and ablation of AF may become difficult. In these cases, the use of multielectrode basket catheter mapping (see Fig. 11-11) or noncontact mapping (EnSite) system can map a single beat and help identify the origin of spontaneously occurring PACs and/or PACs induced following the cardioversion of spontaneous or induced AF.

Following successful ablation of the initially targeted PV triggers, a second PV is usually targeted if there are either significant spontaneous isolated PACs (5/min or more), at least two separate PACs inducing AF, or PACs originating from the same PV inducing AF following cardioversion on at least two occasions.

Electroanatomical Mapping

A quadripolar, deflectable, 4-mm-tip catheter is inserted into the LA via a long sheath for mapping and ablation. Using the CARTO mapping system, the LA anatomy is reconstructed by point-to-point sequential sampling of the endocardial sites (100 to 150 sites) to create a complete 3-D shell of the LA. The LA appendage is demarcated, and three locations are recorded along the mitral isthmus to tag valve orifice. Mapping of each PV is performed by placing the mapping catheter 2 to 4 cm inside each PV and slowly pulling it back to the LA under fluoroscopic guidance. During this course, virtual tubes are created by CARTO to represent the main body of the PVs (Fig. 11-14).

The PV of interest is initially identified based on the earliest activation of triggers in the CS and RA catheters. Subsequently, more detailed mapping of the triggers is performed using a CARTO catheter in the target PV, which is used to measure local activation time compared with a reference electrogram in the CS or RA catheters. The goal of activation mapping is to acquire enough points during the triggers to define an early site surrounded by later activation sites, and thus appropriate for focal ablation (see Fig. 11-14).

Noncontact Mapping

The EnSite system consists of a 7.5-mL array balloon catheter with 64 electrodes that acquires all information necessary to generate isopotential maps from 3300 reconstructed virtual unipolar endocardial electrograms, which are displayed as a 3-D graphic representation of the heart chamber in an isochronal or isopotential mode. It can simultaneously display as many as 32 electrograms as waveforms.

Under fluoroscopic guidance, the 9 Fr multielectrode array is placed in the center of LA after transseptal puncture, a 7 Fr mapping/ablation catheter is positioned at the ostia of all four PVs sequentially, and geometry data are acquired at the ostia and several centimeters inside the veins. The ostia of the PVs are labeled, and the smoothing feature of the EnSite geometry algorithm is applied. PV sites then are tagged on the reconstructed image that is modeled to the LA chamber. The LA appendage, mitral annulus, and septal area are identified and tagged. 3-D mapping of the LA is performed by moving the mapping catheter over the targeted areas.

The first segment of mapping data is recorded during NSR and analyzed to identify LA conduction breakthrough arising from the RA. Subsequently, several recordings are made during successive runs of spontaneous or induced focal ectopy. After data are acquired, isopotential maps are generated during NSR, single ectopic beats, nonsustained runs of focal activity, or onset of AF. Virtual electrograms are applied to verify the isopotential maps. Software filtering produces a bandwidth of 1 to 300 Hz. When overlap occurs with ventricular repolarization, the software filter setting is adjusted to between 2 or 4 and 300 Hz. Morphology of the virtual electrograms and timing of the local atrial activation, as evident from reconstructed electrograms in relation to onset of the P wave on the surface ECG and to conventionally recorded RA electrograms, are analyzed.

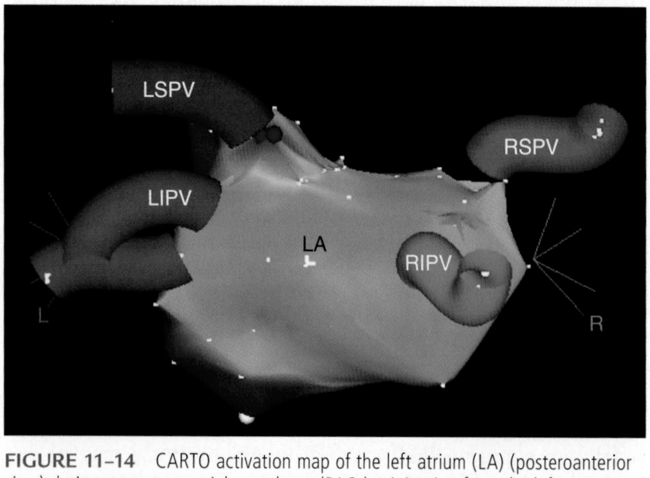

FIGURE 11–14 CARTO activation map of the left atrium (LA) (posteroanterior view) during premature atrial complexes (PACs) originating from the left superior pulmonary vein (LSPV). Focal ablation (red dots) at the PV ostium eliminated those PACs. LIPV = left inferior PV; RIPV = right inferior PV; RSPV = right superior PV.

The system can provide a global simultaneous view of arrhythmia activation, which is of particular importance for the analysis of unstable or nonsustained ectopy. The virtual unipolar electrograms obtained at the earliest site of activation during ectopic activity are characterized by QS or rS morphology, with the intrinsic defection inscribing earlier compared with all adjacent sites, a characteristic comparable to what could be expected with contact unipolar electrograms recorded at the exit site of activation to the LA. Amplitude of the r wave of the virtual electrograms recorded at breakthrough sites and at distant sites is variable. Thus, for correct interpretation of the virtual unipolar electrograms, morphology and timing criteria must be applied. The dV/dt of the virtual unipolar electrograms differs markedly at different recording sites. This phenomenon can be explained in terms of the variable distance and orientation of the center of the EnSite balloon electrode to the recording sites. Subsequently, the mapping-ablation catheter is navigated to the target PV and conventionally recorded electrograms are obtained and analyzed.

The EnSite system has several advantages. Because high-resolution maps of the whole LA can be created simultaneously from a single beat, this technology allows precise mapping, even in patients with rare focal activity. In addition, complex activation sequences caused by ectopic activity arising from different PVs and also extra-PV foci, which may be difficult to map with conventional technologies, can be analyzed and understood. Furthermore, because mapping data are acquired without conventional electrode catheters being in direct contact with the LA endocardium, the use of noncontact mapping avoids the mechanical induction of ectopic activity frequently seen during conventional mapping of the PVs.

On the other hand, the EnSite system has several limitations. Only data segments up to a maximum of 10 seconds in length can be stored retroactively by the EnSite system once the record button is pushed. Thus, continuous recording and storage of all segments of an arrhythmia are not possible at the time of evaluation of the arrhythmia maps. Therefore, it is possible to miss some isolated PACs or PACs inducing AF during evaluation and mapping. Moreover, PV potentials preceding the onset of LA activation during ectopy may not be visualized with virtual electrograms; such PV potentials can be recorded when the balloon electrode is placed close to a PV that displays ectopic activity and not just in the center of LA. Thus, ectopic activity that arises in the PVs but is not conducted to the LA may not be visualized with noncontact mapping. Special attention and care are necessary during placement of the large balloon electrode in a nondilated LA. Additionally, reconstruction of LA geometry limited to the tagging of PVs provides only a rough estimation of true LA geometry and no exact electroanatomical reconstruction of the PV ostia is performed. It is therefore not possible to define target sites for catheter ablation on the basis of the geometry data.

Target of Ablation

If more than one PV is arrhythmogenic, the PV producing the most repetitive ectopy and/or ectopy initiating AF is first targeted. The site showing the earliest atrial activity relative to the reference electrogram or onset of the ectopic P wave is targeted by ablation. If ablation of the ectopic focus fails, electrical isolation of the arrhythmogenic PV should be considered (see later). In addition, ablation may be performed at sites with catheter-induced repetitive ectopy (defined as the acute onset of a burst of rapid PACs on touching the wall, sustained irritability while at the spot, and acute termination of rapid activity on release of the catheter).

Ablation Technique

RF energy is delivered using a 4-mm-tip catheter with a target temperature of 45° to 50°C and a maximal power output of 25 to 30 W to reduce the risk of PV stenosis.[6] The ablation is considered to be delivered at an appropriate site if, during ablation, a rapid burst of PACs originating from that site is seen, or an abrupt disappearance of triggering PACs is observed.

Endpoints of Ablation

The endpoint is elimination of ectopy, spontaneous or induced by provocative maneuvers (using both the same provocative maneuvers and defibrillation protocol as before the ablation). Elimination or dissociation of PV potentials from atrial activity is also a satisfactory endpoint.[6]

Outcome

Early experience with the focal ablation of PV arrhythmias has indicated that the recurrence rate is high and the success rate is only modest, even in experienced laboratories. The suboptimal results can be attributed to the limitations of the technique. Many patients have multiple foci in the same PV or in multiple PVs. Multiple arrhythmogenic PVs are usually associated with older age, longer AF duration, and larger atrial dimensions.[6] In addition, there may be a paucity of spontaneous or inducible arrhythmias during the procedure. The spontaneous occurrence of ectopic beats and paroxysms of AF is unpredictable, and provocative procedures are not consistently effective.[6] Mapping can also be made difficult by frequent recurrences of persistent AF requiring multiple cardioversions. Furthermore, after a successful procedure, new foci may emerge. Remapping usually shows new foci in the ablated vein or in other veins, rather than recurrence of the original focus.

It is also important to recognize that RF ablation inside the PVs carries a significant risk of PV stenosis, which limits the amount of RF energy that can be safely delivered within a PV. PV stenosis was detected by increased PV flow velocity on TEE in 42% of cases in one report. An increased risk of PV stenosis has been associated with the use of RF power more than 45 W.

Focal ablation has been successful only in highly selected patients with frequently recurrent paroxysmal AF. Reported rates of a positive outcome using a focal ablation approach to eliminate AF triggers have varied from 38% to 80%.[6] Haissaguerre and associates[6] have studied 45 patients with frequent episodes of AF (episodes of AF occurring at least once every 2 days; the mean duration of AF was almost 6 hr/day) frequent PACs (more than 700/24 hr), refractory to two or more pharmacological agents. A single point of origin of PACs was identified in 29 patients—9 had two points of origin, and 7 had three or four foci. In that study, 94% of the foci were 2 to 4 cm inside the PVs (31 in the left superior PV, 17 in the right superior PV, 11 in the left inferior PV, and 6 in the right inferior PV); the remaining four foci originated from the RA or LA. After ablation (mean, four to seven RF applications were required; 75% of patients required a second or third procedure) of these foci, 62% of patients had no recurrences at 8 month follow-up in the absence of antiarrhythmic therapy; most episodes of recurrent AF were associated with recurrent PACs. Chen studied 79 patients with frequent PACs and paroxysmal AF; the success rate was 86% at 6 months (only 7% requiring a second procedure) and 75% at 8 months.[49] The success rate of focal ablation is inversely related to the number of arrhythmogenic foci. In a study of 90 patients in whom the majority (69%) had multiple PV foci, the success rates were 93%, 73%, and 55% in patients with one, two, or three or more foci, respectively. Recovery of local PV potential and the inability to abolish it were associated with AF recurrence (90% versus 55% with and without potential abolition).

SEGMENTAL OSTIAL PULMONARY VEIN ISOLATION

Rationale

There are several factors to consider, including the electrical isolation of pulmonary veins and determining which ones to isolate.

Electrical Isolation of Pulmonary Veins

On the basis of the knowledge of the AF initiation mechanism by focal discharges in the PVs, electrical disconnection at the PV ostium is now recognized as a better ablative technique to inactivate focal triggers of AF. Ablation guided by mapping focal ectopy has a high recurrence rate and low long-term success and is limited by unpredictability, inconsistent inducibility, and the risk of inducing AF requiring cardioversion multiple times during the procedure. Moreover, the appearance of multiple sources of AF triggers and the high recurrence rate argue for more extensive ablation strategy. PV isolation has been introduced to address these issues.[6]

PV potentials identify muscular sleeves that extend from the LA into the PVs. These potentials are responsible for transmitting triggering impulses from the vein to the LA. The myocardial fibers that envelop the PVs may not be present along the entire circumference of the PV ostia. Therefore, to eliminate conduction in and out of a PV, ablation along the entire circumference of the ostium may not be necessary. Instead, RF energy can be targeted to the segments of the ostium at which muscle fibers are present, which typically involves RF application to 30% to 80% of the circumference of the PVs. These sites are identified by the presence of high-frequency depolarizations, which likely represent PV muscle potentials.

The major advantages of this technique are that it eliminates the need for detailed mapping of all PV foci and that there is a clear-cut end point of ablation, even when spontaneous arrhythmias are absent.

Which Pulmonary Veins to Isolate

Only Arrhythmogenic Pulmonary Veins. Focal ablation deep in a PV carries a risk of PV stenosis. Restricting RF delivery to the ostium of the arrhythmogenic PV, as in segmental ostial PV isolation, may help reduce this risk. Furthermore, a more limited ablation approach (as compared with isolation of all PVs) requires shorter procedure and fluoroscopy times and may be safer.

All Four Pulmonary Veins. PV isolation of only the arrhythmogenic PV was shown to have limited success rate. Furthermore, identification of the arrhythmogenic PV may be difficult and time-consuming, because focal activity may be difficult to observe or induce during the ablation procedure. Additionally, the prevalence of multiple arrhythmogenic PVs is high (up to 69%). Therefore, isolation of only the culprit PV identified during the procedure may allow the emergence of focal ectopy from other PVs, which may cause AF recurrence after the procedure. Moreover, electrical disconnection may not be achieved by ostial ablation to only the targeted PV in patients with electrical connections between the PVs.

Evidence has suggested that almost all PVs are capable of generating the premature depolarizations that trigger AF, with the upper PVs being responsible for most AF triggers (and the left superior PV is the vein with the longest muscular sleeve); only a minority (0% to 30%) of foci has been identified in the inferior PVs (the right inferior PV being the least important source of triggers).[6] The relatively infrequent importance of the right inferior PV in patients with AF is consistent with prior anatomical studies demonstrating that the muscle sleeves around the right inferior PV are less prominent than the muscle sleeves that surround the other PVs. Although cannulation of the right inferior PV with a distal ring catheter electrode may be challenging in some patients, in most patients this vein can be successfully isolated with little prolongation in the total PV isolation procedural time. Therefore, unless no PV potentials are present at its ostium, all four PVs should be targeted, whenever feasible.

Circumferential Mapping of Pulmonary Vein Potentials

Lasso Catheter Mapping

A deflectable decapolar catheter with a distal ring configuration (Lasso catheter) is advanced sequentially into each PV and is used for ostial mapping (Fig. 11-15). The ring catheter enables circumferential mapping of the PV ostia perpendicular to the axis of the vein.[50] Lasso catheters are of different sizes. The selection of a 15-, 20- or 25-mm diameter Lasso catheter is guided by the estimated size of the PVs angiographically and/or with CT (see Fig. 11-9). Because of the highly variable sizes of PV ostia, fixed-diameter catheters may not always achieve catheter stability and optimal electrogram recordings. In some cases, suboptimal positioning, poor wall contact, and poor stability of an inappropriately sized circumferential catheter underestimates the number of PV potentials and can result in failure to isolate the PV completely because of undetected residual PV-atrial electrical connections.

Some of those issues can be addressed by using an expandable 15- to 25-mm diameter ring catheter (Lasso 2515). The expandable ring catheter is introduced into each PV and withdrawn to the most proximal stable position, with optimal wall contact ensured by progressive loop expansion. These catheters may enable more proximal and stable placement and optimal wall contact at the PV ostia. This is important because the ablation target is not within the ostia, but in the atrial tissue proximal to the LA-PV junction.

The ring catheter is positioned in the left superior PV, left inferior PV, and right superior PV. If accessible, the right inferior PV is usually mapped last because of the technical difficulty and the risk of dislodgment of the mapping catheters from the LA to the RA. The ring catheter is positioned within a PV and gradually withdrawn to within 5 mm of the ostium. It is important to position the ring catheter at the ostium of the PV; when positioned too deeply in the PV, PV potentials can be missed (Fig. 11-16). Subsequently, circumferential mapping of the PV is performed by obtaining 10 bipolar electrograms (1-2, 2-3, up to 10-1 electrode pairs) with the circular arranged electrodes of the ring catheter. The bandpass settings for the bipolar recordings are 30 to 500 Hz. Pacing from each pair of electrodes from the ring catheter has been used by some to ensure appropriate ring

11

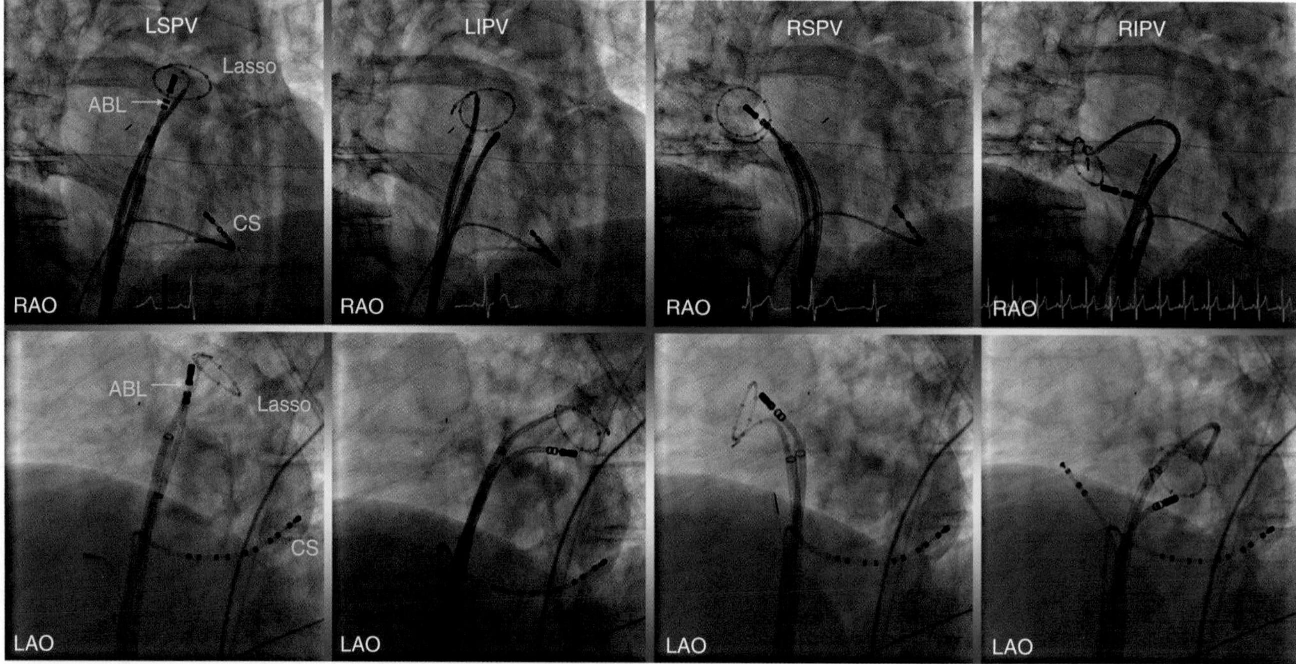

FIGURE 11–15 Fluoroscopy views (right anterior oblique [RAO] and left anterior oblique [LAO]) of the ring catheter positioned at the ostium of the four pulmonary veins (PVs). **Panels from left to right,** Left superior PV (LSPV), left inferior PV (LIPV), right superior PV (RSPV), and right inferior PV (RIPV). Note that during ablation, the ablation catheter is always positioned at the atrial side of the ring catheter.

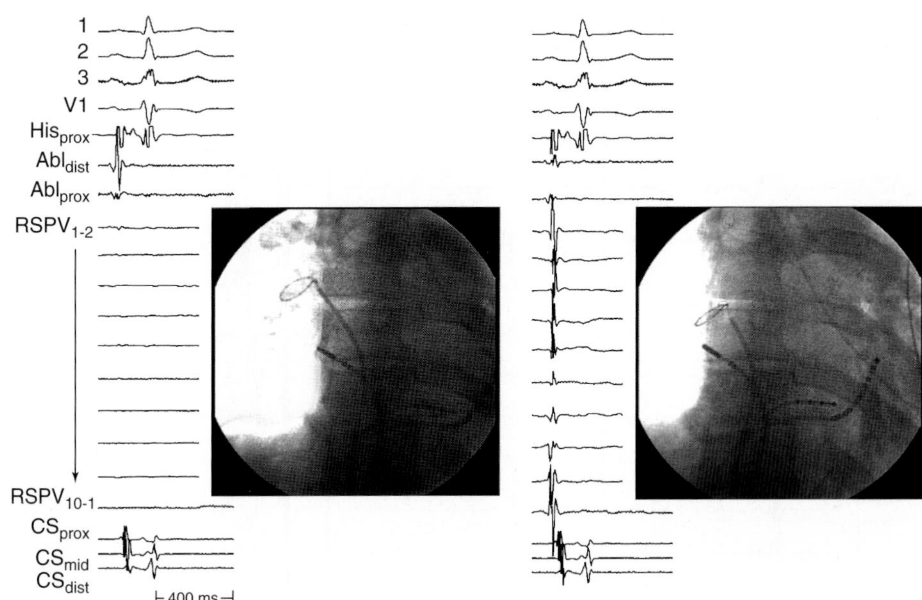

FIGURE 11–16 Recordings from a ring catheter in the right superior pulmonary vein (RSPV). **A,** The ring catheter is situated too deep in vein; recordings suggest no PV potentials. **B,** The ring catheter pulled back 1.5 cm, showing abundant PV potentials.

catheter sizing (80% of electrode pairs resulting in capture) and to demonstrate conduction from the veins to the atrium before ablation.

Ring catheters with 20 poles are also available and can offer higher resolution circumferential mapping and improve the differentiation of PV from LA potentials. The conventional wide bipolar electrograms record the PV potentials as well as the larger LA potentials, which can obscure or mimic the PV potentials. In contrast, the high-resolution electrograms minimize the extent of far-field electrogram detection and display very small or completely absent LA potentials. In the context of PV isolation during sustained AF, improved discrimination between atrial and PV potentials may facilitate the recognition of complete PV disconnection, and possibly limit the number of unnecessary RF applications. On the other hand, when a ring catheter and closely spaced electrodes make poor contact with the PV wall or are placed deep within the PV, near-field potentials may not be seen, which leads to underdetection of PV potentials.

Mapping During Normal Sinus Rhythm

It is preferable to perform PV mapping during NSR or atrial pacing whenever possible, because AF reduces PV potential amplitude, making them harder to identify. Therefore, if the patient is in AF, electrical cardioversion is usually performed to restore NSR. Ibutilide (1 mg) or amiodarone (300 mg) may also be administered intravenously to prevent immediate recurrences of AF after cardioversion.

PV mapping during NSR typically shows double or multiple potentials that are usually recorded in a progressively later temporal sequence, synchronous with the first (right PVs) or second (left PVs) half of the sinus P wave (Fig. 11-17). The first low-frequency potential reflects activation of the adjacent LA. The latest high-frequency potentials indicate PV potentials.

Identification of Pulmonary Vein Potentials Using Pacing Maneuvers. PV potentials often are fused with the far-field LA electrograms but can be identified by their high-frequency appearance. Not uncommonly, an isoelectric interval separates the far-field LA electrogram and the near-field PV potential. The basis for this separation is unclear; however, evidence has suggested that there is an area of slow conduction at the proximal PV. The interval between the far-field electrogram and the PV potential may differ based on the site of pacing. The reasons for this phenomenon may be related to fiber orientation (anisotropy), which may make it easier to enter the vein from certain wavefront directions or because the far-field electrogram is not actually coming from the LA but is arising from a neighboring structure. Therefore, pacing from different atrial sites (most commonly high RA or distal CS) can help separate PV potentials from far-field atrial signals (see Fig. 11-17). Furthermore, incremental rate atrial pacing and premature atrial stimulation from the same atrial site can sometimes result in conduction delay between the LA and PV at the PV ostium, which often exhibits decremental conduction properties (Fig. 11-18). Thus, if a complex electrogram is seen on a PV mapping catheter and, with faster or premature pacing, one of the potentials is seen to occur later after the far-field atrial electrogram, the late potential likely is a PV potential.

Right-sided PVs are typically mapped during NSR or RA pacing. For left PVs, the ostial PV potentials are sometimes not obvious because of the superimposed LA potential during NSR; therefore, pacing from the distal CS (at a CL of 500 to 600 milliseconds) allows their separation and easy recognition of PV potentials (see Fig. 11-17). However, even during CS pacing at a CL of 600 milliseconds, the atrial and PV potentials still may overlap in approximately 50% to 60% of left PVs (see Fig. 11-18). The separation may be less evident in the posterior PV antrum, which is closer to the CS. Pacing from the LA appendage may help in this situation.

Because of the anatomical proximity of the PVs to several other structures that are electrically active, complex signals may be recorded by a catheter placed in the PV. For example, a catheter placed in the left superior PV may record electrical activity in the LA, LA appendage, ipsilateral PV, and vein of Marshall. Similarly, a mapping catheter placed in the right superior PV may record electrical activity in the right middle PV, right inferior PV (particularly a superior branch), RA, LA, and SVC (Fig. 11-19). When a typical PV potential is recorded in a left PV, the far-field electrogram

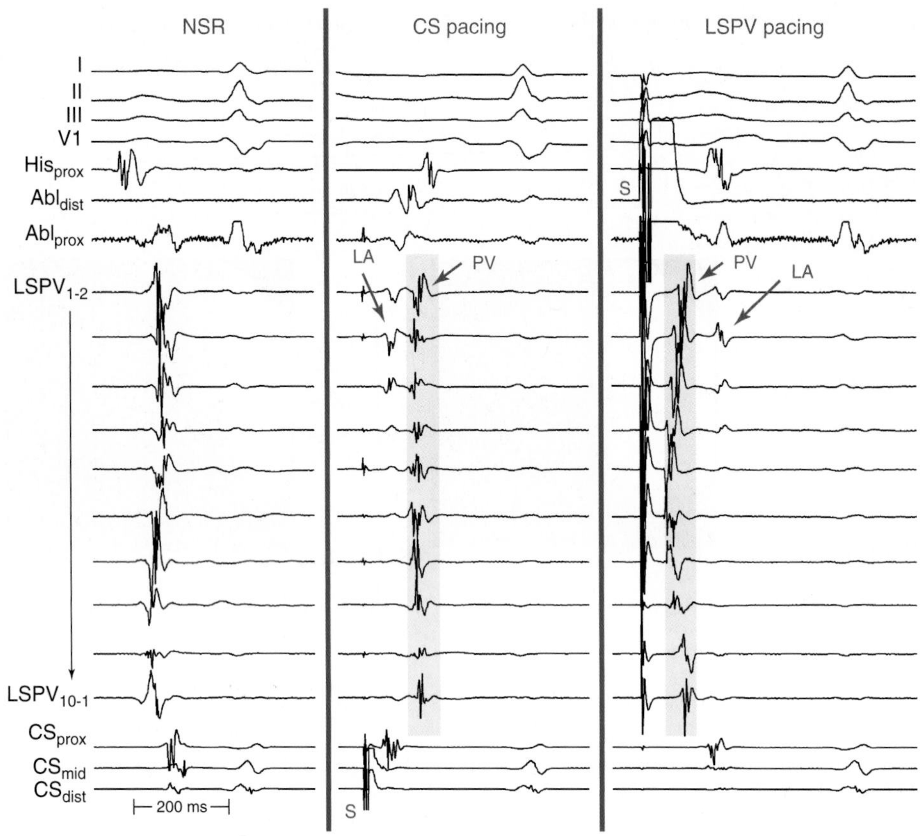

FIGURE 11–17 Differential atrial pacing to identify pulmonary vein (PV) potentials. **Left panel,** During normal sinus rhythm (NSR), the atrial and left superior PV (LSPV) potentials are superimposed and distinction of PV potentials from left atrial (LA) electrograms is difficult, if not impossible. **Middle panel,** During coronary sinus (CS) pacing, PV potentials (shaded area) are delayed relative to LA potentials and are thus readily discerned. **Right panel,** Pacing from within the LSPV also shows a clear delineation of PV versus LA potentials; in this case, PV potentials precede LA potentials.

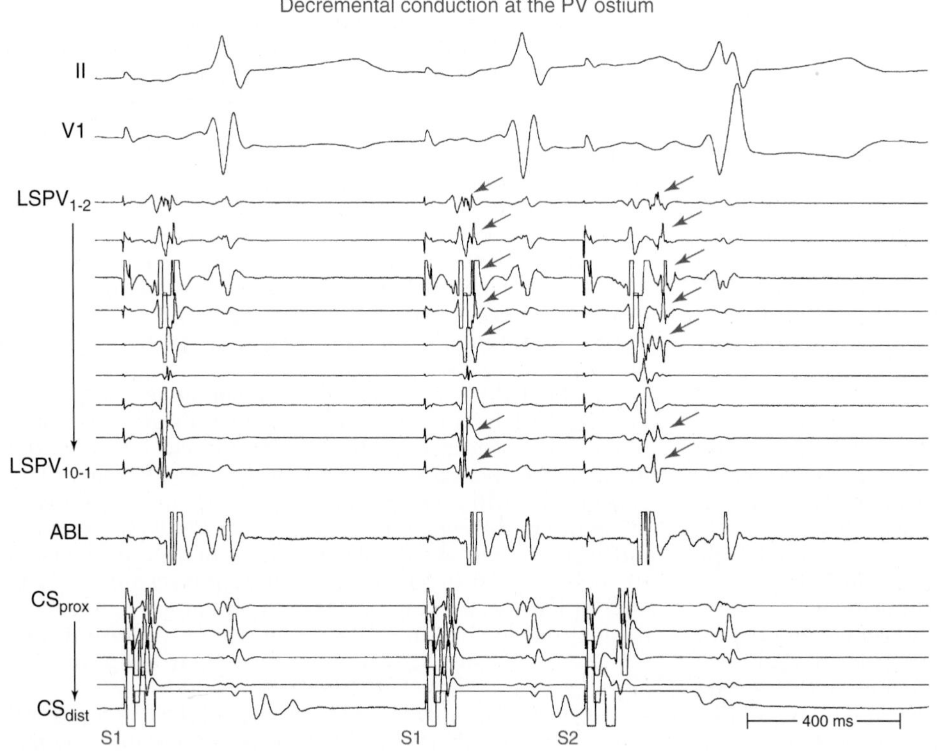

FIGURE 11–18 Decremental conduction at the pulmonary vein (PV) ostium. During coronary sinus (CS) drive pacing, complex electrograms (blue arrows) are recorded by the ring catheter positioned at the ostium of the left superior PV (LSPV). An atrial extrastimulus from the distal CS results in conduction delay between the left atrium (LA) and PV at the PV ostium. Therefore, PV potentials (red arrows) become delayed and separated from atrial electrograms.

usually is coming from the LA. When mapping catheters are placed in the right-sided PV, often the main far-field electrogram is the RA electrogram, and the second far-field electrogram, if seen, is the LA electrogram.[51] In general, only the PV potential itself is near-field; all other structures picked up by the antenna of the mapping catheter are blunted and far-field. However, this criterion alone is insufficient for identifying the true PV potential. For example, if a catheter is deep within the left superior PV, where no PV musculature is present, the LA appendage electrograms will appear relatively near-field. Similarly, when RF ablation has already been performed, edema near the PV os and inadver-

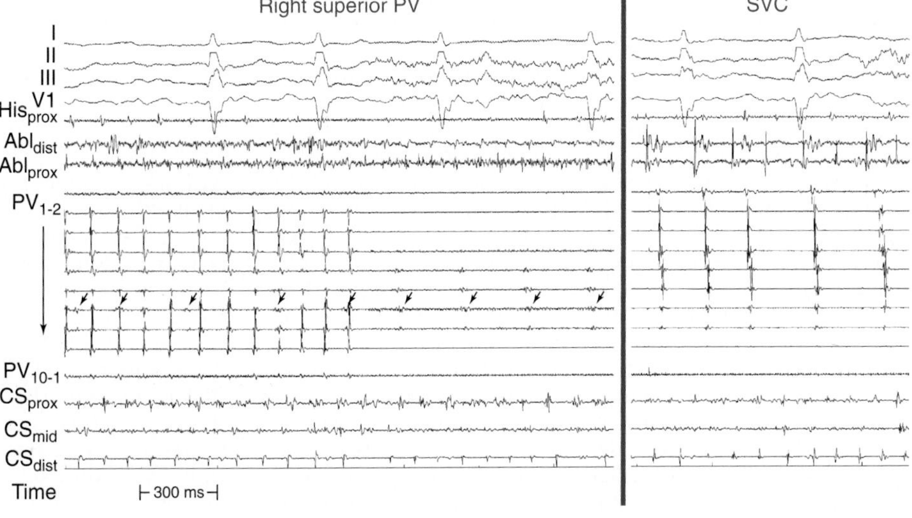

FIGURE 11–19 Superior vena cava (SVC) activity recorded in the right superior pulmonary vein (PV). **Left panel,** Recordings from a ring catheter positioned at the ostium of the right superior PV showing high-amplitude PV potentials that disappear midway through the recording because of isolation of the vein with RF ablation. Another set of lower amplitude signals (arrows) remain and were present prior to PV isolation. **Right panel,** These potentials represent far-field SVC recordings, shown as sharp near-field recordings after the ring catheter is positioned in the SVC.

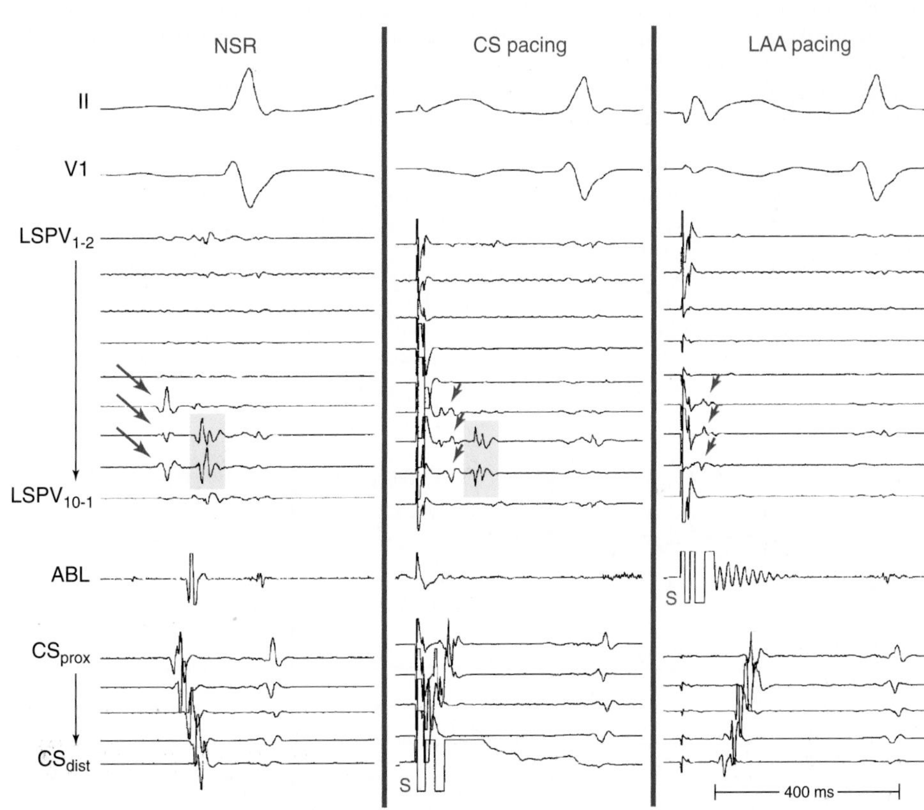

FIGURE 11–20 Differential pacing for identification of pulmonary vein (PV) potentials. During electrical isolation of the left superior PV (LSPV) in normal sinus rhythm (NSR), residual electrograms were persistent despite multiple RF applications. The initial electrograms (red arrows) were consistent with left atrial (LA) far-field activity. However, the late electrograms (shaded area) were suspicious for PV activity. Pacing from the distal coronary sinus (CS) resulted in anticipation of both early and late electrograms. Pacing via the ablation catheter positioned in the LA appendage (LAA) resulted in disappearance of the late electrograms (i.e., those electrograms merged with the saturation artifact related to the pacing spike), suggesting that those electrograms in fact represented LAA activity. Therefore, the presence of PV potentials was excluded, and no further RF ablation was necessary.

tent ablation within the PV (more frequent than generally realized) will cause PV potentials to be less sharp and less near-field in character.[51] Various pacing maneuvers can differentiate from among these possibilities, and can help exclude or prove relationship of various components of the electrogram recorded from a PV to anatomical structures surrounding that particular PV.

One pacing maneuver commonly used when complex electrograms are recorded on a mapping catheter placed in a PV is pacing at specific sites likely to be responsible for the components of the electrogram. The premise of such a maneuver is that pacing performed from a particular site results in the electrogram originating from that site to occur earlier, close to the pacing stimulus. For example, because of the proximity of the LA appendage to the left PVs (especially the left superior PV), far-field LA appendage potentials can be recorded in these PVs, and PV potentials may be confused with LA appendage potentials. These potentials are distinguished from PV potentials by differential pacing from the distal CS and LA appendage. If a pacing catheter is placed in the LA appendage and LA appendage capture is documented, the LA appendage component of the complex electrogram will occur early and will be drawn toward the pacing artifact (Fig. 11-20). Thus, the electrogram that moves the closest to the pacing stimulus can be diagnosed as originating from the LA appendage. Similar reasoning can be applied when pacing in an ipsilateral PV—if a component of the electrogram recorded in the left superior PV is, in fact, a left inferior PV potential—or when pacing in the SVC and vein of Marshall.[51]

LA electrograms, particularly when fragmented secondary to partial ablation, can also be mistaken for a PV potential, and pacing from a site in the LA close, but not within, the PV (perivenous pacing) can help define the LA electrogram component of a complex PV recording. When pacing from a perivenous location, the LA signal will occur very close to, and often will merge with, the saturation artifact related to the pacing spike. However, because pacing is being performed proximal to the site of ostial delay, the PV potential remains unchanged or may occur with slightly more delay. The shift of the LA signal, which now is being captured by perivenous pacing, toward the pacing spike indicates the origin of that component of a complex signal. Differentiation of RA, LA, and PV potentials recorded within right-sided PVs can also be achieved using similar maneuvers (Fig. 11-21).[51]

An extension of the basic concept that pacing from a particular site will cause earlier occurrence of the electrogram arising from that site is multisite simultaneous pacing. For example, pacing from the CS alone is compared with simultaneous pacing from both the CS and LA appendage, with specific attention paid to the transition in the recorded electrogram between single-site (e.g., CS only) and dual-site (e.g., CS and LA appendage) pacing, which can help immediate recognition of the various components of a complex signal recorded within the PV.[51]

Ablation Target Sites. Target sites for ablation are selected by identifying the earliest bipolar PV potentials and/or the unipolar electrograms with the most rapid (sharpest) intrinsic deflection on high-speed recordings (150 to 200 mm/sec) that have equivalent or earlier activation relative to the earliest PV potential recorded on the adjacent ring catheter recording sites (Fig. 11-22).

Electrogram polarity reversal can also be used as an additional indicator of breakthroughs from the LA to the PVs and identify potential ablation targets. Polarity reversal is defined as a sudden change in the main deflection of the PV potential. The reversal occurs as the wavefront of activation propagates radially in the PV from its connection with the LA, thus reaching contiguous bipolar recording electrodes in opposing directions (Fig. 11-23; see also Fig. 11-22).

Mapping During Atrial Fibrillation

Although segmental ostial PV isolation is accomplished most efficiently during NSR, maintenance of NSR during an ablation procedure may not be readily achievable, particularly in patients with chronic AF. During an ongoing episode of AF, PV potentials can be obscured during the chaotic electrical activity of AF. Nevertheless, segmental ostial PV isolation was found to be as feasible and successful during AF as during NSR. An advantage of mapping during AF is that it obviates the need for the administration of antiarrhythmic drugs and for multiple electrical cardioversions in patients with immediately recurrent AF after cardioversion. Two approaches have been described for PV isolation during AF: the first uses intermittent bursts of PV tachycardia to guide PV isolation and the second uses organized PV potentials during AF to guide PV isolation.

Intermittent Pulmonary Vein Tachycardia. Prior studies have demonstrated that rapid rhythms arising in the PVs (intermittent PV tachycardia) are common during AF (recorded during AF in 90% to 97% of PVs) and may play an important role in the maintenance of AF, or may be a marker of an arrhythmogenic PV that triggers AF during NSR. Those intermittent bursts of PV tachycardia indicate the presence of an underlying arrhythmogenic muscle fascicle near the ostial recording sites and, therefore, can be used to guide segmental ostial ablation to isolate the PVs during AF.

During AF, the PVs are sequentially mapped with the ring catheter to assess the presence of intermittent PV tachy-

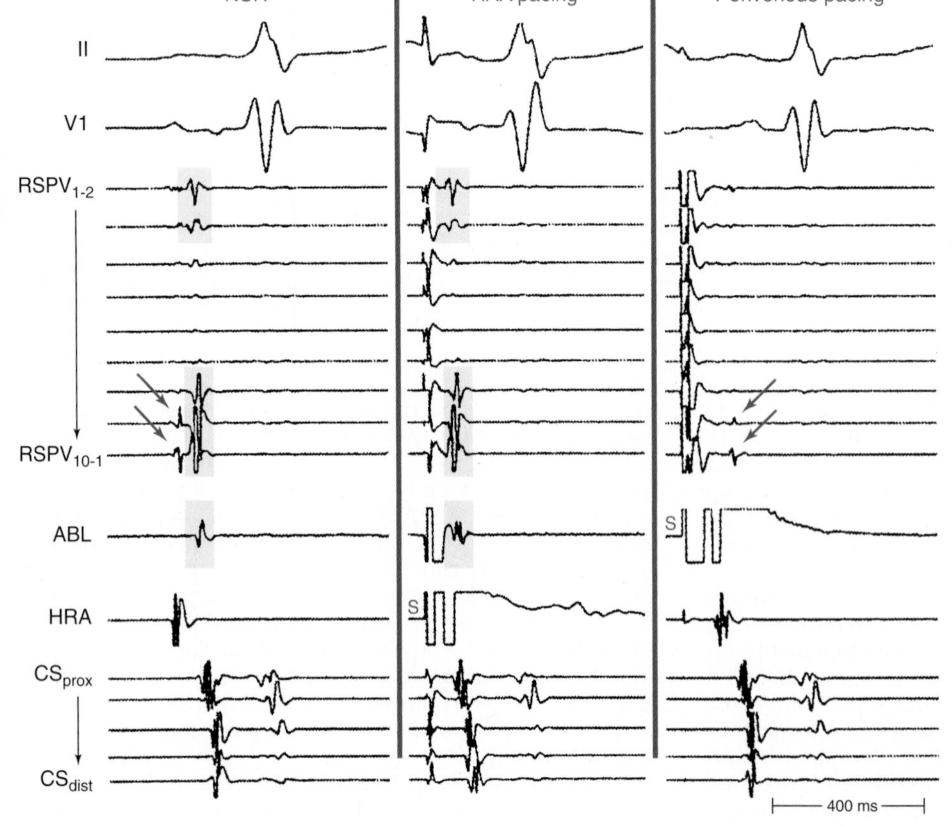

FIGURE 11–21 Differential pacing for identification of pulmonary vein (PV) potentials. During electrical isolation of the right superior PV (RSPV) in normal sinus rhythm (NSR), residual electrograms (blue shaded area and red arrows) were persistent despite multiple RF applications. Pacing from the right atrial (RA) appendage (RAA) resulted in disappearance of the earlier electrograms (red arrows; i.e., those electrograms merged with the saturation artifact related to the pacing spike), suggesting that those electrograms in fact represented RA activity. During pacing just outside the ostium of the RSPV (using the ablation catheter), the second set of electrograms (shaded area) disappeared while the RA electrograms (red arrows) persisted in the ring catheter recordings, indicating that the second set of electrograms in fact represented left atrial (LA) activity. Therefore, the presence of PV potentials was excluded, and no further RF ablation was necessary.

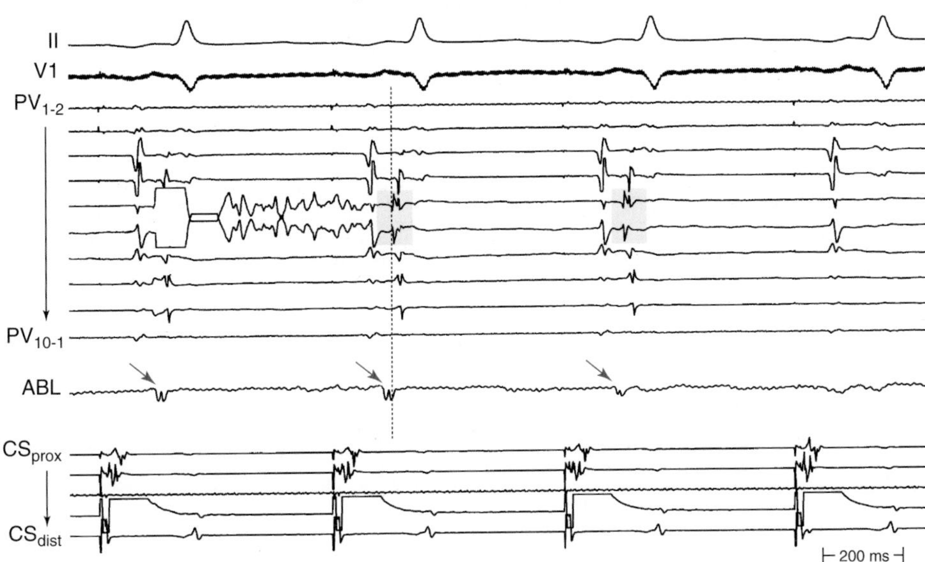

FIGURE 11–22 Segmental ostial pulmonary vein (PV) isolation. During circumferential ostial PV mapping using a ring catheter, electrical connections between the left atrium (LA) and the PV (target sites for ablation) are identified by recording the earliest bipolar PV potentials with electrogram polarity reversal on adjacent poles (shaded electrograms). Note that the distal bipoles of the ablation catheter record even an earlier sharp PV potential (arrows). The presence of ablation artifact on the recording from a specific ring catheter pole confirms the pole the catheter is on and that the catheter is in the same plane as the ring catheter. Catheter ablation at that site results in complete elimination of PV potentials and LA-PV block (last complex).

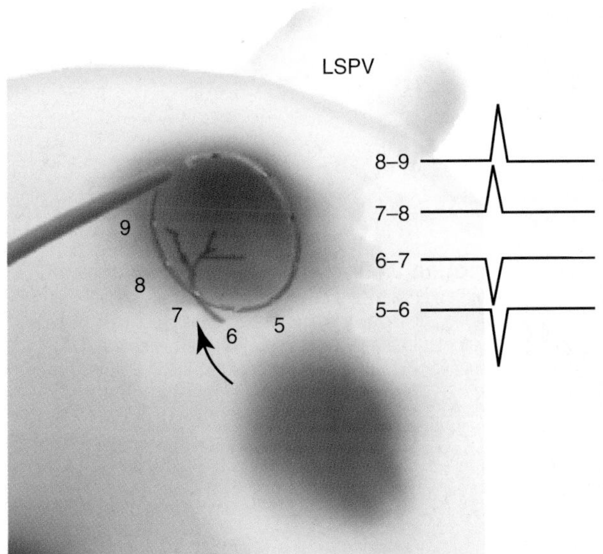

FIGURE 11–23 Bipolar electrogram polarity reversal. The ring electrode catheter (electrodes numbered) is situated in the ostium of the left superior pulmonary vein (LSPV); a strand of atrial muscle crosses from the left atrium (LA) to the PV (red) and branches within the vein. The arrow indicates propagation of the wavefront of activation from the LA to the PV. The strand crosses at electrode 7; recordings from surrounding bipoles indicate the direction of propagation away from (negative deflection) or toward (positive deflection) the bipole. The point at which the polarity reverses from positive to negative is where the strand crosses into the PV.

cardia, defined as a PV rhythm that intermittently has a CL shorter than the AF CL recorded in the adjacent LA. When intermittent PV tachycardia is recorded by several electrodes, the ostial site corresponding to the most rapid intrinsic deflection of the unipolar electrogram should be targeted by RF applications. If PV tachycardia is not observed, ostial sites that display a high-frequency bipolar PV potential and/or rapid unipolar intrinsic deflection during AF can alternatively be targeted for ablation.

If AF terminates during ablation, PV potentials are then assessed during NSR and atrial pacing. If there is evidence of residual conduction over a PV fascicle, RF energy is delivered at these ostial sites during NSR or atrial pacing. On the other hand, if AF is still present after isolation of a PV, electrical cardioversion is performed. If AF recurs, other PVs are isolated during AF and, if NSR is maintained, the remaining PVs are isolated during NSR or atrial pacing.

Organization of Pulmonary Vein Potentials. PV potentials are classified at baseline as organized (have a consistent activation sequence for longer than 10 seconds) or disorganized (activation sequence on the ring catheter varies from beat to beat). Approximately 37% of PVs have organized PV potentials (more for inferior than superior PVs—53% versus 26%; Fig. 11-24). When PV activation pattern is organized (from the beginning or after some anatomically guided RF applications), the area showing the earliest activation and/or demonstrating polarity reversal on the ring catheter is targeted.

For disorganized PV potentials, ablation is performed circumferentially around the ring catheter on the ostial side of the PV. The top and bottom segments of the PV are targeted first because of the high prevalence of LA-PV breakthroughs at these sites. In most cases, initial RF applications result in organization of PV activity; this is probably secondary to progressive reduction of LA-PV breakthroughs that diminishes the mass of fibrillatory conduction within the PV and channel the electrical activity through the last remaining fascicles connecting the LA to the PV, thereby activating the PV in an organized fashion. This consequently enables EP-guided PV isolation.

Organized PV activity may represent fewer LA-PV connections, and therefore may require fewer RF applications than PVs with disorganized activity. This may explain the greater frequency of organized activity in the inferior PVs, presumably because of the presence of less extensive muscular sleeves in these veins as demonstrated by pathological studies.

Basket Catheter Mapping

The basket catheter (Constellation, Boston Scientific, Natick, Mass) is composed of 64 electrodes mounted on eight flexible, self-expanding splines (see Fig. 2-4). Each spline is identified by a letter (from A to H) and each electrode by a number (distal 1 to proximal 8). The 32 bipolar electrograms provide 3-D mapping of PV activation.

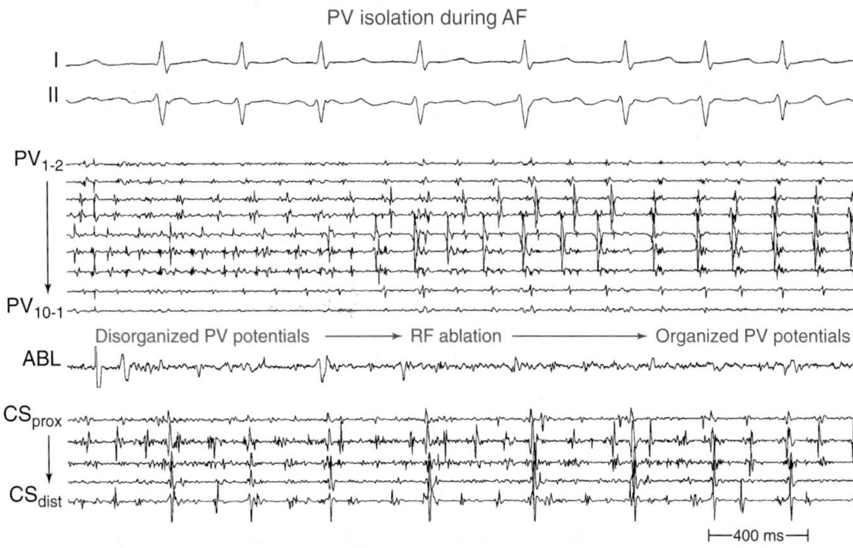

FIGURE 11–24 Pulmonary vein (PV) isolation during atrial fibrillation (AF). Initially (at left), PV potentials are disorganized. During RF application at the PV ostium, the PV potentials become organized. See text for discussion.

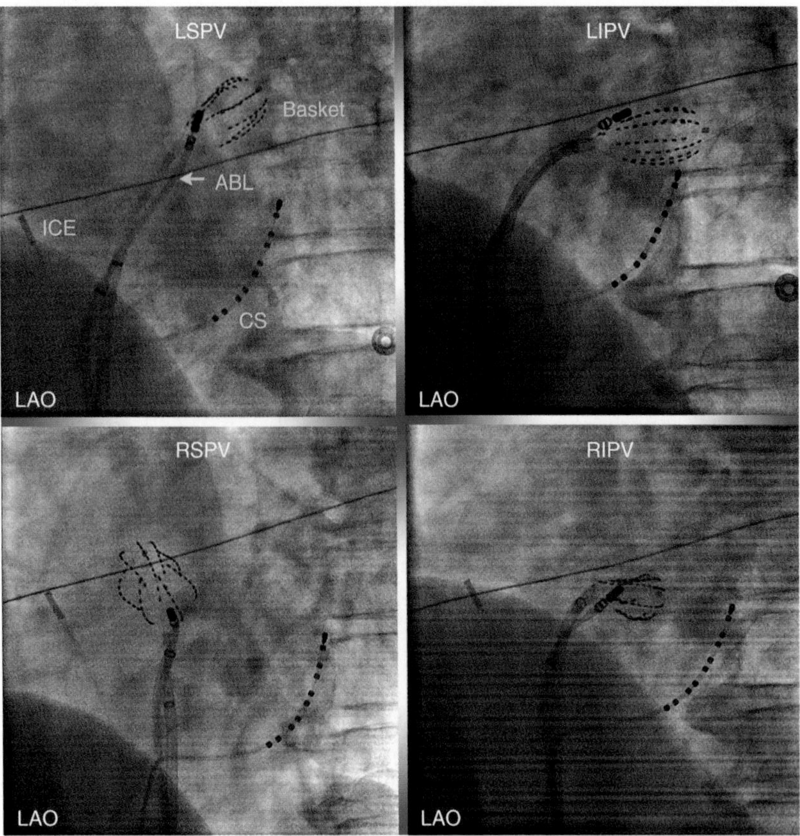

FIGURE 11–25 Left anterior oblique (LAO) fluoroscopic views of basket catheter positioned in the four pulmonary veins (PVs). A long deflectable sheath is used to help position the basket catheter in the different PVs. LIPV = left inferior PV; LSPV = left superior PV; RIPV = right inferior PV; RSPV = right superior PV.

11

Basket Catheter Positioning. After transseptal access is gained, an 8.5 Fr soft-tipped guiding sheath with a 90- or 120-degree curve or, preferably, a deflectable sheath, is introduced into the PVs. The basket catheter is then introduced into the sheath so that the tip of the basket catheter reaches the tip of the sheath; the sheath is then pulled back to allow expansion of the basket catheter (Fig. 11-25). For introduction into the inferior PVs, the sheath is inserted first with the help of the steerable ablation catheter. The ablation catheter is introduced through the sheath and, once it is engaged in the PV, the sheath is advanced over the ablation catheter. Once the sheath is in place in the PV, the steerable catheter is removed and replaced by the basket catheter. The basket catheter is then deployed in the PV by slowly advancing the basket catheter while simultaneously withdrawing the sheath. Alternatively, the basket catheter is inserted directly into the PVs directly with the sheath positioned in the LA; however, although this technique was found to be safe because of the very flexible splines of the basket catheter, extreme caution is required to avoid venous perforation by the stiff catheter tip.

A basket catheter with a diameter of 31 mm is chosen when the diameter of the main PV trunk is 26 mm or less, and a basket catheter with a diameter of 38 mm is used when the PV diameter is more than 26 mm or when there is a common ostium. The PV diameter is determined by MR imaging, CT scanning, or PV angiography. The position of the basket catheter in relation to the PV ostium can be determined by PV angiography (Fig. 11-26). If necessary, the basket catheter is retracted to obtain optimal contact to the main trunk and ostium of the PV.

Basket Catheter Mapping. The basket catheter is deployed within the target PV with its most proximal electrodes positioned at the PV ostium, determined by selective PV angiography. PV activation can be followed during NSR or CS pacing passing the four levels of bipolar electrograms from proximal ostial (7/8) to distal (1/2) inside the PV. During ectopic beats or initiation of AF, the activation can be followed from the source of ectopy to its exit to the LA (see Fig. 11-11).[52]

A computerized 3-D mapping system (QMS2) has been introduced to construct a 3-D color isochronal or isopotential map from a total of 56 bipolar electrograms recorded by the basket catheter. The electrical activity in the space between the splines is estimated by a bicubic spline interpolation to construct a continuous map. This 3-D mapping system has been found useful for identifying a preferential electrical connection and determining its elimination accurately because it enables not only a visualization of the activation sequence of the PV potentials, but also an adequate evaluation of the activation sequence between the splines. An animation of a 3-D potential map, which can reflect a series of electrical activations, is used to reveal the style of breakthrough, distribution of the PV musculature, and activation pattern within the PV. A color setup with a gradation that corresponds to the relative size of the potential amplitude can be arranged variously on the QMS map. For example, in the detection of an AF focus, the color setup needs to be arranged to emphasize the small PV potentials triggering the AF. In contrast, for PV isolation, it is essential to minimize the low-amplitude LA potentials and emphasize the high-amplitude PV potentials to construct a clear 3-D map of the PV potentials. When the small potentials need to be emphasized, the color threshold is decreased to 30% of the largest amplitude of all the related potentials. The short stay of the activation wavefront near the outer frame of the 3-D PV potential map before the longitudinal propagation, which reflects a conduction delay, indicates the LA-PV junction where continuous fractionated potentials connecting the LA potentials and PV potentials are observed. The serial activation patterns moving around the outer frame of the 3-D PV isopotential map before the longitudinal propagation are defined to indicate the LA-PV junction. The onset of a centrifugal activation on the LA-PV junction is identified as an electrical connection.

Basket Catheter–Guided Pulmonary Vein Isolation. With a multipolar basket catheter, ostial PV isolation with disconnection of conduction pathways between the LA and PVs can be performed by RF application to the breakthrough site identified by the 3-D PV potential map. The Astronomer system (Boston Scientific) is used for navigation of the ablation catheter inside the basket catheter.[52] Ablation is performed at the junction between the PV and the LA, as ostial as catheter stability allows at the shortest atrial PV potential delay. The location of the ostium is determined by electrogram morphology and by noting the shape of the basket catheter as it is conformed to the PV and as ostial anatomy can be confirmed by angiography. The QMS recording is performed after every RF application and, if the elimination of a target breakthrough is confirmed, another breakthrough is identified and ablated.

Advantages of the Basket Catheter. The basket catheter is currently the mapping tool with the highest resolution available for endovascular mapping of the LA-PV junction in humans. In addition, the basket catheter provides information about the anatomy of the PV, such as exact ostium localization, because the basket catheter takes the shape of the PV (see Fig. 11-26) and allows 3-D reconstruction of the PV activation from the ostium to deep inside the PV.

The Astronomer navigation system permits precise and reproducible guidance of the ablation catheter tip to areas identified as LA to PV conduction pathways, thereby allowing efficient PV isolation. The distal poles of the basket catheter can be used to monitor changes in the activation sequence in real time and thereby demonstrate the effects of ablation at the ostium as lesions are created. They also provide an immediate indication of successful PV isolation by the disappearance of the distal PV potentials. The system also helps identify areas near the PV ostium with fragmented potentials and with discharging ostial foci, which can be localized in a single beat.

The risk of PV stenosis seems to be low (1.2%) with the use of basket catheter–guided PV isolation. This technology can potentially minimize the risk of PV stenosis, first by reducing the number of RF ablations, and second by avoiding ablations inside the PV, because the basket catheter allows localization of the PV ostium during the entire procedure. Thus, the use of complementary navigation systems or ICE appears to be nonessential when using the basket catheter for PV isolation.

Disadvantages of the Basket Catheter. Carbonizations can form after ablation on the splines of the basket catheter, which can potentially cause embolism. Carbonizations, which appear as dark material attached to the basket catheter electrodes or splines, are thought to be caused by the concentration of RF energy on the thin splines, which results in very high local temperatures that induce denaturization of proteins. However, carbonization can be greatly diminished with the use of an irrigated-tip catheter as opposed to conventional ablation catheters.

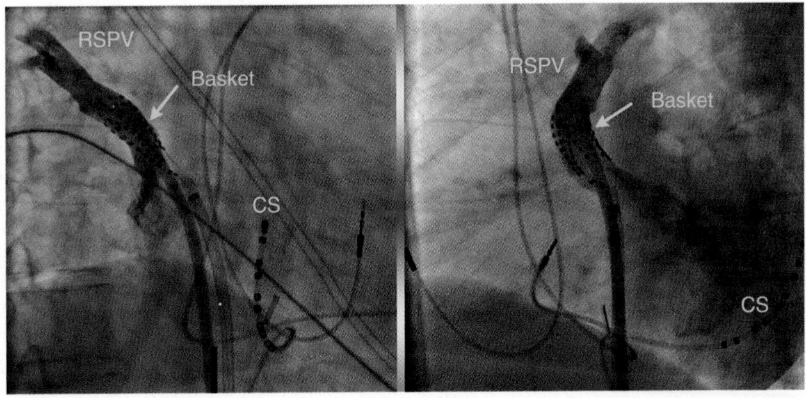

FIGURE 11–26 Fluoroscopic right anterior oblique (RAO) and left anterior oblique (LAO) views of angiography of the right superior pulmonary vein (RSPV) with a basket catheter positioned in the vein. Note that the basket catheter takes the shape of the PV and provides anatomical information about location of the ostium and size of the PV.

Another disadvantage is that the basket catheter is nondeflectable and has limited maneuverability, and it requires a special sheath with a limited number of preshaped curves. Sometimes, it is challenging to introduce a basket catheter into the inferior PVs. The use of a deflectable transseptal sheath can facilitate catheterization of the PVs.

Additionally, the splines may contact one another when the basket catheter is positioned within a relatively small PV, thereby inducing electrical artifact (see Fig. 11-26). Similarly, the splines may not always be equally spaced relative to the circumference of the PV. As a result, areas in which several splines are clustered may be densely mapped, whereas other regions are less densely recorded.

EnSite NavX System

The use of the nonfluoroscopic navigational system (NavX) in ostial segmental PV isolation may offer several potential benefits. Based on the LocaLisa technology (Medtronic, Minneapolis, Minn), the EnSite NavX system (Endocardial Solutions, St. Paul, Minn) combines catheter location and tracking features of LocaLisa with the ability to create an anatomical model of the cardiac chamber using only a single conventional EP catheter and skin patches.

NavX-guided procedures are performed using the same catheter setup as conventional approaches. Standard EP catheters of choice are introduced into the heart. Up to 12 catheters and 64 electrodes can be viewed simultaneously. The system is able to locate the position of the catheters from the moment that they are inserted in the vein. Therefore, all catheters can be navigated to the heart under guidance of the EnSite NavX system and the use of fluoroscopy can be minimized for preliminary catheter positioning. A shadow can be displayed on each of the catheters to record the catheter's spatial position. In case of displacement, the catheter can be returned easily to its original location under the guidance of NavX. In the case of segmental PV isolation, reconstruction of LA anatomy and creation of a 3-D map by the NavX system, which can prolong procedure time, is not necessary.

The ability to visualize and label electrodes on both the ring and the ablation catheters can offer a great benefit in ablation procedures. With the use of the NavX system, fluoroscopy is primarily used to move the ring catheter to the targeted PV. The system allows precise navigation of the ablation catheter to the labeled pole of the ring catheter without the assistance of fluoroscopy. During RF energy delivery, assessment of catheter stability and dragging around the ostium can also be performed without fluoroscopy.

Additionally, the nonfluoroscopic navigation system allows a real-time assessment of wall contact and catheter stability as well as the assessment of the spatial relationship between ablation and ring catheters. Because ablation does not interfere with the localization of the catheters, the operator knows in real time the position of the ablation catheter and can reposition it if required. Therefore, catheter displacement and insufficient wall contact are readily recognized without the use of fluoroscopy, which potentially can help reduce fluoroscopy and procedure duration and also prevent inadvertent ablation inside the PVs.

Furthermore, by the use of NavX technology, with the feature of taking a shadow of the stable position of the ring catheter, repositioning of the catheter after a displacement is much easier than during fluoroscopy guidance, which can facilitate isolation of PVs in which the mapping catheter cannot be completely stabilized.

Target of Ablation

The objective of the mapping and ablation procedure is to identify PV potentials along the circumference of the PV ostium and ablate to eliminate these potentials completely.[41,42,50] Isolation of all PVs is performed without attempting to identify the PVs demonstrating arrhythmogenicity. RF ablation is targeted to the ostial portion of the breakthrough segments (electrical connections) connecting the LA to the PV, which are identified as the earliest PV potentials recorded from the ring catheter. The PV potential reflects the activation of muscular LA bands extending into the PV with longitudinal, oblique, or complex courses and ending in a cul-de-sac or even looping back in the LA. The source, its course within the PV, and its exit into the LA may all be considered appropriate individual targets for ablation. The PV potential is recorded over a broader area proximally, but with great variability. Therefore, a few seconds of energy application may be sufficient at some proximal sites to eliminate downstream PV muscle activity, whereas wide or repeated RF applications may have been required in others.

Once the presence of the PV potentials along the PV circumference is defined on the ring catheter, target sites for ablation are selected by identifying the earliest bipolar PV potentials and/or the unipolar electrograms with the most rapid (sharpest) intrinsic deflection on high-speed recordings (150 to 200 mm/sec) that had equivalent or earlier activation relative to the earliest PV potential recorded on the adjacent ring catheter recording sites (see Fig. 11-22).[41,42,50] The ablation catheter then is maneuvered to a position adjacent to the target electrode pair of the ring catheter and withdrawn to the edge of the ostium (the ostial side of the ring catheter). RF ablation is performed within 5 to 15 mm of the PV ostium; the exact location will usually depend on catheter stability. This would be safer (regarding the risk of PV stenosis) than more distal applications, especially in smaller veins.

Several PV potential electrogram characteristics as recorded by the ablation catheter tip predict a successful ablation site: (1) timing of the (unipolar and bipolar) PV potential electrogram recorded by the ablation catheter equal to or earlier than the earliest PV potential recorded by the ring catheter (see Fig. 11-22); (2) larger (unipolar and bipolar) electrogram amplitude; (3) steeper intrinsic deflection of the unipolar electrogram; and (4) identical morphologies of the unipolar electrograms recorded by the ablation catheter and by the contiguous electrode of the ring catheter.[50]

Ablation Technique

A temperature-controlled, 4- or 8-mm-tip deflectable catheter or a 3.5-mm irrigated-tip ablation catheter can be used. For 8-mm-tip catheters, RF ablation is performed with the maximum temperature set at 45° to 52°C, the power set at 70 W or lower, and for a duration of 20 to 60 seconds. Power limit is usually reduced to 25 W for the case of a left inferior PV and to 20 W if the PV diameter is less than 15 mm. For irrigated-tip catheters, power is set at 50 W or lower and temperature at 40°C or lower. Ablation lesions are delivered for a maximum of 60 seconds to achieve an impedance drop of 5 to 10 Ω at the ablation site. RF application may be repeated or prolonged when a change occurs in activation and/or morphology of the PV potentials, as determined by circumferential mapping recorded downstream. Additional ostial applications targeting fragmented electrograms (more than two deflections) are performed after PV isolation to eliminate any ostial PV potentials, thus reducing the risk of recurrence caused by ostial foci. The presence of ablation artifact on the recording from a specific ring catheter pole confirms the pole the catheter is on and that the catheter is in the same plane as the ring catheter (see Fig. 11-22).

A successful ablation site is defined as a site at which an application of RF energy results in elimination of a PV potential at more than one ring catheter recording sites or delay (shift) of a PV potential by more than 10 milliseconds at more than two ring catheter recording sites (Fig. 11-27). Once a shift or elimination of PV potentials at some ring catheter poles is achieved, the ablation catheter is adjusted to target the new ring catheter pole recording the now earliest PV potential. This maneuver is repeated until the whole PV is electrically isolated. Complete electrical isolation of the PV is defined as complete entrance block into the PV during AF and elimination or dissociation of all ostial PV potentials during NSR and atrial pacing (see Fig. 11-27).

The extent of the circumference ablated is variable among PVs. When ablation is performed proximally to the PV ostium or during AF, more circumferential ablation is often required to achieve PV isolation. Occasionally, electrical connections exist between ipsilateral PVs, and elimination of these connections is important only when isolation of one PV is the goal of the ablation procedure. The electrical connections between PVs are defined as the identification of the earliest activation at the ostium of an untargeted PV during pacing inside the targeted PV; thus, ablation is performed at this untargeted PV ostium to achieve electrical disconnection.[53]

When a multielectrode basket catheter is used for PV mapping, it is recommended to use an irrigated-tip catheter at a maximum temperature of 45°C, maximum power of 30 W, and flow rate during ablation of 17 mL/min.

Cryoablation

Although RF energy has become the gold standard for catheter ablation in most cardiac arrhythmias, PV isolation by heating has potential limitations. RF energy produces tissue disruption, which increases the risk of perforation and thromboembolism. Moreover, RF energy induces inhomogeneous, dense fibrosis and shrinking of the tissue, leading to PV stenosis. Cryothermal energy is a new alternative energy source that may overcome these limitations. Cryothermal energy creates minimal endothelial and endocardial disruption and preserves the underlying tissue architecture. Therefore, the lesions are minimally thrombogenic and arrhythmogenic, and cryoablation of the PV should have a low risk of PV stenosis.

Initial experiences of electrophysiologically guided segmental ostial PV isolation by using cryothermal energy application with a 10.5 Fr (CryoCor, San Diego, Calif) or 7 Fr (Freezor, CryoCath Technologies, Montreal, Canada) focal ablation catheter have shown that PV isolation is feasible with a comparable number of applications and clinical outcome with regard to RF ablation.[54,55] Importantly, the early cryoablation experience has not evidenced, so far, development of PV stenosis following ablation. On the other hand, cryothermal injury is sensitive to surrounding thermal conditions. The high flow of the PVs can present a considerable heat load to cryothermal technologies, which can limit the size and depth of the lesion produced by cryothermal energy at the PV ostium and thus limit the ability of achieving complete and permanent PV isolation. Additionally, the longer application times (2.5 to 5.0 minutes) required when cryothermal energy is used may relevantly reflect on the procedure duration, limiting the clinical use of this theoretically optimal energy source.

Endpoints of Ablation

The main endpoint of the ablation procedure is complete electrical disconnection of the targeted PV(s). Noninducibility of AF is infrequently used to assess the success of the procedure.

Electrical Disconnection of the Pulmonary Vein. Complete PV electrical disconnection is defined as the following: (1) complete entrance block into the PV during AF and the elimination or dissociation of all ostial PV potentials recorded by the ring catheter during NSR and atrial

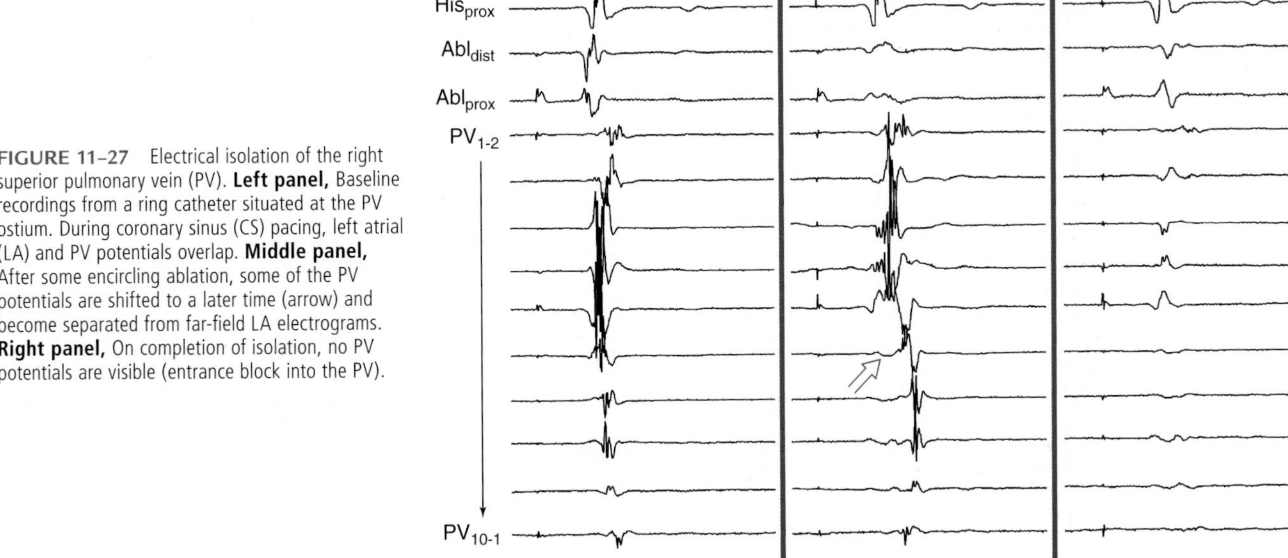

FIGURE 11–27 Electrical isolation of the right superior pulmonary vein (PV). **Left panel,** Baseline recordings from a ring catheter situated at the PV ostium. During coronary sinus (CS) pacing, left atrial (LA) and PV potentials overlap. **Middle panel,** After some encircling ablation, some of the PV potentials are shifted to a later time (arrow) and become separated from far-field LA electrograms. **Right panel,** On completion of isolation, no PV potentials are visible (entrance block into the PV).

pacing (i.e., LA-PV conduction block) (Fig. 11-28; see also Fig. 11-27); and (2) complete exit block from the PV to the PV ostium and LA during intra-PV pacing (i.e., PV-LA conduction block; Fig. 11-29). Demonstration of only entrance block is an insufficient endpoint; evidence has suggested that after achieving entrance block, less than 60% of PVs demonstrate exit block (Fig. 11-30). The fact that tachycardias can be induced in isolated PV segments highlights the importance of achieving PV exit block. This criterion also can unmask electrical connections between ipsilateral PVs, which manifest as intact LA conduction during intra-PV pacing after elimination of all potentials in that PV, indicating unidirectional block. This is relevant when only one (and not all) PV is targeted for isolation. PV pacing is performed from multiple sites in as circumferential a manner as possible using the bipoles of the ring catheter or mapping-ablation catheter, and with the minimal output that constantly captures the PV potential.[41,42,50]

Limited data have suggested the need to reconfirm no recurrence of the PV potentials within all PVs following administration of adenosine during NSR or atrial pacing.[56] One report has shown that after successful ostial PV isolation, electrical activation of the PVs can be transiently reactivated by adenosine (12- to 18-mg rapid intravenous bolus) in 25% of PVs (but not with isoproterenol, beta blockers, or atropine).[56] Additional RF applications to eliminate the adenosine-induced dormant PV conduction have been found to reduce the recurrence rate of AF following PV isolation, which might be caused by the minimization of subsequent PV reconnection.[57]

Early recurrence of PV conduction is thought to be common. Reconfirmation of PV isolation after a 60-minute waiting period after initial PV isolation has been suggested to improve outcome.

Noninducibility of Atrial Fibrillation. Elimination of PV potentials correlates better with clinical success than the acute suppression of AF. However, a successful outcome could be observed without complete PV potential elimination and some supposedly unsuccessfully treated patients were remarkably improved with a previously ineffective drug.

Inducibility of AF is determined by rapid atrial pacing, which is usually attempted several times and at several pacing sites. Alternatively, burst pacing (at 20 mA for 5 to 10 seconds, starting at a pacing CL of 250 milliseconds and decreasing to atrial refractoriness) is performed using ramp pacing three times from three different sites (LA appendage, RA appendage, and CS). AF that terminates spontaneously within 5 minutes of induction is usually considered nonsustained. Sustained AF, thought to indicate the presence of a potential atrial substrate capable of maintaining AF, is defined as AF lasting 10 minutes or longer. Additionally, isoproterenol (4 to 8 μg/min) or dobutamine (20 μg/kg/min) can be administered at the end of the procedure to assess the inducibility of AF.

A significant proportion (up to 57%) of patients with paroxysmal AF has no inducible AF after PV isolation. This subset may represent a group that will benefit from PV isolation alone and do not require additional substrate modification.

Inability to Isolate a Pulmonary Vein. More than 90% of PVs can be electrically isolated from the LA by conventional applications of RF energy along segments of the ostia, guided by PV potentials. The inability to abolish the

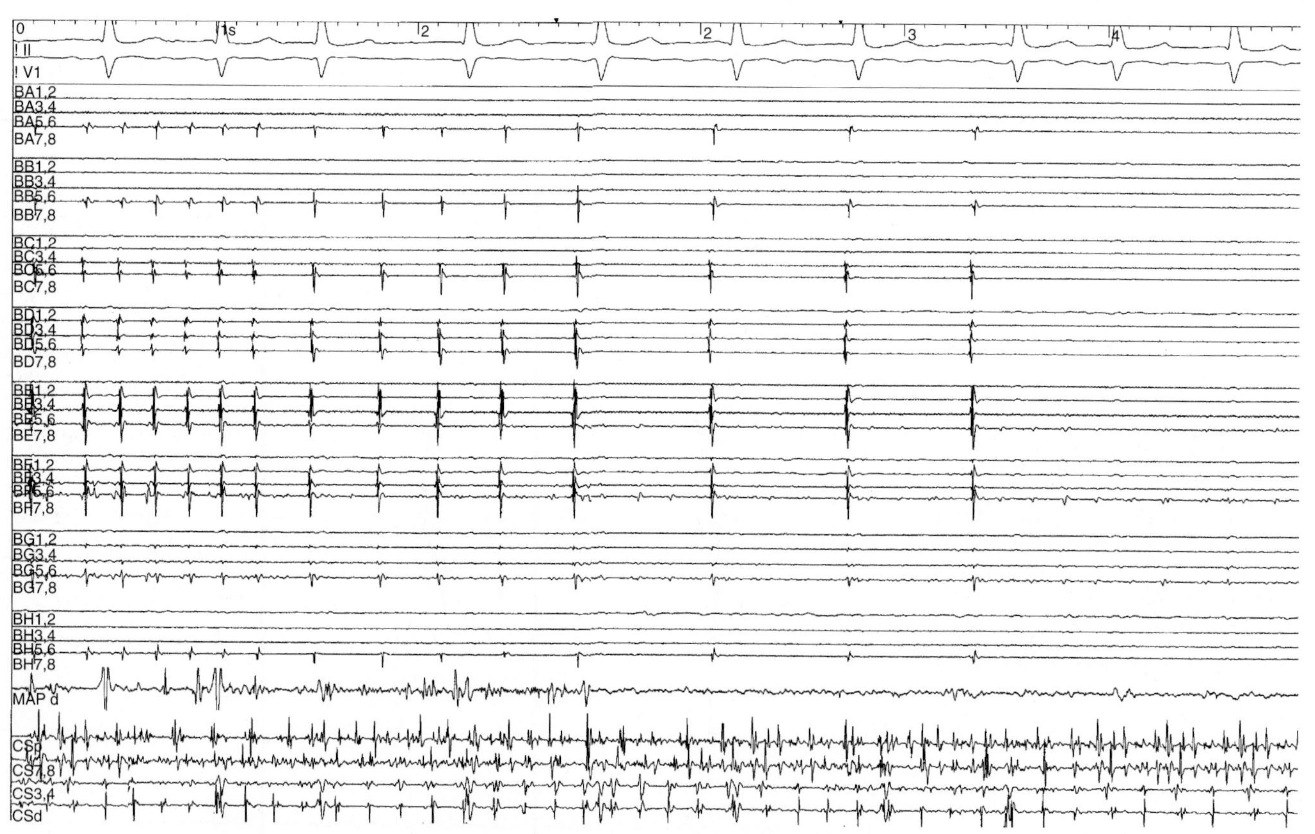

FIGURE 11–28 Pulmonary vein (PV) isolation during atrial fibrillation (AF) using a basket catheter. Bipolar recordings from the eight electrodes (1-2, 3-4, 5-6, 7-8) on each of the eight splines (BA through BH) of the basket catheter positioned in the left superior PV initially show sharp PV potentials. RF ablation during AF results in gradual slowing and then disappearance of all PV potentials and persistence of residual low-amplitude, far-field, left atrial (LA) electrograms, consistent with LA-PV entrance block. AF continues in the coronary sinus (CS) recordings.

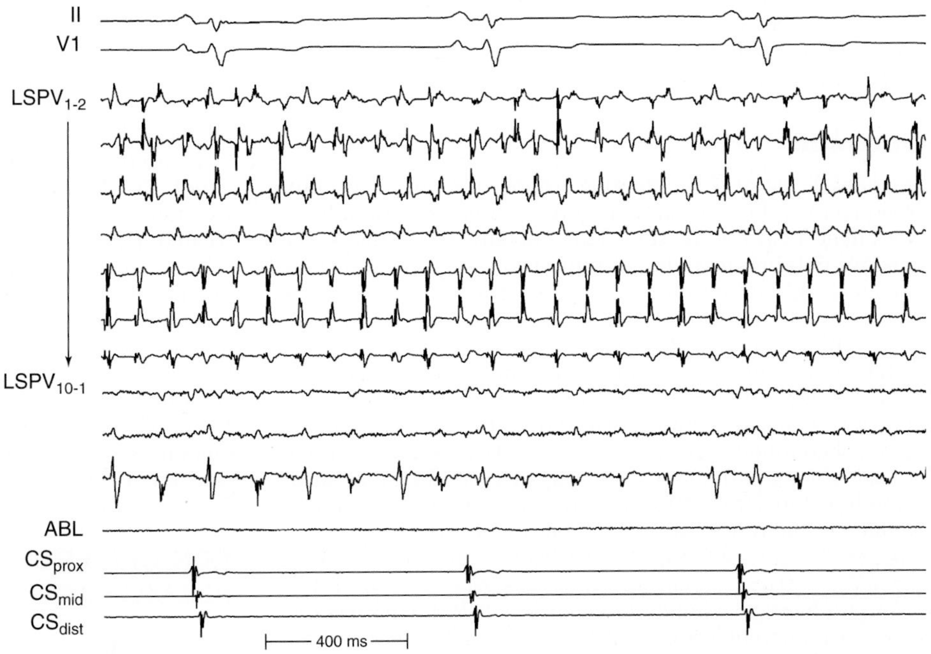

FIGURE 11–29 Electrical isolation of the left superior pulmonary vein (LSPV). Complete electrical isolation of the LSPV resulted in termination of atrial fibrillation (AF) and conversion to normal sinus rhythm (NSR) on the surface ECG and coronary sinus (CS) recordings while AF continued in the LSPV (PV–left atrial exit block).

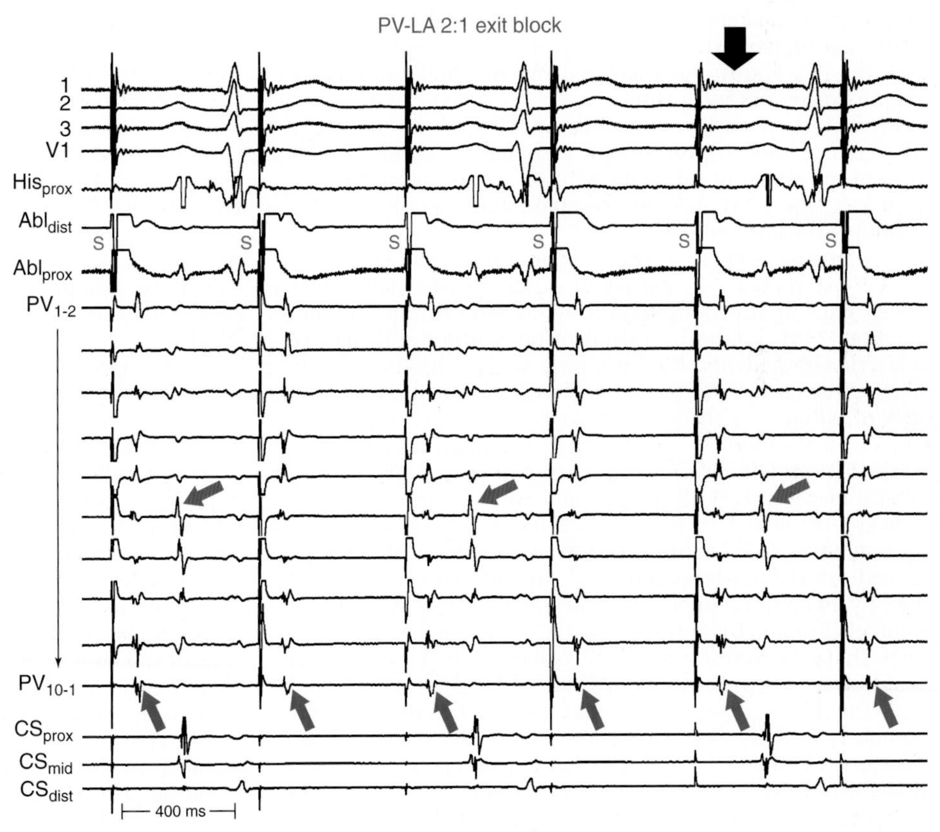

FIGURE 11–30 Pulmonary vein (PV)–left atrium (LA) 2:1 exit block. The ring catheter is positioned at the ostium of the left superior PV. During pacing using the ablation catheter positioned more distally in the vein, consistent capture of PV potentials is shown (blue arrows) but only every other PV potential conducts to LA (red arrows). Note very long delay between the stimulus and P wave of the conducted complex (black arrow).

arrhythmogenic PV potential or its recovery (even in a very discrete area and with a prolonged conduction time) is associated with a higher AF recurrence rate.

The inability to disconnect the PV has been demonstrated in 3% to 24% of targeted PVs in previous studies and may be attributable to anatomical variations in the geometry of the ostia that could limit optimal recording of PV potentials with the ring catheter. Using an expandable ring catheter or using ICE to guide positioning of the ring catheter aids in stabilizing the mapping catheter. Additionally, some fascicles may be too thick to be ablated with conventional RF energy, and the use of high power output or irrigated-tip ablation catheter, which creates deeper lesions than a conventional ablation catheter, may be required to isolate those PVs. Also, the inability to isolate a PV may be caused by the presence of electrical connections between PVs.[53] Approximately 14% of the patients have electrical connections between ipsilateral PVs. In these patients, ostial ablation of an untargeted PV is required for successful disconnection of the targeted PV. Recognition of electrical connections between PVs during ostial ablation of PVs prevents unnecessary or excessive RF applications that probably produce postablation PV stenosis.

Outcome

Segmental ostial PV isolation represents an important advance in catheter treatment of AF and has several advantages over focal PV ablation. This procedure eliminates the need for detailed mapping of spontaneous ectopy and there is a clear-cut endpoint of ablation, even when spontaneous arrhythmias are absent. Importantly, the risk of PV stenosis is less than that with focal PV ablation.

Reconnection of previously isolated PVs, caused by recovery of conduction through inadequately ablated fascicles in the muscle sleeves surrounding the PVs, is probably the most common reason for recurrent AF after PV isolation, at least among patients with paroxysmal AF.[58] Other causes include ectopy from PVs not targeted or that could not be isolated at the initial procedure and the presence of non-PV triggers.[58] In a recent study on the recurrence of AF following PV electrical isolation,[59] most triggers were found to originate from previously targeted PVs (54%), whereas one third of recurrent triggers (32%) originated from PVs that were not ablated during the initial session; 61% of previously isolated PVs in that series had evidence of recovered PV potentials. Therefore, successful PV isolation does not confer permanent disconnection of the PV musculature from the LA, and in most isolated PVs residual conduction remains or recurs with time.

Predictors of early recurrence of AF include older age (65 years or older), presence of associated cardiovascular disease, presence of multiple AF foci, presence of AF foci from LA free wall, LA enlargement, and permanent AF. Predictors of late recurrence of AF include the presence of early recurrence of AF and presence of multiple AF foci.

In most reports, a successful outcome was defined as the absence of any symptomatic atrial arrhythmias beyond the first 2 to 3 months postablation without the use of antiarrhythmic drugs. Medium-term success has reportedly been achieved in 70% of patients with paroxysmal AF and 30% of patients with persistent/permanent AF. A satisfactory clinical outcome, consisting of complete resolution or marked improvement in symptoms, can be achieved in up to 85% of patients with paroxysmal AF.

When three or four PVs are isolated, a satisfactory clinical outcome can be achieved in most patients with a single procedure and without the need for antiarrhythmic drug therapy. In contrast to paroxysmal AF, persistent AF usually is not eliminated by segmental ostial PV isolation. This suggests that intervention with PV isolation in patients with drug-refractory paroxysmal AF should not be postponed until the AF becomes persistent. Once AF has become persistent, it is likely that PV isolation will have to be supplemented by some other type of ablation procedure directed at the atrial myocardium. The less satisfactory outcome of PV isolation in persistent AF suggests that the PVs play a less critical role in generating AF once the AF has become persistent. It is possible that the electrophysiological and anatomical remodeling that occurs during persistent AF often allow the atria to continue fibrillating independently of the PVs.

The overall major complication rate is 6.3%, including stroke (0.7%), pericardial tamponade (1.2%), and significant PV stenosis (4.3%).[42] One important limitation of available data on segmental ostial PV ablation for AF is the paucity of long-term follow-up data for both efficacy and late complications. Mean follow-up of the reported studies has ranged from 4 to 21 months. It is thus difficult to know when a patient may be considered cured of AF. A second limitation is that the definition of success in most of these trials was the elimination of symptomatic AF. It has been recognized that some AF patients have asymptomatic episodes, even those patients who are highly symptomatic with some episodes of AF.

In a study comparing focal PV ablation and segmental ostial PV isolation for treatment of AF in 107 patients,[60] freedom from AF at 1 year was achieved in 80% of patients treated with PV isolation versus 45% of patients treated with focal ablation. This outcome of focal ablation was noted despite aggressive attempts at provoking triggers, use of multipolar catheters to identify a vein of interest, and use of a 3-D mapping system to help localize the origin of triggers within the vein. For the same reason, investigators were soon led to attempt to isolate as many PVs as possible at the initial ablation session. Comparative case series ultimately demonstrated that empirical four-PV isolation led to superior outcomes over isolating fewer veins.

CIRCUMFERENTIAL ANTRAL PULMONARY VEIN ISOLATION

Rationale

The muscular sleeves of the PVs extend proximally to the antral-LA junction and are not restricted to the tubular portion of the PV. This is not surprising, because embryologically the PVs originate from the posterior LA wall, so that a continuum exists between the atrial wall and PVs. Therefore, ablation at the antrum is effective to isolate PVs, assessed by a ring catheter placed around each PV ostium. The preferred ablation target is the outmost atrial side of the PV ostium.[41,61,62] To this effect, a reliable definition of the anatomy is crucial to provide an effective set of lesions. A navigation system is used to provide 3-D anatomical images that allow safe maneuvering of the ablation catheter to complete the lesions at the antrum and eliminate conduction to PVs.[63]

This approach has several advantages over segmental ostial PV isolation.[41,61,62] This technique does not rely on localizing the sites of electrical breakthroughs into the PV, and thus it is easier to perform during AF. Furthermore, this approach reduces the risk of PV stenosis because ablation is performed in the LA, away from the PV ostia (Fig. 11-31). In addition, in some patients with PV anatomical variations, this approach could be more favorable. One such variation is the presence of a common ostium of the left PVs, occurring in up to 32% of patients undergoing PV isolation. Such common ostia typically are too large to allow a stable position of the ring catheter (see Fig. 11-3). Another anatomical variation is the presence of a right middle PV, present in up to 21% of patients, which typically is separated from the right superior PV and right inferior PV by a narrow rim of atrial tissue (see Fig. 11-3). This would predispose to sliding of the ablation catheter into the PV during ablation. Another anatomical finding that renders extraostial PV isolation more favorable is a PV ostial diameter of less than 10 mm. RF application at a small ostium carries a higher risk of PV stenosis.

Circumferential antral PV isolation has been shown to be more effective in preventing AF recurrence than segmental ostial PV isolation. This may be caused by elimination of triggered activity and/or mother waves near the PV ostium that drive AF, or by isolation of relatively large areas that are rendered unavailable for perpetuating AF. Furthermore, a large area of the posterior LA is included inside the ablation lines. This area was shown to harbor foci of high-

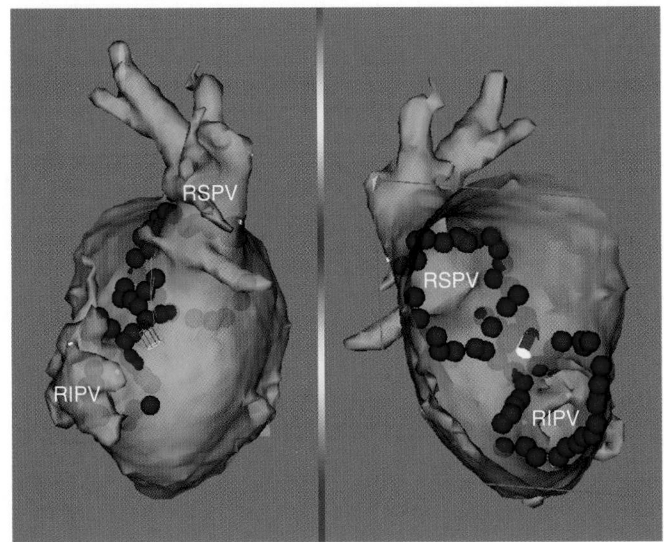

FIGURE 11–31 Circumferential antral pulmonary vein (PV) isolation. Registered 3-D surface reconstructions of the left atrium (LA; right lateral and cardioscopic views) during circumferential antral PV isolation of the right PVs are illustrated. Contiguous RF lesions are deployed in the LA proximal to the ostia of the PVs creating a circumferential line around each PV ostium.

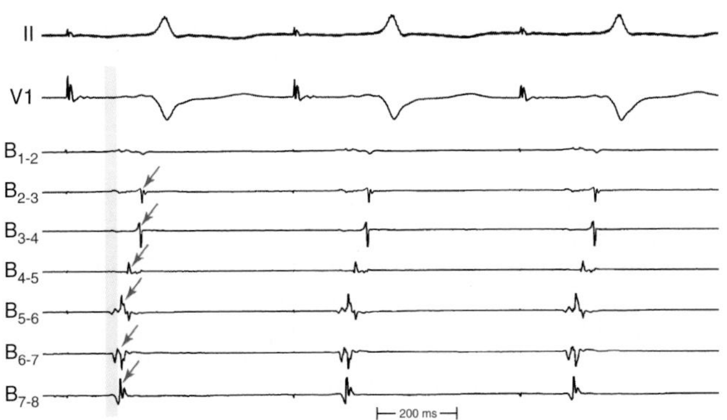

FIGURE 11–32 Identification of the pulmonary vein (PV) antrum using the basket catheter. The basket catheter is positioned in the left superior PV. Shown are seven bipolar recordings obtained from the eight electrodes (1-2, 2-3, to 7-8) on one of the eight splines ($B_{1\text{-}2}$ through $B_{7\text{-}8}$) of the basket catheter. During coronary sinus (CS) pacing, far-field left atrial (LA) potentials are normally recorded almost simultaneously all over the PV (shaded area). In contrast, PV activation propagates from proximal (ostial) to distal, and the interval between the LA potentials and PV potentials is shorter at the proximal PV than at the distal PV. At the transition zone (PV antrum), a total fusion of the PV and LA potentials occurs ($B_{7\text{-}8}$).

frequency activity, which may initiate and maintain AF. Ablation in this area may also result in destruction of endocardial nerve terminals involved in autonomic regulation and leading to AF suppression (i.e., vagal denervation by the ablation lines).

In summary, circumferential antral PV isolation appears to minimize the risk of ablation in the PV ostium and, at the same time, preserve the benefit of PV isolation in addition to modifying the substrate of the periostial LA.

Identification of Pulmonary Vein Antra

The objective of the mapping and ablation procedure is to identify PV potentials along the perimeter of the PV antrum and ablate to eliminate these potentials completely. The technique is guided by ICE or 3-D electroanatomical mapping systems and mapping with a ring catheter. These systems are used to visualize or reconstruct PV antra to help guide RF delivery. However, use of these systems does not prevent or replace the use of circumferential mapping and an EP endpoint to the procedure. More importantly, none of these systems can exclude the risk of RF delivery within the PVs and therefore the risk of PV stenosis.

Lasso Catheter Mapping

The ring catheter is used for circumferential ostial mapping of PV potentials, as described for segmental ostial PV isolation. However, the breakthrough segments (electrical connections) connecting the LA to the PV, identified as the earliest PV potentials recorded from the ring catheter, are not specifically mapped or targeted. Instead, the entire perimeter of the PV ostium is the target for the ablation procedure. Using the ring catheter enables circumferential mapping of the PV ostia perpendicular to the axis of the vein and serves as a landmark for the PV ostium around which RF lesions are delivered. In addition, the ring catheter is vital for confirming complete electrical isolation of the PV, an important endpoint of this ablation strategy.

Basket Catheter Mapping

The technique of positioning the basket catheter into the PVs has been described earlier in this chapter (see Fig. 11-25). For antral PV isolation, the basket catheter is introduced toward the distal PV under fluoroscopy guidance and then pulled back as proximally as possible without dislodgment until its most proximal electrodes are positioned at the PV antrum, which is identified by selective angiography. The basket catheter can help identify the true junction between the PVs and LA anatomically and electrically. Because the basket catheter conforms to the shape of the PV, it provides information about the anatomy of the PV.[52]

Furthermore, longitudinal mapping with a basket catheter can help identify the transition zone between the PV and LA potentials. Far-field LA potentials are normally recorded almost simultaneously all over the PV, whereas the activation sequence of the PV potentials is from proximal to distal when the activation propagates from the LA to the distal PV. Consequently, the interval between the LA potentials and PV potentials is shorter at the proximal PV than at the distal PV. At the transition zone, total fusion of the PV and LA potentials occurs (Fig. 11-32). Therefore, the potential recorded at the transition zone may reflect the activation of the PV antrum. A transverse activation pattern, indicated by simultaneous activation recorded by some neighboring electrode pairs along the spline, sometimes occurs around the LA-PV junction before the longitudinal activation pattern within the PVs; it may reflect the activation of the circle of myocardium at the PV antrum.[52]

On the basis of these findings, PV antrum potentials are defined as single sharp potentials formed by the total fusion of the PV and LA potentials around the PV ostium or single sharp potentials with a transverse activation pattern around the PV ostium (see Fig. 11-32). Targeting those potentials by RF ablation would target the transition zone between the PV ostium and LA. When potentials conforming to the definition of PV antrum potentials are observed from some electrode pairs on the same spline, the antrum potential recorded from the most proximal electrode pair is targeted. RF applications are also delivered to the gap between the targeted electrode pairs on the neighboring splines to produce a continuous RF lesion at the PV antrum.[52]

Electroanatomical Mapping

Different navigation tools, such as NavX and CARTO, have been used to facilitate circumferential PV isolation. These systems help in determining the position of the ablation catheter (anterior, posterior) relative to the mapping electrodes, defining PV ostia and antra, tagging RF ablation lesions, ensuring the continuity of the ablation lines, and reducing fluoroscopy exposure.

CARTO. Initially, a 3-D shell representing the LA is constructed using the ablation catheter as a roving catheter. The LA anatomy is reconstructed by point to point sequential sampling of the endocardial sites. Points are acquired manually when the catheter tip is in good contact with atrial wall. The chamber geometry is reconstructed in real time by interpolation of the acquired points. Usually, 100 points are required to create adequate maps of the LA and PVs. The LA appendage is demarcated, and three locations are recorded along the mitral isthmus to tag the valve orifice.

To acquire the PVs, entry into the vein is clearly identified as the catheter leaves the cardiac shadow on fluoroscopy, the impedance usually rises above 140 to 150 Ω, and electrical activity disappears. Because of the orientation of some veins and the limitations of catheter shape, it can be difficult to enter deep into some veins, but the impedance still rises when the catheter is in the mouth of the vein. To better differentiate between PVs and LA, voltage criteria (fractionation of local bipolar electrogram) and impedance (rise more than 4 Ω above the mean LA impedance) can be used to define the PV ostium. Clearly, the anatomical appearance on CARTO acts as added confirmation of catheter entry into the PV ostium. Mapping of each PV is performed by placing the mapping catheter 2 to 4 cm inside the PV and slowly pulling it back to the LA under fluoroscopy guidance. During this course, virtual tubes are created by CARTO to represent the main body of the PVs. Care should be taken to reconstruct each PV ostium and the transition toward the LA (antrum), posterior free wall, mitral isthmus, and left interatrial septum.

Newer versions of CARTO incorporate the use of CT or MR images to allow verification of the anatomical landmarks and cardiac geometry and help guide the ablation catheter precisely to the different areas of interest. Images from CT angiogram or MR can be superimposed on the electroanatomical imaging created with the CARTO system using custom-designed software (CartoMerge, Biosense Webster, Diamond Bar, Calif; see Fig. 11-31).[64-66] Segmentation of the cardiac image is performed to separate the LA and PVs from the surrounding cardiac structures (see Fig. 3-45). The LA and the PVs are then exported into the real-time mapping system for registration. Registration of the CT image is performed using landmark and surface mapping. Points easily identifiable on fluoroscopy and the CT image at the proximal or first-order venous branches of at least three different PVs are used for landmark registration. The ablation catheter is maneuvered under fluoroscopy guidance to the selected location and a point acquired on the CARTO system. Additionally, selective PV angiography or ICE may be used to define the position of the mapping catheter accurately during the registration process to ensure that the branch point identified during mapping matches that on CT. Afterward, surface registration is performed to refine the match between the CT and true LA geometry further by creating an electroanatomical shell with at least 30 widely spaced points, predominantly from the lateral, septal, roof, inferior and posterior LA walls. Catheter contact is ensured by fluoroscopic visualization of catheter mobility in relation to cardiac motion and a discrete atrial electrogram. Subsequently, the overall closeness of fit can be assessed using customized software that provides a point by point review of registration accuracy. If required, additional landmark and surface registration points are taken to achieve an overall accuracy of less than 3 mm. In addition, each PV is entered with the ablation catheter and the ostium is identified by dragging the catheter back under fluoroscopy guidance to assess the correct representation of the PV-LA junction on the registered CT image.

EnSite NavX. As discussed earlier, the EnSite NavX system combines catheter location and tracking features of LocaLisa technology with the ability to create an anatomical model of the cardiac chamber using only a single conventional EP catheter and skin patches. The EnSite NavX system creates 3-D geometry based on 5.6-kHz electrical fields generated by six skin patches in the x, y, and z axes. The NavX system can provide a high-resolution reconstruction of the PV antrum, its anatomical variations, and the narrow ridge between the LA appendage and left PVs. Additionally, the NavX system allows real-time visualization of the position of up to 64 electrodes on up to 8 standard catheters, and does not need any special catheter. The EnSite Digital Image Fusion (DIF) allows for simultaneously displaying 3-D maps side by side with CT or MR segmented cardiac scans to confirm cardiac structures and guide therapy.

NavX-guided procedures are performed using the same catheter setup as conventional approaches. Any electrode can be used to gather data, create static isochronal and voltage maps, and perform ablation procedures. Standard EP catheters of choice are introduced into the heart. Up to 12 catheters and 64 electrodes can be viewed simultaneously. Once in the heart, one intracardiac catheter is used as a reference for geometry reconstruction. A shadow, to record original position, is placed over this catheter to realize displacement during the procedure. In case of displacement, the catheter can be returned easily to its original location under the guidance of NavX. A shadow can also be displayed on each of the other catheters to record the catheter's spatial position.

Subsequently, 3-D intracardiac geometry is obtained. The NavX approach allows for the rapid creation of detailed models of cardiac anatomy. Initially, fixed anatomical points are acquired at the four PV ostia using the ablation or ring catheter. Subsequently, the system is allowed to create the geometry automatically while moving the ablation (or ring) catheter throughout the LA. Sequential positioning of a catheter at multiple sites along the endocardial surface of the LA establishes that chamber's geometry. The system automatically acquires points from a nominated electrode(s) at a rate of 96 points/sec, which is much faster than the CARTO system. Chamber geometry is created by an estimated several thousand points, a much higher resolution than that created by the CARTO system. Fixed anatomical points are subsequently acquired at the LA roof, LA appendage, posterior wall, septum, and inferior wall to define these regions better. The locations of PVs or even the esophagus are established and readily displayed by the juxtaposition of multiple mapping markers, or sphere stacking, along the length of that vein. The size of each marker is based on size selection rather than actual vessel dimensions.

The system works with most manufacturers' ablation catheters and RF or cryogenerators. Ablation lesions can be tagged, facilitating creation of lines of block with considerable accuracy by serial RF lesion placement, and allowing verification of the continuity of ablation line. The simultaneous visualization of all catheters facilitates immediate control of mapping catheter spatial positioning during RF applications.

Intracardiac Echocardiography–Guided Mapping

Phased array ICE has been used in AF ablation procedures for several purposes—to assist with transseptal puncture, to identify the number and position of PVs, to identify the true border of the PV antrum, to determine the branching patterns of the right PVs needed for total PV isolation, to guide the positioning of the ring and ablation catheters at the antrum of the PV, to verify ablation catheter tip to tissue contact, to assess the degree of PV occlusion during balloon-based ablative interventions, and to detect procedural complications (e.g., pericardial effusion, LA thrombus, and PV stenosis).[41,61,62,67]

For ICE imaging, a 10 or 8 Fr 64-element phased-array ultrasound catheter is positioned in the middle of the RA via an 11 or 9 Fr left femoral venous access. The ICE catheter remains in the RA for the entire procedure to guide transseptal puncture, define PV anatomy, and monitor for microbubble formation during RF ablation. A 7.5- or 8.5-MHz imaging frequency optimizes visualization of LA structures and PVs beyond the interatrial septum. PV imaging is uniformly possible by first visualizing the membranous fossa from a mid to low RA catheter tip position. From this view, clockwise catheter rotation allows visualization of the LA appendage, followed by long-axis views of the left superior and inferior PVs (see Figs. 2-13 and 3-42). Further clockwise rotation of the catheter brings the orifice of the right superior and inferior PVs into view. The LA ostia of these veins are typically viewed "en fas," yielding an owl's eye appearance at the vein's orifice.

As the operator images each vein, the ring and ablation catheters can be positioned at the antral-LA interface for ablation. Because the PV antrum is a large-diameter structure, its circumference cannot be mapped using a stationary ring catheter fixed in one position. Instead, the ring catheter must be sequentially positioned along each segment of the antral circumference to look for PV potentials. ICE can precisely identify the true border of the PV antrum and guide positioning of the ring and ablation catheters. Therefore, the ring catheter is a roving catheter in this procedure. An operator's assistant often must hold the ring catheter in position around the antrum because the ring catheter is not wedged into the tubular ostium for stability. When mapping the anterior segments of the left PVs or septal segments of the right PVs, the ring catheter must be advanced slightly because of the oblique nature of the antral-LA interface.[41,61,62,67]

Target of Ablation

The ablation procedure is based on electrical isolation of all PVs. The objective is to identify PV potentials along the circumference of the PV antrum and ablate to completely eliminate these potentials. However, unlike segmental ostial PV isolation, the ostial portion of the breakthrough segments (electrical connections) connecting the LA to the PV, identified as the earliest PV potentials recorded from the ring catheter, are not the sole target of ablation. Complete encirclement of each PV antrum with ablation lesions is the goal of the ablation procedure, which would consequently result in PV isolation (see Fig. 11-31). All PVs are targeted.[41,61,62]

Ablation lines consist of contiguous focal lesions deployed in the LA at a distance 5 mm or more proximal to the ostia of the PVs, creating a circumferential line of conduction block around each PV (see Fig. 11-31). PV isolation is performed 1 cm from the ostium of the right PVs as well as for the posterior and superior aspects of the left PVs to enhance efficacy and prevent PV stenosis. However, ablation at the anterior portions of the left PVs usually requires energy be delivered less than 5 mm from the ostium of the PV to achieve catheter stability. Ablation is started randomly in the right or left PVs and is performed individually.

When two or three ipsilateral PVs ostia are coalescent, en bloc encirclement of those ostia is performed—that is, one encirclement for the right-sided or left-sided PVs—and no line between the ipsilateral PVs is deployed (Fig. 11-33).[41]

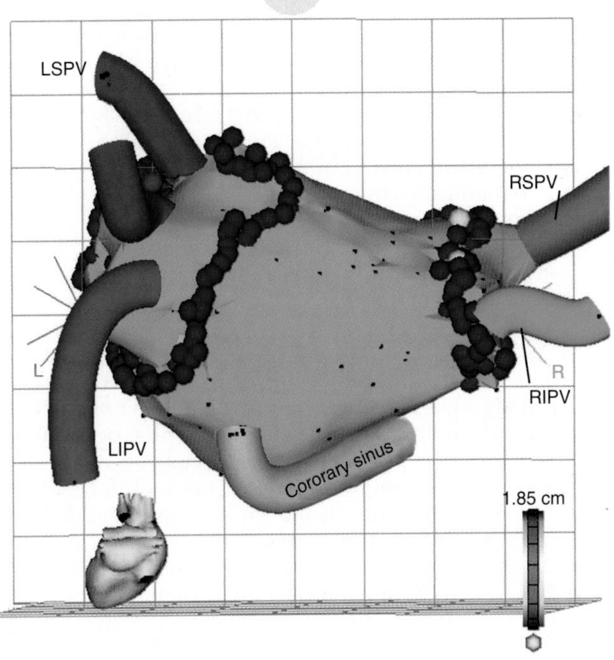

FIGURE 11–33 Circumferential antral pulmonary vein (PV) isolation. This posterior view of the electroanatomical map of the left atrium (LA) at the conclusion of the PV isolation procedure shows closely spaced red dots denoting locations at which RF ablation was performed. En bloc encirclement of the PV ostia (one encirclement for the right-sided and a second encirclement of left-sided PVs) was performed without ablation lines between the ipsilateral PVs.

The use of two ring catheters within the ipsilateral PVs may be considered in such an approach. With this double Lasso technique, electrical isolation of ipsilateral PVs occurs simultaneously in most (more than 80%) of cases. The simultaneous use of two ring catheters provides insights into the electrical interactions of the ipsilateral PVs and helps identify conduction gaps in the complete circumferential ablation lines in case of redoing the ablation procedure for recurrent AF.[56,68,69] Single encirclement of ipsilateral PVs, however, predisposes to breakthrough conduction of both ipsilateral PVs in case of a single gap in the en bloc circle.

Ablation Technique

Ablation is started at the posterior wall of each PV, usually fluoroscopically facing the border of the spine in the anteroposterior projection, and continued around the venous perimeter. The posterior wall of the right PV is reached by counterclockwise torque of the catheter and the left PV by clockwise torque. For ablation at the anterior portions of the left PVs, energy must usually be delivered within a few millimeters of the vein (because of a relatively narrow border between the left PVs and the LA appendage, and the difficulty to balance the catheter tip on the narrow rim of tissue separating these structures) to achieve effective disconnection. RF ablation sites are tagged on the reconstructed 3-D map, which helps ensure coalescence of the ablation lesions to ensure continuity of the ablation line (see Fig. 11-31).

RF energy is delivered using an 8-mm-tip conventional ablation catheter, with a maximum power of up to 70 W and a target temperature of 50° to 55°C. Alternatively, ablation may be performed using an irrigated-tip catheter, with power output limited to 25 to 30 W inside the PV and in the posterior LA wall and 30 to 50 W outside the PV and anterior LA wall, and a target temperature of 40° to 45°C and irrigation rates of 5 to 20 mL/min (0.9% saline).

RF energy is delivered for 30 to 60 seconds at each point, until the maximal local electrogram amplitude is decreased by 50% to 90% or double potentials are observed or to achieve an impedance drop of 5 to 10 Ω at the ablation site. RF application is prolonged for 1 to 2 minutes when a change occurs in the activation and/or morphology of the PV potentials, as determined by circumferential mapping recorded downstream on the ring catheter. Additional ostial applications targeting fragmented electrograms (more than two deflections) are performed after PV isolation to eliminate any ostial PV potentials, thus reducing the risk of recurrence because of ostial foci.

Intracardiac Echocardiography–Guided Ablation

Intracardiac Echocardiography–Guided Catheter Positioning. The ring and ablation catheters are positioned at the antral-LA interface for ablation. The ring catheter is then sequentially positioned along each segment of the antral circumference (guided by ICE) to look for PV potentials. As the ring catheter is moved from one segment of the LA-antral interface to the next, ablation is performed at the poles demonstrating PV potentials. The ablation catheter is moved to the target pole on the ring catheter, taking care to keep the catheter in the same plane as the ring catheter. Ablation is performed only along the specific antral segment that the ring catheter is mapping.[41,61,62,67] Because the PV antrum is a large structure, multiple movements of the ring catheter around the PV antrum are needed. After all segments of a PV are ablated, the ring catheter is used to again map the vein's interface with the LA to confirm the absence of PV potentials at the antral-LA interface. During NSR or CS pacing, the ring catheter is advanced deep into the PV tube to confirm an absence of electrogram recordings, representing entrance block into the PV.

Using ICE to define the PV antrum and guide RF ablation, the anatomical region within the ablation circles typically encompasses the entire posterior wall, LA roof, and anteroseptal extension of the right PVs.

Intracardiac Echocardiography–Guided RF Energy Delivery (Microbubble Monitoring). ICE can help visualize evolving lesions during RF energy delivery and image microbubble formation during tissue heating. The latter is important, because microbubble formation during ablation can indicate excessive tissue heating, which could lead to thrombus or char formation, tissue disruption, or PV stenosis.[41,61,62]

11

Observation by ICE of microbubbles during ablation was previously proposed as a method of titrating RF power delivery.[41] Two types of bubble patterns are seen with ICE, scattered microbubbles (type 1) and a brisk shower of dense microbubbles (type 2) (Fig. 11-34). It has been hypothesized that type 1 microbubbles indicate early tissue overheating (i.e., subcritical heating of the myocardium with imminent risk of steam pop formation), whereas type 2 microbubbles indicate excessive heating. Microbubbles seen on ICE directly correlate to cerebral microembolic events detected by transcranial Doppler, tissue disruption, and char formation. Restricting power output to avoid microbubble formation on ICE increases the efficacy of antral PV isolation while minimizing severe PV stenosis and cerebroembolic complications. Absolute temperature and impedance readings do not correlate with microbubbles and cannot reliably predict tissue disruption and cerebroembolic events.

Using these principles, RF energy is initially set at 30 W and 55°C. Subsequently, RF power is titrated up to a maximum of 70 W by 5-W increments every few seconds while monitoring for microbubble formation on ICE. When type 1 (scattered) microbubbles are seen, energy is titrated down by 5-W decrements every 5 seconds until microbubble generation has subsided. Energy delivery is terminated immediately when type 2 (dense showers) microbubbles are seen. The operator should aggressively avoid any microbubble formation. Ablation is continued in one spot until no more PV potentials are seen. Each lesion typically lasts 30 to 50 seconds.[67]

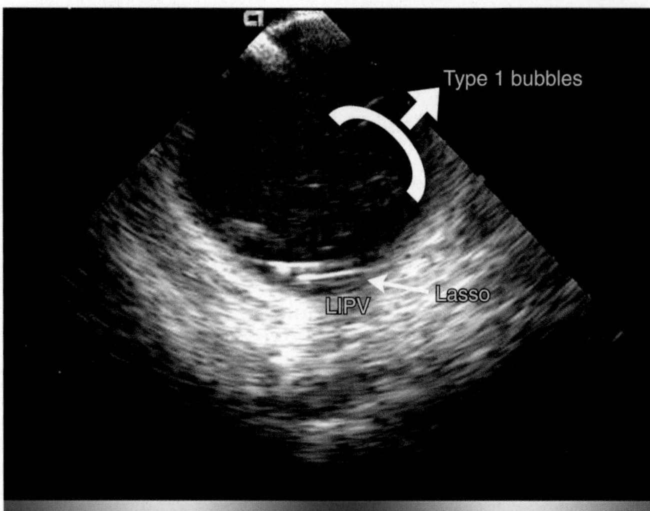

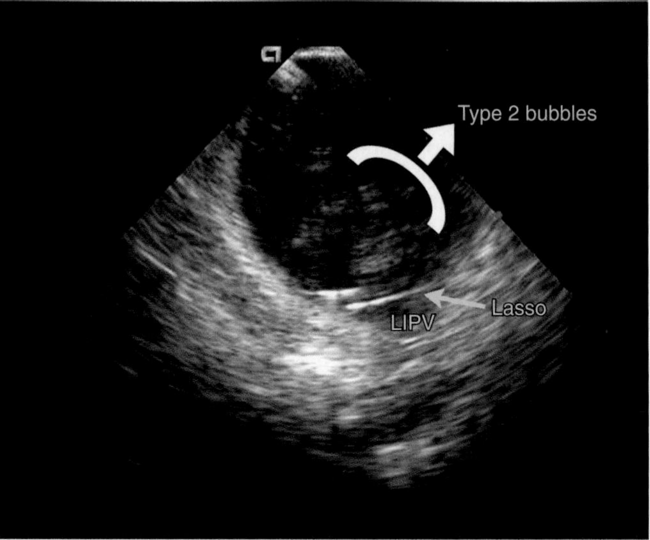

FIGURE 11–34 Intracardiac echocardiography (ICE)–guided RF energy delivery (microbubble monitoring). These are phased-array ICE views of the left atrium (LA) across the interatrial septum with the ring (Lasso) catheter positioned at the ostium of the left inferior pulmonary vein (LIPV). **Upper panel,** Localized microbubbles (type 1 bubbles) are observed during RF delivery. **Lower panel,** Showers of dense microbubbles extending to the LA cavity (type 2 bubbles) are observed during RF delivery. See text for discussion.

Microbubble formation, however, is not a straightforward surrogate for tissue heating. Experimental animal studies have revealed that particularly with the use of an irrigated ablation electrode, the abrupt occurrence of steam popping can occur without prior development of any bubbles on ICE.[70] Thus, caution is warranted in interpretation of the absence of bubble formation on ICE as an indicator of inadequate intramyocardial heating. The absence of microbubble formation does not indicate that tissue heating is inadequate or that the power level should be increased, nor does the presence of scattered microbubbles indicate safe tissue heating. This marker is fairly specific for tissue heating as judged by tissue temperatures, but is not a routinely sensitive one. Specifically, scattered microbubbles are noted to occur over the entire spectrum of tissue temperatures, whereas dense showers of microbubbles occurred only at tissue temperatures higher than 60°C. Scattered microbubbles may represent an electrolytic phenomenon, whereas dense showers of microbubbles suggest steam formation, with associated tissue disruption and impedance rises. Furthermore, it must be recognized that bubbles may be seen during high-output pacing and infusion of saline through the transseptal sheath side port.

Cryoablation

Technological evolution is now aimed at developing new catheter designs for circumferential ostial ablation of the PVs. These devices are to be tested in a large patient cohort to assess whether these technological improvements will lead to optimization of the use of cryothermal energy, maximizing the advantages of this new technology and limiting the drawbacks encountered in its clinical use.

Circular Cryoablation Catheter. A circular linear ablation catheter (Arctic Circler, CryoCath Technologies) was produced to sit within the first few millimeters of the PV to produce circumferential ablation. This catheter is currently undergoing evaluation. The current iteration is a 7 Fr catheter that applies the ablation energy simultaneously at the entire circumference by cooling down to a minimal temperature of −80°C. Within the cooling segment, a nitinol strut causes the circler to self-expand on cooling to engage vein diameters of 18 to 30 mm fully.

Cryoablation Balloon. The highly variable anatomy of the PVs provides a significant challenge for any balloon-based technology. This has been highlighted by the initial use of the over the wire ultrasound balloon experience. By design, this technology works best when the shaft of the catheter sits coaxially to the PV, which can be a significant challenge to any operator, even when assisted by ICE.[63] On the other hand, a cryothermal balloon overcomes this problem, because the entire balloon can freeze and adhere to the adjacent tissue. As such, the perimeter of the balloon in closest apposition to the vein becomes the source of ablation, irrespective of the orientation in the vein. The cryothermal balloon ablation system (CryoCath Technologies) consists of a nondeflectable, over the wire, 10 Fr two-lumen catheter with double inner-outer cooling balloons (outer balloon maximum diameter, 23 mm; total length, 20 mm; see Fig. 4-6). The refrigerant N_2O is delivered under pressure from the console into the inner balloon chamber via a lumen within 2 mm of the catheter tip, where it undergoes a liquid to gas phase change, resulting in inner balloon cooling to temperatures of −80°C or lower. During cryotherapy, temperature is monitored via a thermocouple located at the inner balloon.[71] Preliminary work in a canine preparation has demonstrated feasibility and safety. The lesions were transmural, circumferential, and without overlying thrombus. Moreover, as the heat source of the PV flow is occluded by the balloon, transmural lesions within the thick atrium adjacent to the vein were achieved, unlike with previous nonocclusive technologies.[71] Further safety evaluation and engineering developments are required prior to the successful deployment of such a balloon in humans.

Ultrasound Ablation

The ability of ultrasound to be collimated (i.e., minimization of convergence and divergence with ultrasonic focusing lens) through an echolucent fluid medium (e.g., water, blood) makes it ideal for a balloon delivery system. An 8-MHz cylindrical transducer mounted within a saline filled balloon has been designed for PV isolation using high-intensity focused ultrasound (HIFU) energy. The ablation system (Atrionix, Sunnyvale, Caif) consists of a 0.035-inch diameter luminal catheter with a distal balloon (maximum diameter, 2.2 cm) housing a centrally located ultrasound transducer. The system is advanced over a guidewire into the target PV. Tissue surface temperature monitoring is important and is achieved by thermocouples on the balloon and the ultrasound transducer. The ablation time is 2 minutes, followed by an additional minute before the balloon is deflated. After every ablation with a temperature higher than 55°C, PV isolation is confirmed with ring catheter mapping.

Despite the initial enthusiasm, the long-term report of 33 patients was disappointing, with a chronic cure of about 30%, although electrical isolation was acutely achieved in all but one of the PVs targeted. Surprisingly, several applications were required to achieve PV isolation. The variability of the PV anatomy was the main culprit for the system failure. In larger PV orifices, it was difficult to achieve adequate heating. The system delivered a narrow band of ultrasound energy radially from a centrally located transducer, and it was occasionally challenging to place the catheter in all PVs at the proximal portion. Therefore, foci at the most proximal lip of a PV may not be ablated successfully. More recently, a forward-projecting HIFU balloon catheter (ProRhythm, Ronkonkoma, New York) has been developed for circumferential PV isolation outside the PV ostia to limit the risk of PV stenosis. Radially emitted ultrasound is reflected from the back of the balloon, resulting in forward projection of ultrasound energy with a focal point at the balloon-endocardial interface (see Fig. 4-7). The HIFU balloon is steerable through a pull-wire mechanism integrated in the handle of the catheter, and it has two attached noncompliant balloons. The distal balloon is filled with a mixture of water and contrast medium (6:1 ratio) and contains a 9-MHz ultrasound crystal. The proximal balloon, when filled with carbon dioxide, forms a parabolic surface at the base of the distal (water and contrast) balloon, which reflects the ultrasound in the forward direction, focusing a 360-degree ring of ultrasound energy (sonicating ring) 2 to 6 mm in front of the distal balloon surface to produce a circumferential transmural LA lesion with each application. The distal balloon has three sizes, 24, 28, or 32 mm in diameter, producing sonicating rings of 20, 25, or 30 mm in diameter. The acoustic power of the system is 45 W for all three balloons, with negligible loss of power in the balloon. Once inflated, the water and contrast mixture in the distal balloon is circulated continuously at 20 mL/min to cool the balloon and maintain the balloon surface temperature at 42°C or lower. The pressure of the distal balloon is maintained at 8 psi (0.54 atm) to hold the parabolic shape. The catheter has a central lumen for a guidewire (0.23 inch), which is used to position the catheter over the PV. The central lumen is also used for PV angiography (distal to the balloon).[72,73]

After transseptal LA access is achieved, the transseptal sheath is exchanged for a 16 Fr transseptal sheath to introduce the HIFU balloon catheter into the LA. The HIFU balloon is maneuvered to all PV ostia. When in doubt about the exact location of the inflated balloon and its relation to the PV, the guidewire is temporarily removed and contrast medium is injected into the lumen of the HIFU catheter (occlusion angiogram). After reinsertion of the guidewire, the proximal balloon is inflated with carbon dioxide and HIFU energy (acoustic power, 45 W) is applied for 40 seconds (for the balloon with the 20-mm sonication ring), 60 seconds (for the balloon with the 25-mm sonication ring), or 90 seconds (for the balloon with the 30-mm sonication ring). After every one or two HIFU sonications, PV isolation is evaluated using the ring catheter. If the PV is not isolated, the HIFU balloon is repositioned or switched to another balloon size. To insert the Lasso catheter into the PV, the balloon needs deflation, reinflation, and repositioning. A novel circumferential mapping catheter (ProMap, Pro-

Rhythm) small enough to be placed via the central lumen of the HIFU catheter may overcome this limitation and help shorten the procedure time. Clinical application of this system has recently been evaluated, with successful PV electrical isolation of 89% of patients.[72,73]

A potential advantage of ultrasound is that it does not rely on extensive heating on the vein surface, and heat is not conducted to the cardiac tissue as it is with RF. This may prevent the PV stenosis seen with RF PV isolation. If catheter design limitations are addressed, PV isolation using through the balloon ultrasound can add significantly to the tools available for treating patients with drug-refractory AF. However, patients with common PV ostia with diameters larger than 30 mm may not be eligible because the maximal available balloon size is only 30 mm. Currently, no HIFU catheter is available that can be used for linear (instead of circular) ablation. Thus, if additional linear lesions are required, as proposed for patients with permanent AF, RF catheter ablation should be considered.

Endpoints of Ablation

The endpoint of ablation is electrical isolation of all four PVs, as described for segmental ostial PV isolation. Reconfirmation of PV isolation after a 60-minute waiting period after initial PV isolation has been suggested to detect early recurrence of PV conduction. A recent report has shown that early recurrence of PV conduction is extremely common after circumferential PV isolation, observed in more than 90% of patients and 50% of the PVs. A first recurrence was observed in about one third of PVs at 30 minutes and in another one fifth of PVs at 60 minutes.[74] Some investigators also suggested reconfirmation of PV isolation after administration of IV isoproterenol infusion (1 to 3 μg/min) and adenosine (12- to 30-mg rapid IV bolus).[75]

Inducibility of AF may also be assessed as an endpoint. Inducible sustained AF is thought to indicate the presence of potential atrial substrate capable of maintaining AF. A recent study has found that patients with noninducible AF had a higher success rate than those with inducibility (82% versus 45%; $P = .02$). In addition, the study has demonstrated that the success rate is similar between patients with noninducibility following circumferential antral PV isolation and those after PV isolation plus linear ablation across the LA roof and/or mitral isthmus (83% and 84%, respectively). This suggested that an inducibility test can be used to identify patients in whom additional LA linear ablation should be considered.[76]

Outcome

Studies using ICE-guided circumferential PV isolation have reported a success rate after the first procedure of about 80%, with higher success rates seen in younger patients with paroxysmal AF. This outcome was associated with moderate to severe PV stenosis in only 0.25% of patients, thromboembolic complications in 0.8%, cardiac tamponade in 0.5%, and no cases of atrioesophageal fistula. Almost all patients (more than 80%) with recurrent AF or AT after ablation had recurrent PV conduction at repeat study. Patients with AF recurrence who underwent repeat antral PV isolation alone (without additional linear ablation) had excellent results, with a more than 90% drug-free cure seen over a median follow-up of 8 months.

One study has compared segmental ostial PV isolation and circumferential extraostial PV isolation. With the circumferential extraostial PV isolation approach, a single encirclement was performed around ipsilateral PVs, and complete electrical isolation of all four PVs was used as an endpoint. At 11 ± 3 months' follow-up, 60% of patients in the segmental group were free of AF, compared with 75% of patients in the circumferential group (*P* value was not significant). Isolation of a large area around the PVs (with en bloc encirclement of ipsilateral PVs—i.e., one encirclement for the right-sided or left-sided PVs, and no line between the ipsilateral PVs is deployed) has also been found to be more effective in treating paroxysmal and persistent AF than segmental ostial PV isolation.[77]

CIRCUMFERENTIAL LEFT ATRIAL ABLATION

Rationale

Attempts to replicate the results of the maze procedure in the EP laboratory have consisted of the creation of linear lesions in the LA and/or RA. In the past, multiple catheters with coil electrodes positioned against the atrial wall were used to create the linear lesions without having to reposition the catheter repeatedly. Currently, linear ablation lesions are created with individual contiguous applications of RF energy on a point by point basis. RF ablation is performed circumferentially around the ipsilateral PVs with the endpoint of ablation being the absence or marked reduction (80%) in the amplitude of electrical signals within the encircling lesions.

Whereas the efficacy of PV isolation depends on complete and lasting PV disconnection from the LA, the efficacy of circumferential LA ablation does not. This highlights the fact that circumferential LA ablation (also referred to as wide-area LA ablation and circumferential PV ablation) eliminates AF by mechanisms other than complete PV isolation. Several mechanisms of action may be involved.[42] First, there is substrate modification by LA compartmentalization; about 25% to 30% of the LA myocardium is excluded by the encircling lesions, thereby limiting the area available for circulating wavelets that may be needed to perpetuate AF. The ablation lines may also eliminate anchor points for rotors or mother waves that drive AF, making reentry pathways unsuitable. Autonomic denervation by ablation of vagal inputs to the posterior LA wall is another potential mechanism. A third potential mechanism is damage to the Marshall ligament or Bachmann's bundle, which can be involved in the initiation and maintenance of AF. The vein of Marshall, which has a LA insertion in close proximity to the left superior PV and can be a source of triggers for AF, may be excluded by the ablation line that encircles the left-sided PVs. Additionally, promotion of atrial electroanatomical remodeling involving the LA posterior wall may result, to the point that the substrate for AF is no longer present. Modification of PV arrhythmogenic activity may also be operative. By encircling the PVs, LA ablation may eliminate the triggers and driving mechanisms of paroxysmal AF that arise in the PVs. Although complete conduction block across the encircling lesions may not be achieved, decremental conduction can occur, particularly at shorter CLs, and may impede the conduction of PV tachycardias to the LA.

An advantage of this technique is that the lesion can be tailored to the varying PV-LA junction features, unlike circumferential ablation catheters with a prefixed size and design. These are difficult to accommodate in ostia with larger diameters, eccentric shapes, or a complex proximal PV branching pattern.

There are several differences between circumferential LA ablation and PV isolation strategies.[38,78] From a mechanistic standpoint, segmental ostial ablation electrically isolates the PVs, thereby eliminating the arrhythmogenic activity in the PVs that triggers and/or perpetuates episodes of paroxysmal AF. However, sources of AF that do not originate in the PVs and the substrate that supports the maintenance of AF are not addressed by PV isolation. From a technical aspect, segmental ostial and circumferential antral PV isolation techniques require the insertion of two catheters into the LA, whereas linear LA ablation requires only a single catheter in the LA. Also, a notable difference between the two approaches to ablating AF is that PV isolation requires the identification of PV potentials, which may be difficult to distinguish from atrial electrograms. In contrast, circumferential LA ablation is primarily an anatomical approach to ablation. Furthermore, circumferential LA ablation necessitates the use of a 3-D mapping system, which increases the cost of the procedure. However, the use of the 3-D mapping system has the advantage of limiting radiation exposure to patients and operators. Additionally, the risk of PV stenosis, which is a major concern during ostial PV isolation, is minimized during circumferential LA ablation, because most ablation sites are more than 1 cm away from PV ostia.

Electroanatomical Mapping

Three catheters are used: a standard quadripolar catheter in the RV apex to provide backup pacing; a quadripolar catheter in the CS to allow pacing of the LA; and the ablation catheter, which is passed into the LA following transseptal puncture with a long sheath. A ring catheter is unnecessary; therefore, only one transseptal puncture is required.

A nonfluoroscopic 3-D electroanatomical CARTO or NavX navigation system is used for generating and validating the continuity of the circular ablation lines (Fig. 11-35). CartoMerge incorporates the use of CT or MR scans to allow verification of the anatomical landmarks and cardiac geometry and helps guide the ablation catheter precisely to the different areas of interest (see earlier, under circumferential antral PV isolation). CT integration into the CARTO system improves visualization of complex LA geometries and may improve the safety and success of catheter ablation for AF. Improved visualization of the mapping catheter within the atria may ensure better close apposition or contact with the atrial wall (see Fig. 3-34). CT integration offers the added benefit of displaying the atrial configuration, thus allowing completion of a ring of ablation lesions that follows the patient's own anatomy rather than empirical encirclement. This offers the benefit of displaying skips, in which symmetrical wide encirclement may not follow alterations in atrial architecture. Moreover, accuracy of lesion placement to ensure continuity of linear ablation over complex anatomy is improved.

The ostium of each PV is identified based on the results of selective biplane PV angiography (if performed) and fluoroscopic visualization of the catheter tip entering cardiac silhouette, with a simultaneous decrease in impedance and appearance of the atrial potential.

If validation of the circumferential lesions around PVs and the completeness of conduction block across the ablation lines are to be used as endpoints for the ablation procedure, propagation maps have to be created before and after RF ablation. The CARTO system can create 3-D chamber geometry color-encoded with activation times, and dynamic propagation maps can be displayed as movies of sequential activation. Additionally, the collected data can be displayed as voltage maps, which can be useful to define scar areas and electrically diseased tissues. In patients in NSR at the beginning of the procedure, maps are acquired during pacing from the CS or RA at a CL of 600 milliseconds. In patients in AF, electrical cardioversion to restore NSR is performed at the end of the mapping procedure to allow stimulation maneuvers.

Target of Ablation

The ablation lines are typically created with encircling lesions around the left- and right-sided PVs, 1 to 2 cm from the PV ostia. The circumferential ablation lines may surround each of the PVs or, instead of encircling each PV, one big circle is placed around the PVs of each side (Fig. 11-36; see also Fig. 11-35).[38] An ablation line is also created across the LA roof to connect the two circumferential ablation lines and another ablation line across the mitral isthmus between the inferior portion of the left-sided encircling lesion and the lateral mitral annulus. In some patients, addi-

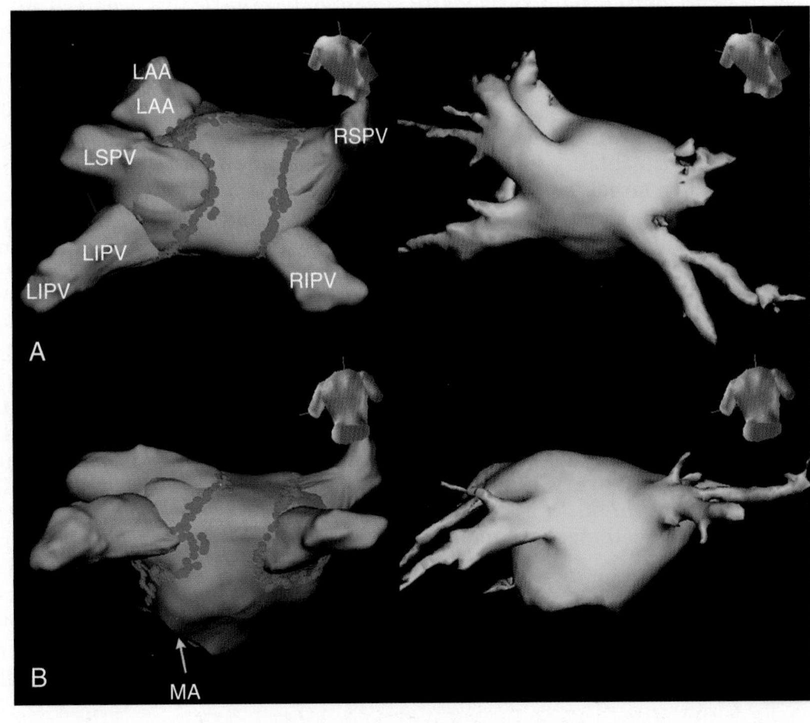

FIGURE 11–35 Wide-area circumferential left atrial (LA) ablation. Shown are cephalic **(A)** and caudal **(B)** posteroanterior views of 3-D reconstruction of the LA and pulmonary veins (PVs) using EnSite NavX (left) and synchronized 3-D reconstruction of the LA and PVs using cardiac CT angiography (right). Red dots indicate the sites of ablation, with circumferential LA ablation in addition to the LA roof and mitral isthmus lines. LAA = LA appendage; LIPV = left inferior PV; LSPV = left superior PV; MA, mitral annulus; RIPV = right inferior PV; RSPV = right superior PV.

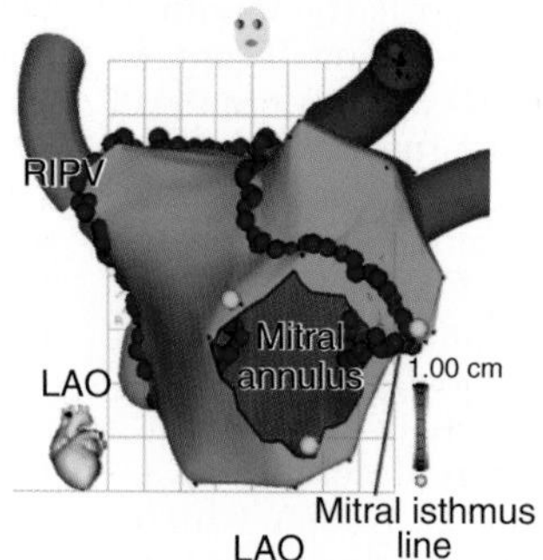

FIGURE 11–36 Wide-area circumferential left atrial (LA) ablation. Shown are multiple (right anterior oblique [RAO], posteroanterior [PA], and left anterior oblique [LAO]) views of anatomical "shell" rendering of the LA anatomy and pulmonary veins (PVs) using CARTO. Red dots indicate sites of ablation. LA roof and mitral isthmus lines, connecting anatomical barriers, are as shown.

tional ablation lines are created in the septum and anterior wall, extending from the roof line to the mitral isthmus. Presently, the number and location of LA linear lesions should be tailored to the individual patient. The ideal configuration would combine technical ease and safety with long-term cure of AF.

Ablation Technique

Once the main PVs and LA have been adequately reconstructed, RF energy is delivered to the atrial endocardium. LA ablation is performed 1 to 2 cm from the PV ostia to encircle the left- and right-sided PVs. However, because there is a narrow rim of atrial tissue between the anterior aspect of the left superior PV and the LA appendage in 50% of patients, ablation can sometimes be performed within 1 cm of the ostium of this vein.

Circumferential ablation lines are usually created starting at the lateral mitral isthmus and withdrawing the ablation catheter tip posteriorly and then anteriorly to the left-sided PVs, passing between the left superior PV and the LA appendage before completing the circumferential line on the posterior wall of the LA. The ridge between the left superior PV and LA appendage can be identified by fragmented electrograms caused by collision of activity from the LA appendage and left superior PV/LA. The LA appendage is identifiable by a significantly higher impedance (more than 4 Ω above the LA mean), a high-voltage local bipolar electrogram, with characteristically organized activity in fibrillating patients. The right PVs are ablated in a similar fashion. Ablation sites are tagged on the model of the LA created with the electroanatomical mapping system, and that system is used for generating and validating the conti-
11 nuity of circular lines.

An 8-mm-tip ablation catheter is typically used, with RF energy set to a target temperature of 55° to 65°C and a power limit of 70 to 100 W. The power and temperature limits are reduced in the posterior LA wall to 50 W and 55°C to reduce the risk of injury to the surrounding structures. A series of RF applications are delivered, each lasting 15 to 40 seconds, and until the maximum local bipolar electrogram amplitude decreases by 80% to 90% or to less than 0.05 to 0.1 mV, or to a maximum RF duration of 40 milliseconds, whichever comes first. Alternatively, RF energy is applied continuously on the planned circumferential ablation lines as the catheter is gradually dragged along the line, with repositioning of the catheter tip every 10 to 20 seconds. Continuous catheter movement, often in a to and fro fashion over a point, helps keep the catheter tip temperature down as a result of passive cooling.

Power, impedance, and electrical activity are monitored continuously during navigation and ablation. Impedance may increase suddenly if a thrombus forms on the catheter tip. A much more useful indicator is a 40% to 50% reduction in the power delivered to reach target temperature. If thrombus formation is suspected, catheter withdrawal from the LA without advancing the transseptal sheath may be necessary to avoid stripping any thrombus present on the catheter tip as the catheter is withdrawn into the sheath, which can result in systemic embolization.

RF application should be immediately terminated when the catheter position deviates significantly from the planned line or falls into a PV, when impedance rises suddenly, or when the patient develops cough, burning pain, or severe bradycardia.

After completion of the circular lesions around the left- and the right-sided PVs, the area within the ablation lines is explored with the ablation catheter. RF energy is applied at sites that have a local electrogram amplitude more than 0.1 mV. In addition, when AF is still present, sites inside the encircling ablation lines where the CL is shorter than the atrial CL in the CS also are ablated.

Endpoints of Ablation

To date, circumferential LA ablation for AF has stood apart from most other types of ablation procedures in that a clear-cut EP endpoint has not been used. The only endpoint of ablation used in most studies has been voltage abatement and, although one study has suggested that complete block across the ablation lines is a useful EP endpoint, this was not confirmed in two other studies.

Voltage Mapping. The primary endpoint for circumferential ablation is more than a 80% to 90% reduction in voltage within the isolated regions or the recording of low (0.05 to 0.1 mV or lower) peak to peak bipolar potentials inside the lesion, as determined by local electrogram analysis and voltage mapping (Fig. 11-37).[42]

Postablation voltage mapping is performed using the preablation map for the acquisition of new points (on the existing LA geometry) to permit accurate comparison of preablation and postablation bipolar voltage maps. After completion of the circular lesions around the left- and right-sided PVs, the area within the ablation lines is explored with the ablation catheter, and RF energy is applied at sites that have a local electrogram amplitude more than 0.1 mV. As an anatomy-based ablation strategy, this may be the only required endpoint.

Activation or Propagation Mapping. Another endpoint used for lesion validation requires the acquisition of two propagation maps during CS and RA pacing for left- and right-sided PVs, respectively. The rationale behind this setting is to pace from a site close to the lesions and shorten conduction time to the ablation site, thereby allowing detection of delayed activation inside the circular line.

Several criteria are used to define line continuity: (1) low peak to peak bipolar potentials (less than 0.1 mV) inside the lesion, as determined by local electrogram analysis and voltage mapping; (2) local activation time delay of more than 30 milliseconds between contiguous points lying in the

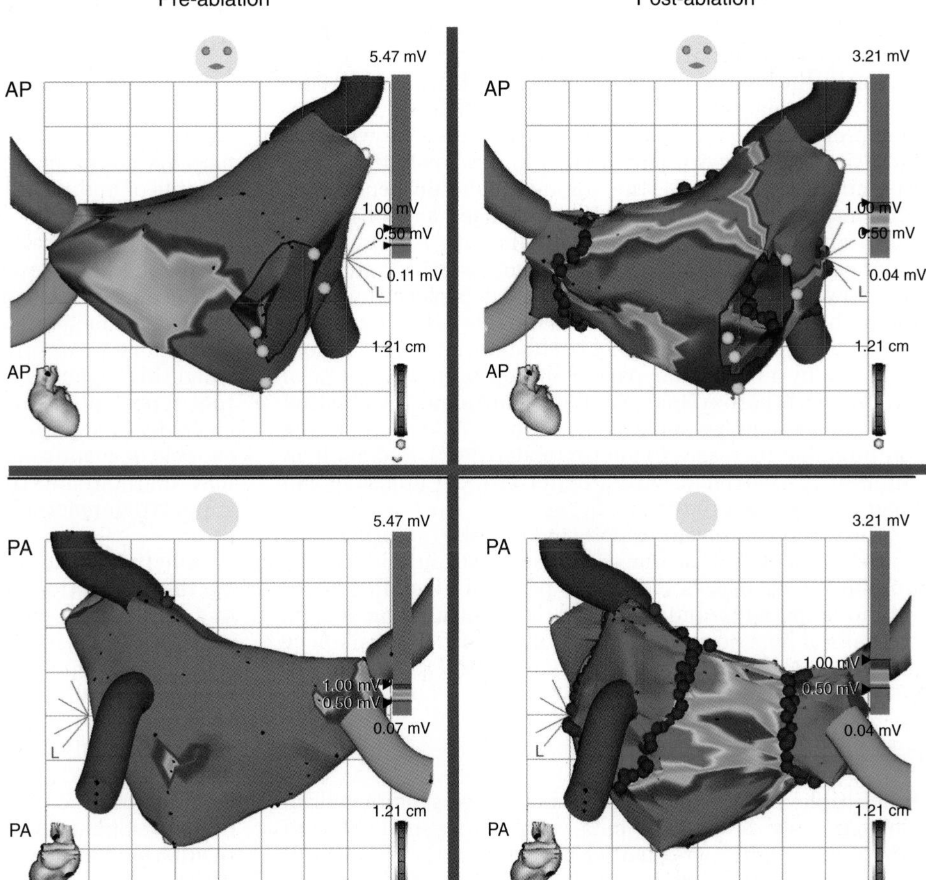

FIGURE 11–37 CARTO voltage map post–wide-area circumferential left atrial (LA) ablation. Anteroposterior (AP) and posteroanterior (PA) views of electroanatomical voltage maps before (left) and after (right) wide-area circumferential LA ablation depict peak to peak bipolar electrogram amplitude. Red represents lowest voltage, purple, highest voltage. In postablation maps, areas within and around the ablation lines, involving to some extent the LA posterior wall, show low-amplitude (<0.5 mV) electrograms.

same axial plane on the external and internal sides of the line, as assessed by activation mapping; and (3) gaps in the ablation lines are defined as breakthroughs in an ablated area and identified by sites with single potentials and by early local activation. Changes in activation spread are also evaluated with propagation mapping. Incomplete block is revealed by impulse propagation across the line; in this case, further RF applications are given to complete the line of block.

Importantly, the only predictive criterion for a successful ablation seems to be the amount of post-RF low-voltage encircled area. Therefore, validation of the circumferential lesions around PVs by pacing maneuvers, the completeness of conduction block across the ablation lines, and the search for gaps in the ablation lines are not routinely performed.

Pulmonary Vein Isolation. Complete PV isolation, as an endpoint for linear LA ablation, is not required. Evidence has shown that complete electrical isolation of the PVs is not necessary for a successful outcome, and freedom from symptomatic AF during follow-up is just as likely when none of the PVs are completely isolated as when all four PVs are isolated. One study has shown that this ablation strategy usually is associated with incomplete PV isolation.[79] However, although PV potentials were still present in one or more PVs in 80% of patients, there usually was a conduction delay between the LA and PVs, and the prevalence of PV tachycardias was markedly reduced after circumferential LA ablation.

Termination of Persistent Atrial Fibrillation. Termination of AF during the procedure occurs in about one third of patients. If AF does not terminate during RF, transthoracic cardioversion is performed at the end of the procedure. If AF recurs immediately after the cardioversion, the completeness of the lines is reassessed and additional ablation lines should be considered.

Additional ablation consists of ablation lines created along the LA septum, roof, posterior mitral isthmus, and/or anterior wall on the basis of the presence of fractionated or rapid atrial activity. Ablation is continued until AF terminates and becomes noninducible (see later discussion).

Organized Atrial Arrhythmias. When LA ablation is performed during an ongoing episode of AF, the AF converts to NSR or to a more organized type of atrial tachyarrhythmia in approximately 20% to 30% of patients.

LA ablation may create macroreentrant circuits in the LA, mediating conversion of AF into AFL. The most common type of macroreentry is mitral isthmus–dependent AFL. Because AF and AFL often occur in the same patient and may induce each other, mitral isthmus–dependent AFL simply may be induced by the AF as it terminates. However, the AFL that coexists with AF is predominantly RA in origin; therefore, it seems more likely that the mitral isthmus–dependent AFL is a direct result of LA ablation. The potential for LA ablation to create mitral isthmus–dependent AFL underscores the importance of an ablation line between the left inferior PV and the mitral isthmus. Mitral isthmus–dependent AFL may occur despite an ablation line in the mitral isthmus, and it is possible that slowed conduction through an area of partial block facilitates macroreentry. Complete block in the mitral isthmus usually can be achieved, although ablation within the CS may be necessary. Occasionally, a macroreentrant circuit can be created by a gap in the ablation line that encircles the right-sided PVs. This AFL can be ablated by RF applications at the gaps in the circumferential ablation lines.

Noninducibility of Atrial Fibrillation. Inducibility of AF after ablation was found to be a significant independent predictor of recurrent AF. Its predictive power was found in patients with paroxysmal and persistent AF and was not dependent on the applied ablation technique. Whether noninducibility of AF can be used as a clinically useful endpoint of ablation in patients with AF who have undergone circumferential LA ablation is still controversial, however. One study has suggested performing additional ablation when AF is still inducible after the initial procedure.[80] Circumferential LA ablation renders AF noninducible by rapid atrial pacing in approximately 40% of patients with paroxysmal AF. With additional LA ablation lines, the percentage of patients in whom AF was rendered noninducible increases to approximately 90%, and such an endpoint is associated with a better clinical efficacy than when AF was still inducible.[80]

Conversely, a recent report has shown a rather low predictive accuracy of the postablation stimulation test,[81] prohibiting its use as a reliable procedural endpoint for individual patients, and suggested that continuation of ablation caused by a positive stimulation test or AF persistence might lead to overtreatment in a substantial proportion of patients.

Outcome

In multiple reports, long-term success was achieved in approximately 74% of patients with paroxysmal AF and 49% of those with persistent or permanent AF. The overall major complication rate was 2.2%, including stroke (0.2%), pericardial tamponade (0.6%), and PV stenosis (0.4%).

One study has suggested that circumferential LA ablation to encircle the PVs is preferable to segmental ostial PV isolation as the first approach in patients with symptomatic paroxysmal AF. In contrast, another prospective randomized study comparing the two strategies has shown opposite results. Not unexpectedly, the opposite results in the two studies were obtained because of the large variability in the success rate observed in patients undergoing circumferential LA ablation (88% versus 47%) whereas the success rates in patients undergoing segmental ostial PV isolation remained unchanged (67% versus 71%).[78,82]

AF ablation may improve mortality in selected patients. A single center report has examined the results of 1171 consecutive patients with AF referred for treatment over a 38-month period who were followed up for a mean of 900 days. Although not randomized, half the patients were treated with circumferential LA ablation, and half were treated medically. Patients treated with catheter ablation were approximately half as likely to die during the follow-up period (6.5% versus 14%) and half as likely to have a stroke or other major adverse cardiovascular events (7.8% versus 16.8%) as those treated medically. Patients treated with ablation, but not those treated medically, enjoyed improvement in quality of life scores to near-normal levels. Although the results need to be confirmed in a multicenter randomized trial, they suggest that adverse events and poor results associated with a medical rhythm control strategy may be related to antiarrhythmic drugs, rather than the strategy itself.

LINEAR ATRIAL ABLATION

Linear atrial ablation may involve the LA roof line, LA mitral isthmus line, and RA cavotricuspid isthmus line.

Left Atrial Roof Line

Rationale

The PVs are a dominant source of triggers initiating AF and PV isolation in patients with paroxysmal AF results in its termination in approximately 75%. However, the remaining patients could sustain AF, suggesting a residual substrate capable of maintaining AF after exclusion of the PV and the PV-LA junction. Several potential mechanisms can coexist to form the substrate for AF after PV isolation; these include localized high-frequency activity (focal or reentrant), meandering multiple wavelet reentry, and macroreentry. Although the exact mechanism by which the LA roof supports the fibrillatory process is unclear, evidence has clearly implicated this region in the substrate for AF. In addition, the LA roof represents a region demonstrating highly fragmented electrograms, perhaps indicating the presence of substrate capable of sustaining localized reentry or focal activity that may maintain fibrillation, and also has the potential for supporting macroreentry around the PVs using the LA roof.

Ablation at the LA roof was found to have a direct effect on the fibrillation process, prolonging the fibrillatory CL and terminating the arrhythmia in some patients and rendering AF noninducible in patients with inducible or sustained arrhythmia after PV isolation, implicating the LA roof in the substrate maintaining AF after PV isolation in humans.

Linear ablation lines were previously performed posteriorly or anteriorly across the LA. However, a posterior ablation line between the two superior PVs carries a higher risk of atrioesophageal fistula.[38] Transection of the anterior LA results in significantly delayed activation of the lateral LA during NSR, which has potentially deleterious hemodynamic consequences.[83] Therefore, these lines are currently substituted with the LA roof line (see Fig. 11-36).

Ablation Technique

Commencing at the encircling lesion at the left superior PV, the sheath and catheter assembly are rotated clockwise posteriorly and dragged toward the right superior PV.[84] To achieve stability along the cranial LA roof, the catheter may be directed toward the left superior PV and the sheath rotated to face the right PVs, or vice versa.[84] Two alternative methods can also be used to reach the LA roof for ablation. First, the catheter can be looped around the lateral, inferior, septal, and then cranial walls, laying the catheter down along the cranial wall of the LA to allow dragging of the catheter by withdrawal from the left to the right superior PV ostia. Second, the catheter can be maximally deflected to form a tight loop near the left superior PV, with the tip facing the right PVs. Releasing the curve positions the catheter tip adjacent to the right superior PV ostia and allows dragging back to the left PV.

The stability of the catheter is monitored during RF applications with the use of the proximal electrograms, intermittent fluoroscopy, and/or a navigation system to recognize inadvertent displacement of the catheter. Electroanatomical mapping (CARTO) or NavX navigation is used for real-time monitoring and to tag the ablation sequence.[84] RF energy is delivered for 60 to 120 seconds at each point while the local atrial electrograms are monitored. Local potential elimination or formation of double potentials during pacing or AF signifies the effectiveness of ablation locally.

Endpoints of Ablation

The electrophysiological endpoint of ablation is the demonstration of a complete line of block joining the two superior PVs. Following the restoration of NSR, complete linear block is defined by point by point mapping of an online corridor of double potentials along the entire length of the roof during pacing of the anterior LA (from the LA appendage or the distal CS),[84] and by demonstration of an activation detour circumventing the right and left PVs to activate the posterior wall caudocranially, with no conduction through the LA roof. The latter is demonstrated by point by point sequential mapping conventionally or by electroanatomical mapping. In some cases, it is difficult to record both double potentials along the ablation line; thus, the second potential is measured at the posterior LA close to the ablation line. When residual conduction is demonstrated, detailed mapping is performed to identify and ablate gaps in the linear lesion.[84]

Outcome

Ablation of the LA roof in conjunction to circumferential antral PV isolation was shown in one study to significantly affect results—improved clinical outcome compared with PV isolation alone in patients with paroxysmal AF. Additional roof line ablation with complete conduction block was associated with 87% of patients being arrhythmia-free without antiarrhythmic medications compared with 69% undergoing PV isolation alone.[84] The clinical benefit was similar to other described lines (e.g., mitral isthmus line); however, the roof line could be achieved with shorter RF application and procedural durations. With a mean of 12 ± 6 minutes of RF energy, complete block at the LA roof could be achieved in 96% of cases.[84]

Although the addition of a complete line of block at the LA roof may result in greater efficacy for the suppression of atrial arrhythmia compared with PV isolation alone, this requires additional ablation and may be associated with a proarrhythmic risk. Whether such linear ablation should be empirically performed in all patients with AF or applied selectively on the basis of clinical or procedural variables, notably persistent inducibility after PV isolation, remains to be determined prospectively.[84]

Left Atrial Mitral Isthmus Line

Emerging evidence has implicated regions of conduction slowing and block associated with atrial remodeling in the substrate predisposing to AF. In the LA, recent studies have demonstrated preferential propagation that is closely correlated with muscle fiber orientation along the posterior LA and circumferentially around the mitral annulus. Such preferential propagation occurring in response to functional or anatomical conduction block (perhaps exacerbated by AF or conditions predisposing to AF) is capable of facilitating reentry, utilizing the mitral isthmus, as recognized with common forms of LA macroreentry, and thus may have a role in the milieu that maintains AF.[85]

Because of the contiguity with the left PVs and LA appendage, ablation of the mitral isthmus results in a long (functional) line of conduction block that transects the lateral LA from the mitral isthmus to the roof. Its electrophysiological consequences can be considered analogous to those produced by cavotricuspid isthmus ablation, in which a short line is amplified by the crista terminalis to result in a long line of functional conduction block. It is thus likely that ablation of the mitral isthmus, as an adjunct to other ablation strategies for AF, helps modify a large region of the LA substrate for AF by eliminating anatomical or functional reentry involving the mitral isthmus or PVs. Additionally, it can eliminate arrhythmogenic triggers arising from the ligament of Marshall.

Macroreentrant LA flutters can develop following catheter ablation of AF in up to 5% of cases. The most common type of macroreentry is mitral isthmus–dependent AFL, and it seems more likely that this type of AFL is a direct result of LA ablation. The potential of this complication underscores the importance of an ablation line across the mitral isthmus. Ablation of the mitral isthmus is discussed in detail in Chapter 10.

In one report, the outcome of 100 consecutive patients with paroxysmal AF undergoing circumferential PV isolation alone was compared with that of an equal number of consecutive patients undergoing circumferential PV isolation and mitral isthmus ablation.[85] Mitral isthmus block was achieved in 92% of patients after 20 ± 10 minutes of endocardial RF application and an additional 5 ± 4 minutes of epicardial RF application from within the CS in 68%. One year after the last procedure, 87% of patients with mitral isthmus ablation and 69% without ablation (P = .002) were arrhythmia-free in the absence of antiarrhythmic drugs. Another study has shown a significant improvement of long-term sinus rhythm maintenance with the combination of bidirectional block along the left mitral isthmus and circumferential PV isolation in patients with both paroxysmal (76% versus 62%) and persistent (74% versus 36%) AF.

Right Atrial Cavotricuspid Isthmus Line

AF and AFL frequently coexist in the same patient. Clinical AFL occurs in more than one third of patients with AF. AF often precedes the onset of AFL and can also develop after the successful catheter ablation of AFL. AFL, usually induced either by atrial pacing or by AF, may be observed in two thirds of patients undergoing PV isolation for AF. Approximately 80% of these episodes are typical AFL.

Although typical AFL and AF frequently coexist, their precise interrelationship is unclear. It may be that the same premature depolarizations that trigger AF also trigger AFL, or the electrophysiological and/or structural remodeling that accompany AF may also promote the occurrence of AFL, or vice versa. Evidence has suggested that AF plays an important role in the genesis of typical AFL. Usually, spontaneous or induced typical AFL does not start immediately after a premature beat or burst rapid atrial pacing. Rather, its onset is generally preceded by a transitional rhythm (AF) of variable duration.[86] AF may promote the formation of intercaval functional line of block in the RA, which may be critical for the initiation of AFL. Additionally, it is also possible that at least some episodes of AFL may degenerate into AF. AFL with a short CL may result in fibrillatory conduction. Class IC and IA antiarrhythmic drugs and amiodarone used to suppress AF commonly promote sustained typical AFL.

Catheter ablation techniques targeting the cavotricuspid isthmus for typical AFL or the initiating triggers within the PVs for AF have been independently shown to offer a potential cure for the two atrial arrhythmias. AF occurrence rates after typical AFL ablation alone have been shown to range from 38% when preprocedural AFL is the dominant arrhythmia over AF to 86% when AF is the dominant arrhythmia. In one study of patients with paroxysmal AF who had periods of AFL, successful elimination of symptomatic AF by PV isolation was not found to be associated with freedom from symptomatic AFL. However, another report has shown that PV isolation, although it does not interrupt the reentrant flutter circuit, can be sufficient to control both arrhythmias, suggesting that AF initiated by PV triggers can be the precursor rather than the consequence of AFL. This is consistent with the observation that AFL commonly starts after a transitional rhythm of variable duration, usually AF.

The occurrence of typical AFL during a PV procedure was shown to be predictive of symptomatic AFL during follow-up after PV isolation, a risk that was lowered by combining AF and AFL ablation in those patients. However, as was shown in another study, although cavotricuspid isthmus ablation may reduce early recurrences of AFL, those early recurrences do not represent a long-term problem in most patients and require only short-term therapy. On the other hand, there is a trend toward a lower incidence of recurrent AF after PV isolation in patients who underwent cavotricuspid isthmus ablation than in those who did not. This suggests that AFL may have been responsible for some episodes of AF. Consistent with a facilitatory role of typical AFL in the pathogenesis of AF, several prior studies have demonstrated that the incidence of AF may be lower after ablation of the cavotricuspid isthmus.

Determining the best ablative approach remains a challenge. Some data suggest that it may be appropriate to ablate the cavotricuspid isthmus whenever typical AFL is observed clinically or in the course of a catheter ablation procedure aimed at elimination of AF. On the other hand, ablation of the cavotricuspid isthmus may be performed on a different occasion only in patients who actually present clinically with typical AFL after AF ablation. This strategy of selective supplementary cavotricuspid isthmus ablation does not seem to be associated with higher rates of AF or typical AFL occurrence after AF ablation. Thus, routinely performing typical AFL ablation in all patients undergoing AF ablation may not provide added clinical benefit but can potentially add time, cost, and risk.[87]

ABLATION OF COMPLEX FRACTIONATED ATRIAL ELECTROGRAMS

Rationale

Atrial electrograms during sustained AF have three distinct patterns—single potential, double potential, and complex fractionated potential(s).[40] Continuous propagation of multiple wavelets in the atria and wavelets as offspring of atrial reentry circuits has been suggested as the mechanism by which AF may be perpetuated without continuous focal discharge. Fractionated and continuous electrical activity may indicate the presence of wave collision, slow conduction, and/or pivot points where the wavelets turn around at the end of the arcs of functional blocks. Thus, areas of complex fractionated atrial electrograms (CFAEs) during AF may represent continuous reentry of the fibrillation waves into the same area or overlap of different wavelets entering the same area at different times.

Such complex electrical activity has a relatively short CL and heterogeneous temporal and spatial distribution. A relatively short CL may indicate the presence of a driver, analogous to the frequency gradient from the drivers or rotors to the rest of the atria observed in experimental models of AF, in which the central core of these rotors may have high-frequency electrical activity, whereas the periphery of the rotors may display complex electrograms because of wave break and fibrillatory conduction.[14] Importantly, the distribution and location of CFAEs seem to remain relatively constant, which is surprising considering the earlier observation that the underlying mechanism for AF is random reentry and that the reentrant wavelets are expected to meander; in turn, the CFAEs should be fleeting.[40] Nevertheless, regional disparities of endocardial atrial activation exist in AF and CFAEs have a propensity to localize in the same areas and do not meander.

Recent data have suggested that areas of CFAEs are critical sites for AF perpetuation and can serve as target sites for AF ablation. Once CFAEs are eliminated by ablation, AF can no longer be sustained because the random reentry paths are altered or eliminated so that the fibrillation wavelets can no longer reenter the ablated areas.[40,88] Whereas PV isolation aims to remove the triggering foci, ablation of CFAEs aims to remove the substrate for AF. However, some connections between both approaches may exist. Data indicate that PVs are the key areas where CFAEs are located; these areas need to be ablated to achieve conversion of AF to NSR. It is thus very likely that many patients may respond to ablation in the PV regions because of both trigger elimination and substrate modification.[40,88]

More evidence is needed to validate this approach as a stand-alone technique for AF ablation or only as an adjunct to other strategies. Nevertheless, this approach should be considered especially in patients with permanent or persistent AF, whose response to other ablation strategies is suboptimal, as well as in patients with recurrent AF undergoing a second ablation procedure.[40,88]

Mapping of Complex Fractionated Atrial Electrograms

Mapping of CFAEs is performed during AF. In patients in NSR at the time of study, AF is induced by isoproterenol infusion and/or rapid atrial pacing. In patients with persistent AF or with induced AF sustained for more than 5 minutes, biatrial electroanatomical (CARTO) mapping is performed.[40,88] The CS or RA appendage recording is used for electrical reference during CARTO mapping. Atrial CLs are monitored and recorded from the reference and mapping catheters. CARTO enables the operator to associate areas of CFAEs with the anatomy of both atria. Relevant sites can thereby be located, tagged, and later revisited. During AF, the local activation time of the arrhythmia is of no value in guiding activation sequence mapping.[89]

CFAEs are defined as (1) atrial electrograms that are fractionated and composed of two deflections or more, and/or have a perturbation of the baseline with continuous deflection of a prolonged activation complex over a 10-second recording period, or (2) atrial electrograms with a very short CL (120 millliseconds or less) averaged over a 10-second recording period (Fig. 11-38).[40,89] CFAEs are tagged and associated with the atrial anatomy created by CARTO, thereby serving as target sites for ablation.

An important limitation of this approach is that the visual appearance of CFAEs is variable and they are often of very low amplitude (<0.25 to 0.5 mV); therefore, their identification by visual inspection can be challenging and is highly investigator-dependent. Additionally, determination of the average atrial CL of a local electrogram in real time is also difficult without stopping the procedure to measure the electrograms offline manually. To improve the accuracy of CFAE mapping, custom software has been developed with algorithms that enable automated detection and tagging of areas of CFAEs with the anatomical shell of both atria, which offers valuable advantages in the detection, quantification, and regionalization of CAFEs. The CFAE complex is identified using an algorithm that quantifies the CFAE phenomena in two parameters. First is the interval confidence level, which is the number of intervals identified between consecutive complexes identified as CFAE. The assumption is that the more complex intervals recorded during the signal recording time (2.5 milliseconds)—that is, the more repetitions in a given time duration—the more confident the categorization of CFAE. Second is the shortest complex interval, which is the shortest interval found in milliseconds out of all the intervals identified between consecutive CFAE complexes. The data for each point are then displayed in the whole-chamber map. CFAE areas are displayed in a color-coded manner according to

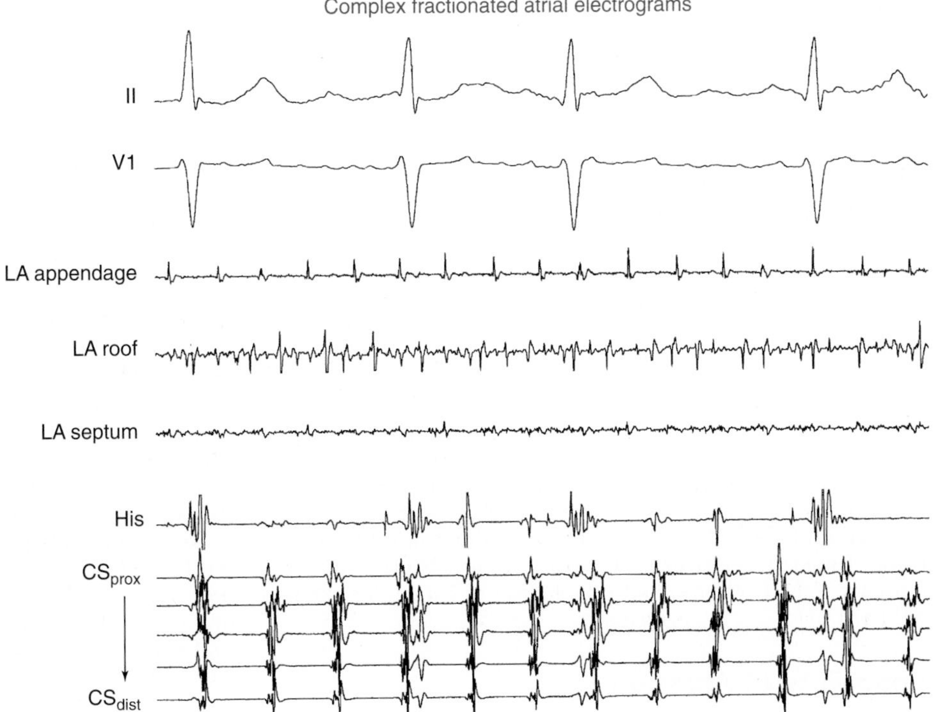

FIGURE 11–38 Examples of complex fractionated atrial electrograms. Fractionated atrial electrograms with a very short cycle length (CL), compared with the rest of the atria, were recorded in the left atrial (LA) roof. In the LA septum, fractionated electrograms with continuous prolonged activation complex were observed. See text for discussion.

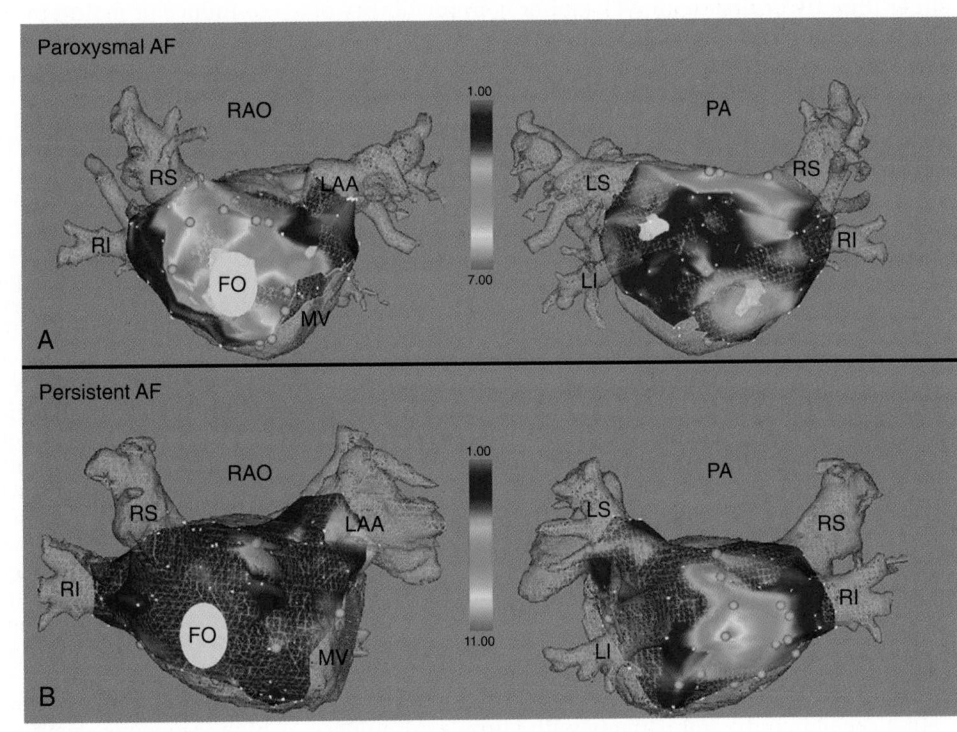

FIGURE 11–39 CARTO maps of complex fractionated atrial electrograms (CFAEs). CFAE maps with registered left atrial (LA) CT surface reconstruction (shown as wire frame), shown in right anterior oblique (RAO) view (left-sided images) and posteroanterior (PA) view (right-sided images), in patients with paroxysmal atrial fibrillation (AF) **(A)** and persistent AF **(B)**. The CFAE maps are color-coded, with red representing the highest interval confidence interval (ICL) and purple representing the lowest ICL. Highly repetitive CFAE sites (ICL ≥ 5) are tagged with light blue dots on the CFAE maps. As shown in this example, the highly repetitive CFAE sites are more likely located at the pulmonary vein (PV) ostia, interatrial septum, and mitral annulus area in paroxysmal AF patients, whereas patients with persistent AF have highly repetitive CFAE sites predominantly identified on the LA posterior wall. FO = fossa ovalis; LAA = LA appendage; LI = left inferior PV; LS = left superior PV; MV = mitral valve; RI = right inferior PV; RS = right superior PV. (From Scherr D, Dalal D, Cheema A, et al: Automated detection and characterization of complex fractionated atrial electrograms in human left atrium during atrial fibrillation. Heart Rhythm 2007;4:1013.)

the degree of fractionated signals and their CLs for easier identification (Fig. 11-39). Using this system, CFAEs were identified in most (80%) areas of the LA but were more predominantly located in the septum, posterior wall, and PV ostia. Compared with patients with paroxysmal AF, persistent AF patients had more highly repetitive CFAE sites identified on the LA posterior wall.[90] Assessment of fractionated electrograms during AF requires a recording duration of 5 seconds or more at each site to obtain a consistent fractionation and accurate analysis.

Target of Ablation

Atrial ablation is performed at all sites displaying continuous electrical activity, complex and fractionated electrograms, regions with a gradient of activation (significant electrogram offset between the distal and proximal recording bipoles on the map electrode), or regions with shorter CL activity compared with the LA appendage.[40] After ablation of CFAEs in the LA, those in the CS and RA are targeted. The atrial septum, followed by the regions of the PVs, is the most common site for complex CFAEs.[40,91] The most common localizations for termination and regularization of AF during CFAE ablation are the regions of the PV ostia, the interatrial septum, and the LA anterior wall close to the roof of the LA appendage.

Ablation Technique

The ablation typically begins at sites at which CFAEs have the shortest interval and preferably also have a high interval confidence level. RF energy is applied at a maximum temperature of 50°C and a maximum power of 35 W around the PV ostia, in the CS, and along the posterior LA and at a maximum temperature of 50° to 60°C and a maximum power of 70 W elsewhere in the atrium.

A mean of 64 ± 36 RF applications was required in one study.[40] In a second study, the mean duration of RF energy application was 36 ± 13 minutes.[91] When the areas with CFAEs are completely eliminated, but the arrhythmia organizes into AFL or AT, the atrial tachyarrhythmias are mapped and ablated (occasionally in conjunction with ibutilide, 1 mg infused over 10 minutes). If the arrhythmias are not successfully terminated by ablation or ibutilide, external cardioversion is performed.

Endpoints of Ablation

The primary endpoints during ablation are complete elimination of the areas with CFAEs or organization and/or slowing of local electrograms, conversion of AF to NSR (either directly or first to an AT), and/or noninducibility of AF (with isoproterenol and atrial pacing).[40,88,91] For patients with paroxysmal AF, the endpoint of the ablation procedure is noninducibility of AF. For patients with persistent AF, the endpoint is termination of AF. When areas with CFAEs are completely eliminated, but arrhythmias continue as organized AFL or AT, those arrhythmias are mapped and ablated.

Outcome

In one study, all patients with persistent AF converted into NSR during the ablation procedure and rendered AF noninducible; 14% required concomitant ibutilide treatment.[40] About 91% of patients with chronic AF converted to NSR during ablation, and 28% required concomitant ibutilide treatment. At the 1-year follow-up, 76% of patients with persistent or permanent AF after one ablative session and
11 91% after a second ablation session were free of arrhythmia, with only a minority requiring antiarrhythmic therapy.[40] Recurrent atrial tachyarrhythmias were common after the first session of ablation (approximately 50% of patients). The majority of the arrhythmias (71%) were typical AFL, atypical AFL, and AT, and 29% were AF. The recurrent atrial tachyarrhythmias were paroxysmal or persistent, and they resolved within 2 months in half of the patients; the other half required a second ablation procedure.[40]

In a second study, 100 patients with chronic AF underwent RF ablation of CFAEs in the LA and CS. AF terminated by RF ablation in only 16%, after the use of ibutilide in an additional 40%, and by DC cardioversion in the rest of patients. During 14 ± 7 months of follow-up after a single ablation procedure, 33% of patients were in sinus rhythm without antiarrhythmic drugs, 38% had AF, 17% had both AF and AFL, 9% had persistent AFL, and 3% had paroxysmal AF on antiarrhythmic drugs. A second ablation procedure was performed in 44% of patients. At 13 ± 7 months after the last ablation procedure, 57% of patients were in sinus rhythm without antiarrhythmic drugs, 32% had persistent AF, 6% had paroxysmal AF, and 5% had AFL.[91]

In another study, ablation of CFAEs was used only if AF was still inducible following PV isolation.[88] During a mean follow-up of 11 ± 4 months after the last ablation procedure, 77% of patients with paroxysmal AF were free from recurrent AF or AFL in the absence of antiarrhythmic drug therapy. LA flutter developed in 19% of patients and was still present in 10% at more than 12 weeks of follow-up. A repeat ablation procedure was performed in 18% of patients.

PULMONARY VEIN DENERVATION

Rationale

Recent studies have provided strong presumptive evidence that hyperactivity of the intrinsic autonomic nervous system constitutes a dysautonomia that can lead to a greater propensity for AF, both the paroxysmal and sustained forms.[17,18] Parasympathetic attenuation by PV denervation was found to confer added benefit in patients undergoing cirumferential LA ablation for paroxysmal AF.[18] Patients free of recurrent AF were characterized by marked and prolonged heart rate variability changes consistent with vagal withdrawal that were more pronounced in those in whom vagal reflexes were elicited and abolished. These changes were absent in patients with recurrent AF. Therefore, targeting autonomic nerves at a few specific sites on the heart that are directly related to arrhythmia formation may help reduce extensive damage to healthy myocardium while curtailing the ability to induce or maintain AF.

Target of Ablation

Ganglionated plexuses are located predominantly in six regions of the atria. In the LA, they are located around the antral regions of the PVs and in the crux. In the RA, they are localized at the junction of the RA and SVC. Ganglionated plexuses also are located at other sites, such as the main pulmonary artery, SVC, and ventricles. During ablation of AF, only LA ganglionated plexuses are targeted. Parasympathetic innervation has been localized around and outside PV areas; the roof junction of the left superior PV, anterosuperior aspect of the right superior PV, and the posteroinferior junction of the left and right inferior PVs are optimal sites for eliciting and eliminating vagal reflexes.[92]

Potential vagal target sites can be identified during the ablation procedure in at least one third of patients.[18] Vagal reflexes are indicated when sinus bradycardia (less than 40 beats/min), asystole, AV block, or hypotension occurs within a few seconds of the onset of RF application (Fig. 11-40). RF ablation in areas adjacent to the ganglionated plexuses has been suggested to result in stimulation causing bradycardia and hypotension when a predominantly vagal response occurs. However, similar responses may be a vagal response caused by pericardial pain. Furthermore, when precisely identifying the location of the ganglionated plexuses using high-frequency stimulation, RF ablation directly over such sites infrequently causes stimulation during ablation, resulting in no specific response to RF energy delivery, followed by no further response to high-frequency stimulation on retesting. The same observation has been made while applying RF energy to the plexuses during epicardial surgical ablation.

The use of high-frequency stimulation to identify ganglionic plexi as target sites for endocardial RF applications has been explored. Elicitation by high-frequency stimulation of a significant slowing of the ventricular response during AF is interpreted as evidence of the presence of a functioning ganglionic plexus.

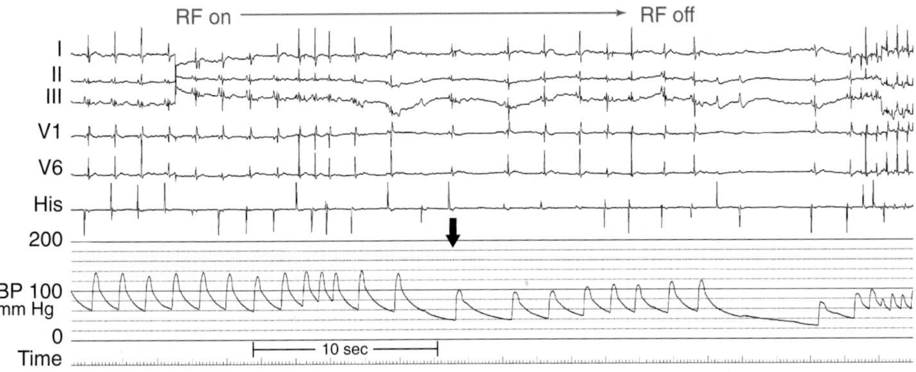

FIGURE 11–40 Vagal reflex during pulmonary vein (PV) isolation. Sinus rhythm is present at the beginning of the tracing; when RF energy is applied ("RF on"), blood pressure (BP) and heart rate decrease markedly (sinus bradycardia and nonconducted P wave). After energy is stopped ("RF off"), a short episode of atrial fibrillation (AF) ensues.

Ablation Technique

High-frequency electrical nerve stimulation is used to study the intrinsic cardiac nervous system. This technique allows for precise determination of the location, threshold, and predominance of parasympathetic or sympathetic response of the ganglionated plexuses. Electrical nerve stimulation requires high rates and strengths of stimulation. The distal electrode of the mapping-ablation catheter is used to deliver typically 1200 beats/min (20 Hz) with a pulse width of 10 milliseconds at 5 to 15 V. Tolerance of the conscious patient to high-frequency stimulation still must be determined, because most reports have described use of this approach in deeply sedated patients.[93]

When high-frequency stimulation is applied during NSR, AF generally occurs and then terminates within the next minute. Repeated stimulation usually results in sustained AF, at least in patients with a clinical history of AF. The predominant vagal response to high-frequency stimulation usually is observed during AF, manifested by AV block and hypotension. This response is elicited within 10 seconds of application of high-frequency stimulation; if no response occurs, the catheter is positioned at adjacent sites. A predominantly efferent sympathetic response to high-frequency stimulation is an increase in blood pressure. Although infrequent, this appears to occur in the region of the left PVs and may be related to stimulation of the Marshall ligament.[94]

The ganglionated plexus of the right superior PV can be mapped precisely and quickly by positioning the catheter anteriorly in the antral region. The ganglionated plexus usually is readily identified using high-frequency stimulation. Near the right inferior PV, the catheter is positioned posteriorly and inferiorly.[94] The ganglionated plexuses of the left PVs are not identified as readily as those of the right PVs, possibly because of a less dense innervation of these regions, especially for the ganglionated plexus of the left inferior PV, which is found posteriorly. The left superior PV generally demonstrates a superior position of the ganglionated plexus, either posteriorly or anteriorly.[94]

When positioning the mapping catheter in the mid body of the LA and deflecting it inferiorly and posteriorly, high-frequency stimulation usually readily provokes an autonomic response with little further catheter manipulation. This region also can be identified from inside the CS using an RA approach, although great care is required to avoid stimulating ventricular myocardium at high stimulation rates.[94]

Endpoints of Ablation

When a vagal reflex is elicited by high-frequency stimulation or during RF application, RF energy should be delivered until such reflexes are abolished, or for up to 30 seconds. Precise targeting of ablation over sites of ganglionated plexus requires only two to four RF applications to eliminate an afferent response to high-frequency stimulation.[93] Failure to reproduce the reflexes with repeat RF applications is considered confirmation of denervation.[18]

Outcome

At present, no reports have suggested that targeting of ganglionated plexuses only will consistently terminate AF or prevent its reinitiation. However, clustering of ablation lesions over regions of ganglionated plexuses and/or complex fractionated electrograms hopefully will result in improved clinical outcomes by including cardiac stomata as part of a comprehensive strategy of AF ablation. Detrimental effects of ablation over such sites have not been specifically reported.[18,93,94]

In a report of 297 patients undergoing circumferential LA ablation for paroxysmal AF, 34% of the patients showed evidence of cardiac vagal denervation during the ablation procedure and in follow-up. Ablation along the posterior LA in the standard lesion set sometimes produced a vagal reflex, resulting in sinus bradycardia and transient AV block. When ablation was continued at these sites, loss of the reflex occurred, suggesting vagal denervation, which was confirmed by indices of heart rate variability on follow-up Holter monitoring. Remarkably, 99% of 100 patients who achieved complete vagal denervation were free of AF at 12 months versus 85% of the remaining patients ($P = .0002$).[18]

ABLATION OF NON–PULMONARY VEIN TRIGGERS

Rationale

Although the PVs are the major site of ectopic foci initiating AF, evidence has demonstrated the important role of non-PV ectopic beats initiating AF. Investigators have debated the frequency of these non-PV sources, with an incidence ranging from 3.2% to 47%; the incidence was found to be higher in chronic AF.[12] Additionally, the presence of non-PV ectopic beats may play an important role in the recurrence of AF after PV isolation. Recently, several investigators have reported focal AT originating from the LA after isolating all four PVs or circumferential LA ablation in up to 3% to 10% of patients. The locations of focal ATs were around the PV ostium, LA appendage, or LA free wall. Those findings support the concept that non-PV triggers actually exist before the AF ablation, and that they become the drivers of the AF or AT after part of the LA tissue is ablated or the

LA-PV conduction is interrupted. Previous studies have also shown that wide-area circumferential LA ablation may be more effective than simple PV isolation, in part because some LA posterior free wall foci may be eliminated and/or isolated during circumferential ablation.[18,42]

The non-PV ectopic beats can arise from the SVC (most common, especially in females), LA posterior free wall (especially in patients with LA enlargement), crista terminalis, CS, ligament of Marshall, interatrial septum, or, rarely, a persistent left SVC.[12,43] Additionally, SVTs such as atrioventricular nodal reentrant tachycardia (AVNRT) and atrioventricular reentrant tachycardia (AVRT) may be identified in up to 4% in unselected patients referred for AF ablation, and can serve as a triggering mechanism for AF (see Fig. 11-2).

At the present time, most PV ablation procedures are performed anatomically by isolating all PV ostia. However, it is currently unclear whether an attempt should be made before and after PV isolation to observe the spontaneous or provoked ectopic beats initiating AF to evaluate for non-PV sources of this ectopy during initial and repeat ablation procedures.

Mapping of Non–Pulmonary Vein Triggers

Provocation of Ectopy

The initial step is to locate the spontaneous onset of ectopic beats initiating AF in the baseline state or after infusion of isoproterenol (up to 4 to 8 μg/min for 5 minutes).[12,43] If spontaneous AF does not develop, intermittent atrial pacing (8 to 12 beats) with a CL of 200 to 300 milliseconds from the high RA or CS is used to facilitate spontaneous initiation of AF after a pause in the atrial pacing. If spontaneous AF does not occur, burst pacing from the high RA or CS is used to induce sustained AF. After an episode of pacing-induced AF is sustained for 5 to 10 minutes, external cardioversion is attempted to convert the AF to NSR and observe the spontaneous reinitiation of AF.[12,43] A bolus of high-dose adenosine (24 to 84 mg) may also be used to provoke the spontaneous onset of AF.

The onset pattern of spontaneous AF is analyzed, and the earliest ectopic site is considered to be the initiating focus of AF. The method used to provoke spontaneous AF is repeated at least twice to ensure reproducibility.

Localization of Ectopy

Mapping of endocardial atrial activation sequences from the high RA, HB, and CS catheters can predict the location of AF initiation foci. The difference in the time interval between the high RA and HB atrial activation obtained during sinus beats and PACs is a good method to identify whether the ectopic focus is from the RA or LA. When the difference in the time interval is less than 0 millisecond, the accuracy for discriminating RA from LA ectopy approximates 100%.[12]

If the initiating focus of the AF is considered to be from the RA, a duodecapolar catheter is placed along the crista terminalis, so that it would reach to the top of the SVC. The polarity of the P wave of the ectopic beat in the inferior leads is a useful method to differentiate the location of the ectopic beats. Ectopy from the SVC and upper crista exhibits upright P waves in the inferior leads, whereas ectopy from the coronary sinus ostium (CS os) exhibits a negative P wave polarity in the inferior leads and ectopy from the mid crista exhibits biphasic P waves. During RA ectopy, the P wave can be biphasic or positive in lead V_1, whereas it is predominantly positive in the case of right superior PV ectopy.

If the RA ectopy cannot be confirmed by the activation time, P wave morphology on the surface ECG, or intracardiac signals, transseptal access is obtained and two multipolar catheters are placed in the right superior PV and at the LA posterior wall simultaneously. Unusual ectopy from the RA septal region also requires biatrial mapping to confirm the location, especially in cases with a shorter activation time (less than 15 milliseconds) preceding P wave onset or a monophasic, narrow, and positive P wave in lead V_1 during ectopy. Multielectrode basket catheter, balloon catheter (EnSite noncontact mapping), and 3-D electroanatomical mapping systems can be of value in localization of the origin of AF triggers, especially in patients with infrequent PACs.[12,43]

Mapping and Ablation of the Ligament of Marshall

Clues to Ligament of Marshall Activation

The ligament of Marshall is an epicardial vestigial fold that marks the location of the embryological left SVC. The ligament of Marshall contains the nerve, vein (vein of Marshall), and muscle tracts, and it encompasses portions of the embryonic sinus venosus and left cardinal vein, running between the left superior and left inferior PVs along the left side of the parietal pericardium. The ligament of Marshall leads to the earliest tributaries of the CS and the transition from a ligamentous structure to a vein occurs in the region between the left superior PV and base of the LA appendage. The proximal portions of the muscle tracts connect directly to the CS myocardial sleeves; the connecting point is the landmark that separates the great cardiac vein from the CS (the origin of the ligament of Marshall corresponds to the location of the tip of a CS catheter advanced to the wedge position as far distally as possible in the CS). The distal portions of the muscle tracts extend upward into the PV region.

The ligament of Marshall as a source of ectopy should be considered when the ectopic beat is located around the posterolateral mitral annulus or the left PV ostium. The P wave morphology associated with vein of Marshall ectopic activity is characterized by an isoelectric P wave in leads I and aVL, positive in leads II, III, aVF, and V_2 to V_5, and similar to that seen with ectopic beats arising from the left PVs.[95]

Additionally, certain observations and pacing maneuvers can indicate vein of Marshall activation, including (1) unexpectedly early exit from PV ectopy, (2) unexpected PV activation sequence during NSR, and (3) unexpected PV activation sequence during low-output CS pacing.[96]

Ectopy or rapid tachycardias arising from the PV typically demonstrate an early near-field potential on catheters placed within the PV and a late far-field electrogram consistent with LA activation. Often, the exit delay (interval between the early near-field potential and late far-field potential) exceeds the entrance delay seen in sinus rhythm with activation from the LA to the PV. Despite this exit delay, however, the earliest atrial activation should be in the perivenous area. If earlier activation is noted in the CS rather than the perivenous LA, direct conduction from the PV to the CS through the musculature of an atrial epicardial vein, usually the vein of Marshall, is likely (Fig. 11-41).[96]

During NSR, PV activation spreads from proximal (PV ostium) to distal. If earlier activation is seen in the mid or distal PV electrodes than near the ostium, a bypass of the ostium with direct activation of the mid or distal PV is likely. One explanation is epicardial activation via the myocardial tissue within the vein of Marshall.[96]

With high-output pacing in the mid-CS, there is capture of both the myocardium of the CS itself and the adjacent LA.

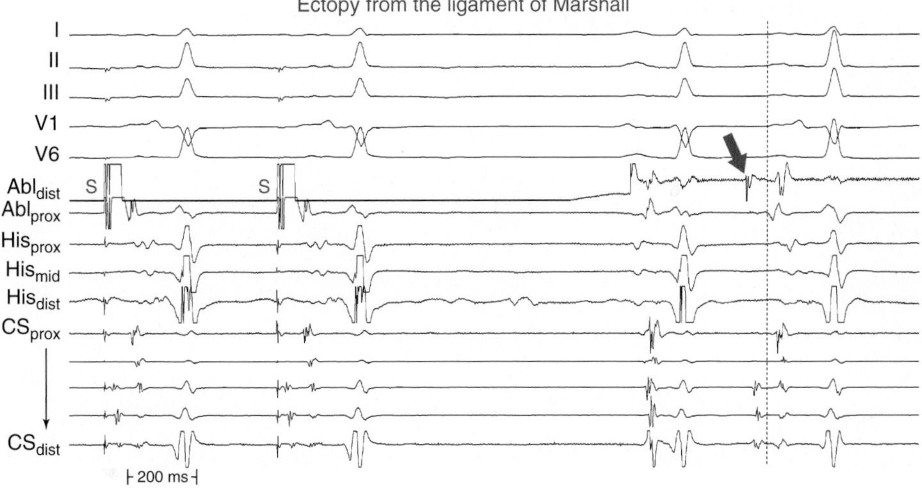

FIGURE 11–41 Ectopy from the ligament of Marshall (LOM)—recordings from a patient with atrial fibrillation (AF) caused by ectopy from the region of the LOM. **Right,** Sinus complex and premature atrial complex (PAC) from the LOM with a very early potential recorded by the ablation catheter in this area. Note the same potential occurring in coronary sinus (CS) recordings. **Left,** Pace mapping replicates atrial activation sequence during ectopy complex.

With lower output pacing, in most cases there will be capture of the myocardium of the CS only, with the LA activated from the CS through a CS-to-LA connection. In some patients, the CS-to-LA connection is small and discrete and, if the connection is not close to the site of pacing within the CS, there can be considerable delay between the CS myocardial electrograms and adjacent LA tissue electrograms (Fig. 11-42). This observation can be used to determine whether PV activation is occurring via the vein of Marshall. During low-output CS pacing, the LA is not directly activated. Because PV activation depends on LA activation, in most cases, when the LA electrogram is delayed, PV potentials also are delayed. When the time from stimulus to PV potential remains fixed regardless of whether direct capture of the LA occurs, PV activation is dependent only on CS muscular activation and a vein of Marshall connection very likely is present (see Fig. 11-42).[96]

Mapping of the Ligament of Marshall

Studies have demonstrated electrical activity within the ligament of Marshall and the two terminal ends of this atrial tract can have insertions into the LA musculature and CS. Also, more recently, the ligament of Marshall has been shown to have focal automatic activity induced by isoproterenol, and it may contribute to the development of AF. It seems that isoproterenol infusion is usually required to provoke ectopy or bursts of AF originating from the ligament of Marshall.[12,97]

The ligament of Marshall can be mapped epicardially or endocardially. The endocardial approach involves obtaining a CS angiogram, followed by insertion of a 1.5 Fr mapping catheter via the CS into the vein of Marshall. However, cannulation of the vein of Marshall is not always successful because of various anatomical and technical reasons. In patients whose vein of Marshall either is not visible on a CS venogram or is visible but cannot be cannulated, the percutaneous (subxyphoid) epicardial approach may result in successful mapping and ablation (Fig. 11-43). This latter approach has the advantage of free catheter movement and is not limited by the size of the vein of Marshall. However, the endocardial approach is the best method for differentiating ligament of Marshall ectopy from other ectopies.[97]

Because the ligament of Marshall can have multiple insertion sites in the LA posterior free wall or near the PV ostium, it is difficult to differentiate ligament of Marshall ectopy from PV or LA posterior free wall ectopy using the

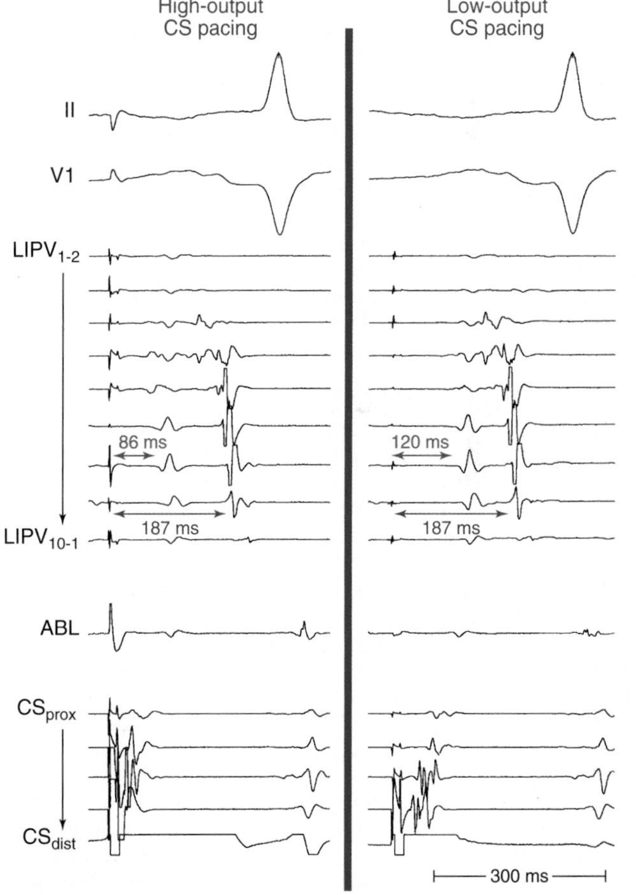

FIGURE 11–42 Identification of vein of Marshall activation using differential-output coronary sinus (CS) pacing. **Left panel,** During high-output CS pacing, both the left atrium (LA) and CS musculature are captured directly. **Right panel,** During low-output CS pacing, only the CS musculature is captured directly; the LA is activated from the CS through a CS to LA connection. In this case, the CS-LA connection is not close to the site of pacing within the CS; therefore, considerable delay is observed between the CS myocardial electrograms and adjacent LA tissue electrograms. Despite the delay in LA activation (as reflected by the interval between the pacing artifact and LA electrograms) during low-output versus high-output CS pacing, the timing of left inferior pulmonary vein (LIPV) activation remains constant (as reflected by the fixed interval between the pacing artifact and PV potentials in both cases), indicating that PV activation is occurring via the vein of Marshall and is independent of LA activation.

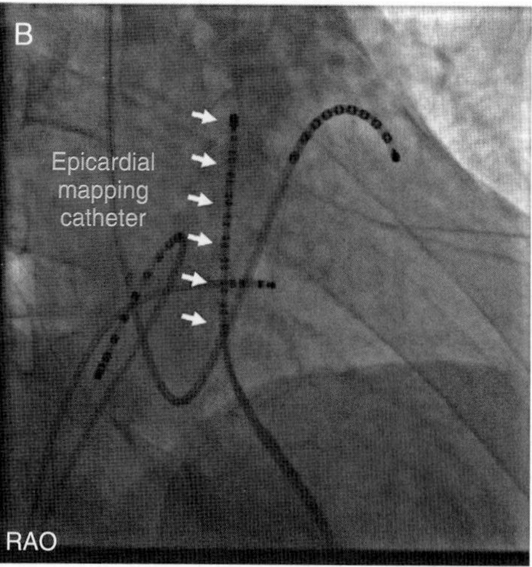

FIGURE 11–43 Two different approaches to mapping of the ligament of Marshall, right anterior oblique (RAO) views. **A,** Vein of Marshall (VOM) visualized by balloon occlusion coronary sinus (CS) angiogram. A 1.5 Fr mapping catheter can be inserted via the CS into this VOM for endocardial mapping. **B,** Epicardial mapping catheter inserted via a subxiphoid pericardial puncture. (From Hwang C, et al: How and when to ablate the ligament of Marshall. Heart Rhythm 2006;3:1505.)

epicardial approach. The possibility of ligament of Marshall ectopy should be considered when the so-called triple potentials (a discrete sharp potential preceding the LA and PV potentials) are recorded around PV ostium.[12] Furthermore, in patients with ectopic beats from the ligament of Marshall, double potentials are present at the orifice of or inside the left PVs, and distal CS pacing can help differentiate the ligament of Marshall potential from the PV musculature potential.[12] If the second deflection of double potentials is attributable to the activation of the ligament of Marshall, the interval between the CS os and the second deflection will be shorter during distal CS pacing compared with NSR. In contrast, if second deflection is attributable to activation of the PV musculature, the interval between the CS os and the second deflection will be longer during distal CS pacing compared with NSR.

Ablation of the Ligament of Marshall

A combined endocardial and epicardial approach can be used to ablate ligament of Marshall ectopy initiating AF, and is associated with a higher success rate. Cannulation of the Marshall vein and direct recording of the ligament of Marshall potentials from the Marshall vein can be used to guide epicardial ablation sites. The catheter inside the vein of Marshall can also be used as the anatomical target for endocardial ablation and to confirm successful elimination
11 of the ligament of Marshall potentials. Additionally, occluding the CS os with injection of contrast medium to visualize, but without cannulation of the Marshall vein, may also be used as an indirect method to trace the possible route of the ligament of Marshall to help guide epicardial ablation (see Fig. 11-43).[97]

The site having the shortest distance from the LA endocardium to the ligament of Marshall is located at the inferior region of the left antrum, just under the left inferior PV ostium. RF energy application (30 W at 55°C) from the endocardium to this region eliminates ligament of Marshall potentials in more than 90% of the cases, as confirmed by the mapping catheter inside the vein of Marshall. To simplify the procedure, a large-diameter (30 to 35 mm) ring catheter can be placed at the antrum of the left inferior PV to guide and then confirm simultaneous isolation of the antrum and ligament of Marshall. Complete isolation or disconnection of the entire left PV and antrum can be confirmed by pacing from the inside of the left PV. If PV potentials are dissociated from the LA potentials, these findings would confirm elimination of all connections to the LA, including the left PVs and ligament of Marshall.[97]

Infrequently, endocardial ablation alone cannot eliminate all connecting fibers, as evidenced by the ability to still record ligament of Marshall potentials. In these situations, most of the remaining connections are located in the ridge between the anterior border of the left PVs and the posterior wall of the appendage. In some patients, the ridge can be as thick as 10 mm. Even using an irrigated-tip catheter and a high-power setting, complete isolation still may not be possible. In these difficult cases, epicardial mapping techniques can be useful for identifying and ablating the remaining connecting fibers between the ligament of Marshall and LA.[97]

Electrical Isolation of the Superior Vena Cava

Rationale

The proximal SVC contains cardiac muscles connected to the RA, and atrial excitation can propagate into the SVC.[43] SVC cardiomyocytes can acquire pacemaker activity, and enhanced automaticity and afterdepolarization play a role in the arrhythmogenic activity of SVC (Fig. 11-44). The SVC myocardial extension harbors most (up to 55%) non-PV triggers of AF (especially in females), and elimination of SVC triggers is associated with improved long-term maintenance of sinus rhythm post–AF ablation.

Electrical isolation of SVC from the RA can be a better strategy than focal ablation of ectopy inside SVC. It obviates the need for detailed mapping of the exact origin of the ectopy focus, as well as the need for RF ablation inside the SVC, which may carry the risk of SVC stenosis. Nevertheless, injury to the sinus node and phrenic nerve remains a concern. The value of empirical isolation of the SVC as an adjunctive strategy for AF ablation needs further evaluation.[98]

Mapping of Superior Vena Cava Ectopy

To localize the accurate site of SVC ectopy, 3-D electroanatomical, ring catheter, or basket catheter mapping can be useful (Fig. 11-45). During NSR or atrial pacing, the intracardiac recordings from inside the lower level of the SVC (near the SVC-RA junction) frequently exhibit a blunted far-field atrial electrogram followed by a sharp and discrete SVC potential. In the higher level of SVC, the SVC potential precedes the atrial electrogram during the SVC ectopic beat (Fig. 11-46).[12,43] Furthermore, the intracardiac recordings in the higher SVC frequently exhibit double potentials. The

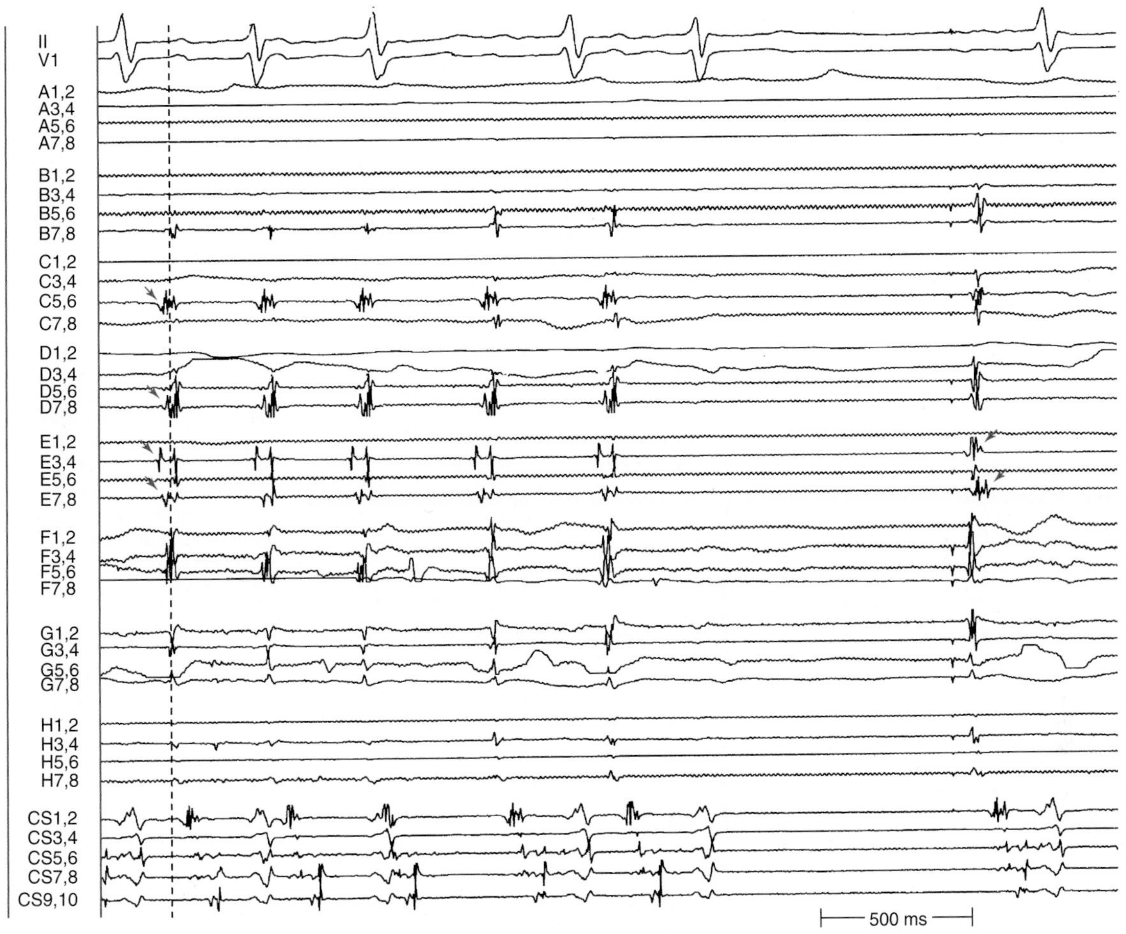

FIGURE 11–44 Focal atrial tachycardia (AT) originating from the superior vena cava (SVC). The basket catheter is positioned in the SVC–right atrial (RA) junction. Bipolar recordings are obtained from the eight electrodes (1-2, 3-4, 5-6, 7-8) on each of the eight splines (A through H) of the basket catheter. During AT (at left), SVC potentials (arrowheads) precede RA potentials and also precede P wave onset on the surface ECG (dashed line). During RA pacing (at right), SVC potentials overlap with or follow RA potentials.

FIGURE 11–45 Superior vena cava (SVC) angiogram. Fluoroscopic right anterior oblique (RAO) views of SVC angiography with the ring (Lasso) catheter (at left) and basket catheter (at right) positioned at the SVC-RA junction (black arrowheads). Note that the size of the ring catheter is usually smaller than the circumference of the SVC, and repositioning of the ring catheter is typically required for circumferential mapping and electrical isolation of the SVC.

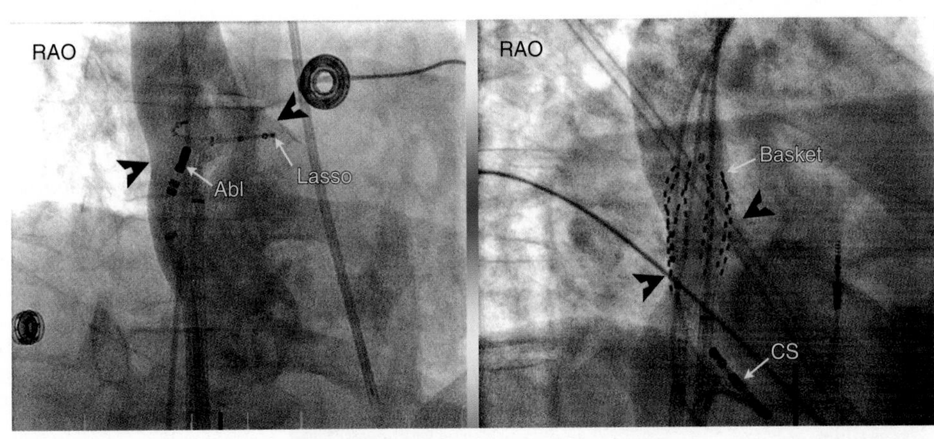

first potential represents the SVC potential, and the second potential represents the far-field right superior PV potential. Simultaneous recordings from the right superior PV also exhibit a double potential during SVC ectopy. The recording from right superior PV shows that the first potential is far-field potential from the SVC, and the second potential is true activation of the right superior PV.[12,43]

Ablation Technique

The SVC is isolated using the same technique and endpoint as used for segmental ostial PV isolation. The SVC-RA junction (defined as the point below which the cylindrical SVC flares into the RA) can be confirmed by SVC venography (see Fig. 11-45), ICE (Fig. 11-47), and/or the electrical signals.

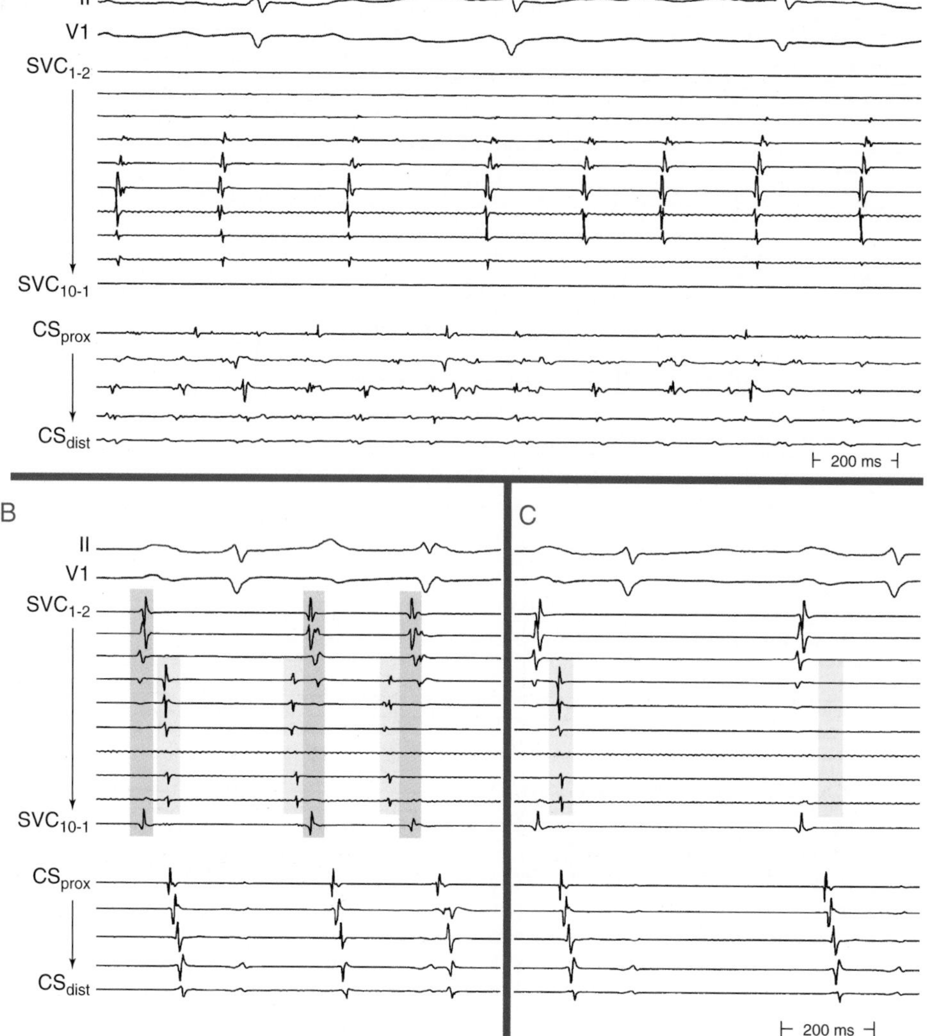

FIGURE 11–46 Electrical isolation of the superior vena cava (SVC). This recording was obtained from a ring catheter positioned at the SVC–right atrium (RA) junction during electrical isolation of the SVC. **A,** During atrial fibrillation (AF), SVC potentials are observed at a cycle length (CL) longer than the atrial CL observed in the coronary sinus (CS) recordings. **B,** The first complex is normal sinus, during which SVC potentials (blue shading) are observed following RA potentials (orange shading). The second and third complexes are premature atrial complexes (PACs) originating from the SVC, during which SVC potentials precede RA potentials. **C,** RF energy application at a single site results in the disappearance of SVC potentials (at right) and complete SVC entrance block.

11

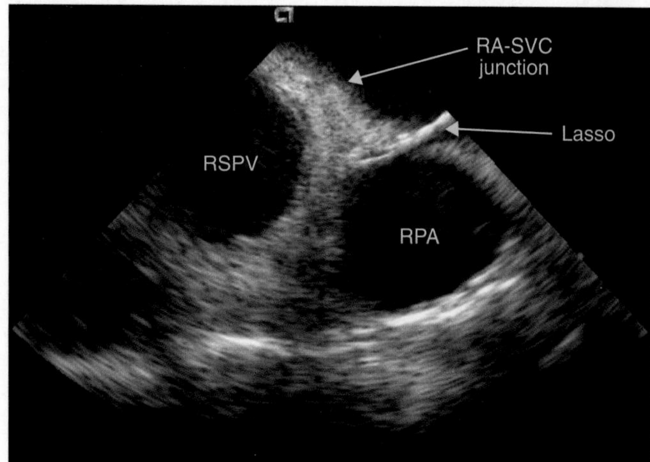

FIGURE 11–47 Electrical isolation of the superior vena cava (SVC). The intracardiac echocardiography (ICE) catheter positioned in the high right atrium (RA) is used to guide positioning of the ring catheter at the RA-SVC junction (at the level of the lower border of the right pulmonary artery, RPA). RSPV = right superior pulmonary vein.

SVC venography can be performed by placing a pigtail catheter at the top of the SVC and using a contrast injector (a total of 40 mL of contrast medium over 2 seconds) and biplane fluoroscopic views (RAO, 30 degrees; LAO 60 degrees).[12,43] The overlapping of the anterior wall of the SVC and RA appendage is near the level of the SVC-RA junction. The ring catheter is placed just above the RA-SVC junction at the level of the lower border of the pulmonary artery, as seen by ICE (see Fig. 11-47). The size of the ring catheter is usually smaller than the circumference of the SVC, and repositioning of the ring catheter is typically required for circumferential mapping and electrical isolation of the SVC (see Fig. 11-45).

In contrast to PV isolation, it is easier to interrupt the conduction between the RA and SVC. Most patients exhibit only two breakthrough sites. A ring or basket catheter can be used for mapping SVC potentials (see Fig. 11-46). The SVC-RA junction exhibits an eccentric shape, not a round shape; thus, the basket or ring catheter may not contact the wall well. Therefore, one needs to manipulate the catheter to contact the whole SVC-RA circumference to confirm the presence or disappearance of SVC potentials. The circumference of the SVC-RA junction is mapped to determine the region of earliest activation during NSR characterized by an initial negative rapid deflection and/or fusion of the major atrial electrogram and the SVC muscular potential. Those regions are then targeted by RF ablation.[12]

RF energy should be applied at the level about 5 mm below the entire circumference of the SVC-RA junction. Although application of RF energy inside the SVC is easier to interrupt the SVC-RA myocardial sleeve, it carries a higher risk of SVC narrowing or stenosis. RF energy is set at a power setting of 45 to 55 W, targeting a temperature of 50° to 55°C and applied for a duration of 20 to 40 seconds. Acceleration of the sinus rate during RF delivery is a sign that heat injury to the sinus node is occurring and should prompt discontinuation of RF application.

The phrenic nerve often courses posterolaterally at the level of the SVC-RA junction. Pacing prior to ablation along the circumference of this vein at an output between 5 and 10 mA is mandatory before energy delivery. The patient should not receive a paralytic agent if general anesthesia is to be used, and both mechanical palpation for diaphragmatic stimulation and fluoroscopy of an entire respiratory cycle should be performed during pacing so that the absence of phrenic nerve stimulation can be determined with certainty. The maneuver should be repeated at each ablation site and, during ablation the catheter should not be moved to sites more than a few millimeters away. If the patient is in AF during the attempted isolation of the SVC, the pacing maneuver still should be performed, but with asynchronous pacing from the ablation catheter.[96]

Electrical Isolation of the Coronary Sinus

The venous wall of the CS is surrounded by a continuous sleeve of atrial myocardium that extends for 25 to 51 mm from the CS os. This muscle is continuous with the RA myocardium proximally but is usually separated from the LA by adipose tissue. This separation can be bridged by muscular strands producing electrical continuity between the CS musculature and the LA. These connections are targeted by RF ablation for electrical isolation of the CS from the LA.

Isolation of the CS is commenced along the endocardial aspect and completed from within the CS, as required. The ablation catheter is dragged along the endocardium of the inferior LA after looping the catheter in such a way as to position it parallel to the CS catheter. After achieving a 360-degree loop in the LA, the catheter is gradually withdrawn initially along the septal area anterior to the right PVs and ablation commenced at the inferior LA along the posterior mitral annulus from a site adjacent to the CS os progressing to the lateral LA (at the 4 o'clock position in the LAO projection). The endpoint is elimination of local endocardial electrograms bordering the mitral isthmus in an attempt to eliminate or prolong the CL of sharp potentials present within the CS (Fig. 11-48).[99] Ablation within the CS is started distally (at the 4 o'clock position in the LAO projection) and pursued along the CS up to the ostium by targeting local sharp potentials at individual sites or as a continuous drag. During AF, ablation within the CS is performed at all sites showing persistent or intermittent rapid activity, either continuous electrograms or discrete electrograms displaying CLs shorter than the CL measured in the LA appendage. Finally, additional RF applications are continued around the CS orifice from the RA. CS disconnection is confirmed by the dissociation or abolition of sharp potentials in its first 3 cm.[99]

Outcome

The success rate of AF elimination varies, depending on the site of ectopy. A higher success rate is noted when the triggering foci are located in the RA, including the SVC and crista terminalis. The LA posterior free wall has a higher recurrence rate because of anatomical limitation and multiple ectopic foci. The success rate of curing ligament of Marshall ectopy initiating AF is low when ablation is limited only to the endocardial area. A combined endocardial and epicardial approach to ablate ligament of Marshall ectopy has a higher success rate (60% to 70%).

OUTCOME OF CATHETER ABLATION OF ATRIAL FIBRILLATION

Success Rates

There are several hypothetical benefits of ablation of AF—improvement in quality of life, reduction of stroke risk, reduction in heart failure risk, and improved survival. However, the only benefit that has been documented so far is improvement of quality of life, and all other potential benefits have not been evaluated systematically. Therefore, the primary justification for an AF ablation procedure at this time is the presence of symptomatic AF.

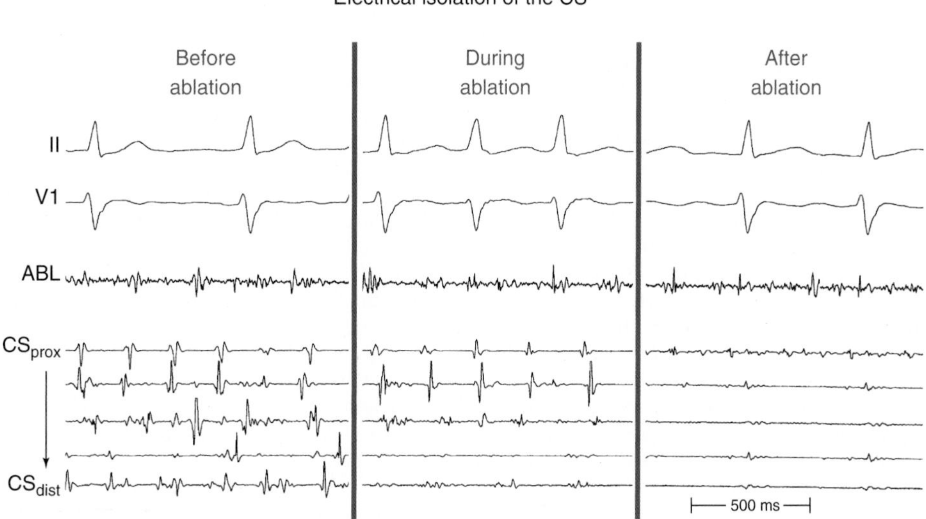

FIGURE 11–48 Electrical isolation of the coronary sinus (CS). Intracardiac recordings illustrating CS electrograms during atrial fibrillation (AF) before, during, and after successful electrical isolation of the CS. Following complete electrical isolation, the local sharp potentials within the CS are eliminated.

With time, operator experience, and greater consistency in the technique, AF ablation has proved itself to be a very effective treatment for AF. Reportedly, current techniques of RF catheter ablation can achieve a 60% to 90% improvement in selected patients with medically refractory AF, with similar success rates being reported by several different groups.[41,42,56,100] Although the cure rates are not 100%, they are two- to threefold better than anything achievable by antiarrhythmic medications.[100] Furthermore, the cures seem to be durable, given the long follow-up (almost 3 years) reported by some groups and the observation that most recurrences tend to occur early in the follow-up period, and rarely occur late after ablation.

In summary, the reported single-procedure efficacy of catheter ablation of AF in nonrandomized clinical trials has varied widely: 38% to 78% for paroxysmal AF (more than 60% in most series), and 22% to 45% for persistent AF (30% or lower in most series). The multiple-procedure success rate of catheter ablation reportedly is 54% to 80% for paroxysmal AF (more than 70% in most series), and 37% to 88% for permanent AF (more than 50% in most series).[45] Only a few randomized clinical trials have evaluated the efficacy of AF catheter ablation; each included 70 to 199 patients. These studies have revealed significant efficacy of catheter ablation compared with antiarrhythmic medications for AF treatment.[101-105]

Variations in success rate for similar procedural techniques for catheter ablation of AF reported by different centers may arise from a number of factors, including variation in study design, different patient population characteristics (age, cardiac disease, LA size), different types of AF (paroxysmal versus persistent versus permanent), differences in follow-up duration and strategy, and differences in definition of success (complete freedom from all atrial arrhythmias versus AF versus symptomatic arrhythmias, with or without antiarrhythmic agents).

Reduction of symptomatic episodes postablation may arise from a placebo effect or autonomic denervation, and exclusive reliance on patient reporting of symptomatic recurrences as the sole endpoint for determination of efficacy may contribute significantly to the variations in clinical outcome reported by different centers. Inclusion or exclusion of early recurrences of AF as procedural failures (blanking period) may also account for the different reported success rates. It is recognized that a transient increase in atrial arrhythmias may be seen in the early postprocedural period (presumably caused by subclinical pericarditis after catheter ablation) and, over time, a significant proportion of such patients become free of AF. Moreover, some studies used Kaplan-Meier curves of freedom from AF recurrence as opposed to incidence of occurrence during predetermined serial time windows on follow-up (e.g., 3, 6, and 12 months postprocedure; use of a Kaplan-Meier curve and time to first recurrence results in a lower success rate being reported). Time to first recurrence has the advantage of being relatively simple to apply and easy to compare with outcomes of antiarrhythmic drug therapy but is clinically less meaningful.

Beyond differences in follow-up and outcome analysis, variations in procedural techniques undoubtedly contribute to the wide range of outcomes reported from different centers. The vast majority of investigators continue to use RF energy as the primary ablation modality. However, there are substantial differences in procedural techniques currently used at different laboratories, including variations in electrode size (4 mm, 8 mm, and irrigated), duration of RF applications (5 to 60 seconds), power settings (30 to 70 W), and temperature limits (40° to 43°C for irrigated and 50° to 70°C for nonirrigated).

Consideration may also need to be given to the adoption of a subclassification of AF based on clinical criteria if the magnitude of therapeutic impact of catheter ablation on patients' quality of life is to be meaningfully assessed. For a patient who is transformed from a predominant pattern of highly symptomatic persistent AF, with occasional spontaneous terminations preablation, to a pattern of asymptomatic or symptomatic short-lived episodes of transient AF (lasting seconds or few minutes) postablation, the procedure could be deemed clinically successful. In contrast, a binary outcome analysis limited to whether a patient has any recurrence of AF at any time or is free of AF recurrence would classify the ablation as a failed procedure and any clinical benefit to the patient would not be recognized. These endpoints extend to pharmacological therapy.

Recurrence of Atrial Fibrillation

Recurrences of AF are common, observed in up to 45% of patients within the first 3 months following catheter ablation, regardless of the ablation technique.[106] The incidence of recurrent AF seems to be higher in patients with persistent AF (47%) as compared with paroxysmal AF (33%), in patients older than 65 years (48%) versus patients younger than 65 years (28%), and in patients with structural heart disease (47% to 74%) versus patients without structural heart disease (29 % to 50%).[45] The incidence of AF recurrences increases with increasing follow-up duration and intensity. Reliance on perception of AF by patients results in an underestimation of recurrence of the arrhythmia. To obtain reliable information about the success of AF ablation, repeated ambulatory monitoring with automatic detection of arrhythmias seems to be necessary.

The mechanism of early postablation transient AF is unclear but seems to be different from that of the patient's clinical arrhythmia; it may be related to a transient inflammatory response to RF thermal injury and/or pericarditis, and a delayed therapeutic effect of RF ablation likely attributable to lesion growth or maturation. Additionally, an inflammatory response or autonomic nerve activation that develops after thermal injury and transiently aggravates the arrhythmogenic activity of the PVs may contribute to an early recurrence of AF.

Administration of antiarrhythmic drug therapy to patients who undergo catheter ablation for AF does not seem to lower the rate of AF early recurrences, although it may increase the proportion of patients with asymptomatic AF episodes. Therefore, continuation of antiarrhythmic drug therapy following AF ablation with a view to prevent arrhythmia recurrences, seems unnecessary.[45] Nevertheless, because early recurrences of AF are common and do not necessarily predict long-term recurrences, some operators choose to treat all patients with suppressive antiarrhythmic drugs during the first 1 to 3 months following ablation. Typically, a class IC agent, sotalol, dofetilide, or amiodarone, is used. In patients discharged on antiarrhythmic drugs therapy, such therapy is discontinued if no recurrence of AF is observed after 1 to 3 months.

In patients discharged without antiarrhythmic drug therapy who develop recurrent AF, antiarrhythmic drug therapy is initiated unless the patient is satisfied with the extent of symptomatic improvement or elects to undergo a repeat ablation procedure. Catheter ablation of AF can be partially effective and allow a patient with AF that was previously refractory to antiarrhythmic drug therapy to become drug-responsive. Therefore, if AF recurs following discontinuation of antiarrhythmic medications, it is common practice to reinitiate the antiarrhythmic drug. Many patients with satisfactory control of AF with drugs prefer to continue antiarrhythmic drug therapy, rather than undergo a repeat ablation procedure, in which case drug therapy is an acceptable long-term management strategy. However, in many patients it is desirable to eliminate all arrhythmias and possibly eliminate antiarrhythmic drug therapy; reablation may be considered in case of AF recurrence following the initial procedure.

Although early recurrence of AF carries an independent risk for ablation failure, its occurrence should not prompt immediate reablation attempts because many patients experiencing this, even within the first months postablation, will not have any further arrhythmias during long-term follow-up. Repeat ablation procedures should be deferred for at least 3 months following the initial procedure, except in patients with poorly tolerated atrial arrhythmias refractory to medical therapy.[45] In general, recurrences of AF or AT after an initial AF ablation procedure lead to a reablation procedure in 20% to 40% of patients.

Beyond the early postablation period, recurrent AF following ostial segmental or circumferential antral PV isolation is predominantly caused by PV ectopy originating from previously isolated PVs rather than non-PV foci. Recurrence of PV-LA conduction is almost universal (more than 80%) in these patients. In contrast, most patients with a drug-free cure show no recovery of PV-LA conduction; substantial delay in PV-LA conduction is seen in patients able to maintain sinus rhythm on antiarrhythmic medication after ablation and in the minority of patients with drug-free cure who have recurrent PV-LA conduction in a single PV. Reisolation of the PVs is recommended in these patients; however, additional linear LA ablation, substrate modification, or targeting non-PV foci should also be considered.

The incidence of very late AF recurrences after long-lasting (longer than 12 months) arrhythmia-free intervals following catheter ablation is approximately 4% to 10%.[107] Such AF appears still to be triggered by foci from reconnected PVs in most cases; however, non-PV triggers may play a more dominant role in AF initiation in this setting. Most studies have reported that patients who fail an initial attempt at ablation and undergo a repeat ablation procedure demonstrate recurrent conduction in previously isolated PVs rather than new arrhythmogenic foci from nontargeted PVs or outside the PVs. In patients with AF caused by reconduction from the PVs, reisolation of the PV is frequently sufficient. Other patients may require targeting non-PV triggers or ablation strategies directed at the AF substrate, including additional linear ablation lesions or ablation of complex fractionated atrial electrograms.

Impact on Cardiac Structure and Function

Recovery of atrial mechanical function is a major goal in the treatment of AF; however, the impact of catheter ablation of AF on LA transport function is still under investigation. Several studies have demonstrated a 10% to 20% decrease in the dimensions of the LA following AF ablation, an observation consistent with reverse modeling, but which may also be secondary to scar formation induced by RF ablation.[108] On the other hand, extensive catheter ablation of atrial tissue replaces myocardium with scar and prolongs intraatrial conduction, which can potentially result in asynchronized contraction of the LA, possibly attenuating atrial contractile performances. Furthermore, in patients in whom the latest activity in the LA occurred after the QRS, LA contribution to LV filling is smaller because of closure of the mitral valve before completion of LA contraction. It is likely that the smaller the surface area occupied by scar tissue, the greater the probable benefit for atrial contractile function. Further refinement of techniques to identify sites crucial for maintenance of AF or subsequent AT on an individual basis is therefore necessary to minimize the extent of LA injury and to maximize the mechanical benefit of catheter ablation therapy for AF. Nevertheless, restoration of sinus rhythm is expected to improve atrial function as compared with AF.[108]

In patients with heart failure and LV ejection fraction lower than 45%, AF ablation was shown to produce significant improvement in LV function, LV dimensions, exercise capacity, symptoms, and quality of life. However, larger studies are needed to determine exactly which component of this improvement in LV function results from improvement in rate control as compared with restoration of sinus rhythm per se.

COMPLICATIONS OF CATHETER ABLATION OF ATRIAL FIBRILLATION

Catheter ablation of AF is one of the most complex interventional EP procedures, and the risk associated with such a procedure is higher than for the ablation of most other arrhythmias. Complications include vascular complications secondary to venous access, cardiac perforation, valvular injury, embolic stroke or systemic embolism, esophageal injury, PV stenosis, and proarrhythmia resulting from reentrant tachycardias arising from incomplete ablative lesions.

In a report of pooled data from 63 clinical studies on AF ablation in 3339 patients between 1994 and 2003, cerebrovascular events occurred in an average of 1% of patients, manifest PV stenosis occurred in 0.9%, and atrial macroreentrant tachycardia occurred in 29%. Recent reports from several groups using ablation of all four PVs outside the tubular portion indicated that transient ischemic attacks occurred in an average of 0.4% of cases, permanent stroke in 0.1%, severe (more than 70%) PV stenosis in 0.3%, moderate (40% to 70%) PV stenosis in 1.3%, cardiac tamponade in 0.5%, and severe vascular access complication in 0.3%.[41,42,56,100]

In a recent multicenter prospective study in an unselected population of 1011 patients undergoing AF catheter ablation (primarily PV isolation), the cumulative complication rate was 3.9%: hemorrhagic complications (cardiac tamponade, pericardial effusion) occurred in 1.4%; peripheral vascular complications in 1.2%; cerebral embolic events in 0.5%; and PV stenosis in 0.4%. Among several clinical and procedural variables, only the presence of coronary artery disease correlated with the occurrence of hemorrhagic events.[109]

Pulmonary Vein Stenosis

Incidence. PV stenosis is one of the most serious complications and has been reported with a wide range of incidence (0% to 42%), mainly because of different ablation sites (left atrial, antral, and ostial ablation) and differing methodology for estimating postablation ostia.[18,42,83] The severity of PV stenosis is generally categorized as mild (lower than 50%), moderate (50% to 70%), or severe (more than 70%). When moderate and mild lesions are included, the overall rate is as high as 15.5% (Fig. 11-49). However, the rate of severe PV stenosis has fallen to as low 1.0 % to 1.4% with increasing experience and improvements in technique, such as performing ablation outside the PVs and the use of ICE. Late progression of PV stenosis to severe stenosis or even complete occlusion can occur in up to 27% of patients (Fig. 11-50), particularly in the smaller PVs.

Circumferential LA ablation, with ablation limited to atrial tissue outside the PV orifice, seems to have less rates

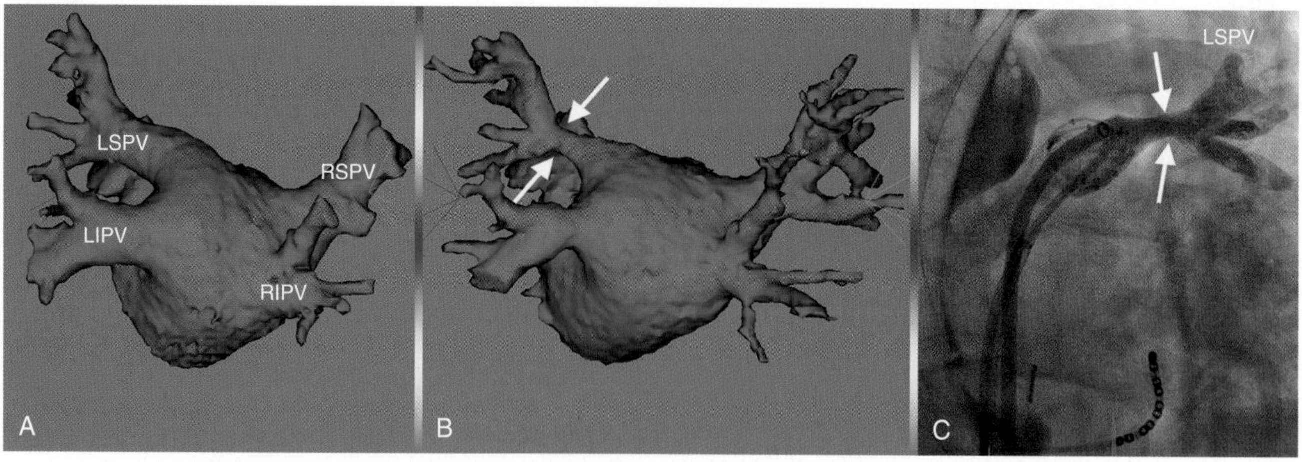

FIGURE 11–49 Pulmonary vein (PV) stenosis. **A,** CT image of the left atrium (LA) and PVs at baseline before segmental ostial PV isolation. **B,** CT image 3 months after the ablation procedure showing moderate stenosis of the left superior PV (arrows), and mild stenosis of the left inferior PV. **C,** Angiogram (left anterior oblique view) of the left superior PV (LSPV) showing moderate degree of stenosis (arrows).

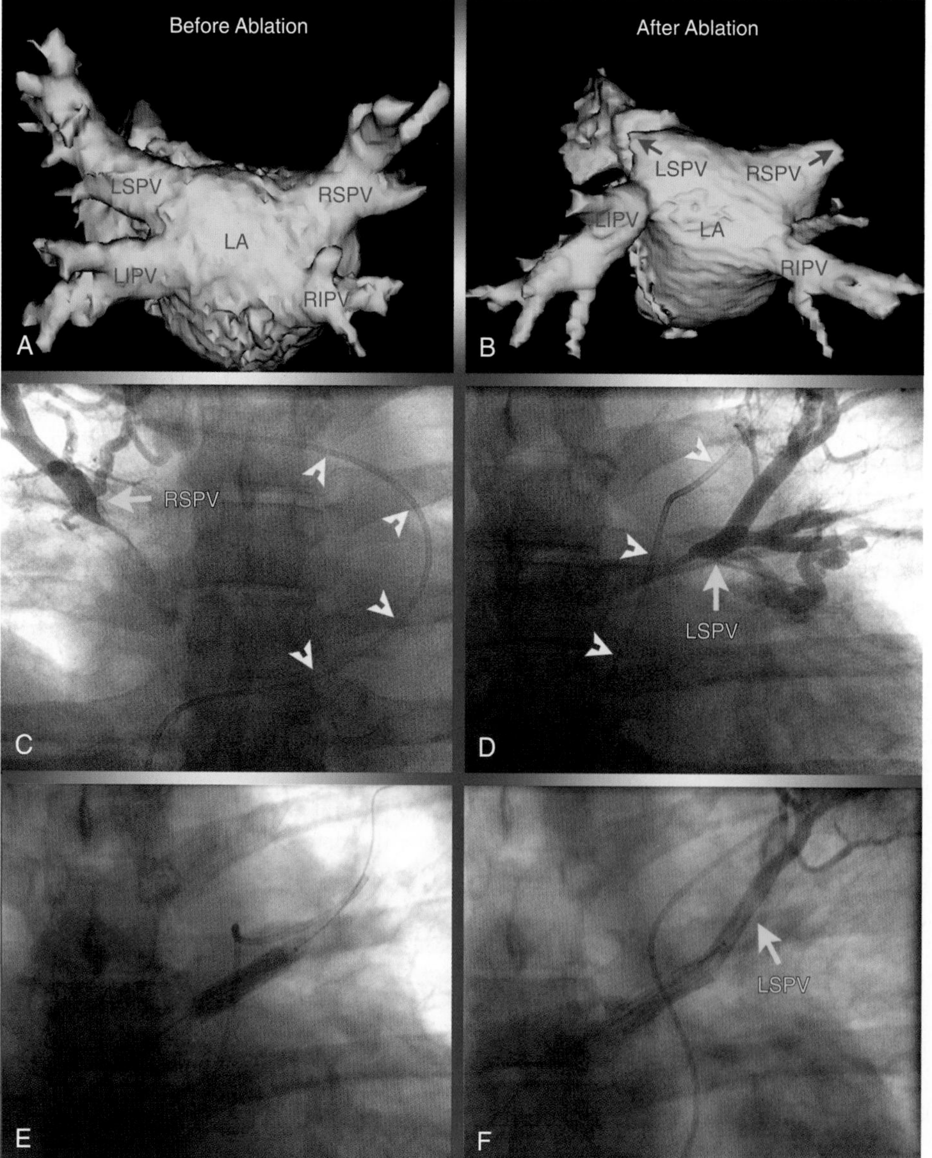

FIGURE 11–50 Pulmonary vein (PV) occlusion. **Upper panel,** CT image of the left atrium (LA) and PVs at baseline before segmental ostial PV isolation **(A)** and 5 months after ablation **(B)**. Following ablation complete occlusion of both superior PVs is observed. **Middle panel,** Fluoroscopic (anteroposterior) views during angiography of the right superior PV (RSPV) **(C)** and left superior PV (LSPV) **(D)** showing severe stenosis-occlusion of both PVs at the ostia. PV angiography is performed with contrast injection via a catheter positioned in the pulmonary artery (arrowheads). **Lower panel,** Fluoroscopic (anteroposterior) views during stenting of the LSPV. **E,** Angioplasty balloon is inflated for stent deployment in the LSPV. **F,** Angiogram of the left superior PV following stenting. LIPV = left inferior PV; RIPV = right inferior PV.

of PV stenosis, whereas focal ablation inside the PV has a higher risk. Moreover, with PV isolation techniques, the use of an individual encircling lesion set that requires RF ablation between the ipsilateral PVs carries a higher risk of PV stenosis.[43] With the focal ablation approach, PV stenosis rate can occur in up to 33% to 42%. Although this figure represents an overestimation of the problem because increased TEE flow velocity was used to establish the diagnosis, it remains a major concern. With PV isolation techniques, the incidence of severe PV stenosis is approximately 1% to 5%. MR and spiral CT scanning have shown that although current PV isolation techniques are associated with minimal reduction of the PV ostial diameter, stenoses exceeding 50% may occur in up to 18% of cases, whereas very severe stenoses (more than 90%) are found in up to 2% of cases. Following circumferential LA ablation, the prevalence of PV stenosis likely ranges between 2% and 7%. In one report, a detectable reduction in PV diameter was present in 38% of PVs; moderate and severe PV stenoses were observed in 3.2% and 0.6% of PVs, respectively.[110]

Stenosis seems to be more common in the left-sided PVs. Delivery of energy inside the PV during ablation, although undesirable, is more likely in the left PVs because the ablation catheter moves easily into them when patients breathe.

Mechanism. The mechanism of the development of PV stenosis remains unclear. Acute reduction of PV diameter (by approximately 30%) has been demonstrated during ablation. It was initially speculated that these changes are caused by edema and spasm. Thermal injury, induced by RF, has recently been shown to produce calcium-mediated irreversible tissue contracture occurring with the production of most if not all RF lesions, and therefore almost certainly contributes to stenosis. It is well known that thermal injury produces denaturation of extracellular proteins, especially collagen. Thermally induced collagen shrinkage has been well documented in animal and human studies. When near-circumferential lesions are produced within the tubular confines of the PVs, the consequences can be easily demonstrated as PV contracture. Thus, PV stenosis likely results from a combination of endothelial disruption with platelet activation and later neointimal proliferation, reversible edema, collagen denaturation, and shrinkage and thermal contracture. The occurrence and degree of PV stenosis correlate with the amount of energy delivered and lesion extension. The high incidence of mild PV stenosis likely reflects PV reverse remodeling rather than pathological PV stenosis. This hypothesis is based on the observation that all the mild PV stenoses were concentric rather than eccentric.

When severe stenosis or occlusion of a PV develops suddenly, gradual decline and then cessation of the arterial flow to the affected lung segment is observed. This is caused by a decline in the arteriovenous gradient as well as compression by the developing tissue edema. As a consequence, the involved alveoli are affected by the resulting ischemia and surrounding edema, leading to atelectasis, infarction, or susceptibility to infections. With the resulting alterations in pulmonary hemodynamics, redistribution of blood flow occurs with the opening of vascular channels or neovascularization in which tissue hypoxia is known to play a role. Hence, the venous drainage of the affected segment becomes mainly dependent on the ipsilateral veins draining the healthy lobes. If the ipsilateral vein(s) is also stenosed, the impedance to the pulmonary flow increases, adding to the hemodynamic burden and the resulting lung pathology.[111]

Clinical Presentation. PV stenosis after ablation is frequently asymptomatic, especially when a mild or moderate degree of PV stenosis is present or a single vein is involved. Severe PV stenosis can be associated with various respiratory symptoms that frequently mimic more common lung diseases, such as asthma, pneumonia, lung cancer, and pulmonary embolism. A high degree of suspicion is necessary to avoid performing misleading diagnostic procedures and to allow proper and prompt management. The onset of symptoms is usually several months after ablation. The initial manifestation is generally dyspnea on exertion, which typically evolves over the course of 1 to 3 months. Persistent cough is a common symptom. Pleuritic chest pain is a late symptom, and hemoptysis is uncommon. Both pleuritic chest pain and hemoptysis are likely related to complete vessel or branch occlusion.

It seems that symptom severity is related not only to the degree of stenosis but also to the number of PVs with stenosis. Symptoms may improve spontaneously over time in a significant percentage of patients. In one report, this improvement occurred in 50% of patients and was always related to improvement in the radiological abnormalities previously detected, although other hemodynamic compensatory mechanisms (e.g., development of collaterals) may also play a role.[110]

Detection. To date, it remains unclear which is the best and most cost-effective noninvasive modality for detecting PV stenosis after ablation. TEE and/or CT scanning are most commonly used; however, no single imaging modality has been able to assess all relevant aspects of PV stenosis. Therefore, complementary methods are used (see Fig. 11-49).[110] Routine follow-up CT or MR imaging for detection of asymptomatic PV stenosis postablation of AF is not mandatory, and it is unknown whether early diagnosis and treatment of asymptomatic PV stenosis provide any long-term advantage to the patient. Nevertheless, it is recommended that follow-up PV imaging be performed to screen for PV stenosis during the initial experience of an AF ablation technique for quality control purposes.[45]

Spiral CT and MR imaging of the PVs are readily available and can reveal the correct diagnosis; they are probably the most helpful in identifying the location and extent of the stenosis (see Fig. 11-49). However, the sensitivity and specificity of these imaging modalities need to be studied further.[110]

Although TEE is useful for providing a good view of the superior PVs, imaging of the right and left inferior PVs is inconsistent. On TEE, PV stenosis is usually indicated by an increased maximum PV Doppler flow velocity or by the presence of turbulence and deformity of the flow signal, as defined by a minimal flow between systolic and diastolic peak flow of 60% of the mean of both peaks.[110] ICE allows straightforward imaging of all PVs and provides a good view into the first 1 to 3 cm of the vein. Color flow contrast imaging is also useful for identifying the location of the orifice of the most tightly stenotic vessels.[110]

Blood gas assessment and pulmonary function testing do not seem to be useful as screening measures for early PV stenosis. Radiographic findings in PV stenosis are nonspecific. Chest radiography often reveals parenchymal consolidation and/or pleural effusion. V/Q scanning can be helpful for establishing the pathophysiology of the stenosis and its progression.[110] In the presence of significant PV stenosis, perfusion abnormalities are usually marked and appear similar to the changes seen in pulmonary embolism.

Prevention. The best way to manage PV stenosis is to avoid it. PV stenosis is independently related to RF lesion location, size, and distribution, and to baseline PV diameter.[110] The prevalence of this complication has decreased because of various factors, including abandonment of in-vein ablation at the site of the AF focus, limiting ablation to the extraostial portion of the PV or PV antrum, use of advanced imaging techniques to guide catheter placement and RF application, reduction in target ablation temperature and energy output, and increased operator experience.[110]

Although PV angiography, electroanatomical mapping, and impedance monitoring have been used in an attempt to avoid delivery of RF energy to the PV ostia or within the PVs, it is important to recognize that these techniques are imperfect. Electroanatomical mapping, for example, relies on the patient's position remaining unchanged throughout the procedure. With patient movement, the 3-D electroanatomical reconstruction of the LA and PVs may not accurately reflect true anatomy. Similarly, PV angiography is typically performed immediately prior to the start of PV ablation. Not only does this provide only a crude 2-D representation of true PV anatomy, but patient movement later in the procedure can also result in misalignment of the true PV anatomy with that reflected by the PV angiograms. Although impedance monitoring provides online feedback to the location of the ablation catheter relative to the PV, a recent study has found no significant difference in impedance between PV ostial and LA sites.[112] Therefore, it is possible for movement of the ablation catheter into the PV ostia to be missed.

Cryothermal ablation has unique characteristics that may prove to be desirable when lesions are required within the PV. Specifically, there is less endothelial disruption, maintenance of extracellular collagen matrix without collagen denaturation, and no collagen contracture related to thermal effects. These characteristics may translate into a reduction in PV stenosis as compared to RF ablation.

Some investigators have suggested that online assessment of PV flow velocities using ICE could serve as a surrogate for acute narrowing. Modest augmentation of acute PV flow velocities (approximately 10 to 50 cm/sec) can be anticipated across the ostia of isolated PVs; however, an increase in PV flow velocity to more than 100 cm/sec should raise concern and force a reassessment of ablation strategy, and flow velocities 158 cm/sec or higher (estimated pressure gradient ≥10 mm Hg) may be associated with an increased risk for significant late PV stenosis.[113] The value of these observations, however, requires further evaluation.

Treatment. Treatment options are currently limited, and restenosis after PV intervention has been described.[110] PV intervention (angioplasty or stenting) is recommended in affected patients because lesions can progress and eventually lead to total occlusion, precluding dilation and potentially resulting in hemodynamic compromise (see Fig. 11-50). ICE can facilitate accurate stent placement by reliably identifying the orifice of the tightly stenotic
11 vessels.

Unfortunately, both in-stent and in-segment restenoses can recur in up to 61% of patients.[110] Those within the body of the stent are likely caused by neointimal hyperplasia and fibrosis. Out-of-stent restenoses are usually observed at bifurcation points beyond the stent into the vessel, also suggesting the progression of PV pathology, despite stent placement. There is no experience to date with the use of sirolimus or paclitaxel drug-eluting stents in this situation, but such a high restenosis rate makes a strong case for the investigation of those devices and larger diameter stents.

Cardiac Tamponade

The incidence of cardiac perforation during ablation of the LA is relatively low but slightly higher than other catheter-based procedures. Previous studies reported the incidence of perforation with catheter-based interventions ranging from 0.8% in all procedures, 1.5% to 4.7% in valvuloplasty, 0.5% to 0.8% in angioplasty-atherectomy, 0.01% in diagnostic catheterization, 0.1% to 0.2% in EP studies to 0.5% to 4.0% for LA ablation.[39] The higher risk of pericardial tamponade during AF ablation (up to 6%) is likely caused by the common need for two or more transseptal punctures, extensive intracardiac catheter manipulation and ablation, and need for prolonged high-dose heparinization during the procedure.

Several factors can affect the risk of developing cardiac tamponade.[114] High RF power output may increase the risk of cardiac perforation. An audible pop associated with an abrupt rise in impedance is heard in many patients who develop tamponade. Popping occurs because of tissue boiling causing endocardial tissue rupture, and is increased by irrigated-tip ablation, high tissue-catheter interface flow, poor or unstable tissue contact, and high catheter tip temperature. Additionally, the atrial dome is susceptible to perforation injury during transitioning the catheter tip between the left and right superior PVs. Mechanical perforation can also occur from inadvertent movement of the catheter inside the LA appendage while it is being positioned during left superior PV or mitral isthmus ablation. In a recent report, pericardial effusion developed in 20% of patients undergoing antral PV isolation using an irrigated-tip ablation catheter at high power (50 W), but none when using lower power (35 W) or a standard 8-mm-tip catheter.[115]

Although the use of ICE may help limit the risk of cardiac perforation by guiding transseptal puncture and visualizing microbubbles in the LA during RF ablation, perforations remain relatively common. New anatomical approaches, such as linear LA ablation or ablation of sites of highly fractionated electrograms that maintain the catheter in the muscular atrium, may affect perforation rates. The thickness of the atrium averages 4 mm, but decreases from 3.7 to 2.5 mm at the venoatrial junction. The PV further decreases in thickness by 1 to 2 mm outside the PV orifice. However, a recent report has shown a higher risk of tamponade during linear LA ablation strategies as compared with PV isolation.[116]

Although most perforations occur in the LA, few (13.3% in one report) require surgical closure. Percutaneous pericardiocentesis effectively restores hemodynamic function. The LA dome seems to be especially susceptible to perforation that may not be responsive to conservative therapy. The atrial dome may be more susceptible to persistent bleeding because the pericardium is not closely adherent to the atrium, and a tight seal of these structures is difficult to achieve by applying negative pressure through the percutaneous pigtail catheter.

Early diagnosis of an effusion should favorably affect the time to evacuation and potentially the consequences of such a complication. Any chest pain that persists beyond the completion of an ablation lesion, especially if associated with hypotension and diaphoresis, should alert the operator to the possible development of pericardial effusion. Assessment of the cardiac silhouette fluoroscopically can provide the first clue, especially if a similar assessment was made at baseline. Furthermore, the use of an arterial line that provides continuous blood pressure monitoring can help detect early hemodynamic compromise. Two-dimensional echocardiography using the transthoracic or substernal approach (or both) is the most definitive method for confirming the development of pericardial effusion. The use of ICE can also facilitate the early detection of pericardial effusions before the emergence of tamponade physiology. Most of the pericardial space is not visualized from the RA imaging venue used to visualize the PVs, but several intrapericardial regions can be visualized with limited catheter rotation, thus allowing ongoing monitoring. Advancing the ICE catheter into the RV and rotating the transducer against the interventricular septum can readily identify pericardial effusions (Fig. 11-51).[41,61,62,113,114]

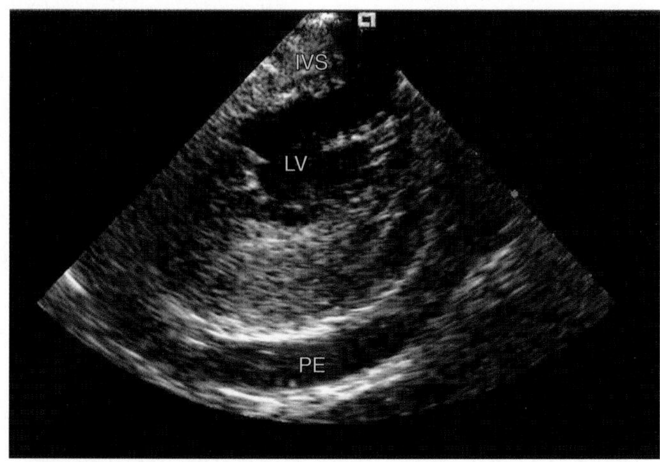

FIGURE 11–51 Intracardiac echocardiography (ICE) imaging of pericardial effusion. The phased-array ICE transducer is positioned in the right ventricle showing a short-axis view of the left ventricle (LV) and a moderate pericardial effusion (PE). IVS = interventricular septum.

Once recognized, the management of pericardial effusion is largely determined by its relative size and hemodynamic effect. Trivial pericardial effusion (3 mm or less), if recognized early during the AF ablation, should be monitored continuously but does not warrant termination of the procedure. For any pericardial effusion that exceeds 3 mm, the procedure should be terminated, and anticoagulation should be reversed and temporarily withheld (for 6 to 12 hours). In most cases, such conservative measures alone are sufficient. Pericardiocentesis typically is indicated for pericardial effusion more than 8 mm and/or smaller pericardial effusion manifesting signs of cardiac tamponade. In most of these patients, an indwelling catheter is generally required for a short interval after initial drainage to confirm that the bleeding has stopped and that no effusion is reaccumulating. In the event of persistence or rapid reaccumulation of the effusion, exploration by open heart surgery may be required, although this is extremely rare.[113]

Early pericarditis after cardiac perforation is common. In one report, 53.3% of such patients had persistent chest pain after effusion evacuation and removal of the pericardial catheter suggestive of pericardial inflammation.[117] All these patients were managed successfully with nonsteroidal anti-inflammatory agents. Subacute reaccumulation of pericardial fluid suggestive of postcardiac injury syndrome or inflammatory pericarditis can also occur, requiring repeat pericardiocentesis.

The occurrence of cardiac perforation is associated with short-term recurrent AF in most patients. These patients probably have a higher rate of arrhythmia recurrence because of pericardial inflammation, but in most patients this appears to be transient. Most patients with completed ablations have favorable long-term rates of AF elimination, although still lower than expected with uncomplicated cases.

Atrioesophageal Fistula

The development of an atrioesophageal fistula is emerging as a significant concern as an early-term potential complication of catheter ablation of AF.[118] Although atrioesophageal fistula formation is a rare complication (less than 0.25%) of RF ablation of AF, it is associated with a high mortality rate.

Mechanism of Fistula Formation. The esophagus is located at the center of the posterior mediastinum and is separated from the LA only by the pericardial sac (oblique sinus), which insinuates itself between the openings of the right and left PVs. The LA posterior wall thickness is 2 to 4 mm and the esophagus thickness is 2 to 3 mm in a cross section on the LA–esophageal area of contact. During RF catheter ablation, lesion depth, extension, and volume are related to the design of ablation electrode and RF power delivered. Theoretically, esophageal damage could occur, even during LA ablation using a regular 4-mm-tip catheter. However, cooled and large-tip ablation catheters induce extended lesions with a volume more than 400 mm^3. Thus, delivering high-power RF applications on the LA posterior wall between left and right PVs might deeply damage the esophagus, precipitating LA fistula formation.

The esophagus does not have a serosal layer and is fixed in the mediastinum, primarily in the pharynx and gastroesophageal junction. Its position within the mediastinum is dynamic, with its mobility caused by peristalsis. In fact, the esophagus often is mobile and shifts sideways by 2 cm or more in most patients undergoing catheter ablation for AF under conscious sedation. Additionally, the position of the esophagus in relation to the LA and PV demonstrates high variability. In many cases, the esophagus is very close to the ostia of the PVs and lies only a short distance from the LA wall. In most subjects (90%), the esophagus courses down beside the ostia of the left PVs with a mean distance of 10.1 mm to the left superior PV and 2.8 mm to the left inferior PV. Therefore, anatomical localization of the esophagus may be critical before or during AF ablation to prevent atrioesophageal fistula, especially as there is a need for transmural atrial lesions.

All reported cases of atrioesophageal fistula had in common attempts to perform deep RF lesions on the LA posterior wall. The precise mechanism of this complication has not yet been determined. Proposed potential mechanisms include direct thermal injury of the esophageal wall in immediate proximity to the posterior LA wall, thermal injury of the arterial blood supply to the esophagus, and mechanical injury to the esophagus during periprocedural TEE as a contributing or predisposing factor.

Clinical Presentation. The clinical course of atrioesophageal fistula formation varies in abruptness of presentation and timing (ranging from 2 days to 3 to 4 weeks), but mostly is manifest after patient discharge from the hospital. The presenting symptoms can include hematemesis, sepsis, or air embolization and stroke. The leading symptom of esophageal perforation is high fever or severe chest or epigastric pain. Fever is not necessarily present.

Leukocytosis is the earliest and most sensitive laboratory marker. Thoracic CT or MR imaging is the most valuable diagnostic examination. The dramatic neurological complications occur with a delay of at least a few hours after the first symptoms. Endoscopy is a diagnostic modality that should be avoided because insufflation of the esophagus with air can result in a devastating cerebrovascular accident and death secondary to a large air embolus. Immediate surgery (within a few hours after the first symptoms) may prevent neurological complications and could possibly result in a high survival rate, without residues. Delay of treatment seems to have devastating results.[45]

Prevention. Various strategies may be used to avoid the development of an atrioesophageal fistula. However, because of the rarity of this complication, it remains unproven whether the use of these approaches lowers or eliminates the risk of esophageal perforation or fistula formation, and the optimal technique has not yet been determined.

Newer imaging techniques have been used to visualize the anatomical relationship between the esophagus and LA during AF catheter ablation. Esophageal imaging is not part of the usual CT or MR angiography of the LA and PVs. Visualization of the esophagus can be achieved during the CT angiogram by the use of barium sulfate or Gastrografin and swallowing instructions, which help the contrast substance to lodge in the middle and distal esophagus rather than the stomach (Fig. 11-52). Visualization of the esophagus during CT or MR imaging can also be achieved by combining the barium sulfate paste with gadolinium diglutamate. The barium cream helps the gadolinium lodge in the esophagus.[119] However, this approach has several limitations. CT and MR imaging scans of the esophagus demand a previous session, and are not real-time images of the esophagus. Furthermore, the esophagus image is obtained with a barium sulfate paste, and the real dimensions of the esophagus depend on the volume of contrast media injected. During ablation the esophagus is empty and the real dimension and probably the exact location could be misinterpreted. Additionally, the esophagus is a mobile structure and static imaging of the esophagus provided by CT or MR may be an unreliable guide to the position of the esophagus during an ablation procedure. This may be particularly true for procedures performed under conscious sedation, when esophageal peristalsis is likely to occur.

The use of 3-D mapping systems that allow the integration of preacquired 3-D CT scans or MR images of LA, PVs, and esophagus, provides a new high-definition visualization tool that permits a rapid understanding of complex cardiac anatomical relationships. The location of the esophagus can also be tagged by the electroanatomical system (CARTO or NavX).[120] A nasogastric tube is inserted into the esophagus. The mapping catheter is coated with lubricant and passed down the nasogastric tube under fluoroscopy guidance. Alternatively, a special catheter (EsophaStar, Biosense Webster) is currently available for esophageal mapping combined with the CARTO system. Acquisition of the catheter tip location is made during pullback of the catheter out of the nasogastric tube; these data points are saved as a separate map in the electroanatomical mapping system. After LA chamber reconstruction is made, the esophageal map is displayed in 3-D space in relation to the LA reconstruction (see Fig. 11-52). The CARTO mapping system, in contrast to NavX, can only show one catheter at a time and hence cannot continuously display an esophageal catheter while the ablation procedure is being performed. However, the EsophaStar catheter can be left in the esophagus and used as a fluoroscopic guide to esophageal location during the ablation procedure (see Fig. 11-52).[120]

Phased-array ICE has been evaluated recently as a diagnostic tool for rapid real-time localization of the esophageal location in relation to the posterior LA wall (Fig. 11-53).[121,122] Location of the esophagus determined by ICE during the ablation procedure was found to correlate well with location determined by MR imaging before the procedure.[121]

Another strategy to limit the risk of esophageal injury is real-time imaging of the anatomical course of the esophagus during the ablation procedure by placement of a radiopaque esophageal monitoring probe or use of a viscous radiopaque contrast paste. Orally administered barium provides a simple, inexpensive, and safe way to keep track of the esophagus accurately during an ablation procedure (Fig. 11-54). In most patients, barium paste coats the wall of the esophagus, and residual barium often allows visualization of the esophagus for 1 to 2 hours after the initial barium

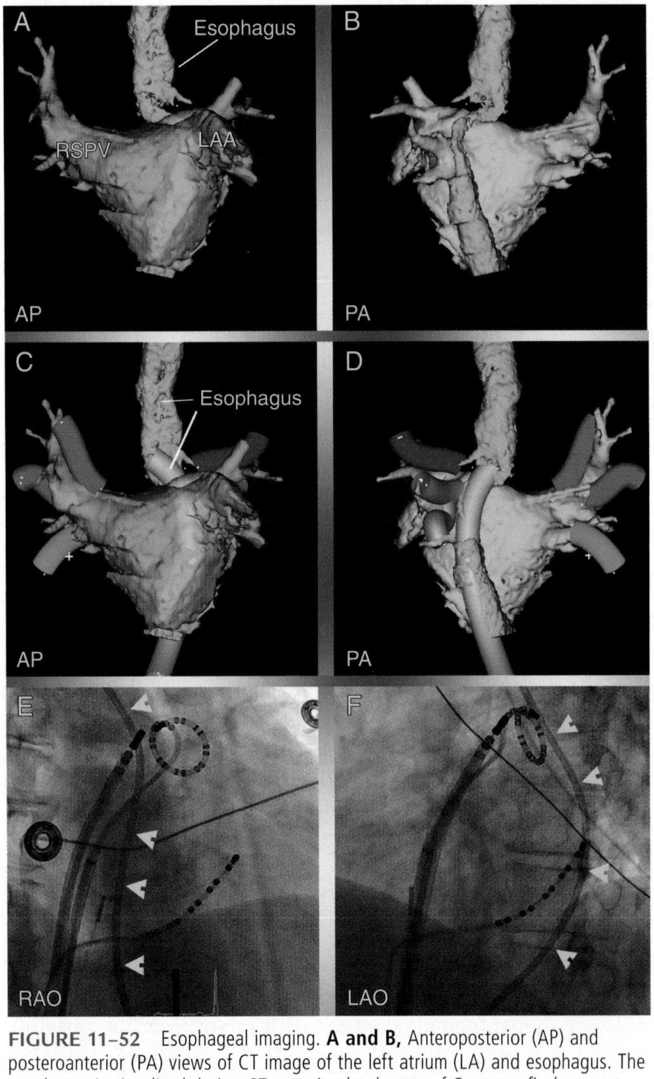

FIGURE 11–52 Esophageal imaging. **A and B,** Anteroposterior (AP) and posteroanterior (PA) views of CT image of the left atrium (LA) and esophagus. The esophagus is visualized during CT scanning by the use of Gastrografin (contrast medium). Note that the real dimensions of the midsegment are not very clear because of peristaltic movements and inadequate filling of the esophagus. **C and D,** AP and PA views of integrated CT image and electroanatomical mapping system (CARTO). The esophagus is tagged by passing the esophageal mapping catheter (EsophaStar) through the esophagus. Note that the position of the esophagus during the ablation procedure (as marked by the CARTO system) correlates well with the position on the preacquired CT image. Note the close proximity of the esophagus to the ostia of the left pulmonary veins (PVs). **E and F,** Fluoroscopic (right anterior oblique [RAO] and left anterior oblique [LAO]) views in the same patient with the esophageal mapping catheter (arrowheads) left in the esophagus during the ablation procedure to provide real-time guide of location of the esophagus.

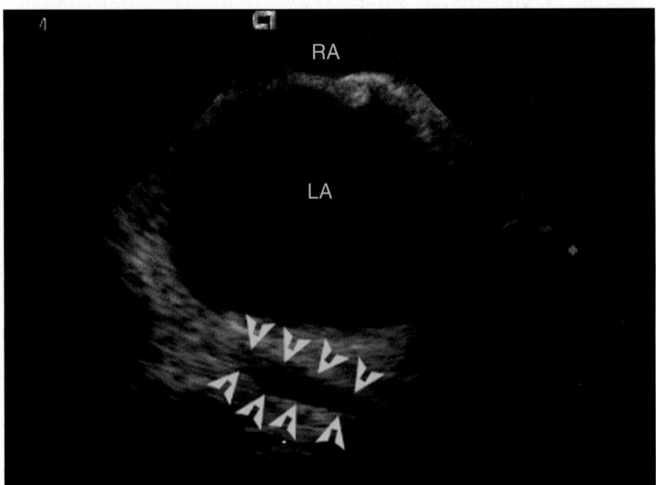

FIGURE 11–53 Intracardiac echocardiography (ICE) imaging of the esophagus. This phased-array ICE image with the transducer placed in the right atrium (RA) showing the esophagus (between arrowheads). Note that the LA posterior wall is contiguous to the esophagus.

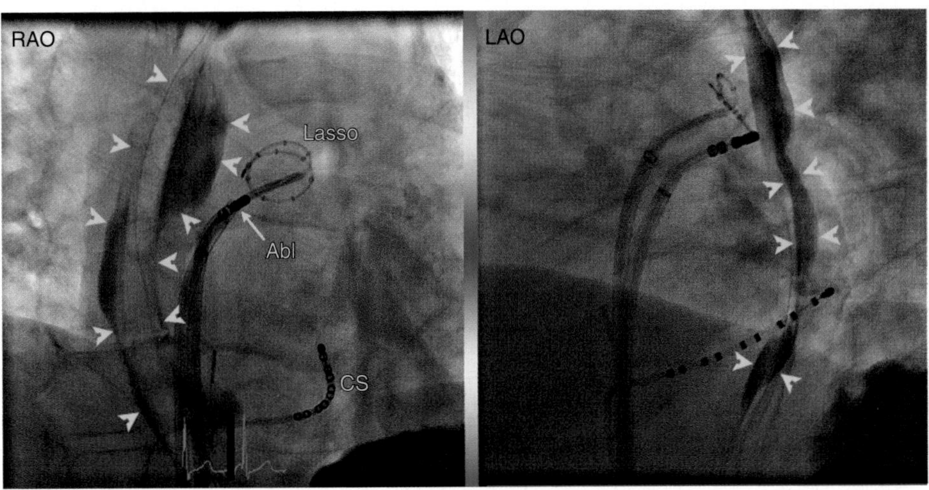

FIGURE 11–54 Esophageal imaging. Fluoroscopic (right anterior oblique [RAO] and left anterior oblique [LAO]) views of the esophagus during catheter ablation of atrial fibrillation. Barium paste was given to the patient just before initiation of sedation for real-time visualization of the esophagus (arrowheads) during the ablation procedure. The ring (Lasso) and ablation (Abl) catheters are positioned at the ostium of the left superior pulmonary vein.

swallow. However, to avoid the risk of aspiration, patients should receive little or no sedation before swallowing the barium.

The ablation procedure may also be performed with the patient under general anesthesia with orotracheal intubation and esophagography during the procedure. General anesthesia guarantees enough esophagus immobilization because the swallow reflex is abolished. Placement of an orogastric tube to allow esophagus localization is carried out before anticoagulation to avoid any risk of trauma and bleeding. At the end of the procedure, the contrast is totally removed. This technique allows visualization of the esophagus position in real time. The operator visualizes any eventual esophageal movement immediately.

Mechanical displacement of the esophagus to the contralateral side from the ablation catheter by an endoscope has also been suggested to reduce the risk of esophageal injury. However, the risk of esophageal perforation by the endoscope should be recognized. This strategy has not yet been successfully performed clinically.

Thermal monitoring of the esophagus during ablation can also be of value.[123] Measurement of esophageal temperature involves the placement of a monotherm temperature probe, which is advanced under fluoroscopy guidance to the lower third of the esophagus directly posterior to the LA. This technique requires general anesthesia to allow tolerability of the esophageal probe. The anatomical course, as visualized fluoroscopically, and baseline temperature in the esophageal lumen are recorded. During each RF lesion, simultaneous esophageal temperature, RF catheter temperature, power output, and lesion location are recorded. The position of the temperature probe is adjusted to the height of the ablation lesion.[123] The probe is used to identify the general location of the esophagus in relation to the posterior LA and PVs based on a 3°-4°C rise in temperature from baseline and assuming a linear degree of heating from the external esophagus relative to the lumen. However, this assumption does not take into account heating of the esophageal wall without recording a change in central luminal esophageal temperature. Similarly, because the esophagus is broad, the lateral position of the temperature probe may not align with the ablation electrode, and the operator may have a false impression of safety. Furthermore, the safety zone of temperature rise from baseline has not been validated. Other limitations of this approach include the potential risk of esophageal perforation caused by insertion of the probe itself. Additionally, the presence of the intraluminal esophageal temperature probe can increase the diameter of the esophagus and increase its contact with the posterior LA wall; this potential risk may be somewhat mitigated by the use of smaller, more flexible temperature monitoring probes.

Modification of RF application parameters at sites close to the esophagus is the most widely used strategy to avoid atrioesophageal fistula formation. Limitation of power and duration of RF applications, particularly in the posterior LA, even if a significant reduction in bipolar electrogram amplitude is not recorded, may be the most important safety consideration at present for the avoidance of fistula formation. Although no data exist on which to make specific recommendations, there is widespread agreement that prolonged RF applications in the posterior LA are to be avoided and that low power settings should be used. When RF energy is to be applied close to the esophagus, the RF power is typically reduced to 20 to 30 W and 55°C for no more than 20 seconds.[118] Additionally, using light conscious sedation during the procedure can allow the use of pain as an assay for potential esophageal injury; if significant or sharp pain occurs during energy delivery, RF application should be interrupted at that site and the catheter moved. Also, direct perpendicular orientation of the ablating electrode and forward pressure against the posterior LA wall should be avoided, particularly if an 8-mm or irrigated electrode is used. Additionally, inclusion of a linear lesion connecting the PV encirclements in the posterior LA wall is no longer advised. If such a connection is thought to be clinically necessary, it should be performed superiorly in the dome of the LA instead of the posterior wall.[118] Lastly, open irrigation RF ablation may be associated with less risk of esophageal injury compared with standard RF ablation using an 8-mm-tip catheter.

Left Atrial Tachyarrhythmias

LA tachycardia or flutter is a known complication of surgical and catheter-based therapies of AF. Originally reported in association with LA scar following mitral valve or maze surgical procedures, several reports have demonstrated LA flutter occurring after linear LA ablation and circumferential and segmental PV isolation, with an incidence ranging between 2% and 31%. The incidence seems to be lower following segmental ostial PV isolation than circumferential PV isolation or linear LA ablation.[42,78,124] Targeting complex fractionated electrograms without linear lesions or PV isolation is associated with a moderate risk (8.3%) for postablation ATs.

LA tachycardias tend to occur at variable time intervals after AF ablation procedures. Early recurrence of AF or AFL after ablation procedures is a common finding after surgical and catheter-based ablation, and does not necessarily portend long-term procedural failure.[106] After catheter-based AF ablation, AFL or focal AT may develop during the procedure or up to 1 year after the procedure, but the most common timing appears to be 1 to 2 months later.[125] This time course suggests that healing of ablation lines may contribute to the substrate for atrial reentry. These tachycardias can be problematic because they frequently are incessant and associated with rapid ventricular rates, and are more likely to require electrical cardioversion when compared with episodes of AF occurring prior to ablation. Although typical AFL should be considered in the differential diagnosis of regular tachycardias observed following AF ablation, most of these arrhythmias arise from the LA.

The three predominant catheter-based techniques for AF ablation appear to be associated with different rates and types of postprocedure atrial tachyarrhythmias. Segmental ostial PV isolation is associated with a lower incidence of atrial tachyarrhythmias (less than 5%).[42,78,124] When they do occur, these arrhythmias tend to be focal ATs, often originating from ostial segments of reconnected PVs. Reisolation of the PV and ablation of non-PV foci are usually sufficient to treat this proarrhythmia. Macroreentrant LA flutter has been reported after segmental PV isolation, but this appears to be significantly less common. Most reentrant circuits use the ablated zone as a central obstacle, resulting in perimitral or peri-PV reentry, with the latter being more prevalent in patients with larger atria.

Circumferential antral PV isolation has also been complicated by LA tachyarrhythmias, and PV-LA conduction recovery is frequently a critical element in these arrhythmias. The area of recovery within an ablated region of the antrum may create a region of slow conduction and the substrate for reentry (Fig. 11-55). When this area is a critical limb of the AFL circuit, reisolation of the PVs by ablation within the antrum terminates the flutter. In some cases, it is also possible that the recovered PV conduction allows PV triggers to induce LA flutter, and the LA flutter circuits do not involve the antra. These patients may also benefit from PV reisolation and subsequent elimination of PV triggers.

Wide-area circumferential LA ablation is the AF ablation approach most frequently complicated by LA flutters, most commonly mitral annular flutter or macroreentry around PV ostia. The vast majority of those ATs are related to gaps in prior ablation lines, which implies that most postablation ATs are avoidable, either by limiting the amount of linear ablation or by confirming complete conduction block across

linear lesions (or both).[126] In one report, more than 30% of patients undergoing circumferential LA ablation developed sustained LA flutter, with a mean of 3.4 different tachycardias per patient.[38,125] The long linear lesions required in this approach to prevent AF also create new fixed obstacles to propagation, adjacent areas of block, and slow conduction, and eventual discontinuities represent ideal substrates for large reentrant circuits. In addition, broad encircling of the PVs can create protected isthmuses with adjacent anatomical structures in the LA, particularly the mitral valve at the mitral isthmus.[38]

Modification of the original circumferential LA ablation technique has involved the addition of linear ablation connecting the left inferior ablation line to the mitral annulus. Whereas some studies have demonstrated a reduction in the incidence of postprocedure LA tachycardias,[38] some actually have raised concern that the addition of linear lesions, if incomplete, could lead to an increased rather than decreased incidence of this problem.[38,100] Therefore, it is still unclear whether these additional ablation lines actually prevent or contribute to macroreentry, and further studies are needed to define their role in the ablation strategy. Focal AT also has been reported following circumferential LA ablation, but gap-related macroreentrant AT is more common. This proarrhythmic effect is likely because circumferential LA ablation prohibits fibrillatory conduction; therefore, even though there may be a focal PV driver, akin to the cause of recurrent AF after segmental PV isolation, the clinical arrhythmia manifests as LA flutter or focal AT.[38]

LA flutter is inducible in a large percentage (38%) of patients immediately after circumferential LA ablation for AF; however, such inducibility does not predict those patients who subsequently develop clinical episodes of LA flutter. Also, the lack of inducibility of such arrhythmias after ablation is not a good predictor of long-term clinical success. Even in patients who develop clinical LA flutter, the flutter usually resolves without the need for chronic medical therapy in approximately two thirds of patients by 4 months or more after ablation of AF. Only a minority of the total patient population (8%) required a second ablation procedure. Furthermore, when performing catheter ablation for AF, it is unadvisable to extend a lengthy procedure by targeting induced LA flutters by mapping and ablation.

There is currently no well-defined standard treatment strategy for LA flutters following AF ablation procedures, and treatment should be tailored to the potential arrhythmia mechanism. It is important to recognize that many of these arrhythmias are self-limited and resolve spontaneously in up to two thirds of patients within the first 3 to 6 months of follow-up. Therefore, efforts should be focused at suppressing these arrhythmias with antiarrhythmic medications or controlling the ventricular response with AVN blocking drugs. Despite the often more severe symptoms associated with these arrhythmias, ablation for LA flutters should be postponed for about 3 to 4 months after diagnosis.[45]

For LA flutters following PV isolation procedures, it has been shown that reisolation of the recovered PVs alone could be attempted to treat these arrhythmias. The septal aspect of ablation lines encircling the right PVs and the area anterior to the left superior PV are particularly vulnerable to recovery of conduction after circumferential PV isolation, predisposing patients to the development of LA tachycardia. Particular attention should be paid at these sites to ensure continuous transmural lesions. For focal ATs, ablation at the site of earliest activation often results in termination of the tachycardia. If the mechanism cannot be determined, reisolation of all reconnected PVs appears to be sufficient in most cases.

Mapping and ablation of LA flutters following circumferential LA ablation or circumferential PV isolation are frequently challenging. Detailed mapping with a high density of points is necessary to elucidate the mechanism of the arrhythmias. Current treatment of LA flutter primarily involves empirical linear lesions within the flutter circuit, often including a line between the mitral annulus and left inferior PV and a line between the superior PVs. However, when the macroreentrant circuit can be mapped, ablation lesions should be tailored to interrupt the path of the reentrant circuit (see Fig. 11-55). The mitral isthmus, LA roof, and septum account for 75% of the ablation target sites for macroreentrant ATs from the LA. Successful catheter ablation has been reported in approximately 85% of macroreentrant ATs arising in the LA in highly experienced laboratories; however, ablation of macroreentrant ATs occurring in the septal wall is challenging and less successful.[126]

Thromboembolism

The risk of thromboembolism associated with AF ablation is reported to be between 0% and 7%. In a worldwide report,

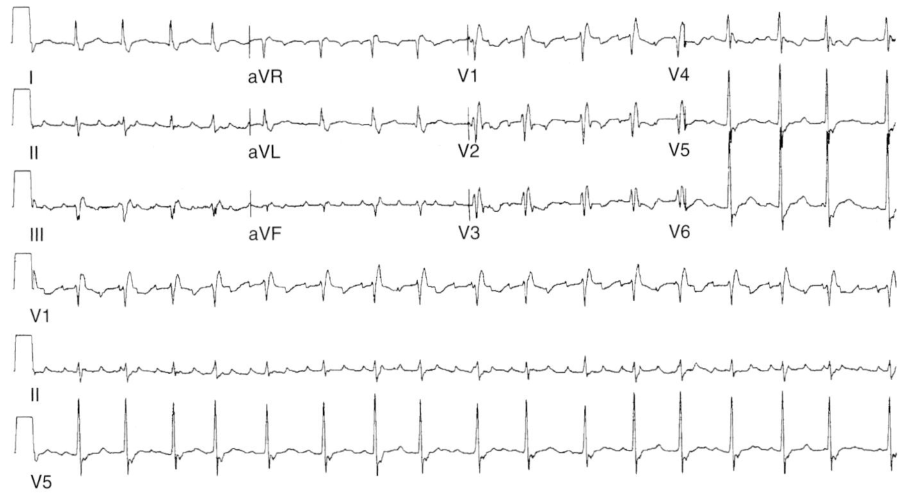

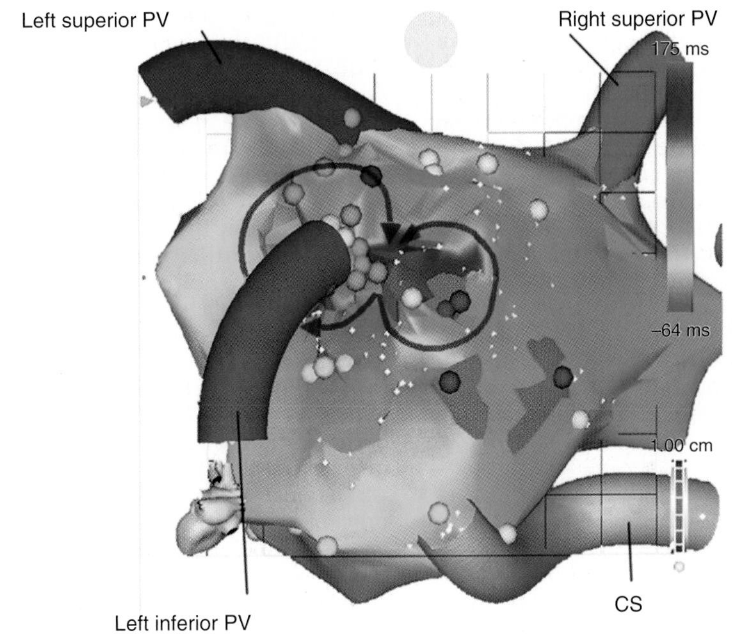

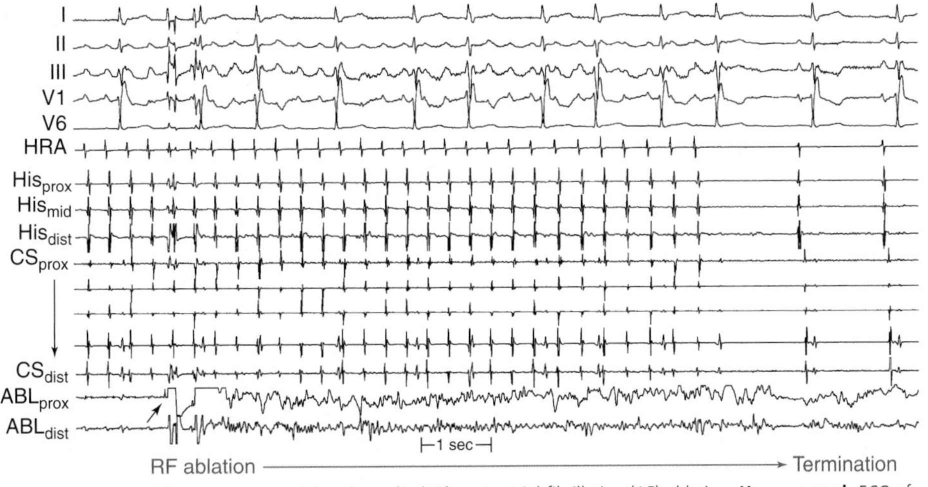

FIGURE 11–55 Macroreentrant atrial tachycardia (AT) post–atrial fibrillation (AF) ablation. **Upper panel,** ECG of incessant AT occurring months following circumferential antral PV isolation. **Middle panel,** Electroanatomical activation map (posterolateral view) of the same AT. Figure-of-8 reentry is seen involving the orifice of the left inferior pulmonary vein (PV) and scar tissue (gray patches) resulting from the prior ablation. **Lower panel,** Intracardiac recordings during the AT. A single RF application at the site of the diastolic potential terminates the AT within a few seconds after onset of power delivery.

the rate of stroke was about 0.25% and that of transient ischemic attacks was 0.66%.[127] Potential sources of emboli include thrombi adherent to catheters and sheaths, char formation at the tip of the ablation catheter or at the site of ablation, endocardial disruption from the ablation lesions, thrombi or air passing through a patent foramen ovale or transseptal access, air introduced through transseptal sheaths, and disruption of a preexistent LA thrombus.

Thromboembolic events typically occur within 24 hours of the ablation procedure, with the high-risk period extending for the first 2 weeks following ablation. Although silent cerebral thromboembolism has been reported, its incidence is unknown.

Prevention remains the best strategy in minimizing cerebrovascular events during AF ablation, and this may be achieved by the following: (1) aggressive anticoagulation, including early heparin administration (before transseptal puncture), followed by continuous infusion to maintain the ACT ≥300 seconds; (2) meticulous attention to sheath management, including constant infusion of heparinized saline and air filters; (3) minimizing char formation during lesion creation by regulating power delivery to prevent abrupt impedance rise; and (4) using ICE for early detection of intracardiac thrombi and accelerated bubble formation consistent with endocardial tissue disruption with RF application. Administration of large doses of protamine on completion of the ablation procedure to reverse heparin abruptly may promote thrombogenesis and warrants further evaluation to confirm its safety.[113] Whether ablation with irrigated-tip catheters or cryoablation can reduce stroke risk further remains to be determined. However, the nature of the procedure with prolonged left-sided catheterization and extensive LA ablation in patients predisposed to stroke precludes eliminating it entirely. Additionally, the reduction in thromboembolic events is counterbalanced by a still-high rate of hemorrhagic events—peripheral vascular complications in 1.3% of cases and pericardial effusion in 0.8%.

Air Embolism

The most common cause of air embolism is introduction of air into the transseptal sheath. Although this may be introduced through the infusion line, it can also occur with suction when catheters are removed. Careful sheath management, including constant infusion of heparinized saline and air filters, should be observed. Whenever catheters are removed, they need to be withdrawn slowly to minimize suction effects and the fluid column within the sheath

should be aspirated simultaneously. The sheath should then be aspirated and irrigated to ascertain that neither air nor blood has collected in the sheath.[45]

Arterial air emboli can distribute to almost any organ, but have devastating clinical sequelae when they enter the end arteries. This can lead to the hypoxic manifestations of myocardial injury and cerebrovascular accidents. A common presentation of air embolism during AF ablation is acute inferior ischemia and/or heart block. This reflects preferential downstream migration of air emboli into the right coronary artery. Air embolism to the cerebral vasculature can be associated with altered mental status, seizures, and focal neurological signs. The central nervous system dysfunction is attributable to both mechanical obstruction of the arterioles and thrombotic-inflammatory responses of air-injured endothelium.

Routine diagnostic modalities to identify air embolism in the terminal arterial circulations lack sensitivity, and diagnosis is typically based on the appropriate clinical scenario, with possible air identified in the antecedent cardiac chambers. Prompt CT or MR scans obtained before the intravascular air is absorbed may show multiple serpiginous hypodensities representing air in the cerebral vasculature, with or without acute infarction.[128]

Therapy for air embolism includes intervention to prevent a recurrence of venous air entry, oxygen therapy for the hypoxia and reduction in the size of the air embolus by establishing a diffusion gradient, cardiopulmonary support in cases of circulatory collapse, and airway protection in comatose patients. Central venous catheter extraction of the residual air embolism if localized in the RA or RV has been described. When cerebral air embolism is suspected, it is important to maximize cerebral perfusion by the administration of fluids and supplemental oxygen, which increases the rate of nitrogen absorption from air bubbles. Treatment with hyperbaric oxygen may reverse the condition and minimize endothelial thromboinflammatory injury if started within a few hours.[45]

Phrenic Nerve Injury

Phrenic nerve damage has been a long-recognized complication during ablation in the RA or LA. Injury to the right phrenic nerve has typically been reported during sinus node modification or ablation of tachycardias on the RA free wall. More recently, right phrenic nerve injury has been described during ablation in and around the right superior PV and electrical isolation of the SVC. The reported incidence of phrenic nerve injury secondary to AF ablation varies from 0% to 0.48%. Although it is much less common, left phrenic nerve injury can also occur during RF delivery at the proximal LA appendage roof.

The intracardiac course of the right phrenic nerve, especially as it approximates the SVC and RA (and not infrequently the right superior PV), is the principal reason for susceptibility to nerve damage from endocardial ablation. Moreover, the atria and great thoracic veins are relatively thin-walled structures (as compared with the ventricle), which increases the possibility of thermal injury to neighboring structures during ablation when lesion depth exceeds myocardial thickness.

The use of a non-RF source of energy is unlikely to prevent this complication because phrenic nerve injury has been reported with ultrasound, laser, and cryotherapy. Furthermore, phrenic nerve injury occurs independently of the strategy of AF ablation used (PV isolation versus wide circumferential LA ablation).[129] Fortunately, phrenic nerve injury has been an infrequent complication of AF catheter ablation. Complete (66%) or partial (17%) recovery of diaphragmatic function was observed in most patients.[129]

Phrenic nerve injury can be asymptomatic in 31% of cases. The most frequent symptom is dyspnea, which is present in all symptomatic patients. Other symptoms or clinical findings are cough or hiccup during ablation and the development of postablation pneumonia or pleural effusion. In asymptomatic patients, the diagnosis is made on the routine chest x-ray (Fig. 11-56) with hemidiaphragm paresis or paralysis (hemidiaphragm elevation with paradoxical movement). There is no active treatment known to aid phrenic nerve healing.

Studies have indicated that transient phrenic nerve injury occurs early and uniformly before permanent injury. Therefore, in areas at high risk of phrenic nerve injury (inferoanterior part of right PV ostium, posteroseptal part of the SVC, and proximal LA appendage roof) that require ablation, high-output pacing should be performed before energy delivery. When diaphragmatic stimulation is observed, energy application at this site should be avoided. Early suspicion of phrenic nerve injury should be considered in the case of hiccup, cough, or decrease in diaphragmatic excursion during energy delivery. Early recognition of phrenic nerve injury during RF delivery allows the imme-

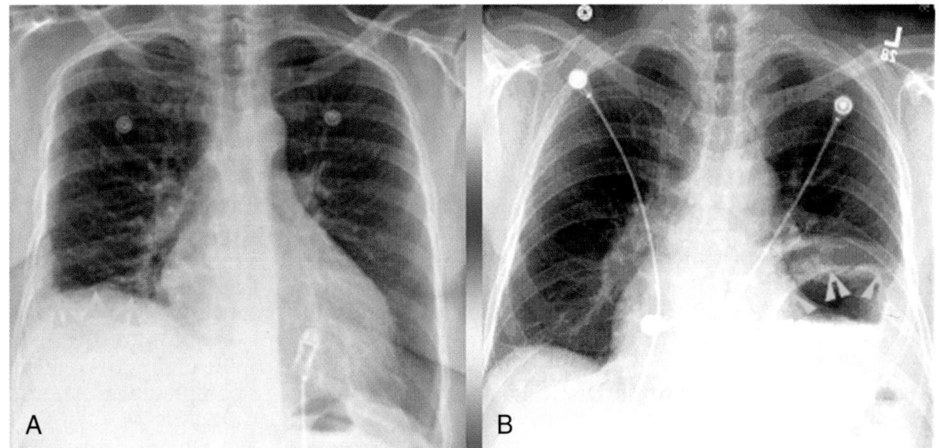

FIGURE 11–56 Chest X-ray (posteroanterior views) showing right hemidiaphragmatic paralysis (arrowheads) caused by right phrenic nerve injury **(A)**, and left hemidiaphragmatic paralysis caused by left phrenic nerve injury **(B)** during catheter ablation of atrial fibrillation.

diate interruption of the application prior to the onset of permanent injury, which is associated with the rapid recovery of phrenic nerve function.[129]

Catheter Entrapment in the Mitral Valve Apparatus

There are several reports of the ring catheter becoming entrapped in the mitral valve apparatus during AF ablation, resulting in valve injury that required open heart surgery and valve replacement.[113,130] The risk of this complication can be minimized by preventing anterior displacement of the ring catheter during the ablation. Catheter position can be monitored using a combination of orthogonal fluoroscopy (ensuring that the ring catheter remains behind the CS on the RAO view) and ICE, as well as paying close attention to the characteristics of the electrograms recorded on the catheter.

Catheters entangled in the valve apparatus may be difficult to free by clockwise and counterclockwise rotation of the shaft, especially after significant tugging has occurred. To prevent this, prior to pulling on the catheter, one may consider instead advancing the catheter toward the LV apex. Advancing the sheath over the catheter may facilitate the effort further and is also recommended so that the catheter can be withdrawn into the sheath and the whole assembly withdrawn to the LA.[113,130]

Forcible traction of the catheter may damage the valve and ultimately lead to mitral valve replacement. Therefore, when gentle manipulation and moderate traction are unsuccessful, removing the catheter by open heart surgery may be preferable.[130]

Radiation Exposure

Catheter ablation of AF is associated with markedly prolonged fluoroscopy duration (60 to 100 minutes of fluoroscopy exposure delivered to patients in both the RAO and LAO projections), which exceeds that of patients undergoing catheter ablation of AFL or AVNRT by approximately fourfold.[131] This finding most likely reflects two main factors. First, ablation of AF is far more complex compared with ablation of AFL and AVNRT, requiring single or double transseptal puncture and extensive mapping and ablation. Second, ablation of AF is a relatively new procedure.

With similar fluoroscopy durations in both projections, the radiation dose is higher in the LAO than in the RAO projection, primarily because of a longer attenuation path for the x-ray beam entering in the LAO projection. Increasing availability and familiarity with 3-D mapping systems should significantly reduce fluoroscopy time and the need for biplane fluoroscopy. The use of remote navigation systems also is likely to reduce fluoroscopy exposure to the patient and operator.

In EP procedures, the patient tissue receiving the greatest radiation dose is the skin area of the back at the entrance point of the x-ray beam, and skin injuries are well-recognized complications for catheter ablation procedures.[131] Acute radiation-induced skin injury ranges from erythema to skin necrosis. The threshold for transient erythema and epilation is 2 to 3 Gy. In one report, only 1 of 15 patients reached a peak skin dose of 2 Gy, despite prolonged fluoroscopy durations (up to 99 minutes).[131] This finding is striking and speaks to the effectiveness of the systems that use several technologies, such as last image hold, pulsed fluoroscopy, and additional filters to reduce radiation exposure. This also explains why radiation skin damage is an extremely rare complication of ablation procedures.

The estimated lifetime risk of a fatal malignancy after PV ablation using a modern low-frame pulsed fluoroscopy system is relatively low (0.15% for females and 0.21% for males in one report) and is higher than, although within the range of, previously reported risk to result from the ablation of standard types of supraventricular arrhythmias (0.03% to 0.26%).[131] It has been estimated that for every 60 minutes of fluoroscopy, the mean total lifetime excess risk of a fatal malignancy is 0.03% to 0.065%.

One study has found that patient body mass index is a more important determinant of the effective radiation dose than total fluoroscopy time, and obese patients receive more than twice the effective radiation dose of normal-weight patients during AF ablation procedures. Therefore, obesity needs to be considered in the risk-benefit ratio of AF ablation and should prompt further measures to reduce radiation exposure (e.g., nonfluoroscopic mapping systems).

RECOMMENDATIONS AND CONTROVERSIES

Curative ablation of AF has two mechanistic goals—elimination of all potential triggers that may initiate or perpetuate AF and substrate modification (i.e., the alteration of the conduction properties of the atria so that AF cannot be sustained, even when triggered).

Elimination of Triggers. The PVs are the predominant source of triggers and PV isolation is the usual procedure performed for symptomatic paroxysmal AF. Potential non-

PV triggers, such as the SVC and CS, can also be isolated at the same procedure if they are spontaneously active. Initial attempts were made to identify from which PV the triggers were arising and ablate the culprits only. It was then recognized, however, that AF may have multiple triggers, and many will be silent during the ablation procedure. Consequently, the current approach aims to ablate all four PVs. Two main techniques have been developed for complete PV electrical isolation: (1) segmental ostial ablation, which involves destroying the muscular connections that link the PVs to the LA; and (2) circumferential antral PV isolation, which involves creating a continuous line of conduction block in the atria that surrounds and completely encloses each of the PVs or in ipsilateral pairs.

Substrate Modification. The initial approach is ablating around the PVs (wide-area circumferential LA ablation), which excludes a large area of the LA that is then not available to support AF. PV isolation is not a goal for this approach. Further improvements have required a strategy closer to the surgical maze—that is, lines to connect the ipsilateral pairs of the PVs and a line to link the left PV to the mitral annulus, which can be described as the catheter maze. This approach was developed to help reduce the high incidence of macroreentrant AT postablation. A novel approach has been the ablation of all fractionated electrograms in the RA and LA, with the hypothesis being that these are consistent sites at which fibrillating wavefronts turn or split. By ablating these areas, the propagating random wavefronts are progressively restricted until the atria can no longer support AF.

Although the methodology of the technique of AF ablation has passed through many phases and modifications, currently there is much greater consistency.[100] Since the role of PVs in the initiation of AF was established, PV electrical isolation has become central to any AF ablation strategy, and the vast majority of centers performing AF ablation are empirically isolating all four PVs, without mapping or specific targeting of the trigger of the focus causing the arrhythmia. Furthermore, most groups are ablating outside the tubular portion of the PV (i.e., antral ablation as opposed to ostial ablation) to avoid the risk of PV stenosis and improve the efficacy of the procedure. The antrum blends into the posterior wall of the LA and, on the posterior wall, there is little space between adjacent antra. Therefore, to encompass as much of the PV structure as possible, ablation needs to be performed around the entire antrum, along the posterior LA wall. Although different groups may refer to ablation in this region by different names, such as LA catheter ablation, circumferential antral PV ablation, or extraostial isolation, the lesion sets produced by the procedures are all similar.

There is less consensus, however, about the distance from the PV ostia at which the optimal circumferential lesions should be placed. The greater the distance, the greater the number of applications and density of lesions required to achieve isolation, but the lower the likelihood of PV stenosis. Furthermore, the greater the distance from the ostia, the larger the area encircled and the greater the potential impact of the lesion set on atrial rotors and sites within the posterior LA, which may contribute to the maintenance of AF. However, it is clear that wide-area circumferential LA ablation minimizes the risk of PV stenosis but at the cost of a higher incidence of macroreentrant ATs.

The optimal method of catheter ablation for AF has been hotly debated. The therapeutic mechanisms of action and target substrates of catheter ablation for AF are now thought to be more complex than previously recognized. More recently, the net has widened substantially to include alternative or supplementary approaches. Several different approaches to catheter ablation of AF are emerging: (1) disruption of the substrate for perpetuating rotors in the antra of the PVs and the posterior LA using extensive or limited linear lesions; (2) targeted ablation of ganglionated autonomic plexi in the epicardial fat pads; and (3) disruption of putative dominant rotors in the left and right atria proper as recognized by high-frequency areas of short CL activity, those demonstrating a frequency gradient, or a source indicated by centrifugal activity.

A recent expert consensus statement[45] has recommended ablation strategies that target the PVs and/or PV antra as the cornerstone for most AF ablation procedures. If the PVs are targeted, complete electrical isolation should be the goal, and careful identification of the PV ostia is mandatory to avoid ablation within the PVs. If a focal trigger is identified outside the PVs, it should be targeted if possible. Furthermore, if additional linear ablation lesions are applied, line completeness should be verified by mapping or pacing maneuvers.

One strategy is to use a hybrid approach. A technique that combines the merits of these rival strategies is to perform wide-area circumferential LA ablation and check for PV isolation using a circular mapping catheter. Such a technique potentially attacks all the possible mechanisms of paroxysmal AF: PV triggers, microreentry in the PV antrum, and denervation of the parasympathetic inputs surrounding the PVs.

However, substrate modification is technically challenging, is associated with increased risk, and can be proarrhythmic. Therefore, it may not be advisable to use such an approach for all patients. A rational approach that targets a particular patient profile, rather than a unified strategy used for all patients, may be advisable. It is recognized that particular AF mechanisms may result in a particular clinical substrate and thus allow the procedure to be tailored so that, for example, in paroxysmal AF only isolation of triggers is attempted, whereas in persistent AF additional and more complex substrate modification may be performed. In addition, substrate modification may be reserved for patients with paroxysmal AF with clinical recurrence after PV isolation. Furthermore, inducibility of sustained AF following PV isolation may indicate the presence of a potential atrial substrate capable of maintaining AF and may identify a subgroup of patients in whom additional substrate modification may be required.[88] For patients with chronic AF, a stepwise ablation approach may be considered, starting with PV isolation, which is then followed by LA roof ablation, CS isolation, ablation of CFAEs, mitral isthmus ablation, and RA-SVC ablation in a stepwise fashion whereby each step is started if AF still persists after completion of earlier steps. It should be recognized, however, that despite the best efforts with various combinations of several ablation strategies, converting chronic AF to sinus rhythm solely by ablation may not occur in a large subset of patients. Hence, an endpoint of acute termination of chronic AF may not be practical. Moreover, whether acute termination of chronic AF by RF ablation is a predictor of long-term clinical efficacy remains to be evaluated.[108,132]

Determination of Candidates for Catheter Ablation

One of the difficulties with counseling patients regarding AF ablation is that published studies are difficult to compare and interpret because they vary in the proportion of patients with persistent or permanent AF, prevalence of structural heart disease, length of follow-up, how sinus rhythm is assessed, use of antiarrhythmic drugs, and need for repeat procedures.[100] Furthermore, studies often emerge from single centers with polarized views on the mechanisms of AF and the best technique of ablation. The reader should be aware of such bias; it is often easier to recommend to patients that they ask for the results of an individual center when they are assessed for AF ablation before they make a final decision as to how they wish to proceed.

The ideal candidate for catheter ablation of AF has symptomatic episodes of paroxysmal or persistent AF, has not responded to one or more class I or III antiarrhythmic drugs, does not have severe comorbid conditions or significant structural heart disease, is younger than 65 to 70 years, has an LA diameter less than 50 to 55 mm and, for those with chronic AF, has had AF for less than 5 years.[133] Catheter ablation of AF is likely to be of little or no benefit in patients with end-stage cardiomyopathy or massive enlargement of the LA (more than 6 cm), or who have severe mitral regurgitation or stenosis and are deemed inappropriate candidates for valvular intervention.[133]

The introduction into clinical practice of the various techniques described earlier has contributed to the expansion of inclusion criteria for catheter ablation of AF. Expanded indications at many centers now include patients with permanent AF and those with cardiomyopathy.[134,135] It is controversial whether patient preference to come off anticoagulation should be considered an indication for AF catheter ablation; however, it is important to recognize that there are still no randomized controlled data demonstrating that a patient's stroke risk is reduced by ablation. It is currently recommended to continue chronic anticoagulation with warfarin in all patients with a $CHADS_2$ score of 2 or higher, even those with successful catheter ablation procedure. Therefore, the patient's desire to eliminate the need for long-term anticoagulation by itself should not be considered an appropriate selection criterion.[45]

Complications of catheter ablation may have catastrophic outcomes in certain patients, including those with severe obstructive carotid artery disease, cardiomyopathy, aortic stenosis, nonrevascularized left main or three-vessel coronary artery disease, severe pulmonary arterial hypertension, or hypertrophic cardiomyopathy with severe LV outflow tract obstruction. Another relative contraindication may be a history of major lung resection because of the severe impact of PV stenosis on a remaining PV. Furthermore, because the risk of thromboembolic events during the procedure and in the early postoperative period may be prohibitive in the absence of systemic anticoagulation, patients who cannot be anticoagulated during and for at least 2 months after the ablation procedure should not be considered for catheter ablation of AF. Also, catheter ablation should not be performed in patients with an LA appendage thrombus or a recently implanted LA appendage occlusion device.[133]

It is also important to realize that surgical intervention can be lifesaving should a severe mechanical complication, such as rupture or massive perforation of the heart or catheter entrapment, occur. Therefore, catheter ablation of AF should not be performed, particularly in higher-risk patients such as the elderly, if surgical backup is not readily available.[133] In addition, catheter ablation of AF should not be performed in patients who are scheduled to undergo cardiac surgery for another indication when surgical ablation of AF also can be performed.

Determination of Whether Complete Electrical Isolation of the Pulmonary Veins Is Necessary for Clinical Success

Several investigators have addressed this question and come to differing conclusions. There is evidence that short-term efficacy can occasionally be observed in the presence of conduction recurrence across all previously disconnected PVs.[10] In such cases, it is possible that the extent of conduction delay developed in response to the changes induced by chronic lesions prevents, at least for some time during follow-up, the occurrence of arrhythmia relapses. One report found a high rate (80%) of recurrent PV conduction from previously disconnected veins in 43 AF patients with serial EP studies. Interestingly, freedom from AF was no more likely in those with recurrent conduction than in those without. Furthermore, 40% of patients who had recurrence of PV conduction were free of AF.

Conversely, patients with recurrence of AF invariably show conduction recurrence across one or more previously disconnected PVs. One study has found that in patients with recurrent AF after initial PV isolation, 86% of recurrent AF triggers come from PVs that had either not been targeted for initial ablation (32%) or had developed recurrent conduction (54%).[68] A recent report has strongly suggested that achievement of complete PV isolation improves outcome with the circumferential LA ablation approach.[136] All patients with early AF recurrence who underwent a second ablation procedure showed recurrent conduction from a previously isolated PV and underwent reisolation of that PV, after which 95% of 41 patients were free of AF without antiarrhythmic drugs. Furthermore, with circumferential LA ablation, isolation of the PVs achieved via the completion of the circumferential ablation lines and ablation of all the gaps, as compared with incomplete circumferential LA ablation lines and achievement of PV isolation by additional ablation at the PV ostia, provides superior outcomes. The superior results related to complete circumferential LA ablation are likely caused by a lower incidence of recovery of PV activation, the importance of the atrial tissue in the antrum or around the PVs in generating AF, or a proarrhythmic effect of incomplete circumferential LA ablation with multiple gaps. Although these results are encouraging and suggest that the additional procedural complexity of PV mapping is justified, further investigation is needed. In particular, it is unknown whether PV isolation adds to the success of circumferential ablation for persistent or permanent AF.[69] Of note, there is no evidence to date of postablation AF recurrence in the presence of documented persistent isolation of all previously disconnected PVs.

In conclusion, although the importance of achieving isolation of the PVs remains unclear, it is acknowledged that electrical isolation of the PVs should be at least as effective as not achieving isolation. Furthermore, it is clear that if wide-area circumferential ablation is performed during NSR, complete PV isolation is also the most desirable endpoint. However, when wide-area circumferential ablation is performed during AF using endpoints of voltage abatement inside the encircling lesions and elimination of sites displaying relatively short CLs, complete PV isolation is not required for a successful outcome. As long as PV stenosis is avoided, there are no deleterious effects of complete PV isolation as an additional endpoint in wide-area circumferential LA ablation techniques. Nevertheless, because complete isolation requires additional time and RF energy delivery, it is useful to know that complete elimination of PV potentials may not be necessary to achieve a successful outcome in such an approach.

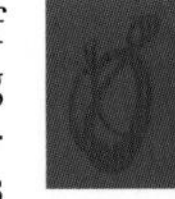

Determination of Necessity of Adding Left Atrial Linear Lesions

Another important issue concerns the safety and efficacy of adding LA linear lesions to the basic ablation lesion set. The two linear lesions most commonly added are a line connecting the right and left superior PVs across the superior aspect of the LA (the so-called roof line) and a line connecting the left inferior PV to the mitral valve annulus (the so-called mitral isthmus line).[84,85] These lesion sets are designed to modify the electrical substrate further to prevent AF as well as to prevent LA flutters that might be formed by the large circumferential lines of block.[84,85] However, continuous linear lesions are difficult to achieve, even under direct visualization during intraoperative ablation, and creating transmural permanent lines of block with a percutaneous approach can be even more challenging. It has been shown that achieving block with the mitral isthmus line in particular is technically challenging and sometimes requires ablation deep within the CS. Gaps within the ablation lines, whether secondary to areas of recovery or areas missed initially, can produce areas of slow conduction and a substrate for macroreentry.[38,100] As noted, although some studies have demonstrated a reduction in the incidence of postprocedure LA tachycardias, some actually have raised concern that addition of linear lesions, if incomplete, could lead to an increased rather than decreased incidence of this problem. Whether these additional lines improve clinical success remains to be determined, but many centers are adding these lesions in patients with persistent or permanent AF or with inducible AF or LA flutter after the standard circumferential lesions are made.

The question is: when and in which patients should one perform additional linear ablation? It is clear that some patients do not need it, and deploying them systematically in all patients may expose them to potential risks without any additional benefit. The clinical picture may help in selection, because patients with structural heart disease and prolonged (more than 24 hours) AF episodes are more likely to have persisting AF or inducible AF after PV isolation. One strategy is to perform PV isolation or wide-area circumferential LA ablation first and, in patients with persisting or inducible AF, to deploy a linear lesion joining both superior PVs (roof line). Ablation at the mitral isthmus is reserved as the final option if AF persists or is still inducible, or if perimitral AFL develops. An alternative strategy is first to isolate the PVs in patients with paroxysmal or persistent AF and, with the persistence of AF after an 8- to 12-week waiting period, to consider linear lesions if recovery of PV conduction is excluded. In patients with long-standing persistent AF, more extensive ablation may be required during the index procedure, including mitral isthmus ablation.

In conclusion, the clinical value of linear lesions created as an adjunct to PV encirclement in patients with persistent or paroxysmal AF appears limited. Although the creation of linear lesions is still performed at many centers, interest has more recently shifted toward the pursuit of other approaches of substrate modification (e.g., autonomic denervation and targeting fractionated electrograms) in patients with persistent AF after PV encirclement.[18,40] The use of linear lesions appears increasingly to be relegated only to those patients who manifest postablation LA flutter.

Future Approaches to Catheter Ablation of Atrial Fibrillation

Use of sources of energy other than radiofrequency is under investigation. Cryoablation may offer several potential advantages, including elimination of coagulum formation, which should reduce stroke risk, and absence of coagulative necrosis of ablated tissue, which may reduce the risk of tamponade, PV stenosis, and pericarditis.[63,71] The use of HIFU will also need further evaluation.

Techniques to deliver simplified circumferential ablation lesions using balloon-tipped catheters have been in development as well, including those using cryoenergy and HIFU energy. Preliminary results of one ultrasound balloon catheter for PV isolation have not been followed by larger studies of efficacy and safety.

Improvement in mapping technology promises to yield important benefits in catheter ablation of AF. 3-D mapping systems capable of CT and MR image integration of the LA and PVs may enhance mapping accuracy and provide greater detail of the PV ostium–LA junction.[64-66] A magnetic guidance system (Niobe, Stereotaxis, St. Louis, Mo) may offer a particular advantage by its capability of remote manipulation of the ablation catheter (discussed in detail in Chap. 3).[137]

ATRIOVENTRICULAR JUNCTION ABLATION

Rationale

AF may not be amenable to ablation procedures and may require multiple pharmacological agents for management. In some of these patients, medical therapy is poorly tolerated or unsuccessful. In these cases, AVN ablation combined with permanent pacemaker implantation (the ablate and pace approach) is a possible treatment strategy, with rate control as the goal. The pacemaker may be single chamber (VVI) for chronic AF or dual chamber (DDD) for paroxysmal or recurrent persistent AF.[29] This procedure is successful in almost 100% of cases and late recovery of AV conduction is rare. However, this procedure still mandates anticoagulation and possibly requires antiarrhythmic therapy to control the AF.

The timing of AVN ablation in relation to pacing is debatable, mainly in the case of paroxysmal AF. In most EP laboratories, permanent pacemaker implantation is performed prior to the ablation procedure. Long-term pacemaker function does not seem to be affected by RF ablation; however, it may develop a transient unpredictable response during RF application in up to 50% of patients, including inhibition, switching to backup mode, oversensing, undersensing, loss of capture, exit block, and electromechanical interference. These responses may argue for the use of an external pacemaker during the ablation procedure. In patients with paroxysmal AF, a dual-chamber pacemaker may be implanted first and the need for AV junction ablation is reassessed after 1 to 3 months of intensification of medical therapy (i.e., AVN blocking drugs).

Target of Ablation

The target site of this approach is located closer to the compact AVN than the HB in the anterosuperior region of the triangle of Koch. This approach selectively ablates the AVN, and not the HB. This ensures ablation of the proximal part of the AV junction to preserve underlying automatism and to avoid pacemaker dependency. Occasionally, when ablation of the AVN is unsuccessful, RF ablation of the HB may be performed using a left or right-sided approach.

Ablation Technique

A 4- or 8-mm-tip ablation catheter is initially positioned at the AV junction to obtain the maximal amplitude of the bipolar His potential recorded from the distal pair of the electrodes. The catheter is then withdrawn while maintaining clockwise torque on the catheter to maintain septal contact until the His potential becomes small or barely visible, or disappears while recording a relatively large atrial electrogram (A/V ratio > 1) or, in patients with AF, until the His potential disappears under the fibrillatory waves (Fig. 11-57).

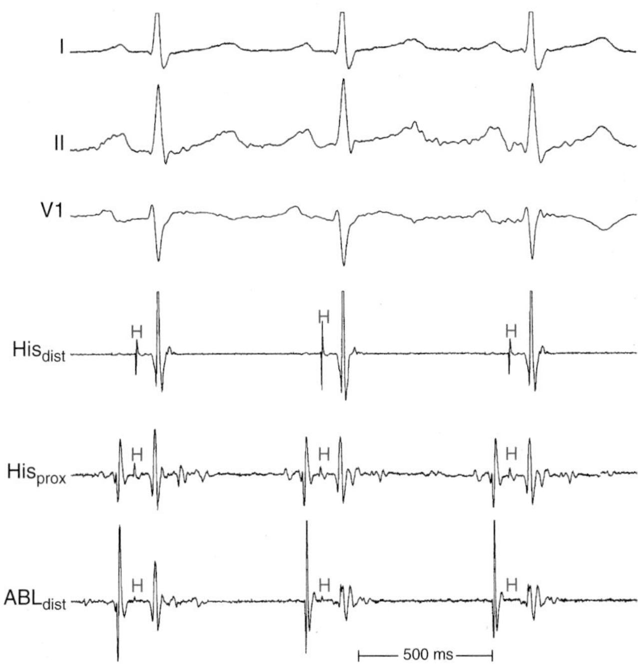

FIGURE 11–57 Optimal ablation site for atrioventricular (AV) junction ablation during normal sinus rhythm (NSR). The distal ablation electrodes record a small His potential and a large atrial electrogram (A/V ratio > 1). More prominent His potentials, such as recorded by the proximal or distal His bundle (HB) catheter bipoles, suggest inappropriate site for ablation.

An alternative approach is to position a quadripolar catheter at the HB position. The tip of the ablation catheter is then withdrawn to about 2 cm below and to the left of the tip of the HB catheter in the RAO view (Fig. 11-58). Occasionally, in 5% to 15% of patients, when the right side approach is undesirable or unsuccessful, a left-sided approach to ablate the HB may be used. The ablation catheter is advanced retrograde through the aorta into the LV, withdrawn so that the catheter tip lies against the membranous septum just below the aortic valve, and records a large HB electrogram and small atrial electrogram (Fig. 11-59). Often, no atrial electrogram is seen. A large atrial electrogram suggests that the catheter tip is close to the LA above the aortic valve; ablation must not be attempted at this site. The left-sided approach typically requires fewer RF applications than the right-sided approach.

A recent report has described the feasibility of AV junction ablation performed from the axillary vein concurrent with the implantation of a dual-chamber pacemaker.[138] This approach involves placing two separate introducer sheaths into the axillary or subclavian vein—the first sheath is used for implantation of the pacemaker ventricular lead, which is then connected to the pulse generator or a temporary pacemaker. Subsequently, a standard ablation catheter is introduced through the second venous sheath and used for ablation of the AV junction. The ablation catheter is advanced into the RV and positioned near the HB region by deflection of the tip superiorly to form a J shape; the catheter is then withdrawn so that it lies across the superior margin of the tricuspid annulus (Fig. 11-60). Alternatively, the catheter

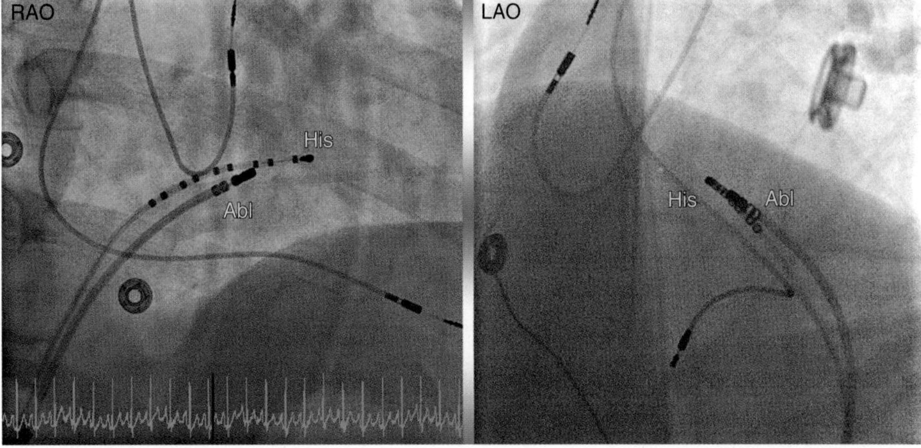

FIGURE 11–58 Fluoroscopic (right anterior oblique [RAO] and left anterior oblique [LAO]) views of the ablation catheter position in relation to the His bundle (HB) catheter at the optimal site of atrioventricular (AV) junction ablation. The distal ablation electrode is positioned just proximal and inferior to the proximal HB electrodes.

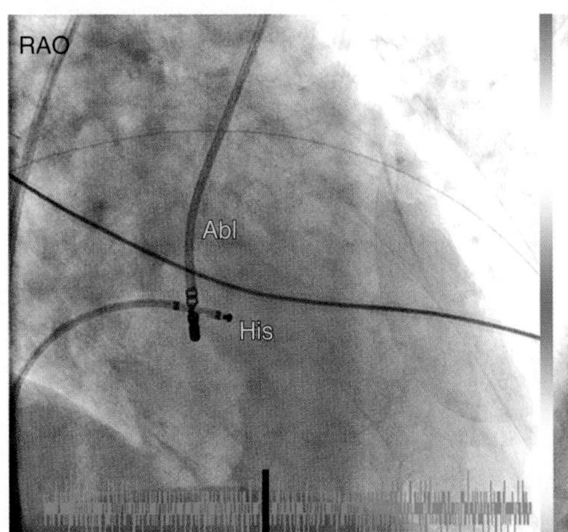

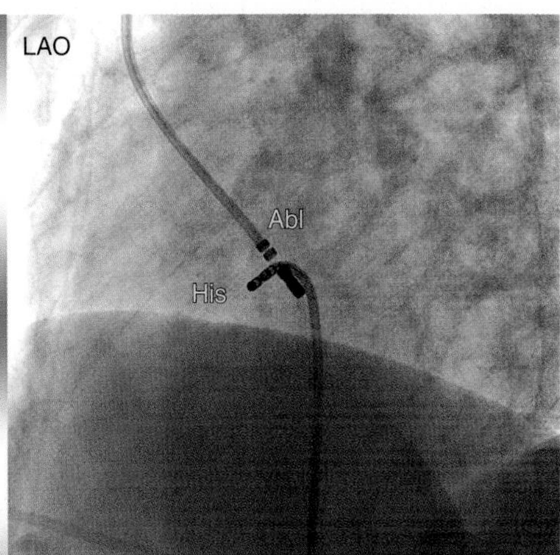

FIGURE 11–59 Fluoroscopic (right anterior oblique [RAO] and left anterior oblique [LAO]) views of the ablation catheter introduced via a transaortic approach in relation to the His bundle (HB) catheter at the optimal site for atrioventricular junction ablation (Abl). The distal ablation electrode is positioned just inferior to the aortic cusp in the left ventricular outflow tract, opposite the HB catheter in the right ventricle.

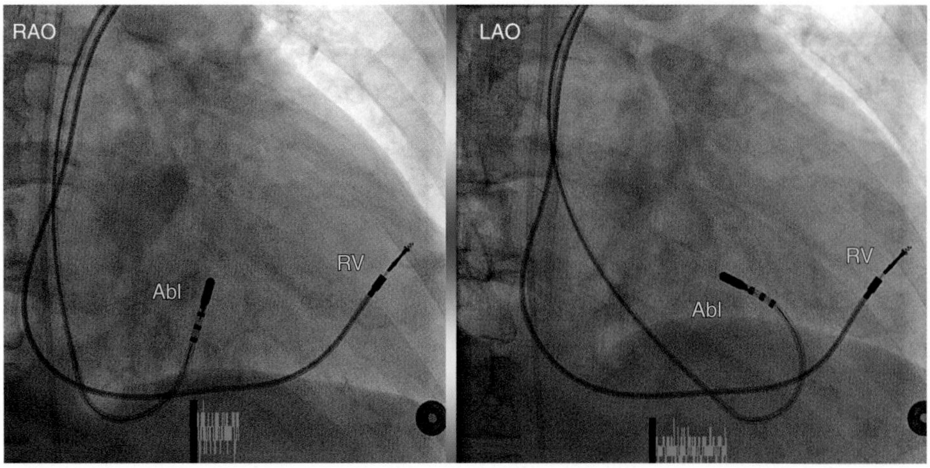

FIGURE 11–60 Fluoroscopic (right anterior oblique) views of the ablation (Abl) catheter introduced via the left axillary vein. Implantation of the pacemaker ventricular lead is initially performed. The ablation catheter is positioned near the His bundle (HB) region by deflection of the tip superiorly to form a J shape and then withdrawing the catheter so that it lies across the superior margin of the tricuspid annulus (at left), or by looping the catheter in the right atrium (RA; figure-of-6) and then advancing the body of the loop into the right ventricle so that the tip of the catheter is pointing toward the RA and lying on the septal aspect of the RA (at right).

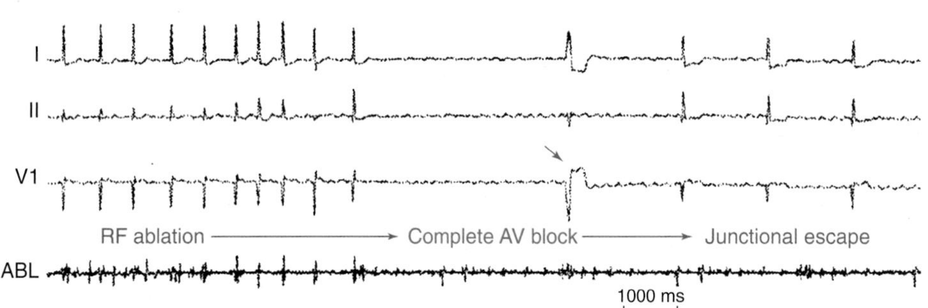

FIGURE 11–61 Atrioventricular (AV) junction ablation during atrial fibrillation (AF). A ventricular pacemaker was implanted prior to ablation and programmed to VVI pacing mode at 30 beats/min. RF application results in complete AV block with an escape ventricular paced complex (blue arrow) followed by the emergence of a junctional escape rhythm at 35 beats/min.

may be looped in the RA (figure-of-6) and the body of the loop advanced in the RV so that the tip of the catheter is pointing toward the RA and lying on the septal aspect of the RA. Gentle withdrawal of the catheter can increase the size of the loop and allow the catheter tip to rest on the HB location (see Fig. 11-60). After successful ablation, the ablation catheter is withdrawn and the pacemaker atrial lead is advanced through that same sheath.[138]

RF energy is delivered with a power output of 50 W, targeting a temperature of 60° to 70°C, and for a duration of 30 to 120 seconds. AV block may appear immediately or after
11 several RF applications. Typically, at good ablation sites, an accelerated junctional rhythm is induced during RF application (Fig. 11-61).

Endpoints of Ablation

The endpoint of ablation is achieving complete AV block. It is preferable to achieve AVN block with a junctional escape rhythm to avoid pacemaker dependency; however, sometimes this is difficult to achieve, and HB ablation with fascicular or no escape rhythm is the end result (see Fig. 11-61).

Outcome

Complete AV block can be achieved in almost 100% of patients, with a 3% risk of recurrence of AV conduction. Achieving complete AVN block specifically, however, is less successful (80% to 90%).[29] Ablation of the AV junction may be difficult to achieve in patients with atrial enlargement or hypertrophy, as seen with long-standing heart failure or hypertension.

Most patients who undergo RF ablation of the AV junction are pacemaker-dependent after the procedure, as defined by lack of an escape rhythm that is faster than 40 beats/min.[29] Following AV junction ablation, an escape rhythm develops in 70% to 100% of cases, and the absence of escape rhythm immediately after ablation seems to be the only predictor for long-term pacemaker dependency. Although the appearance of an escape rhythm does not obviate the need for pacing, it may provide reassurance in case of pacemaker failure.

Malignant ventricular arrhythmias and sudden cardiac death have been observed in the early phase following AV junction ablation.[139] Polymorphic VTs are related to electrical instability caused by an initial prolongation and then slow adaptation of repolarization caused by changes in the heart rate and activation sequence. Most polymorphic VTs, VF, and torsades de pointes that have been reported seem to be consistent with a pause or bradycardia-dependent mechanism. Anomalous dynamics of the paced QT intervals have been observed until the second day after AV junction ablation in patients with rapid refractory AF, resulting in prolongation of the QT interval when the heart rate is less than 75 beats/min. This may explain the ventricular arrhythmias occurring after AV junction ablation and may also explain the beneficial effects of temporary rapid pacing. On the other hand, bradycardia may not be the sole factor. Sympathetic tone augmentation following AV junction ablation has been described in patients paced at 60 beats/min, causing prolongation of action potential duration and RV refractoriness, whereas sympathetic tone was reduced in patients paced at 90 beats/min. Such an increase in sympathetic activity and prolongation in action potential duration may favor early afterdepolarization and triggered activity, which may mediate torsades de pointes and polymorphic VT.[139] To reduce the risk of these arrhythmias, routine pacing at 80 beats/min has been recommended following AV junction ablation. Patients with high-risk factors for arrhythmias, such as congestive heart failure or impaired LV function, may require pacing at higher rates (e.g., at 90 beats/min for 1 to 3 months) as well as in-hospital monitoring for at least 48 hours. Adjustment of the pacing rate, although rarely below 70 beats/min, is usually undertaken after 1 week in most patients, preferably after an ECG evaluation for repolarization abnormalities at the lower rate.

Another adverse effect of the ablate and pace approach is ventricular dyssynchrony induced by RV pacing, which may result in impairment of LV systolic function. Positioning the ventricular pacing electrode over the RV septum, HB pacing, and biventricular pacing are being evaluated to reduce the impact of this potential problem.[140]

ATRIOVENTRICULAR NODAL MODIFICATION

Rationale

AVN modification is performed to injure the AVN to reduce the ventricular rate during AF without producing heart block. As compared with ablation of the AV junction, AVN modification has the advantage in that it results in adequate control of the ventricular rate in most patients while obviating the need for a permanent pacemaker.[141] Therefore, it may be appropriate to attempt first to modify AV conduction in patients with AF and rapid ventricular rates who are appropriate candidates for ablation of the AV junction. Because the risk of inadvertent complete AV block is approximately 20%, the use of the procedure should be limited at present to patients with AF who are symptomatic enough for ablation of the AV junction and implantation of a permanent pacemaker to be justified.

Target of Ablation

The right posteroseptal area along the tricuspid annulus extending from the CS os to the recording site of the HB can be divided into three regions, posterior, medial, and anterior. The conventional technique for ablation of the AV junction uses sites located anteriorly and superiorly on the tricuspid annulus. In contrast, with the technique used to modify AV conduction, the target sites are located inferiorly and posteriorly near the tricuspid annulus close to the CS os—that is, in the posterior or midatrial septum (Fig. 11-62).[141] In the presence of dual AVN physiology, the slow AVN pathway is targeted (as described for ablation of AVNRT).

Ablation Technique

Two quadripolar-electrode catheters are inserted into a femoral vein and positioned at the HB and in the RV. An ablation catheter with a 4-mm tip is used. In patients with no demonstrable dual AVN physiology, RF energy is deliv-

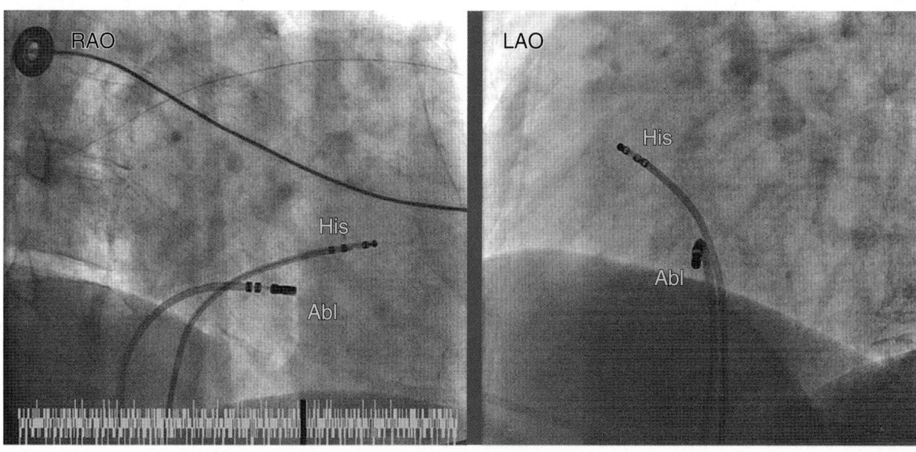

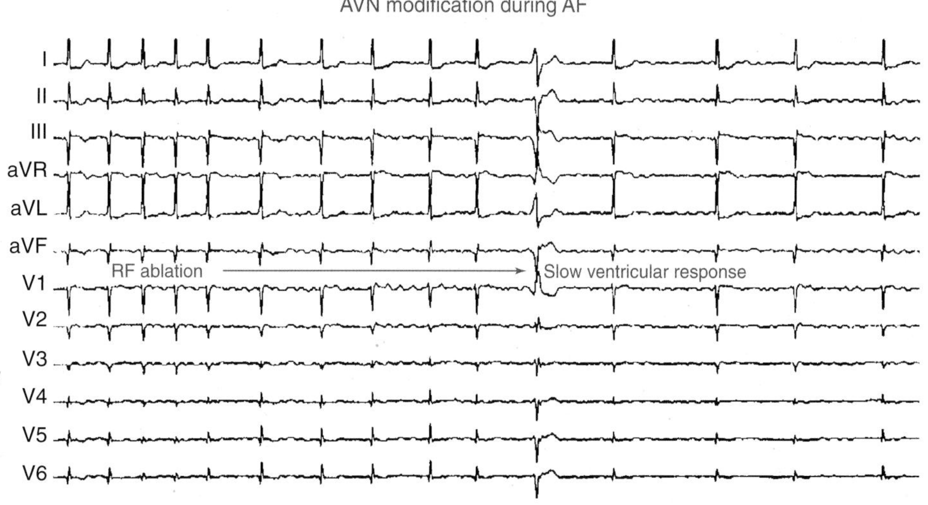

FIGURE 11–62 Atrioventricular node (AVN) modification during atrial fibrillation (AF). **Upper panel,** Fluoroscopic (right anterior oblique [RAO] and left anterior oblique [LAO]) views of the ablation catheter position in relation to the His bundle (HB) catheter at the optimal site of AVN modification. The distal ablation electrode is positioned in the postero- or midatrial septum near the tricuspid annulus, close to the coronary sinus ostium. **Lower panel,** AF with rapid ventricular response is initially observed (at left). RF application results in slowing of the ventricular rate (at right) but not complete AV block, as indicated by irregularity of the rhythm.

ered during AF under continuous infusion of isoproterenol (4 μg /min) to permit immediate assessment of the effect of each RF application. The ventricular rate during AF, obtained after administration of isoproterenol, is presumed to simulate the maximal rate of clinical AF. If NSR is present, AF is induced by rapid atrial pacing before the delivery of RF energy.[141] The ablation catheter is initially positioned against the posterior RA septum, at the level of or lower than the CS os, to record a stable electrogram for at least 10 seconds, with a maximal A/V electrogram amplitude ratio of 0.5 or lower.

RF energy is delivered for 20 seconds at 30 W. If there is no change in the ventricular rate or no accelerating junctional rhythm within 20 seconds, higher energy (an increment of 5 W every 20 seconds, up to 40 W) is delivered to the same site. Whenever there is an abrupt lengthening of the R-R interval or appearance of an accelerated junctional rhythm, the application of energy is immediately discontinued (see Fig. 11-62). If the ventricular rate is still higher than the endpoint ventricular rate (i.e., more than 130 beats/min), higher energy is delivered to the effective site or the ablation site is changed and the catheter is repositioned in progressively upward (more superior and anterior) positions along the tricuspid annulus, until the endpoint is achieved. RF energy should not be delivered at the upper third atrial septum, at which a HB potential is visible.

If the endpoint ventricular rate could not be achieved after RF application to the posterior and midatrial septum, a decision should be made about whether to attempt complete ablation of AVN. In the presence of dual AVN physiology, RF energy is delivered during NSR to eliminate slow AVN pathway. The ablation technique is similar to that described for ablation of AVNRT.

Endpoints of Ablation

The endpoint of the procedure is an average ventricular rate of 120 to 130 beats/min or 70% to 75% of the maximum ventricular rate during infusion of isoproterenol (4 μg/min).

Outcome

Acute Results. The immediate success of AVN modification to control the ventricular rate without inducing pathological AV block is about 75% to 92%.

Long-Term Results. In one report, 92% of patients with paroxysmal AF and uncontrolled ventricular rates refractory to antiarrhythmic drugs achieved adequate slowing of the ventricular rate and were free of symptoms without any antiarrhythmic drug or the need for a permanent pacemaker. The mean resting, ambulatory, and minimal ventricular rates during AF usually remained stable during an interval from 2 days to 3 months after the modification procedure. However, the mean maximal ventricular rate tended to increase (by up to 25%) during this period, which may reflect partial recovery of AV conduction from the immediate effects of RF energy. Nevertheless, the mean maximal ventricular rate during exercise or isoproterenol infusion at 3 months of follow-up still remained approximately 25% lower than at baseline, a degree of attenuation adequate to result in the persistent resolution of symptoms.

Atrioventricular Block. Inadvertent complete AV block occurs in approximately 20% to 25% of patients. Of those patients who develop transient AV block during RF application, about two thirds develop persistent AV block within the first 36 to 72 hours after the procedure. It may be that transient thermal injury to the AV conduction system results in an inflammatory reaction responsible for the delayed occurrence of permanent injury. Regardless of the mechanism, if transient AV block occurs during an attempt to modify AV conduction, continuous ECG monitoring on an inpatient basis is appropriate for 3 to 4 days to watch for a recurrence of AV block.

Limitations. AVN modification approach is only applicable to patients who do not have symptoms caused by irregular heart rhythm. An irregular rhythm may be hemodynamically less efficient than a regular paced rhythm. Additionally, at least 25% of patients in whom AVN modification is attempted develop inadvertent complete AV block that necessitates implantation of a permanent pacemaker.

REFERENCES

1. Fuster V, Ryden LE, Asinger RW, et al American College of Cardiology/American Heart Association/European Society of Cardiology Board: ACC/AHA/ESC guidelines for the management of patients with atrial fibrillation: executive summary. A Report of the American College of Cardiology/ American Heart Association Task Force on Practice Guidelines and the European Society of Cardiology Committee for Practice Guidelines and Policy Conferences (Committee to Develop Guidelines for the Management of Patients With Atrial Fibrillation): Developed in Collaboration With the North American Society of Pacing and Electrophysiology. J Am Coll Cardiol 2001;38:1231.
2. Nattel S, Ehrlich JR: Atrial fibrillation. *In* Zipes DP, Jalife J (eds): Cardiac Electrophysiology: From Cell to Bedside, 4th ed. Philadelphia, WB Saunders, 2004, pp 512-522.
3. Maurits A, Allessie MD, Penelope A, Boyden PA: Pathophysiology and prevention of atrial fibrillation. Circulation 2001;103:769.
4. Schoonderwoerd BA, Van Gelder IC, Van Veldhuisen DJ, et al: Electrical and structural remodeling: Role in the genesis and maintenance of atrial fibrillation. Prog Cardiovasc Dis 2005;48:153.
5. Olgin JE: Electrophysiology of the pulmonary veins: Mechanisms of initiation of atrial fibrillation. *In* Zipes DP, Jalife J (eds): Cardiac Electrophysiology: From Cell to Bedside, 4th ed. Philadelphia, WB Saunders, 2004, pp 355-362.
6. Haissaguerre M, Jais P, Shah DC, et al: Spontaneous initiation of atrial fibrillation by ectopic beats originating in the pulmonary veins. N Engl J Med 1998;339:659.
7. Chen PS, Chou CC, Tan AY, et al: The mechanisms of atrial fibrillation. J Cardiovasc Electrophysiol 2006;17(Suppl 3):S2.
8. Arora R, Verheule S, Scott L, et al: Arrhythmogenic substrate of the pulmonary veins assessed by high-resolution optical mapping. Circulation 2003;107:1816.
9. Chen YJ, Chen SA: Electrophysiology of pulmonary veins. J Cardiovasc Electrophysiol 2006;17:220.
10. Ho SY, Anderson RH, Sanchez-Quintana D: Atrial structure and fibres: Morphologic basis of atrial conduction. Cardiovasc Res 2002;54:325.
11. Jais P, Hocini M, Macle L, et al: Distinctive electrophysiological properties of pulmonary veins in patients with atrial fibrillation. Circulation 2002;106:2479.
12. Lin WS, Tai CT, Hsieh MH, et al: Catheter ablation of paroxysmal atrial fibrillation initiated by non-pulmonary vein ectopy. Circulation 2003;107:3176.
13. Moe GK, Rheinboldt WC, Abildskov JA: A computer model of atrial fibrillation. Am Heart J 1964;67:200-220.
14. Jalife J, Berenfeld O, Mansour M: Mother rotors and fibrillatory conduction: A mechanism of atrial fibrillation. Cardiovasc Res 2002;54:204.
15. Schotten U, Duytschaever M, Ausma J: Electrical and contractile remodeling during the first days of atrial fibrillation go hand in hand. Circulation 2003;107:1433.
16. Nattel S: New ideas about atrial fibrillation 50 years on. Nature 2002;415:219.
17. Scherlag BJ, Po S: The intrinsic cardiac nervous system and atrial fibrillation. Curr Opin Cardiol 2006;21:51.
18. Pappone C, Santinelli V, Manguso F, et al: Pulmonary vein denervation enhances long-term benefit after circumferential ablation for paroxysmal atrial fibrillation. Circulation 2004;109:327.
19. Jayachandran JV, Sih HJ, Winkle W, et al: Atrial fibrillation produced by prolonged rapid atrial pacing is associated with heterogeneous changes in atrial sympathetic innervation. Circulation 2000;101:1185.
20. Oral H, Knight BP, Ozaydin M, et al: Segmental ostial ablation to isolate the pulmonary veins during atrial fibrillation: feasibility and mechanistic insights. Circulation 2002;106:1256.
21. Wu TJ, Ong JJ, Chang CM, et al: Pulmonary veins and ligament of Marshall as sources of rapid activations in a canine model of sustained atrial fibrillation. Circulation 2001;103:1157.
22. Fynn SP, Kalman JM: Pulmonary veins: Anatomy, electrophysiology, tachycardia, and fibrillation. Pacing Clin Electrophysiol 2004;27:1547.
23. Kistler PM, Sanders P, Fynn SP, et al: Electrophysiological and electrocardiographic characteristics of focal atrial tachycardia originating from the pulmonary veins: Acute and long-term outcomes of radiofrequency ablation. Circulation 2003;108:1968.
24. European Heart Rhythm Association; Heart Rhythm Society, Fuster V, Rydén LE, Cannom DS, et al American College of Cardiology; American Heart Association Task Force on Practice Guidelines; European Society of Cardiology Committee for Practice Guidelines; Writing Committee to Revise the 2001 Guidelines for the Management of Patients With Atrial Fibrillation: ACC/AHA/ESC 2006 guidelines for the management of patients with atrial fibrillation–executive summary: a report of the American College of Cardiology/American Heart Association Task Force on

Practice Guidelines and the European Society of Cardiology Committee for Practice Guidelines (Writing Committee to Revise the 2001 Guidelines for the Management of Patients With Atrial Fibrillation). J Am Coll Cardiol 2006;48:854.
25. Van GI, Hagens VE, Bosker HA, et al: A comparison of rate control and rhythm control in patients with recurrent persistent atrial fibrillation. N Engl J Med 2002;347:1834-1840.
26. Wyse DG, Waldo AL, DiMarco JP, et al: A comparison of rate control and rhythm control in patients with atrial fibrillation. N Engl J Med 2002;347:1825-1833.
27. Snow V, Weiss KB, LeFevre M, et al: Management of newly detected atrial fibrillation: A clinical practice guideline from the American Academy of Family Physicians and the American College of Physicians. Ann Intern Med 2003;139:1009.
28. Hylek EM, Go AS, Chang Y, et al: Effect of intensity of oral anticoagulation on stroke severity and mortality in atrial fibrillation. N Engl J Med 2003;349:1019.
29. Ozcan C, Jahangir A, Friedman PA, et al: Long-term survival after ablation of the atrioventricular node and implantation of a permanent pacemaker in patients with atrial fibrillation. N Engl J Med 2001;344:1043.
30. Hohnloser SH, Kuck KH, Lilienthal J: Rhythm or rate control in atrial fibrillation—pharmacological intervention in atrial fibrillation (PIAF): A randomised trial. Lancet 2000;356:1789.
31. Van GI, Hagens VE, Bosker HA, et al: A comparison of rate control and rhythm control in patients with recurrent persistent atrial fibrillation. N Engl J Med 2002;347:1834.
32. Wyse DG, Waldo AL, DiMarco JP, et al: A comparison of rate control and rhythm control in patients with atrial fibrillation. N Engl J Med 2002;347:1825.
33. Khargi K, Hutten BA, Lemke B, Deneke T: Surgical treatment of atrial fibrillation: a systematic review. Eur J Cardiothorac Surg 2005;27:258.
34. O'Neill MD, Jais P, Hocini M, et al: Catheter ablation for atrial fibrillation. Circulation 2007;116:1515.
35. Cox JL, Boineau JP, Scheussler RB: Five year experience with the maze procedure for atrial fibrillation. Ann Thorac Surg 1993;56:814-824.
36. Schuessler RB, Damiano RJ J:. Patient-specific surgical strategy for atrial fibrillation: Promises and challenges. Heart Rhythm 2007;4:1222.
37. Khargi K, Hutten BA, Lemke B, Deneke T: Surgical treatment of atrial fibrillation; A systematic review. Eur J Cardiothorac Surg 2005;27:258-265.
38. Pappone C, Manguso F, Vicedomini G, et al: Prevention of iatrogenic atrial tachycardia after ablation of atrial fibrillation: A prospective randomized study comparing circumferential pulmonary vein ablation with a modified approach. Circulation 2004;110:3036.
39. Pappone C, Rosanio S, Oreto G, et al: Circumferential radiofrequency ablation of pulmonary vein ostia: A new anatomical approach for curing atrial fibrillation. Circulation 2000;102:2619.
40. Nademanee K, McKenzie J, Kosar E, et al: A new approach for catheter ablation of atrial fibrillation: mapping of the electrophysiological substrate. J Am Coll Cardiol 2004;43:2044.
41. Marrouche NF, Martin DO, Wazni O, et al: Phased-array intracardiac echocardiography monitoring during pulmonary vein isolation in patients with atrial fibrillation: Impact on outcome and complications. Circulation 2003;107:2710.
42. Oral H, Scharf C, Chugh A, et al: Catheter ablation for paroxysmal atrial fibrillation: segmental pulmonary vein ostial ablation versus left atrial ablation. Circulation 2003;108:2355.
43. Lee SH, Tai CT, Hsieh MH, et al: Predictors of non-pulmonary vein ectopic beats initiating paroxysmal atrial fibrillation: Implication for catheter ablation. J Am Coll Cardiol 2005;46:1054.
44. Wazni OM, Beheiry S, Fahmy T, et al: Atrial fibrillation ablation in patients with therapeutic international normalized ratio: Comparison of strategies of anticoagulation management in the periprocedural period. Circulation 2007;116:2531.
45. Calkins H, Brugada J, Packer DL, et al: HRS/EHRA/ECAS expert Consensus Statement on catheter and surgical ablation of atrial fibrillation: Recommendations for personnel, policy, procedures and follow-up: A report of the Heart Rhythm Society (HRS) Task Force on catheter and surgical ablation of atrial fibrillation. Heart Rhythm 2007;4:816.
46. Lang CC, Gugliotta F, Santinelli V, et al: Endocardial impedance mapping during circumferential pulmonary vein ablation of atrial fibrillation differentiates between atrial and venous tissue. Heart Rhythm 2006;3:171.
47. Oral H, Chugh A, Ozaydin M, et al: Risk of thromboembolic events after percutaneous left atrial radiofrequency ablation of atrial fibrillation. Circulation 2006;114:759.
48. Sanders P, Jais P, Hocini M, Haissaguerre M: Electrical disconnection of the coronary sinus by radiofrequency catheter ablation to isolate a trigger of atrial fibrillation. J Cardiovasc Electrophysiol 2004;15:364.
49. Chen SA, Hsieh MH, Tai CT, et al: Initiation of atrial fibrillation by ectopic beats originating from the pulmonary veins: Electrophysiological characteristics, pharmacological responses, and effects of radiofrequency ablation. Circulation 1999;100:1879-1886.
50. Tada H, Oral H, Wasmer K, et al: Pulmonary vein isolation: Comparison of bipolar and unipolar electrograms at successful and unsuccessful ostial ablation sites. J Cardiovasc Electrophysiol 2002;13:13.
51. Asirvatham SJ: Pulmonary vein-related maneuvers: part I. Heart Rhythm 2007;4:538.
52. Yamada T, Murakami Y, Okada T, et al: Electrophysiological pulmonary vein antrum isolation with a multielectrode basket catheter is feasible and effective for curing paroxysmal atrial fibrillation: efficacy of minimally extensive pulmonary vein isolation. Heart Rhythm 2006;3:377.
53. Takahashi A, Iesaka Y, Takahashi Y, et al: Electrical connections between pulmonary veins: implication for ostial ablation of pulmonary veins in patients with paroxysmal atrial fibrillation. Circulation 2002;105:2998.
54. Tse HF, Reek S, Timmermans C, et al: Pulmonary vein isolation using transvenous catheter cryoablation for treatment of atrial fibrillation without risk of pulmonary vein stenosis. J Am Coll Cardiol 2003;42:752.
55. Moreira W, Manusama R, Timmermans C, et al: Long-term follow-up after cryothermic ostial pulmonary vein isolation in paroxysmal atrial fibrillation. J Am Coll Cardiol 2008;51:850.
56. Ouyang D, Baensch D, Ernst S: Complete isolation of the left atrium surrounding the pulmonary veins: New insights from the double-lasso technique in paroxysmal atrial fibrillation. Circulation 2004;110:2090.
57. Matsuo S, Yamane T, Date T, et al: Reduction of AF recurrence after pulmonary vein isolation by eliminating ATP-induced transient venous re-conduction. J Cardiovasc Electrophysiol 2007;18:704.
58. Nanthakumar K, Plumb VJ, Epstein AE, et al: Resumption of electrical conduction in previously isolated pulmonary veins: Rationale for a different strategy? Circulation 2004;109:1226.
59. Ouyang F, Antz M, Ernst S, et al: Recovered pulmonary vein conduction as a dominant factor for recurrent atrial tachyarrhythmias after complete circular isolation of the pulmonary veins: Lessons from double Lasso technique. Circulation 2005;111:127-135.
60. Marchlinski FE, Callans D, Dixit S, et al: Efficacy and safety of targeted focal ablation versus PV isolation assisted by magnetic electroanatomic mapping. J Cardiovasc Electrophysiol 2003;14:358-365.
61. Verma A, Marrouche NF, Natale A: Pulmonary vein antrum isolation: Intracardiac echocardiography-guided technique. J Cardiovasc Electrophysiol 2004;15:1335.
62. Schwartzman D: Left heart transducer position. *In* Ren JF, Marchlinski FE, Callans DJ, Schwartzman D (eds): Practical Intracardiac Echocardiography in Electrophysiology. Malden, Mass, Blackwell Futura, 2006, pp 117-149.
63. Ahmed J, Sohal S, Malchano ZJ, et al: Three-dimensional analysis of pulmonary venous ostial and antral anatomy: Implications for balloon catheter-based pulmonary vein isolation. J Cardiovasc Electrophysiol 2006;17:251.
64. Dong J, Calkins H, Solomon SB, et al: Integrated electroanatomical mapping with three-dimensional computed tomographic images for real-time guided ablations. Circulation 2006;113:186.
65. Kistler PM, Earley MJ, Harris S, et al: Validation of three-dimensional cardiac image integration: use of integrated CT image into electroanatomical mapping system to perform catheter ablation of atrial fibrillation. J Cardiovasc Electrophysiol 2006;17:341.
66. Sra J, Krum D, Hare J, et al: Feasibility and validation of registration of three-dimensional left atrial models derived from computed tomography with a noncontact cardiac mapping system. Heart Rhythm 2005;2:55.
67. Kanj MH, Wazni OM, Natale A: How to do circular mapping catheter-guided pulmonary vein antrum isolation: The Cleveland Clinic approach. Heart Rhythm 2006;3:866.
68. Ouyang F, Antz M, Ernst S, et al: Recovered pulmonary vein conduction as a dominant factor for recurrent atrial tachyarrhythmias after complete circular isolation of the pulmonary veins: Lessons from double Lasso technique. Circulation 2005;111:127.
69. Ouyang F, Ernst S, Chun J, et al: Electrophysiological findings during ablation of persistent atrial fibrillation with electroanatomical mapping and double Lasso catheter technique. Circulation 2005;112:3038.
70. Bunch TJ, Bruce GK, Johnson SB, et al: Analysis of catheter-tip (8-mm) and actual tissue temperatures achieved during radiofrequency ablation at the orifice of the pulmonary vein. Circulation 2004;110:2988-2995.
71. Sarabanda AV, Bunch TJ, Johnson SB, et al: Efficacy and safety of circumferential pulmonary vein isolation using a novel cryothermal balloon ablation system. J Am Coll Cardiol 2005;46:1902.
72. Nakagawa H, Antz M, Wong T, et al: Initial experience using a forward directed, high-intensity focused ultrasound balloon catheter for pulmonary vein antrum isolation in patients with atrial fibrillation. J Cardiovasc Electrophysiol 2007;18:136.
73. Schmidt B, Antz M, Ernst S, et al: Pulmonary vein isolation by high-intensity focused ultrasound: first-in-man study with a steerable balloon catheter. Heart Rhythm 2007;4:575.
74. Cheema A, Dong J, Dalal D, et al: Incidence and time course of early recovery of pulmonary vein conduction after catheter ablation of atrial fibrillation. J Cardiovasc Electrophysiol 2007;18:387.
75. Hachiya H, Hirao K, Takahashi A, et al: Clinical implications of reconnection between the left atrium and isolated pulmonary veins provoked by adenosine triphosphate after extensive encircling pulmonary vein isolation. J Cardiovasc Electrophysiol 2007;18:392.
76. Chang SL, Tai CT, Lin YJ, et al: The efficacy of inducibility and circumferential ablation with pulmonary vein isolation in patients with paroxysmal atrial fibrillation. J Cardiovasc Electrophysiol 2007;18:607.
77. Arentz T, Weber R, Burkle G, et al: Small or large isolation areas around the pulmonary veins for the treatment of atrial fibrillation? Results from a prospective randomized study. Circulation 2007;115:3057.
78. Karch MR, Zrenner B, Deisenhofer I, et al: Freedom from atrial tachyarrhythmias after catheter ablation of atrial fibrillation: A randomized comparison between 2 current ablation strategies. Circulation 2005;111:2875.
79. Stabile G, Turco P, La RV, et al: Is pulmonary vein isolation necessary for curing atrial fibrillation? Circulation 2003;108:657-660.
80. Oral H, Chugh A, Lemola K, et al: Noninducibility of atrial fibrillation as an end point of left atrial circumferential ablation for paroxysmal atrial fibrillation: a randomized study. Circulation 2004;110:2797.
81. Richter B, Gwechenberger M, Filzmoser P, et al: Is inducibility of atrial fibrillation after radio frequency ablation really a relevant prognostic factor? Eur Heart J 2006;27:2553-2559.

82. Schmitt C, Deisenhofez I, Schzeieck J: Symptomatic and asymptomatic recurrence of atrial fibrillation after ablation: Randomized comparison of segmental pulmonary vein ablation with circumferential pulmonary vein ablation. Eur Heart J 2004;25:277.
83. Sanders P, Jais P, Hocini M, et al: Electrophysiological and clinical consequences of linear catheter ablation to transect the anterior left atrium in patients with atrial fibrillation. Heart Rhythm 2004;1:176.
84. Hocini M, Jais P, Sanders P, et al: Techniques, evaluation, and consequences of linear block at the left atrial roof in paroxysmal atrial fibrillation: A prospective randomized study. Circulation 2005;112:3688.
85. Jais P, Hocini M, Hsu LF, et al: Technique and results of linear ablation at the mitral isthmus. Circulation 2004;110:2996.
86. Waldo AL, Feld GK: Inter-relationships of atrial fibrillation and atrial flutter mechanisms and clinical implications. J Am Coll Cardiol 2008;51:779.
87. Shah DC, Sunthorn H, Burri H, Gentil-Baron P: Evaluation of an individualized strategy of cavotricuspid isthmus ablation as an adjunct to atrial fibrillation ablation. J Cardiovasc Electrophysiol 2007;18:926.
88. Oral H, Chugh A, Good E, et al: A tailored approach to catheter ablation of paroxysmal atrial fibrillation. Circulation 2006;113:1824.
89. Nademanee K, Schwab M, Porath J, Abbo A: How to perform electrogram-guided atrial fibrillation ablation. Heart Rhythm 2006;3:981.
90. Scherr D, Dalal D, Cheema A, et al: Automated detection and characterization of complex fractionated atrial electrograms in human left atrium during atrial fibrillation. Heart Rhythm 2007;4:1013.
91. Oral H, Chugh A, Good E, et al: Radiofrequency catheter ablation of chronic atrial fibrillation guided by complex electrograms. Circulation 2007;115:2606.
92. Tan AY, Li H, Wachsmann-Hogiu S, et al: Autonomic innervation and segmental muscular disconnections at the human pulmonary vein-atrial junction: Implications for catheter ablation of atrial-pulmonary vein junction. J Am Coll Cardiol 2006;48:132.
93. Lemery R, Birnie D, Tang AS, et al: Feasibility study of endocardial mapping of ganglionated plexuses during catheter ablation of atrial fibrillation. Heart Rhythm 2006;3:387.
94. Lemery R: How to perform ablation of the parasympathetic ganglia of the left atrium. Heart Rhythm 2006;3:1237.
95. Higa S, Tai CT, Chen SA: Catheter ablation of atrial fibrillation originating from extrapulmonary vein areas: Taipei approach. Heart Rhythm 2006;3: 1386.
96. Asirvatham SJ. Pacing maneuvers for nonpulmonary vein sources: Part II. Heart Rhythm 2007;4:681.
97. Hwang C, Fishbein MC, Chen PS: How and when to ablate the ligament of Marshall. Heart Rhythm 2006;3:1505.
98. Arruda M, Mlcochova H, Prasad SK, et al: Electrical isolation of the superior vena cava: An adjunctive strategy to pulmonary vein antrum isolation improving the outcome of AF ablation. J Cardiovasc Electrophysiol 2007;18:1261.
99. Haissaguerre M, Hocini M, Takahashi Y, et al: Impact of catheter ablation of the coronary sinus on paroxysmal or persistent atrial fibrillation. J Cardiovasc Electrophysiol 2007;18:378.
100. Verma A, Natale A: Should atrial fibrillation ablation be considered first-line therapy for some patients? Why atrial fibrillation ablation should be considered first-line therapy for some patients. Circulation 2005;112:1214.
101. Pappone C, Augello G, Sala S, et al: A randomized trial of circumferential pulmonary vein ablation versus antiarrhythmic drug therapy in paroxysmal atrial fibrillation: The APAF Study. J Am Coll Cardiol 2006;48:2340.
102. Oral H, Pappone C, Chugh A, et al: Circumferential pulmonary-vein ablation for chronic atrial fibrillation. N Engl J Med 2006;354:934.
103. Wazni OM, Marrouche NF, Martin DO, et al: Radiofrequency ablation vs antiarrhythmic drugs as first-line treatment of symptomatic atrial fibrillation: A randomized trial. JAMA 2005;293:2634.
104. Stabile G, Bertaglia E, Senatore G, et al: Catheter ablation treatment in patients with drug-refractory atrial fibrillation: A prospective, multi-centre, randomized, controlled study (Catheter Ablation For The Cure Of Atrial Fibrillation Study). Eur Heart J 2006;27:216.
105. Jais P, Cauchemez B, Macle L: Atrial fibrillation ablation vs antiarrhythmic drugs: A multicenter randomized trial. Heart Rhythm 2006;3:1126.
106. Tanner H, Hindricks G, Kobza R, et al: Trigger activity more than three years after left atrial linear ablation without pulmonary vein isolation in patients with atrial fibrillation. J Am Coll Cardiol 2005;46:338.
107. Hsieh MH, Tai CT, Lee SH, et al: The different mechanisms between late and very late recurrences of atrial fibrillation in patients undergoing a repeated catheter ablation. J Cardiovasc Electrophysiol 2006;17:231.
108. Takahashi Y, O'Neill MD, Hocini M, et al: Effects of stepwise ablation of chronic atrial fibrillation on atrial electrical and mechanical properties. J Am Coll Cardiol 2007;49:1306.
109. Bertaglia E, Zoppo F, Tondo C, et al: Early complications of pulmonary vein catheter ablation for atrial fibrillation: A multicenter prospective registry on procedural safety. Heart Rhythm 2007;4:1265.
110. Packer DL, Keelan P, Munger TM, et al: Clinical presentation, investigation, and management of pulmonary vein stenosis complicating ablation for atrial fibrillation. Circulation 2005;111:546.
111. Di BL, Fahmy TS, Wazni OM, et al: Pulmonary vein total occlusion following catheter ablation for atrial fibrillation: Clinical implications after long-term follow-up. J Am Coll Cardiol 2006;48:2493.
112. Cheung P, Hall B, Chugh A, et al: Detection of inadvertent catheter movement into a pulmonary vein during radiofrequency catheter ablation by real-time impedance monitoring. J Cardiovasc Electrophysiol 2004;15:674-678.
113. Dixit S, Marchlinski FE: How to recognize, manage, and prevent complications during atrial fibrillation ablation. Heart Rhythm 2007;4:108.
114. Hsu LF, Jais P, Hocini M, et al: Incidence and prevention of cardiac tamponade complicating ablation for atrial fibrillation. Pacing Clin Electrophysiol 2005;28(Suppl 1):S106.
115. Kanj MH, Wazni O, Fahmy T, et al: Pulmonary vein antral isolation using an open irrigation ablation catheter for the treatment of atrial fibrillation: a randomized pilot study. J Am Coll Cardiol 2007;49:1634.
116. Hsu L, Jais P, Hocini M, et al: Incidence and prevention of cardiac tamponade complicating ablation for atrial fibrillation. PACE 2005;28:S106-S109.
117. Bunch TJ, Asirvatham SJ, Friedman PA, et al: Outcomes after cardiac perforation during radiofrequency ablation of the atrium. J Cardiovasc Electrophysiol 2005;16:1172-1179.
118. Pappone C, Oral H, Santinelli V, et al: Atrioesophageal fistula as a complication of percutaneous transcatheter ablation of atrial fibrillation. Circulation 2004;109:2724.
119. Piorkowski C, Hindricks G, Schreiber D, et al: Electroanatomical reconstruction of the left atrium, pulmonary veins, and esophagus compared with the "true anatomy" on multislice computed tomography in patients undergoing catheter ablation of atrial fibrillation. Heart Rhythm 2006;3:317.
120. Sherzer AI, Feigenblum DY, Kulkarni S, et al: Continuous nonfluoroscopic localization of the esophagus during radiofrequency catheter ablation of atrial fibrillation. J Cardiovasc Electrophysiol 2007;18:157.
121. Kenigsberg DN, Lee BP, Grizzard JD, et al: Accuracy of intracardiac echocardiography for assessing the esophageal course along the posterior left atrium: A comparison to magnetic resonance imaging. J Cardiovasc Electrophysiol 2007;18:169.
122. Ren JF, Lin D, Marchlinski FE, et al: Esophageal imaging and strategies for avoiding injury during left atrial ablation for atrial fibrillation. Heart Rhythm 2006;3:1156.
123. Cummings JE, Schweikert RA, Saliba WI, et al: Assessment of temperature, proximity, and course of the esophagus during radiofrequency ablation within the left atrium. Circulation 2005;112:459.
124. Gerstenfeld EP, Callans DJ, Dixit S, et al: Mechanisms of organized left atrial tachycardias occurring after pulmonary vein isolation. Circulation 2004;110: 1351.
125. Chugh A, Oral H, Lemola K, et al: Prevalence, mechanisms, and clinical significance of macroreentrant atrial tachycardia during and following left atrial ablation for atrial fibrillation. Heart Rhythm 2005;2:464.
126. Chae S, Oral H, Good E, et al: Atrial tachycardia after circumferential pulmonary vein ablation of atrial fibrillation: Mechanistic insights, results of catheter ablation, and risk factors for recurrence. J Am Coll Cardiol 2007;50:1781.
127. Cappato R, Calkins H, Chen SA, et al: Worldwide survey on the methods, efficacy, and safety of catheter ablation for human atrial fibrillation. Circulation 2005;111:1100.
128. Wazni OM, Rossillo A, Marrouche NF, et al: Embolic events and char formation during pulmonary vein isolation in patients with atrial fibrillation: Impact of different anticoagulation regimens and importance of intracardiac echo imaging. J Cardiovasc Electrophysiol 2005;16:576.
129. Sacher F, Monahan KH, Thomas SP, et al: Phrenic nerve injury after atrial fibrillation catheter ablation: Characterization and outcome in a multicenter study. J Am Coll Cardiol 2006;47:2498.
130. Kesek M, Englund A, Jensen SM, Jensen-Urstad M: Entrapment of circular mapping catheter in the mitral valve. Heart Rhythm 2007;4:17.
131. Lickfett L, Mahesh M, Vasamreddy C, et al: Radiation exposure during catheter ablation of atrial fibrillation. Circulation 2004;110:3003.
132. Morady F: Patient-specific ablation strategy for atrial fibrillation: Promises and difficulties. Heart Rhythm 2007;4:1094.
133. Oral H, Morady F: How to select patients for atrial fibrillation ablation. Heart Rhythm 2006;3:615.
134. Earley MJ, Abrams DJ, Staniforth AD, et al: Catheter ablation of permanent atrial fibrillation: Medium-term results. Heart 2006;92:233.
135. Hsu LF, Jais P, Sanders P, et al: Catheter ablation for atrial fibrillation in congestive heart failure. N Engl J Med 2004;351:2373.
136. Liu X, Dong J, Mavrakis HE, et al: Achievement of pulmonary vein isolation in patients undergoing circumferential pulmonary vein ablation: A randomized comparison between two different isolation approaches. J Cardiovasc Electrophysiol 2006;17:1263-1270.
137. Pappone C, Vicedomini G, Manguso F, et al: Robotic magnetic navigation for atrial fibrillation ablation. J Am Coll Cardiol 2006;47:1390.
138. Issa ZF: An approach to ablate and pace: AV junction ablation and pacemaker implantation performed concurrently from the same venous access site. Pacing Clin Electrophysiol 2007;30:1116.
139. Ozcan C, Jahangir A, Friedman PA, et al: Sudden death after radiofrequency ablation of the atrioventricular node in patients with atrial fibrillation. J Am Coll Cardiol 2002;40:105.
140. Manolis AS: The deleterious consequences of right ventricular apical pacing: Time to seek alternate site pacing. Pacing Clin Electrophysiol 2006;29:298.
141. Rokas S, Gaitanidou S, Chatzidou S, et al: Atrioventricular node modification in patients with chronic atrial fibrillation: role of morphology of RR interval variation. Circulation 2001;103:2942.

CHAPTER 12

Inappropriate Sinus Tachycardia

PATHOPHYSIOLOGY

Inappropriate sinus tachycardia is a nonparoxysmal tachyarrhythmia characterized by a persistent increase in resting sinus rate unrelated to, or out of proportion with, the level of physical, emotional, pathological, or pharmacological stress, and/or an exaggerated heart rate response to minimal exertion or a change in body posture.[1] Inappropriate sinus tachycardia is neither a response to a pathological process (e.g., heart failure, hyperthyroidism, hypovolemia, anemia, infection, diabetic autonomic dysfunction, pheochromocytoma, orthostatic hypotension, or drug effects) nor a result of physical deconditioning.

The underlying mechanism of inappropriate sinus tachycardia is not well understood. Several potential mechanisms have been suggested, including enhanced automaticity of the sinus node, disorder of autonomic responsiveness of the sinus node, manifest as enhanced sympathetic tone (either directly or via increased sympathetic receptor sensitivity or blunted parasympathetic tone), and primary abnormality of sinus node function as evidenced by higher intrinsic heart rate (after total autonomic blockade) than that found in normal controls or blunted response to adenosine with less sinus cycle length (CL) prolongation than control subjects (with and without autonomic blockade).[2,3] In addition, impaired baroreflex sensitivity and autonomic neuritis or autonomic neuropathy can play a role in some cases. The extent to which each of these mechanisms contributes to tachycardia and associated symptoms is unknown. In some patients, there can be an overlap between inappropriate sinus tachycardia and disorders such as chronic fatigue syndrome and neurocardiogenic syncope, and in others there can be a psychological component of hypersensitivity to somatic input.[4] Other groups with similar or overlapping laboratory findings and clinical course include hyperadrenergic syndrome, idiopathic hypovolemia,[5] orthostatic hypotension, and mitral valve prolapse syndrome.[2,3]

CLINICAL CONSIDERATIONS

Epidemiology

Almost all patients afflicted with inappropriate sinus tachycardia are young women (mean age, 38 ± 12 years), and many of them are hypertensive. Inappropriate sinus tachycardia affects people working in health care in disproportionate numbers. The explanation for these findings is lacking.[3,6]

Clinical Presentation

The most prominent symptoms are palpitations, fatigue, and exercise intolerance. Inappropriate sinus tachycardia can also be associated with a host of other symptoms, including chest pain, dyspnea, lightheadedness, dizziness, and presyncope. The degree of disability can vary tremendously, from totally asymptomatic patients identified during routine medical examination to individuals with chronic, incessant, and debilitating symptoms.[2,6]

Initial Evaluation

Inappropriate sinus tachycardia is an ill-defined clinical syndrome with diverse clinical manifestations. There is no gold standard to make a definitive diagnosis of inappropriate sinus tachycardia, and the diagnosis remains a clinical one after exclusion of other causes of symptomatic tachycardia. Clinical examination and routine investigations allow elimination of secondary causes for the tachycardia but are generally not helpful in establishing the diagnosis.[1-3]

The syndrome of inappropriate sinus tachycardia is characterized by the following: (1) a relative or absolute increase in sinus rate out of proportion to the physiological demand (there can be an increased resting sinus rate of more than 100 beats/min or an exaggerated heart rate response to minimal exertion or change in body posture); (2) P wave axis and morphology during tachycardia are similar or identical to that during normal sinus rhythm (NSR); (3) no secondary causes of sinus tachycardia can be diagnosed; and (4) markedly distressing symptoms of palpitations, fatigue, dyspnea, and anxiety during tachycardia, with absence of symptoms during normal sinus rates.[1-3,7,8]

Ambulatory Holter recordings characteristically demonstrate a mean heart rate of more than 90-95 beats/min (Fig. 12-1). However, some patients have either a physiological or normal heart rate at rest (less than 85 beats/min) with an inappropriate tachycardia response to a minimal physiological challenge, or moderately elevated resting heart rate (more than 85 beats/min) with accentuated (inappropriate) heart rate response to minimal exertion.[2,3,9] However, this quantitative definition of inappropriate is arbitrary, and validation of the reproducibility of the heart rate and activity correlation can be challenging.[7,10]

Exercise ECG testing typically shows an early and excessive increase of heart rate in response to minimal exercise (heart rate more than 130 beats/min within 90 seconds of exercise; Bruce protocol). This heart rate response is differentiated from physical deconditioning by chronicity and the presence of associated symptoms.[2]

Isoproterenol provocation helps demonstrate sinus node hypersensitivity to beta-adrenergic stimulation. Isoproterenol is administered as escalating intravenous boluses at 1-minute intervals, starting at 0.25 μg, with doubling of the dose every minute, until a target of heart rate increase by 35 beats/min above baseline or a maximum heart rate of 150 beats/min is reached. In patients with inappropriate sinus tachycardia, the target heart rate is reached with an isoproterenol dose of 0.29 ± 0.1 μg (versus 1.27 ± 0.4 μg in normal controls).[2]

Invasive electrophysiological (EP) testing may be considered when other arrhythmias are suspected or when a decision to proceed with catheter ablation is undertaken. It is important to recognize that sinus node modification to target inappropriate sinus tachycardia is a clinical decision, and it must be made prior to the invasive EP study itself. The diagnosis of inappropriate sinus tachycardia and the treatment approach have to be established before bringing the patient to the EP laboratory.[2,3]

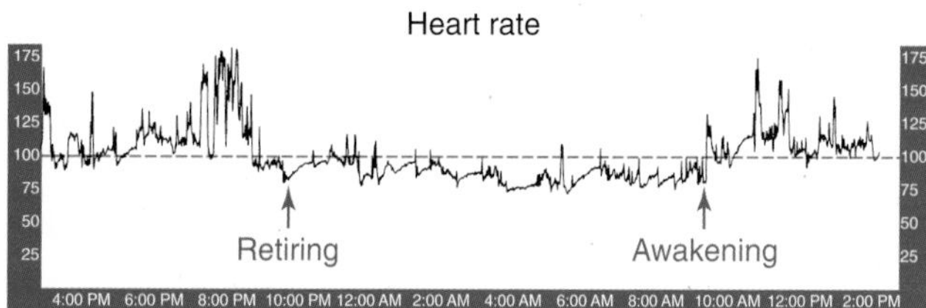

FIGURE 12–1 A 24-hour trend of the long-term ECG showing inappropriate sinus tachycardia throughout usual activity and on awakening.

Principles of Management

The treatment of inappropriate sinus tachycardia is predominantly symptom driven. Medical management remains the mainstay of therapy. Beta blockers can be useful and should be prescribed as first-line therapy for most of these patients. Verapamil and diltiazem can also be effective.[1] Sinus node modification by catheter ablation remains a potentially important therapeutic option in the most refractory cases of inappropriate sinus tachycardia.[1,2] The risk of tachycardia-induced cardiomyopathy in untreated patients is unknown but is likely to be low.[1,6]

ELECTROPHYSIOLOGICAL TESTING

The goals of EP testing in patients with inappropriate sinus tachycardia are to exclude other tachycardias that can mimic sinus tachycardia, such as atrial tachycardia (AT) originating near the superior aspect of the crista terminalis or right superior pulmonary vein (PV), and to ensure that the tachycardia occurring spontaneously or, more likely with isoproterenol infusion, acts in a manner consistent with an exaggeration of normal sinus node physiology.[2,3]

For activation sequence mapping, a multipolar crista catheter (20-pole) is placed along the crista terminalis in addition to the catheters used for a routine EP evaluation (coronary sinus [CS], His bundle [HB], and right ventricular [RV] apex). The crista catheter is positioned on the crista terminalis from the superomedial aspect originating at the junction of the superior vena cava (SVC) and right atrial (RA) appendage inferolaterally, with continuation along the crista toward the junction of the inferior vena cava (IVC) and RA. Catheter contact with the crista terminalis can be enhanced by using a long sheath (Fig. 12-2). Intracardiac echocardiography (ICE) can also be used to identify the crista terminalis and guide mapping catheter positioning as well as RF ablation.[2,3]

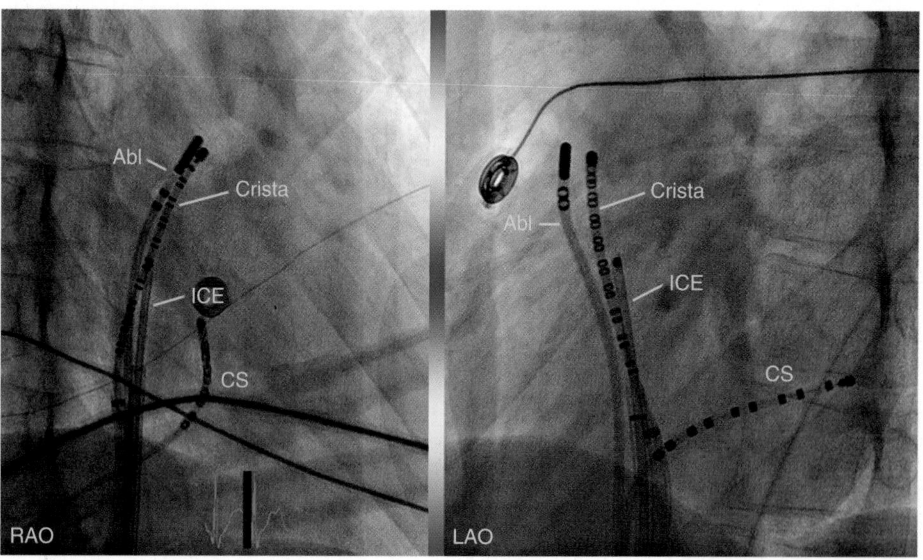

FIGURE 12–2 Right anterior oblique (RAO) and left anterior oblique (LAO) fluoroscopic view during sinus node modification. Multipolar (crista) catheter is placed along the crista terminalis with intracardiac echocardiography (ICE) guidance. CS = coronary sinus.

Induction of Tachycardia

Programmed electrical stimulation is performed before and after isoproterenol infusion. Isoproterenol infusion is started at 0.5 to 1.0 μg/min and titrated every 3 to 5 minutes to a maximum of 6 μg/min. Atropine (1 mg) can also be administered to assess maximum sinus CL. It is important to document failure to induce AT and other supraventricular tachycardias (SVTs) during programmed stimulation. Inappropriate sinus tachycardia cannot be initiated with atrial rapid pacing or extrastimulation, but can be induced by adrenergic stimulation. Initiation of inappropriate sinus tachycardia is associated with a gradual increase of the sinus rate, with a gradual shift of the earliest atrial activation site up the crista terminalis.

EP phenomena such as dual atrioventricular node (AVN) physiology or AVN echo beats should be cautiously evaluated in patients in whom the only documented symptomatic tachycardia appears to have a sinus mechanism, and the relevance of these phenomena should be carefully assessed.

Tachycardia Features

Atrial activation sequence during inappropriate sinus tachycardia is characterized by a craniocaudal activation sequence along the crista, with the site of earliest atrial activation shifting up the crista at faster rates and down the crista at slower rates. The earliest atrial activation site always occurs along the crista terminalis (as confirmed by the multipolar catheter placed on the crista) despite a changing tachycardia rate or autonomic modulation (isoproterenol and atropine).

There is a gradual increase and decrease in heart rate, in contrast to patients with focal AT, with changes in autonomic tone or at the initiation and termination of the tachycardia. Additionally, adrenergic stimulation reproducibly causes an increase in inappropriate sinus tachycardia rate and a cranial shift in atrial activation along the crista terminalis, whereas vagal stimulation causes slowing of the inappropriate sinus tachycardia rate with caudal shift.

Exclusion of Other Arrhythmia Mechanisms

Both sinus node reentrant tachycardia and focal AT have to be excluded. Sinus node reentry is easily and reproducibly initiated with atrial extrastimulation (AES), and AT can be initiated with AES, burst pacing, or adrenergic stimulation, whereas inappropriate sinus tachycardia cannot be initiated with programmed electrical stimulation. Furthermore, AT and the sinus node reentrant tachycardia rate can shift suddenly at initiation, although AT can then warm up over few beats, as opposed to the gradual increase of the inappropriate sinus tachycardia rate over seconds to minutes.

Atrial activation sequence shifts suddenly at the onset of AT or sinus node reentrant tachycardia, as opposed to a gradual cranial shift of the earliest atrial activation up the crista terminalis with adrenergic stimulation as the sinus rate increases during inappropriate sinus tachycardia. Although the rate of focal AT can continue to increase with continued adrenergic stimulation, this is not associated with a further shift in the atrial activation sequence.

Sinus node reentry is easily and reproducibly terminated with programmed stimulation, whereas inappropriate sinus tachycardia cannot be terminated with programmed stimulation. Termination of focal AT and sinus node reentry is sudden, as opposed to gradual slowing (cool down) of the inappropriate sinus tachycardia rate (Fig. 12-3). Vagal maneuvers result in abrupt termination of sinus node reentry and in either no effect or abrupt termination of AT, as opposed to gradual slowing and inferior shift down the crista terminalis of the site of origin of inappropriate sinus tachycardia. Abrupt termination of the tachycardia with a single radiofrequency (RF) application suggests AT, because inappropriate sinus tachycardia originates from a widespread area involving the superior crista terminalis.

ABLATION

Target of Ablation

The sinus node region is a distributed complex characterized by rate-dependent site differentiation (i.e., there is ana-

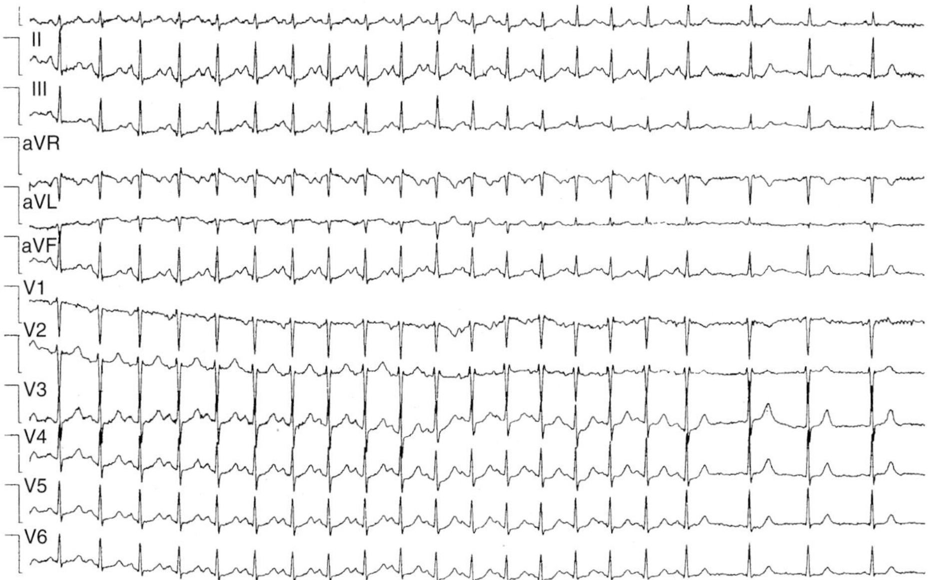

FIGURE 12–3 A 12-lead ECG showing perinodal focal atrial tachycardia (AT) (or sinus node reentrant tachycardia) with abrupt termination and restoration of normal sinus rhythm. Note the similarities between the tachycardia and sinus P wave morphology.

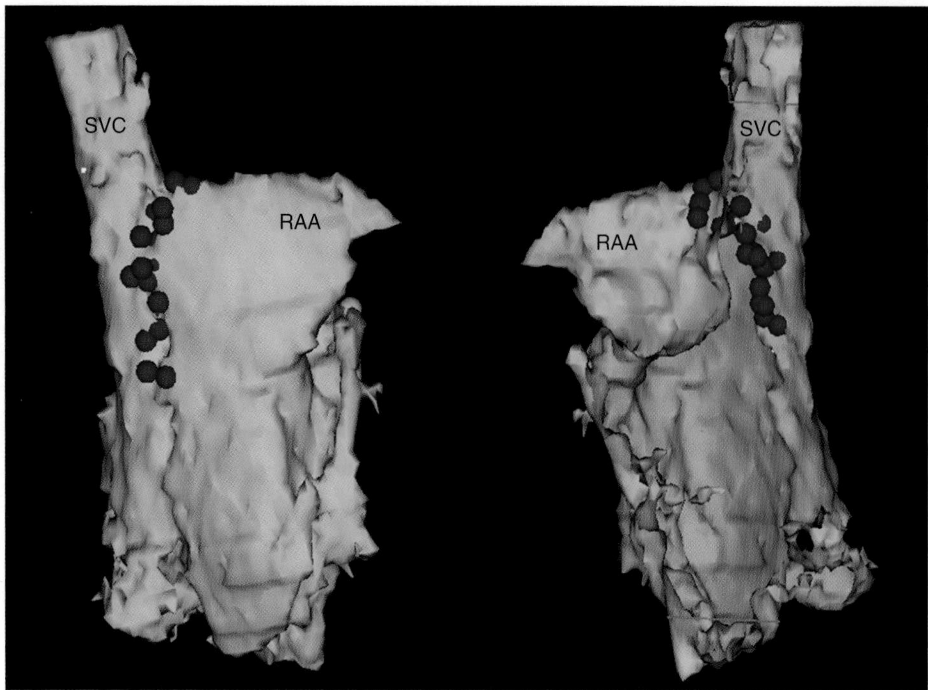

FIGURE 12–4 Integrated CT and electroanatomical (CARTO) map of the right atrium acquired during sinus node modification. Right anterior oblique and cardioscopic views of the CT scan are shown. Note the area targeted by radiofrequency ablation (red dots) starting cranially at the medial portion of the crista as it courses in front of the superior vena cava (SVC). RAA = right atrial appendage.

tomical distribution of impulse generation with changes in sinus rate), which allows for targeted ablation to eliminate the fastest sinus rates while maintaining some degree of sinus node function.[11]

Sinus node modification targets the site of most rapid discharge, generally at the superior aspect of the crista terminalis. One must recognize, however, that sinus node modification is not a focal ablation, but requires complete abolition of the cranial portion of the sinus node complex (Fig. 12-4). This eliminates the areas of the sinus node responsible for rapid rates while preserving some chronotropic competence.

Ablation Technique

The crista terminalis is not visible on fluoroscopy and has a varied course among patients. Therefore, some operators prefer using ICE to help identify the crista, position the tip of the ablation catheter with firm contact on the crista, and assess the RF lesion (see Fig. 8-13).[12,13]

A 3-D mapping system (CARTO, NavX, RPM) can also help delineate relevant anatomical structures (SVC, boundaries of atrium), define the extent of earliest site of activation during inappropriate sinus tachycardia, delineate the course of the phrenic nerve (sites at which pacing stimulates diaphragm), and catalogue sites of ablation.[14,15]

A multipolar (20-pole) catheter is placed along the crista terminalis (with or without ICE guidance; see Fig. 12-2). An ablation catheter with a 4- or 8-mm tip is used for RF application. RF power is adjusted to achieve a tip temperature of 50° to 60°C and/or an impedance drop of 5 to 10 Ω. RF lesions are applied as guided by the earliest atrial activation sequence, usually along superior regions of the crista terminalis using the guidance of the crista catheter (with or without ICE). The local endocardial activation time recorded by the ablation catheter at successful sites typically precedes the onset of the surface P wave during the tachycardia by 25 to 45 milliseconds (Fig. 12-5).

RF ablation is performed under maximal adrenergic stimulation with isoproterenol (with or without parasympathetic blockade with atropine) to reveal the superior portions of the crista terminalis as the earliest sites of atrial activation. The medial portion of the crista as it courses in front of the SVC is the site of earliest activation for the fastest sinus rates; this portion of the crista should be targeted by RF ablation first. Progressively inferior portions of the crista are then ablated until target heart rate reduction is achieved. This often requires ablating an estimated area of 12 ± 4 × 195 mm.[14] Pacing from the ablation catheter tip at high output (5 to 10 mA) before each RF application to verify absence of diaphragmatic stimulation is necessary to avoid phrenic nerve injury.[2,3,13,15]

Acceleration of the sinus rate followed by a marked subsequent rate reduction or the appearance of a junctional rhythm during ablation is an indicator for successful ablation sites, and thereafter delivery of RF energy should be continued for at least 60 to 90 seconds. Most patients demonstrate a stepwise reduction in sinus rate during the course of ablation, associated with migration of the site of earliest atrial activation in a craniocaudal direction along the crista terminalis (see Fig. 12-5); however, it is not uncommon to observe an abrupt reduction in the sinus rate in response to RF ablation at a focal site of earliest atrial activation (Fig. 12-6).[15] Echocardiographic lesion characteristics using ICE can also provide a guide for directing additional RF lesions. The effective RF lesion has an increased and/or changed echodensity completely extending to the epicardium with the development of a trivial linear low echodensity or echo-free interstitial space, which suggests a transmural RF lesion.[16]

Endpoints of Ablation

Acute procedural success is defined as the following: (1) abrupt reduction of the sinus rate by 30 beats/min or more during RF delivery or a 30% decline in maximum heart rate during infused isoproterenol and atropine; (2) persistence of reduced sinus rate; (3) maintenance of a superiorly directed P wave (negative P wave in lead III); and (4) inferior shift of the site of earliest atrial activation down the crista terminalis, even with maximal adrenergic stimulation.[2,3,15]

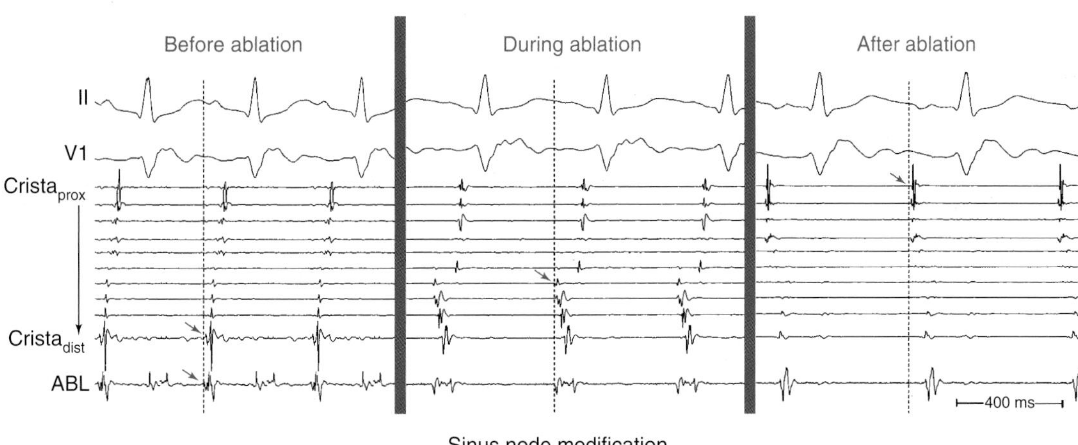

FIGURE 12–5 Intracardiac recordings during sinus node modification. **Left panel,** Before ablation and under adrenergic stimulation, sinus tachycardia is observed, with the earliest local activation (red arrows) recorded by the most distal (cranial) electrodes of crista catheter, just anterior to the superior vena cava–right atrial junction. Note that local activation recorded by the ablation catheter (blue arrow) precedes the onset of the P wave (indicated by the vertical dashed line) by 20 to 30 msec. **Middle panel,** Following ablation of the most cranial part of the sinus node, the sinus rate becomes slower and activation sequence shifts toward more proximal (caudal) electrodes 7-8 on the crista catheter. **Right panel,** Following successful sinus node modification, sinus rate (under constant adrenergic stimulation) is reduced by more than 30% and the atrial activation sequence shifts to the most proximal (caudal) crista catheter electrodes. Note the P wave is now inverted in lead II.

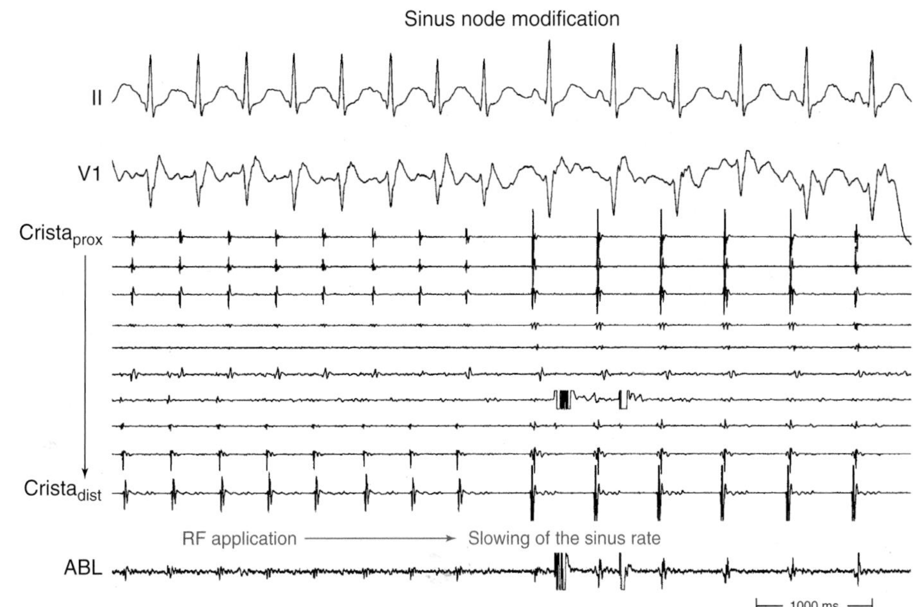

FIGURE 12–6 Intracardiac recordings during sinus node modification. An abrupt reduction in the sinus rate is observed in response to radiofrequency (RF) ablation at a focal site of earliest atrial activation.

RF ablation of inappropriate sinus tachycardia often is difficult and requires multiple RF applications; a mean of 12 RF applications (range, 6 to 92) was required in one study (see Fig. 12-4).[12] The resilience of the sinus node to endocardial catheter ablation can be explained, in part, by the architectural features of the node—the dense matrix of connective tissue in which the specialized sinus node cells are packed; the cooling effect of the nodal artery; the subepicardial nodal location; and the thick terminal crest, particularly in relation to the nodal portion caudal to the sinus node artery.[11] Additionally, the length of the sinus node, the absence of an insulating sheath, the presence of nodal radiations, and caudal fragments offer a potential for multiple breakthroughs of the nodal wavefront.[11]

Outcome

Prior to undertaking ablation of the sinus node for inappropriate sinus tachycardia, the physician and patient should have realistic expectations and understanding of the goals of ablation and potential outcomes. Relatively few patients will achieve the desired combination of relief of symptoms and normal resting heart rate and chronotropic response without the need for implantation of a permanent pacemaker. In some patients, symptoms persist despite an acceptable technical result.[2,3]

Radiofrequency ablation is at best only a modestly effective technique for managing patients with inappropriate sinus tachycardia. The long-term success rate is low, ranging between 23% and 83%.[4] Complete ablation of the sinus node resulting in junctional rhythm has a better long-term success (72%) but requires pacemaker insertion. Most recurrences occur 1 to 6 months after the procedure, and are typically related to electrophysiological and tachycardic recurrence after an initially successful procedure. However, symptomatic recurrence or persistence of symptoms in the absence of documented inappropriate sinus tachycardia and despite persisting evidence of a successful electrophysiological outcome has been observed in some cases. Persistent symptoms despite heart rate reduction can be suggestive of a more global dysautonomia that also happens to affect the sinus node.[2,3,13-15]

Complications of sinus node modification include cardiac tamponade, SVC syndrome, diaphragmatic paralysis, and sinus node dysfunction.[17] Cardiac tamponade is rare, and is usually caused by penetration of an unattended RV catheter in a thin female patient with rapid and vigorous heart action because of high-dose isoproterenol infusion. Transient SVC syndrome can develop because of extensive lesion creation and edema at the SVC-RA junction. This can rarely cause permanent SVC stenosis. More targeted ablation using ICE can help avoid this complication. Diaphragmatic paralysis secondary to damage to the phrenic nerve should be minimized if ablative lesions are confined to the crista itself or placed just anterior to it. Using ICE to guide ablation makes this complication unlikely because the phrenic nerve is a posterior structure. If concern still exists, pacing with a high output of 10 mA should be performed before delivery of RF energy. Additionally, suspicion of phrenic nerve injury should be considered in the case of hiccup, cough, or decrease in diaphragmatic excursion during energy delivery. Early recognition of phrenic nerve injury during RF delivery allows the immediate interruption of the application prior to the onset of permanent injury, which is associated with the rapid recovery of phrenic nerve function. Persistent junctional rhythm requiring pacemaker insertion is rare. Such junctional rhythm usually disappears with the return of sinus rhythm within several days.[2,3,15]

REFERENCES

1. Blomström-Lundqvist C, Scheinman MM, Aliot EM, et al; American College of Cardiology; American Heart Association Task Force on Practice Guidelines; European Society of Cardiology Committee for Practice Guidelines. Writing Committee to Develop Guidelines for the Management of Patients With Supraventricular Arrhythmias: ACC/AHA/ESC guidelines for the management of patients with supraventricular arrhythmias: Executive summary—a report of the American College of Cardiology/American Heart Association Task Force on Practice Guidelines and the European Society of Cardiology Committee for Practice Guidelines. Circulation 2003;108:1871.
2. Line D, Callans D: Sinus rhythm abnormalities. *In* Zipes DP, Jaliffe J (eds): Cardiac Electrophysiology: From Cell to Bedside, 4th ed. Philadelphia, WB Saunders, 2004. pp 479-484.
3. Desh M, Karch M, Kalman J, et al: Ablation of inappropriate sinus tachycardia. *In* Huang S, Wilber D (eds): Radiofrequency Catheter Ablation of Cardiac Arrhythmias: Basic Concepts and Clinical Applications, 2nd ed. Armonk, NY, Futura, 2000, pp 165-174.
4. Shen WK, Low PA, Jahangir A, et al: Is sinus node modification appropriate for inappropriate sinus tachycardia with features of postural orthostatic tachycardia syndrome? Pacing Clin Electrophysiol 2001;24:217.
5. Goldstein DS, Holmes C, Frank SM, et al: Cardiac sympathetic dysautonomia in chronic orthostatic intolerance syndromes. Circulation 2002;106:2358.
6. Still AM, Raatikainen P, Ylitalo A, et al: Prevalence, characteristics and natural course of inappropriate sinus tachycardia. Europace 2005;7:104.
7. Shen WK: Modification and ablation for inappropriate sinus tachycardia: Current status. Cardiol Electrophysiol Rev 2002;6:349.
8. Leon H, Guzman JC, Kuusela T, et al: Impaired baroreflex gain in patients with inappropriate sinus tachycardia. J Cardiovasc Electrophysiol 2005;16:64.
9. Brady PA, Low PA, Shen WK: Inappropriate sinus tachycardia, postural orthostatic tachycardia syndrome, and overlapping syndromes. Pacing Clin Electrophysiol 2005;28:1112.
10. Vatasescu R, Shalganov T, Kardos A, et al: Right diaphragmatic paralysis following endocardial cryothermal ablation of inappropriate sinus tachycardia. Europace 2006;8:904.
11. Sanchez-Quintana D, Cabrera JA, et al: Sinus node revisited in the era of electroanatomical mapping and catheter ablation. Heart 2005;91:189.
12. Ren JF, Marchlinski FE, Callans DJ, Zado ES: Echocardiographic lesion characteristics associated with successful ablation of inappropriate sinus tachycardia. J Cardiovasc Electrophysiol 2001;12:814.
13. Mantovan R, Thiene G, Calzolari V, Basso C: Sinus node ablation for inappropriate sinus tachycardia. J Cardiovasc Electrophysiol 2005;16:804.
14. Marrouche NF, Beheiry S, Tomassoni G, et al: Three-dimensional nonfluoroscopic mapping and ablation of inappropriate sinus tachycardia. Procedural strategies and long-term outcome. J Am Coll Cardiol 2002;39:1046.
15. Man KC, Knight B, Tse HF, et al: Radiofrequency catheter ablation of inappropriate sinus tachycardia guided by activation mapping. J Am Coll Cardiol 2000;35:451.
16. Ren JF, Callans D: Intracardiac echocardiography imaging in radiofrequency catheter ablation for inappropriate sinus tachycardia and atrial tachycardias. *In* Ren JF, Marchlinski FE, Callans D (eds): Practical Intracardiac Echocardiography in Electrophysiology. Malden, Mass, Blackwell Futura, 2006, pp 74-87.
17. Leonelli FM, Pisano E, Requarth JA, et al: Frequency of superior vena cava syndrome following radiofrequency modification of the sinus node and its management. Am J Cardiol 2000;85:771.

CHAPTER 13

Atrioventricular Nodal Reentrant Tachycardia

PATHOPHYSIOLOGY

Anatomy and Physiology of the Atrioventricular Node

The AV junction is a complex structure, located within an area called the triangle of Koch (Fig. 13-1).[1,2] The triangle of Koch is bounded by the coronary sinus ostium (CS os) posteriorly, the tricuspid annulus (the attachment of the septal leaflet of the tricuspid valve) inferiorly, and the tendon of Todaro anteriorly and superiorly. The triangle of Koch is septal in location, and constitutes the right atrial (RA) endocardial surface of the muscular atrioventricular (AV) septum. The compact atrioventricular node (AVN) lies just beneath the RA endocardium, at the apex of the triangle of Koch, anterior to the CS os, and directly above the insertion of the septal leaflet of the tricuspid valve, where the tendon of Todaro merges with the central fibrous body. Slightly more anteriorly and superiorly is where the His bundle (HB) penetrates the AV junction through the central fibrous body and the posterior aspect of the membranous AV septum.[3]

Histological studies have demonstrated that two different areas connect the atrial myocardium to the HB, the transitional cell zone and compact AVN. The compact AVN is a dense network of nodal tissue composed of "typical" AVN (midnodal) cells. The transitional cell zone represents the inferior, more open portion of the AVN into which atrial bands gradually merge (i.e., the approaches from the working atrial myocardium to the AVN). The connections between atrial and transitional cells are so gradual that no clear anatomical demarcations can be detected.[4,5]

Based on activation times during antero-grade and/or retrograde propagation and on the action potential characteristics, the cells of the AVN region are frequently described as AN (atrionodal), N (nodal), and NH (nodal-His). The AN region corresponds to the cells in the transitional region, which are activated shortly after the atrial cells. The N region corresponds to the region where the transitional cells merge with midnodal cells. The NH region corresponds to the lower nodal cells, typically distal to the site of Wenckebach block, and their action potentials are closer in appearance to the fast-rising and long action potentials of the HB. The transition from one cell area to the other is gradual, with intermediate cells exhibiting intermediate action potentials with great changes related to the autonomic tone.[3,6,7]

The N cells represent the most typical of the nodal cells, because they are characterized by a less negative resting membrane potential and low action potential amplitude (mediated by the L-type Ca^{+2} current), slow rates of depolarization and repolarization, few intercellular connections such as gap junctions, and reduced excitability compared with surrounding cells. The N cells in the compact AVN appear to be responsible for the major part of AV conduction delay. Fast pathway conduction through the AVN apparently bypasses many of the N cells by transitional cells, whereas slow pathway conduction traverses the entire compact AVN. Importantly, the recovery of excitability after conduction of an impulse is faster for the slow pathway than for the fast pathway for reasons that are unclear.[6-8]

AVN conduction involves funneling of atrial depolarization into the compact AVN via discrete AVN inputs (approaches). In humans and animals, two such inputs are commonly recognized in the right septal region—the anterior (superior) approaches, which travel from the anterior limbus of the fossa ovalis and merge with the AVN closer to the apex of the triangle of Koch, and the posterior (inferior) approaches located in the inferoseptal RA and which serve as a bridge with the atrial myocardium at the CS os. Although both inputs have traditionally been assumed to be right atrial structures, growing evidence has supported the AV conduction apparatus as a transseptal structure that reaches both atria. A third, middle group of transitional cells has also been identified to account for the nodal connections with the septum and left atrium (LA).[3,6,9-11]

Tachycardia Circuit

The concept of AVN reentry is related, but not identical, to the so-called dual pathway electrophysiology. It is well established that dual AVN physiology is the underly-

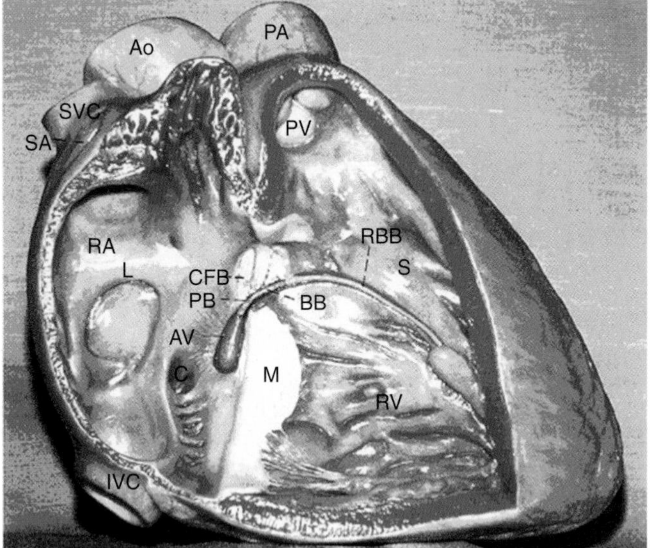

FIGURE 13–1 Right lateral view of the right atrium (RA). Ao = aorta; AR = anterior radiation of the left bundle branch; BB = bundle of His, branching portion; C = coronary sinus; CFB = central fibrous body; CM = central fibrous body and membranous portion of the interventricular system; L = limbus of the fossa ovalis; M = medial (septal) leaflet of the tricuspid valve; MLB = main left bundle branch; MS = midseptal fibers of the left bundle branch; MV = mitral valve; P = peripheral Purkinje fibers; PA = pulmonary artery; PB = bundle of His, penetrating portion; PR = posterior radiation of the left bundle branch; PT = pulmonary trunk; PV = pulmonary valves = septal band of the crista supraventricularis. (From Saffitz J, Zimmerman F, Lindsay B: *In* Braunwald E, McManus BM [eds]: Atlas of Cardiovascular Pathology for the Clinician. Philadelphia, Wiley-Blackwell, 2000, p 21.)

ing substrate for atrioventricular nodal reentrant tachycardia (AVNRT); however, it is important to recognize that dual AVN physiology characterizes the normal AVN electrophysiology, and the presence of dual (or multiple) AVN pathways does not result inevitably in the formation of a reentry loop and initiation of an atrial echo beat or sustained AVNRT. Nevertheless, the presence of dual AVN physiology provides the natural substrate for the occurrence of AVN reentry. In the absence of an animal model, however, the exact pathophysiological substrate for AVNRT is still uncertain.

The AVNRT circuit does not involve the ventricles, but whether the circuit is confined to the compact AVN (subatrial) or involves a component of atrial myocardium is still controversial. There is good evidence that the distal junction of the slow and fast pathways is located in the AVN, with the existence of a region of AVN tissue extending between the distal junction of the two pathways and the HB (called the lower common pathway) at least in a subset of patients (Table 13-1). However, the nature of the proximal link between these pathways is unclear, and the existence of an upper common pathway is still a matter of controversy (Tables 13-2 and 13-3). Based on rare cases of dissociation of atrial activation from the tachycardia and on similarities between fast-slow AV conduction and longitudinal-transverse conduction in nonuniform anisotropy, early studies have proposed that AVNRT results from reentry within the compact AVN as a result of functional longitudinal dissociation within the AVN into fast and slow pathways.[8] Current evidence, derived from multielectrode recordings and optical mapping studies, supports the role of perinodal tissue and suggests that the fast and slow pathways involved in the reentrant circuit of AVNRT represent conduction over different atrionodal connections, making the atrium a necessary part of the reentrant circuit.[12,13]

As noted, the compact AVN is surrounded by transitional cells whose structure and function are intermediate between those of atrial and compact nodal cells. If one considers the compact AVN and the surrounding transitional cells as a functional AVN unit, which implies that the AVN tissue occupies the bulk of the triangle of Koch, then the AVN reentrant circuit may be considered as confined to the AVN. Therefore, much of the disagreement on the presence or absence of an upper common pathway and the role of the atrium in the genesis of the reentrant circuit may, in part, be related to the definition of the extent of the AVN.[14]

Nevertheless, the understanding of the AVN as having superior (anterior) and inferior (posterior) inputs that form the fast and slow pathways, respectively, is a simple conceptual framework that seems to enable the clinician to confront most cases. Reentry occurring along these pathways is the basic mechanism for the various subtypes of AVNRT. The proximal atrial insertions of the fast and slow pathways are anatomically distinct during retrograde conduction, and several important functional differences exist between the two pathways (Table 13-4).[4,8]

Multiple slow pathways (as demonstrated by multiple discontinuities in the AVN function curves; see later) are present in up to 14% of patients with AVNRT, although not

TABLE 13–1 Evidence Against Necessity of Ventricle in Reentrant Circuit*

VA Wenckebach CL during ventricular pacing longer than the tachycardia CL
HA interval during ventricular pacing at the tachycardia CL longer than that during AVNRT
AV block occurring without interruption of AVNRT
AES during AVNRT resulting in changes in the relative activation of HB and atrium (i.e., varying HA intervals)
VES during AVNRT prematurely depolarizing the HB without affecting the tachycardia

From Josephson ME: Supraventricular tachycardias. *In* Josephson ME [ed]: Clinical Cardiac Electrophysiology, 3rd ed. Philadelphia, Lippincott, Williams & Wilkins, 2002, pp 168-271.

AES = atrial extrastimulation; AVNRT = atrioventricular nodal reentrant tachycardia; CL = cycle length; HA = His bundle–atrial; HB = His bundle; VA = ventricular-atrial; VES = ventricular extrastimulation.

*Supporting the presence of a lower common pathway.

TABLE 13–2 Evidence for Necessity of Atrium in Reentrant Circuit*

AES delivered to the inferior atrial septum close to the CS os during AVNRT just before the expected time of retrograde fast pathway conduction can activate the slow pathway and advance the SVT
Cure of AVNRT can be produced by placing ablative lesions in the perinodal atrial myocardium, as much as 10 mm or more from the compact AVN
Differences in the site of earliest atrial activation between retrograde conduction over the fast and slow pathway
Microelectrode and extracellular recordings and optical mapping of AVN reentrant echo beats in animals

From Josephson ME: Supraventricular tachycardias. *In* Josephson ME [ed]: Clinical Cardiac Electrophysiology, 3rd ed. Philadelphia, Lippincott, Williams & Wilkins, 2002, pp 168-271.

AES = atrial extrastimulation; AVN = atrioventricular node; AVNRT = atrioventricular nodal reentrant tachycardia; CS os = coronary sinus ostium; SVT = supraventricular tachycardia.

*That is, against the presence of an upper common pathway.

TABLE 13–3 Evidence Against Necessity of Atrium in Reentrant Circuit*
Initiation of AVNRT in the absence of an atrial echo
AV Wenckebach CL during atrial pacing longer than the tachycardia CL
AH interval during atrial pacing at the tachycardia CL longer than that during AVNRT
Retrograde VA block occurring without interruption of AVNRT
AVNRT occurrence in the presence of AF
Depolarization of the atria surrounding the AVN without affecting the tachycardia
Resetting of the tachycardia by ventricular stimulation in the absence of atrial activation
Heterogeneous atrial activation during AVNRT which is incompatible with atrial participation
Changing V-A relationship with minimal or no change in the tachycardia CL (suggesting that atrial activation is determined by the functional output to the atrium from the tachycardia and not causally related to it)

From Josephson ME: Supraventricular tachycardias. *In* Josephson ME [ed]: Clinical Cardiac Electrophysiology, 3rd ed. Philadelphia, Lippincott, Williams & Wilkins, 2002, pp 168-271.
AF = atrial fibrillation; AH = atrial-His bundle; AVN = atrioventricular node; AVNRT = atrioventricular nodal reentrant tachycardia; CL = cycle length; VA = ventricular-atrial.
*Supporting the presence of an upper common pathway.

TABLE 13–4 Functional Differences Between Fast and Slow Atrioventricular Node Pathways
The fast pathway forms the normal physiological conduction axis, and the AH interval during conduction over the fast pathway is usually no longer than 220 msec. Longer AH intervals can be caused by conduction over the slow pathway.
Anterograde ERP of the fast pathway is usually longer than that of the slow pathway. However, many exceptions exist.
Adrenergic stimulation tends to shorten the anterograde and retrograde ERP of the fast pathway to a greater extent than that of the slow pathway. Conversely, beta blockers tend to prolong ERP of the fast pathway more than that of the slow pathway.
Earliest atrial activation site during retrograde conduction over the fast pathway is in the anterior apex of the triangle of Koch at the same site recording the proximal His potential (although some studies showed the earliest site of atrial activation occurring in the anterior interatrial septum above the tendon of Todaro, outside the triangle of Koch), whereas that over the slow pathway is in the base of the triangle of Koch.

AH = atrial-His bundle; ERP = effective refractory period.

all of them are involved in the initiation and maintenance of AVNRT.[15,16] Whether these pathways represent discrete anatomically distinct circuits or are functionally present because of nonuniform anisotropy is unclear. Frequently, multiple slow pathways are in close proximity within the triangle of Koch, and elimination of multiple slow pathways with radiofrequency (RF) ablation at one site is observed in approximately 42% of cases. Slow pathways with longer conduction times have a more inferior location in the triangle of Koch when compared with locations producing a shorter atrial-His bundle (AH) interval.

Types of Atrioventricular Nodal Reentry

Slow-Fast (Typical, Common) Atrioventricular Nodal Reentrant Tachycardia

Typical AVNRT accounts for 90% of AVNRTs. The reentrant circuit uses the slow AVN pathway anterogradely and the fast pathway retrogradely. The earliest atrial activation during typical AVNRT is usually in the apex of the triangle of Koch; however, retrograde atrial activation over the fast pathway is heterogeneous and may be found at the CS os or on the left side of the septum in up to 9% of patients.[8,10,17-19]

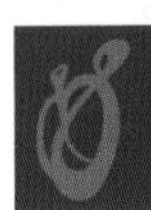

During typical AVNRT, atrial and ventricular activations occur almost simultaneously. The AH interval is relatively long (more than 200 milliseconds) and the HA interval is relatively short (less than 70 milliseconds), resulting in a short RP tachycardia.

The presence of a lower common pathway in typical AVNRT remains controversial. Although some studies have suggested the existence of a lower common pathway in most patients with typical AVNRT, others have demonstrated that most patients with AVNRT without evidence of a substantial lower common pathway had typical AVNRT (lower turnaround within the proximal HB) and that the presence of a lower common pathway was strongly associated with the atypical variants of AVNRT. Nevertheless, it is recognized that the lower common pathway in typical AVNRT, if present, is very short (as assessed by the degree of HB prematurity required for a ventricular extrastimulus [VES] to reset the tachycardia, and by comparing the His bundle-atrial (HA) interval during AVNRT with that during ventricular pacing at the tachycardia cycle length [CL]).[10,19,20]

Fast-Slow (Atypical, Uncommon) Atrioventricular Nodal Reentrant Tachycardia

In this variant of AVNRT, the reentrant circuit uses the fast AVN pathway anterogradely and the slow pathway retrogradely. Although fast-slow AVNRT is thought of as using the same circuit as typical AVNRT but in the reverse direction, two previous studies have reported different anatomical sites for the anterograde and retrograde slow pathways, and the fast-slow form of AVNRT may not be exactly the reverse form of the slow-fast form of AVNRT in some patients.[19]

The earliest retrograde atrial activation is usually in the inferoposterior part of the triangle of Koch. The AH interval is shorter than the HA interval (30 to 185 versus 135 to 435 milliseconds), resulting in a long RP tachycardia. The lower common pathway is relatively long.[10,20,21]

Slow-Slow (Posterior-Type) Atrioventricular Nodal Reentrant Tachycardia

In slow-slow AVNRT, the reentrant circuit uses the slow or an intermediate pathway anterogradely and a second slow pathway retrogradely. The earliest retrograde atrial activation occurs along the roof of the proximal CS or, less commonly, at the inferoposterior part of the triangle of Koch.[19]

The AH interval is long (more than 200 milliseconds). The HA interval is often short, but has a much wider range than that in typical AVNRT (−30 to 260 milliseconds, usually more than 70 milliseconds). The ventricular-atrial (VA) interval (as measured from the onset of ventricular activity to the onset of atrial activity by whichever electrode recorded the earliest interval) may be prolonged, ranging from 76 to 168 milliseconds. The AH/HA ratio, however, remains more than 1. Therefore, this type is sometimes called slow-intermediate AVNRT. The lower common pathway is significantly longer than that in typical AVNRT, which explains the short HA interval seen in many patients with slow-slow AVNRT. These patients often exhibit multiple AH interval jumps during atrial extrastimulus (AES) testing, consistent with multiple slow pathways.[10,20]

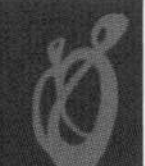

Left Variant of Atrioventricular Nodal Reentrant Tachycardia

It has been known for some time that the slow pathway may be composed of both rightward and leftward posterior nodal extensions. The rightward extensions travel anatomically in the triangle of Koch between the tricuspid annulus and CS os. The leftward extensions travel within the myocardial coat of the proximal CS leftward (transseptally) toward the left inferoseptal region and mitral annulus. These leftward extensions can then connect with the rightward extensions in the triangle of Koch anterior to the CS os. The leftward inferior extension can provide an LA input to the AVN, as suggested by functional studies showing preferential access to the AVN from the left inferior septum.[22,23] Clinically, the leftward inferior nodal extension can behave as the slow pathway and lead to AVNRT. In typical (fast-slow) forms of AVNRT, this would render ablation in the usual inferoseptal RA ineffective and lead to the necessity of ablating inside the CS.[10] In atypical forms of AVNRT, if the leftward inferior extension serves as the slow pathway conducting retrogradely, then the earliest atrial activation would be recorded in the LA, leading to eccentric CS activation.[11,24]

Eccentric retrograde atrial activation sequences that are suggestive of leftward atrionodal extensions of the slow AVN pathway have been described in AVNRT, but the exact incidence is unknown. Various reports have shown a higher incidence of the eccentric CS activation pattern among those with atypical (14% to 80%) than those with typical (0% to 8%) forms of AVNRT.[10,18,20,23-29] However, even in the presence of eccentric retrograde atrial activation during AVNRT, the significance of such leftward extensions to the AVNRT circuit has been debated. Whether the retrograde left-sided atrionodal connection constitutes the critical component of the reentrant circuit or is only an innocent bystander in atypical AVNRT with the eccentric CS activation pattern is controversial. It may be possible for both the leftward and rightward extensions, either together or separately, to participate in nodal reentry. Right-sided ablation is probably sufficient for most of these patients. However, in some patients, the slow pathway participating in the reentrant circuit cannot be ablated from the posteroseptal RA or the CS os, but can be eliminated by ablation along the roof of the CS os, as much as 5 to 6 cm from the CS os, or mitral annulus. In a recent report, direct left-sided ablation to the earliest retrograde activation site inside the CS (without ablation at the conventional site of the slow pathway) rendered the tachycardias noninducible in all 18 patients, which suggests that the left-sided slow pathway constituted critical parts of the reentrant circuit.[10,30]

CLINICAL CONSIDERATIONS

Epidemiology

AVNRT is the most common form of paroxysmal supraventricular tachycardia (SVT). The absolute number of patients with AVNRT and its proportion of paroxysmal SVT increase with age, which may be related to the normal evolution of AVN physiology over the first 2 decades of life, as well as to age-related changes in atrial and nodal physiology observed in later decades.[31] AVNRT often becomes manifest in the teenage years. There is also a striking 2:1 predominance of women, which remains without clear physiological or anatomical explanation.[31]

CLINICAL PRESENTATION

Patients with AVNRT typically present with the clinical syndrome of paroxysmal SVT. This is characterized as a regular rapid tachycardia of abrupt onset and termination. Patients commonly describe palpitations and dizziness. Rapid ventricular rates can be associated with complaints of dyspnea, weakness, angina, or even frank syncope and can at times be disabling. Neck pounding during tachycardia in patients with AVNRT is caused by simultaneous contraction of the atria and ventricles against closed mitral and tricuspid valves. This clinical feature has been reported to distinguish paroxysmal SVT resulting from AVNRT from that caused by orthodromic AVRT. Episodes can last from seconds to several hours. Patients often learn to use certain maneuvers such as carotid sinus massage or the Valsalva maneuver to terminate the arrhythmia, although many require pharmacological treatment. There is no significant association of AVNRT with other types of structural heart disease. The physical examination is usually remarkable only for a rapid, regular heart rate. At times, because of the simultaneous contraction of atria and ventricles, cannon A waves can be seen in the jugular venous waveform.[10]

Initial Evaluation

History, physical examination, and 12-lead ECG constitute an appropriate initial evaluation. In patients with brief, self-terminating episodes, an event recorder is the most effective way to obtain ECG documentation. An echocardiographic examination should be considered in patients with documented sustained SVT to exclude the possibility of structural heart disease.[32] Further diagnostic studies are indicated only if there are signs or symptoms that suggest structural heart disease.[10]

The diagnosis of AVNRT as the mechanism of SVT can be strongly suspected based on the surface ECG but is often difficult to confirm, especially when only single-lead rhythm strips are available during the SVT. Electrophysiological (EP) testing, however, is not indicated unless a decision to proceed with catheter ablation is undertaken.

Principles of Management

Acute Management

Because maintenance of AVNRT is dependent on AVN conduction, maneuvers or drugs that slow AVN conduction can be used to terminate the tachycardia. Initially, maneuvers that increase vagal tone (e.g., Valsalva maneuvers, gagging, carotid sinus massage) are used.[32] When vagal maneuvers are unsuccessful, termination can be achieved with antiarrhythmic drugs whose primary effects increase refractoriness and/or decrease conduction (negative dromotropic effect) over the AVN. Adenosine is the drug of choice and is successful in almost 100% of cases.[32] Verapamil, diltiazem, and beta blockers can also terminate AVNRT and prevent induction. Digoxin, which has a slower onset of action than the other AVN blockers, is not favored for the acute termination of AVNRT, except if there are relative contraindications to the other agents. Class IA and IC sodium-channel blockers can also be used in treating an acute event of AVNRT, a strategy that is rarely used when other regimens have failed. If AVNRT cannot be terminated with intravenous drugs, DC cardioversion can always be used. Energies in the range of 10 to 50 J are usually adequate.[10]

Chronic Management

Because AVNRT is generally a benign arrhythmia that does not influence survival, the primary indication for its treatment relates to its impact on a patient's quality of life. Factors that contribute to the therapeutic decision include the frequency and duration of tachycardia, tolerance of symptoms, effectiveness and tolerance of antiarrhythmic drugs, the need for lifelong drug therapy, and the presence of concomitant structural heart disease. Patients who develop a highly symptomatic episode of paroxysmal SVT, particularly if it requires an emergency room visit for termination, can elect to initiate therapy after a single episode. In contrast, a patient who presents with minimally symptomatic episodes of paroxysmal SVT that terminate spontaneously or with Valsalva maneuvers may elect to be followed clinically without specific therapy.[10,32]

Once it is decided to initiate treatment for AVNRT, the question arises of whether to initiate pharmacological therapy or use catheter ablation. Because of its greater than 95% efficacy and low incidence of complications, catheter ablation has become the preferred therapy over long-term pharmacological therapy, and can be offered as an initial therapeutic option. It is reasonable to discuss catheter ablation with all patients suspected of having AVNRT. Patients considering RF ablation must be willing to accept the risk, albeit low, of AV block and pacemaker implantation. For patients in whom ablation is not desirable or available, long-term pharmacological therapy can be effective.[32]

Most pharmacological agents that depress AVN conduction (including beta blockers and calcium channel blockers) can reduce the frequency of recurrences of AVNRT. If those agents are ineffective, class IA, IC, or III antiarrhythmic agents may be considered. In general, drug efficacy is in the range of 30% to 50%.[10]

Outpatients can use a single dose of verapamil, propranolol, or flecainide to terminate an episode of AVNRT effectively. This so-called pill in the pocket approach (i.e., administration of a drug only during an episode of tachycardia for the purpose of termination of the arrhythmia when vagal maneuvers alone are not effective) is appropriate to consider for patients with infrequent episodes of AVNRT that are prolonged but yet well tolerated, and obviates exposure of patients to chronic and unnecessary therapy between their rare arrhythmic events. This approach necessitates the use of a drug that has a short onset of action (i.e., immediate-release preparations).[32,33] Candidate patients should be free of significant left ventricular (LV) dysfunction, sinus bradycardia, and preexcitation. Single-dose oral therapy with diltiazem (120 mg) plus propranolol (80 mg) has been shown to be superior to both placebo and flecainide in terminating AVNRT.[10,32]

ELECTROCARDIOGRAPHIC FEATURES

P Wave Morphology. In typical (slow-fast) AVNRT, the P wave is usually not visible because of the simultaneous atrial and ventricular activation. The P wave can distort the initial portion of the QRS (mimicking a q wave in the inferior leads), lie just within the QRS (inapparent), or distort the terminal portion of the QRS (mimicking an s wave in the inferior leads or an r wave in lead V_1) (Fig. 13-2).[10,25] When apparent, the P wave is significantly narrower than the sinus P wave and is negative in the inferior leads, consistent with concentric retrograde atrial activation over the fast AVN pathway.[10] In atypical (fast-slow) AVNRT, the P wave is relatively narrow, negative in the inferior leads and positive in lead V_1 (see Fig. 13-2).[10,25]

QRS Morphology. QRS morphology during AVNRT is usually the same as in normal sinus rhythm (NSR). The development of prolonged functional aberration during AVNRT is uncommon, and it usually occurs following induction of AVNRT by ventricular stimulation more frequently than by atrial stimulation, or following resumption of 1:1 conduction to the ventricles after a period of block below the tachycardia circuit.[10,25] At times, alternans of QRS amplitude can occur when the tachycardia rates are rapid. Occasionally, AVNRT can coexist with ventricular preexcitation over an AV bypass tract (BT), whereby the BT is an innocent bystander.[10]

P-QRS Relationship. In typical (slow-fast) AVNRT, the RP interval is very short (−40 to 75 milliseconds).[10,25,34] Variation of the P-QRS relation with or without block can occur during AVNRT, especially in atypical or multiple-form

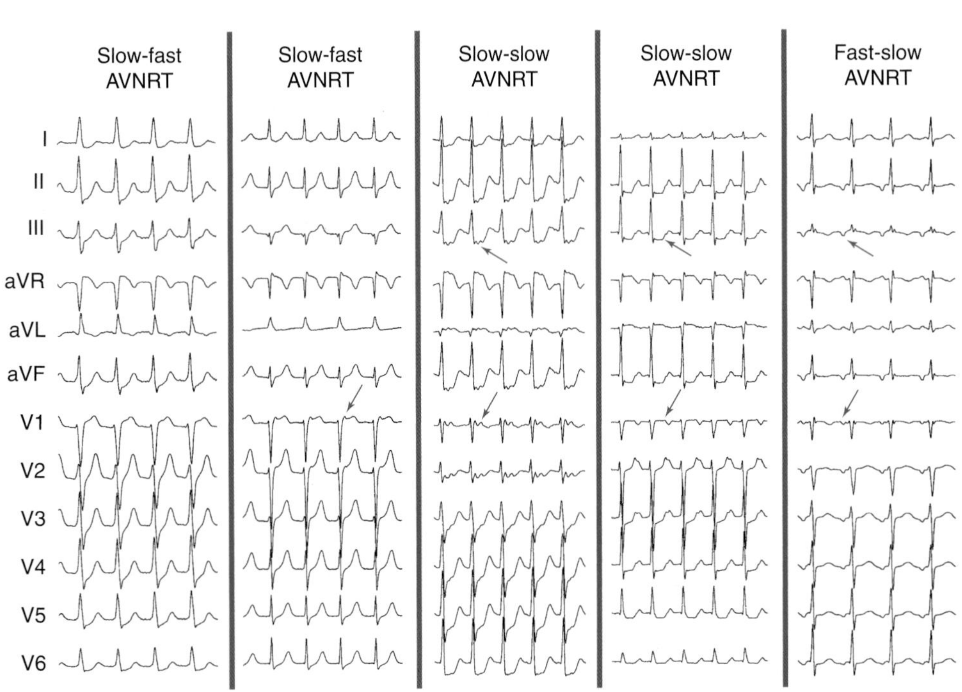

FIGURE 13-2 Surface ECG of the different types of atrioventricular nodal reentrant tachycardia (AVNRT). Arrows mark the P waves. In slow-fast (typical) AVNRT, the P wave may lie within the QRS (invisible, first panel) or distort the terminal portion of the QRS (mimicking an r wave in V_1, second panel). In slow-slow AVNRT, the P wave lies outside the QRS in the ST-T wave, and the RP interval is longer than that in slow-fast AVNRT. In fast-slow AVNRT, the P wave lies before the QRS with a long RP interval. In all varieties of AVNRT, the P wave is relatively narrow, negative in the inferior leads and positive in V_1.

tachycardias.[10,25] This phenomenon usually occurs when the conduction system and/or reentry circuit are unstable during initiation or termination of the tachycardia, likely secondary to decremental conduction in the lower common pathway. The ECG manifestation of P-QRS variations with or without AV block during tachycardia, especially at the initiation of tachycardias or in cases of nonsustained tachycardias, should not be misdiagnosed as atrial tachycardias (ATs)—they could be atypical or, rarely, typical forms of AVNRT. Moreover, the variations can be of such magnitude that a long RP tachycardia can masquerade for brief periods of time as a short RP tachycardia. Usually, the A/V ratio is equal to 1; however, 2:1 AV block can be present because of block below the reentry circuit (usually below the HB and, infrequently, in the lower common pathway). In such cases, narrow, inverted P wave morphology in the inferior leads inscribed exactly between QRS complexes strongly suggests AVNRT (Fig. 13-3). The incidence of reproducible sustained 2:1 AV block during induced episodes of AVNRT is approximately 10%. Rarely, VA block can occur because of block in the upper common pathway.[10]

In atypical (fast-slow) AVNRT, the RP interval is longer than the PR interval and, in slow-slow AVNRT, the RP interval is usually shorter than, and sometimes equal to, the PR interval. Occasionally, the P wave is inscribed in the middle of the cardiac cycle, mimicking atrial flutter (AFL) or AT with 2:1 AV conduction (Fig. 13-4).[21] Slow-slow AVNRT can be associated with RP interval and P wave morphology similar to that during orthodromic atrioventricular reentrant tachycardia (AVRT) using a posteroseptal AV BT. However, although both SVTs have the earliest atrial activation in the posteroseptal region, conduction time from that site to the HB region is significantly longer in AVNRT than orthodromic AVRT, resulting in a significantly longer RP interval in V_1 and a significantly larger difference in the RP interval between V_1 and inferior leads during AVNRT.

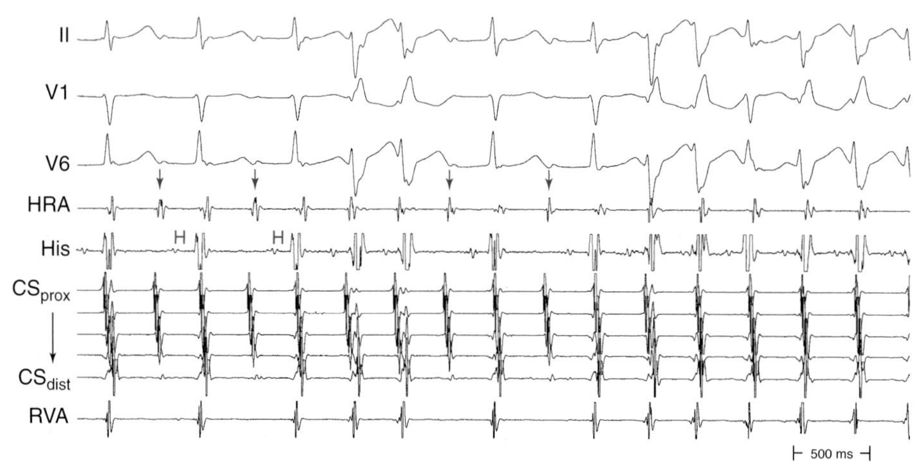

FIGURE 13–3 Typical atrioventricular nodal reentrant tachycardia (AVNRT) with intermittent 2:1 AV block. A His potential (H) is observed following conducted atrial impulses, but not after blocked atrial impulses, indicating AV block in the lower common pathway or in the portion of the His bundle (HB) proximal to the recording site. Note that intermittent AV block results in long-short cycle sequences associated with a right bundle branch block (RBBB) pattern during complexes conducted following a short cycle. RBBB is also observed intermittently during supraventricular tachycardia (SVT) with 1:1 AV conduction. Note the lack of effect of RBBB on the tachycardia cycle length (CL) (A-A interval) or ventricular-atrial (VA) interval.

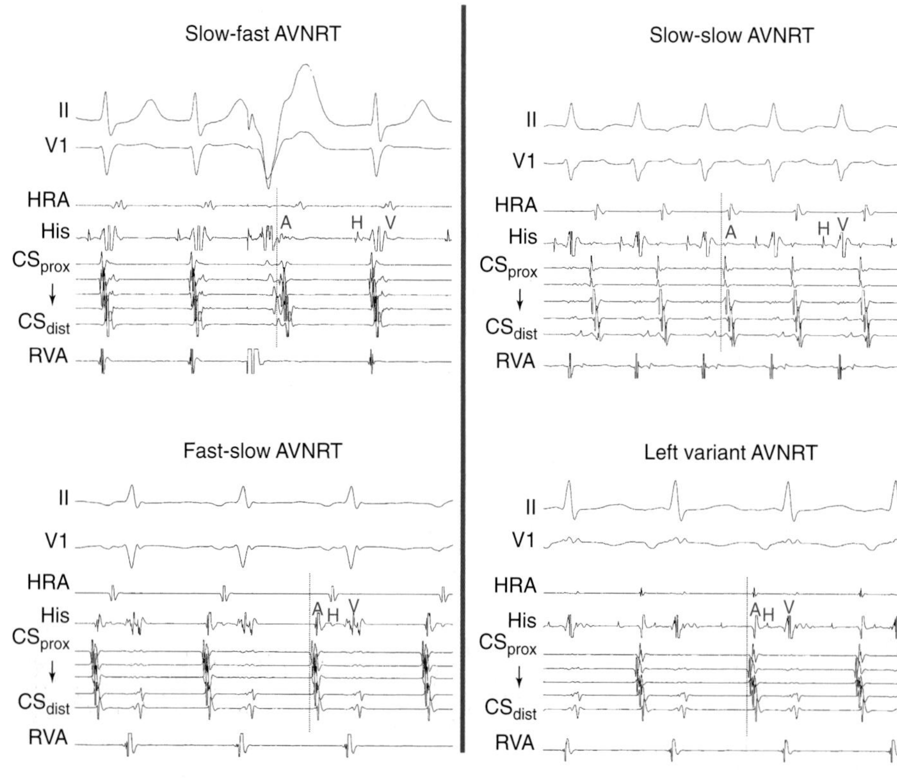

FIGURE 13–4 Surface ECG leads II and V_1 and endocardial recordings of the different types of atrioventricular nodal reentrant tachycardia (AVNRT). The dashed line marks the site with the earliest atrial activation. In slow-fast (typical) AVNRT, the initial site of atrial activation is usually recorded in the His bundle (HB) catheter. In slow-slow AVNRT, the P wave lies outside the QRS in the ST-T wave, and the RP interval is longer than that in slow-fast AVNRT. The earliest retrograde atrial activation is usually in the inferoposterior part of the triangle of Koch. Slow pathways with longer conduction times have a more inferior location in the triangle of Koch. In fast-slow AVNRT, the earliest site of retrograde atrial activation is usually recorded at the base of the triangle of Koch or coronary sinus ostium (CS os). An eccentric retrograde atrial activation sequence with the earliest retrograde activation site inside the CS can be observed in the left variant of AVNRT, more common in atypical than typical forms of AVNRT.

Therefore, ΔRP interval (V_1 – III) more than 20 milliseconds suggests slow-slow AVNRT (sensitivity, 71%; specificity, 87%).

ELECTROPHYSIOLOGICAL TESTING

EP testing is used to study inducibility and mechanism of the SVT and to guide catheter ablation. Typically, three quadripolar catheters are positioned in the high RA, right ventricular (RV) apex, and HB region, and a decapolar catheter is positioned in the CS (see Fig. 2-7).

Baseline Observations During Normal Sinus Rhythm

Atrial Extrastimulation and Atrial Pacing During Normal Sinus Rhythm

Anterograde Dual Atrioventricular Node Physiology. Demonstration of anterograde dual AVN pathway conduction curves requires a longer effective refractory period (ERP) of the fast pathway than the slow pathway ERP and atrial functional refractory period (FRP), as well as a sufficient difference in conduction time between the two pathways. Dual AVN physiology can be diagnosed by demonstrating the following: (1) a jump in the AH interval response to progressively more premature AES; (2) two ventricular responses to a single atrial impulse; (3) PR interval exceeding the R-R interval during atrial pacing; and/or (4) different PR or AH intervals during NSR or fixed-rate atrial pacing.[16]

Atrial-His Interval Jump. In contrast to the normal pattern of AVN conduction, in which the AH interval gradually lengthens in response to progressively shorter AES coupling intervals, patients with dual AVN physiology usually demonstrate a sudden increase (jump) in the AH interval at a critical AES (A_1-A_2) coupling interval (Fig. 13-5). Conduction with a short PR or AH interval reflects fast pathway conduction, whereas conduction with a long PR or AH interval reflects slow pathway conduction. The AH interval jump signals block of anterograde conduction of the progressively premature AES over the fast pathway (once the AES coupling interval becomes shorter than the fast pathway ERP) and anterograde conduction over the slow pathway (which has an ERP shorter than the AES coupling interval), with a longer conduction time (i.e., longer A_2-H_2 interval). A jump in A_2-H_2 (or H_1-H_2) interval of 50 milliseconds or more in response to a 10- millisecond shortening of A_1-A_2 (i.e., AES coupling interval) or of A_1-A_1 (i.e., pacing CL) is defined as a discontinuous AVN function curve and is considered as evidence of dual anterograde AVN pathways (see Fig. 2-23).[10,25]

1 : 2 Response. Rapid atrial pacing or AES can result into two ventricular responses to a single paced atrial impulse; the first ventricular response is caused by conduction over the fast AVN pathway, and the second one by conduction over the slow AVN pathway (Fig. 13-6). This response requires unidirectional retrograde block in the slow AVN pathway. Typically, in the presence of dual AVN pathways, conduction proceeds over both fast and slow AVN pathways; however, the wavefront conducting down the fast pathway reaches the distal junction of the two pathways before the impulse conducting down the slow AVN pathway and, subsequently, it conducts retrogradely up the slow pathway to collide with impulse conducting anterogradely down that pathway, thus preventing that anterograde impulse from reaching the HB and ventricle. Rarely, the slow pathway conducts anterogradely only or has a very long retrograde ERP. In this case, the wavefront traveling anterogradely down the fast pathway blocks (but does not conceal) in the slow pathway retrogradely and fails to retard the impulse traveling anterogradely down that pathway. Consequently, the wavefront traveling down the slow pathway can reach the HB and ventricle to produce a second His potential and QRS in response to a single atrial impulse. Because retrograde block in the slow pathway is a prerequisite to a 1 : 2 response, when such a phenomenon is present, it indicates that the slow pathway cannot support a reentrant tachycardia using the slow pathway as the retrograde limb (i.e., atypical AVNRT cannot be operative). This 1 : 2 response should be differentiated from pseudo–simultaneous fast and slow pathway conduction, which is a much more common phenomenon during rapid atrial pacing. In the latter case, the paced atrial impulses conduct down the slow pathway with prolonged AH intervals, so that the last paced atrial impulse falls before the His potential of the preceding paced beat and is followed by two His potentials and ventricular responses. The last response is then followed by induction of AVN echo beats or AVNRT, mimicking simultaneous fast and slow pathway conduction (Fig. 13-7).[10,35]

PR Interval Longer than Pacing Cycle Length During Atrial Pacing. The PR interval gradually prolongs as the atrial pacing rate is increased. When a critical pacing rate is reached, the PR interval typically exceeds the R-R

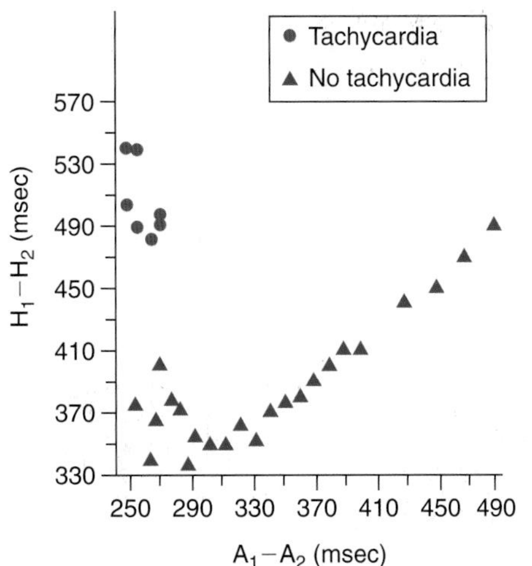

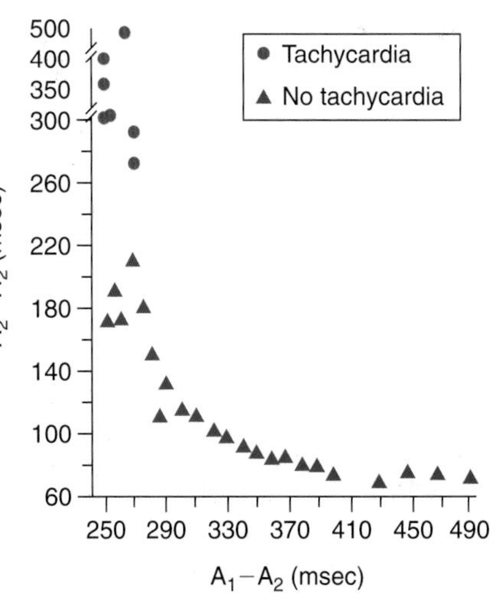

FIGURE 13–5 Dual atrioventricular node (AVN) physiology. H_1-H_2 intervals (left) and A_2-H_2 intervals (right) are at various A_1-A_2 intervals, with a discontinuous AVN curve. At a critical A_1-A_2 interval, the H_1-H_2 and A_1-H_2 intervals increase markedly. At the break in the curves, atrioventricular nodal reentrant tachycardia (AVNRT) is initiated. (From Olgin JE, Zipes DP: Specific arrhythmias: Diagnosis and treatment. *In* Libby P, Bonow RO, Mann DL, Zipes DP (eds): Braunwald's Heart Disease: A Textbook of Cardiovascular Medicine, 7th ed. Philadelphia, WB Saunders, 2008, p 880.)

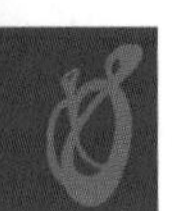

13

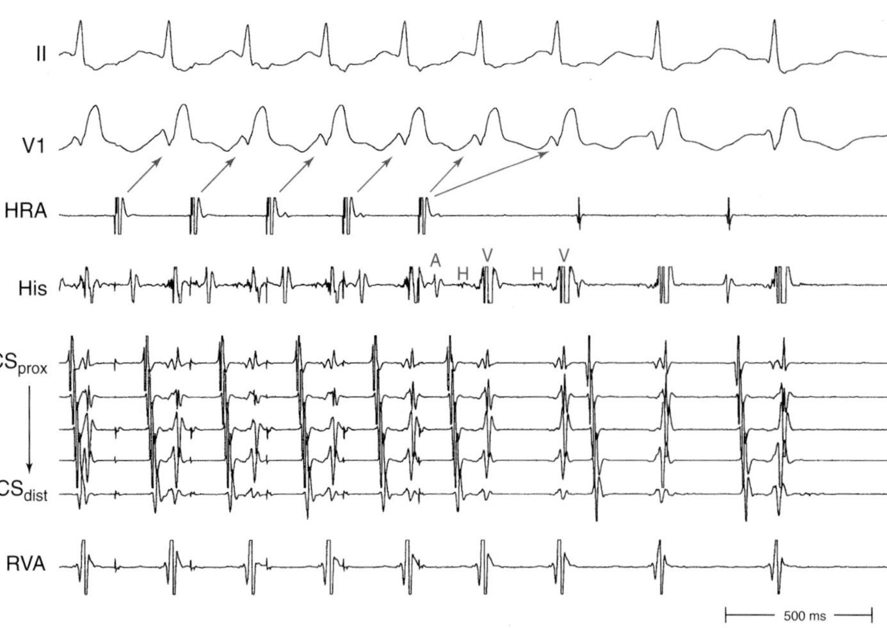

FIGURE 13–6 Rapid atrial pacing during normal sinus rhythm (NSR). Each paced atrial impulse conducts anterogradely over the fast atrioventricular node (AVN) pathway (red arrows). The last paced impulse, however, conducts anterogradely over both the fast (red arrow) and slow (blue arrow) pathways, resulting in two His bundle (HB) and ventricular responses.

interval, with all AVN conduction over the slow AVN pathway (see Fig. 13-7). This manifests as crossing over of the pacing stimulus artifacts and QRSs—that is, the paced atrial complex is conducting not to the QRS immediately following it, but to the next QRS, because of a very long PR interval. There should be consistent 1 : 1 AV conduction for this observation to be interpreted (i.e., without Wenckebach block). Such slow AVN conduction is seen only when conduction proceeds over a slow AVN pathway, and is not seen in the absence of dual AVN physiology. This sign is diagnostic of the presence of dual AVN physiology, even in the absence of an AH interval jump and, therefore, is very helpful in patients with smooth AVN function curves. In fact, 96% of patients with AVNRT and smooth AVN function curves have a PR interval/RR interval ratio more than 1 (i.e., PR interval > pacing CL) during atrial pacing at the maximal rate with consistent 1 : 1 AV conduction (versus 11% in controls).[25]

Different PR or Atrial-His Intervals During Normal Sinus Rhythm or at Identical Atrial Pacing Cycle Lengths. This phenomenon can occur when the fast pathway anterograde ERP is long relative to the sinus or paced CL (Fig. 13-8). Such a phenomenon also requires a long retrograde ERP of the fast pathway. Otherwise, AVN echo beats or AVNRT would result, because once the impulse blocks anterogradely in the fast pathway and is conducted down the slow pathway, it would subsequently conduct retrogradely up the fast pathway if the ERP of the fast pathway is shorter than the conduction time (i.e., shorter than the AH interval) over the slow pathway.[10]

Multiple Atrioventricular Node Pathways. Multiple AVN pathways in response to AES can be observed in up to 14% of patients. These are characterized by multiple AH interval jumps of 50 milliseconds or more in response to an increasingly premature AES. In these patients, a single AES may initiate multiple jumps in only 68%, whereas double AESs or atrial pacing is required in 32%. Such patients can have AVNRT with longer tachycardia CLs and longer ERP and FRP of the AVN. It is uncommon for multiple AVNRTs with different tachycardia CLs and P-QRS relationship to be present in the same patient.

Prevalence of Dual Atrioventricular Node Physiology. The presence of dual AVN pathways can usually be demonstrated using a single AES or atrial pacing in 85% of patients with clinical AVNRT, and in 95% using multiple AESs, multiple-drive CLs (typically 600 and 400 milliseconds) and multiple pacing sites (typically high RA and CS). Failure to demonstrate dual AVN physiology in patients with AVNRT can be caused by similar fast and slow AVN pathway ERPs. Dissociation of refractoriness of the fast and slow AVN pathways may then be required; this can be achieved by introduction of an AES at a shorter pacing drive CL, introduction of multiple AESs, burst atrial pacing, and/or administration of drugs such as beta blockers, verapamil, or digoxin. In general, if fast pathway conduction is suppressed in the baseline (as evidenced by a long AH interval at all atrial pacing rates or VA block during ventricular pacing), isoproterenol infusion and occasionally atropine usually facilitates fast pathway conduction. In contrast, if the baseline ERP of the fast pathway is very short, conduction over the slow pathway can be difficult to document; increasing the degree of sedation or infusion of esmolol can prolong the fast pathway ERP and allow recognition of slow pathway conduction. Another potential reason for the inability to demonstrate dual AVN physiology is block of the fast AVN pathway at the pacing drive CL (i.e., pacing drive CL is shorter than fast pathway ERP). Additionally, atrial FRP can limit the prematurity of the AES; consequently, the AVN activation cannot be adequately advanced to produce block in the fast pathway, because a more premature AES would result in more intraatrial conduction delay and less premature stimulation of the AVN. This can be overcome by the introduction of an AES at shorter pacing drive CL, introduction of multiple AESs, burst atrial pacing, and/or stimulation from multiple atrial sites.[25] The usual programmed electrical stimulation protocol used for EP testing in patients with AVNRT is outlined in Table 13-5.

Ventricular Extrastimulation and Ventricular Pacing During Normal Sinus Rhythm

Retrograde Dual Atrioventricular Node Physiology. Demonstration of retrograde dual AVN pathway conduction curves requires a longer retrograde ERP of the fast pathway than slow pathway ERP and ventricular and His-Purkinje system (HPS) FRP, as well as a sufficient difference in con-

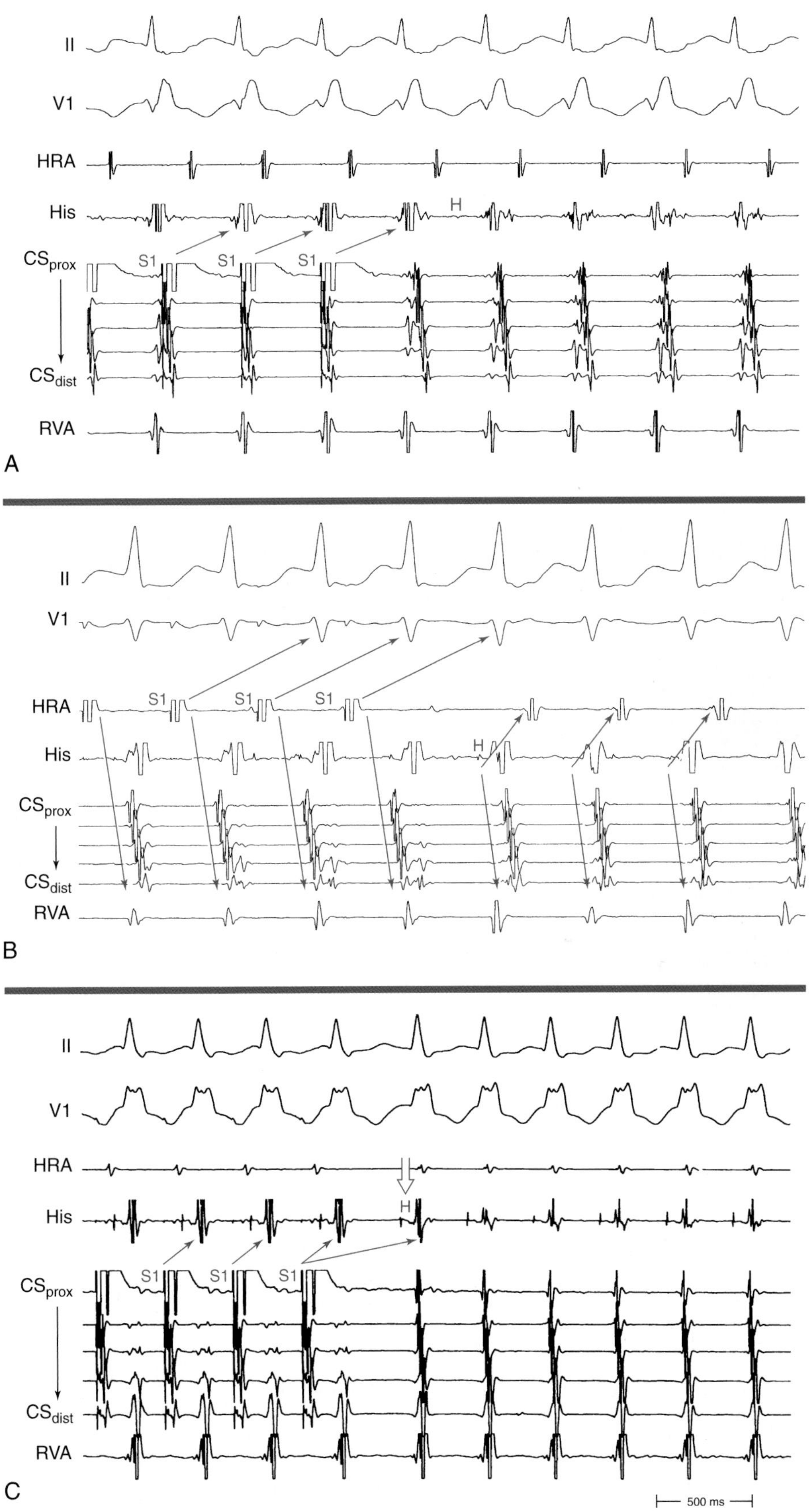

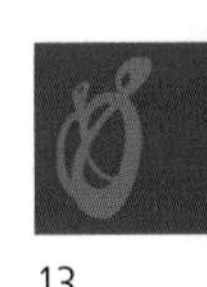

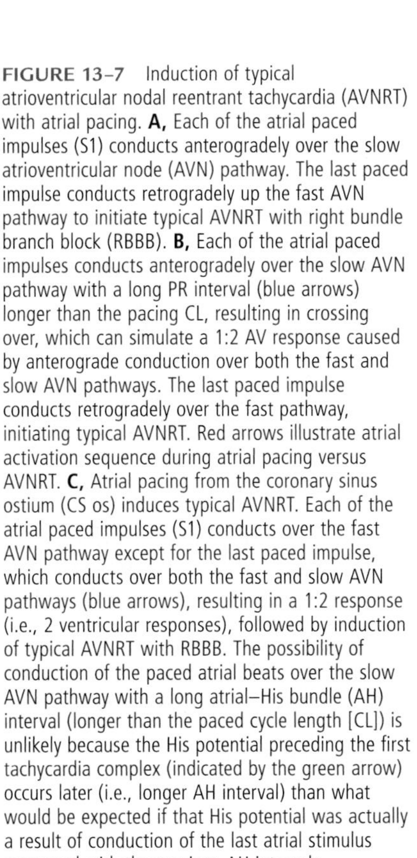

FIGURE 13–7 Induction of typical atrioventricular nodal reentrant tachycardia (AVNRT) with atrial pacing. **A,** Each of the atrial paced impulses (S1) conducts anterogradely over the slow atrioventricular node (AVN) pathway. The last paced impulse conducts retrogradely up the fast AVN pathway to initiate typical AVNRT with right bundle branch block (RBBB). **B,** Each of the atrial paced impulses conducts anterogradely over the slow AVN pathway with a long PR interval (blue arrows) longer than the pacing CL, resulting in crossing over, which can simulate a 1:2 AV response caused by anterograde conduction over both the fast and slow AVN pathways. The last paced impulse conducts retrogradely over the fast pathway, initiating typical AVNRT. Red arrows illustrate atrial activation sequence during atrial pacing versus AVNRT. **C,** Atrial pacing from the coronary sinus ostium (CS os) induces typical AVNRT. Each of the atrial paced impulses (S1) conducts over the fast AVN pathway except for the last paced impulse, which conducts over both the fast and slow AVN pathways (blue arrows), resulting in a 1:2 response (i.e., 2 ventricular responses), followed by induction of typical AVNRT with RBBB. The possibility of conduction of the paced atrial beats over the slow AVN pathway with a long atrial–His bundle (AH) interval (longer than the paced cycle length [CL]) is unlikely because the His potential preceding the first tachycardia complex (indicated by the green arrow) occurs later (i.e., longer AH interval) than what would be expected if that His potential was actually a result of conduction of the last atrial stimulus compared with the previous AH intervals.

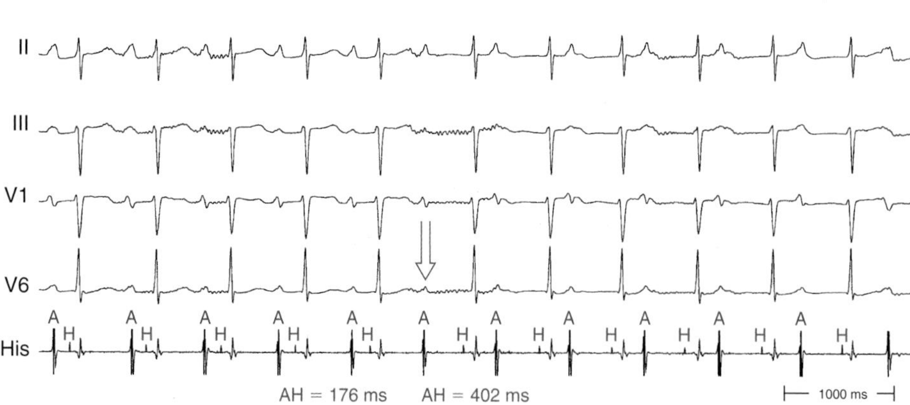

FIGURE 13–8 Dual atrioventricular node (AVN) physiology manifesting as two different PR intervals during normal sinus rhythm (NSR). Note the shift in AV conduction from the fast to the slow AVN pathway (arrow) occurs without any changes in the sinus cycle length (CL) (680 msec). This phenomenon indicates that the fast pathway anterograde effective refractory period (ERP) is long relative to the sinus CL.

TABLE 13–5 Programmed Stimulation Protocol for Electrophysiology Testing of Atrioventricular Nodal Reentrant Tachycardia
Atrial burst pacing from the RA and CS (down to AV Wenckebach CL)
Single and double AESs at multiple CLs (600-400 msec) from the high RA and CS (down to atrial ERP)
Ventricular burst pacing from the RV apex (down to VA Wenckebach CL)
Single and double VESs at multiple CLs (600-400 msec) from the RV apex (down to ventricular ERP)
Administration of isoproterenol infusion as needed to facilitate tachycardia induction (0.5-4 μg/min)

AES = atrial extrastimulus; AV = atrioventricular; CL = cycle length; CS = coronary sinus; ERP = effective refractory period; RA = right atrium; RV = right ventricle; VA = ventricular-atrial; VES = ventricular extrastimulus.

duction time between the two pathways. In a pattern analogous to that of anterograde dual AVN physiology, ventricular stimulation can result in discontinuous retrograde AVN function curves, manifesting as a jump in the H_2-A_2 (or A_1-A_2) interval of 50 milliseconds or more in response to a 10-millisecond decrement of the VES coupling interval (V_1-V_2) or ventricular pacing CL (V_1-V_1). This must be distinguished from sudden VA prolongation caused by VH interval (but not HA interval) increase related to retrograde functional block in the right bundle branch (RB) and transseptal activation of HB via the left bundle branch (LB) (see Fig. 2-27). A 1:2 response (i.e., two atrial responses to a single ventricular stimulus) can also be observed.

Failure to demonstrate retrograde dual AVN physiology in patients with atypical AVNRT can be caused by similar fast and slow AVN pathway ERPs. Dissociation of refractoriness of the fast and slow AVN pathways may be required; this can be achieved by introduction of VESs at a shorter pacing drive CL, introduction of multiple VESs, burst ventricular pacing, and/or administration of drugs such as beta blockers, verapamil, or digoxin. In addition, retrograde block in the fast AVN pathway at the pacing drive CL (i.e., the pacing CL is shorter than the fast pathway ERP) and ventricular or HPS FRP interval limiting the prematurity of the VES can also account for such failure.

Induction of Tachycardia

Initiation by Atrial Extrastimulation or Atrial Pacing

Typical (Slow-Fast) Atrioventricular Nodal Reentrant Tachycardia. Clinical AVNRT almost always can be initiated with an AES that blocks anterogradely in the fast pathway, conducts down the slow pathway, and then retrogradely up the fast pathway. Only when anterograde conduction down the slow pathway is slow enough (critical AH interval) to allow for recovery of the fast pathway to conduct retrogradely does reentry occur (see Fig. 13-5).[25] This critical AH interval is not a fixed interval; it can change with changes in pacing drive CL, changes in autonomic tone, or after drug administration, reflecting changes in the retrograde fast pathway ERP.[25,36]

There is a zone of AES coupling intervals (A_1-A_2) associated with AVNRT induction called the tachycardia zone. This zone usually begins at coupling intervals associated with marked prolongation of the PR and AH intervals. This AVN conduction delay (AH interval prolongation), and not the AES coupling interval, is of prime importance for the genesis of AVNRT.

Atrial pacing can initiate AVNRT at pacing CLs associated with sufficient AVN conduction delay (see Fig. 13-7), especially during the atypical Wenckebach periodicity when anterograde block occurs in the fast pathway and conduction shifts to the slow pathway.

Rarely (2%), AES or atrial pacing can produce a 1:2 response with anterograde conduction over both the fast and slow pathways, as explained earlier (see Fig. 13-7).[35] Such a response predicts easy induction of slow-fast AVNRT by ventricular stimulation because poor slow pathway retrograde conduction would make it easy for the ventricular stimulus to block in the slow pathway and conduct up the fast pathway to return down the slow pathway and initiate AVNRT.

The site of atrial stimulation can affect the ease of inducibility of AVNRT, probably because of different atrial inputs to the AVN or different atrial FRPs. Therefore, it is important to perform atrial stimulation from both the high RA and CS.[25]

Atrial echoes and AVNRT usually occur at the same time that dual pathways are revealed (see Fig. 2-23). In 20%, the dual AVN pathway AH interval jump occurs without echo beats or AVNRT because of failure of retrograde conduction up the fast pathway, which can be caused by the absence of distal connection between the two AVN pathways, long retrograde ERP of the fast AVN pathway, and/or concealment of the AES anterogradely into the fast AVN pathway (i.e., the AES propagates some distance into the fast pathway before being blocked). The latter event results in anterograde postdepolarization refractoriness, which would consequently make the fast pathway refractory to the wavefront invading it in a retrograde direction. The latter phenomenon can be diagnosed by demonstrating that the AH interval following the AES that fails to produce an echo beat is longer than the shortest ventricular pacing CL with 1:1 retrograde conduction; such a pacing CL is a marker of the fast pathway retrograde ERP. This implies that an AES blocking in the fast pathway and conducting over the slow pathway, with an AH interval exceeding fast pathway ERP and still not conducting retrogradely over the fast pathway, is caused by anterograde concealment (and not just block) into the fast pathway.[25]

Markers of poor retrograde conduction over the fast AVN pathway predict low inducibility of AVNRT. These markers include the absence of VA conduction, poor VA conduction (manifest as retrograde AVN Wenckebach CL more than 500 milliseconds), and retrograde dual pathways (indicating long retrograde ERP of the fast pathway, because it has to exceed the refractoriness of the slow pathway for retrograde dual pathways to be demonstrable).[25] In fact, retrograde fast AVN pathway characteristics (i.e., ERP) is the major determinant of whether reentry (AVN echoes and/or AVNRT) occurs, whereas conduction delay anterogradely over the slow pathway (i.e., "critical AH interval" determines when reentry is to occur.[25]

Although isolated AVN echoes can occur as long as VA conduction is present, the ability to initiate sustained AVNRT also requires the capability of the slow pathway to sustain repetitive anterograde conduction. Typically, for AVN reentry to occur, the fast pathway should be able to support 1:1 VA conduction at a ventricular pacing CL less than 400 milliseconds (i.e., retrograde Wenckebach CL less than 400 milliseconds)[25] and the slow pathway should be able to support 1:1 AV conduction at an atrial pacing CL less than 350 milliseconds (i.e., anterograde Wenckebach CL less than 350 milliseconds).[25] The shorter the AH interval with anterograde conduction over the fast pathway, the better the retrograde conduction over the same pathway (i.e., the shorter the HA interval), and the better inducibility of AVNRT.[25] Furthermore, sustenance of AVNRT requires that the tachycardia CL be longer than the ERP of all components of the circuit. It is important to recognize that during EP testing, these criteria are dependent on the cardiac autonomic tone at that moment, and can change dramatically on changes in autonomic tone by changing the level of patient sedation or the use of isoproterenol, which will then affect inducibility of AVNRT.[25]

Atypical (Fast-Slow) Atrioventricular Nodal Reentrant Tachycardia. Anterograde dual AVN physiology is usually not demonstrable in patients with atypical AVNRT.[25] Additionally, as noted, the presence of a 1:2 response to AES predicts noninducibility of atypical AVNRT, because it indicates failure of the slow pathway to support retrograde conduction, a prerequisite for an atypical AVNRT circuit.[21]

With atrial stimulation, atypical AVNRT is usually initiated with modest prolongation of the AH interval along the fast pathway with anterograde block in the slow pathway, followed by retrograde slow conduction over the slow pathway (Fig. 13-9). Therefore, a critical AH interval delay is not obvious.[21]

Initiation by Ventricular Extrastimulation or Ventricular Pacing

Typical (Slow-Fast) Atrioventricular Nodal Reentrant Tachycardia. Ventricular stimulation induces typical AVNRT by different mechanisms; the most common mechanism involves retrograde block of the ventricular stimulus in the slow pathway and retrograde conduction up the fast pathway, followed by anterograde conduction down the slow pathway. This occurs when the retrograde ERP of the slow pathway exceeds that of the fast pathway (no critical VA or HA interval is required for induction). This means that induction occurs without the demonstration of retrograde dual AVN physiology. Occasionally, an interpolated premature ventricular complex (PVC) can block in the slow pathway retrogradely and penetrate into the fast pathway and cause concealment, so that the fast pathway will be refractory when the next sinus beat occurs; the sinus beat would then block in the fast pathway and conduct down the slow pathway and initiate typical AVNRT. This mechanism is uncommon; retrograde VA conduction over the fast AVN pathway is usually good, and VA block rarely occurs in patients with typical AVNRT initiated by ventricular stimulation.[25]

Ventricular stimulation is less effective than atrial stimulation in inducing typical AVNRT (success rate is about 10% with VES and 40% with ventricular pacing), whereas atypical AVNRT can be induced almost as frequently by ventricular stimulation as by atrial stimulation. It is difficult for VES to induce typical AVNRT because the prematurity with which the VES arrives at the AVN can be limited by conduction delay in the HPS or in the lower common

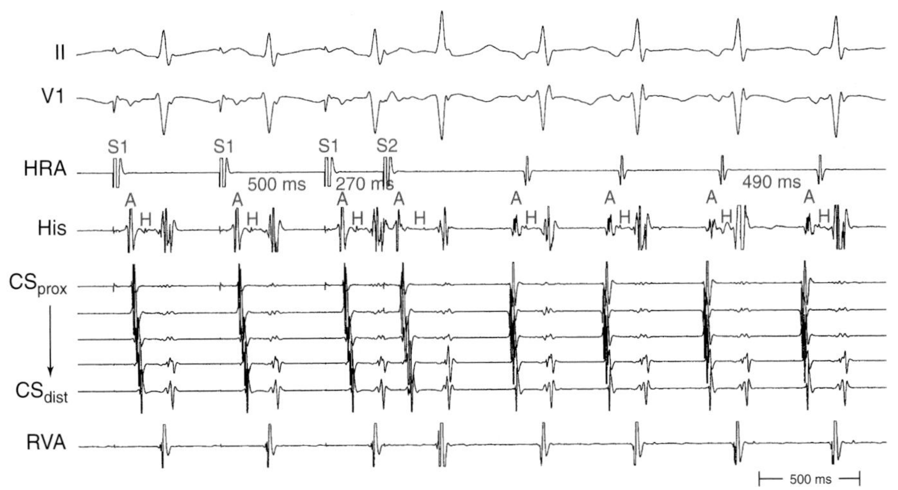

FIGURE 13-9 Induction of atypical atrioventricular nodal reentrant tachycardia (AVNRT) with atrial extrastimulation (AES). AES delivered from the high right atrium (RA) at a coupling interval of 270 msec after a drive cycle length (CL) of 500 msec initiated atypical AVNRT with a CL of 490 msec. Note that the AES conducted with only a modest prolongation of the atrial–His bundle (AH) interval. Additionally, comparing the AH interval between atrial drive pacing and that during the SVT (because the tachycardia CL approximates the pacing CL) reveals that ΔAH ($AH_{atrial\ pacing} - AH_{SVT}$) is more than 40 msec, which favors AVNRT over AT and orthodromic atrioventricular reentrant tachycardia (AVRT).

pathway. The ERP of the HPS may exceed that of the slow AVN pathway. This limitation can usually be overcome by the introduction of multiple VESs, use of a shorter drive CL, or ventricular pacing, which results in adaptation and shortening of the HPS ERP. Additionally, anterograde ERP of the slow pathway may exceed the ventricular pacing CL so that the slow pathway is incapable of anterograde conduction of the ventricular impulse conducting retrogradely over the fast pathway. Similar retrograde ERPs of the slow and fast pathways also can limit the successful initiation of AVNRT by ventricular stimulation. As noted, manipulation of the autonomic tone with vagal maneuvers or drugs can help dissociation of those ERPs. Another explanation for the lower success rate of AVNRT induction by ventricular stimulation is that the ventricular stimulus can penetrate (and not just block) in the slow pathway retrogradely, causing concealment that renders that pathway refractory and incapable of anterograde conduction of the ventricular impulse traveling retrogradely over the fast pathway.

Ventricular pacing can overcome many of the problems imposed by HPS refractoriness in the induction of typical AVNRT (Fig. 13-10). During ventricular pacing, the AVN is the primary site of conduction delay. However, block in the lower common pathway and repetitive concealment (not just block) in the slow AVN pathway can still limit the success of ventricular pacing in inducing typical AVNRT.

Of note, a VES that initiates an SVT with an HA interval longer than the HA (or VA) interval during the SVT, despite the fact that the H-H interval following that particular VES is longer than the H-H interval during the SVT, indicates that the SVT is AVNRT and not orthodromic AVRT, because both the HA interval during orthodromic AVRT and that following the VES represent sequential conduction duration from the HB up the lower common pathway and fast pathway to the atrium (Fig. 13-11). In contrast, during AVNRT, the HB and the atrium are activated in parallel, resulting in a shortened HA interval.

Atypical (Fast-Slow) Atrioventricular Nodal Reentrant Tachycardia. Ventricular stimulation can induce atypical AVNRT by different mechanisms.[25] The ventricular impulse can block in the fast pathway and conduct retrogradely over the slow pathway, with a long HA interval, allowing for recovery of the fast pathway and subsequent anterograde conduction down this pathway, initiating atypical AVNRT (see Fig. 13-11). This requires the retrograde ERP of the fast pathway to exceed that of the slow pathway. In this case, dual retrograde AVN pathways would be demonstrated with ventricular stimulation. Both VES and ventricular pacing are equally effective in inducing atypical AVNRT by this mechanism. Occasionally, a VES can conduct over both AVN pathways, producing a 1:2 response, which is subsequently followed by the induction of atypical AVNRT. Ventricular pacing can initiate atypical AVNRT at pacing CLs associated with sufficient retrograde AVN conduction delay, especially during Wenckebach cycles when retrograde block occurs in the fast pathway and conduction shifts to the slow pathway.[21]

Inducibility of atypical AVNRT is mostly determined by the retrograde slow pathway conduction, because the anterograde fast pathway conduction is usually fast enough and its ERP is short enough to mediate anterograde conduction of the impulse arriving from the slow pathway.

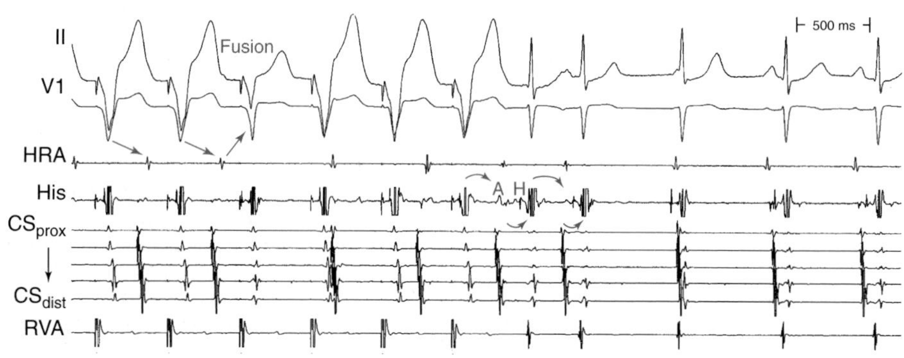

FIGURE 13–10 Ventricular pacing inducing atrioventricular nodal (AVN) echo beats. Note that ventriculoatrial conduction during ventricular pacing is occurring up the slow AVN pathway (red arrows). This results in AVN echo beats caused by anterograde conduction over the fast pathway, which results in occasional QRS fusion (i.e., fusion between the echo beat and the paced impulse) during the pacing drive. Cessation of ventricular pacing is followed by double AVN echo beats (blue arrows).

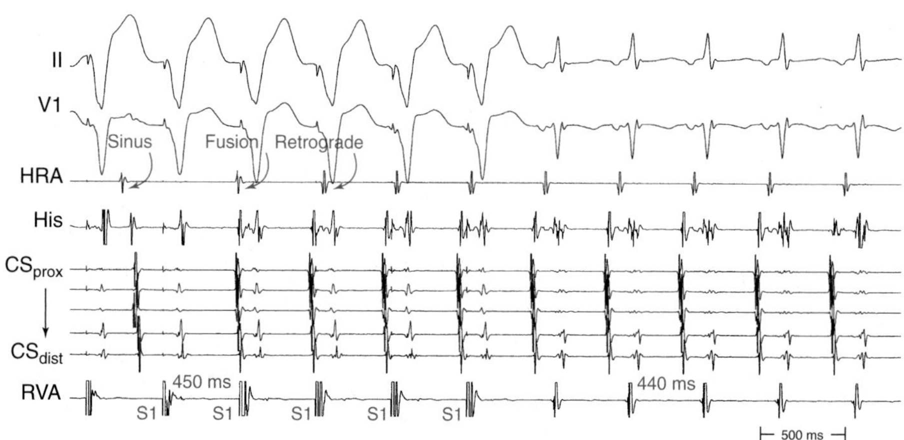

FIGURE 13–11 Induction of atypical atrioventricular nodal reentrant tachycardia (AVNRT) with ventricular pacing. Right ventricle (RV) apical pacing (cycle length [CL] = 450 msec) induces atypical AVNRT (CL = 440 msec). Retrograde atrial activation sequence during ventricular pacing is similar to that during the supraventricular tachycardia (SVT), and the ventriculoatrial (VA) interval during ventricular pacing is longer than during the SVT; both criteria favor AVNRT over orthodromic atrioventricular reentrant tachycardia (AVRT). Note that the first atrial complex on the left of the tracing is actually a sinus P wave, and the second is a fusion between retrograde VA conduction and a sinus impulse; pure retrograde atrial activation sequence is observed only after the third ventricular stimulus.

Tachycardia Features

Typical (Slow-Fast) Atrioventricular Nodal Reentrant Tachycardia

Atrial Activation Sequence. The initial site of atrial activation is usually recorded in the HB catheter at the apex of the triangle of Koch. In general, the shorter the HA interval, the more likely the earliest atrial activation is recorded in the HB electrograms; as the HA interval prolongs, the earliest atrial activation moves closer to the base of the triangle of Koch or in the CS. However, significant heterogeneity in atrial activation exists, with multiple breakthrough points (unlike AT or orthodromic AVRT) and, in approximately 60% of patients, retrograde atrial activation during typical AVNRT can be slightly discordant quantitatively and qualitatively from that during ventricular pacing. Subsequently, the wave of atrial activation propagates radially cephalad and laterally to activate both atria (i.e., concentric atrial activation). This results in a relatively narrow P wave. In fact, the narrowest P wave during any arrhythmia is seen when the atrial activation begins at the apex of triangle of Koch. The site of earliest atrial activation is not always obvious during AVNRT because of superimposition of atrial and ventricular electrograms. Delivering a VES that advances ventricular activation but does not reset atrial activation usually helps unmask atrial activation sequence.[10]

Atrial-Ventricular Relationship. The onset of atrial activation appears before or coincides with the onset of the QRS in about 70% of cases. The RP interval is very short (−40 to 75 milliseconds); however, variation of the A/V relationship (with changes in AH, HA, and AH/HA interval ratio) can occasionally occur during initiation or termination of the tachycardia, likely because of decremental conduction in the lower common pathway. Usually, the A/V ratio equals 1; however, AV block can be present because of block below the reentry circuit (usually below the HB and infrequently in the lower common pathway), which can occur especially at the onset of the SVT, during acceleration of the SVT, and following a PVC or VES. Moreover, Wenckebach-type block can occur in the lower common pathway, resulting in a changing relationship between the His potential and atrial electrogram (i.e., retrograde atrial electrogram moves closer to or actually precedes the His potential, until block occurs with no His potential apparent). Reproducible, sustained 2:1 AV block during induced episodes of AVNRT can be observed in approximately 10% of cases (see Fig. 13-3). The His potential is absent in blocked beats in about 40% of patients who have 2:1 AV block and, in the remaining patients, the His potential can range from being rudimentary to large in amplitude. However, irrespective of whether a His potential is present in blocked beats, the AV block persists after the administration of atropine, suggesting that the site of block is not in the AVN. In addition, a VES introduced during the 2:1 AV block consistently results in 1:1 conduction, indicating that the AV block is functional and that the level of block is infranodal. Therefore, what was previously thought to be 2:1 AVN block in the lower common pathway of the AVNRT circuit (because of the absence of visible His potentials) is more likely to be intra-Hisian block. Rarely, VA block can occur during AVNRT because of block in the upper common pathway (see Fig. 13-10).[10]

Oscillation in the Tachycardia Cycle Length. Analysis of tachycardia CL variability can provide useful diagnostic information for discrimination among the different types of SVT, even when the episodes of SVT are nonsustained. SVT CL variability of 15 milliseconds or more in magnitude occurs commonly in typical AVNRT, and generally is caused by changes in anterograde conduction over the slow AVN pathway. Because retrograde conduction through the fast AVN pathway generally is much less variable, the changes in the ventricular CL that result from variability in anterograde AVN conduction precede the subsequent changes in the atrial CL (Fig. 13-12), and changes in the atrial CL do not predict changes in the subsequent ventricular CL, as is the case in orthodromic AVRT.[37]

Effect of Bundle Branch Block. The development of prolonged functional aberration during AVNRT is uncommon, and it usually occurs at initiation of the tachycardia or after resumption of 1:1 AV conduction after a period of block in the HB or lower common pathway (see Fig. 13-3). When BBB does occur during AVNRT, it does not influence the tachycardia CL (A-A or H-H intervals) because the ventricles are not required for the tachycardia circuit.[25,38]

Termination and Response to Physiological and Pharmacological Maneuvers. The tachycardia CL is correlated best to the conduction time down the slow pathway. Spontaneous or pharmacologically mediated changes in the tachycardia CL are also more closely associated with changes in slow pathway conduction.[25] Spontaneous termination of typical AVNRT occurs because of block in the fast or the slow pathway; however, the better the retrograde fast pathway conduction, the less likely it is the site of block. Carotid sinus massage and vagal maneuvers can terminate typical AVNRT with gradual anterograde slowing and then block in the slow pathway, whereas block in the fast pathway is uncommon.[25] AVN blockers (digoxin, calcium channel blockers, and beta blockers) prolong the refractoriness of the fast and slow pathways to similar or different degrees. Such effects mediate termination of AVNRT but can occasionally

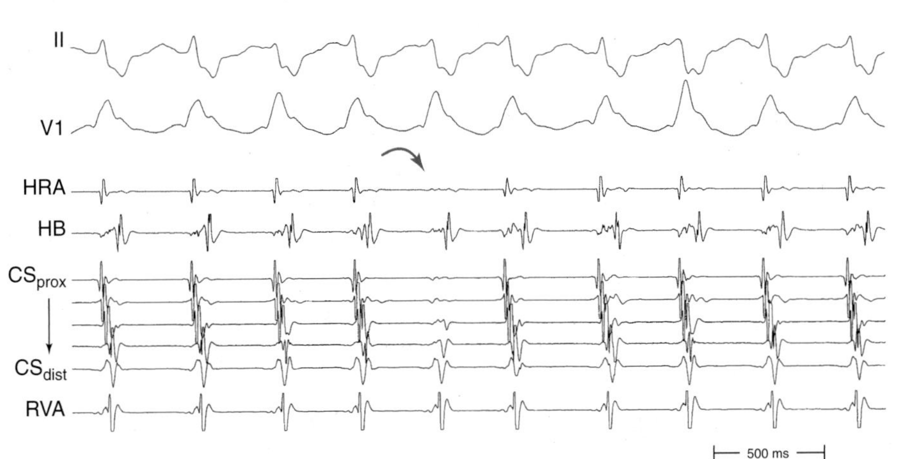

FIGURE 13–12 Typical atrioventricular nodal reentrant tachycardia (AVNRT) with right bundle branch block (RBBB). Intermittent ventricular-atrial (VA) block is observed (arrow) secondary to block in the upper common pathway. Oscillation of the tachycardia cycle length (CL) is observed before the block. Note the changes in the H-H and V-V intervals preceding similar changes in the A-A interval. Both atrial tachycardia (AT) and orthodromic atrioventricular reentrant tachycardia (AVRT) are excluded by the fact that the atrium is not necessary for continuation of the tachycardia.

help dissociate the ERP of the fast and slow pathways and unmask dual AVN physiology, and can also make the AVNRT easily inducible. Adenosine blocks the slow pathway and terminates AVNRT, but it does not affect the fast pathway. Class IA and IC agents and amiodarone affect the fast and the slow pathways.

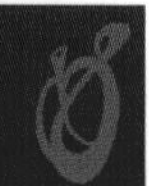

Atypical (Fast-Slow) Atrioventricular Nodal Reentrant Tachycardia

13 The earliest site of retrograde atrial activation during atypical AVNRT is usually recorded at the base of the triangle of Koch or CS os, and a CS breakthrough is observed in most patients. The CS breakthrough is likely part of or very close to the reentry circuit, as demonstrated by entrainment mapping.[27]

The RP interval during atypical AVNRT is longer than the PR interval. Additionally, the PR and AH interval are shorter during AVNRT than during NSR because the atrium and ventricle are activated in parallel with simultaneous conduction up the upper common pathway and down the anterograde fast pathway in atypical AVNRT, but in sequence during NSR (Fig. 13-13).

Usually, the A/V ratio equals 1 and, as is the case for typical AVNRT. BBB can occur but does not influence the tachycardia CL.[25] In contrast to typical AVNRT, CL variability during atypical AVNRT is usually caused by changes in retrograde conduction over the slow AVN pathway. Anterograde conduction occurs over the more stable fast AVN pathway and is less subject to variability (see Fig. 13-13). Therefore, during atypical AVNRT, changes in the atrial CL predict changes in the subsequent ventricular CL (as is the case in AT).[37]

Carotid sinus massage, vagal maneuvers, adenosine, and AVN blockers (e.g., digoxin, calcium channel blockers, and beta blockers) generally terminate the AVNRT by gradual slowing and then block in the retrograde slow pathway (see Fig. 13-13). Termination of atypical AVNRT with adenosine can also result from block in the fast AVN pathway; however, the value of this observation in distinguishing between atypical AVNRT and orthodromic AVRT using a slow retrograde BT is questionable.[25]

Diagnostic Maneuvers During Tachycardia

Atrial Extrastimulation and Atrial Pacing During Supraventricular Tachycardia

A late-coupled AES usually fails to reach the AVN with adequate prematurity and thus fails to affect the tachycardia, and a full compensatory pause results. However, the AES can anterogradely conceal in the upper common pathway, retarding conduction of the impulse traveling retrogradely up the fast pathway and resulting in a delay in the timing of the next atrial activation. This is usually manifested by an AES that delays the subsequent atrial activation but without affecting the timing of the subsequent His potential.[25]

In typical AVNRT, an early-coupled AES frequently penetrates the AVN and resets the reentry circuit, resulting in a compensatory pause that is less than, equal to, or greater than a full compensatory pause, depending on the degree of anterograde conduction delay that the AES encounters down the slow pathway (because of the decremental conduction properties of the AVN). The AES orthodromically propagates through the anterograde slow pathway, resulting in alteration of the subsequent H-H' interval, whereas it antidromically collides with the preceding tachycardia wavefront traveling retrogradely up the fast pathway. Progressively premature AESs encounter progressive anterograde conduction delay in the slow pathway, resulting in an increasing resetting response pattern. Theoretically, the degree of conduction delay in the slow pathway can exactly compensate for the prematurity of the AES, producing a pause that is equal to a full compensatory pause. To verify whether that pause was full compensatory because the AES failed to penetrate the AVN or because the degree of anterograde conduction delay in the AVN was exactly enough to compensate for the prematurity of the AES, the return cycles are evaluated after delivery of additional AESs with different coupling intervals. Similarly, a delay in the slow pathway causes delay in the subsequent His potential timing, and such delay can be enough, more, or less than what is needed to compensate for the prematurity of the AES. Therefore, the His potential following an AES can occur early, late, or on time relative to the expected tachycardia His potential. An early-coupled AES can also impinge on the relative refractory period of the lower common pathway, causing slowed conduction and delay in the timing of the next His potential (i.e., longer A_2-H_2 than the baseline tachycardia A_1-H_1). This can occur even without affecting the timing of the next atrial activation, if conduction delay occurs only in the lower common pathway but not in the slow pathway.[25]

In atypical AVNRT, an early-coupled AES can reset the SVT in a similar fashion as for typical AVNRT; however, the delay in conduction that the AES will endure is mainly in the retrograde limb of the circuit (i.e., the slow pathway).[25]

Resetting with fusion (a hallmark of macroreentrant tachycardias) cannot be demonstrated in AVNRT. For atrial fusion (i.e., fusion of atrial activation from both the tachy-

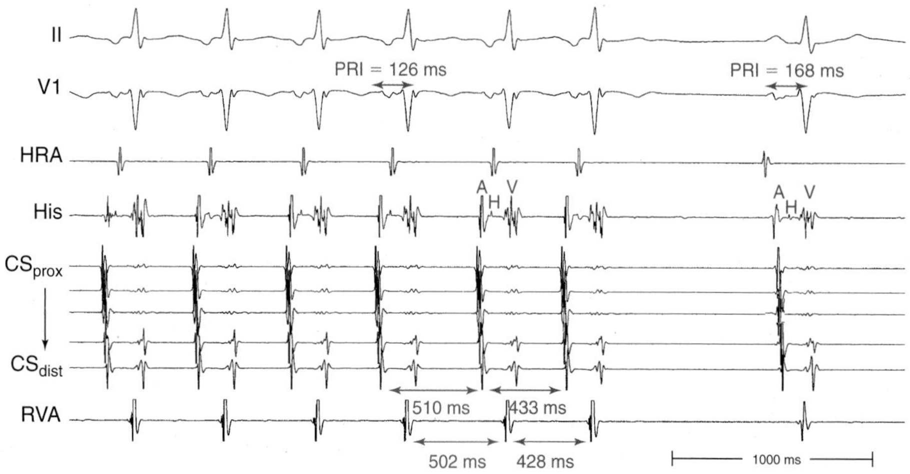

FIGURE 13–13 Atypical (fast-slow) atrioventricular nodal reentrant tachycardia (AVNRT) terminating spontaneously. Oscillation of the tachycardia cycle length (CL) is observed just before termination. Note that changes in the atrial CL predict changes in the subsequent ventricular CL because CL variability during atypical AVNRT is usually caused by changes in retrograde conduction over the slow atrioventricular node (AVN) pathway, whereas anterograde conduction occurs over the more stable fast AVN pathway and is less subject to variability. Additionally, the PR (PRI) and atrial–His bundle (AH) intervals are shorter during AVNRT than those during normal sinus rhythm (NSR) because both the atrium and the ventricle are activated in parallel with simultaneous conduction up the upper common pathway and down the anterograde fast pathway in atypical AVNRT but in sequence during NSR.

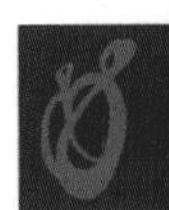

cardia wavefront and the AES) to occur, the AES should be able to enter the reentrant circuit while at the same time the tachycardia wavefront should be able to exit the circuit. This requires spatial separation between the entry and exit sites to the reentrant circuit, a condition that seems to be lacking in the case of AVNRT. Once the tachycardia wavefront exits the reentry circuit to activate the atrium, any AES delivered beyond that time and results in atrial fusion would not be capable of reaching the reentry circuit because the entry/exit site is already refractory because of activation by the exiting wavefront, and the AES has no alternative way of reaching the circuit. Similarly, once an AES is capable of reaching the reentry circuit, the shared entry-exit site will be made refractory and incapable of allowing a simultaneous exit of the tachycardia wavefront.

During typical AVNRT, a very early-coupled AES can block anterogradely in the slow pathway, and it usually collides with a retrograde wavefront in the fast pathway to terminate the SVT. However, if the tachycardia CL is long enough, with a wide fully excitable gap, and the AES is appropriately timed, the AES can block anterogradely in the slow pathway and still conduct down the fast pathway to capture the HB and ventricle and terminate the SVT before the SVT wavefront traveling down the slow pathway reaches the lower turnaround point. Therefore, the last HB and ventricular electrograms before termination are advanced and premature, in contrast to termination secondary to an AES blocking anterogradely in the slow and fast pathways, whereby the last HB and ventricular electrograms of the SVT occur on time. This phenomenon occurs more commonly in atypical AVNRT.

In atypical AVNRT, a very early-coupled AES can conduct down the fast pathway during retrograde slow pathway activation and block retrogradely in the slow pathway. In this case, the AES will result in a premature HB and ventricular activation, and the AVNRT will be terminated before the expected atrial activation.

Termination. The ability of an AES to terminate AVNRT depends on the following: (1) the tachycardia CL (AVNRT with a CL less than 350 milliseconds is rarely terminated by a single AES, unless atrial stimulation is performed close to the AVN); (2) the distance of the site of atrial stimulation from the AVN (which would influence the ability of the AES to arrive to the AVN with adequate prematurity); (3) the refractoriness of the intervening atrial tissue, which can be overcome by delivery of multiple atrial extrastimuli ; (4) atrial conduction velocity resulting from the AES; and (5) the size of the excitable gap in the reentrant circuit.

Entrainment. Atrial pacing at a CL approximately 10 to 30 milliseconds shorter than the tachycardia CL is usually able to entrain AVNRT.[25] In contrast to orthodromic AVRT, entrainment with atrial fusion cannot be demonstrated during AVNRT, suggesting that the reentrant circuit in AVNRT does not have separate atrial entry and exit sites. Therefore, during entrainment of AVNRT by atrial pacing, atrial activation sequence and P wave morphology are always that of pure paced morphology. The inability to demonstrate entrainment with manifest atrial fusion suggests a purely intranodal location of the AVNRT circuit. On the other hand, one study has shown orthodromic capture of the atrial electrogram at the HB recording site (i.e., the bipolar HB electrogram morphology is identical to that during the tachycardia and is unaffected by pacing, and the first post-pacing interval [PPI] is identical to the pacing CL) during entrainment from the CS os region, consistent with intracardiac atrial fusion. This suggests the absence of an upper common pathway between a reentrant circuit confined to the AVN and atrial tissue surrounding the AVN, and supports the concept that the reentrant circuit in AVNRT incorporates the atrial tissue surrounding the AVN. The AH interval during entrainment is usually longer than that during AVNRT, since the atrial and the His electrograms are activated in parallel during AVNRT and in sequence during atrial pacing entraining the AVNRT (due to the presence of intervening atrial tissue and, potentially, an upper common pathway separating the site of atrial stimulation from the reentry circuit).

Ventricular Extrastimulation and Ventricular Pacing During Supraventricular Tachycardia

For a VES to reset the AVNRT circuit, it needs to advance (prematurely activate) the HB timing by a degree that is dependent on the following: (1) tachycardia CL; (2) local ventricular ERP; (3) the time needed for the VES to reach the HB; and (4) length of the lower common pathway. The longer the lower common pathway, the more the timing of HB activation must be advanced. Therefore, in slow-fast and slow-slow AVNRT, which typically has a long lower common pathway, the HB activation must be advanced by more than 30 to 60 milliseconds. In contrast, in slow-fast AVNRT, the lower common pathway is shorter and the tachycardia is typically reset by the VES as soon as the HB activation is advanced.[25]

A late-coupled VES may block in the HPS or lower common pathway and may not affect the SVT (Fig. 13-14A). A late-coupled VES that resets the SVT without first retrogradely activating the HB (i.e., VES delivered at, after, or within 50 milliseconds of the expected inscription of the anterograde His potential) excludes AVNRT.

An early-coupled VES can reset the SVT, especially when the tachycardia CL is relatively long (more than 350 milliseconds). The resetting VES antidromically collides with the preceding tachycardia wavefront traveling anterogradely and is conducted through the retrograde pathway to reset the tachycardia (see Fig. 13-14C).[25] Resetting of AVNRT with fusion of the QRS cannot be demonstrated because of the shared entry-exit site from the ventricle to the circuit, as discussed earlier. A VES that resets the SVT without atrial activation (i.e., advances the subsequent His potential and QRS and blocks in the upper common pathway) excludes AT and orthodromic AVRT, because it proves that the atrium is not part of the SVT circuit.[25]

Termination. Termination of AVNRT with VES is difficult (more so than termination with AES), and is rare when the tachycardia CL is less than 350 milliseconds, and such termination favors the diagnosis of orthodromic AVRT.[25] In typical AVNRT, when termination occurs it is usually caused by block of the VES in the anterograde or retrograde limb of the AVNRT circuit. The slower the SVT, the more likely the block will be in the anterograde slow pathway. Ventricular pacing can terminate AVNRT easier than VES, because rapid ventricular pacing can modulate and overcome the refractoriness of the intervening HPS. VES always terminates atypical AVNRT by blocking retrogradely in the slow pathway.

Entrainment. Ventricular pacing at a CL approximately 10 to 30 milliseconds shorter than the tachycardia CL is usually able to entrain AVNRT. Visualization of the His potential before atrial activation during entrainment helps differentiate AVNRT from orthodromic AVRT.[25] If the His potential cannot be visualized during ventricular pacing, two other parameters can be helpful to distinguish AVNRT from orthodromic AVRT: the VA interval during ventricular pacing and the PPI after entrainment. The VA interval during ventricular pacing is significantly longer than that during AVNRT (ΔVA [$VA_{pacing} - VA_{SVT}$] is usually more than 85 milliseconds), because both the ventricle and atrium are activated in parallel during AVNRT but in sequence during

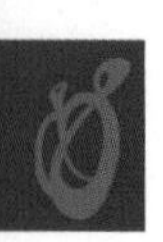

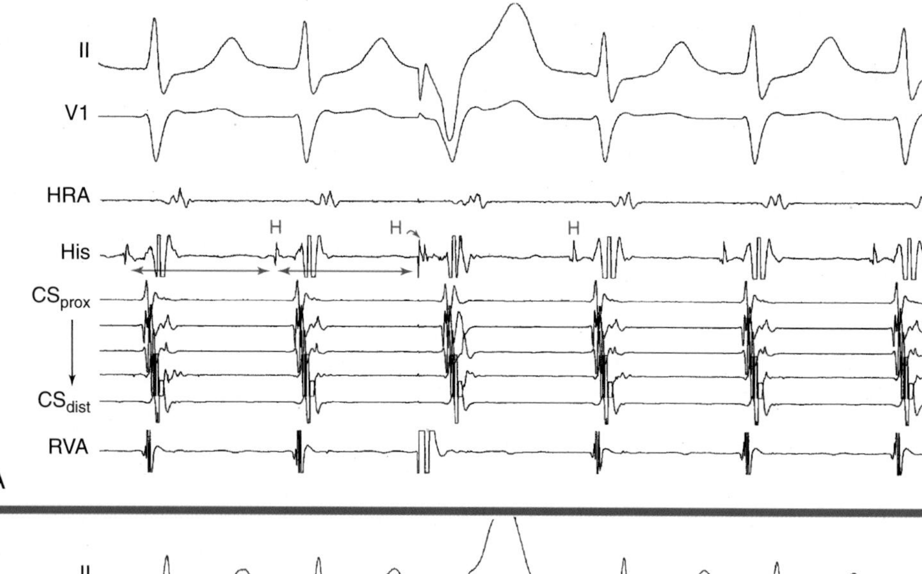

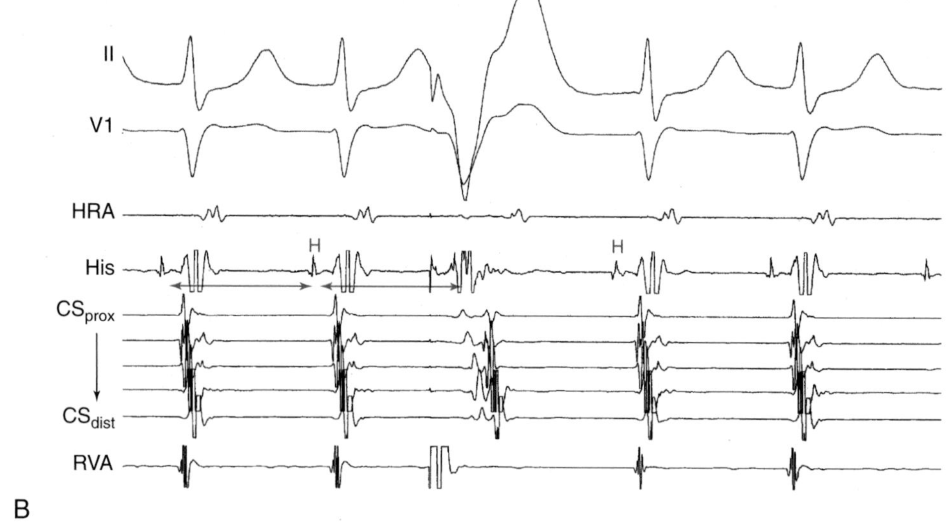

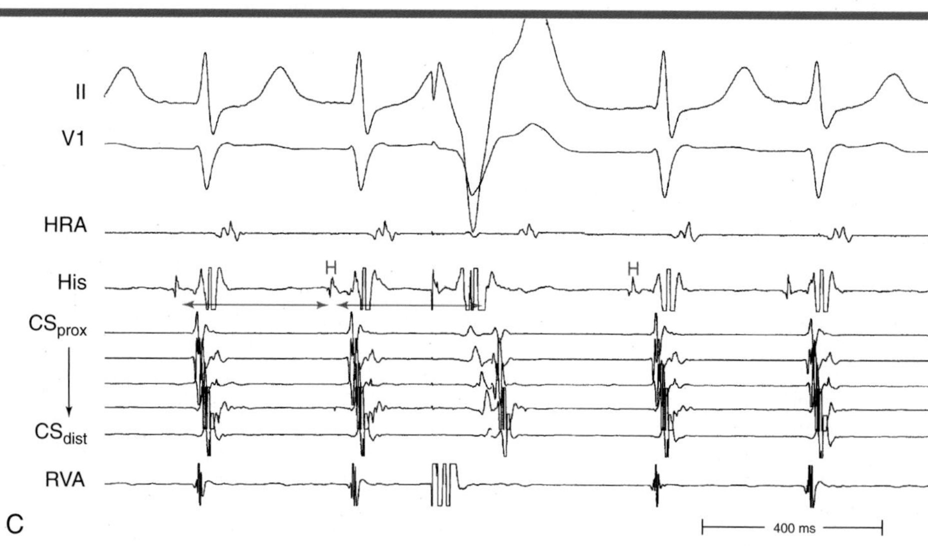

FIGURE 13–14 Resetting of atrioventricular nodal reentrant tachycardia (AVNRT) with ventricular extrastimulation (VES) at different coupling intervals. **A,** Late-coupled VES delivered when the His bundle (HB) is refractory fails to reset the AVNRT. In fact, the anterograde His potential (H) is visualized shortly after the pacing artifact (arrow), occurring at the expected timing (the tachycardia cycle length is indicated by the red lines). **B,** An early VES is delivered well before the expected time of the anterograde His potential fails to reset the supraventricular tachycardia (SVT). The fact that this VES advances ventricular activation at all recorded sites by approximately 70 msec and still fails to reset the SVT excludes orthodromic atrioventricular reentrant tachycardia (AVRT). **C,** Earlier VES results in resetting of the SVT as indicated by earlier timing of the following atrial activation.

ventricular pacing entraining the AVNRT (Figs. 13-15 and 13-16). The PPI after entrainment of AVNRT from the RV apex is significantly longer than the tachycardia CL ([PPI – SVT CL] is usually more than 115 milliseconds), because the reentrant circuit in AVNRT is above the ventricle and far from the pacing site. In AVNRT, the PPI reflects the conduction time from the pacing site through the RV muscle and HPS, once around the reentry circuit and back to the pacing site. Therefore, the [PPI – SVT CL] reflects twice the sum of the conduction time through the RV muscle, the HPS, and the lower common pathway. In orthodromic AVRT using a septal BT, the PPI reflects the conduction time through the RV to the septum, once around the reentry circuit and back. In other words, the [PPI – SVT CL]

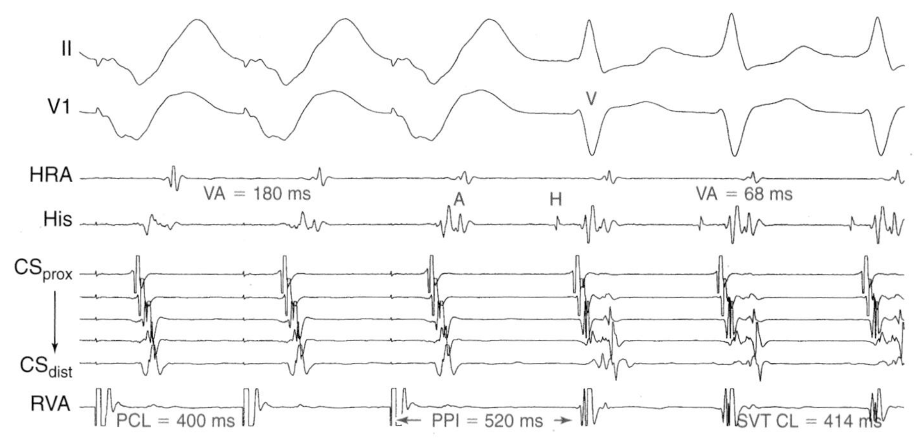

FIGURE 13–15 Entrainment of typical atrioventricular nodal reentrant tachycardia (AVNRT) with right ventricular (RV) apical pacing. The post-pacing interval supraventricular tachycardia cycle length (PPI – SVT CL) is more than 115 msec, and the ΔVA interval ($VA_{pacing} - VA_{SVT}$) is more than 85 msec. The atrial activation sequence during ventricular pacing is identical to that during AVNRT. No QRS fusion is observed. Cessation of ventricular pacing is followed by an A-V response. PCL = pacing CL.

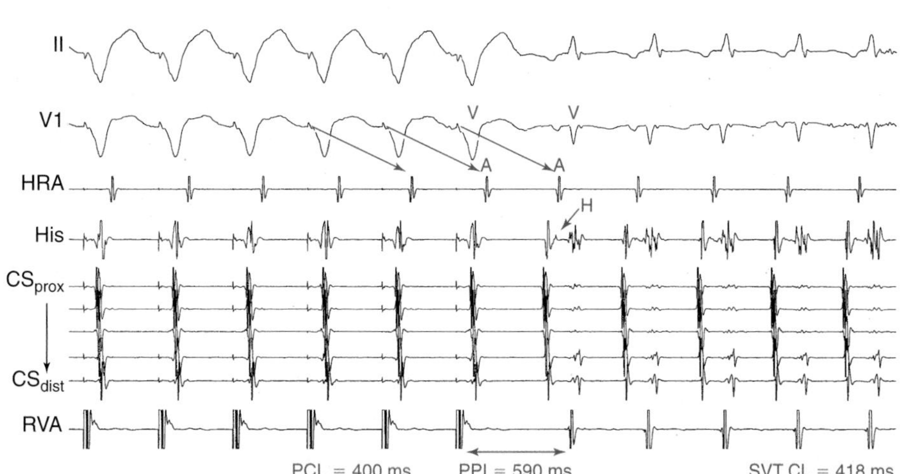

FIGURE 13–16 Entrainment of atypical atrioventricular nodal reentrant tachycardia (AVNRT) with right ventricular (RV) apical pacing. The post-pacing interval minus supraventricular tachycardia cycle length (PPI – SVT CL = 172 msec) is long, and the ΔVA interval is also long (188 msec), both criteria favoring AVNRT over orthodromic atrioventricular reentrant tachycardia (AVRT). Note that atrial activation sequence during RV pacing is similar to that during the SVT, again favoring AVNRT over other types of SVT. Additionally, a pseudo–A-A-V response is observed following cessation of ventricular pacing because retrograde conduction occurs through the slow pathway during ventricular pacing with a long VA interval (red arrows), longer than the pacing CL; hence, the last ventricular paced impulse is followed first by the P wave conducted slowly from the previous paced QRS, and then by the P wave resulting from the last paced QRS, mimicking an A-A-V response. This is confirmed by the observation that the last atrial activation resulting from conduction of the last paced ventricular complex follows the preceding P wave with an A-A interval equal to the ventricular pacing CL.

reflects twice the conduction time from the pacing catheter through the ventricular myocardium to the reentry circuit. Therefore, the PPI more closely approximates the SVT CL in orthodromic AVRT using a septal BT, compared with AVNRT. This maneuver was studied specifically for differentiation between atypical AVNRT and orthodromic AVRT, but the principle also applies to typical AVNRT (see Figs. 13-15 and 13-16). For borderline values, ventricular pacing at the RV base can help exaggerate the difference between the PPI and tachycardia CL in the case of AVNRT, but without significant changes in the case of orthodromic AVRT, because the site of pacing at the RV base is farther from the AVNRT circuit than the RV apex, but still close to an AVRT circuit using a septal BT (and in fact it is closer to the ventricular insertion of the BT).[39]

However, there are several potential pitfalls to those criteria. The tachycardia CL and VA interval are often perturbed for a few cycles after entrainment. For this reason, care should be taken not to measure unstable intervals immediately after ventricular pacing. In addition, spontaneous oscillations in the tachycardia CL and VA intervals can be seen. The discriminant points chosen may not apply when the spontaneous variability is more than 30 milliseconds. Also, it is possible to mistake isorhythmic VA dissociation for entrainment if the pacing train is not long enough or the pacing CL is too slow. Finally, the criteria may not apply to BTs with significant decremental properties, although small decremental intervals are unlikely to provide a false result.

Again, no QRS fusion would be manifest during ventricular entrainment of AVNRT, and QRS morphology is that of pure paced morphology. Fusion during resetting or entrainment of AVNRT with ventricular stimulation would require the paced ventricular wavefronts to enter the circuit propagating through the HB at the time that impulses are exiting through this structure; the HB is also the site of exit of the tachycardia circuit to the ventricular tissue. Under such circumstances, constant fusion during entrainment is almost impossible (unless a second connection exists between the atria and ventricles—i.e., an innocent bystander BT). On the other hand, fusion during resetting and/or entrainment can occur during orthodromic AVRT, and this maneuver can help distinguish orthodromic AVRT from AVNRT.

A-V Versus A-A-V Response. The electrogram sequence following cessation of ventricular entrainment of AVNRT can help exclude AT as the mechanism of SVT. When the ventricle is paced during AVNRT at a pacing CL shorter than the tachycardia CL and all electrograms are advanced to the pacing rate without terminating the tachycardia, 1:1 VA conduction occurs through the retrograde limb of the circuit (similar to the case for orthodromic AVRT).

Therefore, after the last paced QRS, the anterograde limb of the tachycardia circuit is not refractory, and the last retrograde P wave is able to conduct to the ventricle down that limb. This results in an A-V response (see Fig. 13-15). Conversely, when the ventricle is paced during AT and 1:1 VA conduction is produced, retrograde conduction occurs through the AVN. In this case, the last retrograde P wave resulting from ventricular pacing is unable to conduct to the ventricle because the AVN is still refractory to anterograde conduction, and the result is an A-A-V response.

Although this maneuver is helpful in distinguishing AT from AVNRT and orthodromic AVRT, it would not be useful when 1:1 VA conduction during ventricular pacing is absent. Thus, when determining the response after ventricular pacing during SVT, the presence of 1:1 VA conduction must be verified. Isorhythmic VA dissociation can mimic 1:1 VA conduction when the pacing train is not long enough or the pacing CL is too slow (see Fig. 8-8). Additionally, a pseudo–A-A-V response can occur during atypical AVNRT because retrograde conduction occurs through the slow pathway during ventricular pacing. This can result in a VA interval longer than the pacing CL; hence, the last ventricular paced impulse will be followed first by the P wave conducted slowly from the previous paced QRS, and then by the P wave resulting from the last paced QRS, mimicking an A-A-V response (see Fig. 13-16). Careful identification of the last atrial electrogram that resulted from VA conduction during ventricular pacing will avoid this potential pitfall. The last atrial activation resulting from conduction of the last paced ventricular complex will follow the preceding P wave with an A-A interval equal to the ventricular pacing CL. A pseudo–A-A-V response can also occur during typical AVNRT with long HV and/or short HA intervals, where atrial activation precedes ventricular activation. Replacing ventricular activation with HB activation (i.e., characterizing the response as A-A-H or A-H instead of A-A-V or A-V, respectively) can be more accurate and can help eliminate the pseudo–A-A-V response in patients with AVNRT and long HV intervals and/or short HA intervals.[40]

Diagnostic Maneuvers During Normal Sinus Rhythm After Tachycardia Termination

Atrial Pacing at the Tachycardia Cycle Length

Atrial pacing at the tachycardia CL results in an AH interval during atrial pacing longer than the AH interval during AVNRT. The AH interval during AVNRT is shortened because both the atrium and the HB are activated in parallel with simultaneous conduction up the upper common pathway and down the anterograde AVN pathway (the slow pathway in typical AVNRT, and the fast pathway in atypical AVNRT). In contrast, during AT and orthodromic AVRT, the atrium and HB are activated in sequence, and consequently the AH interval during SVT will approximate that during atrial pacing.

Under comparable autonomic tone status, 1:1 AV conduction over the AVN may or may not be maintained during atrial pacing at the tachycardia CL. AV block can occur during atrial pacing but not during AVNRT because of anterograde block in the upper common pathway. Retrograde conduction properties of the upper common pathway may allow 1:1 conduction from the AVNRT circuit up to the atrium but its anterograde conduction properties may not allow 1:1 anterograde conduction from the atrium down to the ventricle during atrial pacing at a similar CL. In contrast, 1:1 AV conduction, under comparable autonomic tone status, is typically maintained during atrial pacing at the tachycardia CL in the case of AT and orthodromic AVRT.

Ventricular Pacing at the Tachycardia Cycle Length

Ventricular pacing at the tachycardia CL results in HA and VA intervals that are longer during pacing than those during AVNRT. The ΔHA interval ($HA_{pacing} - HA_{SVT}$) is more than −10 milliseconds, because the HA interval during AVNRT is shortened because of parallel activation of both the HB and the atrium during AVNRT, whereas the HB and the atrium are activated sequentially during ventricular pacing. The ΔHA interval is even more pronounced in atypical AVNRT, because the lower common pathway is longer in atypical AVNRT than in typical AVNRT.

When pacing the atrium or ventricle at the tachycardia CL, it is important that the autonomic tone be similar to its state during the tachycardia, because alterations of autonomic tone can independently influence the AV or VA conduction. Under comparable autonomic tone, 1:1 VA conduction over the AVN may or may not be maintained during ventricular pacing at the tachycardia CL because of retrograde block in the lower common pathway. Anterograde conduction properties of the lower common pathway may allow 1:1 conduction from the AVNRT circuit down to the ventricle, but its retrograde conduction properties may not allow 1:1 retrograde conduction from the ventricle up to the atrium during ventricular pacing at a CL similar to the tachycardia CL. If VA block is present, orthodromic AVRT is excluded, and AT or AVNRT with lower common pathway physiology is more likely.

Atrial activation sequence during ventricular pacing is similar to that during AVNRT. Different atrial activation sequence suggests the presence of a retrogradely conducting BT that may or may not be related to the SVT.

Para-Hisian Pacing

This maneuver helps exclude the presence of a septal AV-BT, which can mediate an orthodromic AVRT with retrograde atrial activation sequence similar to that during AVNRT. Overdrive ventricular pacing is performed at a long pacing CL (more than 500 milliseconds) and high output from the pair of electrodes on the HB catheter that record the distal HB potential. During pacing, direct HB capture is indicated by shortening of the width of the paced QRS complex. The pacing output and pulse width are then decreased until the paced QRS widens, indicating loss of HB capture. The pacing output is increased and decreased to gain and lose HB capture, respectively, while local ventricular capture is maintained.

When the ventricle and HB are captured simultaneously, the wavefront travels down the HPS and results in a relatively narrow, normal-looking QRS. The wavefront may also travel retrogradely over the AVN to activate the atrium with an S-A interval (the interval from the paced impulse to the atrial electrogram on the HB recording) that represents conduction time over the proximal part of the HB and AVN (i.e., S-A interval = HA interval), because the onset of ventricular activation is simultaneous to that of HB activation (i.e., S-H interval = 0). When the ventricle is captured but not the atrium or HB, the paced wavefront travels through the ventricle via muscle-to-muscle conduction, resulting in a wide QRS with left bundle branch block (LBBB) morphology because of pacing in the RV. Once the wavefront reaches the RV apex, it conducts retrogradely up the RB and then over the HB and AVN to activate the atrium. In this case, the S-A interval represents conduction time from the RV base to the HB (S-H interval) plus conduction time over the HB and AVN (HA interval).

Thus, in the absence of a BT, para-Hisian pacing results in a shorter S-A interval when the HB is captured (S-H = 0 and S-A = HA) than the S-A interval when only the ventricle is captured (S-A = S-H + HA) with no change in the atrial activation sequence or HA interval. This response to para-Hisian pacing is termed *pattern 1* or *AVN/AVN pattern*. However, in the presence of a septal AV-BT, the S-A interval remains fixed as long as the local ventricular capture is maintained, regardless of whether the HB is being captured, because the paced impulse travels in both cases retrogradely over the AV-BT, with constant conduction time to the atrium. Atrial activation in this case can be secondary to conduction over the BT, especially when only the ventricle is captured, or a result of fusion of conduction over both the AV-BT and AVN, especially when the HB is captured.

Therefore, a change in retrograde atrial activation sequence with loss of HB-RB capture indicates the presence of retrograde conduction over both a BT and AVN, whereas an identical atrial activation sequence indicates that retrograde conduction is occurring over the same pathway (either the AVN or a BT) during HB-RB capture and noncapture. On loss of HB-RB capture, a constant S-A interval or local VA interval combined with shortening of the H-A interval indicates that retrograde conduction is occurring only over a BT. Lengthening of the S-A interval combined with a constant H-A interval indicates that retrograde conduction is occurring only over the AVN. See Chapter 14 for more detailed discussion.

Differential Right Ventricular Pacing

The response to differential RV pacing can be evaluated by comparing two variables between RV basilar and RV apical pacing, the VA interval and atrial activation sequence. In the absence of a septal AV-BT, pacing at the RV apex results in rapid access of the paced wavefront to the RB, HB, and AVN, and a shorter VA interval compared with pacing at the RV base. In the presence of a retrogradely conducting septal AV-BT, pacing at the RV base allows the wavefront to access the BT rapidly and activate the atrium with a shorter VA interval than during RV apical pacing that is farther from the BT ventricular insertion site.

Occurrence of right bundle branch block (RBBB) (but not LBBB) can alter the significance of the VA interval criterion, especially when VA conduction proceeds over the HPS-AVN. In the presence of retrograde RBBB, VA conduction occurs over the LB-HB; therefore, the VA interval depends on the distance between the pacing site and the LB rather than the RB, and access of the paced wavefront to the LB can be faster for RV basilar or septal pacing compared with pacing from the RV apex (Fig. 13-17).

Atrial activation sequence will be similar during RV apical and RV basilar pacing in the absence of a retrogradely conducting AV-BT because the atrium is activated over the AVN in both cases. In contrast, in the presence of a septal AV-BT, atrial activation sequence may or may not be similar during pacing from the RV apex and RV base. Atrial activation may proceed only over the AV-BT in both cases or it may proceed over the AV-BT during RV basilar pacing, and over the AVN (or a fusion of conduction over both the AVN and AV-BT) during RV apical pacing. See Chapter 14 for more detailed discussion.

Exclusion of Other Arrhythmia Mechanisms

ATs arising from the anteroseptal region and orthodromic AVRT using superoparaseptal BTs can mimic typical AVNRT. Additionally, ATs arising from the posteroseptal region and orthodromic AVRT using posteroseptal BTs can mimic atypical AVNRT. The various EP testing maneuvers used to exclude these tachycardias are outlined in Tables 13-6 and 13-7.

ABLATION

Target of Ablation

Ablation of the slow pathway is indicated in patients with documented AVNRT during EP testing, but also can be performed in patients with documented SVT that is morphologically consistent with AVNRT but in whom only dual AVN physiology (but not tachycardia) is demonstrated during an EP study. Slow pathway ablation may be considered at the discretion of the physician when sustained (more than 30 seconds) AVNRT is induced incidentally during an ablation procedure directed at a different clinical tachycardia.

Historically, the initial approach of RF ablation of AVNRT was modification of AVN conduction by lesions created near the anterosuperior aspect of the triangle of Koch (fast pathway ablation or anterior approach). However, because the fast pathway constitutes the physiological conduction

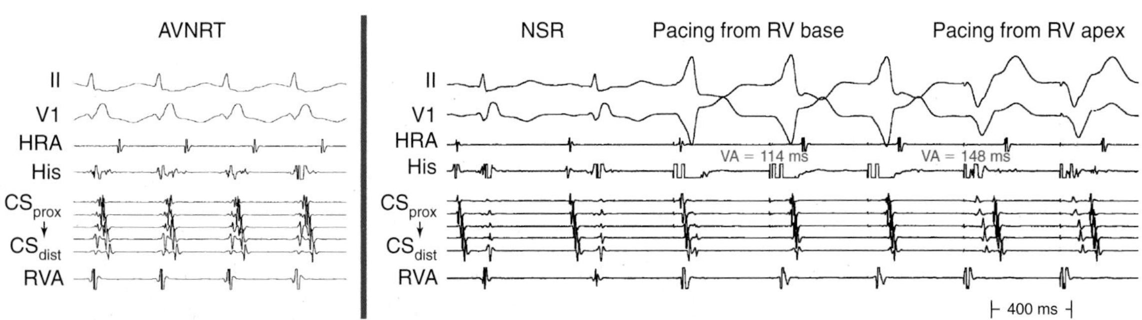

FIGURE 13–17 Comparison between right ventricular (RV) basilar versus apical pacing in a patient with typical atrioventricular nodal reentrant tachycardia (AVNRT) and right bundle branch block (RBBB) (left panel) but no bypass tracts (BTs). RBBB is also observed during normal sinus rhythm (NSR). In the absence of a retrogradely conducting BT, pacing from the RV apex is expected to result in a shorter VA interval than pacing from the RV base. However, in this case, the presence of RBBB produces misleading results, because retrograde VA conduction occurs over the left bundle branch (LB)–His bundle, and the VA interval depends on the distance between the pacing site to the LB, as opposed to the right bundle branch.

13

TABLE 13–6 Exclusion of Atrial Tachycardia (AT)

VES delivered during SVT	· VES that terminates the SVT without atrial activation excludes AT
Entrainment of SVT by ventricular pacing	· If atrial activation sequence during entrainment is similar to that during the SVT, AT is less likely. · Presence of A-V electrogram sequence following cessation of pacing is consistent with AVNRT and generally excludes AT.
Entrainment of SVT by atrial pacing	· ΔAH ($AH_{atrial\ pacing} - AH_{SVT}$) > 40 msec excludes AT. · If the VA interval of the return cycle after cessation of atrial pacing is fixed and similar to that of the SVT (with <10-msec variation) after different attempts at SVT entrainment (the so-called V-A linking), AT is unlikely.[36]
Ventricular pacing during NSR at tachycardia CL	· If retrograde atrial activation sequence during ventricular pacing is similar to that during SVT, AT is less likely, but cannot be excluded.
Atrial pacing during NSR at tachycardia CL	· ΔAH ($AH_{atrial\ pacing} - AH_{SVT}$) > 40 msec excludes AT. · If AV block develops during atrial pacing, AT is excluded.

AH = atrial-His bundle; AV = atrioventricular; A-V = atrium-ventricle; AVNRT = atrioventricular nodal reentrant tachycardia; CL = cycle length; NSR = normal sinus rhythm; SVT = supraventricular tachycardia; VA = ventricular-atrial; VES = ventricular extrastimulation.

axis and is located in close proximity to the compact AVN and HB, such a procedure was associated with an unacceptable risk of AV block and was consequently abandoned. Later on, selective ablation of the slow AVN pathway by lesions created near the posteroinferior base of the triangle of Koch between the CS os and tricuspid annulus (posterior approach) has proved to be a more successful and safer procedure. Additionally, in patients with multiple slow pathways, ablation of the fast pathway can be associated with persistently inducible AVNRT with anterograde conduction over a second slowly conducting pathway. In contrast, successful ablation of the slow pathway can eliminate all variants of AVNRT.[41,42]

Despite the lack of precise knowledge of the pathophysiological substrate for AVNRT, ablation procedures have been successful, with very good outcomes. How ablation works to cure AVNRT is not clear.

The target for the posterior approach is the site of the slow pathway. This target can be defined by one of two approaches, a purely anatomical approach and an electroanatomical approach.

Anatomical Approach. The target of ablation is the isthmus of tissue between the tricuspid annulus and CS os (Fig. 13-18).[25,43,44] The sequence of ablation sites chosen for RF delivery is related to the probability of successful slow pathway ablation at each site and the risk of impairing AV conduction. The most common site for effective and safe ablation is along the tricuspid annulus immediately anterior to the CS os, which has a success rate of 95%. Occasionally, successful ablation can require the catheter positioned along the tricuspid annulus inferior to the CS os. If ablation is not successful at these locations, the catheter is then moved more cephalad along the tricuspid annulus superior to the CS os. Finally, if those sites are unsuccessful, RF delivery at more superior sites (more than halfway between the CS os and HB) can be considered only if the risk of complete AV block can be justified by the severity of clinical symptoms.[25,43,44]

TABLE 13–7 Exclusion of Orthodromic Atrioventricular Reentrant Tachycardia (AVRT)

Parameter	Description
VA interval	VA interval < 70 msec or V-high RA interval < 95 msec during SVT excludes orthodromic AVRT.[25,36]
AV block	Spontaneous or induced AV block with continuation of the SVT excludes orthodromic AVRT.
VES delivered during the SVT	Failure to reset (advance or delay) atrial activation with early-coupled VES on multiple occasions and at different VES coupling intervals, despite advancement of the local ventricular activation at all sites (including the site of the suspected BT) by >30 msec, orthodromic AVRT and presence of AV BT are excluded.
Entrainment of the SVT by ventricular pacing	ΔVA ($VA_{ventricular\ pacing} - VA_{SVT}$) > 85 msec excludes orthodromic AVRT.[61] PPI - SVT CL > 115 msec excludes orthodromic AVRT.[61] Ventricular fusion during entrainment indicates AVRT and excludes AVNRT.
Entrainment of SVT by atrial pacing	ΔAH ($AH_{atrial\ pacing} - AH_{SVT}$) > 40 msec excludes orthodromic AVRT.
Ventricular pacing during NSR at the tachycardia CL	ΔHA ($HA_{ventricular\ pacing} - HA_{SVT}$) >–10 msec excludes orthodromic AVRT.
Atrial pacing during NSR at the tachycardia CL	ΔAH ($AH_{atrial\ pacing} - AH_{SVT}$) > 40 msec excludes orthodromic AVRT. If AV block develops during atrial pacing, orthodromic AVRT is excluded.
Differential RV pacing during NSR	Pacing at the RV base producing a longer VA interval and identical atrial activation sequence compared with that during pacing at the RV apex excludes the presence of a septal AV-BT mediating an orthodromic AVRT.
Para-Hisian pacing	Loss of HB-RB capture resulting in an increase in the S-A interval in all electrograms (equal to the increase in the S-H interval), with no change in the atrial activation sequence or HA interval, excludes the presence of a septal AV-BT mediating an orthodromic AVRT.

AH = atrial-His bundle; AV = atrioventricular; BT = bypass tract; CL = cycle length; HA = His bundle-atrial; HB-RB = His bundle-right bundle branch; NSR = normal sinus rhythm; PPI = post-pacing interval; RA = right atrium; RV = right ventricle; SVT = supraventricular tachycardia; VA = ventricular-atrial; VES = ventricular extrastimulation.

If slow pathway ablation cannot be achieved in the posteroseptal RA, it may be worthwhile to deliver RF energy at sites within the proximal CS, close to the os, with the ablation catheter pointing toward the LV with counterclockwise torque. Rarely, successful slow pathway ablation may require an application of energy on the left side of the posterior septum, along the mitral annulus.[41,45]

Catheter-induced AVN block occasionally occurs during mapping (approximately 2%). This may indicate the presence of a relatively small compact AVN that might be more susceptible to heart block during ablation. Catheter-induced AV block typically resolves after seconds to minutes. Careful catheter positioning to avoid sites at which catheter-induced block occurs generally results in successful ablation without AV block.

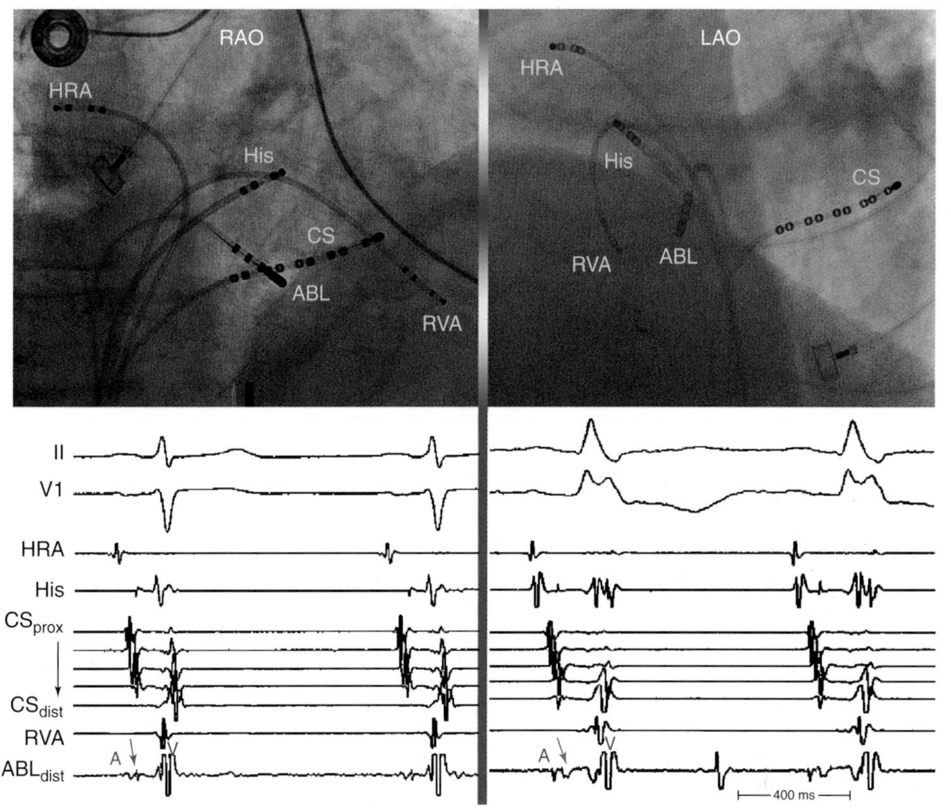

FIGURE 13–18 Ablation of the slow atrioventricular node (AVN) pathway. **Upper panel,** Right anterior oblique (RAO) and left anterior oblique (LAO) fluoroscopic views of typical catheter setup during atrioventricular nodal reentrant tachycardia (AVNRT) ablation. The ablation catheter (ABL) is positioned at the slow pathway location in the lower portion of the triangle of Koch, away from the His bundle (HB) and anterior to the coronary sinus (CS) (those landmarks are defined by the HB and CS catheters, respectively). **Lower panel,** Intracardiac recordings during ablation of the slow pathway. Note the sharp (blue arrow, left lower panel) and broad (red arrow, right lower panel) potentials recorded between the atrial and ventricular electrograms at the ablation sites. Those potentials were suggested to reflect activation of the slow pathway (slow pathway potentials).

Electroanatomical Approach (Slow Pathway Potentials). The electroanatomical approach is guided by the identification of slow pathway potentials in conjunction to anatomical landmarks. These potentials have been used by some to define the site of slow pathway within the triangle of Koch, and can be used effectively as a guide for the ablation target.[25,43,44]

It has been suggested that activation of the slow pathway is associated with inscription of discrete electrical potentials, often referred to as slow pathway potentials. The origin of these potentials is uncertain; whether they represent nodal tissue activation or anisotropic conduction through muscle bundles in various sites in the triangle of Koch or a combination of both is unclear. The electrogram morphology of the slow potentials has been variously described as sharp and rapid (representing the atrial connection to the slow pathway described by Heidbuchel and Jackman[19]; see Fig. 13-18), or slow and broad with low amplitude (representing slow potentials described by Haissaguerre and associates[45]; see Fig. 13-18). The timing of slow potentials during NSR was reported to follow closely (within 10 to 40 milliseconds) local atrial activation near the CS os, or to span the AH interval (and can occur as late as the His potential). However, such potentials are neither specific to the triangle of Koch nor to patients with AVNRT and can be recorded near the tricuspid annulus at sites distant from the slow pathway. Despite these observations, the probability of recording putative slow potentials at the site of effective slow ablation is more than 90%.

For ablation of slow-slow and fast-slow AVNRT, the slow pathway used for retrograde conduction during the tachycardia should be targeted by ablation, which can be different from the slow AVN pathway used for anterograde conduction. Therefore, ablation can be guided by the site of earliest retrograde atrial activation during AVNRT or ventricular pacing, which is usually localized to the isthmus of tissue between the tricuspid annulus and the CS os in fast-slow AVNRT, and along the anterior aspect of the CS in slow-slow AVNRT.[42,46]

Ablation Technique

For slow pathway ablation, a quadripolar, 4-mm-tip, deflectable ablation catheter is advanced via a femoral vein. Rarely, a superior vena cava (SVC) approach (via the internal jugular or subclavian vein) is required because of inferior vena cava (IVC) obstruction or barriers, and a recent report has demonstrated the feasibility of this approach.[47] The target site can be mapped using the anatomical or electroanatomical approach. Large-tip and irrigated-tip catheters have no role in catheter ablation of the slow pathway, because the larger lesions they create can increase the risk of AV block.

Anatomical Approach. The target of slow pathway ablation is the isthmus of tissue between the tricuspid annulus and CS os.[2,25,43,44] Using the right anterior oblique (RAO) view, which best displays the triangle of Koch in profile, the ablation catheter is advanced into the RV, moved inferiorly so that it lies anterior to the CS os, and then withdrawn until the distal pair of electrodes records small atrial and large ventricular electrograms (with an A/V electrogram amplitude ratio during NSR of 0.1 to 0.5). Gentle clockwise torque is maintained to keep the catheter in contact with the low atrial septum. This will position the catheter along the tricuspid annulus immediately anterior to the CS os (see Fig. 13-18). Positioning is best performed during NSR, because the atrial and ventricular electrograms at the tricuspid annulus are more easily discerned. If the catheter does not easily reach far enough into the ventricle, yielding an A/V ratio of only 1:1, or if catheter stability is inadequate, a long sheath with a slight septal angulation can be helpful. Moreover, some ablation catheters have asymmetrical bidirectional deflection curves, an option that can prove to be of value for catheter reach and stability in these cases.[41]

Electroanatomical Approach. The target site is identified by slow pathway potentials (see Fig. 13-18).[25,48] Initially, the triangle of Koch is mapped from the apex (where the HB is recorded) and then moved toward the CS os. This also helps evaluate the extension of the zone recording a His potential. Slow pathway potentials are usually recorded at the midanteroseptal position, where they are located in the middle of the isoelectric line connecting the atrial and ventricular electrograms. Moving the mapping catheter inferiorly, the slow pathway potential moves towards the atrial electrogram, and when the optimal site for slow pathway ablation is reached, it merges with the atrial electrogram. Because electrograms with these characteristics can be recorded near the tricuspid annulus at sites distant from the slow pathway, the region explored with the ablation catheter should be limited to the posterior septum, near the CS os.[25,48] In the left anterior oblique (LAO) view, using the HB and CS os positions (as defined by the HB and CS catheters) as landmarks, the most common area where the slow potentials are recorded is in the posterior third of the line connecting those two landmarks.[46]

Validation of slow pathway potentials can be useful and can be achieved by demonstrating that they represent slow and decremental conduction properties. Typically, brief runs of incremental atrial pacing or AES produce a decline in the amplitude and slope, an increase in the duration, and a separation of the slow potential from the preceding atrial electrogram until disappearance of any consistent activity. This is especially helpful in the presence of a sharp slow pathway potential, to distinguish it from a proximal HB recording. Catheter-induced junctional ectopy, when present, indicates that the catheter tip is at a good ablation site. In patients with slow-slow and slow-fast AVNRT, mapping during AVNRT often shows a discrete potential 20 to 40 milliseconds prior to the earliest atrial electrogram; this may indicate the slow pathway and signify a good target site.[46]

Radiofrequency Energy Delivery. Catheter stability should be optimized before starting RF energy application to avoid inadvertent AV block. This may require cessation of isoproterenol infusion if hyperdynamic contractility is present. Additionally, good positioning of the other EP catheters defining the anatomical landmarks demarcating the triangle of Koch and the location of HB is mandatory.

Ablation should be performed during NSR, when it is easier to maintain a stable catheter position. When ablation is carried out during AVNRT, sudden termination of the tachycardia during RF delivery can result in dislodgment of the ablation catheter, inadvertent AV block, and an incomplete RF lesion.[25,43,44]

Typical RF settings consist of a maximum power of 50 W and a maximum temperature of 55° to 60°C, continued for 30 to 60 seconds, or until the junctional rhythm extinguishes (see later).[25,43,44] Impedance and ECG should be carefully monitored throughout RF application. However, in the case of slow pathway ablation, the decrement in impedance associated with successful energy applications is usually small (approximately 2.5 Ω); such a small change precludes the clinical usefulness of impedance monitoring.

Junctional Rhythm. An accelerated junctional rhythm typically develops within a few seconds of RF delivery at the effective ablation site (Fig. 13-19). The mechanism of this rhythm is unclear but is likely to be secondary to enhanced automaticity in AVN tissue because of thermal injury; it is usually associated with subtle but definite changes in retrograde atrial activation sequence (compared with that during AVNRT). Occurrence of this rhythm is strongly correlated to and sensitive for successful ablation sites; it occurs more frequently (94% versus 64%) and for a longer duration (7.1 versus 5.0 seconds) during successful compared with unsuccessful RF applications. Such a rhythm is, however, not specific for slow pathway ablation and is routinely observed during intentional fast pathway and AVN ablation. Junctional tachycardia, on the other hand, is probably caused by thermal injury of the HB and heralds impending AV block (Fig. 13-20).[42,49-51]

When an accelerated junctional rhythm occurs, careful monitoring of VA conduction during this rhythm is essential and atrial pacing should be performed to ensure maintenance of 1:1 anterograde AV conduction (see Fig. 13-19). Occasionally, atrial pacing at a rate fast enough to override the junctional rhythm results in AV Wenckebach block at baseline, even before the onset of RF energy delivery; in this case, isoproterenol can be used to shorten the AV block CL and maintain 1:1 AV conduction during pacing.[51]

The absence of junctional rhythm during RF application corresponds to an unsuccessful ablation site, and when an accelerated junctional rhythm does not develop within 10 to 20 seconds of RF delivery, RF application is stopped and the catheter tip is repositioned to a slightly different site or better contact is verified and a new RF application attempted. Nevertheless, a junctional rhythm may not occur in several situations, including atypical forms of AVNRT (fast-slow and slow-slow) and some cases of typical (slow-fast) AVNRT undergoing repeat ablation.

After an RF application that results in an accelerated junctional rhythm, programmed electrical stimulation (atrial and ventricular stimulation) is performed to determine the presence or absence of slow pathway conduction, AVN echoes, or inducible AVNRT. If the result is unsatisfactory, the catheter is moved to a slightly different site (usually a few millimeters anteriorly), and RF is reapplied.[42,51]

Several observations should prompt immediate discontinuation of RF application, including sudden impedance rise (more than 10 Ω), prolongation of the PR interval (during NSR or atrial pacing), development of AV block, fast junctional tachycardia (CL < 350 milliseconds), and retrograde conduction block during junctional ectopy (see Fig. 13-20).

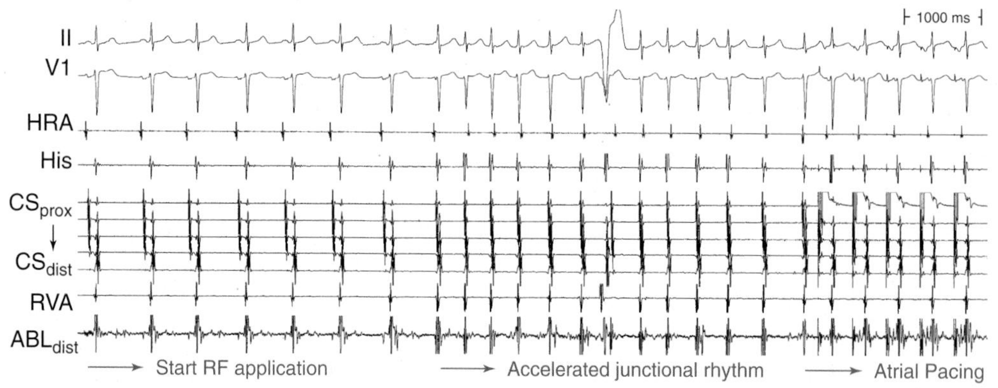

FIGURE 13–19 Catheter ablation of the slow atrioventricular nodal (AVN) pathway. Radiofrequency (RF) energy delivery during normal sinus rhythm (NSR) results in accelerated junctional rhythm with intact ventriculoatrial (VA) conduction. Overdrive atrial pacing at a rate faster than the junctional rhythm rate was started and confirmed intact atrioventricular (AV) conduction. This observation can indicate a good ablation site, with no injury to the fast pathway.

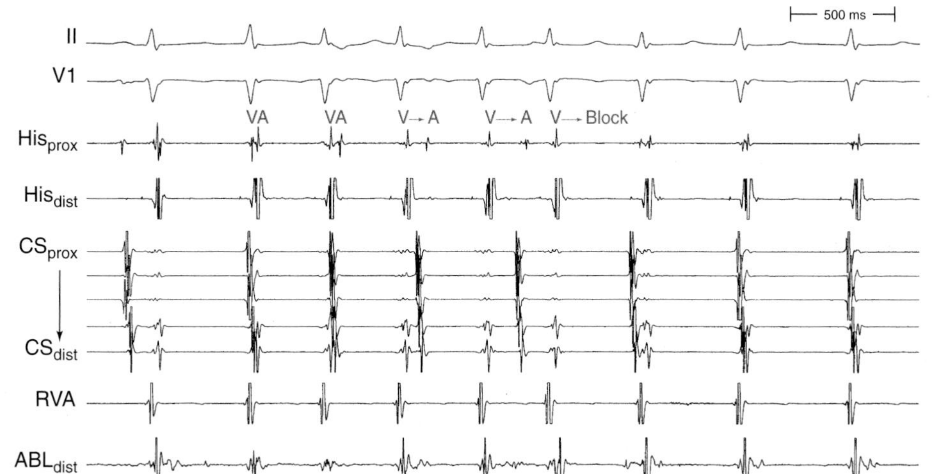

FIGURE 13–20 Junctional tachycardia observed during slow pathway ablation. Wenckebach ventriculoatrial (VA) block is observed during the junctional rhythm, a sign that heralds injury to the His bundle and should prompt immediate termination of radiofrequency application.

Although the latter observation may herald anterograde AV bock in the case of typical AVNRT and necessitates immediate discontinuation of RF delivery, retrograde block over the fast pathway is a common occurrence in patients with atypical AVNRT, even before ablation. In this case, the occurrence of junctional rhythm with no VA conduction may not be such an ominous sign and, in fact, such occurrence may indicate successful ablation of the slow pathway and thus should prompt ongoing RF delivery.[25,43,44,50,52]

Endpoints of Ablation

The optimal endpoint for slow pathway ablation is the complete elimination of slow pathway conduction and dual AVN physiology without impairing the fast pathway. This is evidenced by loss of conduction over the slow pathway (i.e., disappearance of discontinuous AV conduction curves), alteration of Wenckebach CL (shorter or longer), an increase in the ERP of the AVN, and preservation of intact anterograde and retrograde AVN (fast pathway) conduction.[53-55] In many cases, the ERP of the fast pathway can actually shorten, likely secondary to the withdrawal of electrotonic inhibition imposed on the fast pathway by the slow pathway. For atypical AVNRT, elimination of retrograde fast pathway conduction (i.e., complete VA block) is an important additional endpoint.[20,41,42]

However, elimination of all evidence of slow pathway conduction is not a necessary requirement for a successful slow pathway ablation procedure.[25,43,44,53,56] It suffices to eliminate inducibility of AVNRT and 1:1 anterograde conduction over the slow pathway, with and without isoproterenol infusion. Complete elimination of all anterograde slow conduction is not essential for clinical success, and is actually associated with a slightly higher risk of AV block. In patients with a successful slow pathway ablation procedure, 40% to 50% will still have dual AVN pathways, and 75% of those will have AVN echoes, but AVNRT is not inducible (these patients are said to have undergone slow pathway modification). In most patients who no longer have inducible AVNRT post ablation in the slow pathway region, residual discontinuous AVN function curves and single AVN echoes do not predict an increased risk for AVNRT recurrence. Reassessment of inducibility should be repeated 30 minutes after the last successful RF application.

Therefore, noninducibility of AVNRT (with and without isoproterenol infusion) with residual evidence of dual AVN pathways (AH interval jump) and single AVN echoes with an echo zone less than 30 milliseconds is an acceptable endpoint. However, double AVN echoes or single echoes produced over a wide range of coupling intervals predict the inducibility of AVNRT with the addition of isoproterenol or atropine as well as late clinical recurrence of SVT and, therefore, additional RF applications are recommended.[41]

When AVNRT and/or dual AVN physiology is rarely inducible at baseline, it may not be possible to confirm the efficacy of the RF delivery. In this case, other parameters can be indicative of a successful ablation, including the disappearance of a PR/RR ratio more than 1 during rapid atrial pacing with 1:1 AV conduction, prolongation of the Wenckebach CL, and decrease in fast pathway ERP.[10,25,41,43,44]

If isoproterenol was required for initiation of SVT prior to ablation, isoproterenol should be discontinued during ablation and readministered afterward to assess the efficacy of ablation adequately. If isoproterenol was not necessary for SVT initiation prior to ablation, it need not be used for postablation testing. However, if single AVN echoes are accepted as an endpoint, isoproterenol infusion may then be required during postablation testing to verify noninducibility of double echoes or AVNRT.[41,42]

Outcome

Acute success rates of AVNRT ablation using the posterior approach exceed 95%, and are similar whether the ablation is guided anatomically or electroanatomically.[48,54,56,57] The recurrence rate after apparently successful ablation is approximately 2% to 5%. In 40% of patients with AVNRT recurrences, slow pathway conduction recovers after initial evidence of its abolition. Most AVNRT recurrences take place within the first days to months after ablation.[42,48,54,56,57]

The most important complication of AVNRT ablation is AV block.[48,50,52] AV block occurs in about 0.2% to 0.6% of slow pathway ablation using the posterior approach, generally occurs during RF delivery or within the first 24 hours postablation, and is almost always preceded by junctional ectopy with VA block. The level of block is usually in the AVN. Predictors of AV block include proximity of the anatomical ablation site to the compact AVN, occurrence of fast junctional tachycardia (CL < 350 milliseconds) during RF application, occurrence of junctional rhythm with VA block, the number of RF applications (related to the amount of tissue damage), and significant worsening of anterograde AV conduction during the ablation procedure.[48,54,56,57]

Palpitations occur in 20% to 30% of patients following ablation of AVNRT. These are generally transient, and usually not caused by recurrent AVNRT. Most are caused by premature atrial complexes (PACs) or PVCs, which subside spontaneously and require no treatment other than reassurance. Inappropriate sinus tachycardia can develop in some patients after AVN ablation, suggesting disruption of the parasympathetic and/or sympathetic inputs into the sinus and AV nodes.

Subclinical activation of the coagulation system (e.g.,
13 elevated plasma levels of the D-dimer) is common during RF ablation. Nevertheless, clinically detectable embolic events are uncommon (0.7%). Aspirin is usually recommended for 6 to 8 weeks following ablation to minimize the risk of thrombus formation in the RA and/or vena cavae. Other complications include cardiac tamponade, which occurs in 0.2%, hematoma (in 0.2%), and femoral artery pseudoaneurysm (in 0.1%).[42]

There are several advantages of selective slow pathway ablation over fast pathway ablation, including significantly lower risk of AV block, and avoidance of a long postablation PR interval, which can cause symptoms similar to the pacemaker syndrome. Furthermore, in patients with multiple slow pathways, as demonstrated by AVN function curves, ablation of the fast pathway can be associated with persistently inducible AVNRT, with anterograde conduction over a second slowly conducting pathway.[42]

Selective slow pathway ablation can be technically challenging in several clinical situations. For example, in patients with evidence of impaired fast pathway conduction (usually older patients with tachycardia CL > 400 milliseconds), ablation of the slow pathway can result in mandatory conduction via the impaired fast pathway and Wenckebach block during rest. Whether the fast pathway should be targeted by ablation instead of the slow pathway in these patients is controversial.[20,52] Similarly, some patients with AVNRT have first-degree AV block during NSR, suggesting the possibility of absent anterograde fast pathway conduction and a high risk of complete AV block if the slow pathway is ablated. However, in such patients, the fast pathway can be affected by an electrotonic interaction with the slow pathway, and elimination of this effect by slow pathway ablation often shortens the ERP of the fast pathway. In fact, in many of these patients, the AH interval remains stable or even shortens after slow pathway ablation.[20,52] Another challenging situation may be experienced in patients with prior unsuccessful attempts at fast pathway ablation, with persistent AVNRT. Slow pathway ablation may then result in high-degree AV block because of impairment of the fast pathway related to the prior ablation attempt. In such patients, it is wise to confine further ablation efforts to the pathway originally targeted for ablation.[41,42]

It is also important to know that in some cases of typical AVNRT, the fast pathway can have a more posterior location, and the earliest atrial activation site during the tachycardia is near the CS os. In such cases, ablation should be performed with caution, because RF application at the usual slow pathway anatomical site can result in PR interval prolongation or heart block. Cryoablation can be of advantage in these situations.

Fast Pathway Modification (Anterior Approach)

Target of Fast Pathway Ablation

The target site of this approach is located closer to the compact AVN and HB in the anterosuperior region of the triangle of Koch.[2] The anterior approach selectively ablates or modifies the retrograde fast pathway conduction; however, it can also cause damage to the anterograde fast or slow pathway conduction.[41,42]

Fast Pathway Ablation Technique

The ablation catheter is initially positioned at the AV junction to obtain the maximal amplitude of the bipolar His potential recorded from the distal pair of electrodes. The catheter is then withdrawn while a firm clockwise torque is maintained until the His potential becomes small or barely visible, or disappears while recording a relatively large atrial electrogram (with A/V electrogram amplitude ratio more than 1; see Fig. 11-57). At the optimal ablation site, retrograde atrial activation timing occurs earlier or simultaneously with the atrial electrogram in the catheter at the HB position. At this point, the ablation catheter is held steadily and RF energy is applied (starting at low power outputs of 5 to 10 W) until one of the following events occurs: impedance rise, transient high-grade AV block, prolongation of the PR interval by more than 30 % to 50%, or appearance of very rapid junctional rhythm associated with retrograde conduction block. Overdrive atrial pacing is performed to monitor AV conduction in case a junctional escape rhythm occurs during RF application.[41,42]

Endpoints of Fast Pathway Ablation

The endpoint of ablation is noninducibility of AVNRT or development of AV block. Frequently, fast pathway ablation is associated with retrograde VA block over both the slow and fast pathways. Occasionally, dual AVN physiology can still be present.

Outcome of Fast Pathway Ablation

Acute success rates are above 95%. However, the anterior approach has a small safety margin and is associated with a higher risk of inadvertent complete AV block (approximately 10%, but ranging from 2% to 20%). Careful monitoring of AV conduction during RF application and prompt discontinuation of energy delivery on evidence of AV block are the keys to minimize the incidence of AV block.

Cryoablation of the Slow Pathway

Target of Cryoablation

The target of ablation is the region of the slow pathway, and it is identified anatomically or electroanatomically, in a similar fashion as described for standard RF ablation. The target site should be identified during NSR whether cryoablation is to be performed during NSR or AVNRT, because the A/V ratio and electrogram morphology usually are obscured during AVNRT.[58,59]

Cryoablation Technique

Cryomapping. Cryomapping (ice mapping) is designed to verify that ablation at the chosen site will have the desired effect (i.e., block in the slow pathway) and to reassure the absence of complications (i.e., AV block). Cryomapping is performed at a temperature of −30°C. At this temperature, the cryolesion is reversible (for up to 60 seconds) and the catheter is stuck to the atrial endocardium within an ice ball that includes the tip of the catheter (cryoadherence). Formation of an ice ball at the catheter tip and adherence to the underlying myocardium are signaled by the appearance of electrical noise recorded from the ablation catheter's distal bipole. In the cryomapping mode, the temperature is not allowed to drop below −30°, and the duration of energy application is limited to 60 seconds. Once an ice ball is formed, various pacing protocols are performed to test the modification or disappearance of slow pathway conduction.[58-60]

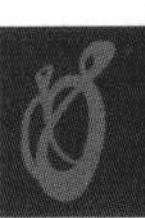

Cryomapping is usually performed during NSR in patients with discontinuous anterograde dual AVN conduction curve. For patients without a clear discontinuity in the AVN conduction curve, cryomapping can be performed during AVNRT, which is feasible without the risk of catheter dislodgment on termination of the tachycardia (because of cryoadherence).[60]

During cryoablation of the slow pathway, no junctional rhythm is observed. Thus, other parameters must be used to validate the potential effectiveness of the ablation site. In fact, the absence of junctional rhythm can be advantageous because it allows the maintenance of NSR during ablation and enables monitoring of the PR interval throughout the procedure. Additionally, the maintenance of NSR during cryoablation allows various pacing maneuvers to be performed during ongoing cryoenergy application to evaluate the effect of the ablation on slow pathway conduction. Disappearance of the dual AVN physiology, noninducibility of AVNRT, and modification of the fast pathway ERP predict a successful ablation site. When cryoablation is performed during AVNRT, progressive AH interval lengthening followed by termination of AVNRT indicates slow pathway block.[60]

Slow pathway block usually occurs quickly (within 10 to 20 seconds) at the optimal target site. If cryomapping does not yield the desired result within 20 to 30 seconds or results in unintended AV conduction delay or block, cryomapping is interrupted and, after a few seconds, allowing the catheter to thaw and become dislodged from the tissue, the catheter is moved to a different site and cryomapping repeated.[60]

Cryoablation. When sites of successful cryomapping are identified by demonstrating satisfactory slow pathway block or modification with no modification of the basal anterograde AV conduction, the cryoablation mode is activated, during which a target temperature below −75°C is sought (a temperature of about −75° to −80°C is generally achieved). The application is then continued for 4 minutes, creating an irreversible lesion.[58,59] If the catheter tip is in close contact with the endocardium, a prompt drop in catheter tip temperature should be seen as soon as the cryoablation mode is activated. A slow decline in temperature or very high flow rates of refrigerant during ablation suggests poor catheter tip tissue contact; in such cases, cryoablation should be interrupted and the catheter repositioned.[60]

The successful site for cryomapping and cryoablation of the slow pathway frequently is found in the midseptal region of Koch's triangle, more superiorly than the usual site of successful RF ablation. Rarely, AV block does not appear during cryomapping at a particular site but occurs during cryoablation at the same site. Fortunately, this resolves quickly if the cryoablation is interrupted promptly.

Endpoints of Cryoablation

The goal of cryoablation is the complete elimination of slow pathway function. This usually requires delivery of several cryoapplications at closely adjacent sites.[58,59] If a discontinuity in the anterograde AVN conduction curve and single AVN echoes persist despite multiple cryoapplications, this is still a reasonable endpoint, provided that multiple echoes or SVT are not inducible, even during isoproterenol infusion. If acute procedural success cannot be achieved with a standard 4-mm-tip catheter, a 6-mm-tip catheter can be used, which can help yield larger and deeper cryolesions.[60]

Advantages of Cryoablation

One of the distinct advantages of cryothermal technology is the ability to demonstrate loss of function of tissue with cooling reversibly (ice mapping or cryomapping), thereby demonstrating the functionality of prospective ablation sites without inducing permanent injury.[58,59] Furthermore, once the catheter tip temperature is reduced below 0°C, progressive ice formation at the catheter tip causes adherence to the adjacent tissue (cryoadherence), which maintains stable catheter contact at the site of ablation and minimizes the risk of catheter dislodgment during changing cardiac rhythm.[58-60]

Cryoablation can be of particular advantage in AVNRT cases with posterior displacement of the fast pathway or AVN, small space in the triangle of Koch between the HB and the CS os, and when ablation must be performed in the midseptum.[43,44,58,59] However, given the high success rate and low risk of RF slow pathway ablation, it may be difficult to demonstrate a clinical advantage of cryoablation over RF ablation of unselected AVNRT cases. A disadvantage of cryoablation is that the cryocatheter is not yet as steerable as the conventional RF catheter, which can potentially limit proper positioning of the catheter tip.[60]

Outcome of Cryoablation

The acute and long-term success rates of cryoablation are slightly less than those with RF ablation (85% to 90%).[58,59] The recurrence rate is 6%. The higher recurrence rate observed in cryoablation suggests that, unlike RF ablation, prolonged cryoenergy applications (up to 480 seconds) and postablation waiting time (up to 60 minutes) are necessary when cryothermal ablation is used.[58,59] The safety of cryoablation is indisputable, without a single case of persistent AV block reported. Temporary first-degree or higher AV block, observed in 4.3% of cases during cryomapping at −30°C or during cryoablation at −75°C, has always been reversible.[58,59] The procedure is also slightly longer than standard RF ablation. Therefore, the use of cryoablation may be recommended in specific circumstances in which the use of RF can be more likely to cause AVN damage. These include patients with unusual cardiac anatomy that makes safe RF delivery difficult, those with evidence of impaired AV conduction at baseline, or those who need ablation in the close vicinity of the compact AVN following unsuccessful RF ablation at more posterior sites.[60]

REFERENCES

1. Tawara S: Das Reitzleitungssystem des Saugetierherzens. *In* Fischer G (ed): Handbuch der vergleichenden und experimentellen entwicklungslehre der wirbeltiere. Semper Bonis Artibvs, Jena, Germany, 1906, pp 136-137.
2. Wu D, Taniguchi Y, Wen MS: Evolving concepts of atrioventricular nodal reentrant tachycardia: Insights into the anatomy and physiology. *In* Huang D, Wilber DJ (eds): Radiofrequency Catheter Ablation of Cardiac Arrhythmias: Basic Concepts and Clinical Applications, 2nd ed. Armonk, NY, Futura, 2000, pp 387-414.
3. Anderson RH, Ho SY: The anatomy of the atrioventricular node (http: //www.hrsonline.org/ Education/SelfStudy/Articles/Anderson_ho1.cfm).
4. Wu J, Olgin J, Miller JM, Zipes DP: Mechanisms for atrioventricular nodal reentry and ventricular tachycardia determined from optical mapping of isolated perfused preparations. *In* Zipes DP, Haissaguerre M (eds): Catheter Ablation of Arrhythmias, 2nd ed. Armonk, NY, Futura, 2002, pp 1-29.
5. Luc PJ: Common form of atrioventricular nodal reentrant tachycardia: Do we really know the circuit we try to ablate? Heart Rhythm 2007;4:711.
6. Mazgalev T: AV nodal physiology (http: //www.hrsonline.org/Education/SelfStudy/Articles/mazgalev.cfm).
7. Shryock J, Belardinelli L: Pharmacology of the AV node. (http: //www.hrsonline.org/ Education/SelfStudy/Articles/shrbel.cfm).
8. Katritsis DG, Becker A: The atrioventricular nodal reentrant tachycardia circuit: A proposal. Heart Rhythm 2007;4:1354.
9. Cosio FG, Anderson RH, Kuck KH, et al: Living anatomy of the atrioventricular junctions. A guide to electrophysiological mapping. A Consensus Statement from the Cardiac Nomenclature Study Group, Working Group of Arrhythmias, European Society of Cardiology, and the Task Force on Cardiac Nomenclature from NASPE. Circulation 1999;100:e31.
10. Lockwood D, Otomo K, Wang Z, et al: Electrophysiological characteristics of atrioventricular nodal reentrant tachycardia: Implications for the reentrant circuit. *In* Zipes DP, Jaliffe J (eds): Cardiac Electrophysiology: From Cell to Bedside, 4th ed. Philadelphia, WB Saunders, 2004, pp 537-557.
11. Valderrabano M: Atypical atrioventricular nodal reentry with eccentric atrial activation. Is the right target on the left? Heart Rhythm 2007;4:433.

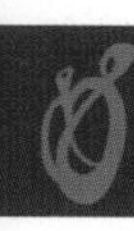

12. Wu J, Wu J, Olgin J, et al: Mechanisms underlying the reentrant circuit of atrioventricular nodal reentrant tachycardia in isolated canine atrioventricular nodal preparation using optical mapping. Circ Res 2001;88:1189.
13. Nikolski VP, Jones SA, Lancaster MK, et al: Cx43 and dual-pathway electrophysiology of the atrioventricular node and atrioventricular nodal reentry. Circ Res 2003;92:469.
14. Otomo K, Okamura H, Noda T, et al: Unique electrophysiological characteristics of atrioventricular nodal reentrant tachycardia with different ventriculoatrial block patterns: effects of slow pathway ablation and insights into the location of the reentrant circuit. Heart Rhythm 2006;3:544.
15. Wu J: Nondiscrete functional pathways and asymmetric transitional zone: A new concept for AV nodal electrophysiology. J Cardiovasc Electrophysiol 2001;12:487.
16. Kuo CT, Luqman N, Lin KH, et al: Atrioventricular nodal reentry tachycardia with multiple AH jumps: Electrophysiological characteristics and radiofrequency ablation. Pacing Clin Electrophysiol 2003;26:1849.
17. Katritsis DG, Ellenbogen KA, Becker AE: Atrial activation during atrioventricular nodal reentrant tachycardia: Studies on retrograde fast pathway conduction. Heart Rhythm 2006;3:993.
18. Otomo K, Okamura H, Noda T, et al: "Left-variant" atypical atrioventricular nodal reentrant tachycardia: Electrophysiological characteristics and effect of slow pathway ablation within coronary sinus. J Cardiovasc Electrophysiol 2006;17:1177.
19. Heidbuchel H, Jackman WM: Characterization of subforms of AV nodal reentrant tachycardia. Europace 2004;6:316.
20. Heidbuchel H, Jackman WM: Catheter ablation of atypical atrioventricular nodal reentrant tachycardia. *In* Zipes DP, Haissaguerre M (eds): Catheter Ablation of Arrhythmias, 2nd ed. Armonk, NY, Futura, 2002, pp 249-276.
21. Lee PC, Hwang B, Tai CT, et al: The electrophysiological characteristics in patients with ventricular stimulation inducible fast-slow form atrioventricular nodal reentrant tachycardia. Pacing Clin Electrophysiol 2006;29:1105.
22. Gonzalez MD, Contreras LJ, Cardona F, et al: Demonstration of a left atrial input to the atrioventricular node in humans. Circulation 2002;106:2930.
23. Katritsis DG, Becker AE, Ellenbogen KA, et al: Right and left inferior extensions of the atrioventricular node may represent the anatomical substrate of the slow pathway in humans. Heart Rhythm 2004;1:582.
24. Chen J, Anselme F, Smith TW, et al: Standard right atrial ablation is effective for atrioventricular nodal reentry with earliest activation in the coronary sinus. J Cardiovasc Electrophysiol 2004;15:2.
25. Josephson ME: Supraventricular tachycardias. *In* Josephson ME (ed): Clinical Cardiac Electrophysiology, 3rd ed. Philadelphia, Lippincott, Williams & Wilkins, 2002, pp 168-271.
26. Verma A: "Guilty culprit or innocent bystander?" J Cardiovasc Electrophysiol 2006;17:1184.
27. Nam GB, Rhee KS, Kim J, et al: Left atrionodal connections in typical and atypical atrioventricular nodal reentrant tachycardias: Activation sequence in the coronary sinus and results of radiofrequency catheter ablation. J Cardiovasc Electrophysiol 2006;17:171.
28. Sorbera C, Cohen M, Woolf P, Kalapatapu SR: Atrioventricular nodal reentry tachycardia: Slow pathway ablation using the transseptal approach. Pacing Clin Electrophysiol 2000;23:1343.
29. Gupta N, Kangavari S, Peter CT, Chen PS: Mechanism of eccentric retrograde atrial activation sequence during atypical atrioventricular nodal reciprocating tachycardia. Heart Rhythm 2005;2:754.
30. Otomo K, Nagata Y, Uno K, et al: Atypical atrioventricular nodal reentrant tachycardia with eccentric coronary sinus activation: Electrophysiological characteristics and essential effects of left-sided ablation inside the coronary sinus. Heart Rhythm 2007;4:421.
31. Porter MJ, Morton JB, Denman R, et al: Influence of age and gender on the mechanism of supraventricular tachycardia. Heart Rhythm 2004;1:393.
32. Blomström-Lundqvist C, Scheinman MM, et al: American College of Cardiology; American Heart Association Task Force on Practice Guidelines; European Society of Cardiology Committee for Practice Guidelines. Writing Committee to Develop Guidelines for the Management of Patients With Supraventricular Arrhythmias: ACC/AHA/ESC guidelines for the management of patients with supraventricular arrhythmias—executive summary: A report of the American College of Cardiology/American Heart Association Task Force on Practice Guidelines and the European Society of Cardiology Committe for Practice Guidelines. Circulation 2003;108:1871.
33. Ferguson JD, DiMarco JP: Contemporary management of paroxysmal supraventricular tachycardia. Circulation 2003;107:1096.
34. Oh S, Choi YS, Sohn DW, et al: Differential diagnosis of slow/slow atrioventricular nodal reentrant tachycardia from atrioventricular reentrant tachycardia using concealed posteroseptal accessory pathway by 12-lead electrocardiography. Pacing Clin Electrophysiol 2003;26:2296.
35. Kertesz NJ, Fogel RI, Prystowsky EN: Mechanism of induction of atrioventricular node reentry by simultaneous anterograde conduction over the fast and slow pathways. J Cardiovasc Electrophysiol 2005;16:251.
36. Knight BP, Ebinger M, Oral H, et al: Diagnostic value of tachycardia features and pacing maneuvers during paroxysmal supraventricular tachycardia. J Am Coll Cardiol 2000;36:574.
37. Crawford TC, Mukerji S, Good E, et al: Utility of atrial and ventricular cycle length variability in determining the mechanism of paroxysmal supraventricular tachycardia. J Cardiovasc Electrophysiol 2007;18:698.
38. Yang Y, Cheng J, Glatter K, et al: Quantitative effects of functional bundle branch block in patients with atrioventricular reentrant tachycardia. Am J Cardiol 2000;85:826.
39. Platonov M, Schroeder K, Veenhuyzen GD: Differential entrainment: Beware from where you pace. Heart Rhythm 2007;4:1097.
40. Yaraman PV, Lee BP, Kalahasty G, et al: Reanalysis of the "pseudo A-A-V" response to ventricular entrainment of supraventricular tachycardia: Importance of His bundle timing. J Cardiovasc Electrophysiol 2006;17:25.
41. McElderry H, Kay GN: Ablation of atrioventricular nodal reentrant tachycardia and variants guided by intracardiac recordings. *In* Huang S, Wood MA (eds): Catheter Ablation of Cardiac Arrhythmias. Philadelphia, WB Saunders, 2006, pp 347-367.
42. Strickberger A, Morady F: Catheter ablation of atrioventricular nodal reentrant tachycardia. *In* Zipes DP, Jaliffe J (eds): Cardiac Electrophysiology: From Cell to Bedside, 4th ed. Philadelphia, WB Saunders, 2004, pp 1028-1035.
43. Gaita F, Riccardi R, Marco S, Caponi D: Catheter ablation of typical atrioventricular nodal reentrant tachycardia. *In* Zipes DP, Haissaguerre M (eds): Catheter Ablation of Arrhythmias, 2nd ed. Armonk, NY, Futura, 2002, pp 225-248.
44. Taylor GW, Kay GN: Ablation of atrioventricular nodal reentrant tachycardia with the posterior approach. *In* Huang S, Wilber DJ (eds): Radiofrequency Catheter Ablation of Cardiac Arrhythmias: Basic Concepts and Clinical Applications, 2nd ed. Armonk, NY, Futura, 2000, pp 423-464.
45. Altemose GT, Scott LR, Miller JM: Atrioventricular nodal reentrant tachycardia requiring ablation on the mitral annulus. J Cardiovasc Electrophysiol 2000;11:1281.
46. Gonzalez MD, Rivera J: Ablation of atrioventricular nodal reentry by the anatomical approach. *In* Huang S, Wood MA (eds): Catheter Ablation of Cardiac Arrhythmias. Philadelphia, WB Saunders, 2006, pp 325-346.
47. Salem YS, Burke MC, Kim SS, et al: Slow pathway ablation for atrioventricular nodal reentry using a right internal jugular vein approach: a case series. Pacing Clin Electrophysiol 2006;29:59.
48. Morady F; Radiofrequency ablation as treatment for cardiac arrhythmias. N Engl J Med 1999;340:534.
49. Lee SH, Tai CT, Lee PC, et al: Electrophysiological characteristics of junctional rhythm during ablation of the slow pathway in different types of atrioventricular nodal reentrant tachycardia. Pacing Clin Electrophysiol 2005;28:111.
50. Lipscomb KJ, Zaidi AM, Fitzpatrick AP, Lefroy D: Slow pathway modification for atrioventricular node re-entrant tachycardia: Fast junctional tachycardia predicts adverse prognosis. Heart 2001;85:44.
51. McGavigan AD, Rae AP, Cobbe SM, Rankin AC: Junctional rhythm—a suitable surrogate endpoint in catheter ablation of atrioventricular nodal reentry tachycardia? Pacing Clin Electrophysiol 2005;28:1052.
52. Li YG, Gronefeld G, Bender B, et al: Risk of development of delayed atrioventricular block after slow pathway modification in patients with atrioventricular nodal reentrant tachycardia and a pre-existing prolonged PR interval. Eur Heart J 2001;22:89.
53. Lukac P, Buckingham TA, Hatala R, et al: Determination of repetitive slow pathway conduction for evaluation of the efficacy of radiofrequency ablation in AVNRT. Pacing Clin Electrophysiol 2003;26(Pt 1):827.
54. Estner HL, Ndrepepa G, Dong J, et al: Acute and long-term results of slow pathway ablation in patients with atrioventricular nodal reentrant tachycardia—an analysis of the predictive factors for arrhythmia recurrence. Pacing Clin Electrophysiol 2005;28:102.
55. Weismuller P, Kuly S, Brandts B, et al: Is electrical stimulation during administration of catecholamines required for the evaluation of success after ablation of atrioventricular node re-entrant tachycardias? J Am Coll Cardiol 2002;39:689.
56. Clague JR, Dagres N, Kottkamp H, et al: Targeting the slow pathway for atrioventricular nodal reentrant tachycardia: Initial results and long-term follow-up in 379 consecutive patients. Eur Heart J 2001;22:82.
57. Willems S, Shenasa H, Kottkamp H: Temperature controlled slow pathway ablation for the treatment of Long-term outcome following slow pathway ablation. Eur Heart J 2001;22:1092.
58. Rodriguez LM, Geller JC, Tse HF, et al: Acute results of transvenous cryoablation of supraventricular tachycardia (atrial fibrillation, atrial flutter, Wolff-Parkinson-White syndrome, atrioventricular nodal reentry tachycardia). J Cardiovasc Electrophysiol 2002;13:1082.
59. Zrenner B, Dong J, Schreieck J, et al: Transvenous cryoablation versus radiofrequency ablation of the slow pathway for the treatment of atrioventricular nodal reentrant tachycardia: a prospective randomized pilot study. Eur Heart J 2004;25:2226.
60. Friedman PL: How to ablate atrioventricular nodal reentry using cryoenergy. Heart Rhythm 2005;2:893.
61. Michaud GF, Tada H, Chough S, et al: Differentiation of atypical atrioventricular node re-entrant tachycardia from orthodromic reciprocating tachycardia using a septal accessory pathway by the response to ventricular pacing. J Am Coll Cardiol 2001;38:1163.

CHAPTER 14

Atrioventricular Reentrant Tachycardia

TYPES OF BYPASS TRACTS

Bypass tracts (BTs) are remnants of the atrioventricular (AV) connections caused by incomplete embryological development of the AV annulus and failure of the fibrous separation between the atria and ventricles. There are several types of BTs. Atrioventricular BTs are strands of working myocardial cells connecting atrial and ventricular myocardium across the electrically insulating fibrofatty tissues of the AV junction bypassing the atrioventricular node–His-Purkinje system (AVN-HPS). In the older literature, these BTs were called Kent bundles, although incorrectly (Kent described AVN-like tissue in the right atrium [RA] free wall that did not connect to the ventricle). Thus, the use of the term *bundle of Kent* should be discouraged.[1] Atrionodal BTs connect the atrium to the distal or compact AVN. They have been called James fibers and are of uncertain physiological significance. Atrio-Hisian BTs connect the atrium to the His bundle (HB); these BTs are rare.[2,3] Atypical BTs include various types of Hisian-fascicular BTs, which connect the atrium (atriofascicular pathways), AVN (nodofascicular pathways), or HB (fasciculoventricular) to distal Purkinje fibers or ventricular myocardium, in addition to slowly conducting short atrioventricular BTs and long atrioventricular BTs. These BTs are sometimes collectively referred to as Mahaim fibers, a term to be discouraged because it is more illuminating to name the precise BT according to its connections.[4]

TYPES OF PREEXCITATION SYNDROMES

Several patterns of preexcitation occur, depending on the anatomy of the BT and the direction in which impulses are conducted. Conduction from the atria to the ventricles normally occurs via the AVN-HPS. Patients with preexcitation have an additional or alternative pathway, the BT, which directly connects the atria and ventricles and bypasses the AVN. The term *syndrome* is used when the anatomical variant is responsible for tachycardia.

In the Wolff-Parkinson-White (WPW) syndrome, AV conduction occurs, partially or entirely, through an AV BT, which results in earlier activation (preexcitation) of the ventricles than if the impulse had traveled through the AVN.[1] In the case of Lown-Ganong-Levine (LGL) syndrome, preexcitation purportedly occurs via atrio-Hisian BTs or, alternatively, no BT is present and enhanced AVN conduction accounts for the ECG findings. The net effect is a short PR interval without delta wave or QRS prolongation. It is important to stress, however, that LGL is not a recognized syndrome with an anatomical basis, but only an ECG description, and the use of the term should be discouraged.[2,3] The Mahaim variant of preexcitation does not typically result in a delta wave, because these pathways, which usually terminate in the conducting system or in the ventricular myocardium close to the conducting system, conduct slowly and the AVN-HPS has adequate time to activate the ventricle predominantly.[4] Concealed AV BTs refer to AV BTs that do not manifest anterograde conduction and therefore do not result in ventricular preexcitation. Because they do not result in alteration of the QRS complex in the ECG, they cannot be detected by inspection of the surface ECG; they are called concealed. However, the concealed BT can conduct in a retrograde fashion, thereby creating a reentrant circuit with impulses traveling from the atrium to the AVN, HPS, ventricle, and then back to the atrium via the BT.[5-7]

PATHOPHYSIOLOGY

Wolff-Parkinson-White Syndrome

WPW pattern refers to the constellation of ECG abnormalities related to the presence of an AV BT (short PR interval, delta wave) in asymptomatic patients.[1] WPW syndrome refers to a WPW ECG pattern associated with tachyarrhythmias.

Because the AV BT typically conducts faster than the AVN, the onset of ventricular activation is earlier than if depolarization occurred only via the AVN, resulting in a shortened PR (P-delta) interval. Additionally, because the BT exhibits nondecremental conduction, the early activation (P-delta interval) remains constant at all heart rates. Preexcited intraventricular conduction in WPW spreads from the insertion point of the AV BT in the ventricular myocardium via direct muscle to muscle conduction. This process is inherently slower than ventricular depolarization resulting from rapid HPS conduction. Thus, although the initial excitation of the ventricles (via the BT) occurs earlier, it is followed by slower activation of the ventricular myocardium than occurs normally. The net effect is that the QRS complex consists of fusion between the early ventricular activation caused by preexcitation with the later ventricular activation resulting from transmission through the AVN and HPS to the ventricles. The initial part of ventricular activation resulting in the upstroke of the QRS complex is slurred because of slow muscle to muscle conduction; this is termed a *delta wave*. The more rapid the conduction along the BT in relation to the AVN, the greater the amount of myocardium depolarized via the BT, resulting in a more prominent or wider delta wave, and increasing prolongation of the QRS complex.

Atrioventricular Bypass Tracts

The AV junctions are the areas of the heart where the atrial musculatures insert into the circumferences of the mitral and tricuspid valves; the latter structures guard the orifices that join together the atrial and ventricular cavities. The septal component of the junctions is the site of the only muscular structure that in the normal heart, conducts the cardiac impulse from the atriums to the ventricles.

AV BTs connect the atria to the ventricle and can cross the AV groove anywhere along the mitral and tricuspid annulus, except between the left and right fibrous trigones, where the left atrial (LA) myocardium is not in direct juxtaposition with the left ventricular (LV) myocardium (the region of the aortomitral continuity, at which site no LV myocardium lies below the LA). The remainder of the AV groove may be divided into quadrants consisting of the left free wall, right free wall, posteroseptal, and anteroseptal spaces. The distribution of BTs within these regions is not homogeneous—46% to 60% of BTs are found within the left free wall space; 25% are within the posteroseptal space; 13% to 21% of BTs are within the right free wall space; and 2% are within the right superoparaseptal (formerly called anteroseptal) space (Fig. 14-1).[5]

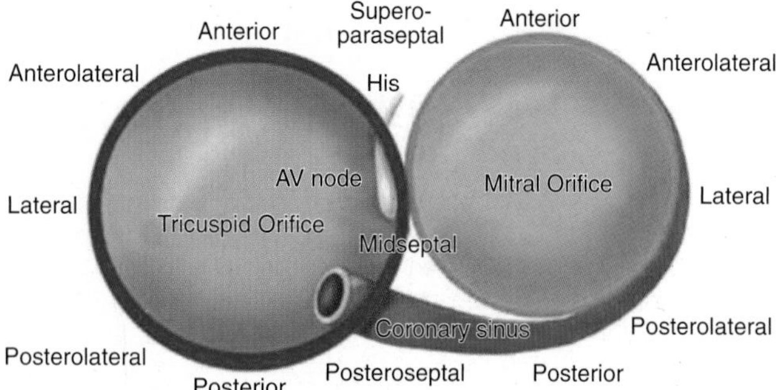

FIGURE 14–1 Locations of atrioventricular bypass tracts (AV BTs) by anatomical region. Tricuspid and mitral valve annuli are depicted in a left anterior oblique view. Locations of the coronary sinus, atrioventricular node, and His bundle are shown. AV BTs may connect atrial to ventricular myocardium in any of the regions shown. (From Miller JM, Zipes DP: Therapy for cardiac arrhythmias. *In* Libby P, Bonow R, Mann DL, Zipes DP [eds]: Braunwald's Heart Disease: A Textbook of Cardiovascular Medicine, 8th ed. Philadelphia, WB Saunders, 2007, pp 779-830.)

BTs are usually very thin muscular strands (rarely thicker than 1 to 2 mm) but can occasionally exist as broad bands of tissue. The AV BT can run in an oblique course rather than perpendicular to the transverse plane of the AV groove. As a result, the fibers can have an atrial insertion point that is transversely several centimeters removed from the point of ventricular attachment.[8] Some posteroseptal pathways insert into coronary sinus (CS) musculature rather than atrium and can be associated with the coronary venous system or diverticula from a CS branch vein.

Multiple AV BTs occur in 5% to 10% of patients. BTs are defined as multiple when they are separate by more than 1 to 3 cm. The most common combination of widely spaced multiple BTs is posteroseptal and right free wall BTs. The incidence of multiple BTs is particularly high in patients with antidromic atrioventricular reentrant tachycardia (AVRT) (50% to 75%), patients in whom AF resulted in ventricular fibrillation (VF), and patients with Ebstein's anomaly.

Although the majority (approximately 60%) of AV BTs conduct both anterogradely and retrogradely (i.e., bidirectionally), some AV BTs are capable of propagating impulses in only one direction.[5,6] BTs that conduct only in the anterograde direction are uncommon (less than 5%), often cross the right AV groove, and frequently possess decremental conduction properties.[3] On the other hand, BTs that conduct only in the retrograde direction occur more frequently, with an incidence of 17% to 37%. When the BT is capable of anterograde conduction, ventricular preexcitation is evident during normal sinus rhythm (NSR), and the BT is referred to as manifest. BTs capable of retrograde only conduction are referred to as concealed.

Because working myocardial cells make up the vast majority of AV BTs, propagation is caused by the rapid inward sodium current, similar to normal His-Purkinje tissue and atrial and ventricular myocardium. Therefore, AV BTs have rather constant anterograde and retrograde conduction at all rates until the refractory period is reached, at which time conduction is completely blocked (nondecremental conduction). Thus, conduction over the AV BT usually behaves in an all-or-none fashion. In contrast, the AVN, which depends on the slow inward calcium current for generation and propagation of its action potential, exhibits what has been called decremental conduction in which the conduction time of the impulse propagating through the AVN increases as the atrial cycle length (CL) shortens. Thus, AV conduction is more rapid through the AV BT than through the AVN, a difference that is increased at a fast heart rate. This difference has potentially great clinical importance. A primary function of the AVN is to limit the number of impulses conducted from the atria to the ventricles, which is particularly important during fast atrial rates (e.g., AF or atrial flutter [AFL]) when only a fraction of impulses are conducted to the ventricles, whereas the remainder are blocked in the AVN. However, in the presence of nondecrementally conducting AV BTs, these arrhythmias can lead to very fast ventricular rates that can degenerate into VF.

Atrioventricular Reentry

AVRT is a macroreentrant tachycardia with an anatomically defined circuit that consists of two distinct pathways, the normal AV conduction system and an AV BT, linked by common proximal (atrial) and distal (ventricular) tissues. If sufficient differences in conduction time and refractoriness exist between the normal conduction system and the BT, a properly timed premature impulse of atrial or ventricular origin can initiate reentry. AVRTs are the most common (80%) tachycardias associated with WPW syndrome. AVRT is divided into orthodromic and antidromic according to the direction of conduction in the AVN-HPS (Fig. 14-2). Orthodromic indicates normal direction (anterograde) of conduction over AVN-HPS during the AVRT.

Orthodromic Atrioventricular Reentrant Tachycardia. In orthodromic AVRT, the AVN-HPS serves as the anterograde limb of the reentrant circuit (i.e., the pathway that conducts the impulse from the atrium to the ventricle), whereas an AV BT serves as the retrograde limb (see Fig. 14-2). Approximately 50% of BTs participating in orthodromic AVRT are manifest (able to conduct bidirectionally) and 50% are concealed (able to conduct retrogradely only). Therefore, a WPW pattern may or may not be present on surface ECG during NSR. When preexcitation is present, the delta wave seen during NSR is lost during orthodromic AVRT, because anterograde conduction during the tachycardia is not via the BT (i.e., the ventricle is not preexcited) but over the normal AV conduction system. Orthodromic AVRT accounts for approximately 95% of AVRTs and 35% of all paroxysmal supraventricular tachycardias (SVTs).

Antidromic Atrioventricular Reentrant Tachycardia. In antidromic AVRT, an AV BT serves as the anterograde limb of the reentrant circuit (see Fig. 14-2). Consequently, the QRS complex during antidromic AVRT is fully preexcited (i.e., the ventricles are activated totally by the BT with no contribution from the normal conduction system). The BT involved in the antidromic AVRT circuit must be capable of anterograde conduction and, therefore, preexcitation is typically observed during NSR. During classic antidromic AVRT, retrograde VA conduction occurs over the AVN-HPS. Other less frequent, nonclassic forms of antidromic AVRT can use a second BT as the retrograde limb of the reentrant circuit or a combination of one BT plus the AVN-HPS in either direction (Fig. 14-3). AVRT occurs in 5% to 10% of patients with WPW syndrome. Susceptibility to antidromic AVRT appears to be facilitated by a distance of at least 4 cm between the BT and the normal AV conduction system. Consequently, most antidromic AVRTs use a lateral (right or left) BT as the anterograde route for conduction. Because posteroseptal BTs are in close proximity to the AVN, those BTs are less commonly part of antidromic AVRT if the other limb is the AVN and not a second free wall BT.[3,5] Up to 50% to 75% of patients with spontaneous antidromic AVRT have multiple BTs (manifest or concealed) whether or not they are used as the retrograde limb during the tachycardia.

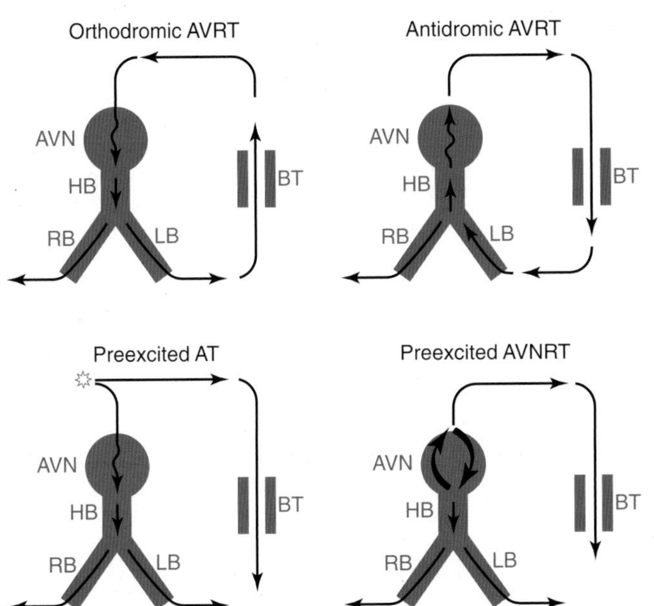

FIGURE 14–2 Schematic representation of the reentrant circuit during orthodromic atrioventricular reentrant tachycardia (AVRT), antidromic AVRT, preexcited atrial tachycardia (AT), and preexcited AVNRT using a left-sided bypass tract (BT). HB = His bundle; LB = left bundle branch; RB = right bundle branch.

Permanent Junctional Reciprocating Tachycardia. Permanent junctional reciprocating tachycardia (PJRT) is an orthodromic AVRT mediated by a concealed, retrogradely conducting AV BT that has slow and decremental conduction properties. The conduction properties of this retrograde BT are slower compared with the anterograde properties of the AVN and with the typical fast BTs found in patients with AVRT. The BT in PJRT is most often located in the posteroseptal region, although other portions of the AV groove can also harbor this unusual pathway. Because these BTs are almost always concealed and have slow conduction, all elements necessary for reentry are present at all times, and thus PJRT can be present much of the time, with only short interludes of sinus rhythm (incessant SVT).

Other Arrhythmias Associated with Wolff-Parkinson-White Syndrome

Atrial tachycardia (AT), AFL, AF, and atrioventricular nodal reentrant tachycardia (AVNRT) can all coexist with a BT. In these settings, the BT serves as a bystander route for ventricular or atrial activation, and is not required for the initiation or maintenance of the arrhythmia.

Atrioventricular Nodal Reentrant Tachycardia and Atrial Tachycardia. Physiology consistent with dual AVN physiology has been reported in 8% to 40% of patients

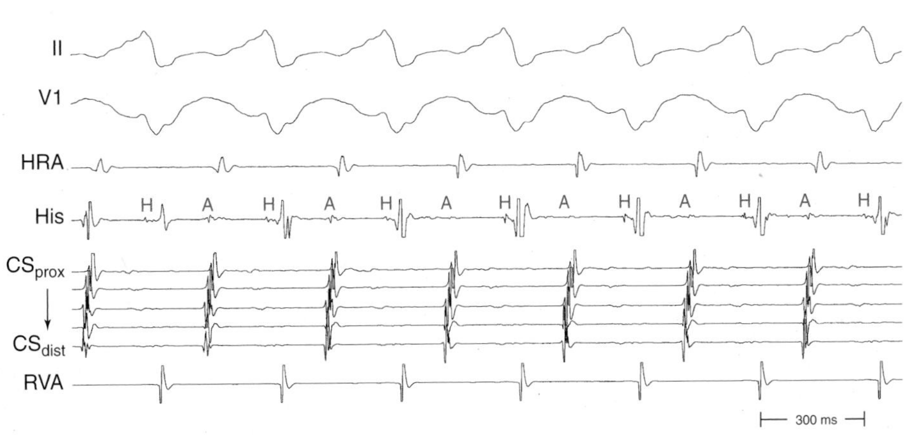

FIGURE 14–3 The presence of multiple bypass tracts (BTs) is indicated by eccentric atrial activation sequence during antidromic atrioventricular reentrant tachycardia (AVRT) using a right lateral BT anterogradely and a left lateral BT retrogradely. A = atrial electrogram; H = His bundle potential.

with WPW syndrome, although spontaneous sustained AVNRT is less frequent. Both AVNRT and AT can use the bystander BT to transmit impulses to the ventricle (see Fig. 14-2). When AVNRT occurs in the WPW syndrome, the arrhythmia can be difficult to distinguish from AVRT without electrophysiological (EP) testing.

Atrial Fibrillation. Paroxysmal AF occurs in 50% of patients with WPW, and is the presenting arrhythmia in 20%. Chronic AF, however, is rare in these patients.[3] Spontaneous AF is most common in patients with antero-grade conduction through the BT.[9] Patients with antidromic AVRT, multiple BTs, and BTs that have short anterograde ERP are more liable to develop AF.[3] In individuals with WPW, AF is often preceded by AVRT that degenerates into AF.

Preexcitation and Predisposition to Atrial Fibrillation. The frequency with which intermittent AF occurs in patients with the WPW syndrome is striking because of the low prevalence of coexisting structural heart disease, which is a major predisposing factor for AF in subjects without a BT. This observation suggests that the AV BT itself can be related to the genesis of AF.

The mechanisms by which AVRT precipitates AF are not well understood. The rapid atrial rate can cause disruption in atrial activation and reactivation, creating an electrophysiological substrate conducive to AF. The observation that most patients with BT and AF who undergo BT ablation are cured of both AVRT and AF is compatible with this hypothesis. Another possibility is that the complex geometry of networks of BTs predisposes to AF by fractionation of the activation wavefronts. Localized reentry has been recorded in some patients using direct recordings of the activation of the BTs. Hemodynamic changes, atrial stretch caused by atrial contraction against closed AV valves during ventricular systole, can also play a role. One report has suggested that an intact BT is not necessary for the initiation of AF but might facilitate its perpetuation. Ablation of the BT can cure AF in more than 90% of patients; however, vulnerability to AF persists in up to 56%, and the response to atrial extrastimulation (AES) is also unaltered by ablation.

Atrial Flutter. AFL is the most common (60%) regular preexcited tachycardia in patients with WPW syndrome. AFL is caused by a reentrant circuit within the RA and therefore exists independently of the BT, and AFL does not have the same causal association to AV BTs as AF. In some patients with WPW syndrome who develop AFL, AVRT is the initiating event. This relationship can be mediated by contraction-excitation feedback into the atria during the AVRT.

AFL, like AF, can conduct anterograde via a BT causing a preexcited tachycardia. Depending upon the various refractory periods of the normal and pathological AV conduction pathways, AFL potentially can conduct 1:1 to the ventricles during a preexcited tachycardia making the arrhythmia difficult to distinguish from ventricular tachycardia (VT) (see Fig. 9-4).

Ventricular Fibrillation and Sudden Cardiac Death. In most cases, VF occurring in patients with the WPW syndrome results from the rapid ventricular response during AF. Although the frequency with which AF with rapid AV conduction via a BT degenerates into VF is unknown, the incidence of sudden cardiac death in patients with the WPW syndrome is rather low, ranging from 0% to 0.39% annually in several large case series. Some series have found that no sudden deaths occurred in individuals who were asymptomatic at the time they were initially found to have preexcitation on their ECGs. However, one report has noted three cases in 162 initially asymptomatic patients followed for 5 years; all three patients developed symptomatic AF before the episode of sudden cardiac death.[10,11]

Several factors can help identify the patient with WPW who is at increased risk for VF including symptomatic SVT, septal location of the BT, presence of multiple BTs, short BT refractoriness, and male gender. Most patients who have been resuscitated from VF secondary to preexcitation have previous history of AVRT and/or AF. However, preexcitation and arrhythmias have been previously undiagnosed in up to 25% of such individuals. Most patients will have inducible AVRT in the EP laboratory; lack of inducibility suggests a relatively low risk.[11] In addition, most patients have a rapid ventricular response to spontaneous or induced AF. If the BT has a very short anterograde effective refractory period (ERP < 250 milliseconds), a rapid ventricular response can occur with degeneration of the rhythm to VF. A short preexcited RR interval during AF of 220 milliseconds or less appears to be a sensitive clinical marker for identifying patients at risk for sudden death in children, although its positive predictive value in adults is only 19% to 38%.[12]

Drug therapy can be an additional determinant of the risk of VF in patients with preexcitation. As an example, intravenous verapamil can increase the ventricular response to AF and has resulted in VF in some patients. Several mechanisms are probably involved; hypotension produced by verapamil-induced vasodilation is followed by a sympathetic discharge that enhances BT conduction. Furthermore, verapamil slows AVN conduction directly and increases AVN refractoriness, resulting in less concealed penetration of the BT by normally conducted beats. Additionally, the increased rate, irregular rate, hypotension, and sympathetic discharge probably result in fractionation of the ventricular wavefront and VF. For these reasons, intravenous verapamil is contraindicated for the acute treatment of AF in patients with WPW. Other intravenous drugs that block the AVN also should be avoided, including beta blockers, adenosine, diltiazem, and digoxin. Both oral and intravenous digoxin have been associated with the degeneration of AF into VF in patients with preexcitation syndromes. A number of these patients had a history of previously benign AF. How digitalis might promote the development of VF is uncertain. One possible mechanism is that shortening of the atrial and BT ERP, plus increasing AVN block, results in decreased concealed retrograde penetration of the BT by normally conducted beats, thereby preventing its inactivation.

Intravenous adenosine, given appropriately to treat orthodromic AVRT, can also precipitate AF episodes. This is unusual and should not be viewed as a contraindication to adenosine use, but one should be prepared for emergency cardioversion before administering adenosine to SVT patients. Lidocaine, for reasons that are unclear, has also been associated with degeneration of AF into VF. It is occasionally used in patients with WPW who have a wide QRS complex tachycardia that might be interpreted as VT.

Ventricular Tachycardia. Coexisting VT is uncommon because patients with WPW syndrome infrequently have structural heart disease.

CLINICAL CONSIDERATIONS

Epidemiology of Wolff-Parkinson-White Syndrome

Wolff-Parkinson-White Pattern. The prevalence of a WPW pattern on the surface ECG is 0.15% to 0.25% in the general population. The prevalence is increased to 0.55% among first-degree relatives of affected patients, suggesting a familial component. The yearly incidence of newly diagnosed cases of preexcitation in the general population was substantially lower, 0.004% in a diverse population of residents from Olmsted County, Minnesota, 50% of whom were asymptomatic.[12a] The incidence in males is twice that in females and highest in the first year of life, with a secondary peak in young adulthood.

The WPW pattern on the ECG can be intermittent and can even disappear (in up to 40% of cases) permanently over time.[13] Intermittent and/or persistent loss of preexcitation can indicate that the BT has a relatively longer baseline ERP, which makes it more susceptible to age-related degenerative changes and variations in autonomic tone. Consistent with this hypothesis is the observation that, compared with patients with a persistent WPW pattern, those in whom anterograde conduction via the BT disappeared were older (50 versus 39 years) and had a longer ERP of the BT at initial EP study (414 versus 295 milliseconds).

Wolff-Parkinson-White Syndrome. The prevalence of the WPW syndrome is substantially lower than that of the WPW ECG pattern. In a review of 22,500 healthy aviation personnel, the WPW pattern on an ECG was seen in 0.25%; only 1.8% of these patients had documented arrhythmia. In another report of 228 subjects with WPW followed for 22 years, the overall incidence of arrhythmia was 1% per patient year.

The occurrence of arrhythmias is related to the age at the time preexcitation was discovered.[13] In the Olmsted County population, one third of asymptomatic individuals younger than 40 years at the time WPW was identified eventually had symptoms, compared with none of those who were older than 40 years at diagnosis.

Associated Cardiac Abnormalities. Most patients with AV BTs do not have coexisting structural cardiac abnormalities, except for those that are age-related. Associated congenital heart disease, when present, is more likely to be right-sided than left-sided in location. Ebstein's anomaly is the congenital lesion most strongly associated with WPW syndrome. As many as 10% of such patients have one or more BTs; the most of these are located in the right free wall and right posteroseptal space. An association between mitral valve prolapse and left-sided BTs has also been reported. However, this association may simply reflect the random coexistence of two relatively common conditions.

Familial Wolff-Parkinson-White Syndrome. Among patients with the WPW syndrome, 3.4% have first-degree relatives with a preexcitation syndrome. A familial form of WPW has infrequently been reported and is usually inherited as an autosomal dominant trait.

The genetic cause of a rare form of familial WPW syndrome has been described.[14-17] The clinical phenotype is characterized by the presence of preexcitation on the ECG, frequent SVTs, including AF, progressive conduction system disease, and cardiac hypertrophy. The patients present in late adolescence or third decade with syncope or palpitations. Premature sudden cardiac death occurred in 10% of the patients. Paradoxically, by the fourth decade of life, progression to advanced sinus node dysfunction or AV block (with the loss of preexcitation) requiring pacemaker implantation was common. Approximately 80% of the patients older than 50 years had chronic AF. Causative mutations in the *PRKAG2* gene were identified in these families. The *PRKAG2* gene codes the gamma-2 regulatory subunit of the adenosine monophosphate (AMP)–activated protein kinase, which is a key regulator of metabolic pathways, including glucose metabolism. The penetrance of the disease for WPW syndrome was complete, but the expression was variable. The described phenotype of this syndrome is similar to the autosomal recessive glycogen storage disease, Pompe's disease. Given the function of the AMP-activated protein kinase and this similarity, the PRKAG2 syndrome is likely a cardiac-specific glycogenosis syndrome. This syndrome thus rather belongs to the group of genetic metabolic cardiomyopathies, than to the congenital primary arrhythmia syndromes.

Concealed Bypass Tracts. The true prevalence of concealed BTs is unknown because, unlike the situation with WPW syndrome, these BTs are concealed on the surface ECG and are only expressed during AVRT; only symptomatic patients undergo EP testing. As noted, orthodromic AVRT accounts for approximately 95% of AVRTs and 35% of all paroxysmal SVTs, and 50% of the BTs that participate in orthodromic AVRT are concealed. SVTs using a concealed BT have no gender predilection and tend to occur more frequently in younger patients than those with AVNRT; however, significant overlap exists. PJRT most often occurs in early childhood, although clinically asymptomatic patients presenting later in life are not uncommon.

Clinical Presentation

Most patients with preexcitation are asymptomatic and are discovered incidentally on an ECG obtained for unrelated reasons. When symptomatic arrhythmias occur in the WPW patient, the disorder is called the WPW syndrome. The two most common types of arrhythmias in the WPW syndrome are AVRT and AF. Patients with AVRT experience symptoms characteristic of paroxysmal SVT with sudden onset and termination, including rapid and regular palpitations, chest pain, dyspnea, presyncope and, rarely, syncope. Symptoms are usually mild and short-lived and terminate spontaneously or with vagal maneuvers. However, occasionally patients present with disabling symptoms, especially in the presence of structural heart disease. Of note, clinical symptoms are not usually helpful in differentiating AVRT from other forms of paroxysmal SVT.

An AVRT that in general is well tolerated by the patient when additional heart disease is absent can deteriorate into AF. AF can be a life-threatening arrhythmia in the WPW syndrome if the BT has a short anterograde ERP, resulting in very fast ventricular rates, with possible deterioration into VF and sudden death.

The incidence of sudden cardiac death in patients with the WPW syndrome has been estimated to range from 0.15% to 0.39% over a 3- to 10-year follow-up. It is unusual for cardiac arrest to be the first symptomatic manifestation of WPW syndrome. Conversely, in about 50% of cardiac arrest cases in WPW patients, it is the first manifestation of WPW.

PJRT commonly presents as a frequently recurring tachycardia.[5] The tachycardia is typically incessant and refractory to drug therapy and can lead to cardiomyopathy and congestive heart failure symptoms.

Initial Evaluation

History, physical examination, and 12-lead ECG constitute an appropriate initial evaluation. In patients with brief, self-terminating episodes of palpitations, an event recorder is the most effective way to obtain ECG documentation. Echocardiographic examination is required to exclude structural heart disease.

Several other noninvasive and invasive tests have been proposed as useful for evaluating symptomatic patients and risk-stratifying patients for sudden death risk. Invasive EP testing may be considered in patients with arrhythmias and those with a WPW ECG pattern when noninvasive testing does not lead to the conclusion that a relatively long anterograde ERP of the BT is present.

Methods for Evaluation of Bypass Tract Refractory Period

Demonstration of Intermittent Preexcitation. Intermittent preexcitation is generally correlated with a long BT ERP and slower ventricular rate during AF. Intermittent preexcitation has to be distinguished from inapparent preexcitation (see later) and from a bigeminal ventricular rhythm with a long coupling interval.

Assessing Ability of Antiarrhythmic Agents to Produce Anterograde Block in Bypass Tracts. When, during NSR, the intravenous injection of ajmaline (1 mg/kg over 3 minutes) or procainamide (10 mg/kg over 5 minutes) results in complete block of the BT, a long anterograde ERP (more than 270 milliseconds) of the BT is likely. The shorter the BT ERP, the less likely it would be blocked by these drugs. Furthermore, the amount of ajmaline required to block conduction over the BT correlates with the duration of the anterograde ERP of the BT. However, the incidence of BT block in response to these drugs is low and, although the occurrence of block predicts a long ERP of the BT, failure to produce block does not necessarily suggest a short ERP. Moreover, pharmacological testing is carried out at rest and therefore does not indicate what effect the drug will have on the BT ERP during sympathetic stimulation, such as exercise, emotion, anxiety, and recreational drug use.[11,18,19]

14

Response of Preexcitation to Exercise. Demonstration of a sudden loss of preexcitation (indicated by abrupt loss of the delta wave associated with prolongation of the PR interval and normalization of the QRS) during exercise is consistent with block in the BT and is indicative of a long BT ERP (more than 300 milliseconds). This is a good predictor that the patient is not at risk for VF, even during sympathetic stimulation. However, the frequency of block in the BT during exercise is low (approximately 10%), and thus sensitivity of this test is poor.

Evaluation of Ventricular Response During Atrial Fibrillation. During spontaneous or induced AF, the propensity for rapid AV conduction can be judged by the interval between consecutively preexcited QRS complexes. A mean preexcited RR interval of more than 250 milliseconds and a shortest preexcited RR of more than 220 milliseconds predict low risk for sudden cardiac death, with a negative predictive value of >95%; however, the positive predictive value is low (20%).

Response of Preexcitation to Transesophageal Atrial Stimulation. There is good correlation between the value of the anterograde ERP of the BT obtained during single-test programmed atrial stimulation and atrial pacing at increasing rates and the ventricular rate during AF. Programmed electrical stimulation of the atrium can be performed by the transesophageal route and the value of the anterograde ERP of the BT can be determined.

Electrophysiological Testing. Programmed atrial stimulation is used to evaluate the BT ERP. Because BT refractoriness shortens with decreasing pacing CL, the ERP should be determined at multiple pacing CLs (preferably 400 milliseconds or less). Atrial stimulation should be performed close to the BT atrial insertion site to obviate the effect of intraatrial conduction delay. Incremental rate atrial pacing is performed to determine the maximum rate at which 1:1 conduction over the BT occurs. Induction of AF should be performed to determine the average and the shortest RR interval during preexcited AF.

Principles of Management

Management of Asymptomatic Patient with Preexcitation

The role of EP testing and catheter ablation in asymptomatic patients with preexcitation is controversial. Guidelines of the American College of Cardiology and European Society of Cardiology on the management of asymptomatic WPW patients suggest restricting catheter ablation of BTs to those in high-risk occupations (e.g., school bus drivers and pilots) and professional athletes—that is, to advise on the basis of individual considerations.[20] Catheter ablation in asymptomatic preexcitation was classified as a IIA indication with a B level of evidence. According to the NASPE Expert Consensus Conference, asymptomatic WPW pattern on the ECG without recognized tachycardia is a class IIB indication for catheter ablation in children older than 5 years and a class III indication in younger children.[21] This approach has several justifications; one third of asymptomatic individuals younger than 40 years when preexcitation was identified eventually developed symptoms, whereas no patients in whom preexcitation was first uncovered after the age of 40 years developed symptoms. Additionally, most patients with asymptomatic preexcitation have a good prognosis; cardiac arrest is rarely the first manifestation of the disease. The positive predictive value of invasive EP testing is considered to be too low to justify routine use in asymptomatic patients.

Some studies, however, have questioned this approach.[11,18,19] Those studies have shown that in the asymptomatic WPW population, a negative EP study with no AVRT or AF inducibility identifies subjects at very low risk for the development of spontaneous arrhythmias. Inducibility of sustained preexcited AF with a fast ventricular response, particularly in the presence of multiple BTs, may help select asymptomatic WPW subjects at definite risk for dying suddenly, and catheter ablation of the BT(s) appears to be required to prevent sudden death. Because extensive studies have reported no fatal complications from EP testing and radiofrequency (RF) ablation in experienced centers, it has been suggested that all asymptomatic patients with WPW pattern should undergo EP testing for risk stratification, and those with inducible AVRT or AF should undergo catheter ablation of the BT.[22] This argument is further supported by the fact that assessment of the future VF risk in an asymptomatic patient with WPW is not easy. Noninvasive markers of lower risk such as intermittent loss of preexcitation, sudden loss of BT conduction on exercise stress testing, and loss of BT conduction after treatment with antiarrhythmic drugs are limited by inadequate sensitivity or specificity and the low incidence of future adverse events. With this approach, prophylactic ablation of BTs in high-risk subjects may be justified but is not an acceptable option for low-risk individuals.

In summary, the potential value of EP testing in identifying high-risk patients who may benefit from catheter ablation must be balanced against the approximately 2% risk of a major complication associated with catheter ablation.[23] If RF catheter ablation were a totally risk-free procedure, one would logically advise such a procedure to the asymptomatic WPW patient with a short anterograde ERP. However, certain risks are associated with RF ablation. Although complications of a diagnostic EP study are minor and non–life-threatening and are less common than those of catheter ablation, if routine EP testing of all asymptomatic WPW patients was considered, many patients would proceed immediately to RF ablation and, in others, there would be a strong temptation to ablate when catheters are in place. This greatly increases the risk to the patient. Furthermore, invasive EP assessment has drawbacks, because no single factor has both a high sensitivity and specificity for identifying at-risk individuals. For example, a shortest preexcited RR interval of less than 250 milliseconds during sustained induced AF is a very sensitive but not specific marker of the risk of VF in WPW patients, because approximately one third of patients will have a shortest RR interval of less than 250 milliseconds during induced AF. In view of those considerations, it may be more appropriate to start with noninvasive studies (e.g., exercise, Holter, effect of pharmacological intervention) to identify the low-risk patient because of a long anterograde ERP of the BT.[20,23]

For the low-risk patient, no measures are advised other than an explanation to the patient of the ECG findings. It is advisable to give the patient a copy of his or her ECG and a short note about the fact that the WPW pattern is present to prevent the misdiagnosis of myocardial infarction (MI) and to explain the basis of cardiac arrhythmias in case they develop later. Patients should also be encouraged to seek medical expertise whenever arrhythmia-related symptoms occur. In patients not showing block in their BT during noninvasive studies, esophageal pacing can be performed to determine the anterograde ERP of the BT and the ability to induce sustained arrhythmias. If arrhythmias can be induced, the benefits and risk of an invasive investigation and catheter ablation should be based on individual considerations such as age, gender, occupation, and athletic involvement. This should be discussed with the patient or, in the case of a child, with the parents. Because knowledge about the success and complication rate at the EP center plays a major role in decision making, that information should be made available so that the appropriate place for invasive diagnosis and treatment can be selected. If an EP study is performed for risk stratification, the combination of inducible AVRT and a shortest preexcited RR interval during AF of less than 250 milliseconds provide the most compelling indications for ablation. The key is a clear understanding by the patient of the relative merits of each strategy. The well-informed patient needs to choose between a very small risk over a long period of time and a one-time risk over a short span (i.e., ablation). Certain patients such as athletes and those in higher risk occupations will generally choose ablation. Others, especially older patients (older than 30 years), may prefer the small risk of a conservative strategy.[22,23]

Management of the Symptomatic Patient

Acute Management. Patients with AVRT are treated in a similar fashion as those with paroxysmal SVT. In patients with orthodromic and antidromic AVRT, drug treatment can be directed at the BT (ibutilide, procainamide, flecainide) or at the AVN (beta blockers, diltiazem, verapamil) because both are critical components of the tachycardia circuit. Adenosine should be used with caution because it can induce AF with a rapid ventricular rate in patients with preexcited tachycardias.[20]

AVN blocking drugs are ineffective in patients with antidromic AVRT who have anterograde conduction over one BT and retrograde conduction over a separate BT because the AVN is not involved in the circuit.[20] Additionally, caution is advised against AVN blocking agents for the treatment of preexcited tachycardias occurring in patients with AT, AFL, or AF with a bystander BT. Antiarrhythmic drugs such as ibutilide, procainamide, or flecainide, which prevent rapid conduction through the bystander pathway, are preferable, even if they may not convert the atrial arrhythmia. When drug therapy fails or hemodynamic instability is present, electrical cardioversion should be considered.

Chronic Management. The NASPE Policy Statement on Catheter Ablation states that catheter ablation is considered first-line therapy (class I) and the treatment of choice for patients with WPW syndrome—that is, patients with manifest preexcitation along with symptoms.[21] It is curative in more than 95% of patients and has a low complication rate. It also obviates the unwanted side effects of antiarrhythmic agents. For patients with preexcitation who are not candidates for ablation, antiarrhythmic drugs to block BT conduction should be used, such as sodium or potassium channel blockers.[24] However, there have been no controlled trials of pharmacological therapy in patients with AVRT, but small nonrandomized trials have reported the safety and efficacy of drug therapy. Despite the absence of data from clinical trials, chronic oral beta blocker therapy can be used for the treatment of patients with WPW syndrome, particularly if their BT has been demonstrated during EP testing to be incapable of rapid anterograde conduction. Verapamil, diltiazem, and digoxin, on the other hand, generally should not be used as the sole long-term therapy for patients with BT that might be capable of rapid conduction during AF.

Catheter ablation is also considered first-line therapy (class I) for patients with paroxysmal SVT involving a concealed BT. However, because concealed BTs are not associated with an increased risk of sudden cardiac death in these patients, catheter ablation can be presented as one of a number of potential therapeutic approaches, including pharmacological therapy and clinical follow-up alone.[20] When pharmacological therapy is selected for patients with concealed BTs, it is reasonable to consider a trial of beta blocker therapy, calcium channel blocker therapy, or class IC antiarrhythmic agent.

ELECTROCARDIOGRAPHIC FEATURES

Electrocardiography of Preexcitation

Anterogradely conducting AV BTs produce the classic WPW ECG pattern characterized by a fusion between conduction via the BT and the normal AVN-HPS: (1) short PR (P-delta) interval (less than 120 milliseconds); (2) slurred upstroke of the QRS (delta wave); and (3) wide QRS (more than 120 milliseconds) (Fig. 14-4).

The degree of preexcitation depends on several factors, including AVN-HPS conduction, conduction time from the sinus node to the atrial insertion site of the BT, which depends on the distance, conduction, and refractoriness of the intervening atrial tissue, and conduction time through the BT, which depends on the length, thickness, and conduction properties of the BT.

Pharmacological and/or physiological maneuvers (e.g., carotid sinus massage, Valsalva maneuvers, and adenosine) that alter AVN conduction can be used to alter the degree of preexcitation, thereby confirming the diagnosis of the presence of an AV-BT.

The ECG pattern displayed by some patients with the WPW syndrome can simulate the pattern found in other cardiac conditions and can alter the pattern seen in the presence of other cardiac disease. A negative delta wave (presenting as a Q wave) can mimic an MI pattern. Conversely, a positive delta wave can mask the presence of a previous MI. Intermittent WPW can also be mistaken for frequent premature ventricular complexes (PVCs). If the WPW pattern persists for several beats, the rhythm can be misdiagnosed as an accelerated idioventricular rhythm. The WPW pattern is occasionally seen on alternate beats and may suggest ventricular bigeminy. An alternating WPW and normal pattern can occasionally suggest electrical alternans.

Inapparent Versus Intermittent Preexcitation

Inapparent Preexcitation. With inapparent preexcitation, preexcitation is absent on the surface ECG despite the presence of an anterogradely conducting AV BT, because conduction over the AVN-HPS reaches the ventricle faster than that over the BT. In this case, the PR interval is shorter

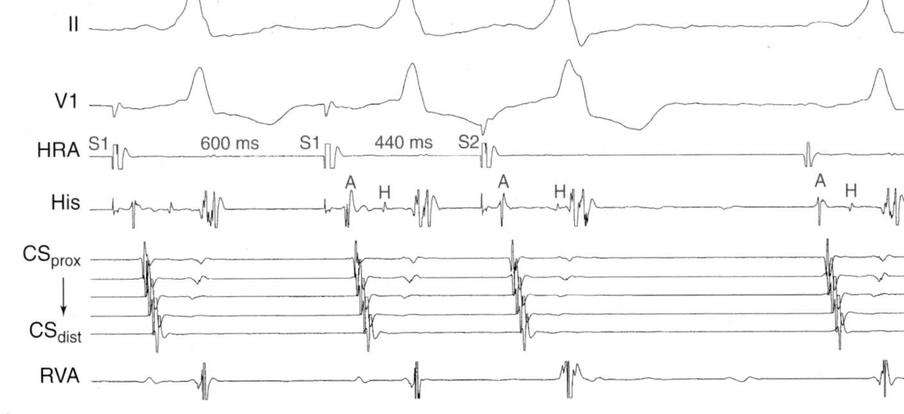

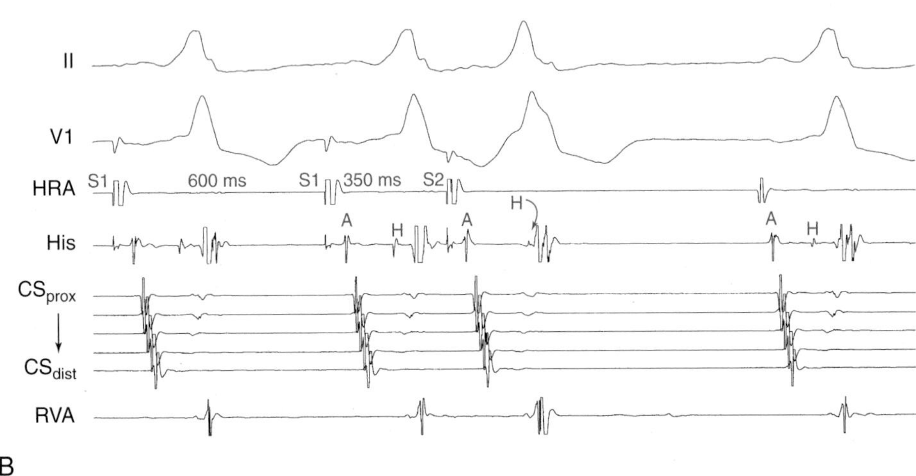

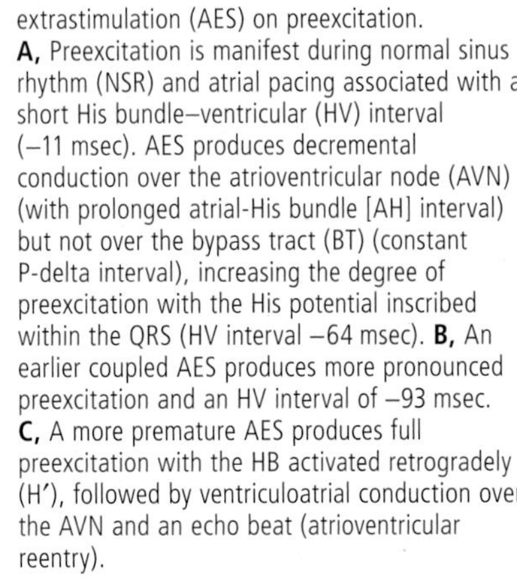
FIGURE 14–4 Effect of atrial extrastimulation (AES) on preexcitation. **A,** Preexcitation is manifest during normal sinus rhythm (NSR) and atrial pacing associated with a short His bundle–ventricular (HV) interval (−11 msec). AES produces decremental conduction over the atrioventricular node (AVN) (with prolonged atrial-His bundle [AH] interval) but not over the bypass tract (BT) (constant P-delta interval), increasing the degree of preexcitation with the His potential inscribed within the QRS (HV interval −64 msec). **B,** An earlier coupled AES produces more pronounced preexcitation and an HV interval of −93 msec. **C,** A more premature AES produces full preexcitation with the HB activated retrogradely (H′), followed by ventriculoatrial conduction over the AVN and an echo beat (atrioventricular reentry).

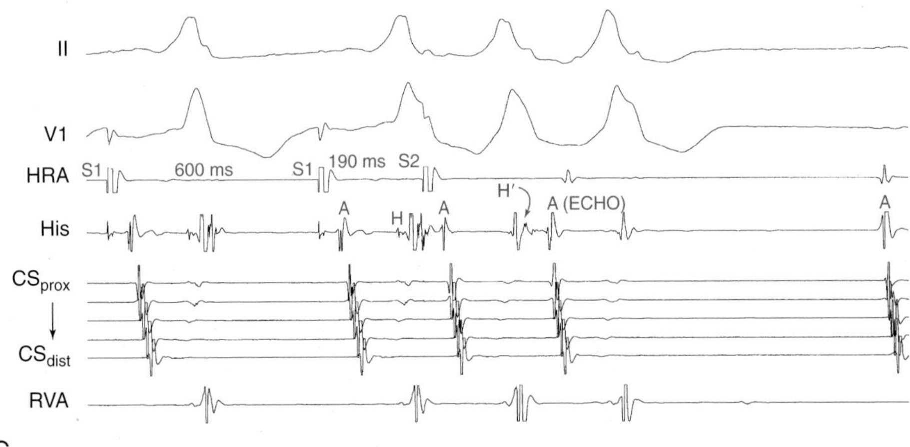

than what the P delta interval would be if preexcitation were present. Therefore, when preexcitation becomes inapparent, the PR interval becomes shorter, reflecting the now better AVN-HPS conduction.[3]

Inapparent preexcitation is usually caused by the following: (1) enhanced AVN conduction, so that it is faster than conduction over the BT; (2) prolonged intraatrial conduction from the site of atrial stimulation to the atrial insertion site of BT (most often left lateral), favoring anterograde conduction over the AVN-HPS; and/or (3) prolonged conduction over the BT, so that it is slower than AVN-HPS conduction.

Intermittent Preexcitation. Intermittent preexcitation is defined as the presence and absence of preexcitation on the same tracing (Fig. 14-5). True intermittent preexcitation is characterized by an abrupt loss of the delta wave (independently of how fast or slow is AVN conduction), with prolongation (normalization) of the PR interval (reflecting the loss of the faster BT conduction, and the subsequent conduction over the slower AVN-HPS), and normalization of the QRS in the absence of any significant change in heart rate.

Intermittent preexcitation is usually caused by the following: (1) phase 3 (i.e., bradycardia-dependent) or phase 4 (i.e., tachycardia-dependent) block in the BT; (2) anterograde or retrograde concealed conduction produced by PVCs, premature atrial complexes (PACs), or atrial arrhythmias; (3) BTs with long ERP and the gap phenomenon in response to PACs, and/or (4) BTs with long ERP and supernormal conduction.

Intermittent preexcitation is generally a reliable sign that the AV BT has a relatively long anterograde ERP and is not capable of excessively rapid impulse conduction, such as during AF. Maneuvers that slow AVN conduction (e.g., carotid sinus massage, AVN blockers) would unmask inapparent preexcitation but would not affect intermittent preexcitation.

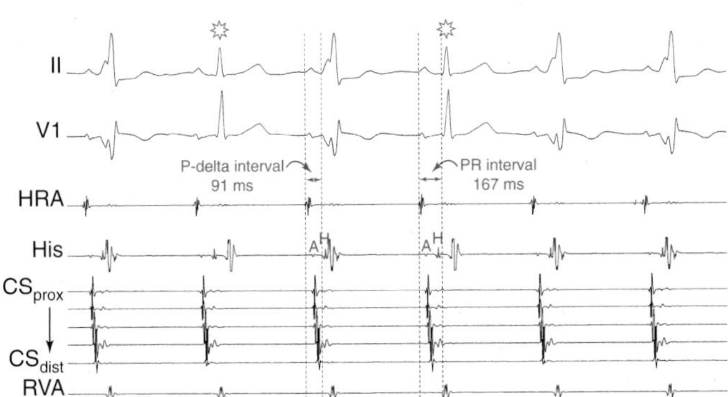

FIGURE 14–5 Intermittent preexcitation. Surface ECG leads II and V_1 and intracardiac recordings in a patient with Wolff-Parkinson-White syndrome and a right anterior bypass tract (BT). Note the intermittent abrupt loss of delta wave (stars) associated with prolongation of the PR interval and normalization of the His bundle–ventricular (HV) interval, despite the presence of a constant atrial–His bundle (AH) interval (atrioventricular node [AVN] conduction) and a stable sinus rate, indicating that loss of preexcitation is secondary to anterograde block in the BT (i.e., intermittent preexcitation) rather than enhanced AVN conduction.

Preexcitation alternans is a form of intermittent preexcitation in which a QRS complex manifesting a delta wave alternates with a normal QRS complex. Concertina preexcitation is another form of intermittent preexcitation in which the PR intervals and QRS complex durations show a cyclic pattern; that is, preexcitation becomes progressively more prominent over a number of QRS complex cycles followed by a gradual diminution in the degree of preexcitation over several QRS cycles, despite a fairly constant heart rate.

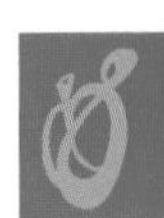

Differentiation between intermittent preexcitation and inapparent preexcitation on an ECG showing QRS complexes with and without preexcitation can be performed by comparing the P-delta interval during preexcitation and the PR interval when preexcitation is absent. Loss of preexcitation associated with a PR interval longer than the P-delta interval is consistent with intermittent preexcitation (see Fig. 14-5), whereas loss of preexcitation associated with a PR interval shorter than the P delta interval is consistent with inapparent preexcitation.

Supraventricular Tachycardias Associated with Wolff-Parkinson-White Syndrome

Orthodromic Atrioventricular Reentrant Tachycardia. The ECG during orthodromic AVRT shows P waves inscribed within the ST-T wave segment with an RP interval that is usually less than half of the tachycardia RR interval (i.e., RP interval < PR interval) (Fig. 14-6). The

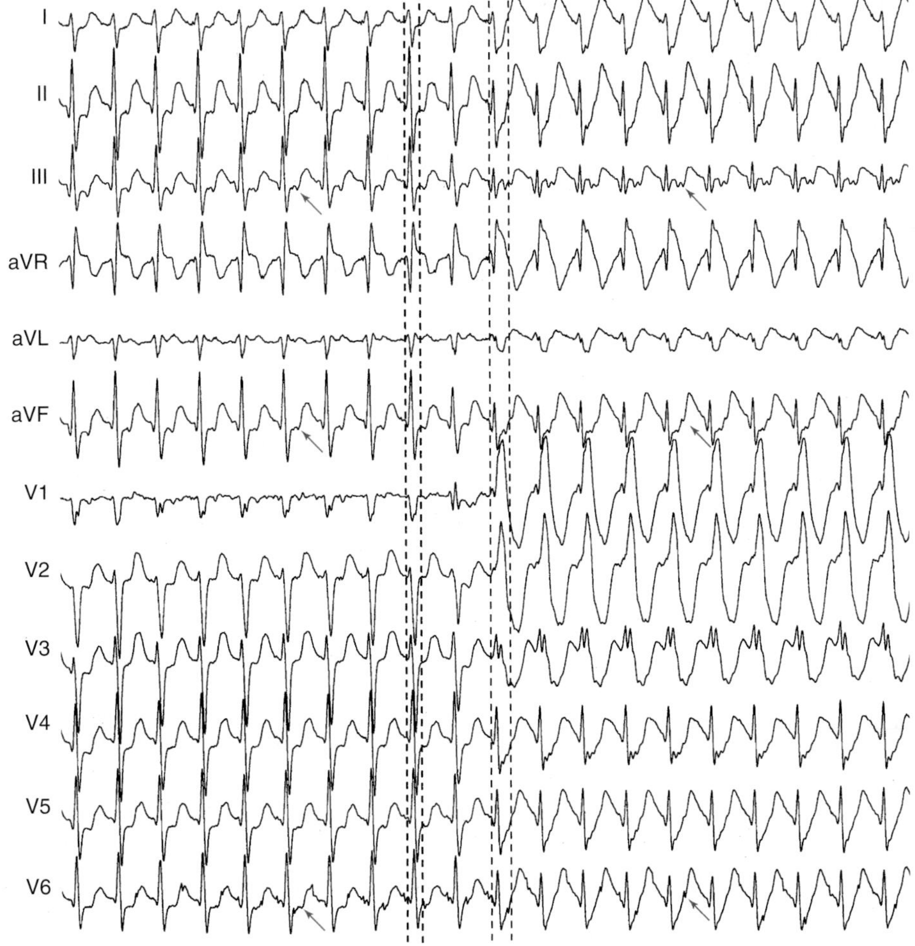

FIGURE 14–6 Surface ECG of orthodromic atrioventricular reentrant tachycardia (AVRT) using a concealed superoparaseptal bypass tract (BT). Note the P waves (arrows) inscribed within the ST-T wave segment (short RP interval). Ischemic-appearing ST segment depression is also observed. Functional right bundle branch block occurs in the right side of the tracing, with prolongation of the RP (ventriculoatrial [VA]) interval, suggesting that retrograde VA conduction during the supraventricular tachycardia is mediated by a right-sided BT. The dashed lines denote the QRS onset and P wave onset.

RP interval remains constant, regardless of the tachycardia CL, because it reflects the nondecremental conduction over the BT. QRS morphology during orthodromic AVRT is generally normal and not preexcited, even when preexcitation is present during NSR. Functional bundle branch block (BBB) can be observed frequently during orthodromic AVRT (see Fig. 14-6).

Orthodromic AVRT tends to be a rapid tachycardia, with rates ranging from 150 to more than 250 beats/min. A beat-to-beat oscillation in QRS amplitude (QRS alternans) is present in up to 38% of cases and is most commonly seen when the rate is very rapid. The mechanism for QRS alternans is not clear but can partly result from oscillations in the relative refractory period of the distal portions of the HPS.[5]

Ischemic-appearing ST segment depression also can occur during orthodromic AVRT, even in young individuals who are unlikely to have coronary artery disease. An association has been observed between repolarization changes (ST segment depression or T wave inversion) and the underlying mechanism of the tachycardia, because such changes are more common in orthodromic AVRT than AVNRT (57% versus 25%). Several factors can contribute to ST segment depression in these arrhythmias. These include changes in autonomic nervous system tone, intraventricular conduction disturbances, a longer ventricular-atrial (VA) interval, and a retrograde P wave of longer duration that overlaps into the ST segment. The location of the ST segment changes can vary with the location of the BT; ST segment depression in leads V_3 to V_6 is almost invariably seen with a left lateral BT, whereas ST segment depression and a negative T wave in the inferior leads is associated with a posteroseptal or posterior BT. A negative or notched T wave in V_2 or V_3 with a positive retrograde P wave in at least two inferior leads suggests an anteroseptal BT. However, ST segment depression occurring during orthodromic AVRT in an older patient mandates consideration of possible coexisting ischemic heart disease.

Antidromic Atrioventricular Reentrant Tachycardia. Antidromic AVRT is characterized by a wide (fully preexcited) QRS complex, usually regular RR intervals, and ventricular rates of up to 250 beats/min. The width of the preexcited QRS complex and the amplitude of the ST-T wave segment usually obscure the retrograde P wave on the surface ECG. When the P waves can be identified, they are inscribed within the ST-T wave segment with an RP interval that may be more than half of the tachycardia RR interval because retrograde conduction occurs slowly via the AVN-HPS. The PR (P-delta) interval remains constant, regardless of the tachycardia CL, because it reflects nondecremental conduction over the BT.[5]

Permanent Junctional Reciprocating Tachycardia. PJRT tends to be incessant, stopping and starting spontaneously every few beats without initiating PACs or PVCs. The heart rate is usually between 120 and 200 beats/min and the QRS duration is generally normal. Slow retrograde conduction over the BT causes the RP interval during PJRT to be long, usually more than half of the tachycardia RR interval (Fig. 14-7). The P waves resulting from retrograde conduction are easily seen on the ECG and are inverted in leads II, III, aVF, and V_3 to V_6.

Atrioventricular Nodal Reentrant Tachycardia and Atrial Tachycardia. Both AVNRT and AT can cause the bystander BT to transmit impulses to the ventricle; therefore, the QRS during these SVTs may be preexcited secondary to anterograde conduction over the BT. When AVNRT occurs in the WPW syndrome, the arrhythmia can be difficult to distinguish from orthodromic AVRT without EP testing.

Atrial Fibrillation. There are several characteristic findings on the ECG in patients with AF conducting over a BT, so-called preexcited AF. The rhythm is irregularly irregular, and can be associated with very rapid ventricular response caused by the nondecremental anterograde AV conduction over the BT. However, sustained rapid ventricular rate of more than 180 to 200 beats/min will often create pseudoregularized RR intervals when the ECG is recorded at 25 mm/sec. Although the QRS complexes are conducted aberrantly, resembling those during preexcited NSR, their duration can be variable and they can become normalized. This is not related to the RR interval (i.e., it is not a rate-related phenomenon), but rather is related to the variable relationship between conduction over the BT and AVN-HPS. Preexcited and normal QRS complexes often appear "clumped." This can result from concealed retrograde conduction into the BT or the AVN.

The QRS complex during preexcitation is a fusion of the impulse that preexcites the ventricles caused by rapid conduction through a BT and of the impulse that takes the usual route through the AVN. The number of impulses that can be transmitted through the BT and the amount of preexcitation depend on the refractoriness of both the BT and AVN. The shorter the ERP of the BT, the more rapid is anterograde impulse conduction and, because of more preexcitation, the wider the QRS complexes. Patients who have a BT with a very short ERP and rapid ventricular rates represent the group at greatest risk for development of VF.

Anterograde block in the BT abolishes retrograde conduction into the AVN, which in turn allows the AVN to recover its excitability and conduct anterogradely. These conducted beats through the AVN can result in retrograde

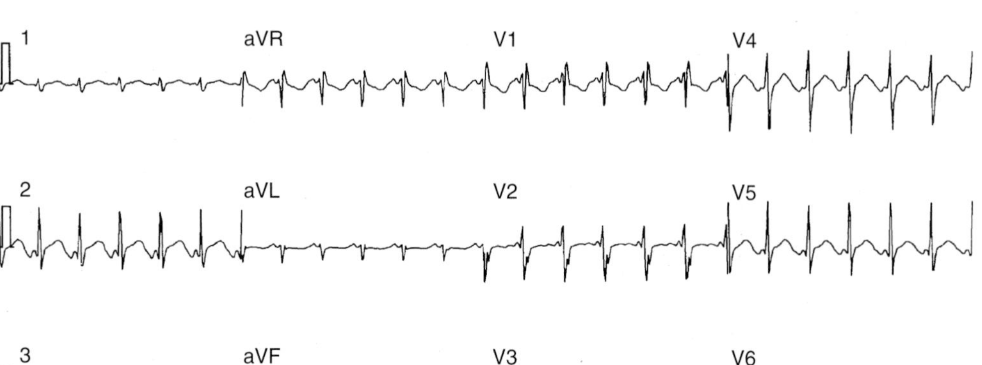

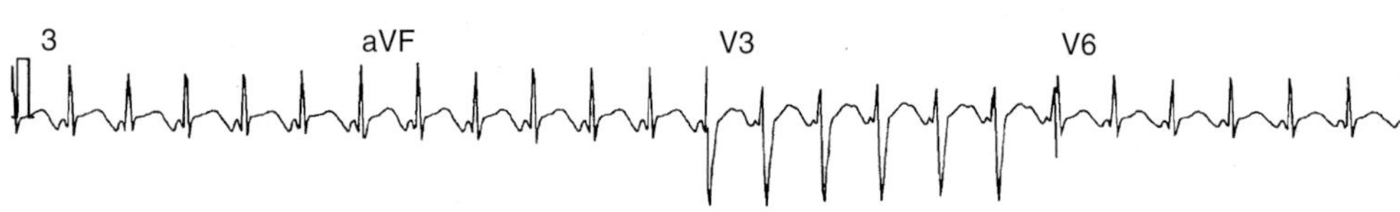

FIGURE 14–7 Surface ECG of a 17-year-old boy with permanent junctional reciprocating tachycardia.

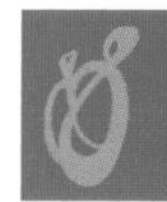

concealment into the BT, causing anterograde block of the BT, thereby slowing the ventricular rate.

Atrial Flutter. AFL, like AF, can conduct anterogradely via a BT causing a preexcited tachycardia. Depending on the various refractory periods of the normal and pathological AV conduction pathways, AFL potentially can conduct 1:1 to the ventricles during a preexcited tachycardia, making the arrhythmia difficult to distinguish from VT.

Electrocardiographic Localization of the Bypass Tract

Localization Using the Delta Wave. Several algorithms have been developed for localization of the BT using the delta wave polarity (Table 14-1; Figs. 14-8 and 14-9).[25,26] The delta wave vector is helpful, especially when maximal preexcitation is present. However, during NSR, the QRS is usually a fusion and total preexcitation is not present, which limits the accuracy of ECG localization of the BT. Therefore, it is important to use only the delta wave for localization (the first 40 milliseconds of the QRS in most cases, unless fully preexcited).[25-29] The accuracy of surface ECG localization of manifest BTs is imperfect and tends to be higher for the diagnosis of left free wall BTs than for BTs in other locations.

Localization Using Polarity of the Retrograde P Wave During Orthodromic Atrioventricular Reentrant Tachycardia. The polarity of the retrograde P waves during orthodromic AVRT is dependent on the location of the atrial insertion of the BT, and is helpful to localize the BT. However, the P wave is usually inscribed within the ST segment and its morphology may not be easily determined.[3,30-33]

In general, P wave morphology in leads I and V_1 and in the inferior leads is most helpful. Negative P wave vector in lead I is highly suggestive of left free wall BTs, whereas a positive P wave is suggestive of right free wall BTs. On the other hand, a negative P wave in V_1 is highly suggestive of right-sided BTs. P wave polarity in the inferior leads, positive or negative, suggests superior or inferior location of the BT, respectively.[3,30-33]

Posteroseptal BTs have positive P waves in V_1, aVR, and aVL and negative P waves in the inferior leads. Left posterior BTs also have negative P waves in the inferior leads, but the P waves are more negative in lead II than in lead III and are more positive in aVR than in aVL, which is often isoelectric. Left lateral BTs have negative P waves in I and aVL, with a tendency for more positive P waves in III than in II and aVF as the location of the BT moves more superiorly.[3,30-33]

TABLE 14–1 Delta Wave Characteristics During Preexcitation According to Bypass Tract (BT) Location

Location / Criteria
Left Lateral/Left Anterolateral BTs
A. R/S $\geq$ 1 in V_2 and positive delta in III, or R/S < 1 in V_2 and positive delta in III and V_1
B. RS transition $\leq V_1$ and > 2 positive delta in the inferior leads or S > R in a VL
C. QS or QR morphology in aVL and no negative QRS in III and V_1
Left Posterior/Left Posterolateral BTs
A. R/S $\geq$ 1 in V_1 & V_2, no positive delta in III and positive delta in V_1
B. R/S transition $\leq V_1$, no $\geq$ 2 positive delta in the inferior leads, no S > R in aVL, in lead I R < (S + 0.8 mV), and the sum of the inferior delta is not negative
C. Positive QRS in aVL and an equiphasic QRS or positive in V_1 and no negative QRS in III
Left Posteroseptal BTs
A. R/S $\geq$ 1 in V_2, no positive delta in III, and positive delta and R/S < 1 in V_1
B. R/S transition $\leq V_1$, no $\geq$2 positive delta in the inferior leads, no S > R in aVL, in lead I R < (S + 0.8 mV), and the sum of the inferior delta was negative
C. Negative QRS in III, V_1, and aVF, tallest precordial R wave in V_2-V_4 and R wave width in V_1 > 0.06 ms
Midseptal BTs
A. R/S < 1 in V_2, no positive delta in III, and negative delta in V_1
B. R/S transition between V_2 and V_3 or between V_3 and V_4 but the delta amplitude in lead II $\geq$ 1.0 mV (septal location), and the sum of delta polarities in inferior leads was −1, 0, or +1 mV
C. Negative QRS in leads III, V_1, and aVF, tallest precordial R in leads V_2-V_4 and R wave width in V_1 < 0.06 ms
Right Posteroseptal BTs
A. R/S $\geq$ 1 in V_2 and no positive delta in III and V_1
B. The sum of delta polarities in inferior leads was $\leq$ −2 mV
C. Negative QRS in leads III, V_1, and AVF and tallest precordial R in V_5 or V_6
Right Posterior/Right Posterolateral BTs
A. R/S < 1 in V_2, no positive delta in III and no negative delta in V_1 and negative delta polarity in aVF
B. R/S transition between V_3 and V_4 with delta amplitude in lead II < 1.0 mV or $\geq V_4$ and the delta axis is < 0 degrees and the R in lead III was $\leq$0 mV
C. Positive QRS in III, negative in V_1, and RS morphology in aVL
Right Lateral/Right Anterolateral BTs
A. R/S < 1 in V_2, no positive delta in III and no negative delta in V_1 and negative or biphasic delta in aVF
B. R/S transition between leads V_3 and V_4 with delta amplitude in lead II < 1.0 mV or > V_4 and the delta axis is < 0 degrees and the R amplitude in lead III is < 0 mV
C. Positive QRS in leads aVL and III and negative in V_1
Right Anterior/Right Superoparaseptal BTs
A. R/S < 1 in V_2, positive delta in III and no positive delta in V_1
B. The sum of delta polarities in inferior leads was $\geq$ +2
C. Positive QRS in aVF and negative in leads III and V_1

From Katsouras CS, Greakas GF, Goudevenos JA, et al: Localization of accessory pathways by the electrogram. Pacing Clin Electrophysiol 2004;27:189.

A, Algorithm of Chiang et al[27]; B, Algorithm of Fitzpatrick et al[25]; C, Algorithm of Xie et al.[28]

ELECTROPHYSIOLOGICAL TESTING

EP testing is used to study the features, location, and number of BTs and the tachycardias, if any, associated with them (Table 14-2). Typically, three quadripolar catheters are positioned in the high RA, right ventricle (RV) apex, and HB region, and a decapolar catheter is positioned in the CS (see Fig. 2-7).

Baseline Observations During Normal Sinus Rhythm

Preexcitation is associated with a short His bundle–ventricular (HV) or H-delta interval during NSR. The HV interval can even be negative or the His potential can be buried in the local ventricular electrogram (see Fig. 14-4). The QRS is a fusion between conduction over the BT and that over the AVN-HPS. The site of earliest ventricular activation is near the ventricular insertion site of the BT (i.e., near the tricuspid annulus or mitral annulus at the base of the heart). Slowing of conduction in the AVN by carotid sinus massage, AVN blockers, or rapid atrial pacing unmasks and increases the degree of preexcitation, because these maneuvers do not affect the conduction over the BT. Dual AVN pathways can be present in 8% to 40% of patients.

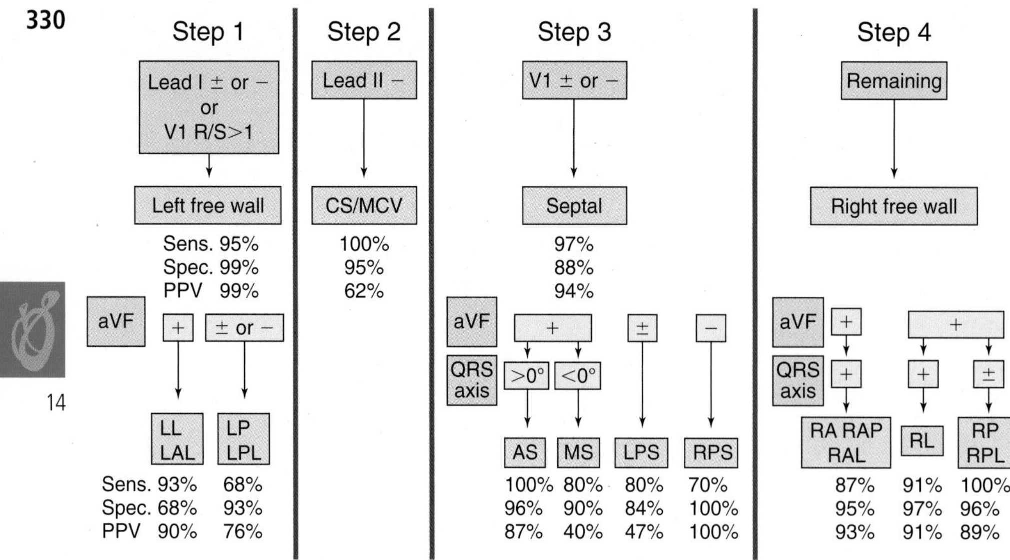

FIGURE 14–8 Algorithm for localization of bypass tract (BT) using delta wave morphology on the surface ECG. + = positive delta wave; ± = isoelectric delta wave; – = negative delta wave; AS = right anteroseptal; CS/MCV = coronary sinus/middle cardiac vein; LL = left lateral; LAL = left anterolateral; LP = left posterior; LPL = left posterolateral; LPS = left posteroseptal; MS = midseptal; PPV = positive predictive value; RA = right anterior; RAL = right anterolateral; RL = right lateral; RPL = right posterolateral; RP = right posterior; RPS = right posteroseptal; R/S = R-S wave ratio; Sens = sensitivity; Spec = specificity. (From Arruda M, Wang X, McClennand J: ECG algorithm for predicting sites of successful radiofrequency ablation of accessory pathways. Pacing Clin Electrophysiol 1993;16:865.)

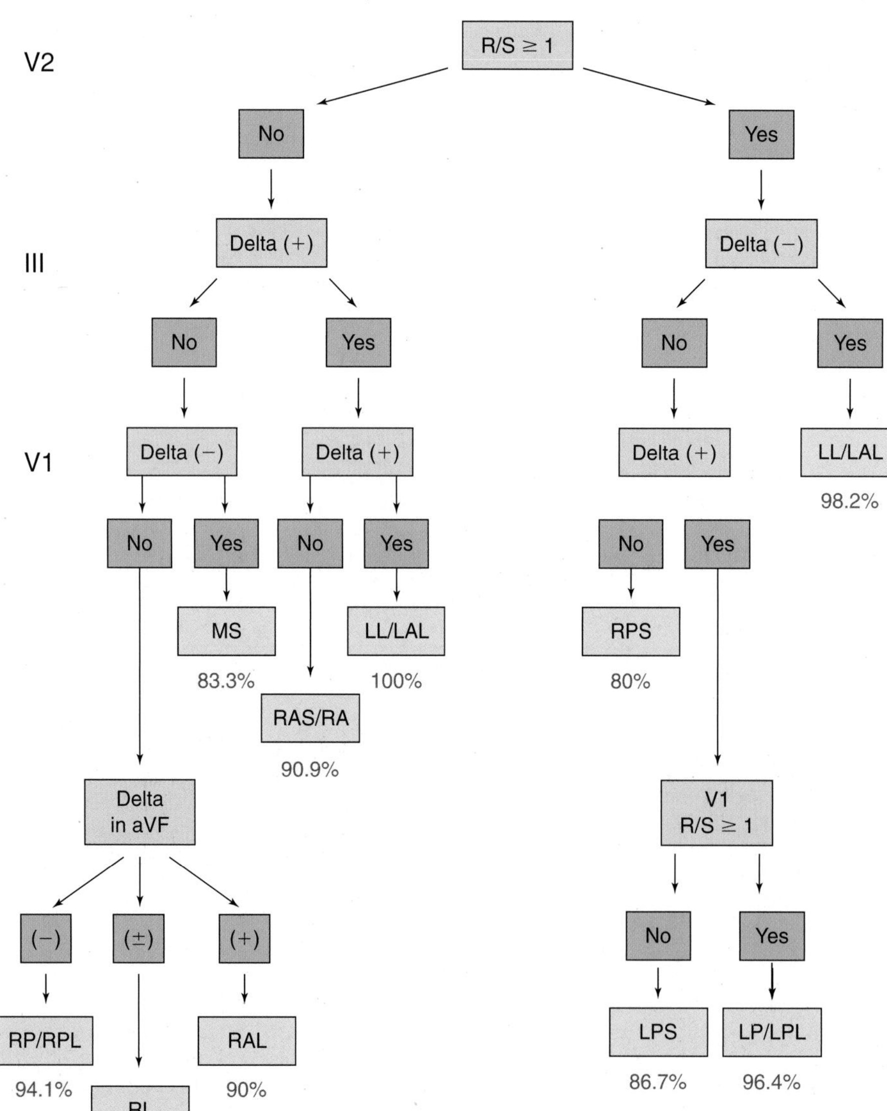

FIGURE 14–9 Stepwise algorithm for localization of the bypass tract (BT) by delta wave polarity. Numbers indicate the accuracy of the algorithm for each BT location. LAL = left anterolateral; LL = left lateral; LP = left posterior; LPL = left posterolateral; LPS = left posteroseptal; MS = midseptal; RA = right anterior; RAL = right anterolateral; RAS = right anteroseptal; RL = right lateral; RP = right posterior; RPL = right posterolateral; RPS = right posteroseptal. (From Chiang CE, Chen SA, Teo WS , et al: An accurate stepwise electrocardiographic algorithm for localization of accessory pathways in patients with Wolff-Parkinson-White syndrome from a comprehensive analysis of delta waves and R/S ratio during sinus rhythm. Am J Cardiol 1995;76:40.)

TABLE 14–2	Goals of Electrophysiology Evaluation in Patients with Wolff-Parkinson-White Syndrome
Confirming the presence of an atrioventricular bypass tract (BT) Evaluation for the presence of multiple BTs Localization of the BT(s) Evaluation of the refractoriness of the BT and its implications for life-threatening arrhythmias Induction and evaluation of tachycardias Demonstration of the BT role in the tachycardia Evaluation of other tachycardias not dependent on the presence of the BT Termination of the tachycardias	

Atrial Pacing and Atrial Extrastimulation During Normal Sinus Rhythm

In the presence of a manifest AV-BT, atrial stimulation from any atrial site can help unmask preexcitation if it is not manifest during NSR caused by fast AVN conduction. Incremental rate atrial pacing and progressively premature AES produce decremental conduction over the AVN (but not over the BT), increasing the degree of preexcitation and shortening the HV interval, until the His potential is inscribed within the QRS. The His potential is still activated anterogradely over the AVN until anterograde block in the AVN occurs; the QRS then becomes fully preexcited, and the His potential becomes retrogradely activated (see Fig. 14-4).

Atrial stimulation close to or at the AV BT insertion site results in maximal preexcitation and the shortest P-delta interval because of the lack of intervening atrial tissue whose refractoriness may otherwise limit the ability of atrial stimulation to activate the AV BT as early (Fig. 14-10). The failure of atrial stimulation to increase the amount of preexcitation can be caused by markedly enhanced AVN conduction, presence of another AV-BT, pacing-induced block in the AV BT because of a long ERP of the BT (longer than that of the AVN), total preexcitation already present at the basal state caused by prolonged or absent AVN-HPS conduction, and/or decremental conduction in the BT.

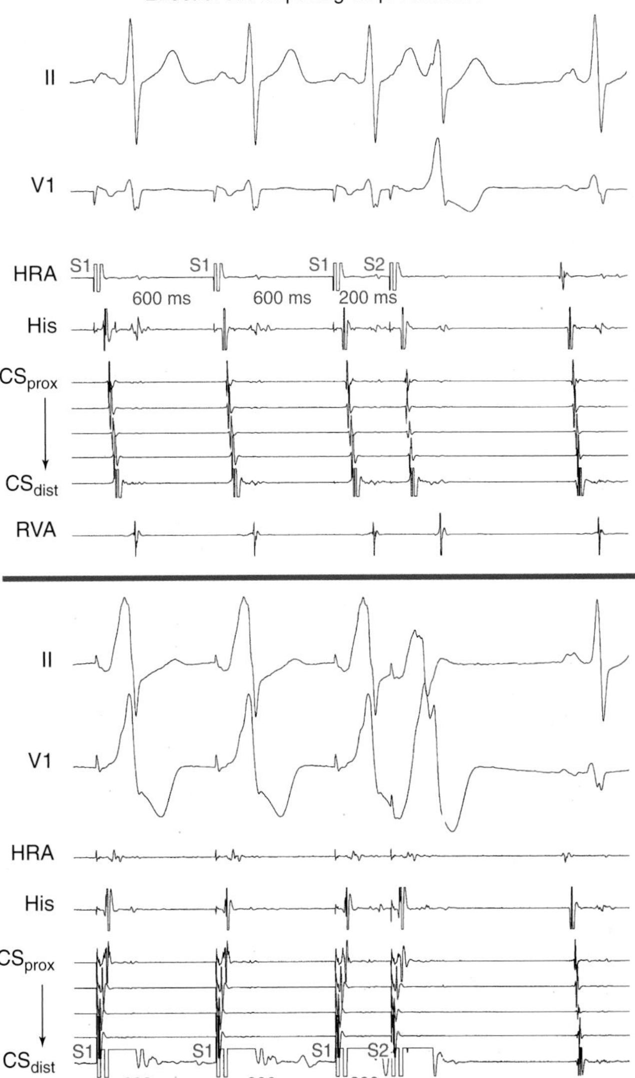

FIGURE 14–10 Effect of site of pacing on preexcitation. **Upper panel,** In the presence of a manifest left lateral bypass tract (BT), pacing from the high right atrium at a cycle length (CL) of 600 msec produces minimal preexcitation. The degree of preexcitation increases with premature stimulation because of delay in atrioventricular nodal conduction. **Lower panel,** In the same patient, pacing at the same CLs from the distal coronary sinus (CS), close to or at the BT insertion site, results in a larger degree of preexcitation and shorter P-delta interval because of the lack of intervening atrial tissue whose refractoriness might otherwise limit the ability of atrial stimulation to activate the BT as early.

Ventricular Pacing and Ventricular Extrastimulation During Normal Sinus Rhythm

In the presence of a retrogradely conducting AV BT (whether manifest or concealed), ventricular extrastimulation (VES) during NSR can result in VA conduction over the BT, AVN, both, or neither (Fig. 14-11). Conduction over the BT alone is the most common pattern at short pacing CLs or short VES coupling intervals. In this case, the VA conduction time is constant over a wide range of pacing CLs and VES coupling intervals, in the absence of intraventricular conduction abnormalities or additional BTs. On the other hand, retrograde conduction over the BT and HPS-AVN is especially common when RV pacing is performed in the presence of a left-sided BT at long pacing CLs or long VES coupling intervals. This occurs because it is easier to engage the right bundle branch (RB) and conduct retrogradely through the AVN than it is to reach a distant left-sided BT. In this case, atrial activation pattern depends on the refractoriness and conduction times over both pathways, and usually exhibits a variable degree of fusion. In addition, VA conduction can proceed over the HPS-AVN alone, resulting in a normal pattern of VA conduction, or can be absent because of block in both the HPS-AVN and BT, which is especially common with short pacing CLs and very early VES.

Ventricular stimulation during NSR also helps prove the presence of a retrogradely conducting AV BT. Ventricular stimulation resulting in retrograde VA conduction not consistent with normal conduction over the AVN (i.e., eccentric atrial activation sequence; see Fig. 14-11) and a VES delivered when the HB is refractory that results in atrial activation are indicators of the presence of a retrogradely conducting AV BT. However, if a VES delivered when the HB is refractory does not result in atrial activation, this does not necessarily exclude the presence of a retrogradely conducting AV-BT, because such a VES can be associated with retrograde block in the BT itself (see Fig. 14-11). Additionally, the lack of such a response does not exclude the presence of unidirectional (anterograde-only) AV BTs.

During retrograde conduction over the BT, the VA interval may increase slightly in response to incremental rate ventricular pacing or progressively premature VES. At short ventricular pacing CLs or VES coupling intervals, intramyo-

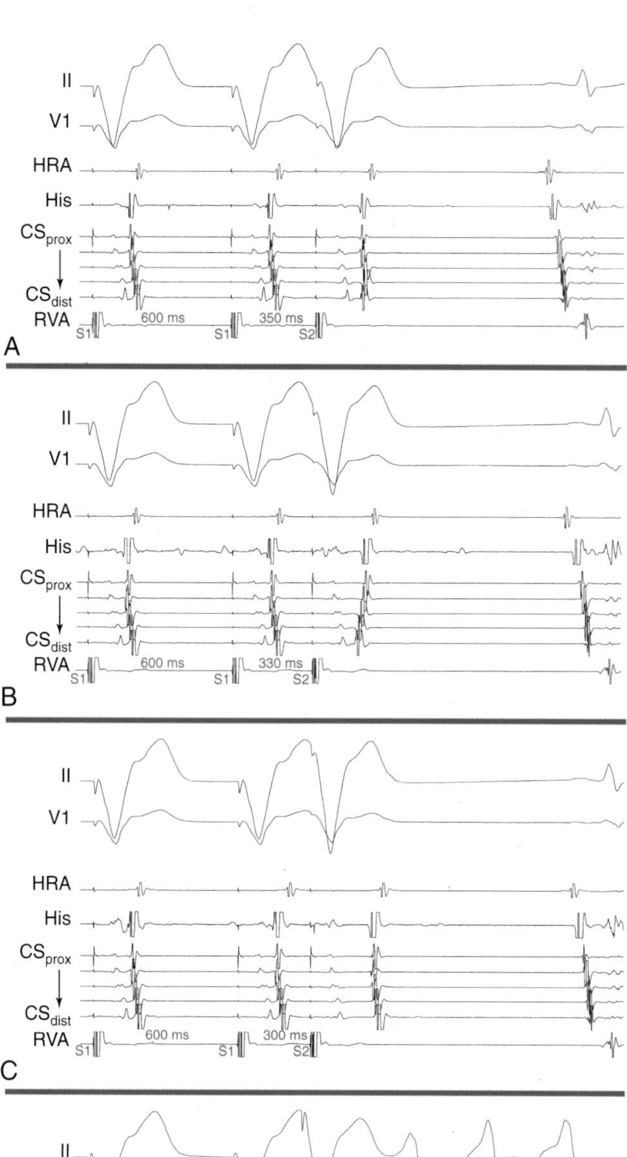

FIGURE 14–11 Retrograde conduction during ventricular extrastimulation (VES) in a patient with a bidirectional left lateral bypass tract (BT). **A,** The ventricular pacing drive is conducted retrogradely over the atrioventricular node (AVN) with a concentric atrial activation sequence. The VES is conducted over both the AVN and BT (atrial fusion). **B,** An earlier VES encounters delay in the His-Purkinje system (HPS)–AVN and conducts solely over the BT with an eccentric atrial activation sequence. **C,** An early-coupled VES blocks retrogradely in the BT and conducts solely over the AVN. **D,** The VES conducts only over the HPS-AVN with more pronounced ventriculoatrial (VA) delay, which allows recovery of the BT and anterograde conduction, initiating antidromic atrioventricular reentrant tachycardia (AVRT). The VA delay is provided by conduction delay, not only within the AVN but also within the HPS. Note that the VES encounters retrograde block in the right bundle branch (RB), and His bundle (HB) activation is mediated by retrograde conduction over the left bundle branch (LB). Consequently, the His potential is visible after the ventricular electrogram. Note that despite the fact that the H_1-H_2 interval following VES approximates the H-H interval during supraventricular tachycardia (SVT), the His bundle–atrial (HA) interval following the initiating VES is shorter than that during the SVT, which favors antidromic AVRT over preexcited atrioventricular nodal reentrant tachycardia (AVNRT) as the mechanism of the SVT.

cardial conduction delay can occur, resulting in prolongation in the VA interval; however, the local VA interval at the BT location remains unchanged. Furthermore, short ventricular pacing CLs or VES coupling intervals can encroach on the BT refractoriness, causing some decremental conduction, with a consequent increase in total and local VA intervals. The VA interval can also change with changing the site of ventricular stimulation, because the VA interval represents the sum of conduction time over the BT and conduction time through the ventricular tissue intervening between the site of stimulation and ventricular insertion site of the BT. BTs with retrograde decremental conduction properties can also exhibit prolongation of conduction time and VA interval with ventricular pacing or VES.

The absence of VA conduction (at long pacing CLs) or the presence of decremental VA conduction at baseline makes the presence of a retrogradely conducting BT unlikely, except for the catecholamine-dependent BTs.

Induction of Tachycardia

Initiation by Atrial Extrastimulation or Atrial Pacing

Orthodromic Atrioventricular Reentrant Tachycardia: Manifest Atrioventricular Bypass Tract. In the presence of a manifest AV-BT, initiation of orthodromic AVRT with an AES requires the following: (1) anterograde block in the AV-BT; (2) anterograde conduction over the AVN-HPS; and (3) slow conduction over the AVN-HPS, with adequate delay to allow for the recovery of the atrium and AV BT and subsequent retrograde conduction over the BT (see Fig. 1-8).[3] The reason this occurs is because, whereas the BT conducts more rapidly than the AVN, it has a longer ERP, so the early atrial impulse blocks anterogradely in the BT but conducts over the AVN. The site of AV delay is less important; it is most commonly in the AVN, but it can occur also in the HB, bundle branches, or ventricular myocardium. Because the coupling intervals of the AES required to achieve anterograde block in the BT are usually short, sufficient AVN delay is usually present so that orthodromic AVRT is initiated once anterograde BT block occurs.

The presence of dual AVN physiology can facilitate the initiation of orthodromic AVRT by providing adequate AV delay by mediating anterograde conduction over the slow AVN pathway. BBB ipsilateral to the AV BT provides an additional AV delay that can facilitate tachycardia initiation. AES can also result in a 1:2 response caused by conduction over both the AV BT and AVN-HPS (i.e., a single AES resulting in two ventricular complexes; the first is fully preexcited and the second is normal). For this response to occur, significant delay in AVN-HPS conduction should be present to allow for recovery of the ventricle after its activation via conduction over the BT. AES can also produce sinus nodal or AVN echo beats that in turn may block in the BT and achieve adequate AV delay to initiate orthodromic AVRT.

Induction of orthodromic AVRT is easier with atrial stimulation from a site near the AV BT insertion site; the closer the stimulation site to the BT, the easier it is to encroach on the refractory period of the BT and achieve block, because it is not limited by the refractoriness of intervening atrial tissue. Furthermore, the earlier the atrial insertion of the BT is activated, the more likely it will recover before arrival of the retrograde atrial activation wavefront to the BT atrial insertion site, thereby facilitating reentry. Thus, one may actually require less anterograde AV delay if recovery of excitability is shifted earlier in time. In addition, different sites of atrial stimulation can produce different AVN conduction velocities and refractoriness (even at the same AES coupling intervals).

If SVT induction fails, the use of multiple AESs, rapid atrial pacing, and pacing closer to the BT would achieve block in the BT and produce adequate AV delay.

Orthodromic Atrioventricular Reentrant Tachycardia: Concealed Atrioventricular Bypass Tract. Orthodromic AVRT in patients with concealed BTs is identical to that in patients with WPW. The only difference is that in patients with concealed BTs anterograde block in the BT is already present. Because the AV BT does not conduct anterogradely, the only condition needed to induce orthodromic AVRT is adequate AV delay (in the AVN or HPS) in order to allow for recovery of the atrium and atrial insertion site of the AV-BT. Therefore, orthodromic AVRT initiation requires less premature coupling intervals of the AESs in patients with concealed BTs than in patients with WPW.

Orthodromic Atrioventricular Reentrant Tachycardia: Slowly Conducting Concealed Atrioventricular Bypass Tract (Permanent Junctional Reciprocating Tachycardia). PJRT is usually incessant and initiated by spontaneous shortening of the sinus CL, without an initiating PAC or PVC. The tachycardia can be transiently terminated by PACs or PVCs but usually resumes after a few sinus beats (Fig. 14-12). This phenomenon has three potential mechanisms: a rate-related decrease in the retrograde ERP of the BT, a rate-related decrease in atrial refractoriness that allows the impulse to reactivate the atrium retrogradely over the BT, or a concealed Wenckebach block with block at the atrial-BT junction terminating the Wenckebach cycle, relieving any anterograde concealed conduction that may have prevented retrograde conduction up the BT. The latter is the most likely mechanism, because such slow BTs actually demonstrate decremental conduction at rapid rates and, in most cases, the atrial ERP at the atrial-BT junction is shorter than the RP (VA) interval. Thus, some sort of anterograde concealment during NSR in the BT must be operative, preventing tachycardia from always occurring.[3] Late-coupled AESs can also readily initiate PJRT.

Antidromic Atrioventricular Reentrant Tachycardia. The initiation of classic antidromic AVRT by an AES requires the following: (1) intact anterograde conduction over the BT; (2) anterograde block in the AVN or HPS; and (3) intact retrograde conduction over the HPS-AVN once the AVN resumes excitability following partial anterograde penetration (see Fig. 14-4). This is usually the limiting factor for the initiation of antidromic AVRT. A delay of more than 150 milliseconds between atrial insertion of the BT and HB is probably required for the initiation of antidromic AVRT.[3,5]

Several mechanisms of antidromic AVRT initiation can be operative.[3] The AES may block in the AVN with anterograde conduction down the BT and subsequent retrograde conduction over the HPS-AVN. In this case, ventricular–His bundle (V-H) delay is required to allow recovery of the AVN. Because antidromic AVRTs have relatively short VA intervals, this mechanism of initiation is probably uncommon, except with left-sided BTs, which would potentially provide sufficient V-H delay to allow retrograde conduction. Tachycardia initiation may be facilitated by a short retrograde AVN ERP, a common finding in patients with these SVTs. Alternatively, the AES may block in the AVN, with anterograde conduction down the BT and subsequent retrograde conduction over a different BT. Subsequent complexes can conduct retrogradely over the AVN-HPS or the second BT. Changing tachycardia CL (and VA interval) may relate to whether retrograde conduction proceeds over the AVN-HPS or the second BT. A third potential mechanism for the initiation of antidromic AVRT involves AES conduction over the BT and simultaneously over the slow pathway of a dual AVN pathway situation, with anterograde block in the fast AVN pathway. Conduction beyond the HB to the ventricle is not possible because of ventricular refractoriness, yet an AVN echo to the atrium can occur, which in turn can conduct anterogradely over the BT, when the ventricle would have recovered excitability, and subsequently back up the now-recovered AVN, initiating antidromic AVRT. AVN reentry may not persist or may be preempted by retrograde conduction up the fast AVN pathway because of the premature ventricular activation over the BT. In this case, the location of the His potential will depend on whether or not it was anterograde or retrograde.

In general, if atrial stimulation induces antidromic AVRT, multiple BTs are often operative. Whether or not they are operative throughout the SVT depends on the relative retrograde activation times over the additional BTs and HPS-AVN and the varying degree of anterograde and/or retrograde concealment into the additional BTs and/or HPS-AVN during the SVT.

The site of atrial stimulation plays an important role in inducibility of AVRT, and can also determine the type of AVRT initiated in patients with bidirectional BTs. The closer the stimulation site to the BT, the more likely anterograde block in the BT will occur and orthodromic AVRT will result. Conversely, antidromic AVRT is more likely to occur with atrial stimulation close to the AVN.

Initiation by Ventricular Extrastimulation or Ventricular Pacing

Orthodromic Atrioventricular Reentrant Tachycardia: Manifest or Concealed Atrioventricular Bypass Tract. Ventricular stimulation is usually able to induce orthodromic AVRT (inducibility rate of 60% with VES and 80% with ventricular pacing), and is similar in patients with manifest or concealed BTs (Fig. 14-13). Initiation of orthodromic AVRT by ventricular stimulation requires the following[3]: (1) retrograde block of the ventricular impulse in the HPS-AVN; (2) retrograde conduction only over the AV-BT; and (3) adequate VA conduction delay to allow for recovery of the AVN-HPS from any concealment produced by ventricular stimulation, so it can support anterograde conduction of the reentrant impulse. Because the BT retrograde ERP is usually very short, the prime determinant of orthodromic AVRT initiation is the extent of retrograde conduction and/or concealment in the HPS-AVN.

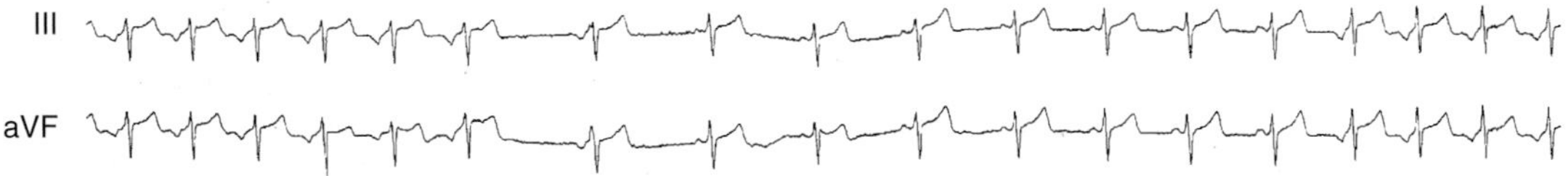

FIGURE 14–12 Two surface ECG leads are shown during permanent junctional reciprocating tachycardia. Carotid sinus pressure is applied at left, resulting in termination of supraventricular tachycardia (SVT) caused by block in the bypass tract (the SVT terminates with a QRS). Several escape and sinus complexes follow, and then the SVT resumes. This phenomenon gives rise to the use of the term *permanent* or *incessant.*

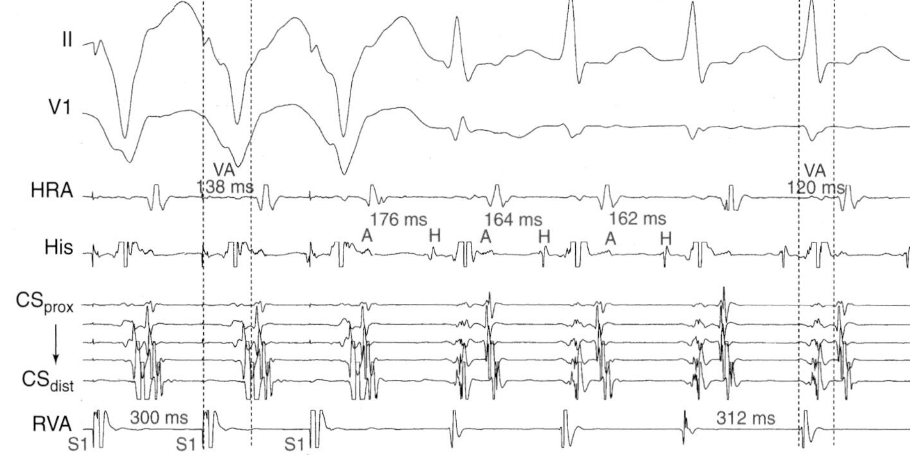

FIGURE 14–13 Induction of an orthodromic atrioventricular reentrant tachycardia (AVRT) using a concealed posteroseptal bypass tract with ventricular pacing. Note that although the ventricular pacing cycle length (CL) approximates the supraventricular tachycardia (SVT) CL, the ventriculoatrial (VA) interval (dashed lines) during ventricular pacing is only slightly longer than that during SVT, which favors orthodromic AVRT over atrioventricular nodal reentrant tachycardia (AVNRT) as the mechanism of the SVT. Additionally, the atrial–His bundle interval of the first SVT complex is longer than that of subsequent beats, indicating retrograde concealment in the AVN produced by the last ventricular stimulus.

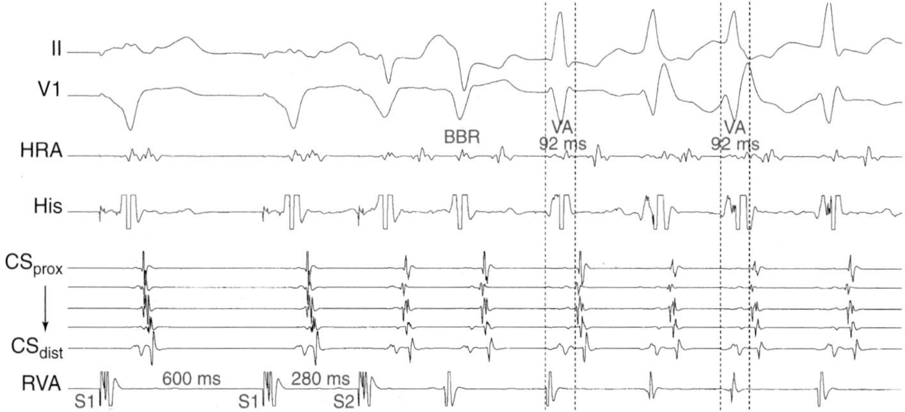

FIGURE 14–14 Induction of an orthodromic atrioventricular reentrant tachycardia (AVRT) using a concealed left posteroseptal bypass tract (BT) with ventricular extrastimulation (VES). The VES conducts retrogradely over the BT, but also results in a bundle branch reentrant (BBR) beat, which in turn conducts to the atrium over the BT and initiates orthodromic AVRT. Note that right bundle branch block (RBBB) develops shortly after initiation of the SVT; however, the ventriculoatrial (VA) interval (dashed lines) remains constant, regardless of the presence or absence of RBBB, because the BT is in the ipsilateral ventricle.

Multiple modes of initiation of orthodromic AVRT can be present, depending on the pacing CL and VES coupling interval, conduction velocities, and refractoriness of the HPS-AVN and BT, in addition to the site of ventricular stimulation. Consequently, the initiation of orthodromic AVRT by ventricular stimulation can be mediated by different mechanisms.[3] A VES with a coupling interval or ventricular pacing at a CL shorter than the ERP of the AVN but longer than that of the HPS and AV BT would block retrogradely in the AVN and conduct over the AV BT to initiate orthodromic AVRT. Block in the AVN, which is more likely to occur with rapid ventricular pacing or VES delivered after a short-drive CL, can cause concealment and subsequent delay in anterograde conduction of the first SVT impulse over the AVN, resulting in longer AH and PR intervals of the first SVT beat compared with subsequent beats (see Fig. 14-13). On the other hand, a VES with a coupling interval or ventricular pacing at a CL shorter than the ERP of the HPS, but longer than that of the AV BT, would block retrogradely in the HPS and conduct over the AV BT to initiate orthodromic AVRT. When block occurs in the HPS, which is more likely to occur with a VES delivered during NSR or after a long-drive CL, the first SVT beat will approach a fully recovered AVN and conduct with short AH and PR intervals equal to subsequent SVT beats. In this case, adequate prolongation of the HV interval may be required to allow for the recovery of ventricular refractoriness for the ventricle to be activated and support reentry, because AVN delay may have not been adequate. When HV interval prolongation is required to initiate orthodromic AVRT, it is almost invariably associated with left bundle branch block (LBBB). A short-coupled VES, especially following a pacing drive with a long CL, that blocks retrogradely in both the AV BT and RB and conducts transseptally and then retrogradely over the left bundle (LB), can result in a bundle branch reentrant (BBR) beat that conducts to the ventricle down the RB, and then retrogradely to the atrium over the AV-BT, mediating the initiation of orthodromic AVRT. The long HV interval often associated with BBR beats, plus the LBBB pattern, facilitate the induction of orthodromic AVRT using a left-sided BT (Fig. 14-14).

Orthodromic Atrioventricular Reentrant Tachycardia: Slowly Conducting Concealed Atrioventricular Bypass Tract (Permanent Junctional Reciprocating Tachycardia). Ventricular stimulation is less effective in initiating PJRT because of the already impaired conduction in the BT, such that an early VES produces block in the BT. A late-coupled VES (when the HB is refractory) can initiate SVT in some cases.

Antidromic Atrioventricular Reentrant Tachycardia. Initiation of classic antidromic AVRT by ventricular pacing and VES requires the following: (1) retrograde block in the BT; (2) retrograde conduction over the AVN or HPS; and (3) adequate VA delay to allow for recovery of the atrium and BT so it can support subsequent anterograde conduction (see Fig. 14-11).[3,5]

When induction of the SVT is achieved by ventricular pacing at a CL similar to the tachycardia CL or by a VES that activates the HB at a coupling interval (i.e., H_1-H_2 interval) similar to the H-H interval during the SVT, the His bundle–atrial (HA) interval following the initiating ventricular stimulus is always equal to or shorter than that during the antidromic AVRT. This is because the His potential and atrium are activated in sequence during antidromic AVRT and in parallel during ventricular stimulation. Therefore, an HA interval of the initiating ventricular stimulus longer than the HA interval during SVT favors AVNRT and excludes antidromic AVRT (see Fig. 14-11). Moreover, because the AVN usually exhibits greater decremental conduction with repetitive engagement of impulses than to a single impulse at a similar coupling interval, the more prolonged the HA interval with the initiating ventricular stimulus, the more likely that the SVT is AVNRT.

Tachycardia Features

Orthodromic Atrioventricular Reentrant Tachycardia: Manifest or Concealed Atrioventricular Bypass Tract

Atrial Activation Sequence. The initial site of atrial activation during orthodromic AVRT depends on the location of the AV BT, but is always near the AV groove, without multiple breakthrough points. Atrial activation sequence during orthodromic AVRT should be identical to that during ventricular pacing at comparable CLs when VA conduction occurs exclusively over the AV BT. However, retrograde conduction during ventricular pacing may proceed over the AVN or over both the BT and AVN, resulting in fusion of atrial activation, depending on the site of ventricular stimulation relative to the BT and HPS, and on retrograde conduction and refractoriness of the HPS-AVN.

Atrial-Ventricular Relationship. Conduction time over the classic (fast) BTs is approximately 30 to 120 milliseconds. Therefore, the RP interval is short, but longer than that during typical AVNRT, because the wavefront has to activate the ventricle before it reaches the AV BT ventricular insertion site close to the AV groove and subsequently conduct to the atrium. A VA interval of less than 70 milliseconds or V–high RA interval of less than 95 milliseconds largely excludes orthodromic AVRT, and is consistent with AVNRT.[34] The RP and VA intervals remain constant regardless of oscillations in tachycardia CL from whatever cause or changes in the PR interval (AH interval); thus, the RP/PR ratio can change (Fig. 14-15). The tachycardia CL is most closely associated with the PR interval (i.e., anterograde slow conduction).

A 1:1 A-V relationship is a prerequisite for maintenance of AVRT, because parts of both the atrium and ventricle are essential components of the reentrant circuit. If an SVT persists in the presence of AV block, orthodromic AVRT is excluded.

When dual AVN pathways are present, the slow AVN pathway functions as the anterograde limb during orthodromic AVRT in most cases. An AH interval of more than 180 milliseconds during orthodromic AVRT suggests a slow AVN pathway mediating the anterograde limb of the reentrant circuit, whereas an AH interval of less than 160 milliseconds suggests a fast AVN pathway mediating anterograde conduction. Obviously, orthodromic AVRT using the slow pathway will have a longer tachycardia CL.

Slow-slow AVNRT is associated with an RP interval and P wave morphology similar to that during orthodromic AVRT using a posteroseptal AV BT. However, although both SVTs have the earliest atrial activation in the posteroseptal region, conduction time from that site to the HB region is significantly longer in AVNRT than in orthodromic AVRT, resulting in a significantly longer RP interval in V_1 and larger difference in the RP interval between V_1 and the inferior leads. Therefore, ΔRP interval (V_1 – III) longer than 20 milliseconds suggests slow-slow AVNRT with a sensitivity of 71%, specificity of 87%, and positive predictive value of 75%.

Effects of Bundle Branch Block. The presence of BBB during SVT is much more common in orthodromic AVRT than AVNRT or AT (90% of SVTs with sustained LBBB are orthodromic AVRTs). Two reasons have been proposed to explain why prolonged aberration occurs less commonly during AVNRT than orthodromic AVRT. First, the induction of AVNRT requires significant AVN delay, which makes the H_1-H_2 interval longer and makes aberration unlikely, whereas

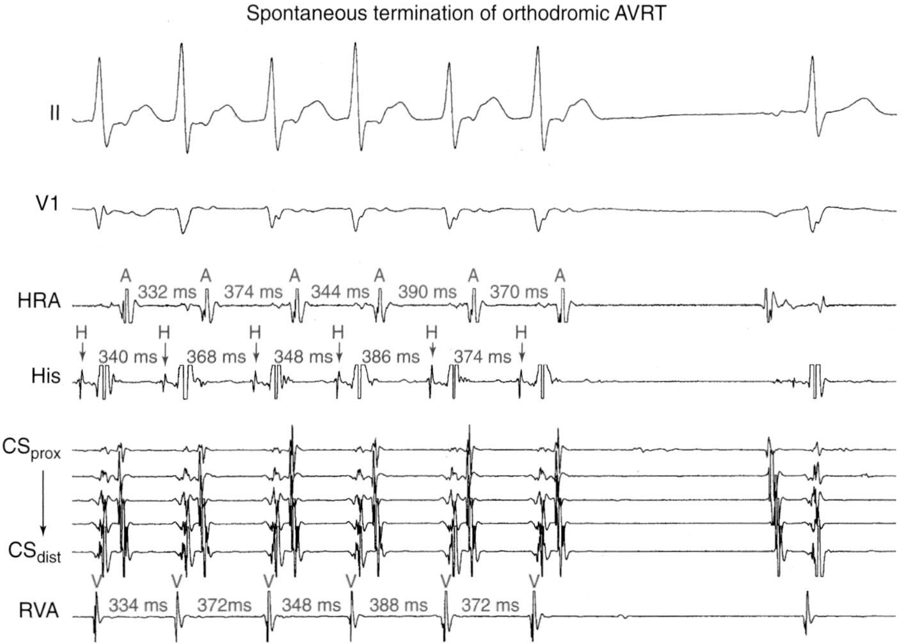

FIGURE 14–15 Spontaneous termination of an orthodromic atrioventricular reentrant tachycardia (AVRT) using a concealed superoparaseptal bypass tract. Note that the supraventricular tachycardia (SVT) terminates with an atrial complex not followed by a QRS, consistent with anterograde block in the atrioventricular node (AVN). Also, note the oscillation in the SVT cycle length (CL) preceding termination. Changes in H-H and V-V intervals precede the subsequent changes in A-A intervals, and the ventriculoatrial (VA) interval remains constant despite oscillation of the CL. This indicates that the variability in the tachycardia CL is secondary to changes in the anterograde conduction over the AVN, whereas VA conduction over the retrograde limb of the reentrant circuit (the BT) remains constant.

in orthodromic AVRT, AVN conduction need not be slow, resulting in a shorter AH interval and an impulse encroaching on HPS refractoriness, in turn resulting in BBB. Second, LBBB facilitates the induction of orthodromic AVRT when a left-sided AV BT is present.[35]

BBB is more common when an AES is delivered during NSR or after long-drive CLs, during which HPS refractoriness is longest and AVN conduction and refractoriness are shortest. During atrial stimulation, right bundle branch block (RBBB) is more common than LBBB (2 : 1). In contrast, during ventricular stimulation, LBBB is much more common than RBBB (because of concealment in the LB). The incidence of BBB is more common with ventricular stimulation than with atrial stimulation (75% versus 50%).

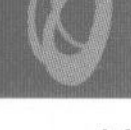

BBB ipsilateral to the AV BT results in prolongation of the surface VA interval because of more time is needed for the impulse to travel from the AVN down the HB and contralateral bundle branch, and transseptally to the ipsilateral ventricle to reach the AV BT and then activate the atrium (Fig. 14-16). However, the local VA interval, measured at the site of BT insertion, remains constant. The tachycardia CL usually increases in concordance with the increase in the surface VA interval as a result of ipsilateral BBB, because of the now-larger tachycardia circuit; however, because the time the wavefront spends outside the AVN is now longer, AVN conduction may improve, resulting in shortening in the AH interval (PR interval), which can be sufficient to overcome the prolongation of the VA interval. This can consequently result in shortening in the tachycardia CL. Thus, the surface VA interval and not the tachycardia CL should be used to assess the effects of BBB on the SVT (Fig. 14-17; see Fig. 14-6).

Prolongation of the surface VA interval during SVT in response to BBB by more than 35 milliseconds indicates ipsilateral free wall AV BT that is present and participating in the SVT (i.e., diagnostic of orthodromic AVRT). Prolongation of more than 25 milliseconds suggests a septal AV BT (posteroseptal AV BT in association of LBBB, and superoparaseptal AV BT in association of RBBB; see Fig. 14-17). Prolongation of the VA interval by more than 45 milliseconds in response to RV pacing entraining the orthodromic AVRT is also diagnostic of a left-sided BT (VA prolongation is secondary to LBBB created by RV pacing). On the other hand, BBB contralateral to the AV BT does not influence the VA interval or tachycardia CL (because the contralateral ventricle is not part of the reentrant circuit; see Figs. 14-14 and 14-16).

Oscillations in the Tachycardia Cycle Length. Analysis of the tachycardia CL variability can provide useful diagnostic information for discrimination among the different types of SVT, even when episodes of SVT are nonsustained. SVT CL variability of 15 milliseconds or more in magnitude occurs commonly in orthodromic AVRT, and generally is caused by changes in the anterograde conduction over the AVN (see Fig. 14-15). Because retrograde conduction through the BT is much less variable, the changes in ventricular CL that result from variability in the anterograde AVN conduction precede the subsequent changes in atrial CL, and changes in atrial CL do not predict changes in subsequent ventricular CL, as is the case during typical AVNRT. In contrast, changes in atrial CL predict the changes in subsequent ventricular CL during atypical AVNRT and AT.[36]

Additionally, orthodromic AVRT in the presence of dual AVN physiology can be associated with retrograde conduction alternating over the slow and fast BT, resulting in a regular irregularity of the tachycardia CL (alternating long and short cycles). Alternatively, the presence of dual AVN pathways can lead to two separate stable tachycardia CLs. In either case, the RP interval during the SVT will remain constant.

QRS Alternans. QRS alternans during relatively slow SVTs is almost always consistent with orthodromic AVRT. On the other hand, although QRS alternans during fast SVTs is most commonly seen in orthodromic AVRT, it can also be seen with other types of SVT.

FIGURE 14–16 Schematic illustration of the effect of bundle branch block (BBB) on the reentrant circuit during orthodromic atrioventricular reentrant tachycardia (AVRT) using a left-sided bypass tract (BT). Block in the left bundle branch (LB) (ipsilateral to the BT) results in prolongation of the reentrant pathway and, therefore, prolongation of the ventriculoatrial (VA) interval. In contrast, block in the right bundle branch (RB) (contralateral to the BT) has no effect on the reentrant circuit.

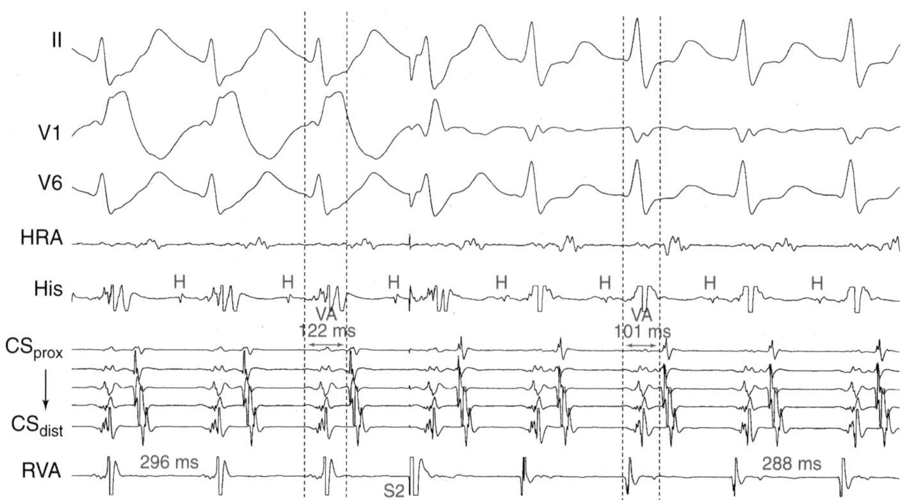

FIGURE 14–17 Effect of right bundle branch block (RBBB) on orthodromic atrioventricular reentrant tachycardia (AVRT). RBBB is initially present during an orthodromic AVRT using a concealed superoparaseptal bypass tract (BT). Introduction of a ventricular extrastimulus (VES [S2]) from the right ventricular (RV) apex during the tachycardia is followed by resolution of RBBB (peeling of refractoriness). Note that the loss of RBBB is associated with shortening of the ventriculoatrial (VA) interval (by 21 msec) and milder degree of shortening of the tachycardia cycle length (by 8 msec), indicating the presence and participation of a septal BT in the reentrant circuit.

Termination and Response to Physiological and Pharmacological Maneuvers. Spontaneous termination of AVRT is usually caused by gradual slowing and then block in the AVN (see Fig. 14-15), sometimes causing initial oscillation in the tachycardia CL, with alternate complexes demonstrating a Wenckebach periodicity before block. However, termination with block in the AV BT without any perturbations of the tachycardia CL can occur during very rapid AVRT or following a sudden shortening of the tachycardia CL.

Carotid sinus massage can terminate orthodromic AVRT by gradual slowing and then block in the AVN. Adenosine, digoxin, calcium channel blockers, and beta blockers terminate orthodromic AVRT by block in the AVN; therefore, the SVT terminates with a P wave not followed by a QRS. Verapamil rarely produces block in the AV BT and, when it does, block is usually preceded by oscillation in the tachycardia CL produced by changes in AVN conduction, leading to long-short sequences. Class IA and IC agents can produce block in the AV BT with variable effect on the AVN-HPS. Amiodarone can terminate AVRT by block in the AVN, HPS, or AV BT. Sotalol affects the AVN with little or no effect on the AV BT.

Orthodromic Atrioventricular Reentrant Tachycardia: Slowly Conducting Concealed Atrioventricular Bypass Tract (Permanent Junctional Reciprocating Tachycardia)

Atrial Activation Sequence. The initial site of atrial activation is most often in the posteroseptal part of the triangle of Koch near the CS os, similar to that in atypical AVNRT (Fig. 14-18).

Atrial-Ventricular Relationship. Because the retrograde limb of the reentry circuit is the slow BT (which is slower than the AVN), the RP interval is longer than the PR interval, similar to atypical AVNRT (see Figs. 14-7 and 14-18). In contrast to the classic fast BTs, the RP interval is not fixed, because this BT has decremental properties. Similar to all types of AVRT, a 1:1 A-V relationship is a prerequisite to sustenance of the tachycardia.

Oscillations in the Tachycardia Cycle Length. The tachycardia rate (100 to 220 beats/min) fluctuates in response to autonomic tone and physical activity, and the rate changes result from modulation of the PR and RP intervals. The tachycardia CL is often just longer than the shortest CL at which the BT can conduct retrogradely.

Effects of Bundle Branch Block. BBB affects PJRT in a manner analogous to that described for orthodromic AVRT.

Termination and Response to Physiological and Pharmacological Maneuvers. Carotid sinus massage and AVN blockers (adenosine, digoxin, calcium channel blockers, and beta blockers) usually terminate PJRT by block in the AVN (two thirds) or in the BT (one third) (see Fig. 14-12). Although the mode of tachycardia termination by adenosine has been suggested to distinguish between PJRT and atypical AVNRT, one report has shown that termination of atypical AVNRT with adenosine can also result from block in the fast AVN pathway and therefore its value in distinguishing between atypical AVNRT and PJRT is questionable.[37]

Antidromic Atrioventricular Reentrant Tachycardia

Atrial Activation Sequence. The initial site of atrial activation in classic antidromic AVRT is consistent with retrograde conduction over the AVN. If the antidromic AVRT is using a second BT for retrograde conduction, then atrial activation sequence will depend on the location of that BT (see Fig. 14-3). Additionally, ventricular activation precedes HB activation during classic antidromic AVRT. Therefore, a positive HV interval or a V-H interval of 10 milliseconds or less, especially when the HA interval is 50 milliseconds or less, favors preexcited AVNRT over antidromic AVRT.

Atrial-Ventricular Relationship. Conduction time over classic (fast) BTs is approximately 30 to 120 milliseconds. Therefore, the PR is short and fixed, regardless of oscillations in the tachycardia CL from whatever cause. Similar to all types of AVRT, the A/V ratio is always equal to 1. If the SVT persists in the presence of AV block, antidromic AVRT is excluded.

Oscillations in the Tachycardia Cycle Length. Antidromic AVRT can be irregular. Tachycardia CL changes are usually caused by changes in retrograde conduction over different fascicles of the HPS with different VA intervals (regardless of the type and degree of changes in the V-H or HA intervals), retrograde conduction over dual AVN pathways (with different HA intervals), different routes of anterograde conduction (with different AV intervals), and/or retrograde conduction over different BTs (with different VA intervals). When the change in the tachycardia CL can be ascribed to a change in the V-H interval and/or the subsequent HA interval, it suggests that retrograde conduction occurs over the HPS AVN and not over a second BT.

The tachycardia CL appears to be shorter during classic antidromic AVRT than orthodromic AVRT when they occur in the same patient. This may be explained by the fact that antidromic AVRT uses the fast AVN pathway (of a dual AVN physiology) retrogradely, whereas orthodromic AVRT uses the slow pathway anterogradely or, in the absence of dual AVN physiology, this may be merely supportive evidence that retrograde conduction during antidromic AVRT uses

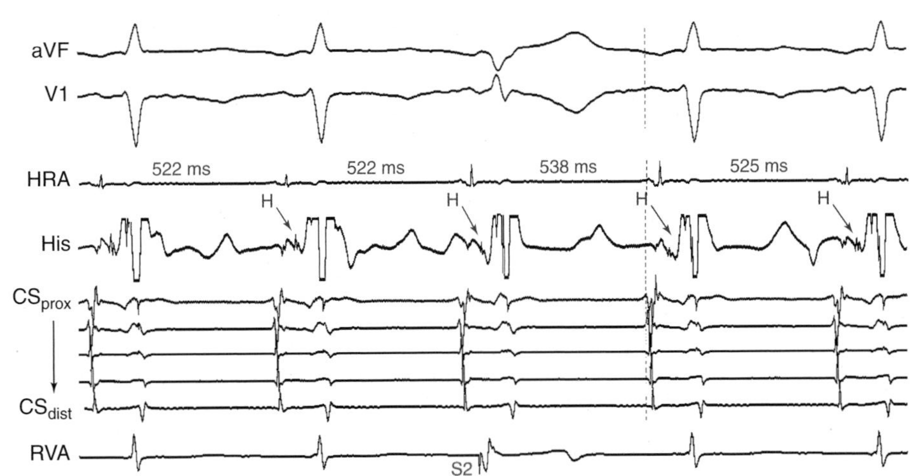

FIGURE 14–18 Ventricular extrastimulation (VES) during permanent junctional reciprocating tachycardia. The supraventricular tachycardia has a stable baseline cycle length (522 msec). A single ventricular extrastimulus (S2) is introduced during His bundle refractoriness and retards the timing of the next atrial complex (538 msec) (postexcitation). The anticipated timing of the high RA electrogram is indicated by the dashed line.

another BT instead of the slow AVN. On the other hand, antidromic AVRTs using two or more BTs tend to have longer tachycardia CLs than orthodromic AVRT or classic antidromic AVRT. This is because the two BTs are typically in opposite chambers and are incorporated in a larger reentrant circuit than one involving a midline AVN.[3]

Effects of Bundle Branch Block. Retrograde BBB affects antidromic AVRT in a manner analogous to that described for orthodromic AVRT.

Termination and Response to Physiological and Pharmacological Maneuvers. Various physiological and pharmacological maneuvers affect the AV BT and AVN during antidromic AVRT in a fashion similar to that described for orthodromic AVRT. Carotid sinus massage and adenosine terminate classic antidromic AVRT after ventricular activation, secondary to retrograde block up the AVN. In contrast, preexcited AVNRT terminates after atrial activation, secondary to anterograde block down the slow AVN pathway.

Termination or prolongation of the VA (and V-H) interval and tachycardia CL with transient RBBB, caused by mechanical trauma or introduction of VES, is diagnostic of antidromic AVRT using a right-sided or septal BT and excludes preexcited AVNRT. Continuation of an SVT at the same tachycardia CL, despite anterograde block in the BT (by drugs, mechanical trauma caused by catheter manipulation, or ablation), excludes antidromic AVRT.

Diagnostic Maneuvers During Tachycardia

Atrial Extrastimulation and Atrial Pacing During Supraventricular Tachycardia

Orthodromic Atrioventricular Reentrant Tachycardia. Atrial pacing at a CL slightly shorter than the tachycardia CL generally can produce entrainment of orthodromic AVRT (Fig. 14-19). If the P waves on the surface ECG can be seen, which usually is not the case, they may appear to be fusion beats resulting from the intraatrial collision of the impulse propagating from the paced site, with the impulse emerging from the BT. In general, when pacing is initiated orthodromically to the zone of slow conduction—the AVN in this case—the conduction time within the area of slow conduction is long enough to allow a wide atrial antidromic wavefront to generate surface ECG fusion (see Fig. 14-19).[38]

VA linking is observed after termination of entrainment during orthodromic AVRT. VA linking refers to a VA interval of the return cycle after cessation of atrial pacing that is fixed and similar to that of the SVT (with less than 10 milliseconds variation) after different attempts at SVT entrainment (see Fig. 14-19). This phenomenon occurs because retrograde VA conduction of the last entrained QRS is mediated by the BT, which is fixed and constant regardless of the duration or the CL of the entraining atrial pacing drive. VA linking can also be observed in typical AVNRT but not AT.[34,38]

It is difficult for AES not to affect the SVT because of the large size and large excitable gap of the reentrant circuit. However, this can be influenced by the distance between the site of atrial stimulation and that of the BT. Because only parts of the atrium ipsilateral to the BT are requisite components of the orthodromic AVRT circuit, AES delivered in the contralateral atrium may not affect the circuit.

AES over a wide range of coupling intervals can reset orthodromic AVRT via conduction down the AVN-HPS. In this case, atrial activation is a fusion of the AES and the SVT impulse traveling retrogradely up the AV-BT. The next QRS can be early or late, depending on the degree of slowing of conduction of the AES anterogradely down the AVN (i.e., the degree of prolongation of the A_2-H_2 interval).

An early-coupled AES can terminate the SVT, usually by block in the AVN-HPS. In this case, the SVT terminates with an AES not followed by a QRS (i.e., AV block). Alternatively, the AES can render the atrium refractory to the SVT impulse incoming up the AV BT, in which case the SVT terminates with an AES followed by a QRS (i.e., VA block). The AES can also anterogradely penetrate the AV BT and collide with the retrogradely conducting SVT wavefront (VA block). Lastly, the AES can conduct down the AVN-HPS and advance the next QRS, which then blocks in the still-refractory AV BT or atrium (VA block).[38]

Antidromic Atrioventricular Reentrant Tachycardia. AES is of value in distinguishing antidromic AVRT from preexcited AVNRT. A late-coupled AES, delivered close to the BT atrial insertion site during SVT when the AV junctional atrium is refractory (i.e., when the atrial electrogram is already manifest in the HB recording at the time of AES delivery) that advances the timing of both the next ventricular activation and the subsequent atrial activation, proves that the SVT is an antidromic AVRT using an AV BT anterogradely, and excludes preexcited AVNRT (Fig. 14-20A). Because the AV junctional atrium is refractory at the time of the AES, the AES cannot penetrate the AVN, and resetting of the SVT by such an AES is therefore incompatible with AVNRT.

Also, an AES delivered during the SVT that advances ventricular activation and does not influence the VA inter-

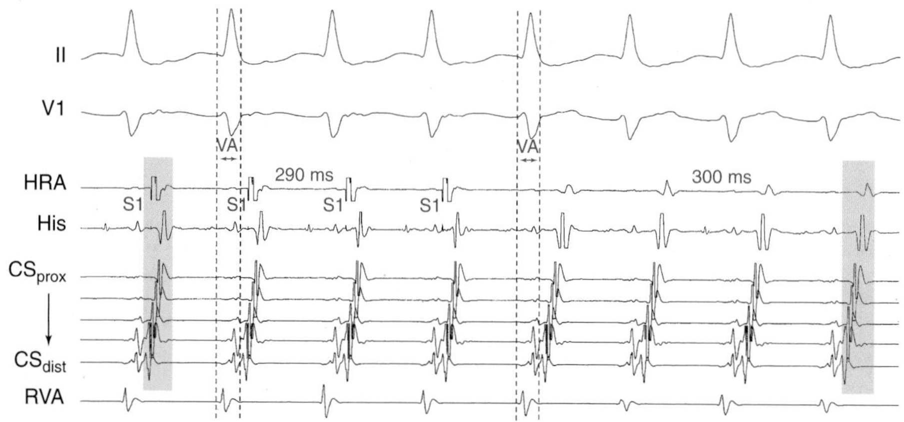

FIGURE 14–19 Atrial entrainment of an orthodromic atrioventricular reentrant tachycardia (AVRT) using a left lateral bypass tract (BT). Atrial fusion (between the paced and tachycardia wavefronts, compare shaded areas) is observed during entrainment, which is consistent with AVRT and excludes both focal atrial tachycardia (AT) and atrioventricular nodal reentrant tachycardia (AVNRT). Note that the ventriculoatrial (VA) interval (dashed lines) of the return cycle after cessation of atrial pacing is similar to that of the supraventricular tachycardia (V-A linking), because retrograde VA conduction of the last entrained QRS is mediated by the BT.

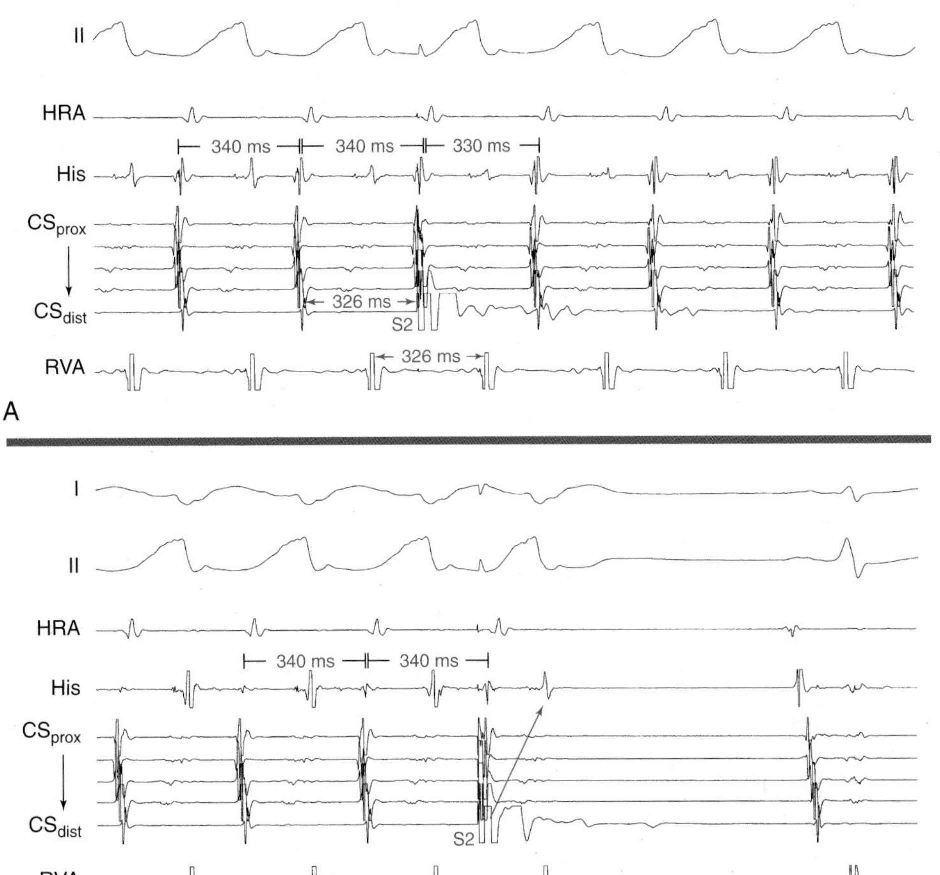

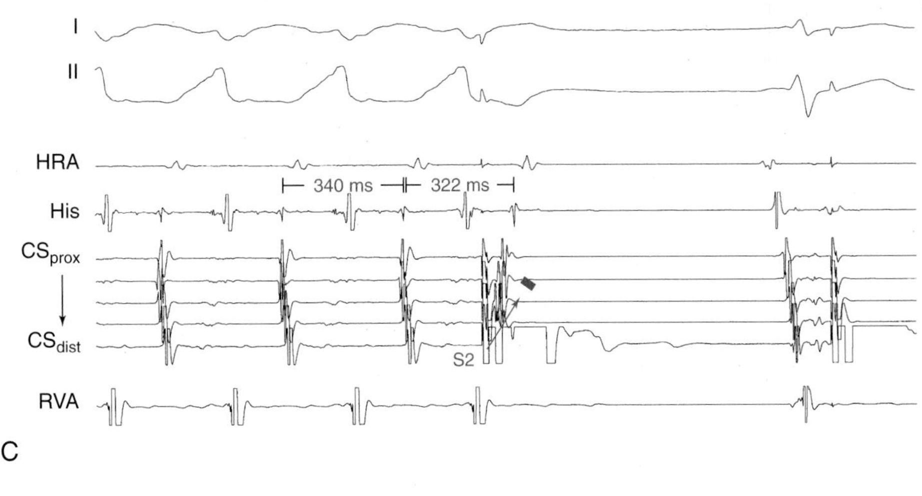

FIGURE 14–20 Atrial extrastimulation (AES) during antidromic atrioventricular reentrant tachycardia (AVRT) using a left lateral bypass tract (BT). **A,** A late-coupled AES delivered when the atrioventricular (AV) junction is refractory, as indicated by lack of advancement of the timing of the local atrial electrogram recording by the His bundle catheter, resets both the next ventricular activation and the subsequent atrial activation. This proves that the supraventricular tachycardia (SVT) is an antidromic AVRT using an AV BT anterogradely, and excludes preexcited atrioventricular nodal reentrant tachycardia (AVNRT). Additionally, the reset ventricular activation occurs at a coupling interval identical to the AES coupling interval (i.e., exact coupling phenomenon), and the ventriculoatrial (VA) interval following the AES remains similar to that during SVT, which is consistent with antidromic AVNRT. **B,** Late-coupled AES delivered when the AV junction is refractory advances the subsequent QRS and terminates the SVT by retrograde block in the His-Purkinje system–atrioventricular node. **C,** An earlier AES terminates the SVT without conduction to the ventricle (i.e., anterograde block in the BT). The AES advances the timing of AV junctional atrial activation.

val excludes preexcited AVNRT and is diagnostic of antidromic AVRT (see Fig. 14-20A). The VA interval should change in the case of preexcited AVNRT because the AES penetrates the AVN, producing slower conduction down the AVN before resumption of the tachycardia, which, in the presence of a fixed AV interval (caused by conduction down the BT) in response to the AES, would lead to a longer VA interval. In addition, the advanced QRS could invade and capture the HB retrogradely and conduct up the fast AVN pathway and reset the AVN. Then, the V-H interval of the advanced QRS plus the HA interval in response to this QRS should add up to the same VA interval on an undisturbed AVNRT, which is clearly unlikely.

Exact atrial and ventricular capture by an AES delivered when the AV junction is depolarized excludes AVNRT (see Fig. 14-20A). An AES that captures the ventricle at the same coupling interval as that of the AES indicates that the atrial stimulation site is inside the reentrant circuit, because if there were intervening atrial tissue involved, the AV interval would increase, and consequently, the V-V interval would exceed the AES coupling interval.[3]

The presence of a fixed and short V-H interval during entrainment of the SVT with atrial pacing suggests antidromic AVRT, and makes AVNRT unlikely (but does not exclude AVNRT). Moreover, failure of entrainment by atrial pacing to influence the VA interval during SVT excludes preexcited AVNRT. An early-coupled AES can terminate the SVT by retrograde block in the AVN-HPS (the SVT terminates with an AES followed by a QRS; i.e., VA block, Fig. 14-20B) or by anterograde block in the BT (the SVT terminates with an AES not followed by a QRS; i.e., AV block, Fig. 14-20C).

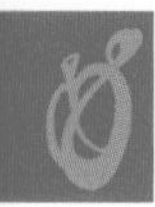

Ventricular Extrastimulation and Ventricular Pacing During Supraventricular Tachycardia

Orthodromic Atrioventricular Reentrant Tachycardia: Manifest or Concealed Atrioventricular Bypass Tract. VES and ventricular pacing can easily reset, entrain, and may terminate orthodromic AVRT (Fig. 14-21).[7,34,39] However, the ability of the VES to affect the SVT depends on the distance between the site of ventricular stimulation to the ventricular insertion site of the BT and on the VES coupling interval. Because only parts of the ventricle ipsilateral to the BT are requisite components of the orthodromic AVRT circuit, a VES delivered in the contralateral ventricle may not affect the circuit.

The preexcitation index analyzes the coupling interval of the VES (delivered from the RV) that resets orthodromic AVRT as a percentage of the tachycardia CL.[39] A relative preexcitation index (the ratio of the coupling interval to the tachycardia CL) of more than 90% of a VES that advances atrial activation during orthodromic AVRT suggests that the BT is close to the site of ventricular stimulation (i.e., RV or septal BT). An absolute preexcitation index (tachycardia CL minus VES coupling interval) of 75 milliseconds or more suggests a left free wall BT, an index of less than 45 milliseconds suggests a septal BT, and an index of 45 to 75 milliseconds is indeterminate.

Resetting and/or Entrainment with QRS Fusion. The relative proximity (conduction time) among the pacing site, site of entrance to a reentrant circuit, and site of exit from the circuit to the paced chamber are critical for the occurrence of fusion during resetting and/or entrainment. A requirement for the presence of fusion, independent of the pacing site, is spatial separation between the sites of entrance to and exit from the reentrant circuit. In orthodromic AVRT, the entrance and exit of the reentrant circuit (to and from ventricular tissue) are separated from each other, the entrance being from the HPS and the exit being at the ventricular insertion site of the BT. Therefore, pacing at a site closer to the BT ventricular insertion site (e.g., LV pacing in case of left free wall BTs, and RV pacing in case of right-sided or septal BTs) than the entrance of the reentrant circuit to ventricular tissue (HPS) would result in fusion of the QRS morphology between the baseline morphology during orthodromic AVRT and that of the fully paced QRS (Fig. 14-22). On the other hand, such phenomena cannot occur during AVNRT. During resetting or entrainment of AVNRT, the stimulated wavefront must conduct retrogradely through the HB to reach the AVN, so that there is no possibility for concomitant anterograde conduction from the AVN to the ventricle. Under such circumstances, the collision between the antidromic wavefront and the orthodromic wavefront from the preceding beat must occur in the AVN, where it is concealed, so that the QRS morphology is always that of a fully paced beat, and constant fusion during entrainment is almost impossible (unless a second connection exists between the atria and ventricles—i.e., an innocent bystander BT).[38]

Termination of orthodromic AVRT by VES can occur secondary to block of the VES retrogradely in the AV BT, conduction of the VES retrogradely over the AVN-HPS with or without conduction up the BT, or retrograde conduction of the VES up the BT and preexcitation of the atrium and subsequent anterograde block in the AVN-HPS (the most common mechanism) (see Fig. 14-21). Termination of SVT with a single VES strongly suggests orthodromic AVRT as the mechanism of SVT in three situations: a late-coupled VES (more than 80% of tachycardia CL), a tachycardia CL less than 300 milliseconds, and a VES delivered when the HB is refractory and associated with no atrial activation.

Maneuvers to Prove Presence of an Atrioventricular Bypass Tract. When VES or ventricular pacing results in eccentric atrial activation sequence, the presence of a BT is indicated. Similarly, a VES delivered when the HB is refractory (i.e., when the His potential is already manifest or within 35 to 55 milliseconds before the time of the expected His potential) that advances the next atrial activation is diagnostic of the presence of a retrogradely conducting BT. Such a VES has to conduct and advance atrial activation via an AV BT because the HPS-AVN is already refractory and cannot mediate retrograde conduction of the VES to the atrium (see Fig. 14-21). Although such an observation excludes AVNRT, it does not exclude AT or prove orthodromic AVRT, and the preexcited atrial activation can reset or even terminate an AT, whereby the AV BT is an innocent bystander. However, if this VES advances atrial activation with an activation sequence identical to that during the SVT, this suggests that the SVT is orthodromic AVRT and the AV BT is participating in the SVT, although it does not exclude the rare example of an AT originating at a site close to the atrial insertion site of a bystander AV-BT. Furthermore, a VES delivered when the HB is refractory may not affect the next atrial activation if the ventricular stimulation site is far from the BT. Conduction from the ventricular stimulation site to the BT, local ventricular refractoriness, and the tachycardia CL all determine the ability of a VES to reach the reentrant circuit before ventricular activation over the normal AVN-HPS.[7,34]

Maneuvers to Prove Presence and Participation of Atrioventricular Bypass Tract in the Supraventricular Tachycardia. One maneuver is a VES delivered when the HB is refractory that delays the next atrial activation. Although such a VES can advance atrial activation during AT through fast retrograde conduction over a bystander BT, it should not be able to delay an AT beat by conduction over the AV-BT. Such delay indicates that the VES was conducted with some delay over the AV BT and that the next atrial activation was dependent on this slower conduction; thus, the AV BT is participating in the SVT, proving orthodromic AVRT. Similarly, a VES delivered when the HB is refractory that terminates the SVT without atrial activation is diagnostic of AVRT. Furthermore, entrainment of the SVT by ventricular pacing that results in prolongation in the surface V-A interval indicates that the SVT is orthodromic AVRT mediated by an AV BT in the ventricle contralateral to the site of ventricular pacing; this is analogous to the influence of ipsilateral BBB on the VA interval during orthodromic AVRT (see Fig. 14-22). Exact and paradoxical capture phenomena are also diagnostic of AVRT. VES that captures the atrium at the same coupling interval as that of the VES (exact capture phenomenon) indicates that the ventricular stimulation site is inside the reentrant circuit, because if there were intervening tissue involved, the V-A interval would increase and, subsequently, the A-A interval would exceed the VES coupling interval. Similarly, a VES that captures the atrium at a shorter coupling interval than that

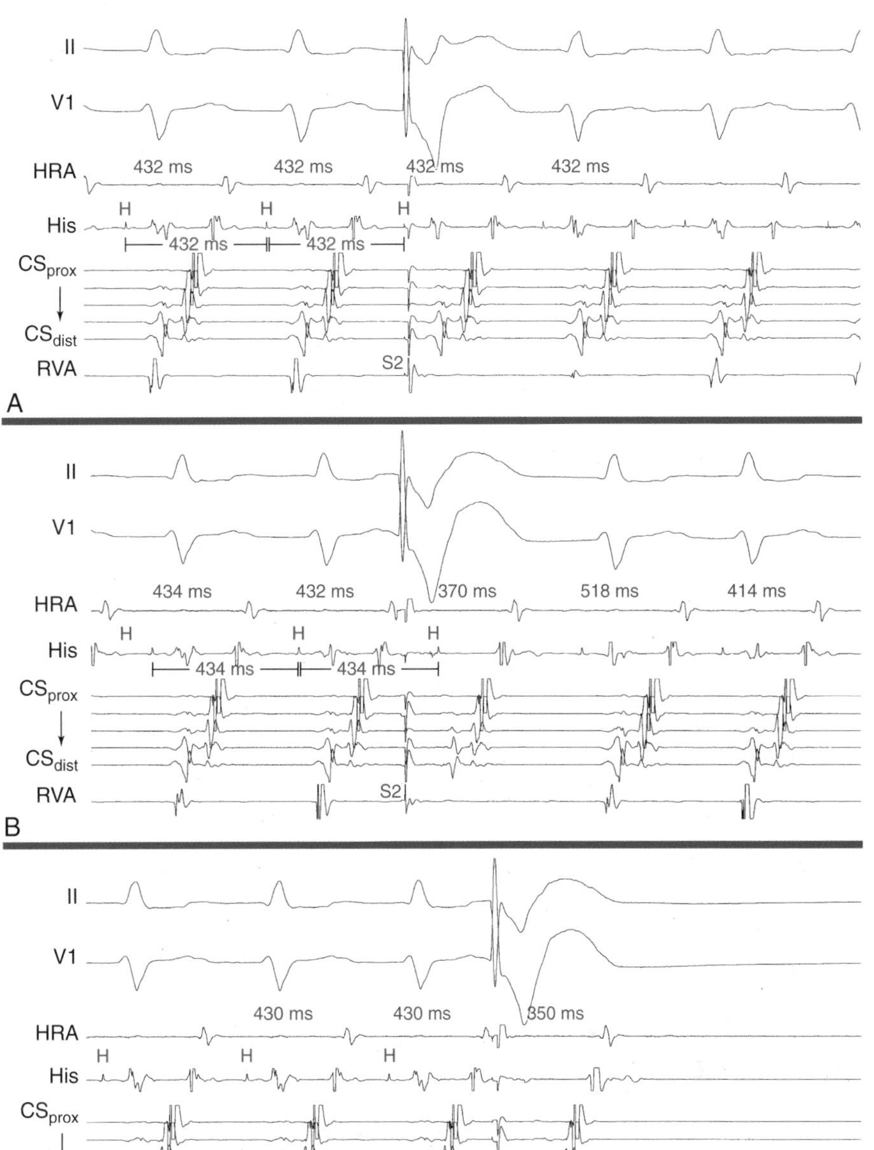

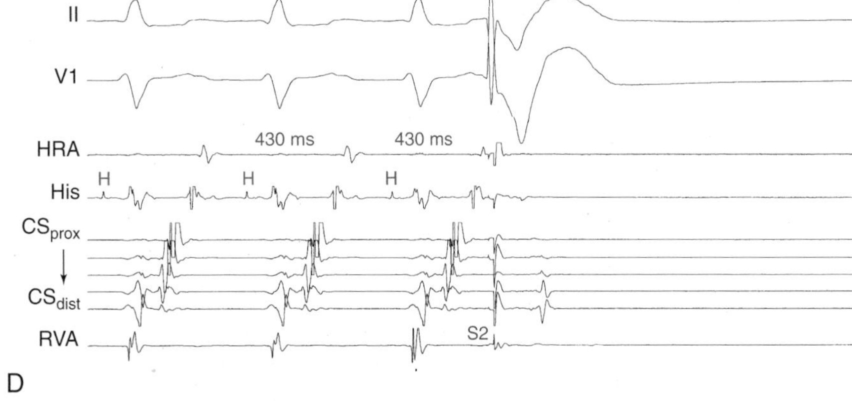

FIGURE 14–21 Ventricular extrastimulation (VES) during orthodromic atrioventricular reentrant tachycardia (AVRT) using a left lateral bypass tract (BT). **A,** A late-coupled VES delivered when the His bundle (HB) is refractory, as indicated by lack of advancement of the timing of the His potential, fails to reset the supraventricular tachycardia (SVT). **B,** An earlier VES fails to advance the timing of the HB but advances the subsequent atrial activation, indicating orthodromic AVRT and excluding atrioventricular nodal reentrant tachycardia (AVNRT). Note that the reset atrial impulse is followed by a prolonged atrial–His bundle (AH) interval caused by decremental anterograde conduction in the atrioventricular node (AVN). However, the local ventriculoatrial (VA) interval (retrograde BT conduction) remains constant. **C,** An earlier VES delivered before the HB is refractory resets the subsequent atrial activation and terminates the SVT by anterograde atrioventricular (AV) block in the AVN. **D,** A more premature VES terminates the SVT by retrograde VA block in the BT, excluding atrial tachycardia (AT), but can still occur in AVNRT because the VES is delivered before anterograde activation of the HB and could potentially penetrate the AVN.

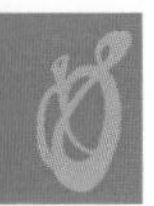

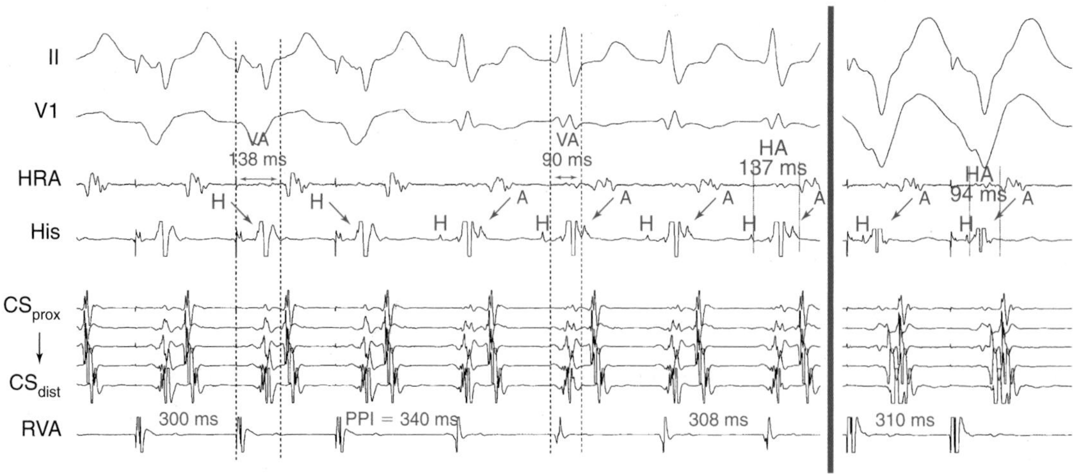

FIGURE 14–22 Ventricular entrainment of an orthodromic atrioventricular reentrant tachycardia (AVRT) using a concealed superoparaseptal bypass tract. Note that the ΔVA interval (ventriculoatrial interval during ventricular pacing minus VA interval during supraventricular tachycardia [SVT]) is <85 msec and the post-pacing interval minus SVT cycle length (CL) [PPI – SVT CL] is <115 msec, both of which favor orthodromic AVRT over atrioventricular nodal reentrant tachycardia (AVNRT). Additionally, ventricular fusion (between the paced and tachycardia wavefronts) is observed during entrainment (the right panel shows pure paced QRS morphology), which is consistent with AVRT and excludes AVNRT. Comparing the His bundle–atrial (HA) interval during the SVT (left panel) with that during ventricular pacing during normal sinus rhythm at the tachycardia CL (right panel) demonstrates that the ΔHA interval (HA interval during ventricular pacing minus HA interval during SVT) is −43 msec, which favors orthodromic AVRT over AVNRT; the HA interval is measured from the end of the His potential to the atrial electrogram in the high RA.

of the VES (paradoxical capture phenomenon) indicates that the ventricular stimulation site is not only inside the reentrant circuit but also closer to the ventricular insertion site of the AV BT than the initial site of ventricular activation over the AVN-HPS during the SVT, so that the V-A interval following the VES is shorter than that during the SVT. This is easier to demonstrate with RV apical pacing during orthodromic AVRT mediated by a right-sided BT.[3,7]

Entrainment of the Supraventricular Tachycardia by Right Ventricular Apical Pacing. This technique can help differentiate orthodromic AVRT from AVNRT. The VA interval during ventricular pacing is compared with that during SVT. The ventricle and atrium are activated in sequence during orthodromic AVRT and during ventricular pacing, whereas during AVNRT the ventricle and atrium are activated in parallel. Therefore, the VA interval during orthodromic AVRT approximates that during ventricular pacing. On the other hand, the VA interval during AVNRT is much shorter than that during ventricular pacing (see Fig. 14-22).[40,41] Therefore, when the ΔVA interval (VA interval during ventricular pacing minus VA interval during SVT) is more than 85 milliseconds, the SVT is AVNRT, and when the ΔVA interval is less than 85 milliseconds, the SVT is orthodromic AVRT. In addition, evaluation of the post-pacing interval (PPI) versus the tachycardia CL is of value. In AVNRT (typical or atypical), the PPI reflects the conduction time from the RV pacing site through the RV muscle and HPS, once around the reentry circuit and back. Therefore, the [PPI – tachycardia CL] represents twice the sum of the conduction time through the RV muscle and HPS. In orthodromic AVRT using a septal BT, the PPI reflects the conduction time through the RV to the septum, once around the reentry circuit and back. Therefore, the PPI more closely approximates the tachycardia CL in orthodromic AVRT using a septal BT compared with AVNRT (see Fig. 14-22). Therefore, when the [PPI – tachycardia CL] is more than 115 milliseconds, the SVT is AVNRT, and when [PPI – tachycardia CL] is less than 115 milliseconds, the SVT is orthodromic AVRT. For borderline values, ventricular pacing at the RV base can help exaggerate the difference between the PPI and tachycardia CL in the case of AVNRT, but without significant changes in the case of orthodromic AVRT, because the site of pacing at the RV base is farther from the AVNRT circuit than the RV apex, but is still close to an AVRT circuit using a septal BT (and in fact is closer to the ventricular insertion of the BT).[42] Another finding excluding AVNRT is entrainment with QRS fusion. As noted, entrainment with fusion can occur with orthodromic AVRT when the pacing site is relatively close to the BT, whereas with AVNRT entrainment with fusion cannot occur (see Fig. 14-22).[38]

Orthodromic Atrioventricular Reentrant Tachycardia: Slowly Conducting Concealed Atrioventricular Bypass Tract (Permanent Junctional Reciprocating Tachycardia). A VES delivered during PJRT can produce decremental conduction in the BT and prolongation of the VA interval, resulting in possible delay of the next atrial activation (i.e., postexcitation or delay of excitation; see Fig. 14-18). Such a response excludes AT, and when this occurs in response to a VES delivered when the HB is refractory, it is diagnostic of orthodromic AVRT, and excludes both AT and AVNRT. Additionally, a late-coupled VES introduced when the HB is refractory frequently blocks retrogradely in the BT and reproducibly terminates the tachycardia without reaching the atrium, again excluding both AT and AVNRT.

The ability to preexcite the atrium with a VES introduced when the HB is refractory is difficult to demonstrate in PJRT because of the long conduction time over the BT, the decremental conduction properties of the BT, and the fact that the tachycardia CL is just longer than the shortest length at which the BT is capable of retrograde conduction. This may be facilitated by introduction of the PVC at a site closer to the BT ventricular insertion.

Antidromic Atrioventricular Reentrant Tachycardia. Failure of entrainment by ventricular pacing to influence the surface VA interval during SVT excludes AVNRT. In addition, when a VES introduced during the SVT results in retrograde RBBB, such RBBB will not change the timing of the next atrial activation in the case of AVNRT. However, in antidromic AVRT using a right-sided BT, such RBBB will increase the size of the circuit, because the impulse cannot reach the HB through the RB and has to travel transseptally and then retrogradely over the LB. This results in prolongation in the VA interval and delay in the timing of the next atrial activation. The increment in the VA interval is caused by prolongation of the VH interval and, if RBBB persists, the SVT will have a long VH.

Antidromic AVRT usually can be terminated by ventricular pacing. Termination occurs by retrograde invasion and concealment in the BT, resulting in anterograde block over the BT following conduction to the atrium through the AVN.

Diagnostic Maneuvers During Normal Sinus Rhythm After Tachycardia Termination

Atrial Pacing at the Tachycardia Cycle Length

Atrial pacing at the tachycardia CL results in PR and AH intervals during atrial pacing comparable to those during orthodromic AVRT, as is the case during AT, but not during AVNRT.

Under comparable autonomic tone, 1:1 AV conduction over the AVN should be maintained during atrial pacing at the tachycardia CL. If AV block develops during atrial pacing, AT and orthodromic AVRT are less likely, and AVNRT is the likely mechanism of the SVT.

Ventricular Pacing at the Tachycardia Cycle Length

ΔHis Bundle-Atrial Interval. Ventricular pacing at the tachycardia CL results in HA and VA intervals that are shorter during ventricular pacing than during orthodromic AVRT, because the HB and atrium are activated sequentially during orthodromic AVRT but in parallel during ventricular pacing (see Fig. 14-22).[43] The HA interval is measured from the *end* of the His potential (where the impulse leaves the HB to enter the AVN) to the atrial electrogram in the high RA recording. When ΔHA interval (HA interval during ventricular pacing minus HA interval during SVT) is less than −10 milliseconds, the SVT is orthodromic AVRT; when ΔHA interval is more than −10 milliseconds, the SVT is AVNRT. This criterion has a 100% specificity and sensitivity and positive predictive accuracy for differentiation between AVNRT and orthodromic AVRT. The main limitation of the ΔHA interval criterion is the ability to record the retrograde His potential during ventricular pacing. The retrograde His potential generally appears before the local ventricular electrogram in the HB tracing, and can be verified by the introduction of a VES that causes the His potential to occur after the local ventricular electrogram. Moreover, pacing from different sites (e.g., midseptum) can allow earlier penetration into the HPS and facilitate observation of a retrograde His potential. Another limitation is that atrial activation during ventricular pacing may not occur over the BT in patients with orthodromic AVRT but proceed preferentially over HPS-AVN, leading to earlier atrial activation over this pathway than over the BT. If this were the case, the HA interval during ventricular pacing would be shorter than that observed if the atrium were activated via the BT. This would yield a more negative ΔHA interval. When the retrograde His potential is not visualized, using ΔVA interval instead of ΔHA interval is not as accurate in discriminating orthodromic AVRT from AVNRT.

Under comparable autonomic tone status, 1:1 VA conduction over the AVN should be maintained during ventricular pacing at the tachycardia CL. If VA block develops during ventricular pacing, orthodromic AVRT is unlikely, and AT and AVNRT are favored.

It is important to recognize that atrial activation sequence during ventricular pacing can be mediated by retrograde conduction over the BT, over the AVN, or a fusion of both, and consequently it can be similar or different from that during orthodromic AVRT.

Para-Hisian Pacing During Normal Sinus Rhythm

Technique. Ideally, two quadripolar catheters (one for pacing and one for recording) or a single octapolar catheter (for both pacing and recording) are placed at the distal HB-RB region. Alternatively, a single quadripolar HB catheter (which is typically used during a diagnostic EP study) is used, taking into account that such an approach would limit the ability to record the retrograde His potential and HA interval.[44]

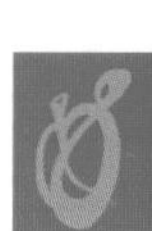

Overdrive ventricular pacing is performed (from the pair of electrodes on the HB catheter which records activation of the distal HB-RB) at a long pacing CL (more than 500 milliseconds) and high output. During pacing, direct HB-RB capture is indicated by shortening of the width of the paced QRS complex. The pacing output and pulse width are then decreased until the paced QRS widens, which is associated with a delay in the timing of the retrograde HB potential, indicating loss of HB-RB capture. The pacing output is increased and decreased to gain and lose HB-RB capture, respectively, while local ventricular capture is maintained. Occasionally, the HB can be captured uniquely (without myocardial capture), resulting in a QRS identical to the patient's normally conducted QRS.[44]

Concept of Para-Hisian Pacing. The para-Hisian pacing site is unique because it is anatomically close but electrically distant from the HB. Para-Hisian pacing at high output simultaneously captures the HB or proximal RB, as well as the adjacent ventricular myocardium. At lower output, direct HB-RB capture is lost and retrograde activation of the HB is delayed because the HB and RB are insulated from the adjacent myocardium and the peripheral inputs to the Purkinje system are located far from the para-Hisian pacing site. By maintaining local ventricular capture while intermittently losing HB-RB capture, retrograde VA conduction can be classified as dependent on the timing of local ventricular activation (BT), HB activation (AVN), or both (fusion).

Para-Hisian pacing can result in capture of the ventricle (indicated by a wide paced QRS), the atrium (indicated by atrial activation in the pacing lead immediately following the pacing artifact), the HB (indicated by narrow paced QRS), or any combination of these (Fig. 14-23).[44] Careful attention must be given to minimize the atrial signal seen on the recording from the pacing electrode pair to ensure that local atrial capture does not occur during pacing.

Response to Para-Hisian Pacing. When the ventricle and HB are captured simultaneously, the wavefront travels down the HPS and results in a relatively narrow, normal-looking QRS. The wavefront can also travel retrogradely over the AVN to activate the atrium with an S-A interval (i.e., the interval from the pacing stimulus to the atrial electrogram) that represents conduction time over the proximal part of the HB and AVN (i.e., S-A interval = HA interval) because the onset of ventricular activation occurs simultaneously to that of HB activation (i.e., S-H interval = 0).

When the ventricle is captured but not the atrium or HB, the wavefront travels through the ventricle by muscle to muscle conduction, resulting in a wide QRS with LBBB morphology caused by pacing in the RV. Once the wavefront reaches the RV apex, it conducts retrogradely up the RB and then over the HB and AVN to activate the atrium. In this case, the S-A interval represents the conduction time from the RV base to the HB (S-H interval) plus the conduction time over the HB and AVN (HA interval). Thus, normally, para-Hisian pacing results in a shorter S-A interval when the HB (or HB + RV) is captured than the S-A interval when

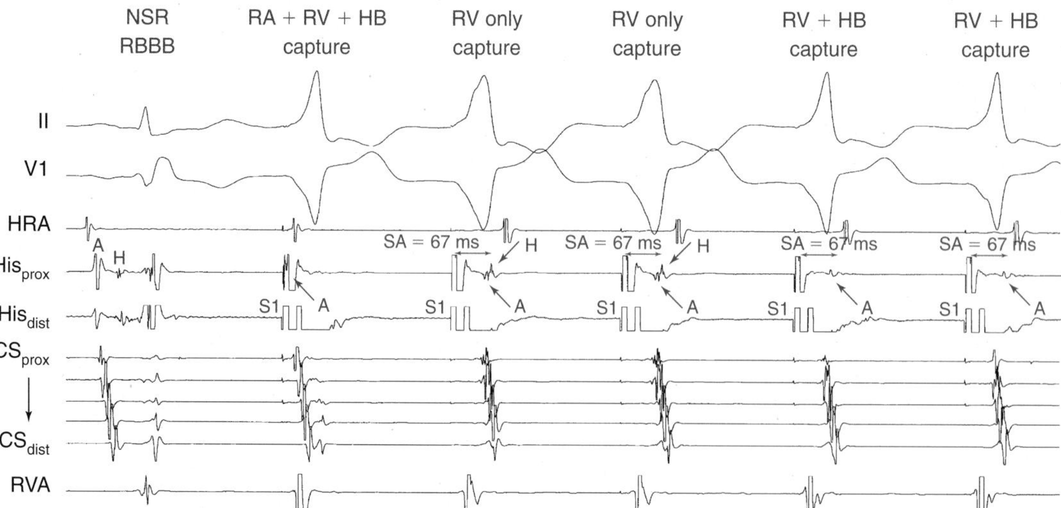

FIGURE 14–23 Para-Hisian pacing in a patient with concealed midseptal bypass tract and right bundle branch block (RBBB). The first complex is a sinus beat with RBBB. The second complex shows capture of the atrium, ventricle, and His bundle–right bundle branch (HB-RB). Atrial capture is indicated by immediate inscription of atrial electrogram following the pacing artifact. It is important to identify this occurrence to avoid erroneous interpretation of the results of para-Hisian pacing. The third and fourth complexes show right ventricle (RV)-only capture, and the last two complexes show RV and HB-RB capture but without atrial capture. Note that the atrial activation sequence and stimulus-atrial (SA) intervals remain unchanged, regardless of whether HB-RB capture occurs because retrograde ventriculoatrial (VA) conduction occurs over the bypass tract in either case. During RV-only capture, the HB activation occurs after atrial activation, indicating that ventriculoatrial (VA) conduction is independent of the atrioventricular node (AVN). Note that para-Hisian pacing could be performed successfully even in the presence of RBBB if capture of the HB-RB is achieved proximal to the site of block. NSR = normal sinus rhythm.

only the ventricle is captured (because of the delayed conduction of the impulse to the HB [i.e., S-H interval] when only the ventricle is captured).

In the presence of a septal AV-BT, the S-A interval usually remains fixed regardless of whether or not the HB is being captured, because in both cases the impulse travels retrogradely over the AV BT, with constant conduction time to the atrium as long as local ventricular myocardium is being captured. Atrial activation in this case can be secondary to activation over the BT, especially when only the ventricle is captured, or a result of fusion of conduction over both the AV BT and AVN, especially when both the ventricle and the HB are captured.

Seven patterns of response to para-Hisian pacing can be observed (Table 14-3, Fig. 14-24; see Fig. 14-23). In patients in whom retrograde conduction occurs over both the AVN and BT during para-Hisian pacing, the amount of atria activated by each of the two pathways (atrial fusion) is dependent on four variables: (1) the magnitude of the delay in retrograde activation of the HB (i.e., S-H interval); (2) the retrograde conduction time over the AVN (H-A interval during HB-RB capture); (3) the intraventricular conduction time from the para-Hisian pacing site to the ventricular end of the BT (S-V_{BT}); and (4) the retrograde conduction time over the BT (V-A_{BT}). The first two variables (S-H plus H-A) form the S-A interval resulting from retrograde conduction time over the AVN, and the latter two variables (S-V_{BT} plus V-A_{BT}) form the retrograde VA conduction time over the BT. The amount of the atria activated by the AVN is greater during HB-RB capture, secondary to a minimal S-H interval. Loss of HB-RB capture results in prolongation of the S-H interval and, therefore, an increase in the amount of atria activated by the BT, resulting in a change in the retrograde atrial activation sequence. Consequently, a change in the retrograde atrial activation sequence with loss of HB-RB capture always indicates the presence of retrograde conduction over both the BT and AVN. There are four such patterns (patterns 4 through 7). In patterns 4 and 5, HB-RB capture is associated with activation of the atria exclusively by retrograde conduction over the AVN. In patterns 6 and 7, HB-RB capture results in atrial activation over both the AVN and the BT.[44]

Interpretation of Results of Para-Hisian Pacing. The response to para-Hisian pacing can be determined by comparing the following four variables between HB-RB capture and noncapture while maintaining local ventricular capture and no atrial capture: (1) atrial activation sequence, (2) S-A interval, (3) local VA interval, and (4) HA interval (see Figs. 14-23 and 14-24).

The S-A interval is defined as the interval between the pacing stimulus and atrial electrogram. It should be recorded at multiple sites, including close to the site of earliest atrial activation during SVT.

The local VA interval is defined as the local ventricular to atrial electrogram interval in the electrode position with the earliest retrograde atrial activation time. For the local VA to be relied on, it actually has to be measured at the site of earliest atrial activation (this requires positioning a catheter at the site of earliest atrial activation recorded during SVT). The high RA catheter, for example, may not be satisfactory for evaluation of the local VA interval in the presence of a septal BT.

The HA interval is recorded in the HB electrogram; however, this measurement can be obtained only if two catheters are placed in the HB position (one for pacing and one for recording) or if an octapolar catheter is used for pacing and sensing around the HB. The use of a single quadripolar HB catheter, which is typically used during a diagnostic EP study, negates the ability to record the retrograde His potential and HA interval during pacing. However, the combination of the S-A and local VA intervals is sufficient to identify the presence of retrograde BT.

If the S-A (and local VA) interval at any site remains fixed, regardless of whether or not HB-RB capture occurs, while the HA interval shortens on loss of HB-RB capture, retrograde conduction is occurring only over an AV-BT. On the other hand, if the S-A (and local VA) interval increases in all electrograms (including the electrode recording the

TABLE 14–3 Response Patterns to Para-Hisian Pacing

Pattern 1 (AVN/AVN Pattern) Retrograde conduction occurs exclusively over the AVN regardless of whether the HB-RB is captured. Loss of HB-RB capture results in an increase in the S-A interval in all electrograms equal to the increase in the S-H interval, with no change in the atrial activation sequence. The HA interval remains essentially the same. This response indicates that retrograde conduction is dependent on HB activation and not on local ventricular activation. This pattern is observed in all patients with AVNRT and is not observed in any patient with a septal or right free wall BT. However, this pattern can be observed in some patients with a left free wall BT or PJRT, in which case retrograde AVN conduction masks the presence of retrograde BT conduction.	**Pattern 4 (AVN-BT Pattern)** Loss of HB-RB capture is associated with atrial activation exclusively over the BT. Loss of HB-RB capture results in an increase in S-A and local VA intervals in all electrograms, with the least increase occurring in the electrogram closest to the BT. The HA interval shortens, indicating that the atrium near the AVN is activated by the BT before retrograde conduction over the AVN is complete. **Pattern 5 (AVN–Fusion Pattern)** Loss of HB-RB capture results in activation of part of the atria by the AVN and part by the BT. Loss of HB-RB capture is associated with an increase in S-A and local VA intervals in all electrograms. The HA interval remains constant, indicating that part of the atria was still activated by the AVN.
Pattern 2 (BT-BT Pattern) Retrograde conduction occurs exclusively over a single BT. The S-A interval is identical during HB-RB capture and noncapture, indicating that retrograde conduction is dependent on local ventricular activation and not on HB activation. This pattern does not exclude the presence of retrograde conduction over the AVN with longer conduction time or a second BT with longer conduction time or located far from the pacing site.	**Pattern 6 (Fusion-BT Pattern)** Loss of HB-RB capture results in atrial activation exclusively over the BT. Loss of HB-RB capture is associated with no change in the S-A or local VA intervals recorded near the BT. In the HB electrogram, the S-A interval increases, but not as much as the S-H interval, leading to a decrease in the H-A interval. This indicates that the atrial myocardium in that region is no longer activated by the AVN.
Pattern 3 (BT-BT_L Pattern) Retrograde conduction occurs exclusively over a BT. Loss of HB-RB capture is associated with a delay in the timing of ventricular activation close to the BT. This results in an increase in the S-A interval in all electrograms, with no change in the atrial activation sequence. The local VA interval, recorded close to the BT, remains approximately the same. The increase in S-A interval is less than the increase in the S-H interval. Therefore, the HA interval is shortened with loss of HB-RB capture, indicating that retrograde conduction cannot be occurring over the AVN. Two mechanisms have been identified accounting for the delay in timing of ventricular activation close to the BT. Activation of the HPS results in earlier ventricular activation near some BTs located far from the para-Hisian pacing site, such as left lateral or anterolateral BTs. Decreasing the pacing output to lose HB-RB capture occasionally results in a small delay in ventricular activation close to the pacing site. Pattern 3 is referred to as the BT-BT_L pattern, where BT_L refers to a lengthening of the S-A interval with loss of HB-RB capture.	**Pattern 7 (Fusion-Fusion Pattern)** The atria continue to be activated by both the AVN and the BT during loss of HB-RB capture, with more of the atria activated by the BT than during HB-RB capture. Like pattern 6, loss of HB-RB capture is associated with minimal change in the S-A or local VA intervals recorded close to the BT; however, the HA interval remains essentially the same, indicating that part of the atria is still activated by the AVN.

AVN = atrioventricular node; AVNRT = atrioventricular nodal reentrant tachycardia; BT = bypass tract; HA = His bundle–atrial; HB-RB = His bundle–right bundle branch; HPS = His-Purkinje system; PJRT = permanent junctional reciprocating tachycardia; S-A = stimulus-atrial; S-H = stimulus–His bundle; VA = ventriculoatrial.

earliest atrial activation) coincident with loss of HB-RB capture, while the HA interval remains essentially the same, retrograde conduction is occurring only over the AVN.

An identical retrograde atrial activation sequence during HB-RB capture and noncapture indicates that retrograde conduction is occurring over the same system (either the BT or AVN) and does not help prove or exclude the presence of a BT (especially a septal BT; see Fig. 14-24). A change in retrograde atrial activation sequence with loss of HB-RB capture, however, indicates the presence of retrograde conduction over both a BT and the AVN. Morphological change in the atrial electrogram recorded at the AV junction without overlapping the ventricular electrogram also seems to have diagnostic significance, indicating the presence of both BT and AVN conduction.

Limitations of Para-Hisian Pacing. The location of the BT, as well as the retrograde conduction time over the BT, must be taken into account when interpreting the results of para-Hisian pacing. For superoparaseptal BTs, the S-V_{BT} interval is short. For BTs located progressively farther from the para-Hisian pacing site, the S-V_{BT} increases progressively. This is not a significant factor for midseptal, posteroseptal, or most right free wall BTs. However, for left free wall BTs, which are located far from the pacing site, the S-V_{BT} interval can be sufficiently long to have the entire atria activated by the AVN, even during loss of HB-RB capture. In this case, para-Hisian pacing can produce an AVN retrograde conduction pattern, regardless of whether or not the HB-RB is captured (pattern 1: AVN-AVN), failing to identify the presence of retrograde BT conduction (because of the long S-V_{BT}). However, a left lateral BT should not be a diagnostic challenge because of the obvious eccentric retrograde atrial activation sequence during orthodromic AVRT, and para-Hisian pacing is performed mainly to prove the presence of a septal BT. Additionally, for BTs located far from the para-Hisian pacing site, it is important to record atrial activation close to the suspected site of the BT. Otherwise, without recording electrograms near the BT, the change in atrial activation sequence may not be identified, incorrectly suggesting that retrograde conduction is occurring over just the AVN. This is most likely to occur in patients with short retrograde AVN conduction (short HA interval) and a BT located far from the pacing site.

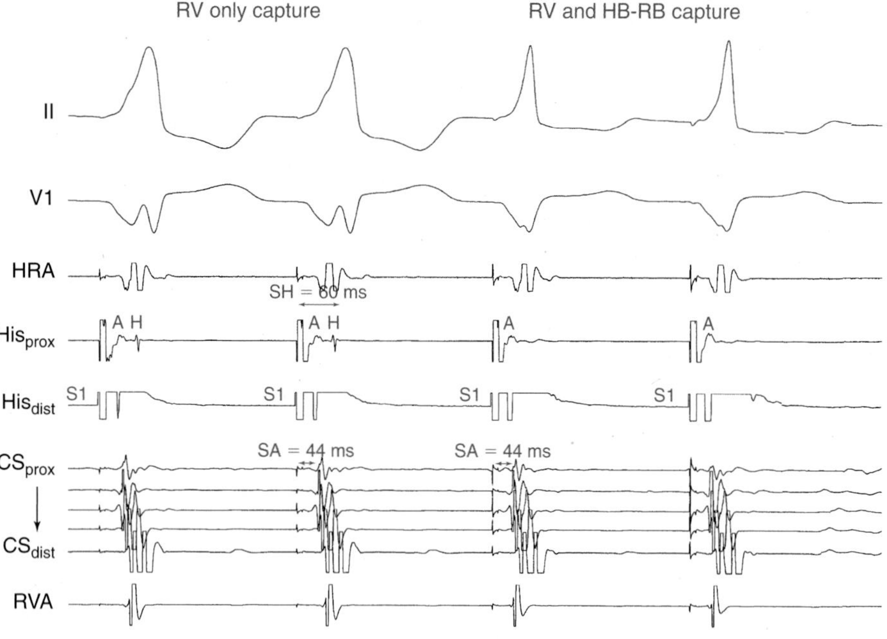

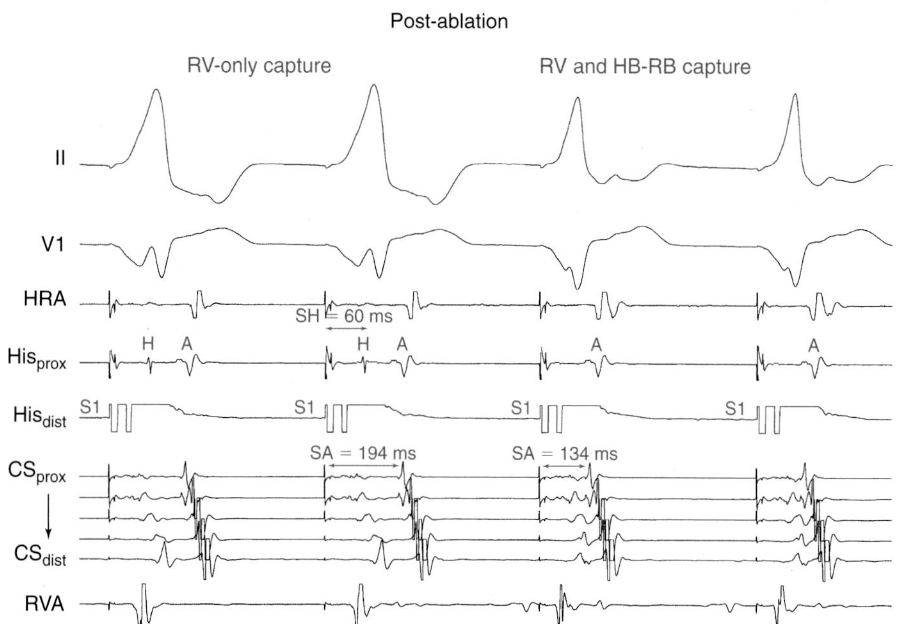

14

FIGURE 14–24 Para-Hisian pacing in a patient with concealed superoparaseptal bypass tract (BT). In each panel, the first two complexes show right ventricle (RV)-only capture, and the last two complexes show RV and His bundle–right bundle branch (HB-RB) capture. The loss of HB-RB capture is identified by delay in the HB activation (S-H interval = 60 msec) and widening of the QRS. The His potential is not visible during HB-RB capture. **Upper panel,** Para-Hisian pacing is performed before ablation of the BT, and the S-A interval remains unchanged regardless of whether HB-RB capture occurs, because retrograde ventriculoatrial (VA) conduction occurs over the BT in either case. In fact, during RV-only capture, the S-A interval is shorter than the S-H interval, indicating that VA conduction is independent of the atrioventricular node (AVN). **Lower panel,** Para-Hisian pacing is performed after successful ablation of the BT; the S-A interval is longer than before ablation, and it prolongs further on loss of HB-RB capture, concomitant with delay in HB activation (i.e., prolongation in the S-H interval) and a constant HA interval, indicating that VA conduction is mediated only by the AVN. Note that the activation sequence before ablation (VA conduction occurring over the BT) is slightly different from after ablation (VA conduction occurring over the AVN). However, in each case, atrial activation sequence occurs over the same pathway and remains constant, regardless of whether HB-RB occurs.

Para-Hisian pacing may fail to identify retrograde conduction over a slowly conducting BT (e.g., PJRT) because of the long $V\text{-}A_{BT}$ interval. Performing para-Hisian entrainment or resetting during SVT can help in these situations (see later). Additionally, although para-Hisian pacing during NSR can help prove the presence of an AV-BT, it does not show whether that BT is operative during the SVT.

In patients with very proximal retrograde RBBB, RB capture may fail to produce early retrograde activation of the HB, limiting the use of para-Hisian pacing in these patients. This observation suggests that HB-RB capture actually represents capture of the proximal RB and not HB capture. This is supported by the observation that, during HB-RB capture, the HB potential is often recorded 10 to 20 milliseconds after the pacing stimulus. Importantly, para-Hisian pacing has been performed successfully in many patients with more distal RBBB (see Fig. 14-23).

Assurance of lack of atrial capture by the pacing stimulus is important to interpret the results of para-Hisian pacing. Atrial capture is indicated by a very short S-A interval in the pacing lead recording.

Para-Hisian Pacing During Supraventricular Tachycardia (Para-Hisian Entrainment or Resetting)

Technique. Entrainment of the tachycardia is performed by pacing at the para-Hisian region using the HB catheter, as described earlier, at a pacing CL 10 to 30 milliseconds shorter than the tachycardia CL. Entrainment is confirmed when the atrial CL accelerates to the pacing CL, without a change in the atrial activation sequence, and the tachycardia continues after pacing is discontinued.[45]

Para-Hisian entrainment is performed by alternately pacing at high-energy output for HB-RB capture or lower energy output for HB-RB noncapture. Entrainment with HB-RB capture is recorded separately from that without HB-RB capture. The S-A and local VA intervals during HB-RB capture and noncapture are then examined.[45]

One must be cautious about performing the para-Hisian entrainment maneuver by simply decreasing the pacing energy output during the same run to achieve HB-RB noncapture. That is, even though the SVT may have been entrained during HB-RB capture, on loss of HB-RB capture, the initial paced complexes typically do not entrain the SVT. This initial failure of entrainment occurs because of the sudden increase in the distance from the pacing site to the actual reentrant circuit. During HB-RB capture of AVNRT, the pacing site is near the circuit (the HB-RB); however, the pacing site (the basal RV myocardium) is well outside the circuit during HB-RB noncapture. This limitation would not apply if HB-RB noncapture is performed *prior* to HB-RB capture. That is, if the pacing output is increased while the SVT is being entrained during HB-RB noncapture, the circuit almost certainly will be entrained on HB-RB capture (unless the SVT terminates).

If para-Hisian entrainment cannot be performed because of repetitive termination of the tachycardia during entrainment attempts, isoproterenol infusion may be used to help sustain the rhythm. Alternatively, single or double VESs can be given to reset the tachycardia (para-Hisian resetting). These VESs are delivered at progressively shorter coupling intervals until the first VES that reliably advances or resets the tachycardia. This is performed alternately with high- or low-energy outputs to achieve HB-RB capture and noncapture, respectively. As with para-Hisian entrainment, the retrograde atrial activation sequence pattern and timing are compared during para-Hisian resetting to characterize the response.

Interpretation of Results of Para-Hisian Entrainment or Resetting. In AVNRT (typical or atypical), the AVN-AVN pattern is observed in response to para-Hisian entrainment/resetting. Both the S-A and the local VA intervals increase during HB-RB noncapture compared with HB-RB capture.[45]

In orthodromic AVRT, the BT-BT pattern or $BT\text{-}BT_L$ pattern is observed. In the case of BT-a BT pattern, the S-A and local VA intervals are usually not significantly different between HB-RB capture and noncapture. Conversely, in the case of a $BT\text{-}BT_L$ pattern, the S-A interval increases on HB-RB noncapture, but without significant change in the local VA interval.[45]

A ΔS-A interval of less than 40 milliseconds was found to be a reasonable guide to separating the AVN-AVN from the BT-BT response; patients with AVNRT uniformly have a ΔS-A interval of more than 40 milliseconds, and only rare patients with AVRT (with a left lateral BT) have a ΔS-A interval less than 40 milliseconds. However, the Δ local VA interval is a more accurate parameter.

An AVN-AVN or fusion pattern during para-Hisian entrainment or resetting has not been observed in patients with AVNRT, a potential advantage over para-Hisian pacing during NSR in identifying the presence of a BT. Because retrograde VA conduction can only proceed over a single route during entrainment of the SVT (assuming that a complex scenario such as multiple BTs is not present), the various forms of retrograde fusion that might be seen during para-Hisian pacing during NSR cannot occur during para-Hisian entrainment or resetting.[45]

Differential Right Ventricular Pacing

The response to differential-site RV pacing can be evaluated by comparing the VA interval and atrial activation sequence during pacing at the RV base versus the RV apex (Fig. 14-25). The RV apex, although anatomically more distant from the atrium than the RV base, is nonetheless electrically closer because of the proximity of the distal RB to the pacing site. Consequently, in the absence of a retrogradely conducting septal AV-BT, pacing at the RV apex allows entry into the rapidly conducting HPS and results in a shorter stimulus to atrial (S-A) interval during pacing from the apex than from the base. Pacing from the RV base requires the paced wavefront to travel a longer distance by muscle to muscle conduction to reach the RV apex and then propagate retrogradely through the RB and HB. In other words, the VH interval is shorter with pacing at the RV apex versus the RV base. In the presence of a septal AV-BT, pacing at the RV base allows the wavefront to access the AV BT rapidly and activate the atrium with a shorter S-A interval than during pacing at the RV apex, which is distant from the AV BT (i.e., because the V-BT interval is shorter with pacing at the RV base versus the RV apex).

In the absence of a retrogradely conducting AV-BT, the atrial activation sequence will be similar during pacing both at the RV apex and the RV base because the atrium is activated over the AVN in both cases. On the other hand, if a septal AV BT is present, atrial activation proceeds over the AV BT during pacing at the RV base, and over either the AVN, AV BT, or both during pacing at the RV apex. Therefore, a variable retrograde atrial activation sequence in response to differential RV pacing (RV base versus RV apex) is indicative of the presence of an AV BT, but a constant atrial activation sequence is not helpful in excluding the presence of an AV BT.

This maneuver, however, does not exclude the presence of a distant right or left free wall AV BT, because the site of pacing is far from the AV BT and atrial activation results from conduction over the AVN in either case (RV apical or RV basilar pacing), and neither does it exclude a slowly conducting BT. The VA interval criterion identifies the actual route of VA conduction and therefore the fastest path of this conduction. Consequently, a slowly conducting BT would be missed in the presence of fast VA conduction over the HPS-AVN.

Conflicting results can also occur if conduction occurs simultaneously over a BT and HPS-AVN or, alternatively, over these two routes, depending on the pacing site. To help in these settings, calculation of the VA interval should be performed at several pacing CLs (the VA index should be independent of the pacing rate and, consequently, different values of the index at different rates would suggest more than one conducting path), after verapamil infusion (which would block the AVN and allow preferential VA conduction over the BT, if one is present), or during entrainment of the SVT (which would then ensure that VA conduction is occurring over the same path as that during the SVT).

The occurrence of RBBB (but not LBBB) also can alter the significance of the VA interval criterion, especially when VA conduction proceeds over the HPS-AVN. In the presence of retrograde RBBB, VA conduction occurs over the LB-HB; therefore, the VA interval depends on the distance between the pacing site and the LB rather than the RB, and access of the paced wavefront to the LB can be faster for RV basilar or septal pacing compared with pacing from the RV apex (see Fig. 13-17).

Exclusion of Other Arrhythmia Mechanisms

AVNRT and AT arising near the AV groove can mimic orthodromic AVRT and, in the presence of a manifest BT, those tachycardias can be associated with ventricular preexcitation mimicking antidromic AVRT, whereby the BT is functioning as an innocent bystander. Therefore, EP testing is required, not just to identify the presence of a BT, but also to define its role in any clinical or inducible arrhythmia. Tables 14-4 and 14-5 summarize the EP findings indicative

Pre-ablation

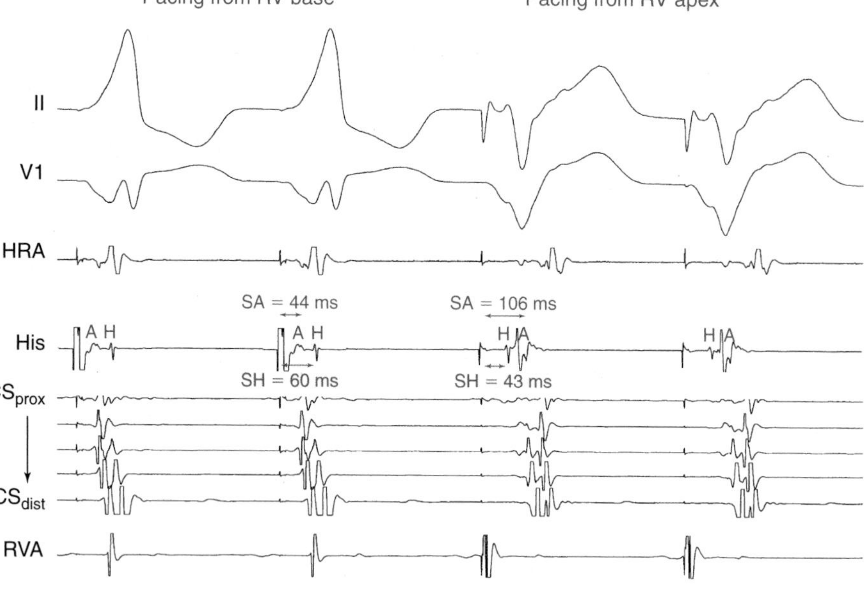

Post-ablation

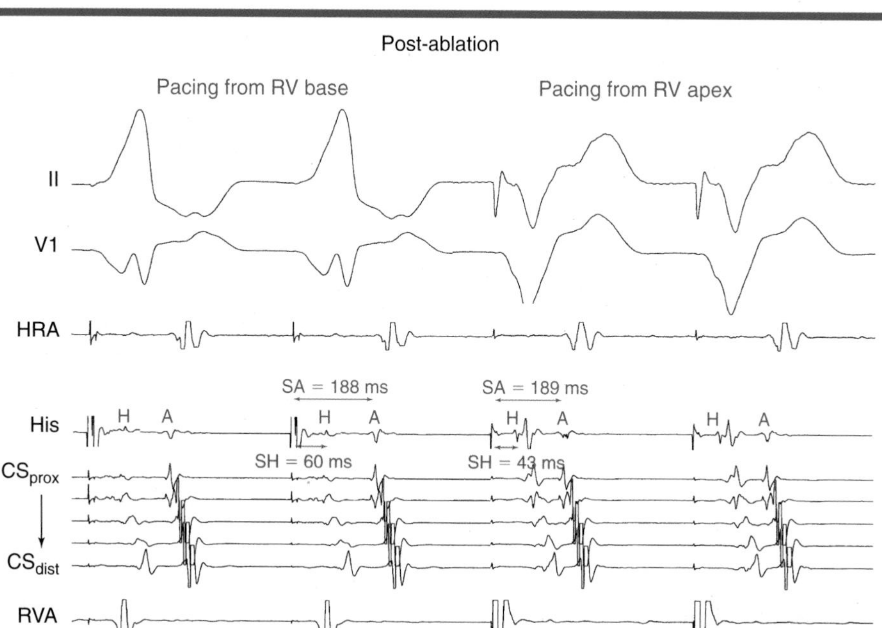

FIGURE 14–25 Differential-site right ventricular (RV) pacing in a patient with concealed superoparaseptal bypass tract (BT). In each panel, the first two complexes show RV basal-septal pacing, and the last two complexes show RV apical pacing. **Upper panel,** RV pacing is performed before ablation of the BT. The S-A (ventriculoatrial [VA]) interval is shorter during pacing at the RV base than during pacing at the RV apex, suggesting VA conduction occurring over a BT. Note that atrial activation occurs even before His bundle (HB) activation during pacing from the RV base, suggesting that VA conduction is independent of the AVN. **Lower panel,** RV pacing is performed after successful ablation of the BT. During pacing from the RV apex, the S-A interval is longer than before ablation, and it prolongs further by pacing at the RV base, consistent with the occurrence of VA conduction exclusively over the AVN. Note that in both panels the S-H (VH) interval during RV apical pacing is shorter than that during RV basilar pacing because of the faster access of the paced wavefront to the right bundle branch–His bundle (RB-HB) during pacing at the RV apex. However, when VA conduction occurs over a BT (upper panel), the S-A interval remains constant; in contrast, in the absence of a BT (lower panel), the S-A interval shortens, coinciding with shortening of the S-H interval during pacing at the RV apex compared with pacing at the RV base.

TABLE 14–4	Electrophysiological Findings Indicating Presence of Retrograde Atrioventricular Bypass Tract Function

Eccentric atrial activation sequence during ventricular pacing
RV apical pacing producing longer VA interval and/or different atrial activation sequence compared with that during RV basilar pacing
Para-Hisian pacing producing similar VA interval with and without HB capture or producing different atrial activation sequence depending on whether the HB is captured
VES delivered when the HB is refractory advances the next atrial activation during SVT

HB = His bundle; RV = right ventricle; SVT = supraventricular tachycardia; VA = ventriculoatrial; VES = ventricular extrastimulus.

TABLE 14–5	Electrophysiological FIndings Indicating Presence and Participation of Atrioventricular Bypass Tract in Supraventricular Tachycardia

VES delivered during SVT when the HB is refractory terminates the SVT without atrial activation.
VES delivered during SVT when the HB is refractory delays the next atrial activation.
VES during SVT captures the atrium at the same coupling interval as that of the VES (exact capture phenomenon).
VES delivered during SVT captures the atrium at a shorter coupling interval than that of the VES (paradoxic capture phenomenon).
Prolongation of VA interval (with or without concomitant prolongation in tachycardia CL) during the SVT secondary to the development of BBB.
Entrainment of the SVT by ventricular pacing results in prolongation of the VA interval ($VA_{ventricular\ pacing} > VA_{SVT}$).

BBB = bundle branch block; CL = cycle length; HB = His bundle; SVT = supraventricular tachycardia; VA = ventriculoatrial; VES = ventricular extrastimulus.

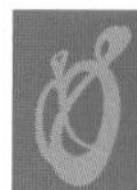

TABLE 14–6 Exclusion of Atrial Tachycardia (AT)

Effects of BBB
If surface VA interval prolongs (with or without tachycardia CL prolongation) on development of BBB, AT is excluded.
Spontaneous Oscillations of Tachycardia CL
Spontaneous changes in tachycardia CL accompanied by constant VA interval excludes AT.
VES Delivered During SVT
VES that terminates the SVT without atrial activation excludes AT. VES that delays next atrial activation excludes AT. VES during SVT that captures the atrium at the same coupling interval as that of the VES (exact capture phenomenon) excludes AT. VES delivered during SVT that captures the atrium at a shorter coupling interval than that of the VES (paradoxic capture phenomenon) excludes AT.
Entrainment of SVT by Atrial Pacing
If the VA interval of the return cycle after cessation of atrial overdrive pacing during SVT is fixed and similar to that of the SVT (with <10-msec variation) after different attempts at SVT entrainment ("V-A linking"), AT is unlikely.
Entrainment of SVT by Ventricular Pacing
If atrial activation sequence during ventricular entrainment is similar to that during the SVT, AT is less likely. Presence of A-V electrogram sequence at cessation of ventricular pacing excludes AT. Ventricular fusion during entrainment indicates AVRT and excludes AT.
Ventricular Pacing During NSR at Tachycardia CL
If retrograde atrial activation sequence during ventricular pacing is similar to that during SVT, AT is less likely.

BBB = bundle branch block; CL = cycle length; NSR = normal sinus rhythm; SVT = supraventricular tachycardia; VA = ventriculoatrial; VES = ventricular extrastimulus.

of the presence of a BT and its potential participation in an inducible SVT. Exclusion of the other SVT mechanisms is necessary, because the mere presence of a BT is not adequate to make a diagnosis and a treatment strategy (Tables 14-6, 14-7, and 14-8).

Furthermore, the presence of multiple BTs is not infrequent, and careful EP testing is required to evaluate this possibility. Several clinical and EP findings are indicative of the presence of multiple BTs (Table 14-9, Fig. 14-26; see Fig. 14-3). However, despite these various methods, many BTs are not identified until after catheter ablation of the first BT. Failure to detect the presence of multiple BTs during EP testing has been reported in as many as 5% to 15% of patients. This may be explained by the fact that changes in the preexcitation pattern can be subtle in shifting from one BT to another. Furthermore, one BT may preferentially conduct during atrial pacing or participate in preexcited tachycardias and another BT can be responsible for the retrograde limb during orthodromic AVRT or ventricular pacing. Additionally, there may be fusion of BT conduction, anterograde or retrograde. Repetitive concealed conduction into the BT during AVRT also may preclude identification of that BT before ablation of the first BT.

LOCALIZATION OF THE BYPASS TRACT

Pacing from Multiple Atrial Sites. The closer the pacing site to the BT atrial insertion, the more rapidly the impulse will reach the BT relative to the AVN and thus the greater the degree of preexcitation and the shorter the P-delta interval. This method is especially helpful when the BT cannot conduct retrogradely, prohibiting localization with atrial mapping during SVT or ventricular pacing.

TABLE 14–7 Exclusion of Atrioventricular Nodal Reentrant Tachycardia (AVNRT)

Atrial Activation Sequence
Eccentric atrial activation sequence during the SVT excludes AVNRT (with rare exceptions of left-sided insertion of fast or slow AVN pathways).
Effects of BBB
If VA interval or tachycardia CL prolongs on development of BBB, AVNRT is excluded.
Spontaneous Oscillations of Tachycardia CL
Spontaneous changes in tachycardia CL accompanied by constant VA interval make AVNRT unlikely.
VES Delivered During SVT
VES delivered during SVT when the HB is refractory that resets or terminates the SVT excludes AVNRT. VES during SVT that captures the atrium at the same coupling interval as that of the VES (exact capture phenomenon) excludes AVNRT. VES delivered during SVT that captures the atrium at a shorter coupling interval than that of the VES (paradoxic capture phenomenon) excludes AVNRT.
Entrainment of SVT by Atrial Pacing
$AH_{atrial\ pacing} - AH_{SVT} < 20$ msec excludes AVNRT.
Entrainment of SVT by Ventricular Pacing
$VA_{ventricular\ pacing} - VA_{SVT} < 85$ msec excludes AVNRT. PPI – tachycardia CL < 115 msec excludes AVNRT. Ventricular fusion during entrainment indicates AVRT and excludes AVNRT.
Atrial Pacing During NSR at Tachycardia CL
$AH_{atrial\ pacing} - AH_{SVT} < 20$ msec excludes AVNRT.
Ventricular Pacing During NSR at Tachycardia CL
$HA_{ventricular\ pacing} - HA_{SVT} < -10$ msec, the SVT excludes AVNRT.
Differential RV Pacing
If atrial activation sequence changes during pacing at the RV apex vs. pacing at the RV base, AVNRT is less likely.
Para-Hisian Pacing
Para-Hisian pacing producing similar VA interval, regardless of whether HB capture occurs, and/or different atrial activation sequence, depending on whether HB capture occurs, makes AVNRT unlikely.

AH = atrial-His bundle; BBB = bundle branch block; CL = cycle length; HA = His bundle–atrial interval; HB = His bundle; NSR = normal sinus rhythm; PPI = post-pacing interval; SVT = supraventricular tachycardia; VA = ventriculoatrial; VES = ventricular extrastimulus.

Preexcitation Index. As noted, the preexcitation index analyzes the coupling interval of the VES (delivered from the RV) that resets orthodromic AVRT as a percentage of the tachycardia CL.[39] A relative preexcitation index (the ratio of coupling interval to the tachycardia CL) of more than 90% of a VES that advances atrial activation during orthodromic AVRT suggests that the BT is close to the site of ventricular stimulation (i.e., RV or septal BT). An absolute preexcitation index (tachycardia CL minus VES coupling interval) of 75 milliseconds or more suggests a left free wall BT, an index of less than 45 milliseconds suggests a septal BT, and an index of 45 to 75 milliseconds is indeterminate.

Effects of Bundle Branch Block During Orthodromic Atrioventricular Reentrant Tachycardia. Prolongation of the tachycardia CL and, more importantly, the surface VA interval by more than 35 milliseconds following the development of BBB is diagnostic of AVRT using a free wall BT ipsilateral to the BBB (LBBB with left-sided BT, and RBBB with right-sided BT).[34,35] Superoparaseptal and posteroseptal BTs are associated with a lesser degree of prolongation of the VA interval (approximately 5 to 25 milliseconds)

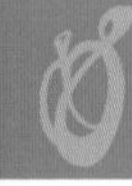

14

TABLE 14–8 Differentiation Between Antidromic AVRT and Preexcited AVNRT

SVT Features

HA_{SVT} < 70 msec excludes antidromic AVRT.
Positive HV or VH interval ≤ 10 msec (especially when HA interval is ≤50 msec) suggests AVNRT.

Termination of SVT

Continuation of the SVT at the same tachycardia CL, despite anterograde block in the BT (by drugs, mechanical trauma, or ablation), is diagnostic of AVNRT and excludes antidromic AVRT.
Block of the BT by drugs and subsequent induction of narrow-complex SVT with the same tachycardia CL, HA interval, and retrograde atrial activation sequence as that of the preexcited SVT induced before the BT block is diagnostic of preexcited AVNRT and excludes antidromic AVRT.
Termination of SVT in response to carotid sinus massage or adenosine:
AVNRT terminates after atrial activation (secondary to anterograde block down the slow pathway).
Classic antidromic AVRT terminates after ventricular activation (secondary to retrograde block up the AVN).

Effects of BBB

If VA interval or tachycardia CL prolongs on development of BBB, AVNRT is excluded.

SVT Induction with Ventricular Stimulation

Induction of the SVT by ventricular pacing at a pacing CL similar to the tachycardia CL or by a VES that advances the timing of the His potential by a coupling interval (i.e., H_1-H_2 interval) similar to the H-H during the SVT, the HA interval following such a VES is compared with that during the SVT:
$HA_{VES\ or\ ventricular\ pacing} > HA_{SVT}$ is diagnostic of AVNRT and excludes antidromic AVRT.
$HA_{VES\ or\ ventricular\ pacing} \leq HA_{SVT}$ is diagnostic of antidromic AVRT and excludes AVNRT.

AES Delivered During SVT

Late-coupled AES is delivered close to the BT atrial insertion site during SVT when the AV junctional atrium is refractory. If it advances the timing of both the next ventricular activation and the subsequent atrial activation, it proves that the SVT is antidromic AVRT using an AV BT anterogradely, and excludes preexcited AVNRT.
AES during the SVT that advances ventricular activation and does not affect VA interval excludes AVNRT and is diagnostic of antidromic AVRT.
Exact atrial and ventricular capture by AES delivered when the AV junction is depolarized excludes AVNRT.

Entrainment of SVT by Atrial Pacing

Failure of entrainment by atrial pacing to influence the VA interval during SVT excludes AVNRT.
The presence of a fixed short VH interval during entrainment of the SVT with atrial pacing suggests antidromic AVRT, and makes AVNRT unlikely (but does not exclude AVNRT).

Entrainment of SVT by Ventricular Pacing

Failure of entrainment by ventricular pacing to influence the VA interval during SVT excludes AVNRT.

Ventricular Pacing During NSR at the Tachycardia CL

Pacing at the RV apex at tachycardia CL is performed and the HA interval during RV pacing vs. HA interval during SVT are compared. (It is important to verify that VA conduction occurred only over the AVN and not over the BT for this analysis to be valid).
$HA_{ventricular\ pacing} > HA_{SVT}$ is diagnostic of AVNRT and excludes antidromic AVRT.
$HA_{ventricular\ pacing} \leq HA_{SVT}$ is diagnostic of antidromic AVRT and excludes AVNRT.
If VA block develops during RV apical pacing, antidromic AVRT is excluded.

A = atrium; AES = atrial extrastimulus; AVNRT = atrioventricular nodal reentrant tachycardia; AVRT = atrioventricular reentrant tachycardia; BBB = bundle branch block; BT = bypass tract; CL = cycle length; HA = His bundle-atrial; HV = His bundle-ventricular; NSR = normal sinus rhythm; RV = right ventricle; SVT = supraventricular tachycardia; VA = ventriculoatrial; VES = ventricular extrastimulus; VH = ventricular-His bundle.

TABLE 14–9 Electrophysiological Findings Indicating Presence of Multiple Atrioventricular Bypass Tracts

During Preexcited Rhythms (NSR, PACs, Spontaneous or Induced AF, RA and LA Pacing)

Changing anterograde delta wave (i.e., variations in preexcited QRS morphology). Atrial pacing from different sites (high RA and CS) may accentuate preexcitation over one BT and not the other, help unmask the changes in the delta wave
Atypical pattern of preexcitation (i.e., does not conform to an expected QRS morphology for a given location)
Changing anterograde delta wave following antiarrhythmic agents (e.g., amiodarone or class I agents) that may block one BT and not the other or following ablation of one BT

During Ventricular Pacing at Different CLs and from Multiple Pacing Sites

Evidence of multiple routes of retrograde atrial activation:
Changing P wave morphology or atrial activation sequence
Multiple atrial breakthrough sites
Changing VA interval
Evidence of mismatch of site of anterograde preexcitation and site of retrograde atrial activation observed during ventricular pacing

During Orthodromic AVRT

Evidence of multiple routes of retrograde atrial activation:
Changing P wave morphology or atrial activation sequence
Multiple atrial breakthrough sites
Changing VA interval
Failure to delay atrial activation at all sites with the development of BBB ipsilateral to the BT
Evidence of multiple routes of anterograde ventricular activation:
Intermittent anterograde fusion (preexcited) complexes
Evidence of mismatch of site of anterograde preexcitation and site of retrograde atrial activation observed during orthodromic AVRT

During Antidromic AVRT

Eccentric atrial activation sequence
Varying degrees of anterograde fusion
Changing VH interval without any change in the tachycardia CL or atrial activation sequence (suggesting that the HPS is not part of the reentrant circuit)
Tachycardia CL during antidromic AVRT slower than orthodromic AVRT in the same patient (in absence of dual AVN pathways)
Anterograde ventricular activation over posteroseptal BT
The mere presence of antidromic AVRT

AF = atrial fibrillation; AVN = atrioventricular node; AVRT = atrioventricular reentrant tachycardia; BBB = bundle branch block; BT = bypass tract; CL = cycle length; CS = coronary sinus; HPS = His-Purkinje system; LA = left atrium; NSR = normal sinus rhythm; PAC = premature atrial complex; RA = right atrium; VA = ventriculoatrial.

on the development of BBB (RBBB with superoparaseptal BT, and LBBB with posteroseptal BT). In an analogous fashion, entrainment of the SVT by ventricular pacing that results in prolongation in the VA interval ($VA_{ventricular\ pacing} > VA_{SVT}$) suggests that the SVT is orthodromic AVRT mediated by an AV BT in the ventricle contralateral to the site of ventricular pacing.

Earliest Ventricular Activation Site During Preexcitation. The earliest site of ventricular activation (preceding the onset of the delta wave) during mapping along the tricuspid and mitral annuli identifies the BT ventricular insertion site. Both bipolar and unipolar recordings on the ablation catheter should be used for mapping (Fig. 14-27). Bipolar electrograms display electrogram components and BT potentials. Unfiltered unipolar electrograms can accurately reflect local ventricular activation (QS complex with an initial steep negative component represents the BT insertion site). In addition, the use of unipolar signals provides directional information and is also important to demonstrate that the distal electrode, which is used

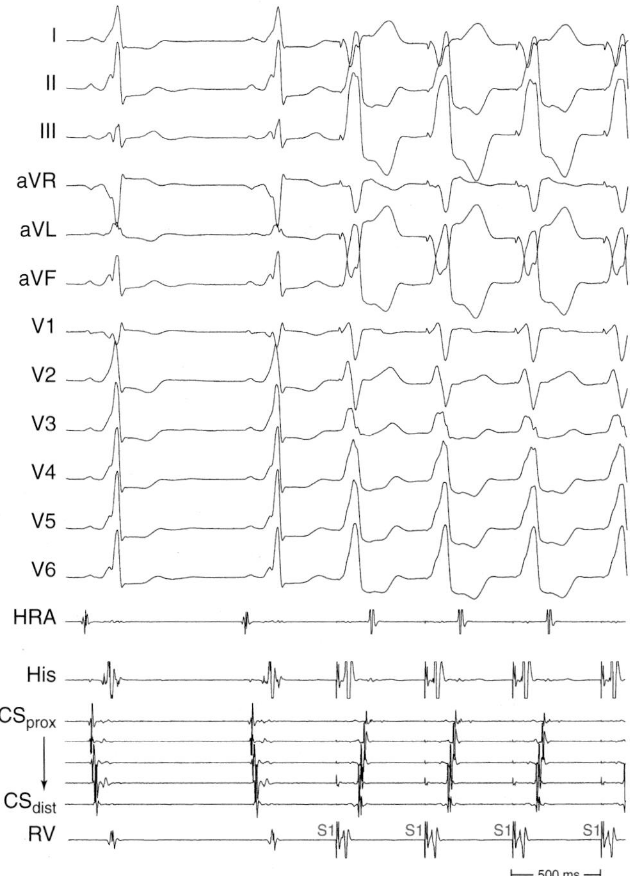

FIGURE 14–26 The presence of multiple bypass tracts (BTs) is indicated by the mismatch of sites of anterograde preexcitation during normal sinus rhythm (the delta wave morphology is consistent with anterograde conduction over a right anterior BT) and site of retrograde atrial activation observed during ventricular pacing (the atrial activation sequence is consistent with VA conduction over a left lateral BT).

for RF delivery, is actually the electrode recording the earliest activity. If only bipolar recordings are used, one does not know which of the two poles is responsible for the earliest component of the bipolar electrogram.[8,46]

The surface ECG lead with the earliest onset of the delta wave, preferably with a relatively sharp delineation of its onset, should be picked. This should always be used as the timing reference when comparing one mapping site with another.

Earliest Atrial Activation Site During Retrograde Bypass Tract Conduction. The site of earliest atrial activation during mapping along the tricuspid and mitral annuli during ventricular pacing or orthodromic AVRT identifies the BT atrial insertion site. When mapping is performed during ventricular pacing, fusion of atrial activation, caused by simultaneous retrograde conduction over both the AVN and the BT, has to be considered, because it can affect the accuracy of mapping. This can be an issue in the case of septal BTs whereby the retrograde atrial activation sequence over the BT may not be very different from that over the AVN. Dissociation of retrograde conduction over the BT from that over the AVN is required in these situations, and can usually be achieved with ventricular stimulation from sites closer to the BT and with the use of AVN blockers (e.g., adenosine) to ensure preferential retrograde conduction over the BT.[3] As with ventricular mapping, both bipolar and unipolar recordings on the distal ablation electrode should be used for atrial mapping (Fig. 14-28).[46]

Mapping Atrial Electrogram Polarity Reversal. The morphology and amplitude of the bipolar electrograms are influenced by the orientation of the bipolar recording axis to the direction of propagation of the activation wavefront. Although the direction of wavefront propagation cannot be reliably inferred from the morphology of the bipolar signal, a change in morphology can be a useful finding, and the unfiltered bipolar electrogram with the electrodes oriented parallel to the axis of the annulus can be used to localize the atrial insertion site of the BT.

During retrograde BT conduction (orthodromic AVRT or ventricular pacing), the atrial insertion is identified as the site where the polarity of the atrial potential reverses. Because the atrial insertion site is usually discrete, atrial

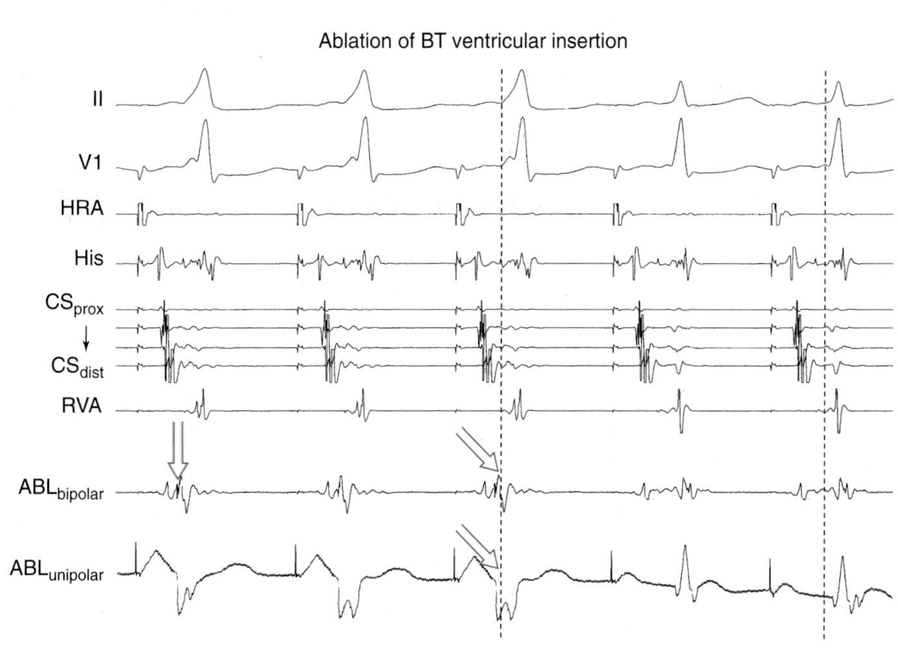

FIGURE 14–27 Catheter ablation of a left anterolateral bypass tract (BT) during anterograde conduction. Ablation is performed during preexcited atrial pacing. Preexcitation is observed during the first three complexes. The dashed line indicates the onset of the delta wave. Note the sharp negative deflection (QS morphology) in the unipolar recording. Also, note the concordance of the timing of the unipolar and bipolar electrograms (blue arrows), which precedes the onset of the delta wave by 10 to 15 msec. A sharp potential (possible BT potential, red arrow) is recorded between the atrial and ventricular electrograms. RF application at this site successfully eliminated preexcitation (last two complexes).

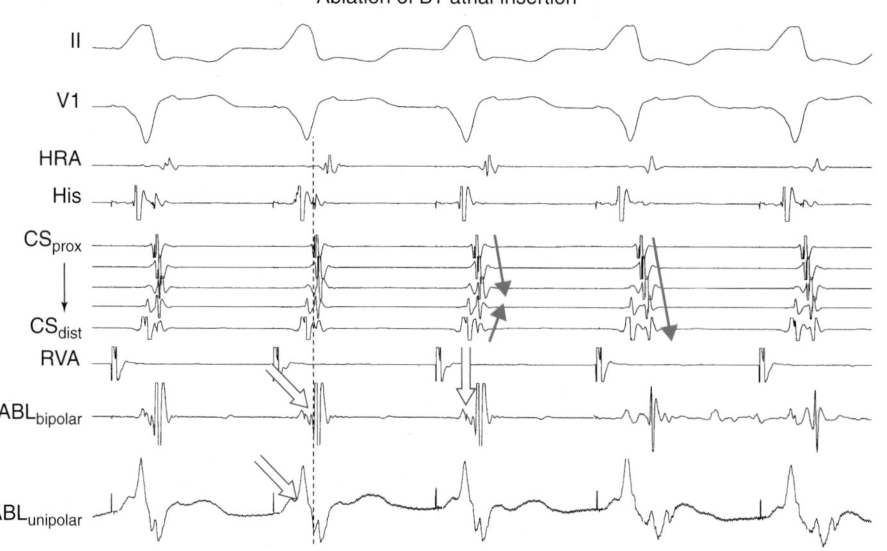

FIGURE 14–28 Catheter ablation of a left lateral bypass tract (BT) during retrograde conduction. Ablation is performed during ventricular pacing with atrial fusion (ventriculoatrial conduction occurring over both the BT and atrioventricular node [AVN]). The dashed line indicates the onset of the earliest atrial activation. Note the sharp negative deflection (QS morphology) in the unipolar recording. The timing of the unipolar electrogram coincides with the bipolar electrogram (blue arrows) and precedes the delta wave by 5 to 10 msec. The atrial and ventricular electrograms merge together, and the true morphology of the ventricular electrogram is unmasked after successful ablation (last two complexes). A sharp potential (possible BT potential, red arrow) is recorded between the two electrograms. After successful elimination of the BT function, atrial activation occurs exclusively over the AVN (last two complexes, green arrows).

14

activation propagates anteriorly and posteriorly along the annulus from the insertion site. Consequently, an RS configuration electrogram will be present on one side of the BT, where the wavefront is propagating from the distal electrode toward the proximal electrode, and a QR morphology electrogram on the other side, where the wavefront is propagating from the proximal electrode toward the distal electrode (see Fig. 3-5).

This technique is typically used for localization of left free wall BTs via the transseptal approach, which allows an electrode orientation parallel with atrial activation along the mitral annulus. As the ablation catheter is moved along the mitral annulus during retrograde BT conduction, the amplitude and polarity of the atrial electrogram are examined. With the tip electrode negative, and the catheter lying on the mitral annulus from anterior to posterior, an upright atrial electrogram indicates a catheter position anterior to the insertion site, whereas a negative electrogram indicates positions posterior to the insertion site. When the bipole approaches and then passes directly over the atrial insertion site, the atrial electrogram becomes diminished in amplitude, isoelectric, and fractionated. As the catheter moves from one side of the insertion site to the other side, reversal of the atrial electrogram polarity is observed. This maneuver has a sensitivity of 97%, specificity of 46%, and positive predictive value of 75%.[24]

Direct Recording of Bypass Tract Potential. The BT potential manifests as a sharp narrow spike on both unipolar and bipolar recordings 10 to 30 milliseconds before the onset of the delta wave during anterograde preexcitation or between the ventricular and atrial electrograms at the earliest site of retrograde atrial activation during orthodromic AVRT or ventricular pacing. The BT potential amplitude averages 0.5 to 1 mV at successful ablation sites (see Figs. 14-27 and 14-28). Similar electrical signals, however, can be a component of the atrial or ventricular electrogram, and proof that an electrical signal actually is a BT potential is difficult, because it needs to be dissociated from the local atrial and ventricular electrograms.

Dissociation of Bypass Tract Potential from Local Atrial Potential. During orthodromic AVRT or ventricular pacing, introduction of a VES may cause retrograde block near the BT-atrial interface. This would result in loss of the atrial potential while maintaining the BT potential, providing evidence that the BT potential does not result from atrial activation. Additionally, during ventricular pacing, introduction of a late-coupled AES can advance the timing of the local atrial potential without affecting the retrograde BT potential, providing evidence that the BT potential does not result from atrial activation.

Dissociation of Bypass Tract Potential from Local Ventricular Potential. During AVRT or ventricular pacing, introduction of a late-coupled VES may block retrogradely in the BT near the ventricular-BT interface. This would result in loss of the BT potential while maintaining the ventricular potential, providing evidence that the BT potential does not result from ventricular activation. Additionally, during preexcited atrial pacing, introduction of a late-coupled VES (occurring at the time of the anterograde BT potential) that advances the local ventricular electrogram but does not alter the BT potential dissociates this potential from the local ventricular activation. Moreover, during ventricular pacing, introduction of a critically timed AES may anterogradely activate the BT, advancing the timing of the BT potential without affecting the timing or morphology of the ventricular potential, providing evidence that the BT potential does not result from atrial activation.

However, these criteria for validation of BT potentials are often difficult to achieve. Therefore, the validation of BT potentials by programmed electrical stimulation is often not practical in clinical settings; instead, such a potential is called *possible* or *probable* BT potential.[47]

Targeting an isolated BT potential has been associated with the highest ablation success. The usefulness of this criterion, however, has been limited by difficulty in locating or validating a BT potential. The difficulty in identifying the BT potential is often related to the oblique course of the BT. A ventricular or atrial wavefront propagating concurrently with the BT can overlap and mask the BT potential. Pacing from the site producing the shorter local VA or local AV helps identify the BT potential in most of these cases.

Local Atrioventricular (or Ventricular) Interval. Although the site of the shortest local VA interval during retrograde BT conduction and the site of the shortest local AV interval during anterograde BT conduction are often considered the optimal target for BT ablation,[8,48,49] the reliability of this criterion has been debated and is misleading in the case of oblique BTs.[3,8] Short local VA intervals can occur at sites along the valve annulus distant from the BT because atrial and ventricular activation wavefronts can propagate circumferentially along the annulus, and the timing of local atrial and ventricular activation can be close to one another at multiple sites along the annulus. Furthermore, with oblique BTs, the shortest local VA interval can be shifted away from the BT in the direction of the ventricular wavefront if the velocity of the ventricular wavefront along the annulus is less than the velocity of the atrial wavefront. Similarly, the site of the shortest local AV interval can be shifted away from the BT in the direction of the atrial wavefront if the atrial wavefront is slower than the ventricular wavefront.

With an oblique course, the local VA and AV intervals at the site of earliest ventricular activation should vary by reversing the direction of the paced ventricular and atrial wavefronts, respectively.[8] During ventricular pacing, a ventricular wavefront propagating from the direction of the ventricular end (concurrently with BT activation) would produce a short local VA interval, because activation along the BT would proceed to the site of earliest atrial activation concomitant with the ventricular wavefront. A ventricular wavefront propagating in the opposite (countercurrent) direction would produce a longer local VA interval because the ventricular wavefront must pass the site of earliest atrial activation before reaching the ventricular end of the BT (Fig. 14-29). This has important implications for localizing oblique AV BTs. With a concurrent wavefront, the ventricular potential may overlap and mask the BT potential and overlap the atrial potential, masking the site of earliest atrial activation. If the velocity of the ventricular wavefront along the annulus were slower than the BT and atrial wavefronts, the shortest local VA interval would be shifted away from the BT. A countercurrent wavefront should expose the atrial activation sequence and BT potential. Similarly, during atrial pacing, a concurrent atrial wavefront would shorten the local AV interval at the site of earliest ventricular activation (local AV) and could mask the BT potential and site of earliest ventricular activation. A countercurrent wavefront should lengthen the local AV and expose the BT potential and ventricular activation sequence (see Fig. 14-29).

Reversing the paced ventricular or atrial wavefronts increases the local VA or local AV interval, respectively, by 15 milliseconds or more in more than 85% of patients, which suggests that most BTs have an oblique course. The increase in the local VA or local AV intervals may facilitate identification of the BT potential.[8] An anterograde or retrograde BT potential can be recorded in more than 85% of patients with oblique BTs, which is much more frequent than that with nonoblique BTs, because fusion of the atrial, BT, and ventricular potentials may be expected with nonoblique BT.

During retrograde BT conduction, the earliest atrial activation may be recorded 3 to 5 mm (or possibly more) from the actual BT insertion. Ablation is likely to be successful if the electrode is located 3 to 5 mm from the atrial insertion in the direction of the ventricular insertion and unsuccessful if located in the opposite direction. During anterograde BT conduction, ablation at a site recording earliest ventricular activation is likely to be successful, even if the electrode is located 3 to 5 mm from the ventricular end but in the direction of the atrial insertion and unsuccessful if located in the opposite direction. This explains the 40% ablation success for the criterion of local ventricular activation preceding the onset of the delta wave by less than 0 millisecond during anterograde BT conduction, even though ventricular activation usually can be recorded as much as 30 milliseconds before the delta wave in right-sided BTs and 15 to 20 milliseconds in left-sided BTs.

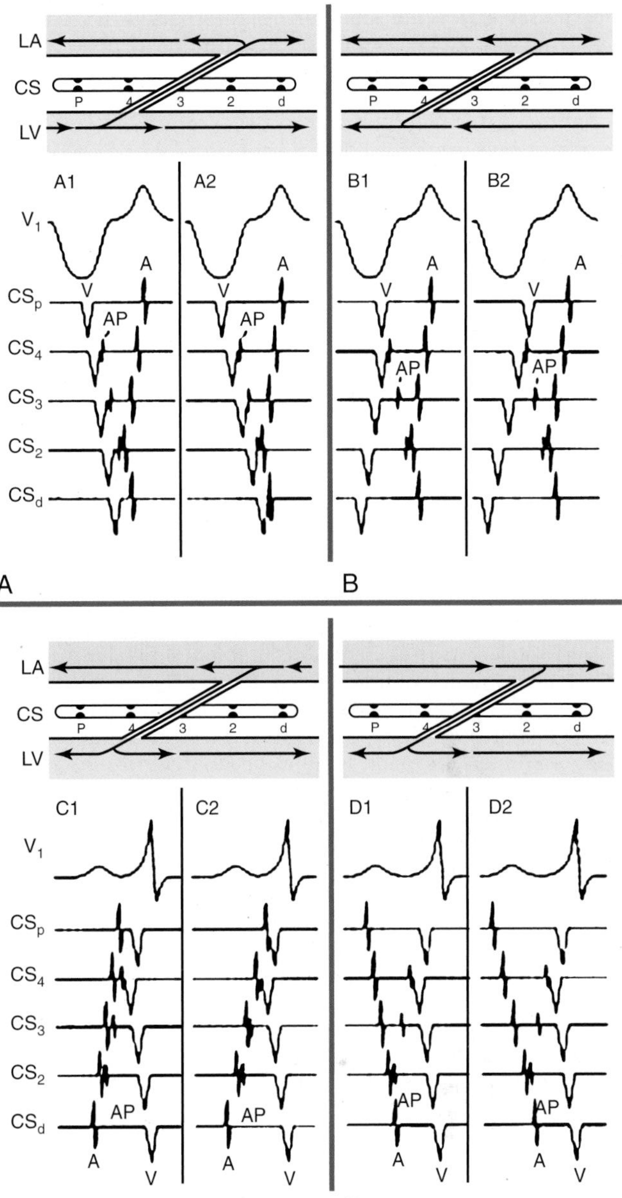

FIGURE 14–29 Schematic representation of anterograde and retrograde activation of a left free wall bypass tract. The oblique course illustrates change in electrogram timing with the reversal of the paced ventricular wavefront **(A, B)** and reversal of the paced atrial wavefront **(C, D)**. AP = accessory pathway potential; p = proximal; d = distal. (From Otomo K, Gonzalez MD, Beckman KJ, et al: Reversing the direction of paced ventricular and atrial wavefronts reveals an oblique course in accessory AV pathways and improves localization for catheter ablation. Circulation 2001;104:550.)

ABLATION

Target of Ablation

The BT is the target of ablation. The best site of ablation of a BT is where it crosses the annulus. Localization of the BT can be achieved with different mapping methods, as described earlier. Ablation should be performed at the same side of the annulus to the one being mapped (i.e., ablation on the atrial side during mapping of the atrial insertion site during retrograde BT conduction, and ablation on the ventricular side during mapping of the earliest ventricular activation during anterograde BT conduction). This is especially important in the case of oblique BTs, whereby the earliest ventricular activation site during anterograde BT conduction from the atrial aspect of the annulus can be distant from the atrial insertion site of the BT, and ablation would not then be successful.

Although BT conduction can be eliminated by ablation anywhere between the atrial and ventricular ends, RF applications targeted to the atrial end (site of earliest atrial activation during retrograde BT conduction) or ventricular end (site of earliest ventricular activation during anterograde BT conduction) can occasionally fail. This observation suggests that the recording range of the 4-mm electrode (unipolar or bipolar configuration) commonly used for RF ablation is greater than the RF lesion radius.

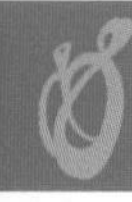

Criteria of successful ablation sites during anterograde or retrograde activation mapping of BTs are presented in Table 14-10 (see Figs.14-27 and 14-28).

TABLE 14–10 Electrophysiological Criteria of Successful Bypass Tract (BT) Ablation Sites

Criteria of Successful Ablation Sites During Anterograde Activation Mapping
Stable catheter position, as confirmed fluoroscopically and by observing a stable electrogram (<10% change in amplitude in atrial and ventricular electrograms over 5-10 beats).
Atrial electrogram amplitude > 0.4 mV, or A/V ratio >0. Both atrial and ventricular electrogram components should be recorded from the ablation (tip) electrode. When ablating from the atrial aspect of the annulus, the atrial electrogram is usually equal to or larger than the ventricular electrogram. Sometimes, the two can merge and it may be difficult to determine whether both components are present. Rapid atrial or ventricular pacing resulting in block in the BT can help eliminate ventricular or atrial electrogram (respectively) so that the exact morphology of the other component can be visualized.
Local AV interval on the ablation catheter is usually short (25-50 msec, except for previously damaged, slowly conducting, oblique, or epicardial BTs).[51]
The local ventricular electrogram on the ablation catheter should precede the onset of the delta wave on the ECG by a mean of 0-10 msec for left-sided BTs and 10-30 msec for right-sided BTs (the local ventricular electrogram is measured from the peak of the bipolar electrogram or the maximal dV/dT in the unipolar electrogram).
QS (or, less preferably, rS) morphology of the unipolar electrogram. Right-sided BTs usually have unipolar recordings that show more pronounced (rapid and deeper) QS configuration than left-sided BTs.[46,51]
Continuous electrical activity (defined as isoelectric interval of <5 msec between ventricular and atrial electrograms).
Presence of BT potential.
Criteria of Successful Ablation Sites During Retrograde Activation Mapping
Stable catheter position, as confirmed fluoroscopically and by observing a stable electrogram (<10% change in amplitude in atrial and ventricular electrograms over 5-10 beats).
Local VA interval during retrograde activation of the BT is short (25-50 msec, except for previously damaged, slowly-conducting, oblique, or epicardial BTs), usually resulting in inscription of the atrial electrogram on the ascending portion of the terminal ventricular electrogram. The "pseudodisappearance" of the atrial electrogram within the terminal portion of the ventricular electrogram (forming a W sign) during orthodromic AVRT is a manifestation of an extremely short local VA interval, which correlates with successful ablation sites.
Surface QRS to local atrial electrogram interval ≤ 70 msec (during orthodromic AVRT).
The local VA interval remains constant regardless of which direction the ventricular wavefront engaging the BT is traveling (i.e., despite pacing from different ventricular sites). If one uses the ventricular approach to ablate a concealed BT, the ventricular insertion site can be identified as one that maintains a constant local VA interval, despite differences in direction of activation to the ventricular site.
Continuous electrical activity (defined as isoelectric interval < 5 msec between ventricular and atrial electrograms).
Presence of BT potential.

A/V = atrium to ventricle; AVRT = atrioventricular reentrant tachycardia; VA = ventriculoatrial.

Ablation Technique: General Considerations

Some investigators have advocated a simplified approach to ablation using one or two catheters. Although often successful, 10% of patients with preexcitation have multiple arrhythmias, and 10% to 20% of such patients have multiple BTs that can result in a very complex procedure. Because it is difficult to know beforehand in any given patient whether the procedure will be straightforward or complex, the single-catheter approach to ablation of arrhythmias should be discouraged.

For most free wall BTs, complete bidirectional block can be achieved with a conventional 4-mm-tip ablation catheter, using a power setting of 50 W and targeting a temperature of 60°C. If the conduction block is transient, permanent BT block can usually be obtained with better and more consistent contact at the same site. It is rare that an 8-mm- or irrigated-tip ablation catheter is necessary, except when ablating in small branches of the CS, at which time irrigated-tip catheters can be helpful.

Radiofrequency Delivery. A temperature of 55° to 60°C should be sought. Transient loss of BT function is seen roughly at 50°C, and permanent loss of function occurs at 60°C. Therefore, sites with favorable electrogram characteristics should not be abandoned until a temperature higher than 50° to 55°C is reached. Conversely, repeated energy applications at the same location after achieving a temperature of 55°C or higher are unlikely to succeed.[50]

Loss of BT conduction is expected within 1 to 6 seconds of RF application (once the target temperature and power delivery have been reached) for most successful lesions. If no effect is seen after 15 seconds of RF delivery, energy delivery should be discontinued because it is unlikely to be beneficial, and mapping criteria and catheter contact should be reexamined. If BT conduction is eliminated during the application, RF delivery should be continued for up to 60 seconds.

If preexcitation is present, ablation should be performed during NSR or, preferably, atrial pacing. For concealed BTs, RF energy is delivered during ventricular pacing, which usually allows for detection of an altered retrograde atrial activation sequence. RF energy delivery during AVRT should be avoided because of potential catheter dislodgment from its critical position on abrupt tachycardia termination. This event can be associated with transient loss of conduction over the BT for a variable period of time without resulting in permanent damage to the BT caused by premature interruption of the RF application. Occasionally, BT conduction may resume hours to days after the procedure; therefore, one may not find a suitable target to complete the RF lesion. Ablation during continuous pacing prevents this problem. For incessant AVRT, energy may be delivered during ventricular pacing entraining the tachycardia. The use of an electroanatomical mapping system can obviate this problem by tagging the initial site of ablation, allowing precise return to that site.[50]

If BT function is not eliminated at a site with apparent favorable electrographic features, catheter contact with the tissue may be inadequate. Adequacy of catheter contact can be verified by evaluating the electrode temperature, catheter stability on fluoroscopy, electrogram stability, and ST elevation on the unipolar electrogram. If electrode temperature is consistently more than 50°C with more than 25 W energy delivered to the tissue during the RF application, good catheter contact is likely; however, if electrode temperature reaches more than 50°C but with very low power (less than 10 W), coagulum may have formed at the catheter tip. Also, catheter "shimmering" on fluoroscopy suggests poor contact. Similarly, changing electrographic amplitudes before or during ablation suggests inadequate catheter contact. Furthermore, ablation-related injury usually yields ST elevation on the unipolar electrogram; if absent, inadequate tissue heating is likely.[50]

Ablation of Left Free Wall Bypass Tracts

Anatomical Considerations

Although the atrial insertion of the BT is typically discrete (1 to 3 mm) in size and close to the mitral annulus, the ventricular insertion site tends to ramify over the region of tissue and may be displaced a small distance away from the mitral annulus, toward the ventricular apex.[51] Most left free wall BTs cross the mitral annulus obliquely, with the atrial insertion typically 4 to 30 mm proximal (posterior) to the more distal (anterior) ventricular insertion site (as mapped from within the CS).[8]

Conduction at the insertion sites of the BT is markedly anisotropic because of almost horizontal orientation of the atrial and ventricular fibers as they insert into the mitral annulus. In addition, the atrial fibers run parallel to the annulus, giving rise to rapid conduction away from the insertion site, parallel to the annulus, and slow conduction to the free wall of the atrium, perpendicular to the annulus.

Although the CS is useful as a guide for mapping the mitral annulus in the left anterior oblique (LAO) view, it has a variable relationship to the mitral annulus. The CS lies 2 cm superior to the annulus as it crosses from the RA to the LA. Anterolaterally, the CS frequently overrides the LV. Thus, depending on the distance from the ostium, the CS can lie above the mitral annulus and be associated with the LA, or can cross over the LV side of the mitral annulus. Therefore, electrograms recorded from the CS can only provide a reference for atrial and/or ventricular insertion sites of the BT and can only be used to guide the ablation catheter to areas in which more detailed mapping may be performed.[51]

Technical Considerations

Transaortic (Retrograde) Approach. The right femoral artery is the most commonly used access. A long vascular sheath may provide added catheter stability, although with a possibly increased risk of thromboembolism. Anticoagulation is started once the LV is accessed (with heparin, 5000 U IV bolus, followed by 1000 U/hr infusion), to maintain the activated clotting time (ACT) between 250 and 300 seconds. The ablation catheter is advanced to the descending aorta and, in this position, a tight J curve is formed with the catheter tip before passage to the aortic root to minimize catheter manipulation in the arch. In a 30-degree right anterior oblique (RAO) view, the curved catheter is advanced through the aortic valve with the J curve opening to the right, so the catheter passes into the LV oriented anterolaterally. The straight catheter tip must never be used to cross the aortic valve, because of the risk of leaflet perforation. Once in the LV, and while maintaining a tight curve, the catheter is rotated counterclockwise and withdrawn in the LA as the tip turns posteriorly. By opening the J curve slightly, the tip can easily map the mitral annulus; clockwise torque moves the tip anteriorly (distally along the CS), and counterclockwise torque returns the tip posteriorly (proximally along the CS). Alternatively, after crossing the aortic valve, the catheter can be straightened and steered directly under the mitral annulus to the BT location or withdrawn in the LV outflow tract, rotated posteriorly with a slight curve, and then advanced under the posterior mitral annulus for left paraseptal or posterior BTs. When the ablation catheter is approximated along the mitral annulus, the catheter tip is simultaneously withdrawn and straightened slightly to slip under the annulus for fine manipulation. For left lateral and anterior BTs, extended-reach catheters may be required.[51]

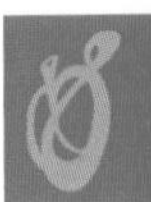

Catheter positions beneath the annulus between the ventricular myocardium and mitral leaflet are most stable and target the ventricular BT insertion for ablation, but manipulation can be constrained by the chordae. Catheter positions above or along the annulus provide more freedom to map along the mitral annulus but are sometimes too unstable for successful energy delivery using the retrograde approach. Initial mapping is performed with the ablation electrode on the annulus. From this general area, the catheter is then positioned beneath the mitral annulus for more precise mapping. Catheter tip positions beneath the mitral annulus are suggested by proximity to the CS catheter, motion concomitant with the CS catheter, and an A/V electrogram ratio < 1.0.

Because the transaortic approach targets the ventricular insertion site of the BT, it is best suited for mapping anterograde BT activation (i.e., preexcitation). Mapping retrograde activation from the subannular position is more difficult than for anterograde mapping because of obscuration of the low-amplitude atrial electrogram following the large ventricular electrogram.

Although BT locations are commonly defined by mapping along the CS catheter, this only approximates localization of the subannular ablation site because of the oblique course of left free wall BTs, displacement of the CS above the mitral annulus, variable basilar-apical ventricular insertion of the BT, and BT location beyond the distal CS electrode.

Transseptal Approach. Transseptal and transaortic approaches are equally effective.[52] The transseptal approach is primarily used for atrial mapping during orthodromic AVRT or ventricular pacing and not for anterograde mapping. On the other hand, ventricular mapping of manifest BTs (during preexcitation) using the transseptal approach is limited.[48-50]

The transseptal approach has several advantages over the transaortic approach.[52,53] The transseptal approach provides better access to far lateral and anterolateral BT locations, easier catheter maneuverability in the LA, and less risk of coronary injury. Additionally, no arterial access is required with the transseptal approach, and vascular recovery is therefore shorter. However, the transseptal approach provides less catheter stability and is associated with a higher risk of cardiac perforation and air embolism. Furthermore, the transseptal approach entails higher cost if intracardiac echocardiography is used.[52]

Before introducing the standard transseptal sheath, its curvature can be modified according to BT location. The curve is left intact for left posterior BTs. The sheath is progressively withdrawn toward the RA for lateral BT locations, and it is almost entirely withdrawn toward the RA for anterior BTs. Alternatively, preformed sheaths can be used.

Once the ablation catheter is positioned on the mitral annulus in a 30-degree RAO view, mapping is performed in the LAO view. In the absence of preformed septal sheaths, gentle clockwise torque is needed to maintain the catheter on the posterior mitral annulus. No torque is needed for lateral positions. As the catheter is moved anteriorly, counterclockwise torque is necessary to keep the catheter tip on the annulus. In the anterior positions, the catheter tip can dislodge into the LA appendage or LV, and attention to intracardiac electrograms is necessary when mapping anterior regions, because the CS catheter rarely provides an accurate fluoroscopic reference in this case. The goal is to maintain the catheter tip on the atrial aspect of the mitral annulus, so that the mitral annulus can be easily mapped by advancing and withdrawing the catheter, causing it to slide along the mitral annulus freely in parallel to the CS catheter. Advancing the catheter moves the tip posteriorly; withdrawing it moves the tip anteriorly. The ventricular aspect of the mitral annulus can be mapped by passing the catheter tip across the mitral valve and deflecting the tip toward the annulus.

The transseptal approach facilitates mapping of the atrial aspect of the mitral annulus. Catheter position on the atrial aspect of the mitral annulus is documented by recording a bipolar A/V electrogram amplitude ratio ≥1, and a unipolar electrogram PR segment displacement from baseline without ST segment displacement. The stability of the catheter can be assessed by PR segment elevation (confirming good atrial tissue contact), consistent local electrographic amplitudes, and concordant motion of the CS and ablation catheters.

Because of the mobility of the ablation catheter and the electrode orientation parallel with atrial activation along the mitral annulus, a unique vectorial mapping technique is possible with the transseptal approach. As noted, this allows mapping atrial electrogram polarity reversal during retrograde BT conduction. Using the unfiltered bipolar electrogram with the electrodes oriented parallel to the axis of the mitral annulus, the atrial insertion is identified as the site at which the polarity of the atrial potential reverses.

Ablation of Right Free Wall Bypass Tracts

Anatomical Considerations

The anatomy of right-sided and left-sided BTs differs somewhat. The tricuspid annulus has a larger circumference than the mitral annulus (12 versus 10 cm) and is not a complete fibrous ring, but can have many regions of discontinuity. In addition, there is a portion of the mitral annulus (the region of the aortomitral continuity) where BTs do not occur. This means that a larger region must be mapped to ablate right free wall versus left free wall BTs. Despite these facts, right-sided BTs are much less common than left-sided BTs (12% versus 59%).[47,54,55]

Ablation of right-sided BTs is often more challenging than that of left free wall BTs, and the recurrence rate after apparent success is higher. However, the complication rate is low. Caused by the unique features of the tricuspid annulus, one can encounter difficulty in maintaining catheter stability, mapping difficulties, increased cooling of the ablation tip by the blood pool, and the possibility of multiple or unusual BTs.[47] The mitral valve attaches to its fibrous annulus at a right angle, whereas the tricuspid valve attaches to its annulus at an acute angle oriented toward the RV, making it more difficult to wedge an ablation catheter underneath the tricuspid valve. Moreover, there is folding over of the RA and RV (but not on the left side of the heart), so that it can be difficult to position the catheter at the tricuspid annulus because of a tendency of the catheter to fall into the folded-over sac. In addition, because BTs can connect between the RA and RV anywhere along the folded sac, the BT can be somewhat removed from the annulus, making accurate localization of the atrial insertion site critical to successful ablation. Atrial insertion of the BT can be as far as 1 cm away from the annulus in the folded-over atrial sac. The folded-over atrium and bizarre angle required for mapping of the inferior and posterolateral aspect of the RA by a catheter passed through the RA from the inferior vena cava (IVC) can make mapping of this region challenging. Thus, sometimes the superior vena cava (SVC) approach is required to allow full exploration of the folded-over atrial sac and the inferior-inferolateral positions around the tricuspid annulus. The standard IVC approach, however, is adequate to map the superior aspects of the tricuspid annulus. If the IVC approach is used, a guiding sheath can be especially helpful for better catheter stability and tissue contact. The use of a Halo catheter or multipolar catheter positioned around the tricuspid annulus can provide good regional localization to guide the ablation catheter.

Transient interruption of BT conduction during RF delivery, with subsequent resumption of conduction within seconds or minutes, and recurrence rates over the first few weeks of BT ablation are more common with right-sided BTs compared with left-sided BTs. This might be related to the fact that some right free wall BTs do not travel as close to the endocardium as left free wall BTs. Furthermore, closely adjacent but anatomically discrete sites of catheter ablation may be necessary to eliminate anterograde and retrograde BT conduction in up to 10% of patients—the incidence is highest (18.6%) with right free wall BTs. The explanation for this phenomenon is not clear but probably relates to the complexity of fiber orientation, possibly branching over 1 to 2 cm along the annulus. This factor emphasizes the importance of identifying atrial and ventricular insertion sites.[47,56]

In Ebstein's anomaly, the posterior leaflet of the tricuspid valve is displaced a variable distance into the RV away from the anatomical tricuspid annulus.[47] Right posteroseptal, posterior, and posterolateral BTs occur commonly and can be manifest or concealed. Echocardiography should be performed to exclude Ebstein's anomaly in patients with ECGs suggestive of BTs in this region. Up to 25% of patients with Ebstein's anomaly and WPW syndrome have multiple BTs. The BTs bridge the true anatomical tricuspid annulus, regardless of where the valve is located. Identification of the true anatomical tricuspid annulus can be difficult, especially because the electrical signal recorded from the endocardium near the tricuspid annulus in these patients is often prolonged and fractionated. Ablation is usually accomplished at the true tricuspid annulus, above the displaced valve leaflet, although some patients may undergo successful ablation from the ventricular side of the tricuspid annulus (but still above the valve leaflet).

Technical Considerations

Characteristics of successful ablation sites for right-sided BTs include the following: the local AV interval is shorter than that for BTs elsewhere, the local ventricular electrogram precedes the onset of the delta wave by an interval longer than that for BTs elsewhere (18 ± 10 milliseconds for right-sided BTs versus 0 ± 5 milliseconds for left-sided BTs), and the unipolar recording shows more pronounced (rapid and deeper) QS configuration.

Most commonly, ablation of the BT is approached from the atrial aspect. The optimal site of ablation is the earliest atrial activation site during retrograde BT conduction (during orthodromic AVRT or ventricular pacing), preferably with a BT potential present. The earliest site of atrial activation is identified using a roving catheter, Halo catheter, or multipolar catheter along the tricuspid annulus. If mapping is performed during ventricular pacing, conduction over both the BT and AVN can occur, resulting in atrial fusion, which can interfere with localization of the BT. Ventricular pacing performed close to the BT ventricular insertion site can accentuate atrial activation over the BT.[47]

Occasionally, the BT may be better approached from the ventricular side. Ventricular activation mapping is performed during preexcited NSR, atrial pacing, preexcited SVT, or antidromic AVRT.[47] The site of the earliest ventricular activation during preexcitation, preferably with a BT potential present, would be the optimal site. The earliest onset of ventricular activation recorded on the ablation catheter (using unipolar or bipolar electrograms) should precede the onset of the delta wave by 10 to 25 milliseconds or more. For concealed BTs, the ventricular insertion site cannot be determined by ventricular activation mapping because of the lack of preexcitation. In this case, recording of a BT potential can be especially useful to help guide ablation.

The tricuspid annulus is usually mapped in the LAO view. Recording from any location around the tricuspid annulus can be obtained, although good catheter-tissue contact is more difficult to obtain than on the left side. The right posterior, posterolateral, and lateral regions are usually best mapped from the IVC approach. The right anterior and anterolateral regions can also often be ablated using the IVC approach, but the SVC approach can obtain better catheter-tissue contact in these areas. The catheter can be prolapsed across the tricuspid valve to help stabilize the tip on the tricuspid annulus. In the LAO view, the HB is located at about 1 o'clock and the CS at 5 o'clock; right free wall BTs span from approximately 6 to 12 o'clock. Right anterior BTs are at the most superior aspect of the tricuspid annulus, right superoparaseptal BTs are located near the HB catheter, and right posterior free wall BTs are located at the most posterior aspect of the tricuspid annulus, whereas right posteroseptal BTs are located near the CS.[47] Although the location of the mitral annulus is reasonably indicated by the CS catheter, the location of the tricuspid annulus is not as easily discerned because there is no analogous venous structure to mark with a catheter. Furthermore, because the mitral and tricuspid annuli are not always in the same plane, the CS catheter is only a rough guide to the location of the tricuspid annulus in the RAO view. Occasionally, a fine angioplasty wire may be passed into the right coronary artery to delineate the location of the tricuspid annulus. To target the ventricular aspect of the tricuspid annulus, the catheter is introduced across the tricuspid valve and looped back on itself in the RV underneath the valve until a small atrial electrogram and a larger ventricular electrogram are recorded, confirming adequate proximity to the tricuspid annulus. A long sheath can be used to stabilize the body of the catheter and direct the catheter to several different locations along the tricuspid annulus.

RF energy may be delivered during NSR, atrial pacing, ventricular pacing, or entrained AVRT. Delivery during AVRT can result in sudden termination of the SVT, which can cause dislodgment of the ablation catheter, resulting in an inadequate RF application. Therefore, if retrograde mapping during orthodromic AVRT is used to determine the optimal atrial ablation site, especially for concealed BTs, it is preferable to entrain the orthodromic AVRT with ventricular pacing at a slightly shorter CL so that block in the BT and termination of the SVT during RF energy delivery will be followed by ventricular pacing at a rate similar to that of the SVT, minimizing catheter movement. If BT function does not disappear despite good catheter stability, adequate catheter-tissue contact, and good temperature rise (more than 50°C), the catheter is probably located at the wrong site. Transient interruption of BT conduction during RF delivery, with subsequent reappearance of conduction within seconds or minutes after energy delivery is completed, is more common with right than left free wall BTs. The use of multisite "insurance lesions" is discouraged, and the use of one or two ablation sites should be the goal, which requires careful mapping to achieve.

3-D electroanatomical mapping systems can help ablation of BTs, and are especially useful in the presence of multiple BTs or complicated anatomy.[57] An electroanatomical color-coded activation map along the tricuspid annulus can be constructed, either along the atrial side, during orthodromic AVRT or ventricular pacing, or the ventricular side, during anterograde preexcitation. Sites of interest can be tagged for further reference, so that the ablation catheter can be returned to any of them with precision. Information with regard to catheter stability and movement can also be provided.

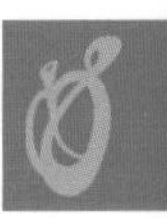

Ablation of Posteroseptal (Inferoparaseptal) Bypass Tracts

Anatomical Considerations

Ablation of posteroseptal BTs is more difficult than other BT locations because of the complexity of the anatomical structures involved and the difficulty to discriminate successful ablation sites on the right versus the left posteroseptal area before ablation.[51,58]

The posteroseptal region corresponds to a region where the four cardiac chambers reach their maximal proximity posteriorly. It spans the area between the central fibrous body (superiorly), the interventricular septum (anteriorly), and the RA and LA posteriorly. Because the interatrial sulcus is displaced to the far left of the interventricular sulcus, and because the AV valves are not isoplanar (the attachment of the septal tricuspid valve leaflet into the most anterior part of the central fibrous body is displaced a few millimeters apically relative to the attachment of the septal mitral valve leaflet), the true septal part of the AV junction (the RA-LV sulcus) actually separates the cavity of RA from that of the LV (left ventricular outflow tract [LVOT]). The undersurface of the CS is about 1 cm above the mitral annulus, and the coronary sinus ostium (CS os) abuts the superior margin of the RA-LV sulcus.[51] The right margin of the posteroseptal space includes the area surrounding the CS os and the inferior portion of the triangle of Koch; the left margin (the junction of the posterior septum and left free wall) lies as far as 2 to 3 cm from the CS os. The posterior septal space at the level of the valve annuli extends a mean of 3.4 ± 0.5 cm around the epicardium. BTs located in the proximal 1.5 cm of the CS are almost always in the posterior septum. Those located between 1.5 and 3 cm from the CS os can be in the left free wall or posterior septum, and those located more than 3 cm from the CS os are almost invariably in the left free wall.[51]

Most posteroseptal BTs are believed to be RA to LV BTs, with the ventricular insertion attaching onto the posterior superior process of the LV, but some posteroseptal BTs are considered to be left paraseptal (connecting the LA to the LV) or right paraseptal (connecting the RA to the RV). Because the posteroseptal region is actually posterior to the septum and not a septal structure, posteroseptal BTs are more appropriately referred to as right- or left-sided inferoparaseptal or posterior paraseptal BTs.

Although epicardial BTs can be found at any location, they are most common in the posteroseptal and left posterior paraseptal regions.[52,59] Approximately 20% of all posteroseptal BTs and 40% of those in patients referred after a failed ablation procedure are epicardial. One hypothesis for this predilection is that those BTs connect the myocardial coat of the CS, which is connected anatomically and electrically to both the RA and LA, to the LV. Not infrequently, BTs connecting the CS muscular coating to the LV occur in association with a CS diverticulum. An epicardial location of the BT is suggested if the earliest site of endocardial ventricular activation does not precede the onset of the delta wave, and if a very large BT potential can be easily recorded on the CS electrodes.

Technical Considerations

Several criteria have been used to differentiate left from right posteroseptal BTs (Table 14-11). Generally, a right-sided endocardial approach is initially adopted for mapping and ablation of BTs in the posteroseptal region.[58] The posteroseptal tricuspid annulus, including the CS os and its most proximal part, and inferomedial RA are carefully mapped. If the ablation site fails or no appropriate ablation site can be obtained, the left posteroseptal area is mapped (with a transaortic or transseptal approach, as described for left-sided BTs). A primary left-sided approach can also be considered if multiple ECG and EP features suggest a left-sided location of the BT. If endocardial mapping fails, an epicardial approach via the CS is then considered (see later).[59]

PJRT is usually caused by a slowly conducting BT, commonly located in the posteroseptal region. In 50% of cases, such BTs can be located in the left posterior or free wall (more than 4 cm inside the CS). In the remaining 50%, it is located between the base of the pyramidal space formed by the points of pericardial deflection that contact the posterior RA and LA. None have been reported in the anteroseptal region.

Ablation of Superoparaseptal and Midseptal Bypass Tracts

Anatomical Considerations

The triangle of Koch is bordered by the CS os posteriorly and the attachment of the septal leaflet of the tricuspid valve inferiorly. The compact AVN is located anteriorly at its apex, where the tendon of Todaro (the superior margin of the triangle of Koch) merges with the central fibrous body. Slightly more anteriorly and superiorly is where the HB penetrates the AV junction through the central fibrous body and posterior aspect of the membranous AV septum (see Fig. 13-1). The triangle of Koch is septal, and constitutes the RA surface of the muscular AV septum. BTs with an atrial insertion in the floor of the triangle of Koch, posteroinferior to the compact AVN and HB and above the anterior portion of the CS os, have been labeled as midseptal, and they are septal structures. In fact, these BTs are the only truly septal BTs; hence, they can be referred to simply as septal BTs.

TABLE 14–11 Criteria for Differentiating Left from Right Posteroseptal Bypass Tracts (BTs)

Negative or isoelectric delta wave in V_1 with abrupt transition to R > S in V_2 or V_3 suggests right-sided location. R/S ratio > 1 in V_1 suggests left-sided approach.
Long RP tachycardia (i.e., slowly conducting posteroseptal BT) suggests a right endocardial approach.
Decrementally conducting posteroseptal BTs suggests a right endocardial approach.
During orthodromic AVRT, a difference in VA interval recorded in HB catheter and that recorded at site of earliest atrial activation of ≥25 msec suggests a left endocardial approach.
Earliest atrial activation during orthodromic AVRT recorded in the CS electrode at the bottom of the mitral annulus suggests a left endocardial approach.
A 10- to 25-msec increase in the VA interval in association with LBBB during orthodromic AVRT suggests a left endocardial approach.

AVRT = atrioventricular reentrant tachycardia; CS = coronary sinus; HB = His bundle; LBBB = left bundle branch block; VA = ventriculoatrial.

The larger parts of the regions anterior and posterior to the true AV septal areas are not septal but are parts of the parietal AV junction. The true septal components of the AV junction are the muscular and membranous AV septal areas. These separate the cavity of the RA from that of the LV. The region previously designated as the anterior septum is part of the right parietal junction. Anterosuperior to the AV septum and compact AVN and HB, the tricuspid annulus diverges laterally away from membranous part of the septum to course along the supraventricular crest of the RV (crista supraventricularis). This muscular structure interposes between the attachments of the leaflets of the tricuspid and pulmonic valves in the roof of the RV. BTs in this area (at the apex of the triangle of Koch) are labeled anteroseptal, but they must be considered superoparaseptal right free wall BTs, because anatomically they do not belong to the septum. There is no atrial septum in the region anterior to the HB recording site; atrial walls are separated here by the aortic root.

Technical Considerations

BTs are classified as superoparaseptal if the BT potential and His potential are simultaneously recorded from the diagnostic catheter placed at the HB region. The precise location of the BT is verified by mapping this space in a 30-degree LAO view using the ablation catheter, advanced via the right internal jugular vein or IVC. The use of a long vascular sheath may help stabilize the catheter tip during mapping and ablation in the superoparaseptal region. The optimal site of ablation is one from which the atrial and ventricular electrograms are recorded in conjunction with a BT potential, but with no or only a tiny His potential (less than 0.1 mV).[60] Preferably, the ventricular insertion site of the BT is targeted with ablation to minimize the risk of damage to the AVN. Rarely, ablation is required in the presence of a marked (more than 0.1 mV) His potential recorded through the ablation catheter (true para-Hisian BTs).

BTs are classified as midseptal if ablation is achieved through the mapping-ablation catheter located in an area bounded superiorly by the electrode recording the His potential, and posteroinferiorly by the CS os, as marked by the vortex of curvature in the CS catheter. The optimal site of ablation for a right midseptal BT is one from which atrial and ventricular electrograms are recorded simultaneously with a BT potential in between. Ablation is first attempted from the right side. If it is ineffective or early recurrence occurs after termination of RF application, then the left side approach is attempted. The combination of a negative delta wave in lead V_1 and R-S transition in leads V_3-V_4 suggest right-sided midseptal BT, whereas a biphasic delta wave in V_1 and earlier QRS transition (V_1-V_2) suggest a left-sided location of the midseptal BT.[61] Midseptal BTs can be differentiated from superoparaseptal and para-Hisian BTs by a negative delta wave in lead III and a biphasic delta wave in lead aVF.[28,62]

Ablation in the region of the triangle of Koch is associated with a 5% incidence of AV block and, to decrease this risk, such BTs should be ablated with the catheter placed on the tricuspid annulus or on the ventricular side of the tricuspid annulus, preferably with the use of lower RF power. Titrated RF energy output can be used for true para-Hisian BTs, starting with 5 W, and increasing by 5 W every 10 seconds of energy application, up to a maximum of 40 W. For other superoparaseptal BTs, ablation can be started at 30 W, targeting a temperature of 50° to 60°C. During RF ablation within the triangle of Koch, the occurrence of junctional tachycardia is not uncommon and is associated with loss of preexcitation; this should not be misinterpreted as successful ablation leading to continuing RF energy delivery. Instead, overdrive atrial pacing should be performed to monitor AV conduction or RF application should be stopped and other sites sought (Fig. 14-30).[60] RF application should be stopped after 10 to 15 seconds if no block in the BT is achieved to minimize potential damage to the AVN-HB.

For manifest BTs, RF application is performed during NSR or atrial pacing. In case of concealed para-Hisian BTs, it is challenging to assess the success of RF application and monitor AV conduction simultaneously, an important parameter when performing RF ablation near the HB. When RF delivery is performed during ventricular pacing, monitoring the success of RF application is not possible because the retrograde atrial activation sequence during ventricular pacing can be similar with BT and AVN conduction. Although atrial pacing during RF delivery helps monitor AV conduction and override junctional rhythms that may occur during RF delivery, it is not helpful for assessing the efficacy of RF application because the BT is retrograde-only. RF delivery during orthodromic AVRT is an option; however, this will certainly have the potential for catheter dislodgment on SVT termination, as stated earlier, and such dislodgment can endanger the AVN-HB. Moreover, application of RF energy during orthodromic AVRT will not allow monitoring of AV conduction. In such a case, monitoring of the mode of termination of orthodromic AVRT during RF delivery is essential. Termination of orthodromic AVRT with an atrial electrogram signifies potential damage to the anterograde limb of the SVT circuit (i.e., the AVN), and therefore RF delivery should be immediately stopped. On the other hand, termination of orthodromic AVRT with a ventricular electrogram suggests successful block in the retrograde limb of the SVT circuit (i.e., the BT), and therefore RF delivery should be continued, with careful monitoring of AV conduction during NSR following termination of the SVT. Another valuable option is RF delivery during atrial-entrained orthodromic AVRT with manifest atrial fusion. This technique enables continuous monitoring of effects of RF application on BT function and also obviates a sudden change in ventricular rate on termination of the SVT. In addition, this technique allows monitoring of AV conduction during RF application once the orthodromic AVRT is terminated, and therefore reduces the risk of damage to the AVN-HB. During successful RF application, termination of orthodromic AVRT will be indicated by transformation from the tachycardia P wave morphology and atrial activation sequence into a fully paced atrial activation sequence at the same rate.

To reduce the risk of AV block, RF delivery should be immediately discontinued when the following occur: (1) the impedance rises suddenly (more than 10 Ω); (2) the PR interval (during NSR or atrial pacing) prolongs; (3) AV block develops; (4) retrograde conduction block is observed during junctional ectopy; or (5) fast junctional tachycardia (tachycardia CL < 350 milliseconds) occurs, which may herald imminent heart block.

Cryoablation of Superoparaseptal and Midseptal Bypass Tracts

Cryothermal ablation of BTs in the superoparaseptal and midseptal areas, both at high risk of complete permanent AV block when standard RF energy is performed, is extremely safe and successful.[63-65]

Cryomapping Cryomapping, or ice mapping, is designed to verify that ablation at the chosen site will have the desired effect (i.e., block in the BT) and to reassure the absence of complications (i.e., AV block). Cryomapping is performed at −30°C in the selected site. At this temperature, the lesion is reversible (for up to 60 seconds) and the catheter is "stuck" to the endocardium in an ice ball that includes the tip of the catheter (cryoadherence). This permits programmed electrical stimulation to test the disappearance of BT conduction during ongoing ablation and also allows ablation to be performed during AVRT without the risk of catheter dislodgment on tachycardia termination.

In the cryomapping mode, the temperature is not allowed to drop below −30°C, and the time of application is limited to 60 seconds. Formation of an ice ball at the catheter tip and adherence to the underlying myocardium are signaled by the appearance of electrical noise recorded from the ablation catheter's distal bipole. Once an ice ball is formed, programmed electrical stimulation is repeated to verify that the BT has been blocked. If cryomapping does not yield the desired result within 30 seconds or results in unintended AV conduction delay or block, cryomapping is interrupted and, after a few seconds, allowing the catheter to thaw and become dislodged from the tissue, the catheter can be moved to a different site and cryomapping repeated. Alternatively, if the test application is unsuccessful, after rewarming, further 30-second applications are tested, decreasing the temperature by 10°C for every step of the application, up to the last application at −70°C. This is because the amount of cryothermal energy required for permanent ablation is individualized, ranging from an application of −40°C for 40 seconds to one of −75°C for 480 seconds; limiting test applications to only −30°C can limit the applicability of cryoablation for these patients. On the other hand, the use of cryothermal energy at temperatures lower than −30°C should be considered safer than RF energy at these critical sites.

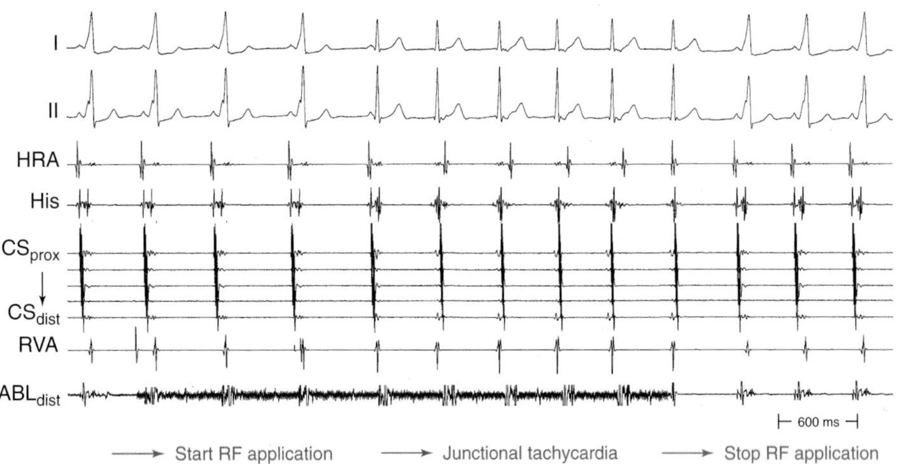

FIGURE 14–30 Junctional tachycardia during radiofrequency (RF) ablation of a superoparaseptal bypass tract. The first few complexes demonstrate normal sinus rhythm with preexcitation. A few seconds after starting RF energy delivery, junctional tachycardia develops, with loss of preexcitation. This prompted immediate termination of RF application, after which preexcitation resumed.

Cryoablation. When sites of successful cryomapping are identified by demonstrating BT block with no modification of the basal AVN conduction, the cryoablation mode is activated, in which a target temperature below −75°C is sought (a temperature of −75° to −80°C is generally achieved). The application is then continued for up to 480 seconds, creating an irreversible lesion. If the catheter tip is in close contact with the endocardium, a prompt drop in catheter tip temperature should be seen as soon as the cryoablation mode is activated. A slow decline in temperature or very high flow rates of refrigerant during ablation suggests poor catheter tip tissue contact and, in such a case, cryoablation is interrupted and the catheter is repositioned.

Advantages of Cryoablation. One of the distinct advantages of cryothermal technology is the ability to demonstrate loss of function of tissue reversibly with cooling (cryomapping), thereby demonstrating the functionality of prospective ablation sites without inducing permanent injury. Furthermore, once the catheter tip temperature is reduced below 0°C, progressive ice formation at the catheter tip causes adherence to the adjacent tissue (cryoadherence). A disadvantage of cryoablation is that the cryocatheter is not yet as steerable as the conventional RF catheter, which can potentially limit proper positioning of the catheter tip.

Outcome of Cryoablation. The success rate is more than 90%. Although transient modifications of the normal AVN conduction pathways can be observed during cooling, no permanent modifications have been observed. In fact, immediate discontinuation of cryothermal energy application at any temperature on observation of modification of conduction over normal pathways results in return to baseline condition soon after discontinuation. Resumption of BT conduction with palpitation recurrences can occur in up to 20% of patients; however, especially in young healthy individuals, a recurrence is more acceptable than permanent complete AV block requiring pacing, which was invariably the case in many series of RF ablation of these pathways.

Ablation of Epicardial Bypass Tracts

Anatomical Considerations

Epicardial BTs can be found at any location, but they are most common in the posteroseptal and left posterior regions.[52,59] Up to 20% of all posteroseptal BTs and 40% of those in patients referred after a failed ablation procedure are epicardial. Epicardial BTs also account for 4% of left lateral ablation cases and 10% of those in patients referred after a failed ablation attempt. ECG predictors of epicardial posteroseptal BTs include the following: (1) steep negative delta wave in lead II; (2) steep positive delta wave in aVR; and (3) deep S wave in V_6.[66]

Epicardial BTs may consist of connections between the muscular coat of the CS and ventricle. These BTs are ablatable only within a branch of the CS, most commonly the middle cardiac vein, on the floor of the CS at the orifice of a venous branch, or within a CS diverticulum.[59] Rarely, a transcutaneous pericardial approach is required to ablate epicardial BTs that are posteroseptal or right-sided. In the presence of CS-ventricular BTs, ventricular activation within a branch of the CS precedes endocardial activation, and CS muscle extension potentials usually are recorded in the venous branch, producing a pattern similar to a BT potential.[52,59] The closer proximity of these BTs to the CS than the mitral annulus results in large BT potentials recorded within the CS and susceptibility to ablation from within the CS. Such large BT potentials usually exceed the local atrial and/or ventricular electrogram amplitude. When no effective sites result from endocardial mapping, the presence of an epicardial BT should be considered. An epicardial location of the BT is suggested if the earliest site of endocardial ventricular activation does not precede the onset of the delta wave.

Other types of unusual BTs that cannot be ablated with a standard endocardial approach at the annulus have been described. These include BTs that connect the RA appendage to the RV, which can be successfully ablated using a transcutaneous pericardial approach or endocardial ablation over a large area.[67,68] Another example is BTs closely associated with the ligament of Marshall, which can be ablated by targeting this ligament.[69]

Technical Considerations

CS venography is typically required to help delineate its anatomy and guide ablation.[59] Also, coronary angiography should be performed before delivering RF energy near or within a branch of the CS to determine whether there are any branches of the right or left coronary artery in proximity to the ablation site. If there is a branch of the right coronary artery within 2 mm of the ablation site, there may be a high risk of coronary artery injury if RF energy is delivered. In this situation, cryoablation can be performed with little or no risk of coronary artery injury.

A 4-mm-tip 7 Fr (for CS) or 6 Fr (for CS branches) ablation catheter is generally used. However, a conventional ablation catheter may completely occlude a branch of the CS, preventing cooling of the ablation electrode and resulting in high impedance when RF energy is delivered. This markedly reduces the amount of power that can be delivered and may result in adherence of the ablation electrode to the wall of the vein. An external saline-cooled ablation catheter allows more consistent delivery of RF energy, with less heating at the electrode-tissue interface.

RF energy of 20 to 30 W and temperature of 55° to 60°C for 30 to 60 seconds is delivered at sites within the CS, with the ablation catheter tip directed toward the ventricle within the CS (by maintaining a gentle counterclockwise torque on the ablation catheter). RF energy is stopped if impedance rises significantly (more than 130 to 140 Ω).[59]

Epicardial posteroseptal BTs are most successfully ablated from the terminal segment of the middle cardiac vein or posterior coronary vein at the site recording the largest, sharpest unipolar BT potential. However, the distal right (or left) coronary artery is frequently located within 2 mm of the ideal ablation site, increasing the risk of acute arterial injury.

Causes of Failed Bypass Tract Ablation

Technical difficulties are the most common cause of failed BT ablation. These difficulties are typically related to catheter manipulation and stability or inability to access the target site, and are occasionally caused by inability to deliver sufficient energy to the target site. They are more common with right-sided BTs because of the smooth atrial aspect of the tricuspid annulus. Such difficulties can be overcome by using preformed guiding sheaths to help stabilize the catheter, using different catheter curvatures and shaft stiffness, changing the approach for ablation (e.g., from transseptal to transaortic, or from IVC to SVC), or changing the ablation modality. Cryoablation can help achieve better catheter stability and target sites that might otherwise be avoided because of the risk of damage to neighboring structures. Large (8-mm) ablation electrodes and cooled RF ablation can also help generate large RF lesions. However, other causes of ablation failure should be considered first before shifting to those approaches, which are only rarely required for BT ablation.

Mapping errors are the second most common cause of failed BT ablation. Mapping pitfalls are largely related to inaccurate localization of a BT that has an oblique course. This is more likely to occur when retrograde atrial activation mapping is performed with the ablation catheter positioned at the ventricular side of the annulus because of the oblique course of the BT, the site of the earliest atrial activation recorded from the ventricular aspect of the annulus does not correspond to the ventricular insertion site. Similar situations can occur when the ablation catheter is positioned on the atrial aspect of the annulus and RF applications are delivered where the earliest ventricular activation is recorded. In these situations, mapping for the earliest atrial activation site with the catheter on the atrial side of the annulus, or mapping for the earliest ventricular activation site with the catheter on the ventricular side of the annulus, should be undertaken.

Failure to recognize that a posteroseptal BT is left-sided rather than right-sided, and epicardial location of a left-sided or a posteroseptal BT, are other potential causes of failed ablation of those BTs. Detailed mapping in the CS should be considered in such situations. Furthermore, some BTs insert in the ventricle at a distance from the annulus, in which case a search for a presumed BT potential within the ventricle adjacent to the region of the earliest ventricular activation recorded at the annulus can be helpful. Unusual BTs (e.g., atriofascicular BTs) and anatomical abnormality (e.g., congenital heart disease) also account for some failures in BT ablation.

Catheter-induced trauma to the BT also can lead to ablation failure. Catheter-induced BT trauma is often persistent, leading to discontinuation of the mapping and ablation procedure in many cases, and the long-term risk for recovery of BT function is high.[70] Superoparaseptal and atriofascicular BTs exhibit the highest incidence of mechanical trauma, followed by left free wall BTs.[70] The outcome can still be improved in these situations by close observation of the ECG recordings to recognize catheter-induced trauma of a BT promptly and, whenever conduction block in the BT does not resolve within 1 minute, by immediate application of RF energy, provided that the catheter has not moved from the site of presumed trauma.[70]

Endpoints of Ablation

Confirmation of complete loss of BT function, and not just noninducibility of tachycardias, is essential. Confirmation of complete loss of anterograde BT function using AES and atrial pacing is achieved by demonstrating lack of preexcitation and marked prolongation of the local AV interval at the ablation site. Atrial stimulation should be performed at sites and rates that were associated with preexcitation before ablation.

Confirmation of complete loss of retrograde BT function using VES and ventricular pacing is achieved by demonstrating concentric and decremental retrograde atrial activation, consistent with VA conduction over the AVN, VA dissociation, and/or marked prolongation of the local VA interval at the ablation site. Ventricular stimulation should be performed at sites and rates that were associated with retrograde VA conduction over the BT before ablation. Para-Hisian pacing and RV apical versus RV basilar pacing can also help confirm the absence of septal and paraseptal BT function.

Outcome

RF ablation is a highly effective and curative treatment for AVRT (more than 90%). Initially successful RF ablation is persistent and late recurrence of BT conduction after ablation is rare (4%).[52,53,71] Short runs of palpitations are frequent, usually caused by isolated or short runs of PACs or PVCs and not by recurrence of BT conduction, and can be easily managed with symptomatic treatment without further investigation. Recurrence of BT-mediated tachycardia is usually observed during the first month after ablation, whereas later symptoms (palpitations appearing more than 3 months after the ablation) are highly suggestive of SVTs not related to the ablated BT and justify thorough evaluation (e.g., event monitoring, long-term ECG monitoring, new EP study).

In a survey of 6065 patients, the long-term success rate was 98% and a repeat procedure was necessary in 2.2% of cases.[52] Serious complication (e.g., cardiac tamponade, AV block, coronary artery injury, retroperitoneal hemorrhage, stroke) occurred in 0.6% of patients, with one fatality (0.02%).[52] Therefore, the one-time risk of catheter ablation is considerably lower than the cumulative annual risk associated with the WPW syndrome. It is clear that the treatment of choice for patients with the WPW syndrome who may be at risk for life-threatening arrhythmias is catheter ablation. In addition, the highly favorable risk-benefit ratio justifies the use of catheter ablation as first-line therapy for any patient with BT-dependent tachycardia requiring treatment.

Success rates and risk of complications vary with different BT locations. Ablation of right free wall BT is associated with a success rate of 93% to 98%, a recurrence rate of 21%, and a complication rate less than that with other BT locations. Ablation of posteroseptal BTs is also associated with a high success rate (98%) and a recurrence rate of 12%. With ablation of superoparaseptal BTs, the reported success rate is up to 97%, with a risk of RBBB in 5% to 10% of cases. Similarly, ablation of midseptal BTs is associated with a success rate of 98%, with an incidence of first-degree AV block in 2% and second-degree AV block in 2%.

The immediate success rate of transaortic ablation of left free wall BTs is 86% to 100% (highest with anterograde BT activation), and the recurrence rate is 2% to 5%, less frequent than for BTs at other locations. Complications of this approach include vascular complications (50% of all complications: groin hematoma, aortic dissection, and thrombosis), cardiac tamponade, stroke, coronary dissection (from direct catheter trauma), injury to the left circumflex coronary artery (from subannular RF application), valvular damage, and systemic embolism (from aortic atherosclerosis, catheter tip coagulum, or ablation site thrombosis). The transseptal approach, on the other hand, is associated with a success rate of 85% to 100%, a recurrence rate of 3% to 6.6%, and a complication rate of 0% to 6%. Such complications include coronary spasm, cardiac tamponade, systemic embolization (0.08%), and death (0.08%).

The ablation of epicardial BTs (within the CS) is associated with a success rate of 62% to 100% and a complication rate of 0% to 6%. Complications associated with this approach include coronary artery spasm, CS spasm, cardiac tamponade, right coronary artery occlusion, and pericarditis.

REFERENCES

1. Wolff L, Parkinson J, White PD: Bundle branch block with a short P-R interval in healthy young people prone to paroxysmal tachycardia. Am Heart J 1930;5:685.
2. Lown B, Ganong WF, Levine SA: The syndrome of short P-R interval, normal QRS complex and paroxysmal rapid heart action. Circulation 1952;5:693.
3. Josephson ME: Preexcitation syndromes. *In* Josephson ME (ed): Clinical Cardiac Electrophysiology, 3rd ed. Philadelphia, Lippincott, Williams & Wilkins, 2002, pp 322-424.
4. Mahaim I: Kent's fiber in the A-V paraspecific conduction through the upper connection of the bundle of His-Tawara. Am Heart J 1947;33:651.
5. Cain ME, Luke RA, Lindsay BD: Diagnosis and localization of accessory pathways. Pacing Clin Electrophysiol 1992;15:801.

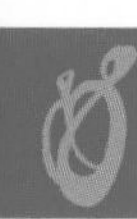

6. Chen SA, Tai CT, Chiang CE, et al: Electrophysiological characteristics, electropharmacological responses and radiofrequency ablation in patients with decremental accessory pathway. J Am Coll Cardiol 1996;28:732.
7. Zipes DP, DeJoseph RL, Rothbaum DA: Unusual properties of accessory pathways. Circulation 1974;49:1200.
8. Otomo K, Gonzalez MD, Beckman KJ, et al: Reversing the direction of paced ventricular and atrial wavefronts reveals an oblique course in accessory AV pathways and improves localization for catheter ablation. Circulation 2001;104:550.
9. Della BP, Brugada P, Talajic M, et al: Atrial fibrillation in patients with an accessory pathway: Importance of the conduction properties of the accessory pathway. J Am Coll Cardiol 1991;17:1352.
10. Fitzsimmons PJ, McWhirter PD, Peterson DW, Kruyer WB: The natural history of Wolff-Parkinson-White syndrome in 228 military aviators: A long-term follow-up of 22 years. Am Heart J 2001;142:530.
11. Pappone C, Santinelli V, Rosanio S, et al: Usefulness of invasive electrophysiological testing to stratify the risk of arrhythmic events in asymptomatic patients with Wolff-Parkinson-White pattern: Results from a large prospective long-term follow-up study. J Am Coll Cardiol 2003;41:239.
12. Priori SG, Aliot E, Blomstrom-Lundqvist C, et al: Task Force on Sudden Cardiac Death of the European Society of Cardiology. Eur Heart J 2001;22:1374.
12a. Munger TM, Packer DL, Hammill SC, et al: A population study of the natural history of Wolff-Parkinson-White syndrome in Olmsted County, Minnesota, 1953-1989. Circulation 1993;87:866-873.
13. Chen SA, Chiang CE, Tai CT, et al: Longitudinal clinical and electrophysiological assessment of patients with symptomatic Wolff-Parkinson-White syndrome and atrioventricular node reentrant tachycardia. Circulation 1996;93:2023.
14. Gollob MH, Green MS, Tang AS, et al: Identification of a gene responsible for familial Wolff-Parkinson-White syndrome. N Engl J Med 2001;344:1823.
15. Gollob MH, Seger JJ, Gollob TN, et al: Novel PRKAG2 mutation responsible for the genetic syndrome of ventricular preexcitation and conduction system disease with childhood onset and absence of cardiac hypertrophy. Circulation 2001;104:3030.
16. MacRae CA, Ghaisas N, Kass S, et al: Familial hypertrophic cardiomyopathy with Wolff-Parkinson-White syndrome maps to a locus on chromosome 7q3. J Clin Invest 1995;96:1216.
17. Blair E, Redwood C, Ashrafian H, et al: Mutations in the gamma(2) subunit of AMP-activated protein kinase cause familial hypertrophic cardiomyopathy: Evidence for the central role of energy compromise in disease pathogenesis. Hum Mol Genet 2001;10:1215.
18. Pappone C, Santinelli V, Manguso F, et al: A randomized study of prophylactic catheter ablation in asymptomatic patients with the Wolff-Parkinson-White syndrome. N Engl J Med 2003;349:1803.
19. Pappone C, Manguso F, Santinelli R, et al: Radiofrequency ablation in children with asymptomatic Wolff-Parkinson-White syndrome. N Engl J Med 2004;351:1197.
20. Blomström-Lundqvist C, Scheinman MM, et al: American College of Cardiology; American Heart Association Task Force on Practice Guidelines; European Society of Cardiology Committee for Practice Guidelines. Writing Committee to Develop Guidelines for the Management of Patients With Supraventricular Arrhythmias: ACC/AHA/ESC guidelines for the management of patients with supraventricular arrhythmias—executive summary: A report of the American College of Cardiology/American Heart Association Task Force on Practice Guidelines and the European Society of Cardiology Committe for Practice Guidelines. Circulation 2003; 108:1871.
21. Scheinman M, Calkins H, Gillette P, et al: NASPE policy statement on catheter ablation: personnel, policy, procedures, and therapeutic recommendations. Pacing Clin Electrophysiol 2003;26:789.
22. Pappone C, Santinelli V: Should catheter ablation be performed in asymptomatic patients with Wolff-Parkinson-White syndrome? Catheter ablation should be performed in asymptomatic patients with Wolff-Parkinson-White syndrome. Circulation 2005;112:2207.
23. Wellens HJ: Should catheter ablation be performed in asymptomatic patients with Wolff-Parkinson-White syndrome? When to perform catheter ablation in asymptomatic patients with a Wolff-Parkinson-White electrocardiogram. Circulation 2005; 112:2201.
24. Knight B, Morady F: Atrioventricular reentry and variants. *In* Zipes DP, Jalife J (eds): Cardiac Electrophysiology: From Cell to Bedside, 4th ed. Philadelphia, WB Saunders, 2004, pp 528-536.
25. Fitzpatrick AP, Gonzales RP, Lesh MD, et al: New algorithm for the localization of accessory atrioventricular connections using a baseline electrocardiogram. J Am Coll Cardiol 1994;23:107.
26. Arruda M, Wang X, McClennand J: ECG algorithm for predicting sites of successful radiofrequency ablation of accessory pathways (abstract). Pacing Clin Electrophysiol 1993;16:865.
27. Chiang CE, Chen SA, Teo WS, et al: An accurate stepwise electrocardiographic algorithm for localization of accessory pathways in patients with Wolff-Parkinson-White syndrome from a comprehensive analysis of delta waves and R/S ratio during sinus rhythm. Am J Cardiol 1995;76:40.
28. Xie B, Heald SC, Bashir Y, et al: Localization of accessory pathways from the 12-lead electrocardiogram using a new algorithm. Am J Cardiol 1994;74:161.
29. Katsouras CS, Greakas GF, Goudevenos JA, et al: Localization of accessory pathways by the electrogram. Pacing Clin Electrophysiol 2004;27:189.
30. Tai CT, Chen SA, Chiang CE, et al: A new electrocardiographic algorithm using retrograde P waves for differentiating atrioventricular node reentrant tachycardia from atrioventricular reciprocating tachycardia mediated by concealed accessory pathway. J Am Coll Cardiol 1997;29:394.
31. Tai CT, Chen SA, Chiang CE, et al: Electrocardiographic and electrophysiological characteristics of anteroseptal, midseptal, and para-Hisian accessory pathways. Implication for radiofrequency catheter ablation. Chest 1996;109:730.
32. Chen SA, Tai CT: Ablation of atrioventricular accessory pathways: Current technique—state of the art. Pacing Clin Electrophysiol 2001 December;24(12): 1795-1809.
33. Fitzgerald DM, Hawthorne HR, Crossley GH, et al: P wave morphology during atrial pacing along the atrioventricular ring. ECG localization of the site of origin of retrograde atrial activation. J Electrocardiol 1996;29:1.
34. Knight BP, Ebinger M, Oral H, et al: Diagnostic value of tachycardia features and pacing maneuvers during paroxysmal supraventricular tachycardia. J Am Coll Cardiol 2000;36:574.
35. Yang Y, Cheng J, Glatter K, et al: Quantitative effects of functional bundle branch block in patients with atrioventricular reentrant tachycardia. Am J Cardiol 2000;85:826.
36. Crawford TC, Mukerji S, Good E, et al: Utility of atrial and ventricular cycle length variability in determining the mechanism of paroxysmal supraventricular tachycardia. J Cardiovasc Electrophysiol 2007;18:698.
37. Glatter KA, Cheng J, Dorostkar P, et al: Electrophysiological effects of adenosine in patients with supraventricular tachycardia. Circulation 1999;99:1034.
38. Saoudi N, Anselme F, Poty H, et al: Entrainment of supraventricular tachycardias: A review. Pacing Clin Electrophysiol 1998 November;21(11 Pt 1):2105-2125.
39. Miles WM, Yee R, Klein GJ, et al: The preexcitation index: an aid in determining the mechanism of supraventricular tachycardia and localizing accessory pathways. Circulation 1986;74:493.
40. Michaud GF, Tada H, Chough S, et al: Differentiation of atypical atrioventricular node re-entrant tachycardia from orthodromic reciprocating tachycardia using a septal accessory pathway by the response to ventricular pacing. J Am Coll Cardiol 2001 October;38(4):1163-1167.
41. Tai CT, Chen SA, Chiang CE, Chang MS: Characteristics and radiofrequency catheter ablation of septal accessory atrioventricular pathways. Pacing Clin Electrophysiol 1999;22:500.
42. Platonov M, Schroeder K, Veenhuyzen GD: Differential entrainment: Beware from where you pace. Heart Rhythm 2007;4:1097.
43. Miller JM, Rosenthal ME, Gottlieb CD, et al: Usefulness of the delta HA interval to accurately distinguish atrioventricular nodal reentry from orthodromic septal bypass tract tachycardias. Am J Cardiol 1991;68:1037.
44. Nakagawa H, Jackman WM: Para-Hisian pacing: Useful clinical technique to differentiate retrograde conduction between accessory atrioventricular pathways and atrioventricular nodal pathways. Heart Rhythm 2005;2:667.
45. Reddy VY, Jongnarangsin K, Albert CM, et al: Para-Hisian entrainment: A novel pacing maneuver to differentiate orthodromic atrioventricular reentrant tachycardia from atrioventricular nodal reentrant tachycardia. J Cardiovasc Electrophysiol 2003;14:1321.
46. Barlow MA, Klein GJ, Simpson CS, et al: Unipolar electrogram characteristics predictive of successful radiofrequency catheter ablation of accessory pathways. J Cardiovasc Electrophysiol 2000;11:146.
47. Miles W: Ablation of right free wall accessory pathways. *In* Huang D, Wilber DJ (eds): Radiofrequency Catheter Ablation of Cardiac Arrhythmias: Basic Concepts and Clinical Applications, 2nd ed. Armonk, NY, Futura, 2000, pp 465-494.
48. Villacastin J, Almendral J, Medina O, et al: "Pseudodisappearance" of atrial electrogram during orthodromic tachycardia: New criteria for successful ablation of concealed left-sided accessory pathways. J Am Coll Cardiol 1996;27:853.
49. Xie B, Heald SC, Camm AJ, et al: Successful radiofrequency ablation of accessory pathways with the first energy delivery: The anatomic and electrical characteristics. Eur Heart J 1996;17:1072.
50. Wood MA, Swartz JF: Ablation of left-free wall accessory pathways. *In* Huang D, Wilber DJ (eds): Radiofrequency Catheter Ablation of Cardiac Arrhythmias: Basic Concepts and Clinical Applications, 2nd ed. Armonk, NY, Futura, 2000, pp 509-540.
51. Chen SA, Chiang CE, Tai CT, Chang MS: Ablation of posteroseptal accessory pathways. *In* Huang D, Wilber DJ (eds): Radiofrequency Catheter Ablation of Cardiac Arrhythmias: Basic Concepts and Clinical Applications, 2nd ed. Armonk, NY, Futura, 2000, pp 495-508.
52. Morady F: Catheter ablation of supraventricular arrhythmias: state of the art. J Cardiovasc Electrophysiol 2004;15:124.
53. Calkins H, Yong P, Miller JM, et al: Catheter ablation of accessory pathways, atrioventricular nodal reentrant tachycardia, and the atrioventricular junction: Final results of a prospective, multicenter clinical trial. The Atakr Multicenter Investigators Group. Circulation 1999;99:262.
54. Guiraudon GM, Klein GJ, Yee R: Surgery for the Wolff-Parkinson-White syndrome: The endocardial approach. *In* Zipes DP, Jalife J (eds): Cardiac Electrophysiology: From Cell to Bedside, 2nd ed. Philadelphia, WB Saunders, 1995, pp 1553-1562.
55. Anderson RH, Ho SY: Anatomy of the atrioventricular junctions with regard to ventricular preexcitation. Pacing Clin Electrophysiol 1997;20(Pt 2):2072.
56. Chen SA, Tai CT, Lee SH, et al: Electrophysiological characteristics and anatomical complexities of accessory atrioventricular pathways with successful ablation of anterograde and retrograde conduction at different sites. J Cardiovasc Electrophysiol 1996;7:907.
57. Shpun S, Gepstein L, Hayam G, Ben-Haim SA: Guidance of radiofrequency endocardial ablation with real-time three-dimensional magnetic navigation system. Circulation 1997;96:2016.
58. Chiang CE, Chen SA, Tai CT, et al: Prediction of successful ablation site of concealed posteroseptal accessory pathways by a novel algorithm using baseline electrophysiological parameters: implication for an abbreviated ablation procedure. Circulation 1996;93:982-991.
59. Sun Y, Arruda M, Otomo K, et al: Coronary sinus-ventricular accessory connections producing posteroseptal and left posterior accessory pathways: Incidence and electrophysiological identification. Circulation 2002;106:1362.

60. Schluter M, Cappato R, Ouyang F, Kuck KH: Ablation of anteroseptal and midseptal accessory pathways. *In* Huang D, Wilber DJ (eds): Radiofrequency Catheter Ablation of Cardiac Arrhythmias: Basic Concepts and Clinical Applications, 2nd ed. Armonk, NY, Futura, 2000, pp 541-558.
61. Chang SL, Lee SH, Tai CT, et al: Electrocardiographic and electrophysiological characteristics of midseptal accessory pathways. J Cardiovasc Electrophysiol 2005;16:237.
62. Haghjoo M, Kharazi A, Fazelifar AF, et al: Electrocardiographic and electrophysiological characteristics of anteroseptal, midseptal, and posteroseptal accessory pathways. Heart Rhythm 2007;4:1411.
63. Skanes AC, Dubuc M, Klein GJ: Cryothermal ablation of the slow pathway for the elimination of atrioventricular nodal reentrant tachycardia. Circulation 2000;102:2856.
64. Skanes AC, Yee R, Krahn AD, Klein GJ: Cryoablation of atrial arrhythmias. Cardiol Electrophysiol Rev 2002;6:383.
65. Kimman GP, Szili-Torok T, Theuns DA, et al: Comparison of radiofrequency versus cryothermy catheter ablation of septal accessory pathways. Heart 2003;89:1091.
66. Takahashi A, Shah DC, Jaïs P, et al: Specific electrocardiographic features of manifest coronary vein posteroseptal accessory pathways. J Cardiovasc Electrophysiol 1998;9:1015.
67. Lam C, Schweikert R, Kanagaratnam L, Natale A: Radiofrequency ablation of a right atrial appendage–ventricular accessory pathway by transcutaneous epicardial instrumentation. J Cardiovasc Electrophysiol 2000;11:1170.
68. Goya M, Takahashi A, Nakagawa H, Iesaka Y: A case of catheter ablation of accessory atrioventricular connection between the right atrial appendage and right ventricle guided by a three-dimensional electroAnatomic mapping system. J Cardiovasc Electrophysiol 1999;10:1112.
69. Hwang C, Peter CT, Chen PS: Radiofrequency ablation of accessory pathways guided by the location of the ligament of Marshall. J Cardiovasc Electrophysiol 2003;14:616.
70. Belhassen B, Viskin S, Fish R, et al: Catheter-induced mechanical trauma to accessory pathways during radiofrequency ablation: incidence, predictors and clinical implications. J Am Coll Cardiol 1999;33:767.
71. Morady F: Radio-frequency ablation as treatment for cardiac arrhythmias. N Engl J Med 1999;340:534.

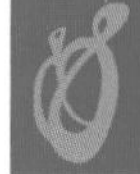

CHAPTER 15

Variants of Preexcitation

MAHAIM FIBERS (ATYPICAL BYPASS TRACTS)

Definition

Mahaim Fibers. In 1937, during pathological examination of the heart, Mahaim and Benatt identified islands of conducting tissue extending from the His bundle (HB) into the ventricular myocardium. These fibers were called Mahaim fibers or fasciculoventricular fibers.[1-3] This description was subsequently expanded to include connections between the atrioventricular node (AVN) and the ventricular myocardium (nodoventricular fibers). Later, it was recognized that bypass tracts (BTs) could arise from the AVN and insert into the right bundle branch (RB; nodofascicular fibers).[2-4] This classification for Mahaim fibers persisted until evidence suggested that the anatomical substrate of tachycardias with characteristics previously attributed to nodoventricular and nodofascicular fibers is actually atrioventricular and atriofascicular BTs with decremental conduction properties (i.e., conduction slows at faster heart rates) (Fig. 15-1).[4] Although these BTs are sometimes collectively referred to as Mahaim fibers, the use of this term is discouraged because it is more illuminating to name the precise BT according to its connections. In this chapter, these BTs are referred to as *atypical* BTs to differentiate them from the more common (*typical*) rapidly conducting atrioventricular (AV) BTs that result in the Wolff-Parkinson-White (WPW) syndrome.[5,6]

Mahaim Tachycardias. The term *Mahaim tachycardia* is used to describe the typical constellation of electrophysiological (EP) features that characterize this unusual form of reentrant tachycardia using an atypical BT, without implication about the underlying anatomical cause. It should be noted that, because the term was originally applied to an anatomical finding and subsequently (incorrectly) applied to physiology that matched what would be expected from this anatomy, it has given rise to more confusion than understanding. Hence, the use of the term *Mahaim tachycardia* should generally be discouraged; instead, one should simply describe the physiological characteristics of the tachyarrhythmia.[5,7]

Types of Atypical Bypass Tracts

Long Decrementally Conducting Atrioventricular Bypass Tracts and Atriofascicular Bypass Tracts. These BTs comprise the majority (80%) of atypical BTs; their atrial insertion site is in the right atrial (RA) free wall.[8,9] These BTs tend (84%) to cross the tricuspid annulus in the lateral, anterolateral, or anterior region. They extend along the right ventricular (RV) free wall to the region where the moderator band usually inserts at the apical third of the RV free wall, inserting into the distal part of the RB (atriofascicular BT) or ventricular myocardium close to the RB (long decrementally conducting atrioventricular BT). The tissue of these BTs is structurally similar to the normal AV junction, with an AVN-like structure leading to a His bundle (HB)–like structure. In essence, those BTs function as an auxiliary conduction system parallel to the normal conduction system (AVN–His-Purkinje system [HPS]).[9] These BTs demonstrate decremental conduction and Wenckebach-type block in response to rapid atrial pacing and are sensitive to adenosine. The conduction delay in these BTs has been localized to the intraatrial portion of the BT (the AVN-like portion); the interval from the inscription of the BT potential at the tricuspid annulus and the onset of ventricular activation (BT-V interval) remains constant.[5,6,9-11]

Short Decrementally Conducting Atrioventricular Bypass Tracts. These BTs are analogous to decrementally conducting concealed BTs responsible for the permanent form of junctional reciprocating tachycardia (PJRT) in that they bridge the AV rings and insert proximally into the RV base near the AV annulus.[8,12,13] These BTs primarily arise from the RA free wall, but can also arise from the posterior or septal region. Although these BTs demonstrate decremental conduction and Wenckebach-type block in response to rapid atrial pacing, they do not consistently appear to be responsive to adenosine, which suggests that their structure is not composed of AVN-like tissue.[13]

Nodoventricular Bypass Tracts and Nodofascicular Bypass Tracts. Nodoventricular BTs arise in the normal AVN

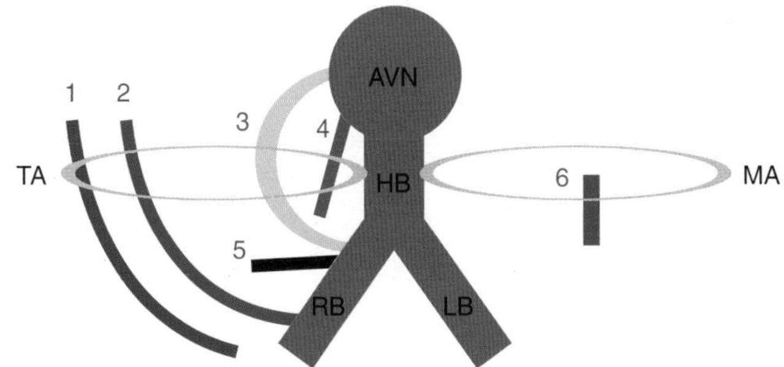

FIGURE 15–1 Schematic of variant endocardial atrioventricular bypass tracts (AV BTs). 1, long atrioventricular BT; 2, atriofascicular BT; 3, nodofascicular BT; 4, nodoventricular BT; 5, fasciculoventricular BT; 6, short AV BT. AVN = atrioventricular node; HB = His bundle; LB = left bundle branch; MA = mitral annulus; RB = right bundle branch; TA = tricuspid annulus.

and insert into the myocardium near the AV junction.[4,8,9,12] Nodofascicular BTs arise in the normal AVN and insert into the RB. These BTs are sensitive to adenosine.[5]

Fasciculoventricular Bypass Tracts. Fasciculoventricular BTs are the rarest form of preexcitation (1.2% to 5.1% of atypical BTs). These BTs have different features from the other atypical BTs, and are discussed separately (see later).[5]

Arrhythmias Associated with Atypical Bypass Tracts

Atypical BTs in patients with clinical arrhythmias have the following characteristics: (1) unidirectional (anterograde-only) conduction (with rare exceptions); (2) long conduction times; and (3) decremental conduction.

The atypical BTs comprise 3% to 5% of all BTs. The incidence is slightly higher (6%) in patients presenting with supraventricular tachycardia (SVT) with a left bundle branch block (LBBB) morphology.[12] Multiple BTs occur in 10% of patients with atypical BTs. In some cases, a typical, rapidly conducting AV BT can mask the presence of an atypical BT, which only becomes apparent after ablation of the typical BT. Dual AVN pathways or multiple BTs occur in 40% of patients with atypical BTs. Atypical BTs can also be associated with Ebstein's anomaly.

Supraventricular Tachycardias Requiring an Atrioventricular Bypass Tract for Initiation and Maintenance. Antidromic atrioventricular reentrant tachycardia (AVRT) can utilize the atypical BT anterogradely and the HPS-AVN retrogradely. Antidromic AVRT can also utilize the atypical BT anterogradely and a second AV BT retrogradely. In the latter case, the AVN can participate as an innocent bystander mediating anterograde or retrograde fusion. Because these atypical BTs almost always conduct anterogradely only, they cannot mediate orthodromic AVRT, but can mediate antidromic AVRT or can be an innocent bystander during other SVTs (e.g., atrioventricular nodal reentrant tachycardia [AVNRT]). However, they can coexist with typical rapidly conducting AV BTs. AVRTs using a nodoventricular or nodofascicular BT as the anterograde limb generally utilize a second AV BT as the retrograde limb of the reentrant circuit.[5]

Supraventricular Tachycardias not Requiring an Atrioventricular Bypass Tract for Initiation and Maintenance. AVNRT, atrial tachycardia (AT), atrial flutter (AFL), or atrial fibrillation (AF) can coexist with atypical BTs, in which case the atypical BTs function as bystanders, wholly or partly responsible for ventricular activation during the tachycardia.[8]

Electrocardiographic Features

Normal Sinus Rhythm

During normal sinus rhythm (NSR), the ECG shows normal QRS or minimal preexcitation in most patients with atypical BTs. Subtle preexcitation can be suspected by the absence of the normal septal forces (small q waves) in leads I, aVL, and V_5-V_6 and the presence of an rS complex in lead III in the setting of a narrow QRS.[14] The amount of preexcitation depends on the relative conduction time over the AVN and BT. Maneuvers that prolong conduction over the AVN (e.g., atrial pacing, vagal maneuvers, or drugs) to a greater degree than BT conduction will increase the degree of preexcitation. Because the atypical BTs exhibit decremental conduction, increasing the atrial pacing rate results in prolongation of the P-delta interval. In contrast, in the presence of typical rapidly-conducting AV BTs, the P-delta interval remains constant regardless of the degree of preexcitation, because the latter depends primarily on the relative conduction time over the AVN. Therefore, prolonging AVN conduction time results in more preexcitation, but with a constant P-delta interval, because conduction over the BT is constant.[5,12,14-16]

Preexcited QRS Morphology

For atriofascicular and nodofascicular BTs, the QRS is relatively narrow (133 ± 10 milliseconds), and its morphology is classic for typical LBBB with a QRS axis between 0 and −75 degrees and a late precordial R/S transition zone (at V_4 or V_5, and sometimes V_6). However, for long decrementally conducting atrioventricular BTs, the QRS is relatively wider (166 ± 26 milliseconds) and the LBBB pattern is less typical (with broad initial r in V_1). The QRS is even wider and the LBBB pattern is less typical with nodoventricular and decrementally conducting short AV BTs than that with atriofascicular or long decrementally conducting AV BTs.[5,14,16]

Supraventricular Tachycardias

Arrhythmias associated with atypical BTs are associated with LBBB and, most often, in case of long decrementally conducting atrioventricular and atriofascicular BTs, left axis deviation on the surface ECG (Fig. 15-2). There are several ECG features that suggest (although are not diagnostic of) atypical BTs as the cause of an SVT with LBBB pattern. These include (1) QRS axis between 0 and −75 degrees, (2) QRS duration of 150 milliseconds or less, (3) R wave in lead 1, (4) rS complex in lead V_1, and (5) precordial R wave transition in lead V_4 or later.[5,14,16]

Electrophysiological Testing

Baseline Observations During Normal Sinus Rhythm

In the baseline state, minimal or no preexcitation can be present; thus, the His bundle–ventricular (HV) interval is normal or slightly short.

Atrial Pacing and Atrial Extrastimulation During Normal Sinus Rhythm. Progressively shorter atrial pacing cycle lengths (CLs) or atrial extrastimulus (AES) coupling intervals produce decremental conduction in both the atypical BT and, to a greater degree, the AVN (Fig. 15-3).[8,12] Consequently, the atrial–His bundle (AH) interval increases, the QRS morphology gradually shifts to a more preexcited LBBB morphology, and the atrioventricular (AV; A-delta) interval increases. However, the AV (A-delta) interval increases to a lesser degree than the AH interval prolongation. This is in contrast to the case of typical rapidly conducting AV BTs, in which the AV (A-delta) interval remains constant despite prolongation of the AH interval and exaggeration of the degree of preexcitation, because the

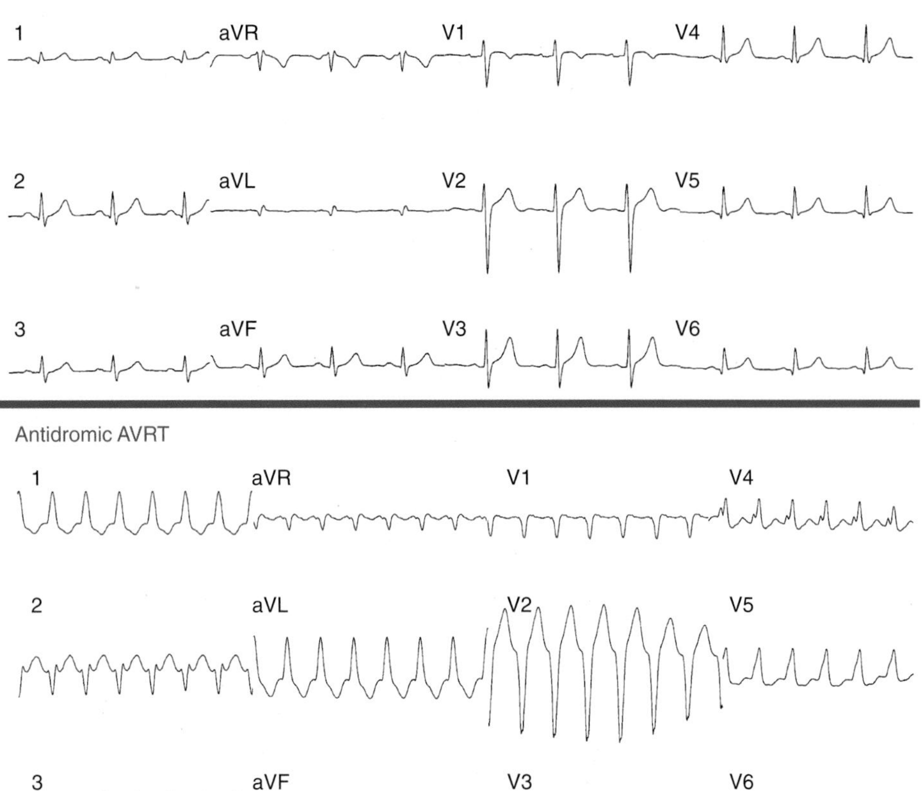

FIGURE 15–2 Atriofascicular bypass tracts (BTs). **Upper panel,** Normal sinus rhythm (NSR) with no evidence of preexcitation. **Lower panel,** Antidromic atrioventricular reentrant tachycardia (AVRT) using an atriofascicular BT. QRS morphology during tachycardia resembles left bundle branch block aberration because of anterograde activation over the atriofascicular BT. Retrograde P waves can be seen after the end of the QRS.

A-delta interval represents the conduction time over the BT. Those BTs maintain constant conduction time during different pacing rates and AES coupling intervals—that is, nondecremental conduction.[5]

With progressively shorter atrial pacing CLs or AES coupling intervals, the HV interval decreases as the His potential becomes progressively inscribed into the QRS (usually within the first 5 to 25 milliseconds after the onset of the QRS). The His potential eventually becomes activated retrogradely as the wavefront travels anterogradely down the BT and then retrogradely up the RB to the HB (see Fig. 15-3). When the His potential is lost within the QRS, it is unclear whether anterograde AV conduction continues to proceed over the HB or block has occurred.[8,12]

At the point of maximal preexcitation, the AV (A-delta) interval continues to prolong with more rapid pacing because of decremental conduction over the BT, and the His potential–QRS relationship remains unaltered because the HB is activated retrogradely until block in the BT occurs. The fixed ventricular–His bundle (VH) interval, despite shorter pacing CLs or AES coupling intervals, suggests that the BT inserts into or near the distal RB at the anterior free wall of the RV with retrograde conduction to the HB. Whenever the VH interval is less than 20 milliseconds, insertion into the RB (i.e., atriofascicular or nodofascicular BT) is likely. On the other hand, with long decrementally conducting atrioventricular BTs, which insert into the ventricular myocardium close to the RB, the VH interval approximates the HV interval minus the duration of the His potential (because the His potential is activated retrogradely).[5,8,12]

For short decrementally conducting BTs, the HB is activated anterogradely, and retrograde conduction to the HB is only seen following AV block or during antidromic AVRT. Decremental conduction (progressive prolongation of the AV interval) and Wenckebach-type block develop in the BT. The conduction delay in these BTs is localized to the intraatrial portion of the BT; the interval from the inscription of the BT potential at the tricuspid annulus to the onset of ventricular activation (BT-V interval) remains constant.[5]

Dual AVN physiology is common in these patients. Sometimes, during AES, a jump from the fast to the slow AVN pathway prolongs the AH interval enough to unmask preexcitation over the BT, at which time the His potential will be inscribed within the QRS.

The site of the earliest ventricular activation during preexcitation is at the RV apex for long, decrementally conducting AV and atriofascicular BTs, but adjacent to the annulus near the base of the RV for short, decrementally conducting AV BTs.

The degree of preexcitation is not influenced by the site of atrial stimulation for nodofascicular and nodoventricular BTs, whereas it increases when atrial stimulation is performed closer to the atrial insertion site of atrioventricular or atriofascicular BTs.

Ventricular Pacing and Ventricular Extrastimulation During Normal Sinus Rhythm. Because these BTs rarely have retrograde conduction, ventricular stimulation cannot help in mapping of the BT location. VA conduction during ventricular pacing should proceed over the HPS-AVN with concentric atrial activation sequence and decremental properties in response to progressively shorter ventricular pacing CLs or VES coupling intervals. If rapid and fixed VA conduction is present, a separate retrogradely

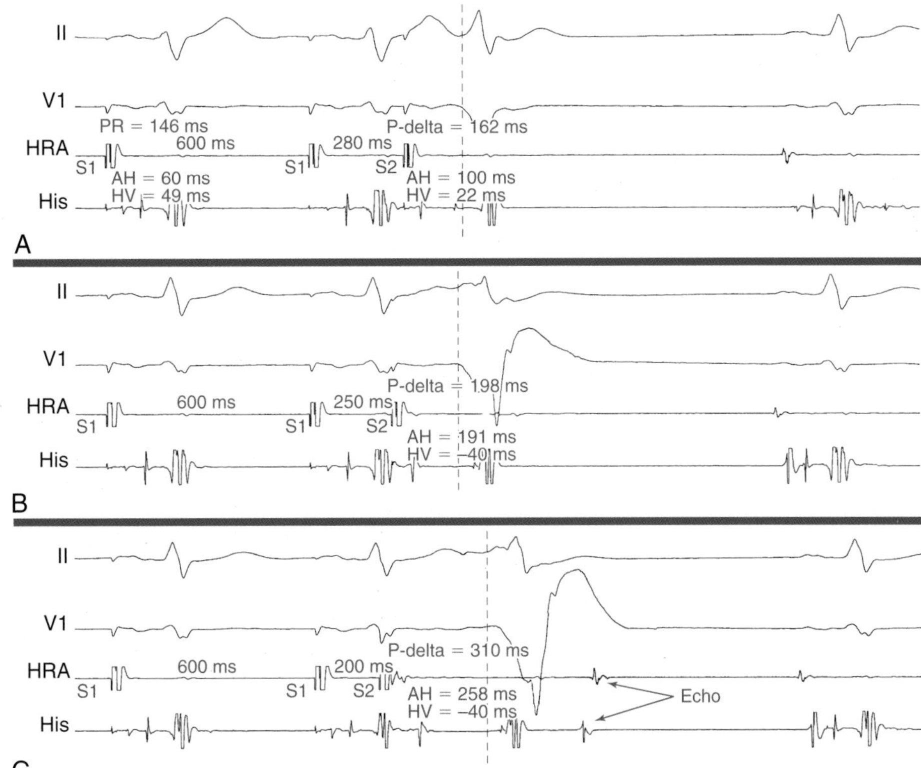

FIGURE 15–3 Effect of atrial extrastimulation (AES) on preexcitation via a long atrioventricular bypass tract (BT). No preexcitation is observed during normal sinus rhythm and during the pacing drive at a cycle length of 600 msec (normal PR and His bundle–ventricular [HV] intervals). **A,** AES produces decremental conduction in the atrioventricular node (AVN) with prolongation of the atrial–His bundle (AH) interval (from 60 to 100 msec), associated with manifest preexcitation and shortening of the HV interval (from 49 to 22 msec). **B, C,** Progressively shorter AES coupling intervals produce decremental conduction in the BT and, to a greater degree, in the AVN. Consequently, the AH interval prolongs, the QRS morphology gradually shifts to a more preexcited left bundle branch block morphology, and the AV (P-delta) interval increases. However, the P-delta interval prolongs to a lesser degree than the AH interval. The HV interval decreases (becomes negative) but remains fixed (**B, C**) although the P-delta interval continues to prolong with more premature AES because of decremental conduction over the BT. The fixed ventricular–His bundle (VH) interval, despite shorter AES coupling intervals, suggests that the BT inserts into or near the distal right bundle branch (RB) at the anterior free wall of the right ventricle, with retrograde conduction to the HB. However, because the VH interval is modestly long (40 msec), a long decrementally conducting atrioventricular BT inserting into the ventricle close to the RB is more likely than an atriofascicular BT. **C,** AV reentrant echo complex (red arrows) secondary to anterograde conduction over the BT and retrograde conduction over the AVN.

conducting rapidly conducting AV BT should be excluded. Retrograde dual AVN pathways can be present.

Effects of Adenosine. Adenosine produces conduction delay in most atypical BTs except for short decrementally conducting atrioventricular BTs. The conduction delay has been localized to the intraatrial portion of the BT; the interval from the inscription of the BT potential at the tricuspid annulus and the onset of ventricular activation remains constant.[12,15] When adenosine administration slows AVN conduction, an increase in the degree of preexcitation is noted in all types of BTs (as long as adenosine does not block the BT).

Induction of Tachycardia

Initiation by Atrial Extrastimulation or Atrial Pacing. Initiation of antidromic AVRT by an AES requires the following: (1) intact anterograde conduction over the BT; (2) anterograde block in the AVN or HPS; and (3) intact retrograde conduction over the HPS-AVN once the AVN resumes excitability following partial anterograde penetration. Whereas the latter is usually the limiting factor for the initiation of antidromic AVRT using typical rapidly conducting AV BTs, it is readily available in case of atypical BTs. This is because of the slow decremental conduction anterogradely over the atypical BT, providing adequate delay for full recovery of the HPS-AVN.

Progressively shorter atrial pacing CLs (especially from the RA) results in progressive AV (A-delta) interval prolongation and a greater degree of preexcitation until maximal. Often, once maximal preexcitation has been achieved, cessation of pacing is followed by preexcited SVT. Progressively shorter AES coupling intervals similarly result in progressive AV (A-delta) interval prolongation and a greater degree of preexcitation until maximal. When anterograde AVN conduction fails but conduction persists over the BT, the HPS-AVN can be activated retrogradely to initiate antidromic AVRT.[12]

The sudden appearance of preexcitation associated with a "jump" from the fast to the slow AVN pathway with a His potential inscribed before ventricular activation or with a VH interval of less than 10 milliseconds strongly favors AVNRT. Although a slowly conducting atriofascicular BT that becomes manifest with a jump to the slow AVN pathway cannot be excluded, a consistent pattern of dual pathway dependence and an HV relationship too short to be retrograde from the distal RB would be unlikely.[12] Induction of AVNRT with AES is always associated with a dual pathway response, which may not be seen if the impulse conducts anterogradely over the BT and captures the HB before it is activated by the impulse traversing the slow AVN pathway anterogradely. In other cases, a jump can be seen so that the anterograde His potential follows the QRS with a typical AVN echo to initiate SVT, analogous to 1:2 conduction initiating antidromic AVRT.

Initiation by Ventricular Extrastimulation or Ventricular Pacing. Initiation of antidromic AVRT by ventricular pacing and VES requires the following: (1) retrograde block in the BT, which is almost always available, because the atypical BTs are usually unidirectional; (2) retrograde conduction over the HPS-AVN; and (3) adequate VA delay to allow for recovery of the atrium and BT so it can support subsequent anterograde conduction.

Ventricular pacing can initiate SVT in 85% of cases. Initiation is almost always associated with retrograde conduction up a relatively fast AVN pathway, followed by anterograde conduction down a slow pathway, which is associated with preexcitation. The anterograde slow pathway can be a BT (i.e., antidromic AVRT) or a slow AVN pathway (i.e., AVNRT with an innocent bystander BT). During induction of the SVT by ventricular pacing at a CL similar to the tachycardia CL or by a VES that advances the His potential by a coupling interval similar to the H-H interval during the SVT, the His bundle–atrial (HA) interval following the ventricular stimulus is compared with that during the SVT—an HA interval that is longer with ventricular pacing or VES initiating the SVT than that during the SVT suggests AVNRT. This occurs despite the fact that the H-H interval of the VES (i.e., the interval between the His potential activated anterogradely by the last sinus beat to the His potential activated retrogradely by the VES initiating the SVT) exceeds the H-H interval during the SVT. Because the AVN usually exhibits greater decremental conduction with repetitive engagement of impulses than in response to a single impulse at a similar coupling interval, the more prolonged the HA with the initiating ventricular stimulus, the more likely the SVT is AVNRT. If the SVT uses the BT for anterograde conduction, the HA interval during ventricular pacing or the VES initiating the SVT, at a comparable coupling interval as the tachycardia CL, should have the same HA interval as during the SVT.

Tachycardia Features

Antidromic Atrioventricular Reentrant Tachycardia Using an Atypical Bypass Tract Anterogradely

Site of Earliest Ventricular Activation. In the case of atriofascicular, nodofascicular, and long decrementally conducting AV BTs, the earliest ventricular activation occurs at or near the RV apex. In contrast, for nodoventricular and short decrementally conducting AV BTs, the earliest ventricular activation occurs adjacent to the tricuspid annulus.

Ventricular–His Bundle Interval. For atriofascicular and nodofascicular BTs, the VH interval is short (16 ± 5 milliseconds), much shorter than the nonpreexcited HV interval and also shorter than the VH interval during ventricular pacing (because the BT inserts into the RB, and the HB and ventricle are activated in parallel, not in sequence). The conduction time to the distal RB is short (V-RB = 3 ± 5 milliseconds).[8,15] For long decrementally conducting AV BTs, the VH interval is short (37 ± 9 milliseconds) but longer than that of atriofascicular BTs because the ventricle and HB are activated in sequence, not in parallel. However, the VH interval is still shorter than the nonpreexcited HV interval (the VH interval would approximate the HV interval minus the duration of the His potential, because the BT inserts close to the RB and the His potential is activated retrogradely). These BTs have a longer conduction time to the distal RB (V-RB = 25 ± 6 milliseconds) than the atriofascicular BTs. During antidromic AVRT using a nodoventricular or a short decrementally conducting AV BT, intermediate VH intervals are observed, whereby the His potential is inscribed in the QRS. The VH interval during the AVRT is longer than the nonpreexcited HV interval and than the VH interval during RV apical pacing, exceeding it by the time it takes the impulse to travel from the ventricular insertion site of the BT at the RV base to the distal RB (i.e., because of long V-RB interval).[12,15] When antidromic AVRT occurs in the presence of retrograde right bundle branch block (RBBB), the VH interval is long (the His potential is inscribed after the QRS and the VH interval is longer than the nonpreexcited HV interval). Retrograde block over the RB results in anterograde conduction over the distal RB (in the case of atriofascicular BTs) or RV and transseptal impulse propagation with subsequent retrograde conduction over the LB into the HB and AVN. This results in an antidromic AVRT with a macroreentrant circuit incorporating the left bundle branch (LB) retrogradely and either an atriofascicular, a long decrementally conducting AV BT, or a short decrementally conducting AV BT anterogradely.[12,15]

Atrial-Ventricular Relationship. For atriofascicular, long decrementally conducting AV, and short decrementally conducting AV BTs, a 1:1 A-V relationship is a prerequisite for the maintenance of antidromic AVRT, because parts of both the RA and RV are incorporated in the reentrant circuit. However, in the case of nodofascicular and nodoventricular BTs, the atrium is not part of or required for the reentrant circuit, and AV block or dissociation can (rarely) be present without disrupting the SVT.[12,15]

Response to Drugs. These SVTs are very responsive to and terminate easily with adenosine, calcium channel blockers, and beta blockers.

Preexcited Atrioventricular Nodal Reentrant Tachycardia Using an Atypical Bypass Tract as an Innocent Bystander. The site of earliest ventricular activation depends on the type of the atypical BT mediating preexcitation (see previous discussion). A positive HV interval or VH interval of 10 milliseconds or less (especially when the HA interval is 50 milliseconds or less) is characteristic of AVNRT, because the HB is usually activated anterogradely. However, the HB can become activated retrogradely when conduction over the anterograde slow AVN pathway is very slow; then the VH interval will depend on the type of the atypical BT mediating preexcitation (see earlier).[12,15]

Diagnostic Maneuvers During Tachycardia

Atrial Extrastimulation and Atrial Pacing During Tachycardia. To prove the presence of a BT and its participation in the SVT, a late-coupled AES is delivered from the lateral RA (close to the BT) when the AV junctional portion of the atrium is refractory, so that the AES does not penetrate the AVN, as indicated by the lack of advancement of local atrial activation in the HB or coronary sinus ostium (CS os) recording. Therefore, such an AES cannot conduct to the ventricle over the AVN; this maneuver is analogous to the introduction of VES when the HB is refractory during orthodromic AVRT. If this AES advances (or delays) the timing of the next ventricular activation, it indicates that an anterogradely conducting AV or atriofascicular BT is present, and excludes nodoventricular and nodofascicular BTs. If the AES advances (or delays) the timing of the next ventricular activation and the advanced (or delayed) QRS morphology is identical to that during the SVT, this proves that the AV or atriofascicular BT also mediates preexcitation during the SVT, either as an integral part of the SVT circuit or as an innocent bystander. On the other hand, if the AES advances the timing of both the next ventricular activation and subsequent atrial activation, it proves that the SVT is

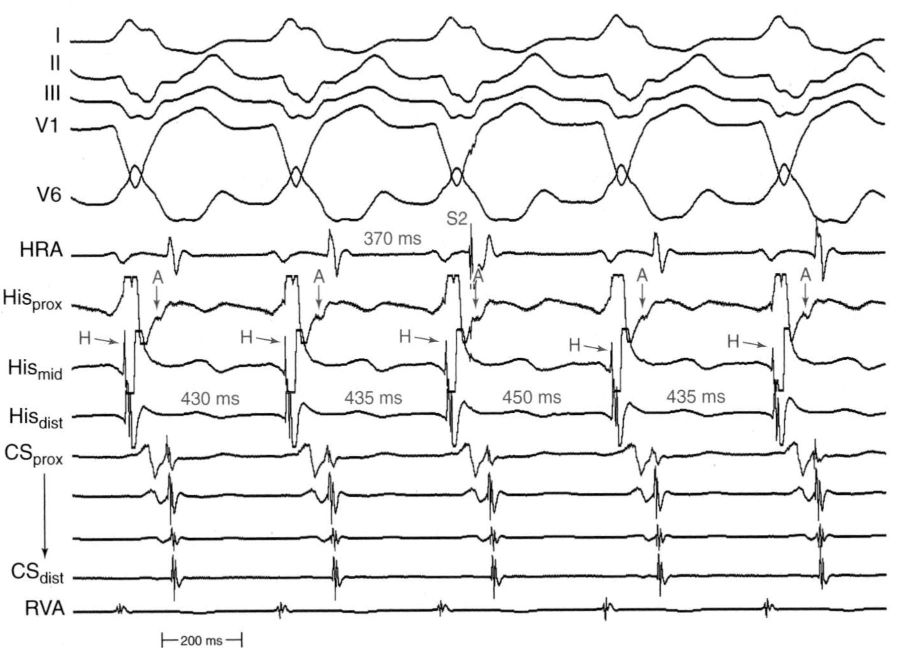

FIGURE 15–4 Atrial extrastimulation (AES) during antidromic atrioventricular reentrant tachycardia (AVRT) using an atriofascicular bypass tract. A late-coupled AES (S2) delivered from the right atrium (RA) when the AV junctional atrium is refractory (as evidenced by the failure of the AES to affect the timing of atrial activation recorded by the proximal His bundle and proximal coronary sinus electrodes) results in a delay in the timing of the next QRS (postexcitation), as well as delay in the timing of the following atrial activation. This confirms the diagnosis of antidromic AVRT and excludes preexcited atrioventricular nodal reentrant tachycardia and ventricular tachycardia as potential mechanisms of this wide QRS complex tachycardia.

an antidromic AVRT using an AV or atriofascicular BT anterogradely, and excludes preexcited AVNRT (Fig. 15-4). Advancement of both ventricular and atrial activation by such an AES requires anterograde conduction over the BT followed by retrograde conduction over the AVN. This can occur during antidromic AVRT but not in AVNRT, because the HB would be refractory because of anterograde activation by the time the advanced ventricular impulse invades the HPS retrogradely, with subsequent failure of the advanced ventricular activation to penetrate the HPS-AVN and affect the timing of subsequent atrial activation.[12,15]

During entrainment of the SVT by atrial pacing at a CL slightly shorter than the tachycardia CL, the presence of a fixed short VH interval suggests antidromic AVRT, but does not exclude AVNRT. SVT can usually be terminated by atrial pacing. Anterograde block is always produced in the AVN, with or without block in the BT. A short-coupled AES can block in the BT, terminating SVT if it is antidromic AVRT or changing to a narrow QRS SVT at the same CL and same HA interval if it is preexcited AVNRT.

Ventricular Extrastimulation and Ventricular Pacing During Tachycardia. Introduction of a VES during the SVT that results in RBBB can be of diagnostic value. In AVNRT, such RBBB will not change the time of the next atrial activation, because the ventricle and HPS are not parts of the AVNRT circuit. Conversely, in antidromic AVRT, such RBBB will increase the size of the reentrant circuit, because the impulse cannot reach the HB through the RB, and it has to travel transseptally and then retrogradely over the LB. This results in prolongation in the VA interval and delay in the timing of the next atrial activation. The increment in the VA interval occurs because of prolongation of the VH interval, and, if RBBB persists, the SVT will have a long VH interval.

The SVT can usually be terminated by ventricular pacing. Termination occurs by retrograde invasion and concealment in the BT, resulting in anterograde block over the BT following conduction to the atrium through the AVN.

Differential Diagnosis

The goals of programmed electrical stimulation during SVT are evaluation of the relationship among the His potential, the QRS, and the VH interval during atrial pacing and during SVT and differentiation between the different types of atypical BTs (Table 15-1). In addition, exclusion of a separate BT is necessary, especially if a rapid and fixed VA interval exists during incremental rate ventricular pacing. Furthermore, it is important to differentiate between antidromic AVRT using the BT anterogradely and preexcited AVNRT in which the BT is an innocent bystander (Table 15-2).

Localization of the Bypass Tract

Mapping principles for typical AV BTs—searching for sites with the earliest atrial activation during retrograde BT conduction and earliest ventricular activation during anterograde BT conduction—are largely inapplicable in the case of atypical BTs because of their unusual course and conduction properties. Therefore, different approaches are used.

Mapping of the ventricular insertion site of atriofascicular and long decrementally conducting AV BTs is difficult because of the long intracardiac course and distal insertion of these BTs, which shows extensive arborization over a wide area of ventricular muscle, with a diameter of up to 0.5 to 2 cm. A propensity to temporary loss of conduction of the atypical BT because of catheter trauma further complicates ventricular mapping.[5]

Mapping of the atrial insertion site can be performed by (1) P-delta interval mapping by stimulation at different atrial sites, (2) recording of the BT potential at the tricuspid annulus, and (3) AES from the RA during antidromic AVRT.[10]

Careful mapping of the tricuspid annulus and the anterior free wall of the RV typically demonstrates discrete potentials with complexes comparable to those recorded at the AV junction. The BT potential is analogous to His potential. Atrial pacing, AES, and adenosine produce delay proximal to BT potential with a constant BT potential to QRS (BT-V) interval. Faster atrial pacing produces Wenckebach block proximal to the BT potential.[15]

Mapping the Atrial Insertion Site

Mapping the Shortest Atrial Stimulus to Delta (S-V) Interval. The mapping catheter is advanced from site to site along the atrial aspect of the tricuspid annulus while

TABLE 15–1 Differentiation Among Different Types of Atypical Bypass Tracts (BTs)

Preexcited QRS Morphology
Atriofascicular BTs: The QRS is relatively narrow (133 ± 10 msec), and is classic for typical LBBB morphology.
Long decrementally conducting atrioventricular BTs: The QRS is relatively wider (166 ± 26 msec) and the LBBB pattern is less typical (with broad initial r in V_1) than that with atriofascicular BTs.
Nodofascicular BTs: Same as for atriofascicular BTs.
Nodoventricular BTs: The QRS is significantly wider and the LBBB pattern is less typical than that with atriofascicular or long decrementally conducting AV BTs.
Short decrementally conducting AV BTs: The QRS is significantly wider and the LBBB pattern is less typical than that with atriofascicular or long decrementally conducting AV BTs.
Site of Earliest Ventricular Activation
Atriofascicular BTs: The earliest ventricular activation occurs at or near the RV apex.
Long decrementally conducting AV BTs: The earliest ventricular activation occurs at or near the RV apex.
Nodofascicular BTs: The earliest ventricular activation occurs at or near the RV apex.
Nodoventricular BTs: The earliest ventricular activation occurs adjacent to the tricuspid annulus.
Short decrementally conducting AV BTs: The earliest ventricular activation occurs adjacent to the tricuspid annulus.
Influence of Site of Atrial Stimulation
Atriofascicular BTs: Preexcitation increases when atrial stimulation is performed closer to the atrial insertion site.
Long decrementally conducting AV BTs: Preexcitation increases when atrial stimulation is performed closer to the atrial insertion site.
Nodofascicular BTs: The degree of preexcitation is not influenced by the site of atrial stimulation.
Nodoventricular BTs: The degree of preexcitation is not influenced by the site of atrial stimulation.
Short decrementally conducting atrioventricular BTs: Preexcitation increases when atrial stimulation is performed closer to the atrial insertion site.
AES Delivered from Lateral RA During Antidromic AVRT when AV Junctional Atrium Is Refractory
Atriofascicular BTs: The AES can advance or delay the next ventricular activation.
Long decrementally conducting AV BTs: The AES can advance or delay the next ventricular activation.
Nodofascicular BTs: The AES cannot advance the next ventricular activation.
Nodoventricular BTs: The AES cannot advance the next ventricular activation.
Short decrementally conducting AV BTs: The AES can advance or delay the next ventricular activation.
VH Interval During Maximal Preexcitation or Antidromic AVRT
Atriofascicular BTs: The VH interval is short (VH interval = 16 ± 5 msec and VRB = 3 ± 5 msec; VH interval < HV interval and < VH interval during RV pacing).
Long decrementally conducting AV BTs: The VH interval is short but longer than that with atriofascicular BTs (VH interval = 37 ± 9 msec and V-RB interval = 25 ± 6 msec).
Nodofascicular BTs: The VH interval is short; as for atriofascicular BTs.
Nodoventricular BTs: The VH interval is intermediate (His potential is inscribed in the QRS, VH interval ≥ HV interval; VH interval > HV interval and > VH interval during RV pacing).
Short decrementally conducting AV BTs: The VH interval is intermediate, as for nodoventricular BTs.
Antidromic AVRT in presence of retrograde RBBB: The VH interval is long (His potential is inscribed after the QRS, VH interval > HV interval).
Presence of VA Block or AV Dissociation
VA block or AV dissociation during the SVT excludes atriofascicular, short decrementally conducting AV BTs, and long decrementally conducting AV BTs, but does not exclude nodofascicular and nodoventricular BTs.
Effects of Adenosine
Adenosine produces conduction delay in most atypical BTs (except for short decrementally conducting BTs).
When adenosine administration slows AVN conduction but not the BT, an increase in the degree of preexcitation is noted in all types of BTs except for fasciculoventricular BTs, whereby the degrees of preexcitation and HV interval remain fixed.

AES = atrial extrastimulation; AV = atrioventricular; AVRT = atrioventricular reentrant tachycardia; HV = His bundle–ventricular; LBBB = left bundle branch block; RA = right atrium; RBBB = right bundle branch block; RV = right ventricle; SVT = supraventricular tachycardia; VA = ventriculoatrial; VH = ventricular–His bundle; V-RB = ventricular–right bundle branch.

pacing from its distal tip. The resulting interval between the stimulus and the onset of the delta wave (S-V interval) should decrease progressively as the BT atrial insertion site is approached, and increase as it is passed. Thus, the atrial pacing site associated with the shortest S-V interval is the site closest to the BT atrial insertion site. It is essential that pacing at different sites be performed at a constant CL to avoid rate-dependent conduction slowing in the BT as a reason for changing the S-V interval. This method is rarely used because of several limitations: (1) a constant distance of the mapping-pacing catheter from the tricuspid annulus must be maintained to reduce the influence of the time spent traversing intervening atrial tissue; (2) catheter manipulation during pacing can result in initiation of tachycardia, which must then be terminated to continue mapping; (3) optimal sites can be overlooked if they cannot be consistently paced because of unstable catheter contact; and (4) this method cannot be applied in the case of incessant tachycardia or when AF is present.[9,15]

Atrial Extrastimulation Mapping During Supraventricular Tachycardias. The BT atrial insertion site is close to the site from which the longest coupled AES during preexcited tachycardia advances the timing of the next ventricular activation. Alternatively, the BT atrial insertion site is close to the site from which the greatest amount of advancement of the next ventricular activation occurs when using a fixed AES coupling interval. This method is rarely used because of several limitations: (1) it is time-consuming, and cannot be used if the SVT is difficult to initiate or nonsustained; (2) it is not particularly useful in cases of true nodofascicular BTs; (3) a constant distance of the mapping-pacing catheter from the tricuspid annulus must be maintained to reduce the influence of the time spent traversing intervening atrial tissue; and (4) optimal sites can be over-

TABLE 15–2 Differentiation Between Antidromic AVRT and Preexcited AVNRT Using an Atypical BT
SVT Induction
Induction of the SVT by ventricular pacing at a CL similar to the tachycardia CL, or by a VES that advances the His potential by a coupling interval similar to the H-H interval during the SVT—the HA interval following such a ventricular stimulus is compared with that during the SVT:
$HA_{VES} > HA_{SVT}$ is diagnostic of AVNRT and excludes antidromic AVRT.
$HA_{VES} \leq HA_{SVT}$ is diagnostic of antidromic AVRT and excludes AVNRT.
Features of the SVT
Positive HV interval or VH interval ≤ 10 msec (especially when HA interval is ≤50 msec) suggests AVNRT.
Continuation of the SVT at the same tachycardia CL, despite anterograde block in the BT (by extrastimuli, drugs, mechanical trauma caused by catheter manipulation, or ablation), is diagnostic of AVNRT and excludes antidromic AVRT.
Termination of the SVT or prolongation of the VA (and VH) interval and tachycardia CL with transient RBBB (caused by mechanical trauma or introduction of VES) is diagnostic of antidromic AVRT and excludes AVNRT.
AES Delivered from Lateral RA when AV Junction Is Refractory
If the AES advances the timing of both the following ventricular activation and the subsequent atrial activation, it proves that the SVT is an antidromic AVRT using an atrioventricular or atriofascicular BT anterogradely, and excludes preexcited AVNRT.
Entrainment of the SVT with Atrial Pacing
The presence of a fixed short VH interval during entrainment of the SVT with atrial pacing suggests antidromic AVRT, and makes AVNRT unlikely (but does not exclude AVNRT).
RV Apical Pacing During NSR
RV apical pacing at the tachycardia CL is performed and the HA interval during RV apical pacing versus the HA interval during SVT are compared:
$HA_{SVT} < HA_{ventricular\ pacing}$ is diagnostic of AVNRT and excludes antidromic AVRT.
$HA_{SVT} \geq HA_{ventricular\ pacing}$ is diagnostic of antidromic AVRT and excludes AVNRT.

AES = atrial extrastimulation; AV = atrioventricular; AVNRT = atrioventricular nodal reentrant tachycardia; AVRT = atrioventricular reentrant tachycardia; BT = bypass tract; CL = cycle length; HA = His bundle–atrial; NSR = normal sinus rhythm; RA = right atrium; RBBB = right bundle branch block; RV = right ventricle; SVT = supraventricular tachycardia; VA = ventriculoatrial; VES = ventricular extrastimulation; VH = ventricular–His bundle.

looked if they cannot be consistently paced because of unstable catheter contact.[9,15]

Mapping the Ventricular Insertion Site

Mapping the Distal Fascicular Insertion Site (for Atriofascicular Bypass Tracts). The distal insertion site of atriofascicular BTs can be localized by careful mapping along the lateral RV wall toward the apex, seeking the earliest site of ventricular activation. A distal RB recording is usually present at this site. This method can be used to map any rhythm during which consistent preexcitation is present (atrial pacing, AF, and preexcited SVT). However, seeking the distal insertion is less precise because a distal RB recording may be localized, but not the portion into which the atriofascicular fiber inserts. It is most useful if the course of the atriofascicular fiber can be traced from the tricuspid annulus to its insertion into the RB. Additionally, ablation at the distal site offers no advantage unless catheter stability is better at that location as opposed to the tricuspid annulus. If the RB is ablated rather than the atriofascicular fiber, RBBB will result. This not only will fail to eliminate the BT function, but can facilitate induction of the SVT by increasing the circuit size.[8-10,15]

Mapping the Distal Ventricular Insertion Site (for Slowly Conducting Atrioventricular Bypass Tracts). Mapping is performed in the same fashion as for typical rapidly conducting AV BTs—seeking the ventricular site with the earliest unipolar or bipolar ventricular electrogram recording. However, there is evidence that a variable degree of arborization of the distal insertion site occurs in some patients. This feature makes the ventricular insertion site a less attractive ablation target because of the potential of requiring ablation of a relatively large amount of ventricular myocardium to be effective.[9,15]

Mapping the Bypass Tracts Potential

Direct recording of the BT potential at the tricuspid annulus is the most precise and preferred method of localizing the atypical BT. The BT potential is usually a low-amplitude, high-frequency recording made at the tricuspid annulus, which resembles a His potential (Fig. 15-5). Only the annular and subannular portions of the BT have been successfully recorded; attempts to record potentials from the atrial portion (corresponding to nodal-like tissue) have been unsuccessful. Distinct atrial, BT, and ventricular potentials can be found at the BT atrial insertion site. Recording a BT potential can be successful during NSR, atrial pacing, or preexcited SVT. However, recording of a BT potential along the tricuspid annulus may not be successful in up to 48% of cases. Furthermore, because of the low amplitude of the BT potential, it is difficult or impossible to record it during AF. Additionally, this technique presents the risk of producing mechanical block in the BT. Nevertheless, this method is less time-consuming and more precise than the previous ones.[10,15]

Mapping Sites of Mechanically Induced Loss of Preexcitation

Atypical BTs are particularly sensitive to mechanical trauma, and catheter manipulation along the tricuspid annulus during mapping of the BT may result in loss of BT function, even as a result of gentle pressure from the catheter tip. When mapping is performed during preexcited atrial pacing or SVT, damage to the BT is indicated by a sudden, transient loss of preexcitation. This phenomenon can be used to localize the BT precisely (bump mapping). Conduction block typically occurs while a BT potential is still recorded; thus, conduction is interrupted within the ventricular course of the BT. Block usually lasts from a few beats to a few minutes but can last for hours, after which preexcitation resumes. This method can be used during any consistently preexcited rhythm (atrial pacing, AF, and antidromic AVRT). However, if it occurs during antidromic AVRT, termination of the antidromic AVRT can result in catheter displacement and loss of the exact location of the BT. Additionally, interruption of BT conduction can occur as the catheter is passing the area, and where the catheter comes to rest may not be the same site as where loss of BT function occurred; in this situation, the target

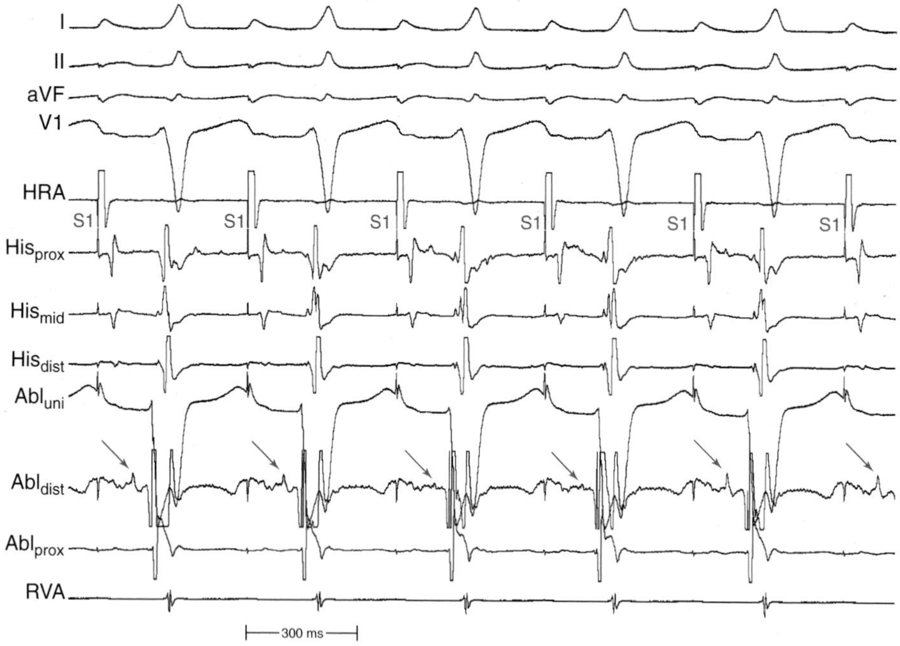

FIGURE 15–5 Ablation of an atriofascicular bypass tract (BT). A discrete potential (arrows) is shown in the ablation recording during atrial pacing, with a small His potential occurring just after the onset of the preexcited QRS. Ablation at this site eliminated this BT in 2 seconds.

cannot be relocated until BT conduction resumes. Delivery of radiofrequency (RF) energy at a site at which catheter pressure caused loss of preexcitation may successfully eliminate conduction in the BT but, because of the possibility that the catheter position may have changed, it is best to wait to deliver energy until preexcitation resumes. Electroanatomical mapping (e.g., CARTO) can help tag sites of interest, facilitating precise relocation of the ablation catheter to these sites if it has been determined that they are a good ablation target. Atriofascicular BTs are more susceptible to mechanically induced block, probably suggesting that these BTs are composed of thinner strands or are located closer to the endocardium.[15]

Ablation

Target of Ablation

Direct recording of the BT potential at the tricuspid annulus is the most precise and preferred method of localizing the BT and serves as the target of ablation (see Fig. 15-5).[8,9,12,15] Ablation at the ventricular insertion site of the BT offers no advantage over targeting the atrial insertion site because there is evidence that a variable degree of arborization of the distal insertion site occurs in some patients, with the potential of requiring ablation of a relatively large amount of ventricular myocardium to be effective.[5,10]

However, when a BT potential along the tricuspid annulus cannot be recorded, ablation of the distal insertion sites of atriofascicular BTs becomes an alternative and has been found to be highly effective, but is commonly (57%) associated with the development of RBBB. Ablation of the RB can carry a proarrhythmic effect and facilitate induction of the SVT or cause incessant tachycardia; however, this not a concern as long as the BT itself is also successfully ablated.[10,15]

Using these methods, the locations of successful ablation of atypical BTs are found to be mostly along the lateral tricuspid annulus, with a minority along the septal aspect of the tricuspid annulus or within the ventricle. Atriofascicular and long decrementally conducting AV BTs tend (84%) to cross the tricuspid annulus in a lateral, anterolateral, or anterior region, whereas short decrementally conducting AV BTs are roughly equally distributed between these and a posterior or septal region.

Ablation Technique

Once an appropriate target site for ablation has been identified, RF energy can be applied during NSR, atrial pacing, or antidromic AVRT. Atrial pacing is preferred to ensure that adequate preexcitation is evident (unlike NSR) to be able to assess the efficacy of ablation, and that the rhythm remains the same after elimination of preexcitation (unlike antidromic AVRT) to prevent catheter dislodgment.[5,10]

The use of long curved sheaths can help achieve good catheter positioning and stability along the tricuspid annulus. Typical RF settings consist of a maximum power of 50 W and a maximum temperature of 55° to 60°C, continued for 30 to 60 seconds after elimination of the BT function (i.e., after disappearance of preexcitation). During RF energy delivery, an accelerated preexcited rhythm is often present. This so-called *Mahaim automatic tachycardia* is analogous to accelerated junctional rhythm observed during AVN modification, presumably because of irritation of the BT caused by heating. RF energy delivery should be continued long enough after termination of this rhythm.[15] Heat-induced automaticity during RF ablation is observed less commonly in short decrementally conducting AV BTs as compared with atriofascicular BTs (50% versus 91%).[17,18]

Endpoints of Ablation

Complete loss of BT function, not just noninducibility of tachycardias, is an essential endpoint. It is confirmed by demonstrating loss of preexcitation with atrial pacing and AES—atrial stimulation should be performed at sites and rates that were associated with preexcitation before ablation—and noninducibility of AVRT.[5]

Outcome

Acute success rate is approximately 90% to 100%, and short-term recurrence rate is less than 5%.[8,9,15]

FASCICULOVENTRICULAR BYPASS TRACTS

General Considerations

Fasciculoventricular BTs are the rarest form of preexcitation (1.2% to 5.1% of atypical BTs). They connect the HB to ventricular myocardium in the anteroseptal location. These fibers do not give rise to any reentrant tachycardia, and appear to be only an ECG and EP curiosity. Even during AF and AFL, a rapid ventricular response is not expected in the presence of a normal AVN proximal to the BT. However, it is important to distinguish fasciculoventricular BTs from superoparaseptal BTs to avoid unnecessary invasive EP procedures and potential harm to the AVN-HB if such a BT is mistakenly targeted for ablation, because this form of preexcitation does not require treatment.[4,12]

Electrocardiographic Features

In patients with fasciculoventricular BTs, preexcitation is always present during NSR. The ECG preexcitation pattern can mimic that of manifest WPW pattern, especially that of superoparaseptal AV BTs, with a normal frontal plane axis between 0 and +75 degrees and precordial RS transitional zone in V_2-V_3. With fasciculoventricular BTs, the PR interval is normal despite the presence of preexcitation (Fig. 15-6). This is in contrast to the superoparaseptal AV BTs, which result in the WPW pattern with significant shortening of the PR interval because of the relative proximity of the BT location to the sinus node.

Several ECG findings in lead V_1 favor fasciculoventricular BTs as the cause of preexcitation, including the following: (1) PR interval > 110 milliseconds; (2) R wave width < 35 milliseconds; (3) S wave amplitude < 20 mm; (4) flat or negative delta wave; and (5) notching in the descending limb of S wave (see Fig. 15-6).[19]

Electrophysiological Testing

With fasciculoventricular BTs, preexcitation is present during NSR with a normal AH interval and short HV interval. The earliest ventricular activation occurs at the HB region (Table 15-3).

Progressively shorter atrial pacing CLs or AES coupling intervals produce progressive prolongation of PR and AH intervals but with fixed degree of preexcitation, constant and short HV interval, and fixed relationship between the His potential and RB potential (Fig. 15-7). AVN Wenckebach block can develop, which is then associated with a fixed degree of preexcitation and a constant, short HV interval. The loss of AV conduction is associated with loss of preexcitation. AES can result in block in the fasciculoventricular BT, producing a sudden loss of preexcitation and prolongation of the HV interval to normal values (see Fig. 15-7).

HB pacing normalizes the HV interval and eliminates preexcitation in all types of BTs except for fasciculoventricular BTs, in which a fixed degree of preexcitation and a constant short HV interval remain unchanged during HB pacing (see Fig. 15-6).

When adenosine administration slows AVN conduction, an increase in the degree of preexcitation is noted in all types of BTs, as long as adenosine does not block the BT, except for fasciculoventricular BTs, in which the degree of preexcitation and HV interval remain fixed. Moreover, adenosine administration can be associated with complete AV block and junctional escape beats and, in the case of fasciculoventricular BTs, these beats are associated with the same degree of preexcitation and the same HV interval as during NSR, even when these ectopic beats are associated with retrograde VA block and no atrial depolarization.

ATRIO-HISIAN BYPASS TRACTS

General Considerations

Patients with palpitations who had a short PR interval but normal QRS complex in the resting ECG were first described in 1938 and then further evaluated by Lown and colleagues in 1952.[20] The latter report consisted of a retrospective examination of 13,500 ECGs and identified a mixed group of 200 subjects with short PR intervals, most of whom had a normal QRS complex (Fig. 15-8). The authors described a "syndrome" characterized by a short PR interval, a narrow QRS complex, and recurrent paroxysmal SVTs. They initially ascribed this syndrome to the presence of an AV nodal BT.[12,20] A variety of explanations were later offered to account for the short PR interval.

Although the incidence of palpitations was significantly higher in these patients with short PR intervals when compared with a control group with a normal PR interval (17% versus 0.5%), most contemporary electrophysiologists do not consider the Lown-Ganong-Levine syndrome as a recognized syndrome of a single entity but an electrocardiographic description. It probably represents one end of the normal spectrum of AVN conduction properties. Therefore, the use of the term is inappropriate and should be discouraged and the mechanism responsible for the short PR interval should be used instead. The persistence of the term probably relates to the appealing parallel with the initials of the WPW syndrome.

The short PR interval can have different mechanisms: (1) enhanced AVN conduction (perhaps using specialized intranodal fibers), which is believed responsible for most cases of short PR interval and is secondary to an anatomically small AVN, enhanced sympathetic tone, or a variant of normal; (2) atrio-Hisian BT (rare), in which case AF or AFL with a rapid ventricular response is the presenting arrhythmia; (3) ectopic atrial rhythm with differential input into the AVN; and (4) isorhythmic AV dissociation, in which case the short PR interval is not caused by a conducted P wave.[12]

Supraventricular Tachycardias in Patients with Short PR Intervals

Patients with Enhanced Atrioventricular Node Conduction. The mechanism(s) of SVTs in patients with enhanced AVN conduction does not appear to differ significantly from those in patients with normal PR intervals (AVNRT being the most common, followed by orthodromic AVRT). The tachycardia CL of AVNRT occurring in patients with short PR intervals is not different from that in patients with normal PR intervals. This is expected, because the tachycardia CL of AVNRT is determined by conduction over the slow AVN pathway, which is similar in these patients and those with a normal PR interval. In contrast, the tachycardia CL of orthodromic AVRT tends to be much shorter in these patients compared with patients with normal PR intervals, which is expected because the circuit of orthodromic AVRT uses the fast AVN pathway for anterograde conduction. In fact, in any SVT with a tachycardia CL shorter than 250 milliseconds, enhanced AVN conduction and orthodromic AVRT should be suspected. In such patients, bundle branch block (BBB) is common during SVT, resulting in wide complex tachycardia.[12]

Patients with Atrio-Hisian Bypass Tracts. These patients primarily present with AF and AFL with rapid ventricular response, and do not develop reentrant SVTs

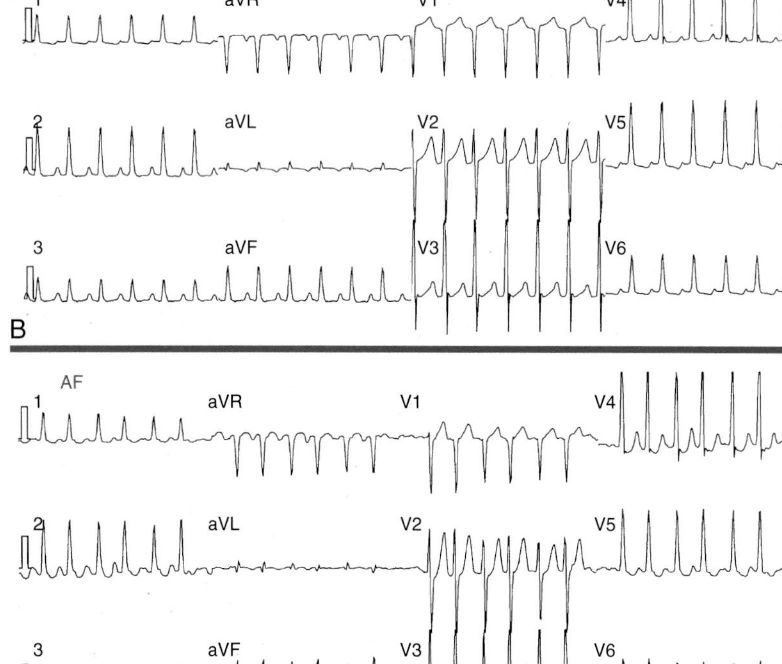

FIGURE 15–6 ECG of fasciculoventricular bypass tracts. **A,** Surface ECG of normal sinus rhythm (NSR) with preexcitation over a fasciculoventricular pathway. Note the short PR and slight slurring of the QRS upstroke in several leads. **B,** Pacing from the right atrium (RA) at the shortest cycle length associated with 1 : 1 AV conduction results in no change in the mild degree of preexcitation compared with NSR despite atrioventricular nodal conduction delay (longer PR interval). **C,** Atrial fibrillation (AF) is present, with no change in the mild degree of preexcitation compared with NSR regardless of the RR interval. **D,** Surface ECG during His bundle (HB) pacing in the same patient. The same degree of preexcitation persists as in NSR. Retrograde P waves are visible (arrows), deforming the end of QRS complexes.

using the AV junction as one limb.[12] Rapid ventricular response during AF depends on refractoriness of the tissue responsible for AV conduction (i.e., AVN or BT) and not on the site of insertion for that tissue.

Electrophysiological Testing

Baseline Observations During Normal Sinus Rhythm

Enhanced AVN conduction is characterized by a short AH interval (≤60 milliseconds) and normal HV interval.[12] In rare cases in which the AVN is completely bypassed by an atrio-Hisian BT, the HV interval is short. The HV interval in these cases is artifactually short because the proximal HB and the ventricle are activated in parallel since the atrio-Hisian BT inserts into the distal HB (i.e., the proximal HB is activated retrogradely).

Atrial Pacing and Atrial Extrastimulation

Patients with Enhanced Atrioventricular Node Conduction. The AH interval prolongs with progressively shorter atrial pacing CLs and AES coupling intervals.[12] The prolongation in the AH interval is smooth, continuous, and blunted, with a maximal increase in the AH interval of 100 milliseconds or less during pacing at a CL of 300 milliseconds compared with the value measured during NSR. The maximum AH interval (at any pacing rate) is rarely longer than 200 milliseconds and 1:1 conduction typically is maintained to pacing rates more than 200 beats/min.

The AH interval response can be characteristic of dual AVN physiology, with an initial blunted small prolongation in the AH interval followed by a significant jump at a critical pacing CL or AES coupling interval, while maintaining 1:1 conduction at a pacing rate more than 200 beats/min. In such patients, the maximum AH interval can be more than 200 milliseconds, and the maximum prolongation in the AH interval can be more than 100 milliseconds.[12] Atrial pacing from the CS is associated with shorter AH intervals, shorter Wenckebach CLs, and shorter AVN effective refractory periods, suggesting a preferential input into the AVN.

Patients with Atrio-Hisian Bypass Tracts. The AH interval remains short with no or minimal prolongation in response to progressively shorter atrial pacing CLs and AES coupling intervals. Block in the BT, which can usually be achieved by antiarrhythmic agents or occasionally by the induction of AF, is associated with simultaneous increase in the PR and AH intervals and normalization of the HV interval.[12]

Ventricular Pacing and Ventricular Extrastimulation

Patients with Enhanced Atrioventricular Node Conduction. Retrograde AVN conduction is extremely rapid. In general, the HA interval is shorter than the AH interval at comparable pacing CLs.[12] The HA interval remains relatively short with little prolongation in response to progressively shorter ventricular pacing CLs and VES coupling intervals.[12] A concealed AV BT mediating retrograde VA conduction should be excluded, which can be achieved by a variety of pacing maneuvers (see Chap. 14).

Patients with Atrio-Hisian Bypass Tracts. VA conduction is unpredictable in these patients. In many cases, VA conduction is absent and, even when present, it is not as good as AV conduction.[12]

Response to Pharmacological and Physiological Maneuvers

Patients with Enhanced Atrioventricular Node Conduction. The AH interval prolongs in response to beta

TABLE 15–3 Features of Fasciculoventricular Bypass Tracts

Preexcitation is present in NSR with normal PR interval with transitional zone in V_2-V_3.
The earliest ventricular activation occurs at the HB region.
The degree of preexcitation is not influenced by the site of atrial stimulation.
Incremental rate atrial pacing results in progressive prolongation in the P-delta interval but the degree of preexcitation is not influenced by the pacing rate.
HB pacing does not change the degree of preexcitation or the HV interval.

HB = His bundle; HV = His bundle–ventricular; NSR = normal sinus rhythm.

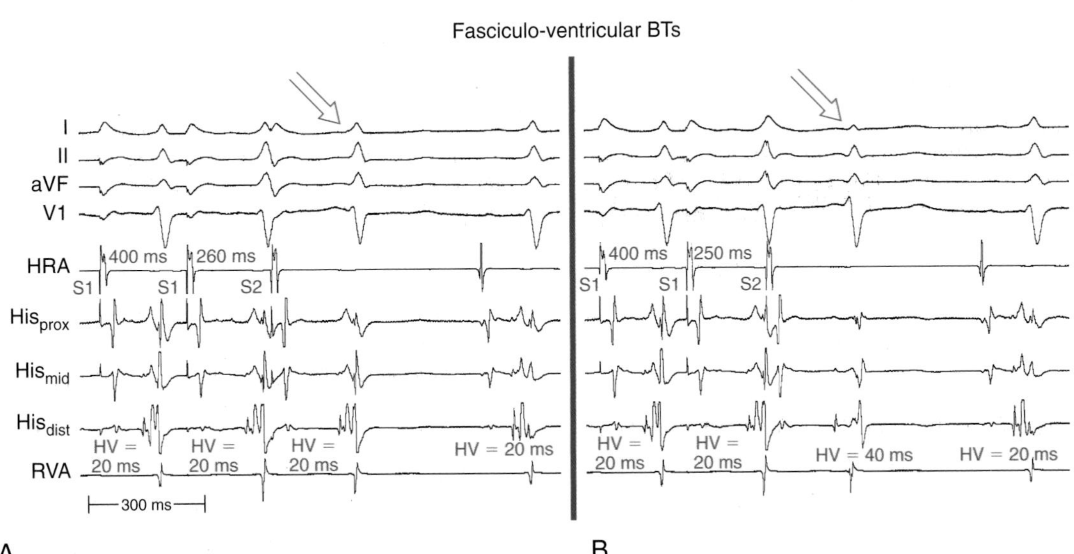

FIGURE 15–7 Effect of atrial stimulation of fasciculoventricular bypass tracts (BTs). **A,** Minimal preexcitation is present during normal sinus rhythm (NSR), with the same during atrial pacing and following an atrial extrastimulus (AES) that lengthens the atrial–His bundle (AH) interval, but the His bundle–ventricular (HV) interval remains fixed at only 20 msec. These features are consistent with a fasciculoventricular pathway. **B,** A more premature AES results in block in the fasciculoventricular pathway, resulting in a narrow QRS complex and normal HV interval (40 msec). Note the difference in QRS complex morphology following the AESs (arrows).

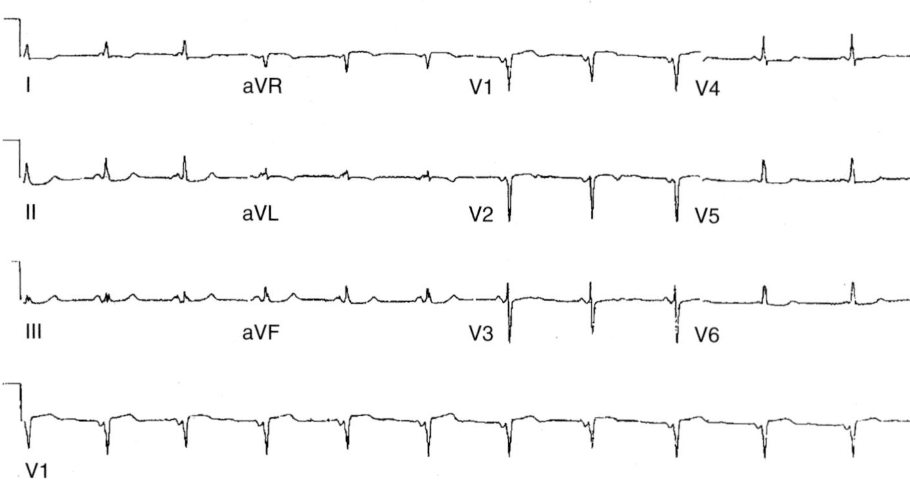

FIGURE 15–8 Surface ECG of an asymptomatic patient with short PR interval and no preexcitation.

blockers, verapamil, digoxin, carotid sinus massage, and vagal maneuvers. Complete autonomic blockade results in increases in the AH interval and AVN functional refractory period, but a minimal change in the AVN effective refractory period (suggesting sympathetic tone predominance in these patients, in contrast to individuals with normal AVN conduction in whom vagal tone predominates).[12]

Patients with Atrio-Hisian Bypass Tracts. AV conduction over the atrio-Hisian BT is not affected by autonomic modulation. Conduction block in the BT requires class IA or IC agents or amiodarone. Conduction block is associated with an immediate, sudden, and marked prolongation of the AH and HV intervals to normal values.

REFERENCES

1. Mahaim I, Benatt A: Nouvelles recherches sur les connexions superieures de la branche gauche du faisceau de His-Tawara avec cloison interventriculaire. Cardiologia 1937;1:61.
2. Mahaim I, Winston MR: Recherches d'anatomie comparee et de pathologie experimentale sur les connexions hautes des His-Tawara. Cardiologia 1941;33:651.
3. Mahaim I: Kent's fiber in the A-V paraspecific conduction through the upper connection of the bundle of His-Tawara. Am Heart J 1947;33:651.
4. Anderson RH, Ho SY, Gillette PC, Becker AE: Mahaim, Kent and abnormal atrioventricular conduction. Cardiovasc Res 1996;31:480.
5. Miller J, Olgin JE: Catheter ablation of free-wall accessory pathways and "Mahaim" fibers. *In* Zipes DP, Haissaguerre M (eds): Catheter Ablation of Arrhythmias. Armonk, NY, Futura, 2002, pp 277-303.
6. Benditt DG, Lu F: Atriofascicular pathways: Fuzzy nomenclature or merely wishful thinking? J Cardiovasc Electrophysiol 2006;17:261.
7. Lee PC, Kanter R, Gomez-Marin O, et al: Quantitative assessment of the recovery property of atriofascicular/atrioventricular-type Mahaim fiber. J Cardiovasc Electrophysiol 2002;13:535.
8. Haissaguerre M, Cauchemez B, Marcus F, et al: Characteristics of the ventricular insertion sites of accessory pathways with anterograde decremental conduction properties. Circulation 1995;91:1077.
9. Klein LS, Hackett FK, Zipes DP, Miles WM: Radiofrequency catheter ablation of Mahaim fibers at the tricuspid annulus. Circulation 1993;87:738.
10. Kothari S, Gupta AK, Lokhandwala YY, et al: Atriofascicular pathways: Where to ablate? Pacing Clin Electrophysiol 2006;29:1226.
11. Davidson NC, Morton JB, Sanders P, Kalman J: Latent Mahaim fiber as a cause of antidromic reciprocating tachycardia: recognition and successful radiofrequency ablation. J Cardiovasc Electrophysiol 2002;13:74.
12. Josephson ME: Preexcitation syndromes. *In* Josephson ME (ed): Clinical Cardiac Electrophysiology, 3rd ed. Philadelphia, Lippincott, Williams & Wilkins, 2002, pp 322-424.
13. Sternick EB, Fagundes ML, Cruz FE, et al: Short atrioventricular Mahaim fibers: Observations on their clinical, electrocardiographic, and electrophysiological profile. J Cardiovasc Electrophysiol 2005;16:127.
14. Sternick EB, Timmermans C, Sosa E, et al: The electrocardiogram during sinus rhythm and tachycardia in patients with Mahaim fibers: the importance of an "rS" pattern in lead III. J Am Coll Cardiol 2004;44:1626.
15. Miller JM, Rothman SA, Hsia HH, Buxton AE: Ablation of Mahaim fibers. *In* Huang SKS, Wilber DJ (eds): Radiofrequency Catheter Ablation of Cardiac Arrythmias: Basic Concepts and Clinical Applications, 2nd ed. Armonk, NY, Futura, 2000, pp 559-578.
16. Sternick EB, Cruz FE, Timmermans C, et al: Electrocardiogram during tachycardia in patients with anterograde conduction over a Mahaim fiber: Old criteria revisited. Heart Rhythm 2004;1:406.
17. Sternick EB, Sosa EA, Timmermans C, et al: Automaticity in Mahaim fibers. J Cardiovasc Electrophysiol 2004;15:738.
18. Sternick EB, Gerken LM, Vrandecic M: Appraisal of "Mahaim" automatic tachycardia. J Cardiovasc Electrophysiol 2002;13:244.
19. Oh S, Choi YS, Choi EK, et al: Electrocardiographic characteristics of fasciculoventricular pathways. Pacing Clin Electrophysiol 2005;28:25.
20. Lown B, Ganong Wf, Levine SA: The syndrome of short P-R interval, normal QRS complex and paroxysmal rapid heart action. Circulation 1952;5:693.

CHAPTER 16

Approach to Paroxysmal Supraventricular Tachycardias

CLINICAL CONSIDERATIONS

Epidemiology

Narrow QRS complex supraventricular tachycardia (SVT) is a tachyarrhythmia with a rate more than 100 beats/min and a QRS duration of less than 120 milliseconds.[1] Narrow QRS complex SVTs include sinus tachycardia, inappropriate sinus tachycardia, sinoatrial nodal reentrant tachycardia, atrial tachycardia (AT), multifocal AT, atrial fibrillation (AF), atrial flutter (AFL), junctional ectopic tachycardia, nonparoxysmal junctional tachycardia, atrioventricular nodal reentrant tachycardia (AVNRT), and atrioventricular reentrant tachycardia (AVRT).[2]

Narrow QRS complex tachycardias can be divided into those that require only atrial tissue for their initiation and maintenance (sinus tachycardia, AT, AF, and AFL), and those that require the AV junction (junctional tachycardia, AVNRT, and AVRT).

Paroxysmal SVT is the term generally applied to intermittent SVT other than AF, AFL, and multifocal AT. The major causes are AVNRT (approximately 50% to 60% of cases), AVRT (approximately 30% of cases), and AT (approximately 10% of cases).[2]

Paroxysmal SVT with sudden onset and termination is relatively common; the estimated prevalence in the normal population is 2.25/1,000, and an incidence of 35/100,000 person-years. Paroxysmal SVT in the absence of structural heart disease can present at any age but most commonly first presents between ages 12 and 30 years. Females have a twofold greater risk of developing this arrhythmia than males.

The mechanism of paroxysmal SVT is significantly influenced by both age and gender. In a large cohort of patients with symptomatic paroxysmal SVT referred for ablation, as patients grew older there was a significant and progressive decline in the number of patients presenting with AVRT, which was the predominant mechanism in the first decade, and a striking increase in AVNRT and AT (Fig. 16-1). These trends were similar in both genders, although AVNRT replaced AVRT as the predominant mechanism much earlier in women.[3] The early predominance of AVRT is consistent with the congenital nature of the substrate and that symptom onset occurs earlier in patients with AVRT than AVNRT, most commonly in the first 2 decades of life. However, a minority of patients have relatively late onset of symptoms associated with AVRT and thus continue to account for a small proportion of ablations in older patients. Men account for a higher proportion of AVRT at all ages. AVNRT is the predominant mechanism overall in patients undergoing ablation and after age 20 accounts for the largest number of ablations in each age group. There is a striking 2 : 1 predominance of women in the AVNRT group, which remains without clear physiological or anatomical explanation. An increase in the proportion and absolute number of patients with AVNRT can be related to the normal evolution of AVN physiology over the first 2 decades of life, as well as age-related changes in atrial and nodal physiology observed in later decades. ATs comprise a progressively greater proportion of those with paroxysmal SVT with increasing age, accounting for 23% of patients older than 70 years. Although there is a greater absolute number of women with AT, the proportion of AT in both genders is similar. Age-related changes in the atrial electrophysiological (EP) substrate (including cellular coupling and autonomic influences) can contribute to the increased incidence of AT in older individuals.

Clinical Presentation

The clinical syndrome of paroxysmal SVT is characterized as a regular rapid tachycardia of abrupt onset and termination. Episodes can last from seconds to several hours. Patients commonly describe palpitations and dizziness. Rapid ventricular rates can be associated with complaints of dyspnea, weakness, angina, or even frank syncope, and can at times be disabling. Neck pounding can occur during tachycardia because of simultaneous contraction of both atria and ventricles against closed mitral and tricuspid valves (as occurs during AVNRT).

Patients often learn to use certain maneuvers such as carotid sinus massage or the Valsalva maneuver to terminate the arrhythmia, although many require

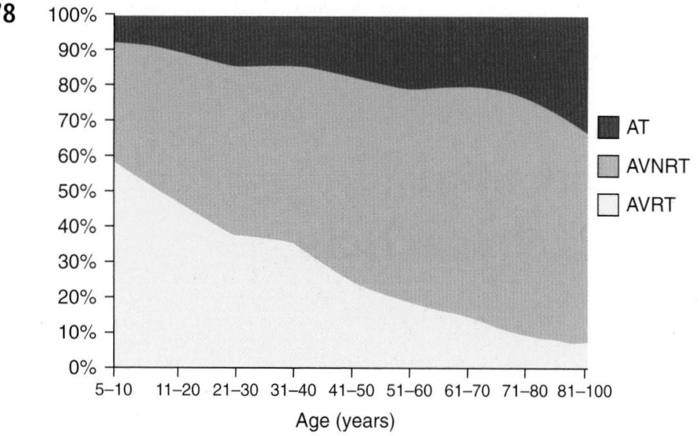

FIGURE 16–1 Proportion of paroxysmal supraventricular tachycardia mechanism by age. AT = atrial tachycardia; AVNRT = atrioventricular nodal reentrant tachycardia; AVRT = atrioventricular reentrant tachycardia. (From Porter MJ, Morton JB, Denman R, et al: Influence of age and gender on the mechanism of supraventricular tachycardia. Heart Rhythm 2004;1:393.)

pharmacological treatment to achieve this. In patients without structural heart disease, the physical examination is usually remarkable only for a rapid, regular heart rate. At times, because of the simultaneous contraction of atria and ventricles, cannon A waves can be seen in the jugular venous waveform. In patients with an AT exhibiting AV block, usually of the Wenckebach type, the ventricular rate is irregular.

Initial Evaluation

History, physical examination, and an ECG constitute an appropriate initial evaluation of paroxysmal SVT. However, clinical symptoms are not usually helpful in distinguishing different forms of paroxysmal SVT. A 12-lead ECG during tachycardia can be helpful for defining the mechanism of paroxysmal SVT. Ambulatory 24-hour Holter recording may be used for documentation of the arrhythmia in patients with frequent (i.e., several episodes per week) but self-terminating tachycardias. A cardiac event monitor is often more useful than a 24-hour recording in patients with less frequent arrhythmias. Implantable loop recorders can be helpful in selected cases with rare episodes associated with severe symptoms of hemodynamic instability (e.g., syncope).

An echocardiographic examination should be considered in patients with documented sustained SVT to exclude the possibility of structural heart disease. Exercise testing is less often useful for diagnosis unless the arrhythmia is clearly triggered by exertion. Further diagnostic studies are indicated only if there are signs or symptoms that suggest structural heart disease.

Transesophageal atrial recordings and stimulation may be used in selected cases for diagnosis or to provoke paroxysmal tachyarrhythmias if the clinical history is insufficient or if other measures have failed to document an arrhythmia. Esophageal stimulation is not indicated if invasive EP investigation is planned. Invasive EP testing with subsequent catheter ablation may be used for diagnosis and therapy in cases with a clear history of paroxysmal regular palpitations. It may also be considered in patients with preexcitation or disabling symptoms.

Principles of Management

Acute Management

Most episodes of paroxysmal SVT require intact 1:1 atrioventricular node (AVN) conduction for continuation and are therefore classified as AVN-dependent. AVN conduction and refractoriness can be modified by vagal maneuvers and by many pharmacological agents and thus are the weak links targeted by most acute therapies. Termination of a sustained episode of SVT is usually accomplished by producing transient block in the AVN.

Vagal maneuvers such as carotid sinus massage, Valsalva maneuvers, or the dive reflex are usually used as the first step and generally terminate the SVT. Valsalva is the most effective technique in adults, but carotid sinus massage can also be effective.[2] Facial immersion in water is the most reliable method in infants. Vagal maneuvers are less effective once a sympathetic response to paroxysmal SVT has become established, so patients should be advised to try them soon after onset. Vagal maneuvers present the advantage of being relatively simple and noninvasive, but their efficacy seems to be lower in comparison with pharmacological interventions, with the incidence of paroxysmal SVT termination ranging from 6% to 22% following carotid sinus massage.

When vagal maneuvers are unsuccessful, termination can be achieved with antiarrhythmic drugs whose primary effects increase refractoriness and/or decrease conduction (negative dromotropic effect) over the AVN. These drugs can have direct (e.g., verapamil blocks the slow inward calcium current of the AVN) or indirect effects (e.g., digoxin increases vagal tone to the AVN). In most patients, the drug of choice is either adenosine or verapamil.

The advantages of adenosine include its rapid onset of action (usually within 10 to 25 seconds via a peripheral vein), short half-life (less than 10 seconds), and high degree of efficacy. The effective dose of adenosine is usually 6 to 12 mg, given as a rapid bolus. Doses up to 12 mg terminate over 90% of paroxysmal SVT episodes. Sequential dosing can be given at 60-second intervals because of adenosine's rapid metabolism. In AVNRT the most common site of termination is the anterograde slow pathway. In AVRT, termination occurs secondary to block in the AVN. Termination can also occur indirectly, i.e., because of adenosine-induced premature atrial complexes (PACs) or premature ventricular complexes (PVCs). Adenosine shortens the atrial refractory period, and atrial ectopy can induce AF. This can be dangerous if the patient has a bypass tract (BT) capable of rapid anterograde conduction. Because adenosine is cleared so rapidly, reinitiation of paroxysmal SVT after initial termination can occur. Either repeat administration of the same dose of adenosine or substitution of a calcium channel blocker will be effective.[2]

The AVN action potential is calcium channel–dependent, and the non–dihydropyridine calcium channel blockers verapamil and diltiazem are effective for terminating AVN-dependent paroxysmal SVT. The recommended dosage of verapamil is 5 mg intravenously over 2 minutes, followed in 5 to 10 minutes by a second 5- to 7.5-mg dose. The recommended dosage of diltiazem is 20 mg intravenously followed, if necessary, by a second dose of 25 to 35 mg. Paroxysmal SVT termination should occur within 5 minutes of the end of the infusion, and over 90% of patients with AVN-dependent paroxysmal SVT respond. As with adenosine, transient arrhythmias, including atrial and ventricular ectopy, AF, and bradycardia, can be seen after paroxysmal SVT termination with calcium channel blockers. Hypotension can occur with calcium channel blockers, particularly if the paroxysmal SVT does not terminate.[2] Adenosine and verapamil have been reported to have a similar high efficacy in terminating paroxysmal SVT, with a rate of success ranging from 59% to 100% for adenosine and from 73% to 98.8% for verapamil, according to the dose and mode of administration. However, data also suggest that the efficacy of adenosine and verapamil is affected by the arrhythmia rate. Increasing SVT rates are significantly associated with higher percentages of sinus rhythm restoration following treatment with adenosine. In contrast, the efficacy of verapamil in restoring sinus rhythm was inversely related to the rate of paroxysmal SVT.[4]

Intravenous beta blockers including propranolol (1 to 3 mg), metoprolol (5 mg), and esmolol (500 μg/kg over 1 minute and 50-μg/kg/min infusion) are also useful for acute termination. Digoxin (0.5 to 1.0 mg) is considered the least effective of the four categories of drugs available, but is a useful alternative when there is a contraindication to the other agents.

AVN-dependent paroxysmal SVT can present with a wide QRS complex in patients with fixed or functional aberration, or if a BT is used for anterograde conduction. Most wide complex tachycardias, however, are caused by mechanisms that can worsen after intravenous administration of adenosine and calcium channel blockers. Unless there is strong evidence that a wide QRS tachycardia is AVN-dependent, adenosine, verapamil, and diltiazem should not be used.

Limited data are available on the acute pharmacological therapy of ATs. Automatic or triggered tachycardias and sinus node reentry should respond to adenosine, verapamil, diltiazem, or beta-adrenergic blockers. Other ATs can respond to class I or III antiarrhythmic drugs given orally or parenterally.[2]

Chronic Management

Because most paroxysmal SVTs are generally benign arrhythmias that do not influence survival, the main reason for treatment is to alleviate symptoms. The threshold for initiation of therapy and the decision to treat SVT with oral antiarrhythmic drugs or catheter ablation depends on the frequency and duration of the arrhythmia, severity of symptoms, and patient preference. The threshold for treatment will also reflect whether the patient is a competitive athlete, a woman considering pregnancy, or someone with a high-risk occupation. Catheter ablation is an especially attractive option for patients who desire to avoid or are unresponsive or intolerant to drug therapy.

For patients requiring therapy who are reluctant to undergo catheter ablation, antiarrhythmic drug therapy remains a viable alternative. For AVN-dependent paroxysmal SVT, calcium channel blockers and beta blockers will improve symptoms in 60% to 80% of patients. In patients who do not respond, class IC and III drugs can be considered. A comparison of verapamil, propranolol, and digoxin has shown equivalent efficacy in a small group of patients. However, in general, calcium channel blockers and beta blockers are preferred to digoxin. Flecainide and propafenone affect the AVN and BTs and will also reduce SVT frequency.[5] Sotalol, dofetilide, and amiodarone are second-line agents. Because sympathetic stimulation can antagonize the effects of many antiarrhythmic agents, concomitant therapy with a beta-adrenergic blocker can improve efficacy.[2]

Patients with well-tolerated episodes of paroxysmal SVT that always terminate spontaneously or with vagal maneuvers do not require chronic prophylactic therapy. Select patients may be treated only for acute episodes. Outpatients can use a single oral dose of verapamil, propranolol, or propafenone to terminate an episode of AVRT or AVNRT effectively. This so-called pill in the pocket or cocktail therapy is a reasonable treatment option for patients who have tachycardia episodes that are sustained but infrequent enough that daily preventive therapy is not desired. Oral antiarrhythmic drug tablets are not reliably absorbed during rapid paroxysmal SVT, but some patients can respond to self-administration of crushed medications.[2]

Pharmacological management of ATs has not been well evaluated in controlled clinical trials. Depending on the mechanism responsible for the arrhythmia, beta blockers, calcium channel blockers, and class I or III antiarrhythmic drugs may reduce or eliminate symptoms.

ELECTROCARDIOGRAPHIC FEATURES

Assessment of Regularity of the Supraventricular Tachycardia

Most SVTs are associated with a regular ventricular rate. If the rhythm is irregular, the ECG should be scrutinized for discrete atrial activity and for any evidence of a pattern to the irregularity (e.g., grouped beating typical of Wenckebach periodicity). If the rhythm is irregularly irregular (i.e., no pattern can be detected), the mechanism of the arrhythmia is either multifocal AT or AF (Fig. 16-2).[1] Multifocal AT is an irregularly irregular atrial rhythm characterized by more than three different P wave morphologies, with the P waves separated by isoelectric intervals and associated with

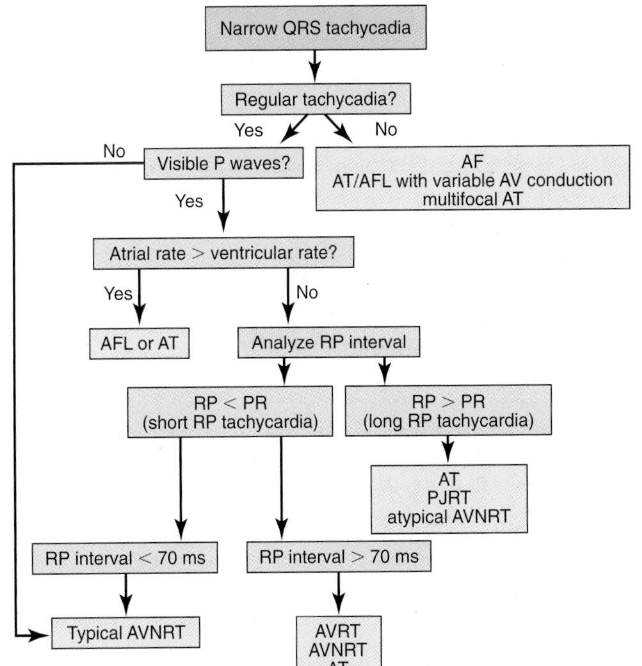

FIGURE 16–2 Differential diagnosis for narrow QRS tachycardia. AF = atrial fibrillation; AFL = atrial flutter; AT = atrial tachycardia; AVNRT = atrioventricular nodal reentrant tachycardia; AVRT = atrioventricular reentrant tachycardia; PJRT = permanent junctional reciprocating tachycardia. (From Blomström-Lundqvist C, Scheinman MM, Aliot EM, et al; American College of Cardiology; American Heart Association Task Force on Practice Guidelines; European Society of Cardiology Committee for Practice Guidelines. Writing Committee to Develop Guidelines for the Management of Patients With Supraventricular Arrhythmias: ACC/AHA/ESC guidelines for the management of patients with supraventricular arrhythmias–executive summary: A report of the American College of Cardiology/American Heart Association Task Force on Practice Guidelines and the European Society of Cardiology Committee for Practice Guidelines (Writing Committee to Develop Guidelines for the Management of Patients With Supraventricular Arrhythmias). Circulation 2003;108:1871.)

varying P-P, R-R, and PR intervals. On the other hand, AF is characterized by rapid and irregular atrial fibrillatory activity and, in the presence of normal AVN conduction, by an irregularly irregular ventricular response. P waves cannot be detected in AF, although coarse fibrillatory waves and prominent U waves can sometimes give the appearance of P waves. At times, the fibrillatory activity is so fine as to be undetectable.

Atrial Activity

Identification

If the patient's rhythm is regular or has a clearly discernible pattern, the ECG should next be assessed for P waves (atrial activity).[6] The P waves may be easily discernible; however, frequently, comparison with a normal baseline ECG is needed and can reveal a slight alteration in the QRS, ST segment, or T or U waves, suggesting the presence of the P wave. If the P waves cannot be clearly identified, carotid sinus massage or the administration of intravenous adenosine may help clarify the diagnosis. These maneuvers may also terminate the SVT.

Carotid Sinus Massage. Carotid sinus massage can produce one of four possible effects:

1. Temporary decrease in the atrial rate in patients with sinus tachycardia or automatic AT.
2. Slowing of AVN conduction and AVN block, which can unmask atrial electrical activity—that is, reveal P waves or flutter waves in patients with AT or AFL by decreasing the number of QRS complexes that obscure the electrical baseline.
3. With some SVTs that require AVN conduction, especially AVNRT and AVRT, the transient slowing of AVN conduction can terminate the arrhythmia by interrupting the reentry circuit; less commonly, carotid sinus massage can cause some ATs to slow and terminate.
4. In some cases, no effect is observed.

Adenosine Administration. Adenosine results in slowing of the sinus rate and AVN conduction. In the setting of SVT, the effects of adenosine are similar to those seen with carotid sinus massage described earlier.[2] For intravenous adenosine administration, the patient should be supine and should have ECG and blood pressure monitoring. The drug is administered by rapid intravenous injection over 1 to 2 seconds at a peripheral site, followed by a normal saline flush. The usual initial dose is 6 mg, with a maximal single dose of 12 mg. If a central intravenous access site is used, the initial dose should not exceed 3 mg and may be as little as 1 mg. Adenosine can precipitate AF and AFL because it shortens atrial refractoriness. In patients with Wolff-Parkinson-White (WPW) syndrome and AF, adenosine can result in a rapid ventricular response that can degenerate into VF. However, this problem has not been observed frequently, and the use of adenosine for diagnosis and termination of regular SVTs, including AVRT, is appropriate as long as close patient observation and preparedness to treat potential complications are maintained.[2]

Termination of the Arrhythmia. Carotid sinus massage or adenosine can terminate the SVT, especially if the rhythm is AVNRT or AVRT. A continuous ECG tracing should be recorded during these maneuvers, because the response can aid in the diagnosis.[6] Termination of the tachycardia with a P wave after the last QRS complex is most common in AVRT and typical AVNRT and is rarely seen with AT (see Fig. 14-15), whereas termination of the tachycardia with a QRS complex is more common with AT, atypical AVNRT, and permanent junctional reciprocating tachycardia (PJRT; see Fig. 14-12). If the tachycardia continues despite development of AV block, the rhythm is almost certainly AT or AFL; AVRT is excluded and AVNRT is very unlikely.

Characterization

Atrial Rate. An atrial rate more than 250 beats/min is almost always caused by AFL. However, overlap exists, and AT and AVRT can occasionally be faster than 250 beats/min.[1] AVRT tends to be faster than AVNRT and AT; again, significant overlap exists and this criterion does not usually help in distinguishing among different SVTs.

P Wave Morphology. A P wave morphology identical to sinus P wave suggests sinus tachycardia, inappropriate sinus tachycardia, sinoatrial nodal reentrant tachycardia, or AT arising close to the region of the sinus node. An abnormal P wave morphology can be observed during AVNRT (P wave is concentric; see Fig. 13-2), AVRT (P wave can be eccentric or concentric; see Fig. 14-6), AT (P wave can be eccentric or concentric), and AFL (lack of distinct isoelectric baselines between atrial deflections is suggestive of AFL, but can also be seen occasionally in AT; see Fig. 9-2).[6]

The P waves may not be discernible on ECG, which suggests typical AVNRT or, less commonly, AVRT (especially in the presence of bundle branch block [BBB] contralateral to the BT).

Characterization of the P/QRS Relationship

RP/PR Intervals. SVTs are classified as short or long RP interval SVTs (see Fig.16-2). During short RP SVTs, the ECG will show P waves inscribed within the ST-T wave with an RP interval that is less than half the tachycardia RR interval. Such SVTs include typical AVNRT (most common), orthodromic AVRT, AT with prolonged AV conduction, and slow-slow AVNRT. A very short RP interval (less than 70 milliseconds) excludes AVRT.[6,7]

In typical AVNRT, the P wave is usually not visible because of the simultaneous atrial and ventricular activation. The P wave may distort the initial portion of the QRS (mimicking a q wave in inferior leads) or lie just within the QRS (inapparent) or distort the terminal portion of the QRS (mimicking an s wave in inferior leads or r′ in V_1; see Fig. 13-2).

Long RP SVTs include AT, atypical (fast-slow) AVNRT, and AVRT using a slowly conducting AV BT (e.g., PJRT). If the PR interval during the SVT is shorter than that during normal sinus rhythm (NSR), AT and AVRT are very unlikely, and atypical AVNRT, which is associated with an apparent shortening of the PR interval, is the likely diagnosis. ATs originating close to the AV junction are also a possibility.

A/V Relationship. SVTs with an A/V ratio of 1 (i.e., equal number of atrial and ventricular events) include AVNRT, AVRT, and AT. On the other hand, an A/V ratio during the SVT of more than 1 indicates the presence of AV block and that the ventricles are not required for the SVT circuit, thereby excluding AVRT and suggesting either AT (most common; see Fig. 8-1) or AVNRT (rare; see Fig. 13-3). A/V dissociation (i.e., complete AV block) can be observed during AT (most common) or AVNRT (rare).

QRS Morphology. The QRS morphology during SVT is usually the same as in NSR. However, functional aberration can occur at rapid rates. Functional aberration occurs frequently in AF, AFL, and AVRT, is less common in AT, and very uncommon in AVNRT.

ELECTROPHYSIOLOGICAL TESTING

Discussion in this section will focus on differential diagnosis of narrow QRS complex paroxysmal SVTs, including AT, orthodromic AVRT, and AVNRT. The goals of EP testing in these patients include the following: (1) evaluation of baseline cardiac electrophysiology; (2) induction of SVT; (3) evaluation of the mode of initiation of the SVT; (4) definition of atrial activation sequence during the SVT; (5) definition of the relationship of the P wave to the QRS at the onset and during the SVT; (6) evaluation of the effect of BBB on the tachycardia CL and ventriculoatrial (VA) interval; (7) evaluation of the SVT circuit and requirement of the atria, His bundle (HB), and/or ventricles in the initiation and maintenance of the SVT; (8) evaluation of SVT response to programmed electrical stimulation and overdrive pacing from the atrium and ventricle; and (9) evaluation of the effects of drugs and physiological maneuvers on the SVT.

Baseline Observations During Normal Sinus Rhythm

The presence of preexcitation during NSR suggests AVRT as the likely diagnosis; however, it does not exclude other causes of SVT during which the AV BT is an innocent bystander. Furthermore, the absence of preexcitation during NSR does not exclude the presence of AV BT or the diagnosis of AVRT mediated by either a concealed or a slowly conducting BT. The presence of intraatrial conduction delay suggests AT, but does not exclude other types of SVT.

Programmed Electrical Stimulation During Normal Sinus Rhythm

The programmed stimulation protocol should include ventricular burst pacing from the right ventricular (RV) apex (down to pacing CL of 300 milliseconds), single and double ventricular extrastimuli (VESs) at multiple CLs (600 to 400 milliseconds) from the RV apex (down to the ventricular effective refractory period, ERP), atrial burst pacing from the high right atrium (RA) and coronary sinus (CS; down to the pacing CL at which 2 : 1 atrial capture occurs), single and double atrial extrastimuli (AESs) at multiple CLs (600 to 400 milliseconds) from the high RA and CS (down to atrial ERP), and administration of isoproterenol infusion (0.5 to 4 µg/min) as needed to facilitate tachycardia induction.

Atrial Extrastimulation and Atrial Pacing During Normal Sinus Rhythm

Dual Atrioventricular Node Physiology. The presence of anterograde dual AVN pathways is indicated by the demonstration of an atrial– His bundle (AH) jump—a jump in the A_2-H_2 or H_1-H_2 interval of more than 50 milliseconds in response to a 10-millisecond shortening of the AES coupling interval (i.e., A_1-A_2) or pacing CL (i.e., A_1-A_1; see Fig. 2-23). Similarly, a 1 : 2 response (i.e., a single atrial stimulus results in two ventricular complexes, the first one because of conduction over the fast AVN pathway, and the second one because of conduction over the slow AVN pathway) also indicates the presence of dual AVN physiology (see Fig. 13-6). Furthermore, the observation of a PR interval that is longer than the pacing CL during atrial pacing, which manifests as crossing over of the pacing stimulus artifact and QRSs (i.e., the paced P wave is conducting not to the QRS immediately following it, but to the next QRS, because of a very long PR interval, also called skipped P waves) is an indication of the presence of anterograde dual AVN pathways (even in the absence of an AH interval jump). There should be 1:1 AV conduction (without Wenckebach block) for this criterion to be valid.[8]

Failure to demonstrate dual AVN physiology does not exclude the possibility of AVNRT, and might be related to similar fast and slow AVN pathway ERPs. Dissociation of refractoriness of the fast and slow AVN pathways might then be necessary. This can be achieved by the introduction of AESs at a shorter pacing drive CL, introduction of multiple AESs, burst atrial pacing, and/or administration of drugs such as beta blockers, verapamil, or digoxin. In general, if fast pathway conduction is suppressed in the baseline, as evidenced by a long AH interval at all atrial pacing rates or VA block during ventricular pacing, isoproterenol infusion (and occasionally atropine) usually facilitates fast pathway conduction. In contrast, if the baseline ERP of the fast pathway is very short, conduction over the slow pathway can be difficult to document and increasing the degree of sedation or infusion of esmolol can prolong the fast pathway ERP and expose slow pathway conduction. Failure to demonstrate dual AVN physiology can also occur because the fast AVN pathway is already blocked at the pacing drive CL (i.e., pacing drive CL is shorter than fast pathway ERP), or because of an atrial functional refractory period limiting the prematurity of the AES. In the latter case, activation of the AVN cannot be adequately advanced to produce block in the fast pathway, because earlier AESs would result in more intraatrial conduction delay and less premature stimulation of the AVN. This can be overcome by the introduction of AESs at shorter pacing drive CL, introduction of multiple AESs, burst atrial pacing, and/or stimulation from multiple atrial sites.

Ventricular Preexcitation. Atrial stimulation can help unmask preexcitation if it is not manifest during NSR because of fast AVN conduction and/or slow BT conduction. AES and atrial pacing from any atrial site result in slowing of AVN conduction and, consequently, unmask or increase the degree of preexcitation over the AV BT (see Fig. 14-4). Moreover, atrial stimulation close to the AV BT insertion site results in maximal preexcitation and the shortest P-delta interval because of the ability to advance the activation of the AV BT down to its ERP from pacing at this site caused by the lack of intervening atrial tissue, whose conduction time and refractoriness can otherwise limit the ability of the AES to stimulate the BT prematurely (see Fig. 14-10).

Failure of atrial stimulation to increase the amount of preexcitation can occur because of markedly enhanced AVN conduction, the presence of another AV BT, pacing-induced block in the AV BT because of the long ERP of the BT (longer than that of the AVN), or total preexcitation is already present at the basal state because of prolonged AVN/His-Purkinje system (HPS) conduction.

Extra Atrial Beats. AES and atrial pacing can trigger extra atrial beats or echo beats. Those beats can be caused by different mechanisms.

Intraatrial Reentrant Beats. These beats usually occur at short coupling intervals, and can originate anywhere in the atrium. Therefore, the atrial activation sequence depends on the site of origin of the beat. The more premature the AES, the more likely it will induce nonspecific intraatrial reentrant beats and short runs of irregular AT or AF.

Catheter-Induced Atrial Beats. These beats usually have the earliest activation site recorded at that particular catheter tip and have the same atrial activation sequence as the atrial impulse produced by pacing from that catheter.

Atrioventricular Nodal Echo Beats. These beats occur in the presence of anterograde dual AVN physiology (see Fig. 2-23). Such beats require anterograde block of the atrial stimulus in the fast AVN pathway, anterograde conduction down the slow pathway, and then retrograde conduction up the fast pathway. AVN echo beats have several features: they appear reproducibly after a critical AH interval, the atrial activation sequence is consistent with retrograde conduction over the fast pathway, with the earliest atrial activation site in the HB, and the VA interval is very short, but it can be longer if the atrial stimulus causes anterograde concealment (and not just block) in the fast pathway.

Atrioventricular Echo Beats. AV echo beats occur secondary to anterograde conduction of the atrial stimulus over the AVN–HPS and retrograde conduction over an AV BT (concealed or bidirectional BT). If preexcitation is manifest during atrial stimulation, the last atrial impulse inducing the echo beat will demonstrate loss of preexcitation because of anterograde block in the AV BT, and atrial activation sequence and P wave morphology of the echo beat will depend on the location of the BT (see Fig. 1-8). These beats have a relatively short VA interval, but always longer than 70 milliseconds. Moreover, the VA interval of the AV echo beat remains constant, regardless of the varying coupling interval of the AES triggering the echo beat (VA linking). Alternatively, AV echo beats can occur secondary to anterograde conduction of the atrial stimulus over a manifest AV BT and retrograde conduction over an AVN.

Ventricular Extrastimulation and Ventricular Pacing During Normal Sinus Rhythm

Retrograde Dual Atrioventricular Nodal Physiology. In a pattern analogous to that of anterograde dual AVN physiology, ventricular stimulation can result in discontinuous retrograde AVN function curves, and retrograde dual AVN physiology can be diagnosed by demonstrating a sudden lengthening (jump) in the H_2-A_2 (or A_1-A_2) of 50 milliseconds or more in response to a 10-millisecond decrement of the VES coupling interval (V_1-V_2) or ventricular pacing CL (V_1-V_1), or a 1 : 2 response (i.e., two atrial responses to a single ventricular stimulus).[8]

Failure to demonstrate retrograde dual AVN physiology in patients with AVNRT can be the result of similar fast and slow AVN pathway ERPs. Dissociation of refractoriness of the fast and slow AVN pathways might be required. It can be achieved by the introduction of VESs at shorter pacing drive CL, introduction of multiple VESs, burst ventricular pacing, and/or administration of drugs such as beta blockers, verapamil, or digoxin. Furthermore, dual AVN physiology cannot be demonstrated when the fast AVN pathway is already blocked at the pacing drive CL (i.e., the pacing CL is shorter than the fast pathway ERP), or when ventricular or HPS functional refractory period limits the prematurity of the VES. The latter limitation can be overcome by the introduction of VESs at a shorter pacing drive CL, introduction of multiple VESs, and/or burst ventricular pacing.

VA block at a ventricular pacing CL more than 600 milliseconds or decremental VA conduction during ventricular pacing makes the presence of a retrogradely conducting BT unlikely, except for decrementally conducting BTs and the rare catecholamine-dependent BTs. In addition, development of VA block during ventricular pacing in response to adenosine suggests the absence of BT.

Retrograde Atrial Activation Sequence. VA conduction over the AVN produces classic concentric atrial activation sequence starting in the anteroseptal or posteroseptal region of the RA because of conduction over the fast or slow AVN pathways, respectively. In the presence of a retrogradely conducting AV BT, atrial activation can result from conduction over the AV BT, over the AVN, or a fusion of both (see Fig. 14-11). An eccentric atrial activation sequence in response to ventricular stimulation indicates the presence of an AV BT mediating VA conduction (see Fig. 14-11). The presence of a concentric retrograde atrial activation sequence, however, does not exclude the presence of a retrogradely conducting BT that could be septal in location or located far from the pacing site, allowing for preferential VA conduction over the AVN.

Extra Ventricular Beats. Ventricular stimulation can trigger extra ventricular beats or echo beats. These beats can be caused by different mechanisms.

Bundle Branch Reentrant Beats. During RV stimulation at close coupling intervals, progressive retrograde conduction delay and block occur in the right bundle branch (RB), so that retrograde HB activation occurs via the left bundle brunch (LB). At this point, the His potential usually follows the local ventricular electrogram. Further decrease in the coupling interval produces an increase in retrograde HPS conduction delay. When a critical degree of HPS delay (S_2-H_2) is attained, the impulse can return down the initially blocked RB and result in a QRS of similar morphology to the paced QRS at the RV apex—specifically, it will look like a typical left bundle branch block (LBBB) pattern with left axis deviation because ventricular activation originates from conduction over the RB. The His bundle–ventricular (HV) interval of the bundle branch reentrant (BBR) beat is usually longer than or equal to the HV interval during NSR. Retrograde atrial activation, if present, follows the His potential (see Fig. 2-27).

Atrioventricular Node Echo Beats. These beats are caused by reentry in the AVN in patients with retrograde dual AVN physiology (see Fig. 13-10). The last paced beat conducts retrogradely up the slow AVN pathway and then anterogradely down the fast pathway to produce the echo beat. AVN echoes appear reproducibly after a critical H_2-A_2 interval (or V_2-A_2 interval, when the His potential cannot be seen), and manifest as extra beats with a normal anterograde QRS morphology, with atrial activity preceding the His potential before the echo beat. This phenomenon can occur at long or short coupling intervals and depends only on the degree of retrograde AVN conduction delay. In most cases, this delay is achieved before the appearance of a retrograde His potential beyond the local ventricular electrogram (i.e., before retrograde block in the RB.

Atrioventricular Echo Beats. These beats occur secondary to retrograde block in the HPS-AVN and VA conduction over an AV BT, followed by anterograde conduction over the AVN, or secondary to retrograde block in the AV BT and VA conduction over the AVN-HPS, followed by anterograde conduction over the AV-BT. In the latter case, the echo beat is fully preexcited (see Fig. 14-11).

Intraventricular Reentrant Beats. This response occurs most commonly in the setting of a cardiac pathological condition, especially coronary artery disease, and usually occurs at short coupling intervals. It can have any QRS morphology, but more often right bundle branch block (RBBB) than LBBB in patients with prior myocardial infarction (MI). These responses are usually nonsustained (1 to 30 complexes) and typically polymorphic. In patients without prior clinical arrhythmias, such responses are of no clinical significance.

Catheter-Induced Ventricular Beats. Such beats usually have the earliest ventricular activation site recorded at that particular catheter tip and have the same QRS morphology as the QRS produced by pacing from that catheter.

Induction of Tachycardia

Initiation by Atrial Extrastimulation or Atrial Pacing

Inducibility. All types of paroxysmal SVTs can be inducible with atrial stimulation (except automatic AT).

Requirement of Atrioventricular Conduction Delay. SVT initiation that is reproducibly dependent on a critical AH interval is classic for typical AVNRT (see Fig. 13-7). Atypical AVNRT is usually initiated with modest prolongation of the AH interval along the fast pathway with anterograde block in the slow pathway, followed by retrograde slow conduction over the slow pathway. Therefore, a critical AH interval delay is not obvious (see Fig. 13-9). AT initiation also can be associated with AV delay, but that is not a prerequisite for initiation. Orthodromic AVRT usually requires some AV delay for initiation; however, the delay can occur anywhere along the AVN-HPS axis. In patients with baseline manifest preexcitation, initiation of orthodromic AVRT is usually associated with anterograde block in the AV BT and loss of preexcitation following the initiating atrial stimulus, which would then allow that BT to conduct retrogradely during the SVT.[9]

Requirement of Catecholamines. Initiation can require catecholamines (isoproterenol) with any type of SVT, and this observation does not help for differential diagnosis.

Warm-up. Progressive shortening of the tachycardia CL for several beats (warm-up) before its ultimate rate is achieved is characteristic of automatic AT, but may occur in other SVTs as well.

Ventriculoatrial Interval. If the VA interval of the first tachycardia beat is reproducibly identical to that during the rest of the SVT, AT is very unlikely, and such "VA linking" is suggestive of AVNRT and AVRT.

Initiation by VES or Ventricular Pacing

Inducibility. Ventricular stimulation commonly induces AVRT, typical and atypical AVNRT, and less frequently AT.

His Bundle–Atrial Interval. During induction of the SVT by ventricular pacing at a CL similar to the tachycardia CL or by a VES that advances the His potential by a coupling interval (i.e., H_1-H_2) similar to the H-H interval during the SVT (i.e., similar to the tachycardia CL), the His bundle–atrial (HA), or VA interval following the initiating ventricular stimulus then can be compared with that during the SVT. During AVNRT, the HA interval of the ventricular stimulus initiating the SVT is longer than that during the SVT, because both the HB and atrium are activated in sequence during ventricular stimulation and in parallel during AVNRT. This is even exaggerated by the fact that the AVN usually exhibits greater decremental conduction with repetitive engagement of impulses than to a single impulse at a similar coupling interval. Therefore, the more prolonged the HA interval with the initiating ventricular stimulus, the more likely the SVT is AVNRT. On the other hand, if the SVT uses an AV BT for retrograde conduction, the HA interval during the initiating ventricular stimulus (at a coupling interval comparable to the tachycardia CL) should approximate that during the SVT, because the atrium and ventricle are activated in sequence in both scenarios (see Fig. 14-11).[9]

Tachycardia Features

Atrial Activation Sequence

During typical AVNRT, the initial site of atrial activation is usually recorded in the HB catheter at the apex of the triangle of Koch.[10] In contrast, the initial site of atrial activation during atypical AVNRT is usually recorded at the base of the triangle of Koch or coronary sinus ostium (CS os) (see Fig. 13-4).[10] On the other hand, in orthodromic AVRT, the initial site of atrial activation depends on the location of the AV BT, but is always near the AV groove, without multiple breakthrough points. It is comparable to that during ventricular pacing when VA conduction occurs exclusively over the AV BT. The atrial activation sequence during AT depends on the origin of the AT, and can simulate that of other types of SVT.[11] In summary, eccentric atrial activation during SVT excludes typical and atypical AVNRT, except for the left variant of AVNRT, during which the earliest atrial activation occurs in the proximal or mid-CS. Moreover, an eccentric atrial activation sequence that originates away from the AV rings is diagnostic of AT and excludes both AVNRT and AVRT.[9]

P/QRS Relationship

PR/RP. During AT, the PR interval is appropriate for the AT rate and is usually longer than that during NSR. The faster the AT rate, the longer the PR interval. Thus, the PR interval can be shorter, longer, or equal to the RP interval. The PR interval can also be equal to the RR and the P wave can then fall within the preceding QRS, mimicking typical AVNRT. During typical AVNRT, the RP interval is very short (−40 to 75 milliseconds); in contrast, during atypical AVNRT, the RP interval is longer than the PR interval. On the other hand, during orthodromic AVRT, the RP interval is short but longer than that in typical AVNRT (more than 70 milliseconds), because the wavefront has to activate the ventricle before it reaches the AV BT and subsequently conduct retrogradely to the atrium. Thus, the ventricle and atrium are activated in sequence, in contrast to AVNRT, during which the ventricle and atrium are activated in parallel, resulting in abbreviation of the VA interval.[7]

Atrioventricular Block. The presence of AV block during SVT excludes AVRT, is uncommon during AVNRT, and strongly favors AT (Fig. 16-3). AV block occurs commonly during AT, with either Wenckebach periodicity or fixed-ratio block. AV block can also be present during AVNRT because of block below the reentry circuit, usually below the HB and infrequently in the lower common pathway, which can occur especially at the onset of the SVT, during acceleration of the SVT, and following a PVC or a VES (see Fig. 13-3). Rarely, VA block can occur during AVNRT, because of block in the upper common pathway (see Fig. 13-12).

Oscillation in the Tachycardia Cycle Length. Analysis of tachycardia CL variability can provide useful diagnostic information that is available even when episodes of SVT are nonsustained. SVT CL variability of 15 milliseconds or more in magnitude occurs in 73% of paroxysmal SVTs and is equally prevalent in AT, AVNRT, and orthodromic AVRT. Changes in atrial CL preceding similar changes in subsequent ventricular CL strongly favor AT or atypical AVNRT (see Fig. 13-13). In contrast, when the change in atrial CL is predicted by the change in preceding ventricular CL, typical AVNRT or orthodromic AVRT is the most likely mechanism (see Fig. 14-15).

The AVN participates either actively or passively in all types of SVT and the AV interval can vary depending on the preceding atrial CL and autonomic tone. A change in anterograde or retrograde AVN conduction can result in tachycardia CL variability in AVNRT or orthodromic AVRT. In contrast, CL variability in AT is a result of changes in the CL of the atrial reentrant or focal tachycardia, or changes in AVN conduction. Therefore, when there is CL variability in both the atrium and ventricle, changes in atrial CL during AT would be expected to precede and predict the changes in ventricular CL. However, ventricular CL variability can be caused by changes in AV conduction instead of changes in the CL of an AT, in which case ventricular CL variability may not be predicted by a prior change in atrial CL during AT. Because there is no VA conduction during AT, ventricu-

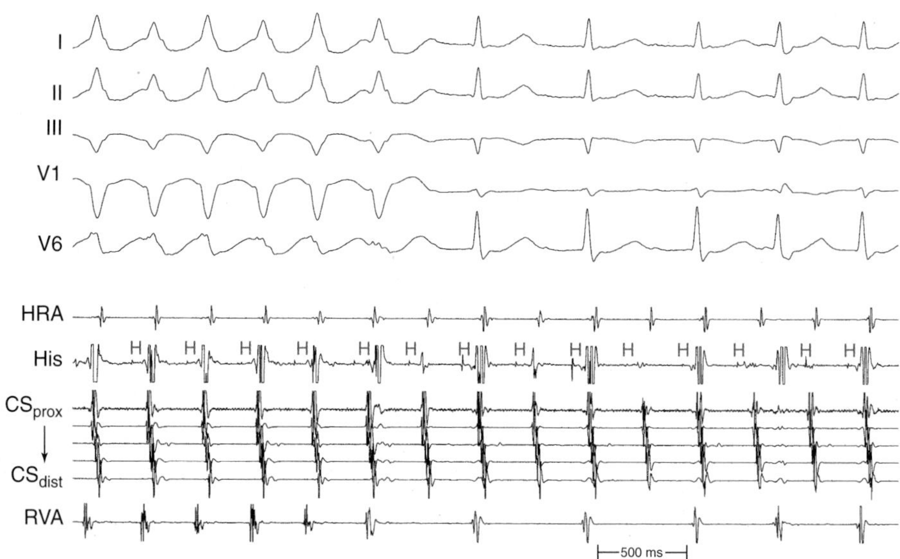

FIGURE 16–3 Supraventricular tachycardia with concentric atrial activation sequence and intermittent atrioventricular (AV) block. At left, a wide complex tachycardia with left bundle branch block (LBBB) pattern and 1 : 1 AV ratio. Simultaneous atrial and ventricular activation is observed, excluding atrioventricular reentrant tachycardia (AVRT) as the mechanism of the tachycardia, and favoring typical atrioventricular nodal reentrant tachycardia (AVNRT) or atrial tachycardia (AT) with a long PR interval. At right, 2 : 1 AV block is observed without disruption of the tachycardia. Normalization of QRS morphology is observed during the period of 2 : 1 AV block, suggesting that wide QRS morphology during 1 : 1 AV conduction was a result of functional LBBB. The development of AV block with continuation of the tachycardia confirms that the ventricle is not part of the tachycardia circuit and, thus, excludes AVRT. The presence of His potentials, even during the blocked beats, suggests that the block is infra-Hisian. The observation of AV block favors AT, but does not exclude AVNRT. The ventriculoatrial (VA) interval remains constant following both the narrow and wide QRS complexes, which suggests AVNRT. Other pacing maneuvers confirmed that this supraventricular tachycardia (SVT) was in fact typical AVNRT.

lar CL variability by itself would not be expected to result in atrial CL variability during AT.

In contrast to AT, typical AVNRT and orthodromic AVRT generally have CL variability because of changes in anterograde AVN conduction. Because retrograde conduction through a fast AVN pathway or a BT generally is much less variable than anterograde conduction through the AVN, the changes in ventricular CL that result from variability in anterograde AVN conduction would be expected to precede the subsequent changes in atrial CL. This explains why the change in atrial CL does not predict the change in subsequent ventricular CL in typical AVNRT and orthodromic AVRT. On the other hand, in atypical AVNRT, anterograde conduction occurs over the more stable fast AVN pathway and retrograde conduction is more subject to variability. This explains the finding that changes in atrial CL predict the changes in subsequent ventricular CL in atypical AVNRT, as was the case in AT.

Variation of the P-QRS relationship (with changes in the AH interval, HA interval, and AH/HA ratio), with or without block, can occur during AVNRT, especially in atypical or slow-slow AVNRT. This phenomenon usually occurs when the conduction system and/or reentry circuit are unstable during initiation or termination of the tachycardia. The ECG manifestation of P-QRS variations, with or without AV block during tachycardia, especially at initiation of tachycardias or in cases of nonsustained tachycardias, should not be misdiagnosed as AT; they can be atypical or, rarely, typical forms of AVNRT. Moreover, the variations could be of such magnitude that a long RP tachycardia can masquerade for brief periods of time as short RP tachycardia.

Spontaneous changes in the PR and RP intervals with fixed A-A interval favor AT and exclude orthodromic AVRT. On the other hand, spontaneous changes in tachycardia CL accompanied by constant VA interval suggest orthodromic AVRT (see Fig. 8-7). During orthodromic AVRT, the RP interval remains fixed, regardless of oscillations in tachycardia CL from whatever cause or changes in the PR (AH) interval. Thus, the RP/PR ratio may change, and the tachycardia CL is most closely associated with the PR interval (i.e., anterograde slow conduction).

Effects of Bundle Branch Block

The development of BBB during SVT that neither influences the tachycardia CL (A-A or H-H interval) nor the VA interval is consistent with AVNRT (see Fig. 13-3), AT, and orthodromic AVRT using a BT in the ventricle contralateral to the BBB (see Fig. 14-14), but excludes orthodromic AVRT using a BT ipsilateral to the BBB.

BBB ipsilateral to the AV BT mediating orthodromic AVRT results in prolongation of the VA interval (see Figs. 14-6 and 14-16). The tachycardia CL usually increases concomitantly with the increase in the VA interval as a result of ipsilateral BBB (because of the now larger tachycardia circuit). However, compensatory shortening in the AH interval can be enough to overcome the prolongation of the VA interval, and consequently result in no change or even shortening in the tachycardia CL. Thus, the VA interval and not the tachycardia CL should be used to assess the SVT response to BBB. Prolongation of the VA interval in response to BBB by more than 35 milliseconds indicates that ipsilateral free wall AV BT is present and participating in the SVT (i.e., diagnostic of orthodromic AVRT). Prolongation of less than 25 milliseconds suggests a septal AV BT (posteroseptal AV BT in association of LBBB, and superoparaseptal AV BT in association with RBBB). The mere presence of LBBB aberrancy during SVT is also suggestive of orthodromic AVRT but can still occur in other types of SVT.[7,9,12]

QRS Alternans

QRS alternans during relatively slow SVTs is almost always indicative of orthodromic AVRT. However, QRS alternans during fast SVTs is most commonly seen in orthodromic AVRT but can also be seen with other types of SVTs as well.

Termination and Response to Physiological and Pharmacological Maneuvers

Spontaneous Termination. Spontaneous termination of orthodromic AVRT usually occurs because of anterograde gradual slowing and then block in the AVN, sometimes causing initial oscillation in the tachycardia CL, with alternate complexes demonstrating a Wenckebach periodicity before block. However, termination with retrograde block in the AV BT can occur without any perturbations of the tachycardia CL during very rapid orthodromic AVRT or with sudden shortening of the tachycardia CL.

Spontaneous termination of AVNRT occurs because of block in the fast or slow pathway. However, the better the retrograde fast pathway conduction, the less likely that it is the site of block. Spontaneous termination of AT is usually accompanied by progressive prolongation of the A-A interval, with or without changes in AV conduction. During AT with 1:1 AV conduction, the last beat of AT is conducted to the ventricle. Spontaneous termination of SVT with a P wave not followed by a QRS practically excludes AT, except in the case of a nonconducted PAC terminating the AT.[9]

Termination with Adenosine. The mere termination of SVT in response to adenosine is usually not helpful in differentiating SVTs. However, the pattern of SVT termination can be helpful in two situations:

1. Reproducible termination of the SVT with a QRS not followed by a P wave excludes orthodromic AVRT using a rapidly conducting AV BT as the retrograde limb (adenosine blocks the AVN and not the BT), is unusual in typical AVNRT (adenosine blocks the slow pathway but does not affect the fast pathway), and is consistent with AT, PJRT, or atypical AVNRT.
2. Reproducible termination of the SVT with a P wave not followed by a QRS excludes AT (Fig. 16-4). Most (50% to 80%) of ATs are terminated by adenosine, typically (80%) prior to the onset of AV block. Response to adenosine does not seem to help differentiate between atypical AVNRT and PJRT.

Termination with Vagal Maneuvers. Carotid sinus massage and vagal maneuvers reproducibly slow or terminate up to 25% of ATs. Orthodromic AVRT usually terminates with gradual slowing and then block in the AVN. Typical AVNRT usually terminates with gradual anterograde slowing and then block in the slow pathway; block in the fast pathway is uncommon. Additionally, carotid sinus massage and vagal maneuvers always terminate atypical AVNRT by gradual slowing and then block in the retrograde slow pathway.[9]

Diagnostic Maneuvers During Tachycardia

Atrial Extrastimulation During Supraventricular Tachycardia

Resetting. An AES can reset AT, AVNRT, and orthodromic AVRT, and demonstration of resetting by itself is not helpful in distinguishing among the different types of SVT. Two responses to resetting, however, can help in the differential diagnosis: (1) resetting with manifest atrial fusion can be demonstrated in orthodromic AVRT and macroreentrant AT, but not with AVNRT or focal AT; and (2) the resetting curve can help differentiate the different subtypes of SVT. Reentrant AT, AVNRT, and orthodromic AVRT are characterized by an increasing or mixed response curve, whereas triggered activity AT exhibits an increasing resetting response curve and automatic AT exhibits a decreasing resetting response curve.[9] It is difficult for an AES not to affect orthodromic AVRT because of the large size of the reentrant circuit, and an AES over a wide range of coupling intervals can reset the SVT via conduction down the AVN-HPS. However, for AVNRT, more premature AESs are needed to demonstrate resetting.[9]

Termination. An AES can reproducibly terminate reentrant AT, AVNRT, and orthodromic AVRT, but not automatic AT. Termination of triggered activity AT is less reproducible. Thus, termination of SVT with an AES is not usually helpful for the differential diagnosis.[9]

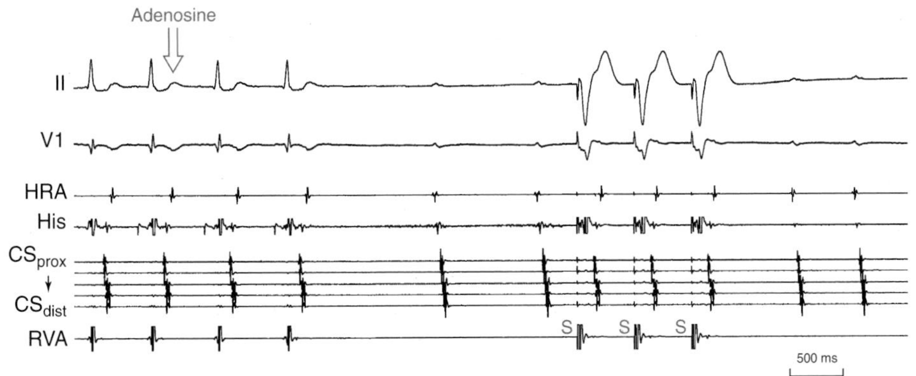

FIGURE 16–4 Termination of supraventricular tachycardia with adenosine. Administration of adenosine during a supraventricular tachycardia (SVT) with concentric atrial activation sequence and short RP interval results in termination of the SVT with an atrial complex not followed by a QRS, which is inconsistent with atrial tachycardia (AT). Following termination of the SVT, complete atrioventricular (AV) block during sinus rhythm is observed; however, ventricular pacing is associated with intact ventriculoatrial (VA) conduction and retrograde atrial activation sequence identical to that during the SVT, which suggests that VA conduction is not mediated by the atrioventricular node (AVN) but by an AV bypass tract (BT). The SVT is in fact an orthodromic AVRT using a concealed septal BT, and termination with adenosine was the result of anterograde block in the AVN. Conduction over the BT was not affected by adenosine.

Atrial Pacing During Supraventricular Tachycardia

Entrainment. Overdrive atrial pacing can entrain reentrant AT, AVNRT, and orthodromic AVRT but not triggered activity or automatic ATs. Entrainment with manifest fusion can be seen only in AVRT and macroreentrant AT, but not with AVNRT or focal AT (see Fig. 14-19).

During entrainment at a pacing CL close to the tachycardia CL, the AH interval during entrainment is longer than that during AVNRT because the atrium and HB are activated in parallel during AVNRT and in sequence during atrial pacing entraining the AVNRT (because of the presence of an upper common pathway). However, for AT and orthodromic AVRT, the AH interval is comparable during SVT and entrainment with atrial pacing.[9]

On cessation of overdrive atrial pacing, if the VA interval following the last entrained QRS is reproducibly constant, despite pacing at different CLs (VA linking) and similar to that during SVT, AT is unlikely. If no VA linking is demonstrable, AT is more likely than other types of SVT (see Fig. 14-19).[7]

Acceleration. Overdrive pacing during triggered activity AT generally produces acceleration of the tachycardia CL.

Overdrive Suppression. Automatic AT cannot be entrained by atrial pacing; however, rapid atrial pacing results in overdrive suppression of the AT rate, with the return CL following the pacing train prolonging with increasing the duration and/or rate of overdrive pacing, in contrast to constant return cycles following entrainment of reentrant circuits, regardless of the length of the pacing drive. The AT resumes following cessation of atrial pacing but at a slower rate, gradually speeding up (warming up) back to prepacing tachycardia CL. On the other hand, overdrive pacing may have no effect on automatic AT.[9]

Termination. Atrial pacing can reproducibly terminate reentrant AT, AVNRT, and orthodromic AVRT, but not automatic AT. Termination of triggered activity AT is less reproducible. Thus, termination of SVT with atrial pacing is not usually helpful for differential diagnosis.

Differential-Site Atrial Pacing. Overdrive pacing during the SVT is performed from different atrial sites (high RA and proximal CS) at the same pacing CL, and the maximal difference in the post-pacing VA intervals (last captured ventricular electrogram to the earliest atrial electrogram of the initial beat after pacing) among the different pacing sites is calculated (ΔVA interval). In a recent report, a ΔVA interval more than 14 milliseconds was diagnostic of AT, whereas a ΔVA interval less than 14 milliseconds favors AVNRT and orthodromic AVRT over AT (with the sensitivity, specificity, and positive and negative predictive values all being 100%).[13]

In orthodromic AVRT and AVNRT, the initial atrial activation following cessation of atrial pacing is linked to the last captured ventricular activation, and therefore cannot be dissociated from the ventricular activation. In contrast, in AT, the first atrial return cycle following cessation of pacing is dependent on the distance between the AT origin and pacing site, atrial conduction properties, and mode of the resetting response of the AT, and is not related to the preceding ventricular activation. Hence, the post-pacing VA intervals vary among pacing sites and the ΔVA interval display is not zero, but a certain value.[13]

Ventricular Extrastimulation During Supraventricular Tachycardia

Resetting. During orthodromic AVRT, a VES can usually reset the SVT. However, the ability of the VES to affect the SVT depends on the distance between the site of ventricular stimulation to the ventricular insertion site of the BT and on the VES coupling interval. Because only parts of the ventricle ipsilateral to the BT are requisite components of the orthodromic AVRT circuit, a VES delivered in the contralateral ventricle may not affect the circuit (see Fig. 14-21). On the other hand, the inability of early single or double VESs to reset the SVT despite advancement of all ventricular electrograms (including the local electrogram in the electrode recording the earliest atrial activation during the SVT, which would be close to the potential BT ventricular insertion site) by more than 30 milliseconds excludes orthodromic AVRT. Several other findings can help confirm the presence of BT function and whether it is participating in the SVT or only a bystander (see Tables 14-4 and 14-5).

The preexcitation index analyzes the coupling interval of the VES delivered from the RV that resets orthodromic AVRT as a percentage of the tachycardia CL. A relative preexcitation index (the ratio of the coupling interval divided by the tachycardia CL) of more than 90% of a VES that advances atrial activation during orthodromic AVRT suggests that the BT is close to the site of ventricular stimulation (i.e., RV or septal BT). An absolute preexcitation index (tachycardia CL minus VES coupling interval) of 75 milliseconds or more suggests a left free wall BT, an index of less than 45 milliseconds suggests a septal BT, and an index of 45 to 75 milliseconds is indeterminate.

For AVNRT, the ability of a VES to affect the SVT depends on its ability to activate the HB prematurely and penetrate the AVN, which in turn depends on the tachycardia CL, local ventricular ERP, and the time needed for the VES to reach the HB. Even when HB activation is advanced by the VES, the ability of the paced impulse to invade the AVN will depend on the length of the lower common pathway; the longer the lower common pathway, the more the timing of HB activation must be advanced. In fast-slow or slow-slow AVNRT, which typically has a long lower common pathway, the HB activation must be advanced by more than 30 to 60 milliseconds. In contrast, in slow-fast AVNRT, the lower common pathway is shorter and the tachycardia is typically reset by the VES as soon as the HB activation is advanced. Therefore, a late VES, delivered when the HB is refractory, would not be able to penetrate the AVN and reset AVNRT. During AT, a VES can advance the next atrial activation when given the chance to conduct retrogradely and prematurely to the atrium. However, it would never be able to delay the next AT beat.

Although resetting the SVT by a VES is not diagnostic by itself of a specific type of SVT, it can be helpful in certain situations. First, the ability of a late VES delivered while the HB is refractory (i.e., when the anterograde His potential is already manifest or within 35 to 55 milliseconds before the time of the expected His potential) to affect (reset or terminate) the SVT excludes AVNRT, because such a VES would not have been able to penetrate the AVNRT circuit (Fig. 16-5; see Fig. 14-21). It also excludes AT, except for cases of AT associated with the presence of innocent bystander BT, in which case the presence of such a BT is usually easy to exclude with ventricular pacing during NSR. Second, the ability of a VES to delay the next atrial activation excludes AT (see Fig. 14-18). Third, the ability of a VES to reset the SVT without atrial activation (i.e., advances the subsequent His potential and QRS and blocks in the upper common pathway) excludes AT and orthodromic AVRT, because it proves that the atrium is not part of the SVT circuit. Fourth, failure of early single or double VESs to reset the SVT, despite advancement of ventricular electrograms in the electrode recording the earliest atrial activation by more than 30 ms, excludes orthodromic AVRT.

Termination. Termination of AVNRT with a single VES is difficult and occurs rarely when the tachycardia CL is

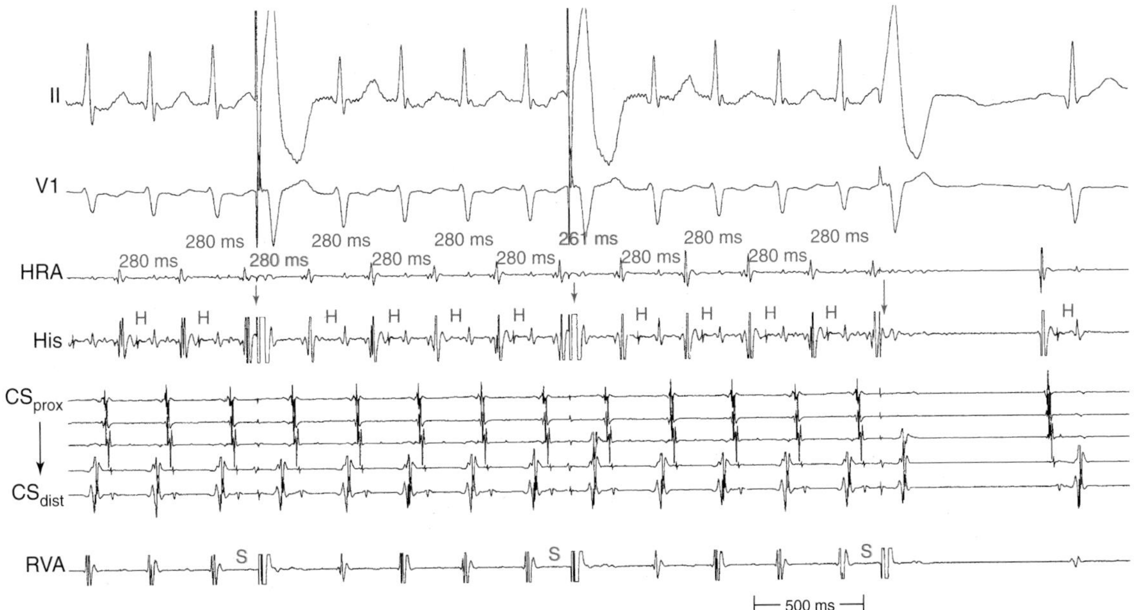

FIGURE 16–5 Ventricular extrastimulation (VES) during supraventricular tachycardia (SVT). VESs were delivered at progressively shorter coupling intervals during a narrow complex SVT with concentric atrial activation sequence. Timing of the anticipated anterograde His bundle (HB) activation is indicated by the blue arrows. The first VES is delivered during HB refractoriness and fails to reset the tachycardia, a phenomenon that does not help in the differential diagnosis. The second VES is delivered slightly earlier but still during HB refractoriness, and it does anticipate the following atrial activation. Atrial activation sequence during the reset atrial complex is identical to that during SVT. This observation excludes atrioventricular nodal reentrant tachycardia (AVNRT), and favors orthodromic atrioventricular reentrant tachycardia (AVRT), but does not exclude the rare example of atrial tachycardia (AT) with a bystander bypass tract (BT) with atrial insertion close to the AT focus. The third VES is delivered during HB refractoriness (within 40 msec before the anticipated anterograde HB activation) and it terminates the tachycardia without conducting to the atrium. This observation, when reproducible, excludes both AVNRT and AT, and proves that the tachycardia is an orthodromic AVRT.

less than 350 milliseconds; such termination favors the diagnosis of orthodromic AVRT, which can usually be readily terminated by single or double VESs. Termination of the SVT with a VES delivered when the HB is refractory excludes AVNRT (see Fig. 16-5). It also excludes AT, except for cases of AT associated with the presence of an innocent bystander BT mediating VA conduction. Reproducible termination of the SVT with a VES not followed by atrial activation excludes AT (see Fig. 14-21) and, if this occurs with a VES delivered while the HB is refractory, it excludes both AT and AVNRT (see Fig. 16-5).

Ventricular Pacing During SVT

Entrainment. Ventricular pacing is almost always able to entrain AVNRT and orthodromic AVRT and, if 1:1 VA conduction is maintained, reentrant AT. Entrainment of the SVT by RV pacing can help differentiate orthodromic AVRT from AVNRT by evaluating the VA interval during SVT versus that during pacing, and also by evaluating the post-pacing interval (PPI).[14] The ventricle and atrium are activated in sequence during orthodromic AVRT and ventricular pacing, but in parallel during AVNRT. Therefore, the VA interval during orthodromic AVRT approximates that during ventricular pacing (see Fig. 14-22). On the other hand, the VA interval during AVNRT would be much shorter than that during ventricular pacing (see Fig. 13-15). In general, if $VA_{ventricular\ pacing} - VA_{SVT}$ is more than 85 milliseconds, the SVT is AVNRT, whereas if $VA_{ventricular\ pacing} - VA_{SVT}$ is less than 85 milliseconds, the SVT is orthodromic AVRT (Fig. 16-6).

Additionally, the PPI after entrainment of AVNRT from the RV apex is significantly longer than the tachycardia CL ([PPI – SVT CL] is usually more than 115 milliseconds), because the reentrant circuit in AVNRT is above the ventricle and far from the pacing site (see Fig. 13-15). In AVNRT, the PPI reflects the conduction time from the pacing site through the RV muscle and HPS, once around the reentry circuit and back to the pacing site. Therefore, the [PPI – SVT CL] reflects twice the sum of the conduction time through the RV muscle, the HPS, and the lower common pathway (see Fig. 16-6). In orthodromic AVRT using a septal BT, the PPI reflects the conduction time through the RV to the septum, once around the reentry circuit and back. In other words, [PPI – SVT CL] reflects twice the conduction time from the pacing catheter through the ventricular myocardium to the reentry circuit. Therefore, the PPI more closely approximates the SVT CL in orthodromic AVRT using a septal BT, compared with AVNRT (see Fig. 14-22). This maneuver was studied specifically for differentiation between atypical AVNRT and orthodromic AVRT, but the principle also applies to typical AVNRT. In general, when [PPI – SVT CL] is more than 115 ms, the SVT is AVNRT, and when [PPI – SVT CL] is less than 115 milliseconds, the SVT is orthodromic AVRT. For borderline values, ventricular pacing at the RV base can help exaggerate the difference between the PPI and tachycardia CL in the case of AVNRT, but without significant changes in the case of orthodromic AVRT, because the site of pacing at the RV base is farther from the AVNRT circuit than the RV apex but still close to an AVRT circuit using a septal BT (and is even closer to the ventricular insertion of the BT).[15]

Furthermore, manifest ventricular fusion during entrainment indicates AVRT and excludes AVNRT and AT (see Fig. 14-22). The relative proximity (conduction time) among pacing site, site of entrance to the reentrant circuit, and site of exit from the circuit to the paced chamber are critical for the occurrence of fusion during resetting and/or entrainment. Another requirement for the presence of fusion, independent of the site of pacing, is spatial separation between the sites of entrance to and exit from the reentrant circuit. For orthodromic AVRT, the entrance and exit of the reentrant circuit (to and from ventricular tissue) are separated from each other; the entrance is from the HPS, and the exit is at the ventricular insertion site of the BT. Therefore, pacing at a site closer to the BT ventricular insertion site

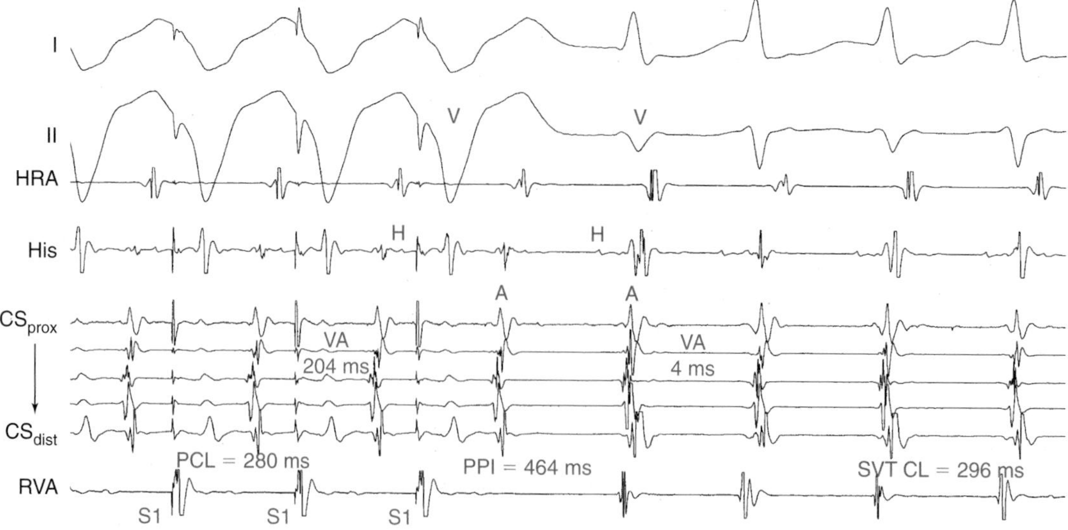

16

FIGURE 16–6 Entrainment of narrow QRS supraventricular tachycardia (SVT) with right ventricular (RV) apical pacing. Several features in this tracing can help in the differential diagnosis of this SVT. First, atrial and ventricular activation occur simultaneously during the SVT, which excludes atrioventricular reentrant tachycardia (AVRT). Second, atrial activation during the SVT is eccentric, with earliest activation in the mid–coronary sinus (CS), which favors atrial tachycardia (AT) over AVNRT. Third, the atrial activation sequence during ventricular pacing is identical to that during SVT, which favors AVNRT and AVRT over AT. Fourth, following cessation over ventricular pacing, the post-pacing interval (PPI) SVT cycle length (CL)—[PPI – SVT CL]—is more than 115 msec, and the ΔVA interval (VA_{pacing} – VA_{SVT}) is more than 85 msec, which favor AVNRT over AVRT. Fifth, although characterization of the activation sequence following cessation of ventricular pacing (A-A-V versus A-V response) is unclear (because of the simultaneous occurrence of atrial and ventricular activation in the first tachycardia complex, replacing ventricular activation with HB activation [i.e., characterizing the response as A-A-H or A-H instead of A-A-V or A-V, respectively]) reveals an A-H response, which favors AVRT and AVNRT over AT. In summary, AVRT can be reliably excluded by the simultaneous atrial and ventricular activation. AT is excluded by the A-H response following cessation of ventricular pacing and by the identical atrial activation sequence during the SVT and ventricular pacing. The left variant of typical AVRT (with an eccentric atrial activation sequence) is the mechanism of the SVT.

(e.g., LV pacing in case of left free wall BTs, and RV apical pacing in case of right-sided or septal BTs) than the entrance of the reentrant circuit to ventricular tissue (HPS) would result in QRS fusion. On the other hand, fusion during resetting or entrainment of AVNRT would require that the paced ventricular wavefronts enter the circuit propagating through the HB when impulses are exiting through this structure (the HB is also the site of exit of the tachycardia circuit to the ventricular tissue). In such a case, constant fusion during entrainment is almost impossible—unless a second connection exists between the atria and ventricles (i.e., an innocent bystander BT).

A-V Versus A-A-V Response. As discussed in detail in Chapter 8, when the ventricle is paced during AVNRT or orthodromic AVRT at a pacing CL shorter than the tachycardia CL, and all electrograms are advanced to the pacing rate without terminating the tachycardia, 1:1 VA conduction occurs through the retrograde limb of the circuit. Therefore, after the last paced QRS, the anterograde limb of the tachycardia circuit is not refractory, and the last retrograde P wave is able to conduct to the ventricle using that limb. This results in an A-V response (see Fig. 8-8). However, when the ventricle is paced during AT and 1:1 VA conduction is produced, retrograde conduction occurs through the AVN. In this case, the last retrograde P wave resulting from ventricular pacing is unable to conduct back to the ventricle because the AVN is refractory to anterograde conduction, and the result is an A-A-V response (see Fig. 8-8).[16]

This pacing maneuver, however, would not be useful when 1:1 VA conduction during ventricular pacing is absent (Fig. 16-7). Furthermore, a pseudo–A-A-V response can occur during atypical AVNRT. Careful examination of the last atrial electrogram that resulted from VA conduction during ventricular pacing will avoid this potential pitfall; the last retrograde atrial complex characteristically occurs at an A-A interval equal to the ventricular pacing CL, whereas the first tachycardia atrial complex usually occurs at a different return CL (see Fig. 8-8). A pseudo–A-A-V response may also occur when 1:1 VA conduction is not present during overdrive ventricular pacing, during typical AVNRT with long or short HA intervals in which atrial activation may precede ventricular activation, and in patients with a bystander BT.

Replacing ventricular activation with HB activation (i.e., characterizing the response as A-A-H or A-H instead of A-A-V or A-V, respectively) can be more accurate and can help eliminate the pseudo–A-A-V response in several situations (see Fig. 16-6).[16]

Termination. Ventricular pacing can easily terminate orthodromic AVRT, and failure to terminate the SVT with ventricular pacing argues against orthodromic AVRT. Termination of AVNRT is also common, but AT is less likely to be terminated with ventricular pacing.

Atrial Activation Sequence. A retrograde atrial activation sequence during ventricular pacing or VES delivered during the SVT is usually similar to that during SVT in the case of AVNRT and orthodromic AVRT, because it should conduct over the tachycardia retrograde limb. On the other hand, for AT, retrograde atrial activation sequence during ventricular pacing is usually different from that during AT, except for ATs originating close to the AV junction. A pitfall of this criterion is the presence of a bystander AV BT, which can provide another retrograde route capable of mediating retrograde conduction of ventricular stimuli without being part of the SVT circuit. In this case, ventricular stimulation can result in a retrograde atrial activation sequence different from that of AVNRT or orthodromic AVRT. The presence of such an AV BT, however, is generally easy to verify with ventricular stimulation during NSR.

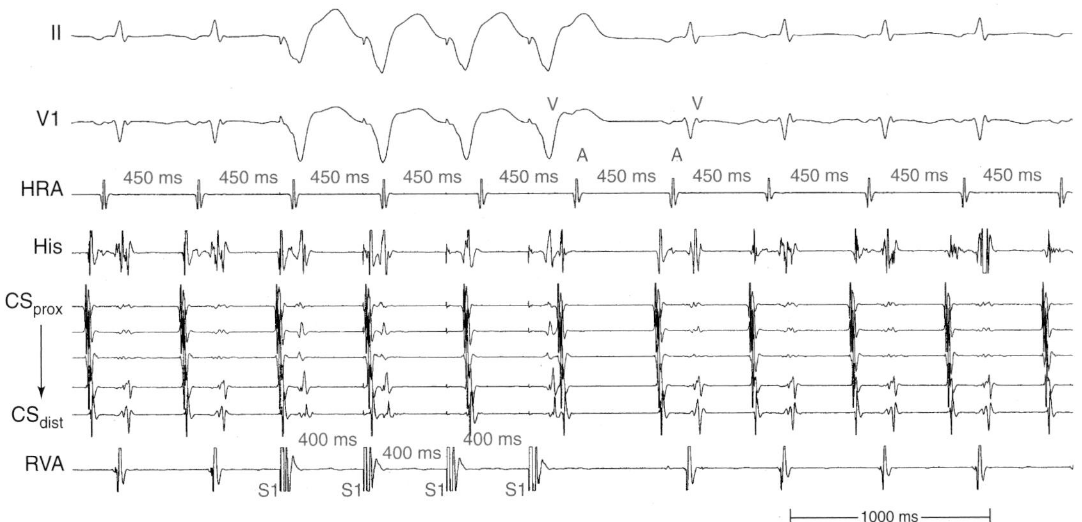

FIGURE 16–7 Overdrive ventricular pacing during a narrow QRS supraventricular tachycardia (SVT). The SVT has a long RP interval and concentric atrial activation sequence, which favors atypical atrioventricular nodal reentrant tachycardia (AVNRT), atrial tachycardia (AT) originating close to the AV junction, or orthodromic AVRT using a slowly conducting septal bypass tract (BT). Overdrive ventricular pacing during the tachycardia fails to entrain the tachycardia or capture the atrium (no ventriculoatrial [VA] conduction), because the tachycardia atrial cycle length (CL; 450 msec) remains stable and unaltered by the faster ventricular pacing CL (400 msec). Therefore, analysis of the post-pacing interval (PPI) or VA interval during pacing versus SVT is invalid. Additionally, analysis of the response sequence following cessation of pacing (A-V versus A-A-A-V response) is also invalid in view of the lack of 1:1 VA conduction during ventricular pacing (resulting in a pseudo–A-A-V response). However, the fact that ventricular pacing has dissociated the atrium from the ventricle excludes AVRT. However, other pacing maneuvers are required for differentiation between atypical AVNRT and AT.

Diagnostic Maneuvers During Normal Sinus Rhythm After Tachycardia Termination

Atrial Pacing at Tachycardia Cycle Length

ΔAH Interval. During AT and orthodromic AVRT, the AH interval during SVT is comparable to that during atrial pacing because the activation wavefront propagates through a similar pathway during SVT and atrial pacing. On the other hand, the AH interval during AVNRT is shorter than that during atrial pacing, because the atrium and HB are activated in parallel during AVNRT (because of the presence of an upper common pathway) but in sequence during atrial pacing. Therefore, a ΔAH ($AH_{atrial\ pacing} - AH_{SVT}$) of more than 40 milliseconds suggests AVNRT and excludes AT and orthodromic AVRT. However, a ΔAH of less than 20 milliseconds suggests that AT and orthodromic AVRT are more likely than AVNRT.

Atrioventricular Block. For AT and orthodromic AVRT, the AVN should be able to conduct 1:1 during atrial pacing and during the SVT, given that the pacing CL is equal to the tachycardia CL and that the same degree of autonomic tone is maintained, as would be expected when pacing is performed shortly after termination of SVT. Therefore, if AV block develops during atrial pacing, it suggests the presence of an upper common pathway and is consistent with AVNRT.

Ventricular Pacing at the Tachycardia Cycle Length

ΔHA Interval. During AVNRT, the HB and atrium are activated in parallel, whereas they are activated in sequence during atrial pacing. Therefore, the HA interval during AVNRT is shorter than that during ventricular pacing. In contrast, the HB and atrium are activated in sequence during orthodromic AVRT and in parallel during ventricular pacing in the presence of a retrogradely conducing BT. Therefore, the HA interval during orthodromic AVRT is longer than that during ventricular pacing (see Fig. 14-22).

Ventriculoatrial Block. If VA block is present during ventricular pacing, orthodromic AVRT and the presence of a retrogradely conducting fast AV BT are practically excluded, but PJRT is not excluded, and AT and AVNRT with a lower common pathway physiology are more likely.

Atrial Activation Sequence. Retrograde atrial activation sequence during ventricular pacing is usually similar to that during SVT for AVNRT and can be similar or different to that during orthodromic AVRT, depending on whether retrograde VA conduction during ventricular pacing proceeds over the AVN, the BT, or both. However, for AT, retrograde atrial activation sequence during ventricular pacing is usually different from that during AT, except for ATs originating close to the AV junction.

Differential RV Pacing

The response to differential RV pacing can be evaluated by comparing the VA interval and atrial activation sequence during pacing at the RV base versus the RV apex. In the absence of a septal AV BT, pacing at the RV apex results in rapid access of the paced wavefront to the RB, HB, and AVN, and a shorter VA interval compared with pacing at the RV base (see Fig. 14-25). In the presence of a retrogradely conducting septal AV-BT, pacing at the RV base allows the wavefront to access the BT ventricular insertion rapidly and activate the atrium with a shorter VA interval than during RV apical pacing, which is farther from the BT.

Additionally, atrial activation sequence will be similar during RV apical and basilar pacing in the absence of a retrogradely conducting AV BT because the atrium is activated over the AVN in both cases. Although atrial activation sequence can be similar during pacing from the RV apex and base if a septal AV BT is present (because atrial activation can proceed only over the AV BT in both cases), it also can be different. This is because atrial activation may proceed over the AV BT during RV basilar pacing and over the AVN (or a fusion of conduction over both the AVN and AV BT) during RV apical pacing.

This maneuver, however, does not exclude the presence of a distant right or left free wall AV BT, because the site of pacing is far from the AV BT and atrial activation results from conduction over the AVN in either case, RV apical or basilar pacing, or a slowly-conducting BT. In the latter case, conduction over the AVN is faster than that over the BT during both RV apical and basilar pacing.

Para-Hisian Pacing

As discussed in detail in Chapter 14, during para-Hisian pacing, when the ventricle and HB are captured simultaneously, the wavefront travels down the HPS and results in a relatively narrow, normal-looking QRS. The wavefront can also travel retrogradely over the AVN to activate the atrium with an S-A interval that represents conduction time over the proximal part of the HB and AVN (i.e., S-A = HA interval) because the onset of ventricular activation is simultaneous to that of HB activation (i.e., S-H interval = 0). When the ventricle is captured, but not the atrium or HB, the wavefront travels through the ventricle by muscle-to-muscle conduction, resulting in a wide QRS with LBBB morphology because of pacing in the RV. Once the wavefront reaches the RV apex, it conducts retrogradely up the RB and then over the HB and AVN to activate the atrium. In this case, the S-A interval represents conduction time from the RV base to the HPS (S-H interval) plus conduction time over the HB and AVN (HA interval).

Thus, normally (in the absence of a retrogradely conducting AV BT), para-Hisian pacing results in a shorter S-A interval when the HB is captured (S-H = 0 and S-A = HA) than the S-A interval when only the ventricle is captured (S-A = S-H + HA). The atrial activation sequence in either case will be the same, because it is mediated by conduction over the AVN. However, in the presence of a septal AV BT, the S-A interval remains fixed regardless of whether or not the HB is being captured, because the impulse travels in both cases retrogradely over the AV BT with constant conduction time to the atrium. Atrial activation in this case may be secondary to conduction over the BT (especially when only the ventricle is captured) or a result of fusion of conduction over both the AV BT and AVN (especially when the HB is captured; see Figs. 14-23 and 14-24).

Therefore, a change in retrograde atrial activation sequence with loss of HB-RB capture indicates the presence of retrograde conduction over both a BT and the AVN, whereas an identical atrial activation sequence indicates that retrograde conduction is occurring over the same pathway (either the AVN or a BT) during HB-RB capture and noncapture. On loss of HB-RB capture, a constant S-A interval (or local VA interval) combined with shortening of the H-A interval indicates that retrograde conduction is occurring only over a BT. Lengthening of the S-A interval combined with a constant H-A interval indicates that retrograde conduction is occurring only over the AVN.

The location of the BT, as well as the retrograde conduction time over the BT, must be taken into account when interpreting the response of para-Hisian pacing. For left free wall BTs located far from the pacing site, the S-V_{BT} can be sufficiently long to have the entire atria activated by the AVN, even during loss of HB capture. In this case, para-Hisian pacing may produce an AVN retrograde conduction pattern, regardless of whether the HB is captured, failing to identify the presence of retrograde BT conduction. Additionally, para-Hisian pacing may fail to identify retrograde conduction over a slowly conducting BT because of a long V-A_{BT}. Moreover, in patients with very proximal RBBB, RB capture may fail to produce early retrograde activation of the HB, limiting the use of para-Hisian pacing in these patients.

PRACTICAL APPROACH TO ELECTROPHYSIOLOGICAL DIAGNOSIS OF SUPRAVENTRICULAR TACHYCARDIA

Maneuvers During Supraventricular Tachycardia

Baseline Supraventricular Tachycardia Features

Atrial Activation Sequence. Eccentric atrial activation sequence excludes AVNRT (except for the left variant of AVNRT). An initial atrial activation site away from the AV groove and AV junction is diagnostic of AT and excludes both AVNRT and orthodromic AVRT.[9-11]

Ventriculoatrial Interval. A VA interval of less than 70 milliseconds or a ventricular to high RA interval of less than 95 milliseconds during SVT excludes orthodromic AVRT, and is consistent with AVNRT, but can occur during AT with long PR interval.[7]

Atrioventricular Block. Spontaneous or induced AV block with continuation of the tachycardia is consistent with AT, excludes AVRT, and is uncommon in AVNRT.

Effects of Bundle Branch Block. BBB does not affect the tachycardia CL or VA interval in AT, AVNRT, or orthodromic AVRT using a BT contralateral to the BBB. BBB that prolongs the VA interval, with or without affecting the tachycardia CL, is diagnostic of orthodromic AVRT using an AV BT ipsilateral to the BBB and excludes AT and AVNRT.[7,9,12]

Spontaneous Oscillations in the Tachycardia Cycle Length. Spontaneous changes in PR and RP intervals with a fixed A-A interval is consistent with AT, and excludes orthodromic AVRT. Spontaneous changes in the tachycardia CL accompanied by a constant VA interval favor orthodromic AVRT. Changes in atrial CLs preceding similar changes in subsequent ventricular CLs strongly favor AT or atypical AVNRT. In contrast, when the change in atrial CL is predicted by the change in the preceding ventricular CL, typical AVNRT or orthodromic AVRT is the most likely mechanism.

Ventricular Extrastimulus During Supraventricular Tachycardia

A VES is delivered when the HB is refractory and then at progressively shorter VES coupling intervals (approximately 10-millisecond stepwise shortening of the VES coupling interval) so as to scan the entire diastole. First, ventricular capture of the VES should be verified, and then the effect of the VES on the following atrial activation (advancement, delay, termination, or no effect) should be evaluated, as well as the timing of the VES in relation to the expected His potential during the SVT. Furthermore, conduction of the VES to the atrium and sequence of atrial activation following the VES should be carefully examined (see Fig. 16-5).

When the Ventricular Extrastimulus Advances the Next Atrial Activation. Advancement (earlier activation) of the next atrial impulse occurring with a VES delivered when the HB is not refractory usually does not help differentiate among the different types of SVT. However, if the advanced atrial activation occurs with similar prematurity (i.e., same coupling interval) to that of the VES (exact coupling phenomenon) or with more prematurity (i.e., shorter coupling interval) than that of the VES (paradoxical coupling phenomenon), orthodromic AVRT is diagnosed. Importantly, if advancement occurs when the HB is refractory, AVNRT is excluded. Furthermore, if advancement occurs with an atrial activation sequence similar to that during SVT, regardless of the timing of the VES, AT is less likely than AVNRT or orthodromic AVRT, but this does not exclude ATs originating near the AV junction. When advancement occurs when the HB is refractory, with an atrial activation sequence similar to that during SVT, AVNRT is excluded, AT is unlikely, and orthodromic AVRT is the most likely diagnosis.

When the Ventricular Extrastimulus Delays the Next Atrial Activation. When the VES causes delay in the next atrial activation, regardless of the timing of the VES, AT is excluded, and when such delay occurs with a VES delivered when the HB is refractory, both AVNRT and AT are excluded.

When the Ventricular Extrastimulus Terminates the Supraventricular Tachycardia. When termination occurs reproducibly with a VES delivered when the HB is refractory, AVNRT is excluded, and presence of a retrogradely conducting AV BT is diagnosed. If atrial activation sequence following the VES is similar to that during the SVT, orthodromic AVRT is indicated and AT is practically excluded, except for the rare case in which AT originates close to the atrial insertion site of an innocent bystander AV BT. When termination occurs reproducibly with a VES that does not activate the atrium, regardless of the timing of the VES in relation to the HB, AT is excluded; when this phenomenon is observed with a VES delivered when the HB is refractory, both AT and AVNRT are excluded and orthodromic AVRT is diagnosed.

When the Ventricular Extrastimulus Fails to Affect the Next Atrial Activation. If resetting does not occur with a relatively late VES, this usually does not help in the differential diagnosis of SVT. However, if resetting does not occur with an early VES, despite advancement of the local ventricular activation at all ventricular sites by more than 30 milliseconds, orthodromic AVRT and the presence of a retrogradely conducting AV BT are excluded.

Ventricular Pacing During Supraventricular Tachycardia

Ventricular pacing is performed at a CL 10 to 30 milliseconds shorter than the tachycardia CL; the pacing CL is then progressively reduced by 10 to 20 milliseconds in a stepwise fashion with discontinuation of ventricular pacing after each pacing CL to verify continuation versus termination of the SVT. The presence of ventricular capture during ventricular pacing should be verified. Additionally, the presence of 1:1 VA conduction and acceleration of the atrial rate to the pacing CL should be carefully examined (see Fig. 16-7). It is also important to verify the continuation of the SVT following cessation of ventricular pacing and whether SVT termination, with or without reinduction of the SVT, during ventricular pacing has occurred.

When acceleration of the atrial CL to the pacing CL during ventricular pacing (with 1:1 VA conduction) is verified, several diagnostic criteria can be applied (see Fig. 16-6).

ΔVA ($VA_{ventricular\ pacing} - VA_{SVT}$) and Post-Pacing Interval. A ΔVA more than 85 milliseconds and [PPI – SVT CL] more than 115 milliseconds favor AVNRT, whereas a ΔVA less than 85 milliseconds and [PPI – SVT CL] less than 115 milliseconds favor orthodromic AVRT.[14]

Entrainment with Ventricular Fusion. Ventricular fusion during entrainment indicates AVRT and excludes AVNRT and AT.

Atrial Activation Sequence During Ventricular Pacing. When overdrive pacing entrains the SVT with an atrial activation sequence different from that during the SVT, AT is indicated and orthodromic AVRT and AVNRT are practically excluded, except for the infrequent case of SVT with a bystander concealed AV BT, which usually can be excluded by programmed ventricular stimulation during NSR. Furthermore, when overdrive pacing entrains the SVT with an atrial activation sequence similar to that during the SVT, AT is less likely than orthodromic AVRT or AVNRT, except for ATs originating close to the AV junction.

Atrial and Ventricular Electrogram Sequence Following Cessation of Ventricular Pacing. The presence of an A-A-V electrogram sequence on cessation of overdrive ventricular pacing immediately after the last *entrained* ventricular and atrial beats indicates AT and excludes AVNRT and orthodromic AVRT. On the other hand, presence of an A-V electrogram sequence is consistent with AVNRT and orthodromic AVRT and excludes AT.[7]

Burst Ventricular Pacing Technique. A burst ventricular pacing technique at a CL of 200 to 250 milliseconds for three to six beats during tachycardia is repeated a few times, or until the maneuver results in tachycardia termination.[7] If the atrial CL is not affected by ventricular pacing—no advancement of any atrial activation and no termination of the SVT, despite dissociation of the ventricles from the tachycardia—orthodromic AVRT is practically excluded. This is analogous to an early VES that fails to affect atrial activation, despite advancement of the local ventricular activation at all ventricular sites by more than 30 milliseconds. When termination occurs during ventricular pacing, it is important to determine whether atrial activation has occurred. Tachycardia termination without depolarization of the atrium (i.e., without VA conduction) following the ventricular stimulus excludes AT. Furthermore, when termination occurs during ventricular pacing, with the ventricular stimulus terminating the SVT occurring while the HB is refractory (as evidenced by a visible anterograde His potential or fusion QRS morphology between that of the ventricular stimulus and anterogradely conducted tachycardia beat, indicating that anterograde activation of the His potential must have occurred), then AVNRT is excluded. If such termination occurs without atrial activation, then AVNRT and AT are excluded.

Atrial Pacing During Supraventricular Tachycardia

Atrial pacing is performed at a CL 10 to 20 milliseconds shorter than the tachycardia CL. The pacing CL is then progressively reduced by 10 to 20 milliseconds in a stepwise fashion, with discontinuation of atrial pacing after each pacing CL to ensure continuation versus termination of the SVT.

Entrainment During Atrial Pacing. Demonstration of entrainment excludes automatic and triggered activity ATs.

Entrainment with Atrial Fusion. Demonstration of entrainment with atrial fusion excludes AVNRT and focal AT.

Overdrive Suppression. Overdrive suppression of the SVT favors automatic AT and excludes AVNRT and orthodromic AVRT.

Ventriculoatrial Interval in Return Cycle Following Cessation of Atrial Pacing. A fixed VA interval (VA linking) equal (within less than 10 milliseconds) to that during the SVT argues against AT, whereas a variable VA interval favors AT over other SVT mechanisms.[7]

ΔAH ($AH_{atrial\ pacing} - AH_{SVT}$). ΔAH more than 40 milliseconds indicates AVNRT, and excludes AT and orthodromic AVRT; however, ΔAH less than 20 milliseconds favors AT and orthodromic AVRT over AVNRT.

Maneuvers After Termination of Supraventricular Tachycardia

Ventricular Pacing from Right Ventriclular Apex at Tachycardia Cycle Length

ΔHA ($HA_{ventricular\ pacing} - HA_{SVT}$). A ΔHA more than –10 milliseconds indicates AVNRT, whereas a ΔHA less than –10 milliseconds indicates orthodromic AVRT.

Retrograde Atrial Activation Sequence During Ventricular Pacing Versus Supraventricular Tachycardia. A retrograde atrial activation sequence during ventricular pacing similar to that during SVT favors orthodromic AVRT and AVNRT over AT, except for the infrequent case when AT originates close to the AV junction or the atrial insertion site of a bystander AV BT.

Presence of Ventriculoatrial Block. The presence of VA block or decremental VA conduction excludes orthodromic AVRT and favors AT and AVNRT with a lower common pathway physiology.

Atrial Pacing from High Right Atrium at Tachycardia Cycle Length

ΔAH ($AH_{atrial\ pacing} - AH_{SVT}$). A ΔAH more than 40 milliseconds indicates AVNRT and excludes AT and orthodromic AVRT, whereas a ΔAH less than 20 milliseconds favors AT and orthodromic AVRT over AVNRT.

Presence of Atrioventricular Block During Atrial Pacing Versus Supraventricular Tachycardia. If AV block develops during atrial pacing, then AT and orthodromic AVRT are excluded, and AVNRT is indicated, given

that the pacing CL is equal to the tachycardia CL and that the same degree of autonomic tone is maintained.

Differential Right Ventriclular Pacing

Evaluation of Ventriculoatrial Interval During Right Ventriclular Apical Versus Basilar Pacing. When the VA interval during RV apical pacing is shorter than that during RV basilar pacing, retrogradely conducting septal BT is excluded. However, this maneuver may not exclude the presence of a free wall or a slowly conducting BT. On the other hand, when the VA interval during RV apical pacing is longer than that during RV basilar pacing, retrogradely conducting AV BT is diagnosed.

Evaluation of Atrial Activation Sequence During Right Ventriclular Apical Versus Basilar Pacing. A retrograde atrial activation sequence that is different depending on the site of ventricular pacing indicates the presence of a BT. However, a constant atrial activation sequence does not help exclude or prove the presence of an AV BT.

Para-Hisian Pacing

Atrial Activation Sequence. An identical retrograde atrial activation sequence, with and without HB capture, indicates that retrograde conduction is occurring over the same system during HB-RB capture and noncapture (either the BT or AVN) and does not help prove or exclude the presence of BT. On the other hand, a retrograde atrial activation sequence that is different depending on whether HB is captured indicates the presence of a BT.

HA and S-A (VA) Intervals. The HA and S-A (VA) intervals are recorded at multiple sites, including close to the site of earliest atrial activation during SVT. An S-A (VA) interval that is constant regardless of whether the HB-RB is being captured indicates the presence of a BT, whereas prolongation of the S-A (VA) interval on loss of HB capture, compared with that during HB capture, excludes the presence of a retrogradely conducting BT, except for slowly conducting and far free-wall BTs.

REFERENCES

1. Saoudi N, Cosio F, Waldo A, et al: A classification of atrial flutter and regular atrial tachycardia according to electrophysiological mechanisms and anatomical bases. A Statement from a Joint Expert Group from the Working Group of Arrhythmias of the European Society of Cardiology and the North American Society of Pacing and Electrophysiology. Eur Heart J 2001;22:1162.
2. Ferguson JD, DiMarco JP: Contemporary management of paroxysmal supraventricular tachycardia. Circulation 2003;107:1096.
3. Porter MJ, Morton JB, Denman R, et al: Influence of age and gender on the mechanism of supraventricular tachycardia. Heart Rhythm 2004;1:393.
4. Ballo P, Bernabo D, Faraguti SA: Heart rate is a predictor of success in the treatment of adults with symptomatic paroxysmal supraventricular tachycardia. Eur Heart J 2004;25:1310.
5. Alboni P, Tomasi C, Menozzi C, et al: Efficacy and safety of out-of-hospital self-administered single-dose oral drug treatment in the management of infrequent, well-tolerated paroxysmal supraventricular tachycardia. J Am Coll Cardiol 2001;37:548.
6. Blomstrom-Lundqvist C, Scheinman MM, Aliot EM, et al: ACC/AHA/ESC guidelines for the management of patients with supraventricular arrhythmias—executive summary. A report of the American College of Cardiology/American Heart Association Task Force on Practice Guidelines and the European Society of Cardiology Committee for Practice Guidelines (Writing Committee to Develop Guidelines for the Management Of Patients with Supraventricular Arrhythmias) developed in collaboration with NASPE–Heart Rhythm Society. J Am Coll Cardiol 2003;42:1493.
7. Knight BP, Ebinger M, Oral H, et al: Diagnostic value of tachycardia features and pacing maneuvers during paroxysmal supraventricular tachycardia. J Am Coll Cardiol 2000;36:574.
8. Kertesz NJ, Fogel RI, Prystowsky EN: Mechanism of induction of atrioventricular node reentry by simultaneous anterograde conduction over the fast and slow pathways. J Cardiovasc Electrophysiol 2005;16:251.
9. Josephson M: Supraventricular tachycardias. *In* Josephson ME (ed): Clinical Cardiac Electrophysiology, 3rd ed. Philadelphia, Lippincott, Williams & Wilkins, 2002, pp 168-271.
10. Lockwood D, Otomo K, Wang Z, et al: Electrophysiological characteristics of atrioventricular nodal reentrant tachycardia: Implications for the reentrant circuit. *In* Zipes D, Jaliffe J (eds): Cardiac Electrophysiology: From Cell to Bedside, 4th ed. Philadelphia, WB Saunders, 2004, pp 537-557.
11. Yamane T, Shah DC, Peng JT, et al: Morphological characteristics of P waves during selective pulmonary vein pacing. J Am Coll Cardiol 2001;38:1505.
12. Yang Y, Cheng J, Glatter K, et al: Quantitative effects of functional bundle branch block in patients with atrioventricular reentrant tachycardia. Am J Cardiol 2000;85:826.
13. Maruyama M, Kobayashi Y, Miyauchi Y, et al: The VA relationship after differential atrial overdrive pacing: a novel tool for the diagnosis of atrial tachycardia in the electrophysiological laboratory. J Cardiovasc Electrophysiol 2007;18:1127.
14. Michaud GF, Tada H, Chough S, et al: Differentiation of atypical atrioventricular node re-entrant tachycardia from orthodromic reciprocating tachycardia using a septal accessory pathway by the response to ventricular pacing. J Am Coll Cardiol 2001;38:1163.
15. Platonov M, Schroeder K, Veenhuyzen GD: Differential entrainment: Beware from where you pace. Heart Rhythm 2007;4:1097.
16. Vijayaraman P, Lee BP, Kalahasty G, et al: Reanalysis of the "pseudo A-A-V" response to ventricular entrainment of supraventricular tachycardia: Importance of His bundle timing. J Cardiovasc Electrophysiol 2006;17:25.

CHAPTER 17

Approach to Wide QRS Complex Tachycardias

CLINICAL CONSIDERATIONS

Cause of Wide Complex Tachycardias

Wide QRS complex tachycardia (WCT) is a rhythm with a rate of more than 100 beats/min and a QRS duration of more than 120 milliseconds. Several arrhythmias can manifest as WCTs (Table 17-1); the most common is ventricular tachycardia (VT), which accounts for 80% of all cases of WCT.[1] Supraventricular tachycardia (SVT) with aberrancy accounts for 15% to 20% of WCTs. SVTs with bystander preexcitation and antidromic atrioventricular reentrant tachycardia (AVRT) account for 1% to 6% of WCTs.

In the stable patient who will undergo a more detailed assessment, the goal of evaluation should include determination of the cause of the WCT (particularly distinguishing between VT and SVT). Accurate diagnosis of the WCT requires information obtained from the history, physical examination, response to certain maneuvers, and careful inspection of the ECG, including rhythm strips and 12-lead tracings. Comparison of the ECG during the tachycardia with that recorded during sinus rhythm, if available, can also provide useful information.

Clinical History

Age. WCT in a patient older than 35 years is likely to be VT (positive predictive value of up to 85%). SVT is more likely in the younger patient (positive predictive value of 70%).

Symptoms. Some patients with tachycardia can have few or no symptoms (e.g., palpitations, lightheadedness, diaphoresis), whereas others can have severe manifestations, including chest pain, dyspnea, syncope, seizures, and cardiac arrest. The symptoms during a WCT are primarily caused by the fast heart rate, associated heart disease, and the presence and extent of left ventricle (LV) dysfunction, and the severity of symptoms is not useful in determining the tachycardia mechanism.[1] It is important to recognize that VT does not necessarily result in hemodynamic compromise or collapse. Misdiagnosis of VT as SVT based on hemodynamic stability is a common error that can lead to inappropriate and potentially dangerous therapy.

Duration of the Arrhythmia. SVT is more likely if the tachycardia has recurred over a period of more than 3 years.[1] The first occurrence of a WCT after an myocardial infarction (MI) strongly implies VT.

Presence of Underlying Heart Disease. The presence of structural heart disease, especially coronary heart disease and a previous MI, strongly suggests VT as the cause of WCT. In one report, over 98% of patients with a previous MI had VT as the cause of WCT, whereas only 7% of those with SVT had had an MI.[2] It should be realized, however, that VT can occur in patients with no apparent heart disease, and SVT can occur in those with structural heart disease.

Pacemaker or Implantable Cardioverter-Defibrillator Implantation. A history of pacemaker or implantable cardioverter-defibrillator (ICD) implantation should raise the possibility of a device-associated tachycardia. Ventricular pacing can be associated with a small and almost imperceptible stimulus artifact on the ECG. The presence of an ICD is also of importance because such a device should identify and treat a sustained tachyarrhythmia, depending on device programming, and because the presence of an ICD implies that the patient is known to have an increased risk of ventricular tachyarrhythmias.

Medications. Many different medications have proarrhythmic effects. The most common drug-induced tachyarrhythmia is torsades de pointes. Frequently implicated agents include antiarrhythmic drugs such as sotalol and quinidine, and certain antimicrobial drugs such as erythromycin. Diuretics are a common cause of hypokalemia and hypomagnesemia, which can predispose to ventricular tachyarrhythmias, particularly torsades de pointes in patients taking antiarrhythmic drugs. Furthermore, class I antiarrhythmic drugs, especially class IC agents, slow conduction and have a property of use dependency, a progressive decrease in impulse conduction velocity at faster heart rates. As a result, these drugs can cause rate-related aberration and a wide QRS complex during any tachyarrhythmia. Digoxin can cause almost any cardiac arrhythmia, especially

TABLE 17–1 Causes of Wide QRS Complex Tachycardia	
Cause	**Description, Examples**
VT	Macroreentrant VT Focal VT
SVT with aberrancy	Functional BBB Preexistent BBB
Preexcited SVT	Antidromic AVRT AT or AVNRT with bystander BT
Antiarrhythmic drugs	Class IA and IC agents, amiodarone
Electrolyte abnormalities	Hyperkalemia
Ventricular pacing	

AT = atrial tachycardia; AVNRT = atrioventricular nodal reentrant tachycardia; AVRT = atrioventricular reentrant tachycardia; BBB = bundle branch block; BT = bypass tract; SVT = supraventricular tachycardia; VT = ventricular tachycardia.

with increasing plasma digoxin concentrations above 2.0 ng/mL (2.6 mmol/L). Digoxin-induced arrhythmias are more frequent at any given plasma concentration if hypokalemia is also present. The most common digoxin-induced arrhythmias include monomorphic VT (often with a relatively narrow QRS complex), bidirectional VT (a regular alternation of two wide QRS morphologies, each with a different axis), and nonparoxysmal junctional tachycardia.

Physical Examination

Most of the elements of the physical examination, including the blood pressure and heart rate, are of importance primarily in determining how severe the patient's hemodynamic instability is and thus how urgent a therapeutic intervention is required. In patients with significant hemodynamic compromise, a thorough diagnostic evaluation should be postponed until acute management has been addressed. In this setting, emergent cardioversion is the treatment of choice and does not require knowledge of the mechanism of the arrhythmia.

Evidence of underlying cardiovascular disease should be sought, including the sequelae of peripheral vascular disease or stroke. A healed sternal incision is obvious evidence of previous cardiothoracic surgery. A pacemaker or defibrillator, if present, can typically be palpated in the left or, less commonly, right pectoral area below the clavicle, although some earlier devices are found in the anterior abdominal wall.

An important objective of the physical examination in the stable patient is to attempt to document the presence of atrioventricular (AV) dissociation. AV dissociation is present, although not always evident, in approximately 20% to 50% of patients with VT, but it is very rarely seen in SVT. Thus, the presence of AV dissociation strongly suggests VT, although its absence is less helpful. AV dissociation, if present, is typically diagnosed on ECG; however, it can produce a number of characteristic findings on physical examination.[1] Intermittent cannon A waves can be observed on examination of the jugular pulsation in the neck, and they reflect simultaneous atrial and ventricular contraction; contraction of the right atrium (RA) against a closed tricuspid valve produces a transient increase in RA and jugular venous pressure. Cannon A waves must be distinguished from the continuous and regular prominent A waves seen during some SVTs. Such prominent waves result from simultaneous atrial and ventricular contraction occurring with every beat. Additionally, highly inconsistent fluctuations in the blood pressure can occur because of the variability in the degree of left atrial (LA) contribution to LV filling, stroke volume, and cardiac output. Moreover, variability in the occurrence and intensity of heart sounds (especially S_1) may also be observed and is heard more frequently when the rate of the tachycardia is slower.

The response to carotid sinus massage can suggest the cause of the WCT. The heart rate during sinus tachycardia and automatic atrial tachycardia (AT) will gradually slow with carotid sinus massage and then accelerate on release. The ventricular rate during AT and atrial flutter (AFL) will transiently slow with carotid sinus massage because of increased atrioventricular node (AVN) blockade. The arrhythmia itself, however, is unaffected. Atrioventricular reentrant nodal tachycardia (AVRNT) and AVRT will either terminate or remain unaltered with carotid sinus massage. VTs are generally unaffected by carotid sinus massage, although this maneuver may slow the atrial rate and, in some cases, expose AV dissociation. VT can rarely terminate in response to carotid sinus massage.

Laboratory Tests

The plasma potassium and magnesium concentrations should be measured as part of the laboratory evaluation. Hypokalemia and hypomagnesemia can predispose to the development of ventricular tachyarrhythmias. Hyperkalemia can cause a wide QRS complex rhythm, usually with a slow rate, with loss of a detectable P wave (the so-called sinoventricular rhythm) or abnormalities of AVN conduction. In patients taking digoxin, quinidine, or procainamide, plasma concentrations of these drugs should be measured to assist in evaluating possible drug toxicity.

Pharmacological Intervention

The administration of certain drugs can be useful for diagnostic, as opposed to therapeutic, purposes. Termination of the arrhythmia with lidocaine suggests, but does not prove, that VT is the mechanism. Infrequently an SVT, especially AVRT, can terminate with lidocaine. On the other hand, termination of the tachycardia with procainamide or amiodarone does not distinguish between VT and SVT. Termination of the arrhythmia with digoxin, verapamil, diltiazem, or adenosine strongly implies SVT. However, VT can also occasionally terminate after the administration of these drugs.

Unless the cause for the WCT is definitely established, however, verapamil, diltiazem, and probably adenosine should not be administered, because they have been reported to cause severe hemodynamic deterioration in patients with VT and can even provoke VF and cardiac arrest. DC cardioversion in unstable patients and intravenous procainamide or amiodarone in hemodynamically stable patients are the appropriate management approach.[2]

ELECTROCARDIOGRAPHIC FEATURES

Ventricular Tachycardia Versus Aberrantly Conducted Supraventricular Tachycardia

Because the diagnosis of a WCT cannot always be made with complete certainty, the unknown rhythm should be presumed to be VT in the absence of contrary evidence. This conclusion is appropriate both because VT accounts for up to 80% of cases of WCT, and because making this assumption guards against inappropriate and potentially dangerous therapy. As noted, the intravenous administration of drugs used for the treatment of SVT (verapamil, adenosine, or beta blockers) can cause severe hemodynamic deterioration in patients with VT and can even provoke VF and cardiac arrest. Therefore, these drugs should not be used when the diagnosis is uncertain.

In general, most WCTs can be classified as having one of two patterns: a right bundle branch block (RBBB)–like pattern (QRS polarity is predominantly positive in leads V_1 and V_2) or left bundle branch block (LBBB)–like pattern (QRS polarity is predominantly negative in leads V_1 and V_2). The determination that the WCT has a RBBB-like pattern or a LBBB-like pattern does not, by itself, assist in making a diagnosis; however, this assessment should be made initially, because it is useful in evaluating several other features on the ECG, including the QRS axis, the QRS duration, and the QRS morphology (Table 17-2).

Rate. The rate of the WCT is of limited value in distinguishing VT from SVT because there is wide overlap in the distribution of heart rates for SVT and VT. When the rate is approximately 150 beats/min, AFL with aberrant conduction should be considered.

Regularity. Regularity of the WCT is not helpful, because both SVT and VT are regular. However, VT is often associated with slight irregularity of the RR intervals, QRS morphology, and ST-T waves. Although marked irregularity strongly suggests atrial fibrillation (AF), VTs can be particularly irregular within the first 30 seconds of onset and in patients treated with antiarrhythmic drugs.[3]

QRS Duration. In general, a wider QRS duration favors VT. In the setting of RBBB-like WCT, a QRS duration more than 140 milliseconds suggests VT, whereas in the setting of LBBB-like WCT, a QRS duration more than 160 milliseconds suggests VT. In an analysis of several studies, a QRS duration more than 160 milliseconds overall was a strong predictor of VT (likelihood ratio more than 20:1). On the other hand, a QRS duration less than 140 milliseconds is not helpful for excluding VT, because VT can sometimes be associated with a relatively narrow QRS complex.

A QRS duration more than 160 milliseconds is not helpful in identifying VT in several settings, including preexisting bundle branch block (BBB), although it is uncommon for the QRS to be wider than 160 milliseconds in this situation, preexcited SVT, and the presence of drugs capable of slowing intraventricular conduction (e.g., class IA and IC drugs). Of note, a QRS complex that is narrower during WCT than during normal sinus rhythm (NSR) suggests VT. However, this is rare, occurring in less than 1% of VTs.[3]

Rarely (4% in one series), VT can have a relatively narrow QRS duration (less than 120 to 140 milliseconds). This can be observed in VTs of septal origin or those with early penetration into the His-Purkinje system (HPS), as occurs with fascicular (verapamil-sensitive) VT.[3,4]

QRS Axis. Generally, the more leftward the axis, the greater the likelihood of VT.[3] A significant axis shift (more than 40 degrees) between the baseline NSR and WCT is suggestive of VT (Fig. 17-1A). A right superior (northwest) axis (axis from −90 degrees to ±180 degrees) is rare in SVT and strongly suggests VT (see Fig. 17-1B).[3]

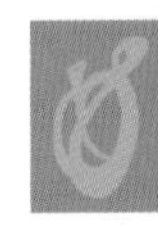

In a patient with an RBBB-like WCT, a QRS axis to the left of −30 degrees suggests VT (see Fig. 17-1A) and, in a patient with an LBBB-like WCT, a QRS axis to the right of +90 degrees suggests VT.[3] Additionally, RBBB with a normal axis is uncommon in VT (less than 3%) and is suggestive of SVT.

Precordial QRS Concordance. Concordance is present when the QRS complexes in the six precordial leads (V_1 through V_6) are either all positive in polarity (tall R waves) or all negative in polarity (deep QS complexes). Negative concordance is strongly suggestive of VT (see Fig. 17-1D). Rarely, SVT with LBBB aberrancy will demonstrate negative concordance, but there is almost always some evidence of an R wave in the lateral precordial leads. Positive concordance is most often caused by VT (see Fig. 17-1A); however, this pattern also occurs in the relatively rare case of preexcited SVT with a left posterior bypass tract (BT). Although the presence of precordial QRS concordance strongly suggests VT (more than 90% specificity), its absence is not helpful diagnostically (approximately 20% sensitivity).[5]

Atrioventricular Dissociation. AV dissociation is characterized by atrial activity (the P wave) that is completely independent of ventricular activity (the QRS complex). The atrial rate is usually slower than the ventricular rate. The detection of AV dissociation is obviously impossible if AF is the underlying supraventricular rhythm.

AV dissociation is the hallmark of VT (specificity is almost 100%; sensitivity is 20% to 50%).[5] However, although the presence of AV dissociation establishes VT as the cause, its absence is not as helpful. AV dissociation can be present but not obvious on the surface ECG because of a rapid ventricular rate. Additionally, AV dissociation is absent in a large subset of VTs; in fact, approximately 30% of VTs have 1:1 retrograde ventriculoatrial (VA) conduction (see Fig. 17-1D) and an additional 15% to 20% have second-degree (2:1 or Wenckebach) VA block (Fig. 17-2).[3]

Several ECG findings are helpful in establishing the presence of AV dissociation, including the presence of dissociated P waves, fusion beats, or capture beats.

Dissociated P Waves. When the P waves can be clearly seen and the atrial rate is unrelated to and slower than the

TABLE 17–2 ECG Criteria Favoring Ventricular Tachycardia

AV Relationship
Dissociated P waves
Fusion beats
Capture beats
A/V ratio < 1
QRS Duration
>160 msec with LBBB pattern
>140 msec with RBBB pattern
QRS during WCT is narrower than in NSR
QRS Axis
Axis shift of >40 degrees between NSR and WCT
Right superior (northwest) axis.
Left axis deviation with RBBB morphology
Right axis deviation with LBBB morphology
Precordial QRS Concordance
Positive concordance
Negative concordance
QRS Morphology in RBBB Pattern WCT
Monophasic R, biphasic qR complex, or broad R (>40 msec) in lead V_1
Rabbit ear sign: Double-peaked R wave in lead V_1 with the left peak taller than the right peak
rS complex in lead V_6
Contralateral BBB in WCT and NSR
QRS Morphology in LBBB-Pattern WCT
Broad initial R wave of ≥40 msec in lead V_1 or V_2
R wave in lead V_1 during WCT taller than the R wave during NSR
Slow descent to the nadir of the S, notching in the downstroke of the S wave in lead V_1
RS interval > 70 msec in lead V_1 or V_2
Q or QS wave in lead V_6

AV = atrioventricular; BBB = bundle branch block; LBBB = left bundle branch block; NSR = normal sinus rhythm; RBBB = right bundle branch block; WCT = wide complex tachycardia.

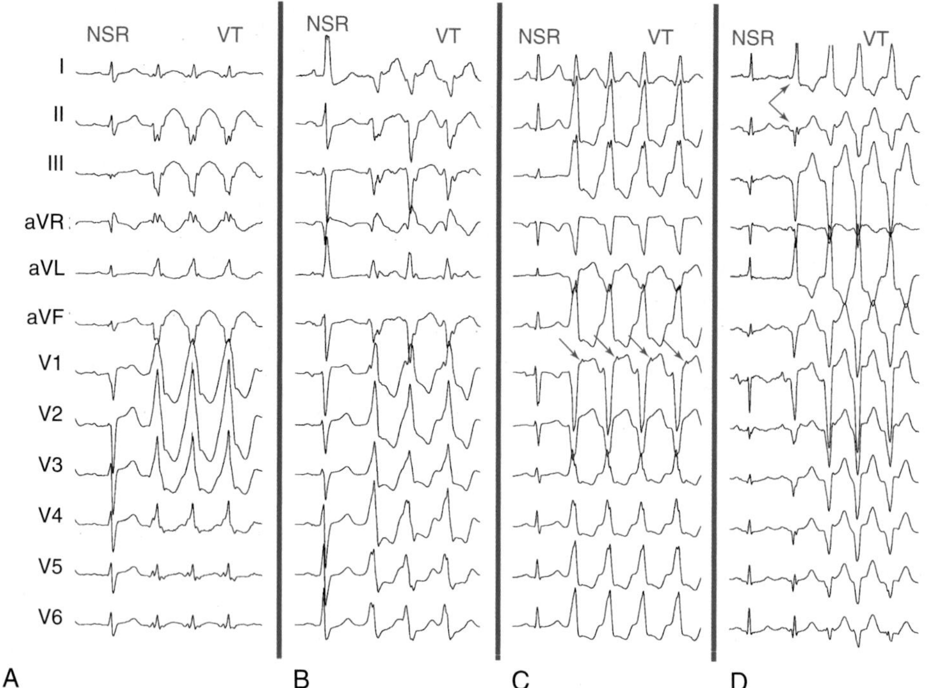

FIGURE 17–1 Surface ECG of four different patients illustrating ECG morphology during normal sinus rhythm (NSR) versus ventricular tachycardia (VT). **A,** VT with right bundle branch block (RBBB) pattern, positive concordance, and long RS interval. Note the monophasic R in lead V_1 during VT and the significant shift in the frontal plane axis in VT versus NSR. **B,** VT with RBBB pattern and long RS interval. Note the superior (northwest) frontal plane axis during VT. **C,** VT with left bundle branch block (LBBB) pattern, long RS interval, and 1 : 1 ventriculoatrial (VA) conduction. Retrograde P waves (red arrows) are visible following the QRSs during VT. **D,** VT with LBBB pattern and negative concordance. Note that the second QRS (blue arrows) is a fusion between the sinus beat and the VT beat.

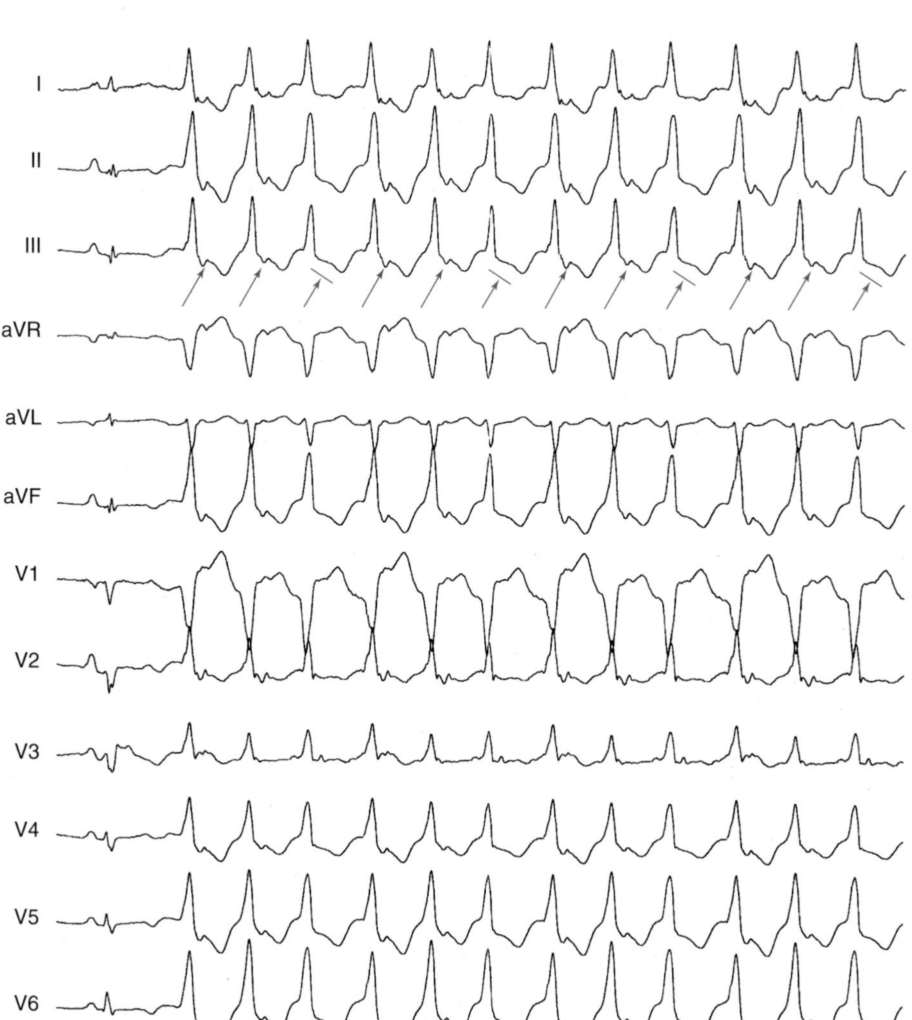

FIGURE 17–2 Ventricular tachycardia (VT) with type 1 second-degree (Wenckebach) ventriculoatrial (VA) block. The first beat is sinus with normal atrioventricular (AV) conduction. VT develops with an initially short VA interval (blue arrows), which then slightly prolongs (red arrows), and then VA block occurs (green arrows). Note that the VT has a right bundle branch block (RBBB) with long RS interval (in lead V_2).

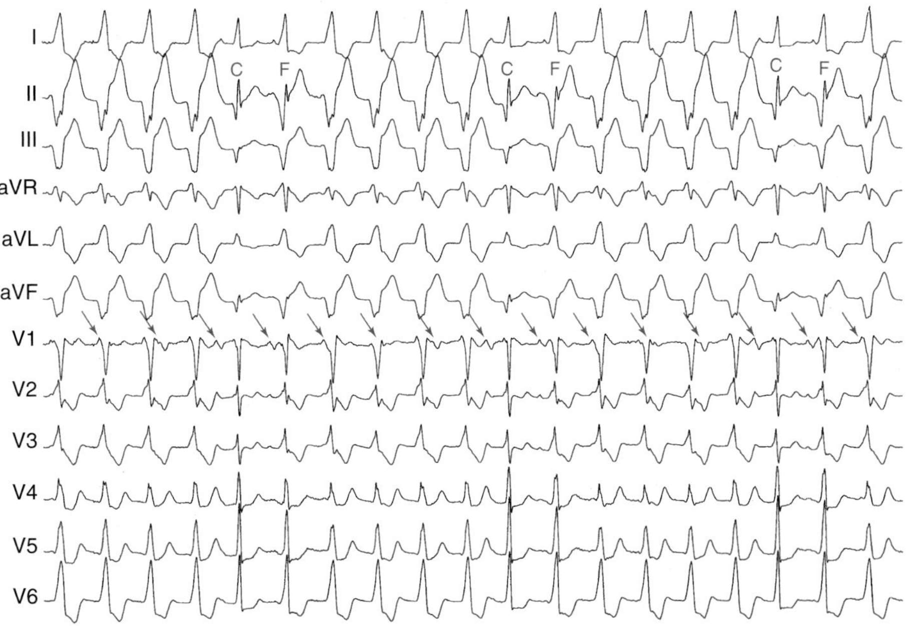

FIGURE 17–3 Ventricular tachycardia (VT) with atrioventricular (AV) dissociation. This is a surface ECG of sustained monomorphic VT at a cycle length (CL) of 488 msec, with AV dissociation and a sinus CL of 616 msec. The P waves can be clearly seen (arrows) marching throughout the different phases of the VT QRS complexes, and the atrial rate is unrelated to and slower than the ventricular rate. Because of the relatively slow VT rate, capture (C) and fusion (F) beats are observed frequently.

ventricular rate, AV dissociation consistent with VT is present (Fig. 17-3). An atrial rate faster than the ventricular rate is more often seen with SVT having AV conduction block. However, during a WCT, the P waves are often difficult to identify; they may be superimposed on the ST segment or T wave (resulting in altered morphology). Sometimes, the T waves and initial or terminal QRS portions can resemble atrial activity. Furthermore, artifacts can be mistaken for P waves. If the P waves are not obvious or suggested on the ECG, several alternative leads or modalities can help in their identification, including a modified chest lead placement (Lewis leads), an esophageal lead (using an electrode wire or nasogastric tube), a right atrial recording (obtained by an electrode catheter in the RA), carotid sinus pressure (to slow VA conduction and therefore change the atrial rate in the case of VT), or invasive electrophysiological (EP) testing.

Fusion Beats. Ventricular fusion occurs when a ventricular ectopic beat and a supraventricular beat (conducted via the AVN and HPS) simultaneously activate the ventricular myocardium. The resulting QRS complex has a morphology intermediate between the appearance of a sinus QRS complex and that of a purely ventricular complex. Intermittent fusion beats during a WCT are diagnostic of AV dissociation and therefore of VT (see Fig. 17-3). It is also possible for premature ventricular complexes (PVCs) during SVT with aberration to produce fusion beats, which would erroneously be interpreted as evidence of AV dissociation and VT.

Dressler Beats. A Dressler beat, or a capture beat, is a normal QRS complex identical to the sinus QRS complex, occurring during the VT. The term *capture beat* indicates that the normal conduction system has momentarily captured control of ventricular activation from the VT focus (see Fig. 17-3). Fusion and capture beats are more commonly seen when the tachycardia rate is slower. These beats do not alter the rate of the VT, although a change in the preceding and subsequent RR intervals may be observed.

QRS Morphology. As a rule, if the WCT is caused by SVT with aberration, then the QRS complex during the WCT must be compatible with some form of BBB that could result in that QRS configuration. If there is no combination of bundle branch or fascicular blocks that could result in such a QRS configuration, then the diagnosis by default is VT.

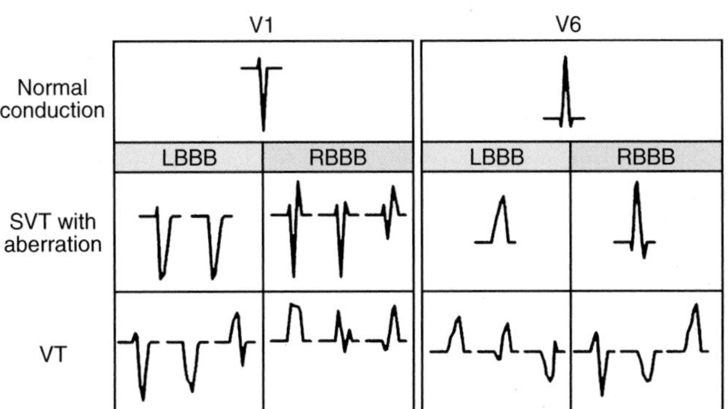

FIGURE 17–4 Diagrammatic representation of common QRS morphologies encountered in ventricular tachycardia (VT) and supraventricular tachycardia (SVT), with aberration in leads V_1 and V_6 for both left bundle branch block (LBBB) and right bundle branch block (RBBB) QRS patterns. Note the initial portions of the QRS complex in normal and aberrant QRS complexes, contrasted with the initial QRS forces in VT complexes. The RS configurations can be designated as an RBBB or LBBB type (grouped with LBBB-type morphologies). (From Miller JM, Das MK, Arora R, Alberte-Lista C: Differential diagnosis of wide QRS complex tachycardia. *In* Zipes DP, Jalife J [eds]: Cardiac Electrophysiology: From Cell to Bedside, 4th ed. Philadelphia, WB Saunders, 2004, pp 747-757.)

As noted, WCTs can be classified as having an RBBB-like pattern or an LBBB-like pattern. Certain features of the QRS complex have been described that favor VT in RBBB-like or LBBB-like WCTs (Fig. 17-4).[3]

In the patient with a WCT and positive QRS polarity in lead V_1 (RBBB pattern), a monophasic R, biphasic qR complex, or broad R (more than 40 milliseconds) in lead V_1 favors VT (Fig. 17-5), whereas a triphasic RSR′, rSr′, rR′, or rSR′ complex in lead V_1 favors SVT (where the capital letter indicates large-wave amplitude and/or duration, and the lower case letter indicates small-wave amplitude and/or duration; see Fig. 7-4). Additionally, a double-peaked R wave in lead V_1 favors VT if the left peak is taller than the right peak (the so-called rabbit ear sign; likelihood ratio more than 50:1). A taller right rabbit ear does not help in distinguishing SVT from VT. On the other hand, an rS complex in lead V_6 is a strong predictor of VT (likelihood ratio more than 50:1), whereas an Rs complex in lead V_6 favors SVT (see Fig. 17-5).

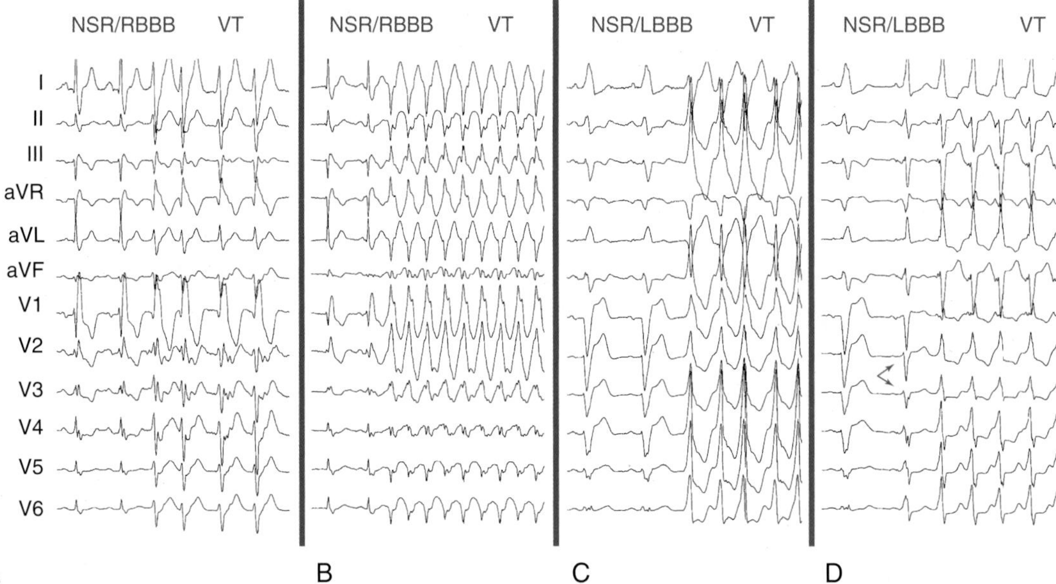

FIGURE 17–5 Surface ECG of four different patients illustrating ECG morphology during normal sinus rhythm (NSR) with bundle branch block (BBB) versus ventricular tachycardia (VT). **A,** NSR with right bundle branch block (RBBB) and VT with RBBB pattern. Note the loss of the initial r wave in V_1 and the larger S wave in V_6 during VT compared with NSR with RBBB. Additionally, note the shift in the frontal plane QRS axis from +90 degrees during NSR with RBBB to the northwest quadrant during VT. **B,** NSR with RBBB and VT with RBBB pattern. Note the change of QRS morphology in V_1 (from rsR′ during NSR with RBBB to R during VT) and V_6 (from RS during NSR with RBBB to QS during VT). Additionally, no RS complexes are observed in the precordial leads during VT. **C,** NSR with LBBB and VT with RBBB pattern. Note the positive precordial concordance during VT. **D,** NSR with LBBB and VT with RBBB pattern. Note the positive precordial concordance during VT. The second QRS is a fusion between the sinus beat and the VT beat, and the fusion QRS is narrower than both the sinus and VT complexes.

In the patient with a WCT and a negative QRS polarity in lead V_1 (LBBB pattern), a broad initial R wave of 40 milliseconds or more in lead V_1 or V_2 favors VT, whereas the absence of an initial R wave (or a small initial R wave of less than 40 milliseconds) in lead V_1 or V_2 favors SVT (see Fig. 7-5). Additionally, an R wave in lead V_1 during a WCT taller than that during NSR favors VT. Furthermore, a slow descent to the nadir of the S wave, notching in the downstroke of the S wave, or an RS interval (from the onset of the QRS complex to the nadir of the S wave) of more than 70 milliseconds in lead V_1 or V_2 favors VT. In contrast, a swift, smooth downstroke of the S wave in lead V_1 or V_2 with an RS interval of less than 70 milliseconds favors SVT. In an analysis of several studies, the presence of any of these three criteria in lead V_1 (broad R wave, slurred or notched downstroke of the S wave, and delayed nadir of S wave) was a strong predictor of VT (likelihood ratio, more than 50:1). The QRS morphology in lead V_6 is also of value; the presence of any Q or QS wave in lead V_6 favors VT (likelihood ratio more than 50:1; see Fig. 17-1D), whereas the absence of a Q wave in lead V_6 favors SVT.

When an old 12-lead surface ECG is available, comparison of the QRS morphology during NSR and WCT is helpful. Contralateral BBB in WCT and NSR strongly favors VT (see Fig. 17-5C, D).[3] It is important to note that identical QRS morphology during NSR and WCT, although strongly suggestive of SVT, can also occur in bundle branch reentrant (BBR) and interfascicular reentrant VTs.

Unfortunately, the value of QRS morphological criteria in the diagnosis of a WCT is subject to several limitations. Most of the associations between the QRS morphology and tachycardia origin are based on statistical correlations, with substantial overlap. Moreover, most of the morphological criteria favoring VT are also present in a substantial number of patients with intraventricular conduction delay present during sinus rhythm, limiting their applicability in these cases. Additionally, morphological criteria tend to misclassify SVTs with preexcitation as VT. However, preexcitation is an uncommon cause of WCT (1% to 6% in most series), particularly if other factors (e.g., age, history) suggest another diagnosis.

Variation in QRS and ST-T Morphology. Subtle, non–rate-related fluctuations or variations in the QRS and ST-T wave configuration suggest VT and reflect variations in the VT reentrant circuit within the myocardium. In contrast, because most SVTs follow fixed conduction pathways, they are generally characterized by complete uniformity of QRS and ST-T shape, unless the tachycardia rate changes.

Algorithms for the ECG Diagnosis of Wide Complex Tachycardia

The various criteria for the diagnosis of WCT listed are difficult to apply in isolation, because most patients will have some, but not all, of the features described. Several algorithms have been proposed to guide integrating ECG findings into a diagnostic strategy. Figure 17-6 illustrates an example of one approach.[2] The effect of history of prior MI, preexcited tachycardias, antiarrhythmic medication usage, precordial lead placement, heart transplantation status, and the presence of congenital heart disease on QRS morphology criteria should be taken into account while applying these elements. Preexcited tachycardias may not be differentiated consistently with the proposed criteria, especially those using epicardial left-sided paraseptal or left-sided inferoposterior BTs.

Algorithm 1. The most commonly used algorithm is the so-called Brugada algorithm or Brugada criteria.[6] The Brugada algorithm consists of four steps (Fig. 17-7). First, all precordial leads are inspected to detect the presence or absence of an RS complex (with R and S waves of any amplitude). If an RS complex cannot be identified in any precordial lead, the diagnosis of VT can be made with 100% specificity. Second, if an RS complex is clearly identified in one or more precordial leads, the interval between the onset of the R wave and the nadir of the S wave (the RS interval)

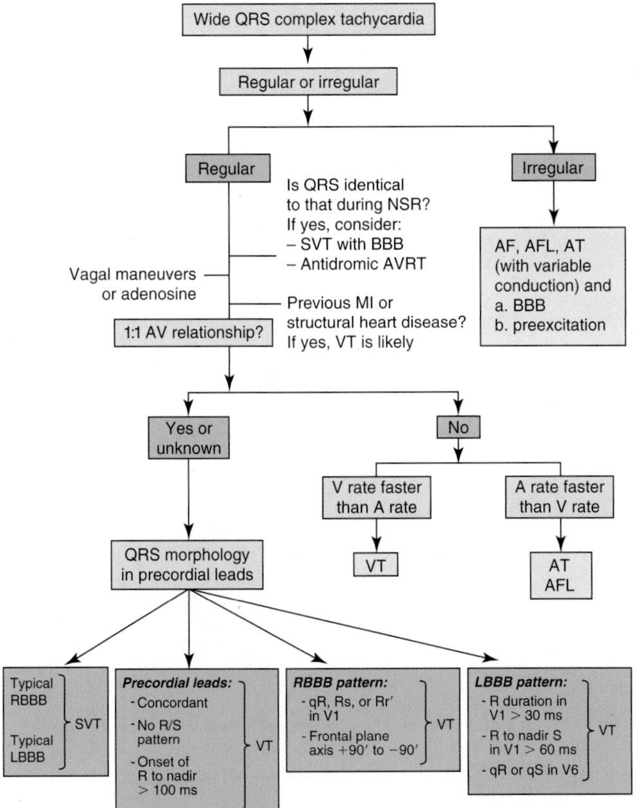

FIGURE 17–6 Differential diagnosis for wide QRS complex tachycardia. A = atrial; AF = atrial fibrillation; AFL = atrial flutter; AT = atrial tachycardia; AVRT = atrioventricular reentrant tachycardia; BBB = bundle branch block; LBBB = left bundle branch block; MI = myocardial infarction; RBBB = right bundle branch block; SVT = supraventricular tachycardia; V = ventricular; VT = ventricular tachycardia. (From Blomström-Lundqvist C, Scheinman MM, Aliot EM, et al; American College of Cardiology; American Heart Association Task Force on Practice Guidelines; European Society of Cardiology Committee for Practice Guidelines. Writing Committee to Develop Guidelines for the Management of Patients With Supraventricular Arrhythmias: ACC/AHA/ESC guidelines for the management of patients with supraventricular arrhythmias—executive summary: A report of the American College of Cardiology/American Heart Association Task Force on Practice Guidelines and the European Society of Cardiology Committee for Practice Guidelines (Writing Committee to Develop Guidelines for the Management of Patients With Supraventricular Arrhythmias). Circulation 2003;108:1871.)

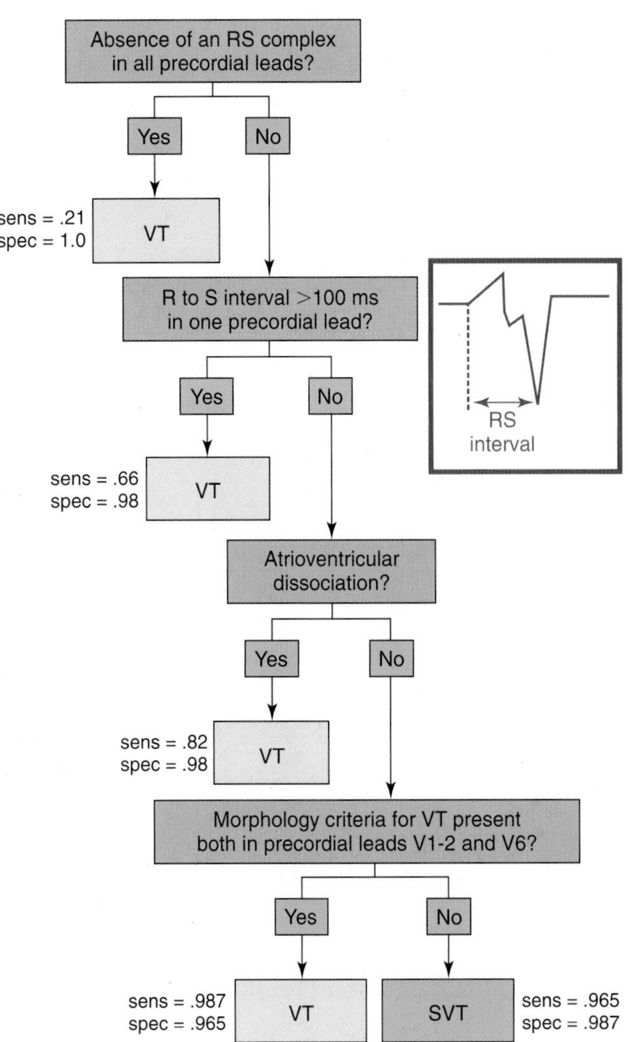

FIGURE 17–7 Brugada algorithm for distinguishing ventricular tachycardia (VT) from supraventricular tachycardia (SVT). As indicated in the inset, the RS interval is between the onset of the R wave and the nadir of the S wave. sens = sensitivity; spec = specificity. (From Brugada P, Brugada J, Mont L, et al: A new approach to the differential diagnosis of a regular tachycardia with a wide QRS complex. Circulation 1991;83:1649.)

is measured. The longest RS interval is considered if RS complexes are present in multiple precordial leads. If the longest RS interval is more than 100 milliseconds, the diagnosis of VT can be made with a specificity of 98% (see Fig. 17-7). Third, if the longest RS interval is less than 100 milliseconds, either VT or SVT still is possible and the presence or absence of AV dissociation must therefore be determined. Evidence of AV dissociation is 100% specific for the diagnosis of VT, but this finding has a low sensitivity. Fourth, if the RS interval is less than 100 milliseconds and AV dissociation cannot clearly be demonstrated, the QRS morphology criteria for V_1-positive and V_1-negative WCTs are considered.

The QRS morphology criteria consistent with VT must be present in leads V_1 or V_2 and in lead V_6 to diagnose VT. A supraventricular site of origin of the tachycardia is assumed if either the V_1 and V_2 or V_6 criteria are not consistent with VT.

The Brugada algorithm was originally prospectively applied to 554 patients with electrophysiologically diagnosed WCTs. The reported sensitivity and specificity were 98.7% and 96.5%, respectively. Other authors also found the Brugada criteria useful, although they reported a lower sensitivity (79% to 92%) and specificity (43% to 70%).

Algorithm 2. A newer algorithm for differential diagnosis of WCT was analyzed in 453 monomorphic WCTs recorded from 287 patients based on the following: (1) the presence of AV dissociation; (2) the presence of an initial R wave in lead aVR; (3) the QRS morphology; (4) estimation of the initial (Vi) and terminal (Vt) ventricular activation velocity ratio (Vi/Vt) by measuring the voltage change on the ECG tracing during the initial 40 milliseconds (Vi) and the terminal 40 milliseconds (Vt) of the same biphasic or multiphasic QRS complex (Fig. 17-8).[7,8]

This algorithm had superior overall total accuracy than that of the Brugada algorithm (90.3% versus 84.8%). The total accuracy of the fourth Brugada criterion was significantly lower (68% versus 82.2%) than that of the Vi/Vt criterion in the fourth step, accounting for most of the difference in outcome between the two methods.

The rationale proposed for the Vi/Vt criterion is that during WCT caused by SVT, the initial activation of the septum should be invariably rapid and the intraventricular conduction delay causing the wide QRS complex occurs in

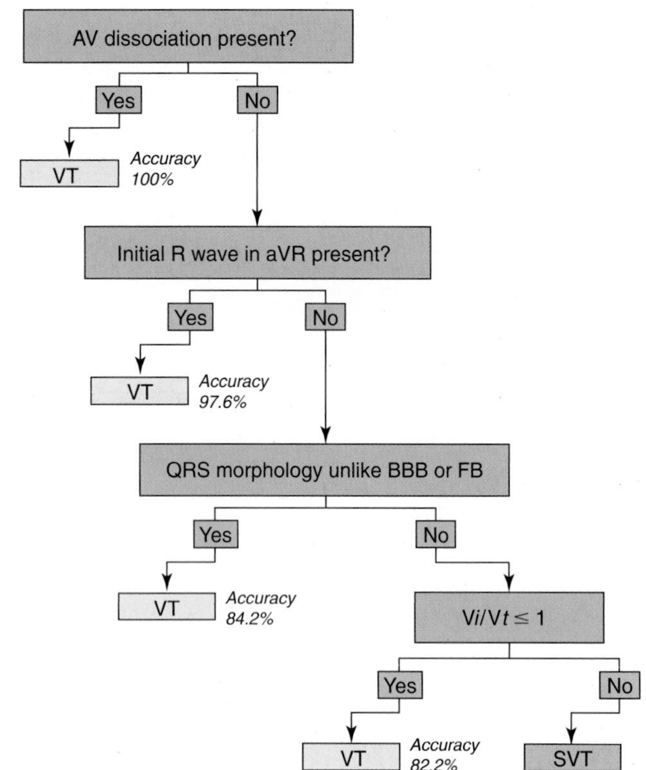

FIGURE 17–8 Stepwise algorithm for distinguishing ventricular tachycardia (VT) from supraventricular tachycardia (SVT). AV = atrioventricular; BBB = bundle branch block; FB = fascicular block. (From Vereckei A, Duray G, Szénási G, et al: Application of a new algorithm in the differential diagnosis of wide QRS complex tachycardia. Eur Heart J 2007;28:589.)

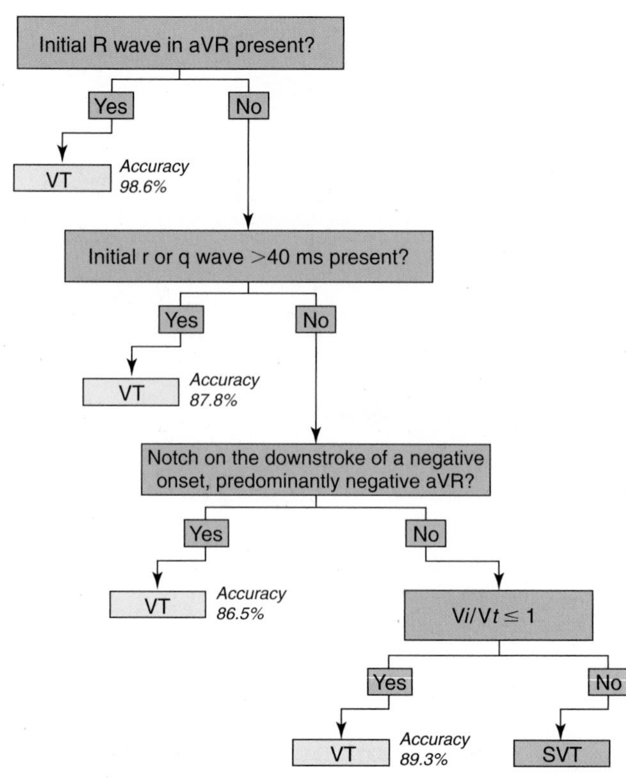

FIGURE 17–9 New algorithm using only lead aVR for differential diagnosis of wide QRS complex tachycardia. SVT = supraventricular tachycardia; VT = ventricular tachycardia. (From Vereckei A, Duray G, Szénási G, et al: New algorithm using only lead aVR for differential diagnosis of wide QRS complex tachycardia. Heart Rhythm 2008;5:89.)

17

the mid to terminal part of the QRS. In contrast, in WCT caused by VT, there is initial slower muscle-to-muscle spread of activation until the impulse reaches the HPS, after which the rest of the ventricular muscle is more rapidly activated.

Antiarrhythmic drugs that impair conduction in the HPS and/or ventricular myocardium (e.g., class I drugs and amiodarone) would be expected to decrease the Vi and Vt approximately to the same degree; therefore, the Vi/Vt ratio should not change significantly. Although the Vi/Vt ratio reflects the electrophysiology of many VTs, there are a number of exceptions to these criteria. First, disorders involving the myocardium locally can alter the Vi or Vt. For example, a decreased Vi with unchanged Vt can be present in the case of an SVT occurring in the presence of an anteroseptal MI, leading to the misdiagnosis of VT. Similarly, a scar situated at a late activated ventricular site can result in a decreased Vt in the presence of VT, leading to the misdiagnosis of SVT. Second, in the case of a fascicular VT, the Vi is not slower than the Vt. Third, if the exit site of the VT reentry circuit is very close to the HPS, it might result in a relatively narrow QRS complex and the slowing of the Vi can last for such a short time that it cannot be detected by the surface ECG.

Algorithm 3. The positive aVR criterion in algorithm 2 suggesting VT was further tested in 483 WCTs in 313 patients, and another algorithm based solely on QRS morphology in lead aVR was developed for distinguishing VT from SVT (Fig. 17-9).[9] The new aVR algorithm is based solely on the principle of differences in the direction and velocity of the initial and terminal ventricular activation during WCT caused by VT and SVT. During SVT with BBB, both the initial rapid septal activation, which can be either left to right or right to left, and the later main ventricular activation wavefront proceed in a direction away from lead aVR, yielding a negative QRS complex in lead aVR. An exception to this generalization occurs in the presence of an inferior MI; an initial r wave (Rs complex) may be seen in lead aVR during NSR or SVT because of the loss of initial inferiorly directed forces. An rS complex also may be present as a normal variant in lead aVR, but with an R/S ratio less than 1. With these considerations, an initial dominant R wave should not be present in SVT with BBB. Because an initial dominant R wave in aVR is incompatible with SVT, its presence suggests VT, typically arising from the inferior or apical region of the ventricles.

Furthermore, VTs originating from sites other than the inferior or apical wall of the ventricles, but not showing an initial R wave in aVR should yield a slow, initially upward vector component of variable size pointing toward lead aVR (absent in SVT), even if the main vector in these VTs points downward, yielding a totally or predominantly negative QRS in lead aVR. Thus, in VT without an initial R wave in lead aVR, the initial part of the QRS in lead aVR should be less steep (slow) because of the slower initial ventricular activation having an initially upward vector component, which may be manifested as an initial r or q wave with a width more than 40 milliseconds, a notch on the downstroke of the QRS, or a slower ventricular activation during the initial 40 milliseconds than during the terminal 40 milliseconds of the QRS (Vi/Vt ≤1) in lead aVR. In contrast, in SVT with BBB, the initial part of the QRS in lead aVR is steeper (fast) because of the invariably rapid septal activation going away from lead aVR, resulting in a narrow (≤40 milliseconds) initial r or q wave and Vi/Vt more than 1.[9]

The overall accuracy of the aVR algorithm was 91.5%, which is similar to algorithm 2 and superior to the Brugada algorithm (90.3% and 84.8%, respectively). The inability of the aVR algorithm to differentiate preexcited tachycardias from VTs, with the possible exception of the presence of initial R wave in lead aVR, is a limitation of the algorithm.[9]

Ventricular Tachycardia Versus Preexcited Supraventricular Tachycardia

Differentiation between VT and preexcited SVT is particularly difficult, because ventricular activation begins outside the normal intraventricular conduction system in both tachycardias (see Fig. 9-4). As a result, algorithms for WCT, like QRS morphology criteria, tend to misclassify SVTs with preexcitation as VT. However, preexcitation is an uncommon cause of WCT, particularly if other factors, such as age and past medical history, suggest another diagnosis. For cases in which preexcitation is thought to be likely, such as a young patient without structural heart disease, or a patient with a known BT, a separate algorithm has been developed by Brugada and colleagues (Fig. 17-10).[6] This algorithm consists of three steps. First, the predominant polarity of the QRS complex in leads V_4 through V_6 is defined as positive or negative. If predominantly negative, the diagnosis of VT can be made with 100% specificity. Second, if the polarity of the QRS complex is predominantly positive in V_4 through V_6, the ECG should be examined for the presence of a qR complex in one or more of precordial leads V_2 through V_6. If a qR complex can be identified, VT can be diagnosed with a specificity of 100%. Third, if a qR wave in leads V_2 through V_6 is absent, the AV relationship is then evaluated. If a 1:1 AV relationship is not present and there are more QRS complexes present than P waves, VT can be diagnosed with a specificity of 100%.

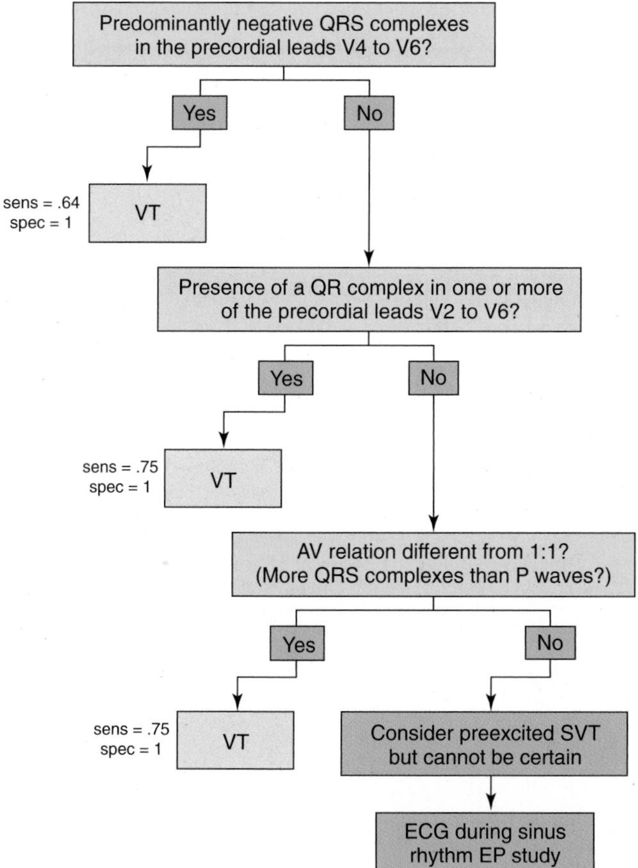

FIGURE 17–10 Brugada algorithm for distinguishing ventricular tachycardia (VT) from preexcited supraventricular tachycardia (SVT). AV = atrioventricular; EP = electrophysiology; sens = sensitivity; spec = specificity. (From Antunes E, Brugada J, Steurer G, et al: The differential diagnosis of a regular tachycardia with a wide QRS complex on the 12-lead ECG. Pacing Clin Electrophysiol 1994;17,1515-1524.)

If the ECG of the WCT does not display any morphological characteristics diagnostic of VT after using this algorithm, the diagnosis of preexcited SVT must be considered. Although this algorithm has a specificity of 100% for VT, it has a sensitivity of only 75% for the diagnosis of preexcited SVT when all three steps are answered negatively (i.e., 25% of such cases are actually VT).

ELECTROPHYSIOLOGICAL TESTING

Baseline Observations During Normal Sinus Rhythm

The presence of preexcitation during NSR or atrial pacing suggests SVT, and the absence of preexcitation during NSR and atrial pacing excludes preexcited SVT.

Induction of Tachycardia

The mode of induction cannot distinguish between SVT and VT. Both atrial and ventricular stimulation may induce SVT or VT. VTs that can be induced with atrial pacing include verapamil-sensitive VT, adenosine-sensitive VT, and BBR VT.[10]

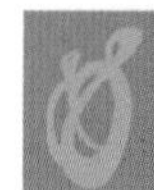

Tachycardia Features

QRS Morphology. As noted, when the QRS configuration of the WCT is not compatible with any known form of aberration, the rhythm is likely to be VT or preexcited SVT. QRS morphology during WCT that is identical to that during NSR may occur in SVT with BBB, preexcited SVT (when NSR is also fully preexcited), BBR VT, and interfascicular VT.

His Bundle–Ventricular Interval. When the His bundle–ventricular (HV) interval is positive (i.e., the His potential precedes the QRS onset), an HV interval during the WCT shorter than that during NSR (HV_{WCT} less than HV_{NSR}) indicates VT or preexcited SVT (see Figs. 14-3 and 18-9). In contrast, an HV_{WCT} equal to or longer than HV_{NSR} indicates SVT with aberrancy, BBR VT, or (rarely) other VTs (see Figs. 14-17 and 20-3).[10-12]

When the HV interval is negative (i.e., the His potential follows the QRS onset), BBR VT and SVT with aberrancy are excluded. However, myocardial VTs and preexcited SVT can have negative HV intervals.

Prolongation of the VA (and VH) interval and tachycardia CL with transient RBBB (caused by mechanical trauma or introduction of a ventricular extrastimulus [VES]) is diagnostic of antidromic AVRT using a right-sided BT and excludes preexcited AVNRT, but can theoretically occur in VT originating in the right ventricle (RV; with LBBB-like morphology). However, continuation of the WCT in the presence of RBBB excludes BBR VT.

Oscillation in the Tachycardia Cycle Length. Variations in the tachycardia CL (the V-V intervals) that are dictated and preceded by similar variations in the H-H intervals are suggestive of SVT with aberrancy or BBR VT. In contrast, variations in the V-V intervals that predict the subsequent H-H interval changes are consistent with myocardial VT or preexcited SVT.

His Bundle–Right Bundle Branch Potential Sequence. When both the His bundle (HB) and right bundle branch (RB) potentials are recorded, a His potential (H)-RB-V activation sequence occurs in SVT with aberrancy and BBR VT with a LBBB pattern. In either case, the H-RB interval during WCT is equal to or longer than that in NSR. On the other hand, an RB-H-V activation sequence occurs in antidromic AVRT using an atriofascicular or right-sided BT, the uncommon type of BBR VT with RBBB pattern, or myocardial VT originating in the RV. An RB-V-H activation sequence occurs in antidromic AVRT using atriofascicular BT, and a V-RB-H or a V-H-RB activation sequence can occur in VT.[10]

Atrioventricular Relationship. A 1 : 1 AV relationship can occur in VT and SVT. When the atrial rate is faster than the ventricular rate, VT is unlikely, except in the rare case of coexistent atrial and ventricular tachycardias (Fig. 17-11). In contrast, when the ventricular rate is faster than the atrial rate, VT is more likely, except for the rare case of junctional tachycardia or AVNRT with VA block in the upper common pathway.

Atrial Activation Sequence. Concentric atrial activation sequence can occur in SVT and VT, whereas eccentric atrial activation sequence practically excludes VT.

Effects of Adenosine. Termination of WCT with adenosine can occur in SVT and adenosine-sensitive VT. AV block with continuation of the WCT can occur in aberrantly conducted AFL, AF, or AT. Adenosine can also have no effect on the WCT, whether it is a VT or SVT.

Diagnostic Maneuvers During Tachycardia

Atrial Extrastimulation. An atrial extrastimulus (AES), regardless of its timing, that advances the next ventricular activation with similar QRS morphology to that of the WCT excludes VT (see Fig. 14-20). Also, an AES (regardless of its timing) that delays the next ventricular activation excludes VT (see Fig. 15-4).

With a late-coupled AES delivered when the AV junctional portion of the atrium is refractory, if the AES advances the next ventricular activation, it proves the presence of an anterogradely conducting AV BT and excludes any arrhythmia mechanism that involves anterograde conduction over the AVN. Moreover, if the AES advances the next ventricular activation with similar QRS morphology as that of the WCT, it proves that the BT is mediating ventricular activation during the WCT (as an integral part of the SVT circuit or as a bystander) and that the WCT is a preexcited SVT, and VT is excluded. Additionally, if the AES advances the timing of both the next ventricular activation and the subsequent atrial activation, it proves that the SVT is an antidromic AVRT using an atrioventricular or atriofascicular BT anterogradely, and excludes preexcited AVNRT and VT (see Fig. 14-20). Also, if the AES delays the next ventricular activation, it proves that the SVT is an antidromic AVRT using an atrioventricular or atriofascicular BT anterogradely, and excludes preexcited AVNRT and VT (see Fig. 15-4).[10]

Atrial Pacing. The ability to entrain the WCT with atrial pacing can occur in VT and SVT. However, the ability to entrain the WCT with similar QRS morphology to that of the WCT (i.e., entrainment with concealed QRS fusion) excludes myocardial VT, but can occur in BBR VT and is typical for SVT.

The ability to dissociate the atrium with rapid atrial pacing without influencing the tachycardia CL (V-V interval) or QRS morphology suggests VT and excludes preexcited SVTs, AT with aberrancy, and orthodromic AVRT with aberrancy. However, it does not exclude the rare case of AVNRT with aberrancy associated with anterograde block in the upper common pathway during rapid atrial pacing.

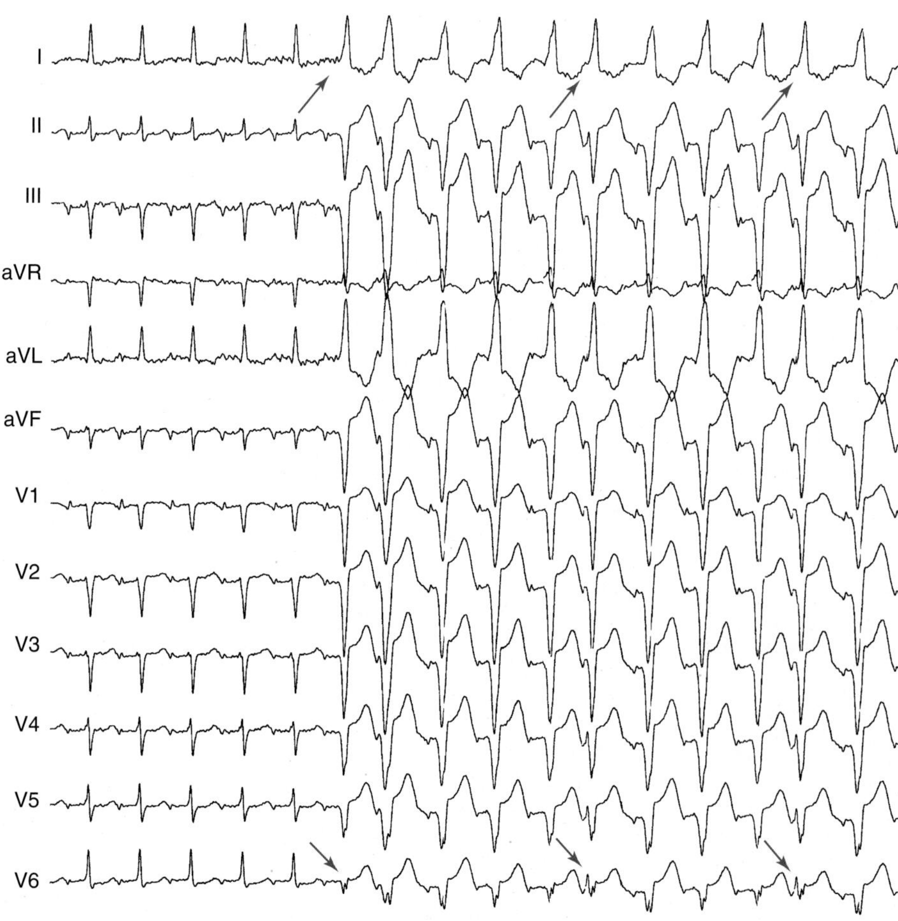

FIGURE 17–11 Surface ECG of atrial tachycardia (AT) with a narrow QRS complex with the development of ventricular tachycardia (VT) with a left bundle branch block (LBBB)–like pattern. Although the atrial rate is faster than the ventricular rate, aberrant conduction during AT as the mechanism of the widening of the QRS can be excluded by observation of QRS morphology in lead V_6 (QS) inconsistent with LBBB aberrancy, a significant shift in the frontal plane QRS axis between AT and VT, and the presence of fusion beats (arrows). Additionally, the atrial rate continues unperturbed, whereas the ventricular rate is slightly irregular.

Ventricular Extrastimulation. A VES that resets (advances or delays) the next QRS without affecting the A-A interval is consistent with VT and practically excludes SVT. Furthermore, a VES that terminates the WCT without conduction to the atrium excludes AT and AVRT, is consistent with VT, and can occur in AVNRT. In addition, a VES delivered when the HB is refractory that terminates the WCT without atrial activation excludes SVT and is consistent with VT, although it can occur in orthodromic AVRT with aberrant conduction or in antidromic AVRT using a second BT as the retrograde limb of the circuit.[10]

Ventricular Pacing. Entrainment with manifest QRS fusion can occur in VT or AVRT but excludes AT and AVNRT, whereas entrainment with concealed fusion excludes SVT with aberrancy.

Entrainment from the RV apex followed by a postpacing interval (PPI) equal (within 30 milliseconds) to the tachycardia CL excludes AVNRT, AT, and myocardial VT, but can occur with BBR VT and AVRT using a right-sided BT.

REFERENCES

1. Gupta AK, Thakur RK: Wide QRS complex tachycardias. Med Clin North Am 2001;85:245.
2. Blomström-Lundqvist C, Scheinman MM, Aliot EM, et al; American College of Cardiology; American Heart Association Task Force on Practice Guidelines; European Society of Cardiology Committee for Practice Guidelines. Writing Committee to Develop Guidelines for the Management of Patients With Supraventricular Arrhythmias: ACC/AHA/ESC guidelines for the management of patients with supraventricular arrhythmias—executive summary: A report of the American College of Cardiology/American Heart Association Task Force on Practice Guidelines and the European Society of Cardiology Committee for Practice Guidelines. Circulation 2003;108:1871.
3. Miller JM, Das MK, Arora R, Alberte-Lista C: Differential diagnosis of wide QRS complex tachycardia. *In* Zipes DP, Jalife J (eds): Cardiac Electrophysiology: From Cell to Bedside, 4th ed. Philadelphia, WB Saunders, 2004, pp 747-757.
4. Miller JM: The many manifestations of ventricular tachycardia. J Cardiovasc Electrophysiol 1992;3:88.
5. Wellens HJ. Electrophysiology: Ventricular tachycardia: Diagnosis of broad QRS complex tachycardia. Heart 2001;86:579.
6. Brugada P, Brugada J, Mont L, et al: A new approach to the differential diagnosis of a regular tachycardia with a wide QRS complex. Circulation 1991;83:1649.
7. Vereckei A, Duray G, Szenasi G, et al: Application of a new algorithm in the differential diagnosis of wide QRS complex tachycardia. Eur Heart J 2007;28:589.
8. Dendi R, Josephson ME: A new algorithm in the differential diagnosis of wide complex tachycardia. Eur Heart J 2007;28:525.
9. Vereckei A, Duray G, Szénási G, et al: New algorithm using only lead aVR for differential diagnosis of wide QRS complex tachycardia. Heart Rhythm 2008;5:89.
10. Josephson ME: Recurrent ventricular tachycardia. *In* Josephson ME (ed): Clinical Cardiac Electrophysiology, 3rd ed. Philadelphia, Lippincott, Williams & Wilkins, 2002, pp 425-610.
11. Daoud EG: Bundle branch reentry. *In* Zipes DP, Jalife J (eds): Cardiac Electrophysiology: From Cell to Bedside, 4th ed. Philadelphia, WB Saunders, 2004, pp 683-686.
12. Fisher JD: Bundle branch reentry tachycardia: Why is the HV interval often longer than in sinus rhythm? The critical role of anisotropic conduction. J Interv Card Electrophysiol 2001;5:173.

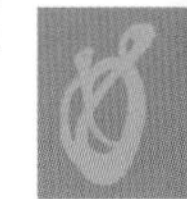

CHAPTER 18

Postinfarction Sustained Monomorphic Ventricular Tachycardia

PATHOPHYSIOLOGY

Classification of Ventricular Tachycardia

Classification According to Tachycardia Morphology. Monomorphic ventricular tachycardia (VT) has a single stable QRS morphology from beat to beat, indicating repetitive ventricular depolarization in the same sequence (Fig. 18-1).[1] Polymorphic VT has a continuously changing or multiform QRS morphology (i.e., no constant morphology for more than five complexes, no clear isoelectric baseline between QRS complexes, or QRS complexes that have different morphologies in multiple simultaneously recorded leads), indicating a variable sequence of ventricular activation and no single site of origin (see Fig. 18-1).[1] Torsades de pointes is a polymorphic VT associated with a long QT interval, and electrocardiographically characterized by twisting of the peaks of the QRS complexes around the isoelectric line during the arrhythmia.[2] Bidirectional VT is associated with a beat to beat alternans in the QRS frontal plane axis, often associated with digitalis toxicity. Ventricular flutter is a regular (cycle length [CL] variability less than 30 milliseconds), rapid (approximately 300 beats/min) ventricular arrhythmia with a monomorphic appearance but no isoelectric interval between successive QRS complexes (see Fig. 18-1). Ventricular fibrillation (VF) is a rapid, usually more than 300 beats/min, grossly irregular ventricular rhythm with marked variability in QRS CL, morphology, and amplitude (see Fig. 18-1).[2]

Classification According to Tachycardia Duration. Sustained VT lasts for more than 30 seconds or requires termination in less than 30 seconds because of hemodynamic compromise, whereas nonsustained VT is VT lasting for three or more complexes at more than 100 beats/min but for less than 30 seconds.[1,3] However, during electrophysiological (EP) testing, nonsustained VT is defined as more than five or six complexes of non–bundle branch reentrant (BBR) VT, regardless of morphology.[1] BBR complexes are frequent (50%) in normal individuals in response to a ventricular extrastimulation (VES) and have no relevance to clinical nonsustained VT. Repetitive polymorphic responses are also common (up to 50%), especially when multiple (three or more) VESs are used with very short coupling intervals (less than 180 milliseconds). The clinical significance of induced polymorphic nonsustained VT is questionable.[1] Incessant VT is a VT that repeatedly recurs and persists for more than half of a 24-hour period, despite repeated attempts to terminate the arrhythmia.[4] Usually, incessant VT manifests as a sustained VT that is recurrent following termination by electrical cardioversion. The time between cardioversion and recurrence can be seconds, minutes, or more.[4] Less commonly, incessant VT manifests as repeated bursts, with runs of VT that spontaneously terminate for a few intervening sinus beats, followed by the next tachycardia burst. The latter form is more common with the idiopathic VTs (see Fig. 19-1).[4]

Classification According to QRS Morphology in V1. VT with left bundle branch block (LBBB)–like pattern has a predominantly negative QRS polarity in V_1 (QS, rS, qrS), whereas VT with right bundle branch block (RBBB)–like pattern has a predominantly positive QRS polarity in V_1 (rsR′, qR, RR bundle branch block, R, RS).[1,3]

Mechanism of Postinfarction Ventricular Tachycardia

The majority of sustained monomorphic VTs (SMVTs) are caused by reentry involving a region of ventricular scar. The scar is most commonly caused by an old myocardial infarction (MI), but right ventricular (RV) dysplasia, sarcoidosis, Chagas' disease, other nonischemic cardiomyopathies, surgical ventricular incisions for repair of tetralogy of Fallot, other congenital heart diseases, or ventricular volume reduction surgery (Batista procedure) can also cause scar-related reentry. Dense fibrotic scar creates areas of anatomical conduction block, and fibrosis between surviving myocyte bundles decreases cell to cell coupling and distorts the path of propagation causing areas of slow conduction and block, which promotes reentry. In post-MI VT, a variety of different circuit configurations are possible. Generally, the reentrant circuit arises in areas of fibrosis

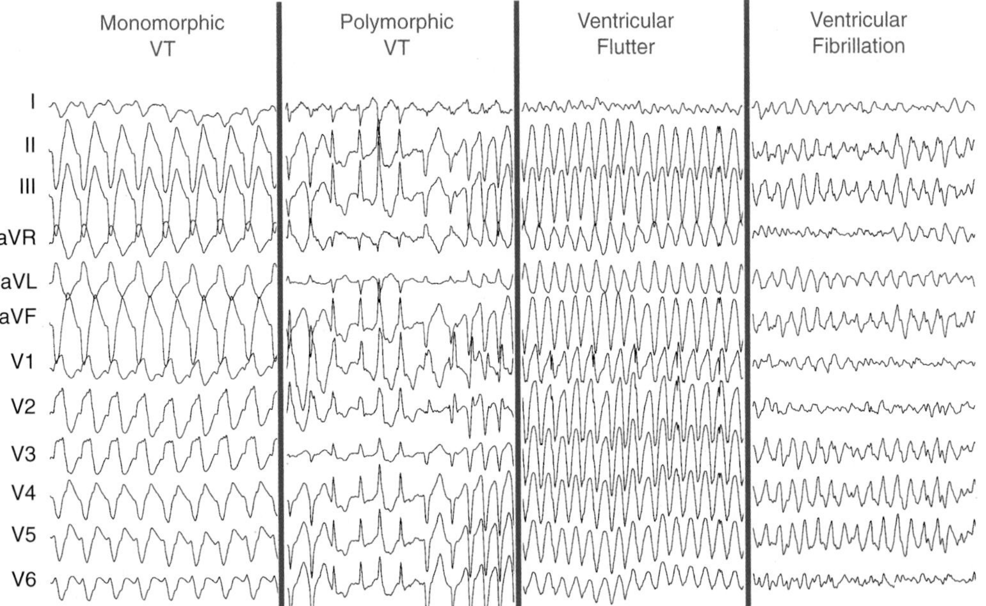

FIGURE 18–1 Surface ECG of different types of ventricular tachycardias. VT = ventricular tachycardia.

that contain surviving myocardial strands, producing a zigzag course of activation leading to inhomogeneous anisotropy (see Fig. 1-16). Buried in the arrhythmogenic area is the common central pathway, the critical isthmus, causing slowing of impulse conduction, allowing reentry to occur. The isthmus itself can be surrounded by dead ends or branches that do not participate in the common pathway of the main reentrant circuit (bystander).[5]

The critical isthmus contained in these reentry circuits often is a narrow path of tissue with abnormal conduction properties. Depolarization of the small mass of tissue in the isthmus is usually not detectable on the surface ECG and constitutes electrical diastole between QRS complexes. The wavefront leaves the isthmus at the exit site and propagates out to depolarize the remainder of the ventricles, producing the QRS complex. After leaving the exit of the isthmus, the reentrant wavefront can return back to the entrance of the isthmus through an outer or inner loop (see Fig. 3-14).[6,7] An outer loop is a broad sheet of myocardium along the border of the infarct. Depolarization of the outer loop can be detectable on the surface ECG. Reentrant circuits can have one or more outer loops. An inner loop is contained within the scar. Inner loop pathways can serve as potential components of a new reentrant circuit should the central common pathway be ablated. If multiple loops exist, the loop with the shortest conduction time generally determines the VT CL and is therefore the dominant loop. Any loop with a longer conduction time behaves as a bystander. Those bystander loops can serve as a potential component of a new reentrant circuit if the dominant loop is ablated.

The critical isthmus in post-MI VT is typically bounded by two approximately parallel conduction barriers that consist of a line of double potentials, a scar area, or the mitral annulus. The endocardial reentrant VT rotates around the isthmus boundaries and propagates slowly through the critical isthmus, which harbors diastolic potentials and measures approximately 30 mm long by 16 mm wide (on average). The axis of a critical isthmus is typically oriented parallel to the mitral annulus plane in perimitral circuits and perpendicular to the mitral annulus plane in other circuits.[6] Ablation lesions produced with standard radiofrequency (RF) ablation catheters are usually less than 8 mm in diameter, relatively small in relation to the entire reentry circuit, and can be smaller than the width of the reentry path at different points in the circuit. Successful ablation of a large circuit is achieved by targeting an isthmus where the circuit can be interrupted with one or a small number of RF lesions, or by creating a line of RF lesions through a region containing the reentry circuit.

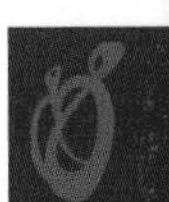

CLINICAL CONSIDERATIONS

Epidemiology

The incidence of SMVT in patients with an acute MI varies with the type of MI. Among almost 41,000 patients with an ST elevation (Q wave) MI treated with thrombolysis in the GUSTO-1 trial, 3.5% developed VT alone and 2.7% developed both VT and VF. A pooled analysis of four major trials of almost 25,000 patients with a non-ST elevation acute coronary syndrome (non–ST elevation MI and unstable angina) noted a lower incidence of VT—0.8% developed VT alone and 0.3% developed both VT and VF.[8]

SMVT within the first 2 days of acute MI is uncommon, occurring in up to 3% of patients as a primary arrhythmia and with VF in up to 2%, and is associated with an increase in in-hospital mortality compared to those without this arrhythmia. However, among 21- to 30-day survivors, mortality at 1 year is not increased, suggesting that the arrhythmogenic mechanisms can be transient in early SMVT. On the other hand, the typical patient with SMVT occurring during the subacute and healing phases beginning more than 48 hours after an acute MI, has had a large, often complicated infarct with a reduced left ventricular (LV) ejection fraction, and such VT is a predictor of a worse prognosis.[9] SMVT within 3 months following an MI is associated with a 2-year mortality rate of 40% to 50%, with most deaths being sudden.[9] Predictors of increased mortality in these patients are an anterior wall MI, frequent episodes of sustained and/or nonsustained VT, heart failure, and multivessel coronary disease, particularly in individuals with residual ischemia.

Most episodes of SMVT associated with MI occur during the chronic phase. The first episode can be seen within the first year post-MI, but the median time of occurrence is about 3 years and SMVT can occur as late as 10 to 15 years after an MI. Late SMVT often reflects significant LV dysfunction and the presence of a ventricular aneurysm or scarring. Late arrhythmias can also result from new cardiac events. The annual mortality rate for SMVT that occurs after the first 3 months following acute MI is approximately 5% to 15%. Predictors of VF include residual ischemia in the setting of damaged myocardium, LV ejection fraction less than 40%, and electrical instability, including inducible or spontaneous VT, particularly in those who present with cardiac arrest.

The relationship between SMVT and VF is uncertain, and it is not clear how often VF is triggered by SMVT rather than occurring de novo. SMVT can simply be the company kept by VF in a number of patients or, in the appropriate setting such as recurrent ischemia, it can provide a rapid wavefront that becomes fractionated, leading to VF.

Clinical Presentation

In chronic ischemic heart disease, VT results in a wide spectrum of clinical presentations, ranging from mild symptoms (palpitations) to symptoms of hypoperfusion (lightheadedness, altered mental status, presyncope, and syncope), exacerbation of heart failure and angina to cardiovascular collapse. Hemodynamic consequences associated with VT are related to ventricular rate, duration of VT, presence and extent of LV dysfunction, ventricular activation sequence (i.e., site of origin of VT), and loss of atrioventricular (AV) synchrony.

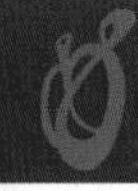

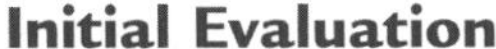

Initial Evaluation

Initial testing in patients with post-MI VT should evaluate for reversible causes of the arrhythmia. These include electrolyte imbalances, acute ischemia, heart failure, hypoxia, hypotension, drug effects, and anemia. Subsequent diagnostic evaluation for acute or persistent ischemia and LV dysfunction is warranted. This may include echocardiographic examination, cardiac catheterization, and exercise testing.

Principles of Management

Acute Management

The degree of hemodynamic tolerance should dictate the initial therapeutic strategy. VTs causing severe symptoms of angina or hemodynamic collapse almost always respond to synchronized DC cardioversion. Treatment of pulseless VT is the same as that for VF and should follow the ACLS protocol. In patients with difficult to control or recurrent VT, intravenous amiodarone is the drug of choice. Intravenous procainamide and sotalol (where available) are alternatives. Lidocaine is less effective in the absence of acute ischemia; however, it can be considered in combination with either procainamide or amiodarone if the latter drugs are ineffective alone. Beta blockers offer additional benefit in patients with ischemic heart disease. Treatment of underlying conditions (e.g., acute ischemia, decompensated heart failure, electrolyte abnormalities) is also necessary.

Chronic Management

Implantation of an implantable cardioverter-defibrillator (ICD) is recommended for secondary prevention, even in patients undergoing catheter ablation of the VT. Although one report has questioned the benefit from an ICD compared with pharmacological therapy in patients with LV ejection fraction more than 40%, the guidelines did not stratify their recommendations based upon the LV ejection fraction.[2,10,11] This seems appropriate for two reasons: the prognostic importance of the LV ejection fraction was based on subset analysis and, given the current ease of ICD implantation, the consequences of choosing a possibly less effective therapy are too great.

Antiarrhythmic drugs can be considered in two main settings, as adjunctive therapy in patients with an ICD and as preventive therapy in patients who do not want or are not candidates for an ICD (e.g., because of marked comorbidities). Because an ICD does not prevent arrhythmias, patients who have frequent symptoms or device discharges triggered by these arrhythmias may benefit from adjunctive drug therapy. There are three main indications for antiarrhythmic drug therapy along with an ICD: to reduce the frequency of ventricular arrhythmia in patients with unacceptably frequent ICD therapy, to reduce the rate of VT so that it is better tolerated hemodynamically and more amenable to pace termination or low-energy cardioversion, and to suppress other arrhythmias (e.g., sinus tachycardia, AF, nonsustained VT) that cause symptoms or interfere with ICD function, resulting in inappropriate discharges. When long-term antiarrhythmic therapy is required, amiodarone is the drug of choice; sotalol is an alternative. For patients who cannot tolerate amiodarone or sotalol, dofetilide has been suggested as an alternative.

Catheter ablation of post-MI VT is indicated in two situations, recurrent VT causing frequent ICD shocks and refractory to antiarrhythmic medications and VT storm or incessant VT refractory to antiarrhythmic medications. Most patients with post-MI VT have multiple types of monomorphic VT, and elimination of all VTs is often not a realistic goal. Furthermore, because the recurrence of an ablated VT or the onset of a new VT can be fatal, RF ablation is rarely used as the sole therapy for VT. Instead, it is usually used for patients with coronary artery disease as an adjunct to an implantable ICD or, less commonly, to antiarrhythmic drug therapy.

ELECTROCARDIOGRAPHIC FEATURES

In general, QRS patterns are less accurate in localizing the site of origin of reentrant VTs in patients with prior MI and wall motion abnormalities than they are for focal VTs in patients with normal hearts.[1,3,12] Nevertheless, the ECG is capable of regionalizing the VT to areas smaller than 15 to 20 cm^2, even in the most abnormal hearts. The site of origin of VT is the source of electrical activity producing the VT QRS. Although this is a discrete site of impulse formation in automatic and triggered (i.e., focal) rhythms, during reentrant VT it represents the exit site from the diastolic pathway (isthmus) to the myocardium giving rise to the QRS. The pattern of ventricular activation and hence the resultant QRS depends on how the wavefront propagates from the site of origin to the remainder of the heart; this can be totally different during VT than during pacing from the same site in NSR.

A sophisticated algorithm has been developed using eight different patterns of R wave progression in the precordium in addition to relationship with prior anterior or inferior MI, axis deviation, and bundle branch block (BBB) morphology. This algorithm has a predictive accuracy of more than 70% for a specific QRS morphology to identify for a particular endocardial region of 10 cm^2 or less (Fig. 18-2). A recent report indicated that the 12-lead surface ECG characteristics can reliably predict the LV VT exit site region in 71% of clinical VTs without prior knowledge of infarct location. That report described a new algorithm that was used independently of the sustainability of VT and could be applied over a wide range of tachycardia CLs and to patients with posterior and/or multiple sites of infarction (Figs. 18-3 and 18-4).[13]

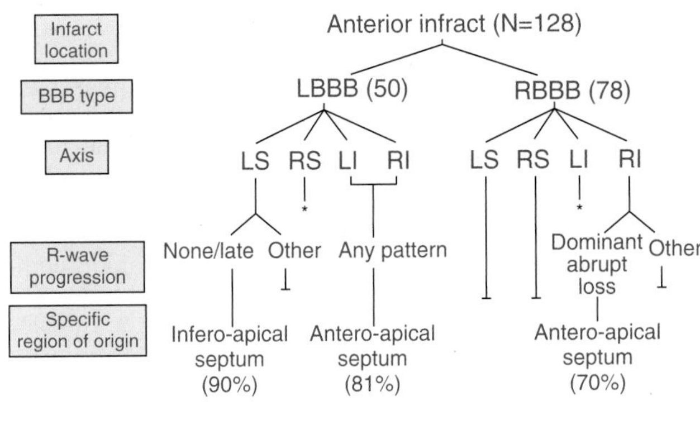

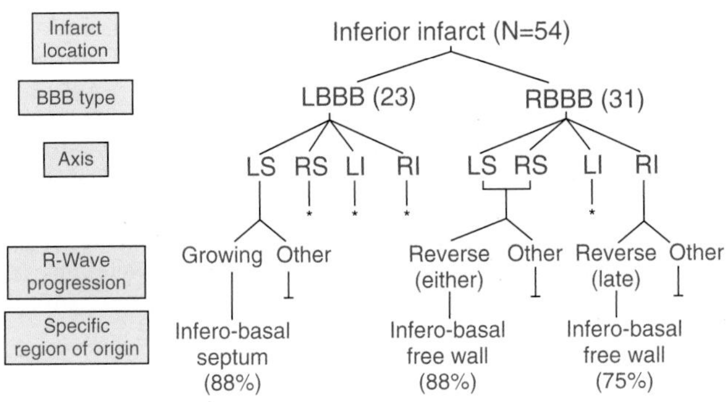

Precordial R-wave progression patterns

PATTERN	V1	V2	V3	V4	V5	V6
Increasing						
None or late						
Regression/growth (not QS)						
Regression/growth (QS)						
Dominant						
Abrupt loss						
Late reverse						
Early reverse						

FIGURE 18–2 Algorithm correlating region of origin to 12-lead ECG of ventricular tachycardia (VT), derived from the retrospective analysis. **Upper panel,** Anterior infarct-associated VTs. **Middle panel,** Inferior infarct-associated VTs. The first branch point is bundle branch block (BBB) configuration, followed by QRS axis and R wave progression. When possible, a specific region of origin is indicated. The number of VTs in each group is indicated in parentheses. A vertical line ending in an asterisk indicates inadequate numbers of VT for analysis; a vertical line terminating in a horizontal bar indicates adequate numbers for analysis, but no specific patterns. **Lower panel,** Precordial R wave progression patterns. Eight different patterns are listed, with the number of examples in parentheses. Typical R wave patterns for V_1 through V_6 are shown. I = inferior; L = left; LBBB = left bundle branch block; R = right; RBBB = right bundle branch block; S = superior. (From Miller JM, Marchlinski FE, Buxton AE, Josephson ME: Relationship between the 12-lead electrocardiogram during ventricular tachycardia and endocardial site of origin in patients with coronary artery disease. Circulation 1988;77:759.)

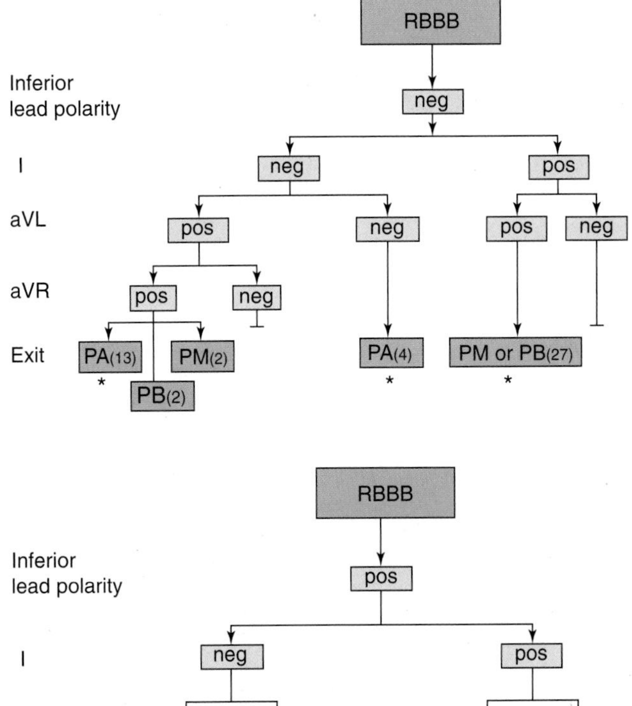

FIGURE 18–3 Algorithm correlating 12-lead ECG morphology of right bundle branch block (RBBB) ventricular tachycardia (VT) with exit site region, derived from retrospective analysis. **A,** VT with negative (neg) polarity in the inferior leads. **B,** VT with positive (pos) polarity in the inferior leads. A vertical line ending a horizontal bar indicates no VT with this ECG pattern was identified. Exit sites with positive predictive value (PPV) ≥70% are marked by asterisks. The numbers of VTs for each ECG pattern and exit site region identified in retrospective analysis are shown in brackets. AA = anteroapical; AB = anterobasal; AM = midanterior; PA = posteroapical; PB = posterobasal; PM = midposterior. (From Segal OR, Chow AW, Wong T, et al: A novel algorithm for determining endocardial VT exit site from 12-lead surface ECG characteristics in human, infarct-related ventricular tachycardia. J Cardiovasc Electrophysiol 2007;18:161.)

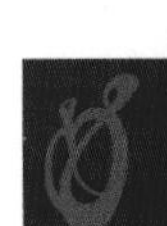

ECG Clues to the Underlying Substrate

VTs arising from normal myocardium typically have rapid initial forces, whereas slurring of the initial forces is frequently seen when the VT arises from an area of scar or from the epicardium. Additionally, VTs originating from very diseased hearts usually have lower amplitude complexes than those arising in normal hearts, and the presence of notching of the QRS is a sign of scar tissue.[1,3,12]

Whereas QS complexes can be seen in a variety of disorders, the presence of qR, QR, or Qr complexes in related leads is highly suggestive of the presence of an infarct. Sometimes it is easier to recognize the presence of MI during VT than during NSR.

General Principles in Localizing the Origin of Post–Myocardial Infarction Ventricular Tachycardias

Post-MI VTs almost always arise in the LV or interventricular septum. Septal VTs generally have QRS durations that are narrower than free wall VTs.[1,3,12]

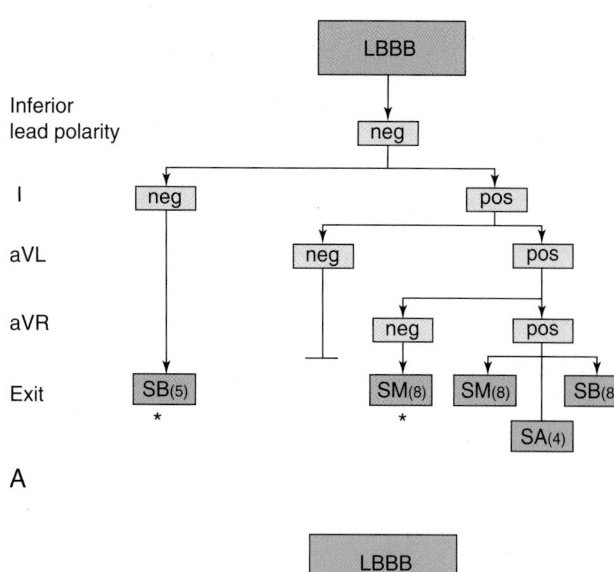

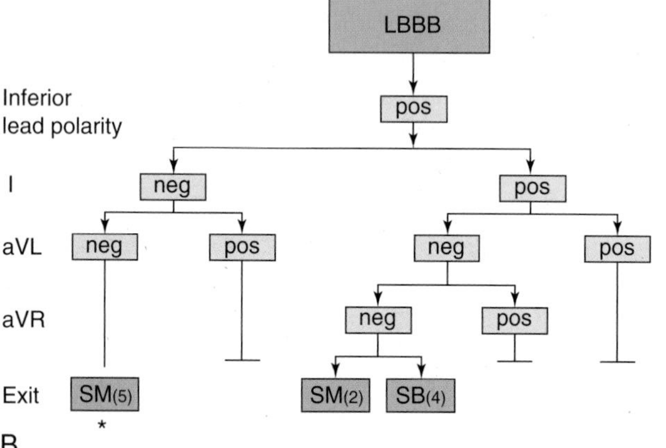

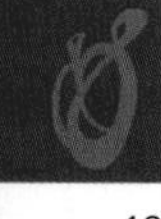

18

FIGURE 18–4 Algorithm correlating 12-lead ECG morphology of left bundle branch block (LBBB) ventricular tachycardia (VT) with exit site region, derived from retrospective analysis. **A,** VT with negative (neg) polarity in the inferior leads. **B,** VT with positive (pos) polarity in the inferior leads. A vertical line ending with a horizontal bar indicates that no VT with this ECG pattern were identified. SA = anteroseptal; SB = basal septum; SM = midseptum. Exit sites with positive predictive value (PPV) ≥70% are marked by asterisks. Numbers of VT for each ECG pattern and exit site region identified in retrospective analysis are shown in brackets. (From Segal OR, Chow AW, Wong T, et al: A novel algorithm for determining endocardial VT exit site from 12-lead surface ECG characteristics in human, infarct-related ventricular tachycardia. J Cardiovasc Electrophysiol 2007;18:161.)

QRS Axis. The right superior axis suggests apical septal or apical lateral sites of origin, often demonstrating QS in leads I, II, and III and QS or rS in leads V_5 and V_6. The right inferior axis suggests a high basal origin (high LV septum, or high lateral LV). A left inferior axis is occasionally associated with VTs arising from the top of the LV septum. Sometimes, the QRS axis is inappropriate for the exit site. This almost always occurs with large apical MIs. Typically, discrepancies occur in VTs with LBBB or RBBB with a right or left superior axis. Such discrepancies can be related to abnormalities of conduction out of the area of the reentrant circuit toward the rest of the myocardium.[1,3,12]

Bundle Branch Block Pattern. VTs with RBBB patterns always arise in the LV, and VTs with LBBB patterns almost always arise in or adjacent to the LV septum. Therefore, LBBB patterns, which all cluster on or adjacent to the septum, have a higher predictive accuracy (regardless of the presence of anterior versus inferior MI) than RBBB patterns, which could be septal or located on the free wall. Most VTs with RBBB patterns associated with inferior MI are clustered in a small region, but are more widely disparate with anterior MI (Figs. 18-5 and 18-6).[1,3,12]

Concordance. VTs with positive concordance arise only at the base of the heart (left ventricular outflow tract [LVOT], along the mitral or aortic valves, or in the basal septum), whereas negative concordance is seen only in VTs originating near the apical septum, most commonly seen with anteroseptal MI.[1,3,12]

Presence of QS Complexes. The presence of QS complexes in any lead suggests that the wavefront is propagating away from that site. Therefore, QS complexes in the inferior leads suggest that the activation is originating in the inferior wall, whereas QS complexes in the precordial leads suggest activation moving away from the anterior wall; QS complexes in leads V_2 to V_4 suggest anterior wall origin, QS complexes in leads V_3 to V_5 suggest apical location, and QS complexes in leads V_5 to V_6 suggest lateral wall. The presence of Q waves in leads I, V_1, V_2, V_6 is seen in VTs with RBBB pattern originating near the apex, but not those originating in the inferobasal parts of the LV. R waves in leads I, V_1, V_2, V_6 are specific for VTs with RBBB or LBBB pattern of posterior origin. Additionally, the presence of Q waves in leads I and V_6 in VTs with an LBBB pattern is seen with an apical septal location, whereas the presence of R waves in leads I and V_6 is associated with inferobasal septal locations.[1,3,12]

Inferior Myocardial Infarction Ventricular Tachycardias

The precordial pattern in VTs associated with inferior MIs always has large R waves that usually are present in leads V_2 to V_4 with the persistence of an r or R wave through lead V_6. In VTs with an RBBB pattern, the R waves can persist across the precordium (positive concordance). When the VT originates near the posterior basal septum and when it arises more laterally (or posteriorly), there can be a decrease in the R wave amplitude across the precordium because the infarct can extend to the posterolateral areas (see Fig. 18-5).[1,3,12]

Left axis deviation is seen in inferior MI VTs when the exit site is near the septum. The more the VT moves from the midline toward the lateral (i.e., posterior) wall, the more right or superior the axis will become. VTs with LBBB (especially when left axis deviation is present) have a characteristic location at the inferobasal septum (see Fig. 18-6). As the VT axis shifts to a more normal axis, the exit site moves higher up along the septum. Rarely, inferior MI VTs can have exit sites as high as the aortic valve along the septum. Very rarely, the VT can only be ablated from the RV or epicardial sites.[1,3,12]

The mitral isthmus (between the mitral annulus and inferior infarct scar) contains a critical region of slow conduction in some patients with VTs following inferior MI, providing a vulnerable and anatomically localized target for catheter ablation. This critical zone of slow conduction is activated parallel to the mitral annulus in either direction, resulting in two distinct QRS configurations not seen in VTs arising from other sites: LBBB (rS in lead V_1, R in lead V_6) and left superior axis morphology, and RBBB (R in lead V_1, QS in lead V_6) and right superior axis morphology.

Anterior Myocardial Infarction Ventricular Tachycardias

Anterior MIs are usually associated with more extensive myocardial damage. Therefore, the accuracy of the ECG in localizing the origin of VTs associated with anterior MI is less than those with inferior MI.

VTs with an LBBB pattern and left axis deviation usually originate from the inferoapical septum, but occasionally there is a discrepancy, with the exit site being more superior than expected for the QRS axis. LBBB VTs associated with anteroseptal MI can present with QS complexes across the

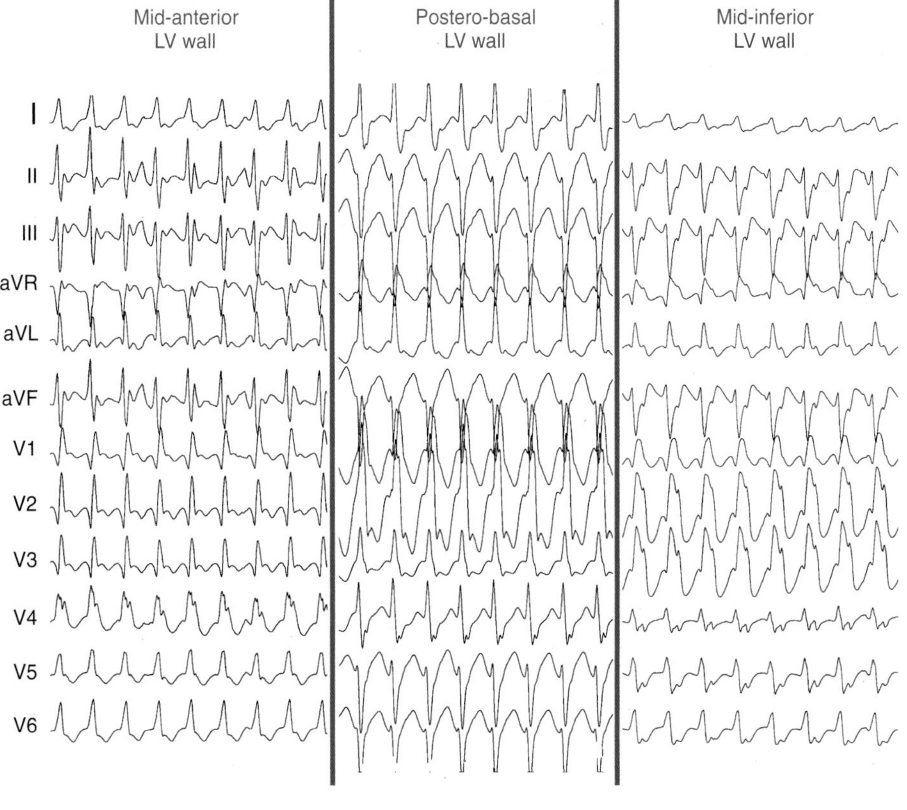

FIGURE 18–5 Surface ECG of sustained monomorphic ventricular tachycardia (SMVT) with right bundle branch block (RBBB) pattern. **Left panel,** Ventricular tachycardia (VT) with RBBB pattern and normal axis in a patient with prior anterior myocardial infarction (MI). The site of origin was mapped to the midanterior left ventriclular (LV) wall. Note the qR pattern in leads V_1-V_3, consistent with anterior infarct. **Middle panel,** VT with RBBB pattern and left superior axis in a patient with prior inferior MI. The site of origin was mapped to the posterobasal LV free wall. **Right panel,** VT with left bundle branch block (LBBB) pattern and left superior axis in a patient with prior inferior MI. The site of origin was mapped to the midinferior LV wall.

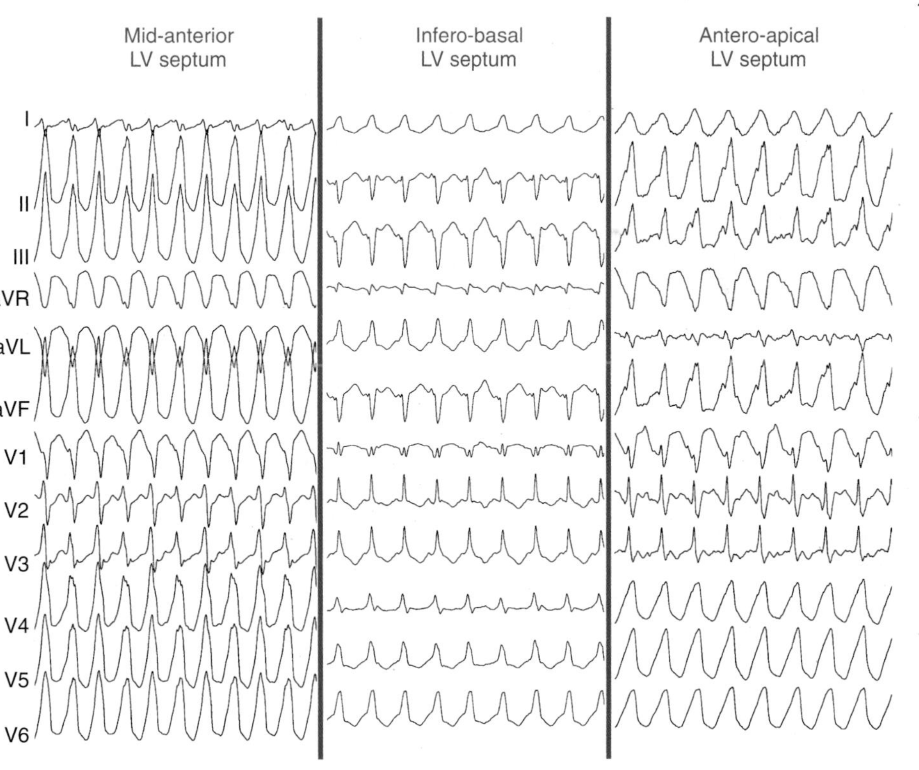

FIGURE 18–6 Surface ECG of sustained monomorphic ventricular tachycardia (SMVT) with left bundle branch block (LBBB) pattern. **Left panel,** Ventricular tachycardia (VT) with LBBB pattern and right inferior axis in a patient with prior anterior myocardial infarction (MI). The site of origin was mapped to the midanterior left ventriclular (LV) septum. **Middle panel,** VT with LBBB pattern and left superior axis in a patient with prior inferior MI. The site of origin was mapped to the inferobasal LV septum. **Right panel,** VT with LBBB pattern and left inferior axis in a patient with prior anterior MI. The site of origin was mapped to the anteroapical LV septum.

precordium (i.e., negative concordance), and they are always associated with a Q wave in leads I and aVL. If an R wave is seen in lead V_1 along with the Q wave in lead aVL, the location of the exit site is more posterior on the septum, closer to the middle third (see Fig. 18-6). LBBB VTs with right inferior axis arise on the upper half of the mid or apical septum but occasionally can be off the septum (see Fig. 18-6).[1,3,12]

RBBB VTs originating from the apex usually have a right and superior axis. Lead V_1 usually has a qR or, occasionally, a monophasic R wave, but there is almost always a QS or QR complex in leads V_2, V_3, and/or V_4. More commonly, when there is a QS complex in leads I, II, and III, there is also a QS complex across the precordium from lead V_2 through V_6. RBBB VTs with right inferior axis arise on the septum but also can be seen across the apex superiorly on the free wall. In both cases, there is a negative deflection in leads aVR and aVL. VTs with LBBB or RBBB patterns and a marked inferior right axis arise superiorly on what usually is the edge of an anterior aneurysm.[1,3,12]

The most difficult VTs to localize are VTs with RBBB and right superior axis associated with anterior MI. QS complexes in the lateral leads (V_4 to V_6) reflect origin near the apex, regardless of whether it is septal or lateral. It is almost impossible to distinguish VTs arising from the apical septum and the apical free wall based on the ECG alone. It is only when the VT location moves more posterolaterally that a difference can be appreciated as the R wave in lead aVR becomes dominant over the R wave in lead aVL. This is usually associated with a large apical aneurysm, but occasionally also can be seen with a posterolateral MI.[1,3,12]

High Posterolateral Myocardial Infarction Ventricular Tachycardias

VTs associated with high posterior MI (left circumflex artery territory) are characterized by a prominent R wave in leads V_1 to V_4 and right inferior axis.[1,3,12]

Epicardial Ventricular Tachycardias

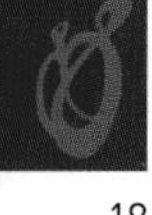

Epicardial origin of VT (i.e., the VT can only be ablated from epicardial surface) is rare in post-MI VT, ranging from 0% to 2% of cases. but more common in dilated cardiomyopathy. With all other factors being equal, the epicardial origin of ventricular activation widens the initial part of the QRS complex (pseudo–delta wave). When the initial activation
18 starts in the endocardium, rapid depolarization of the ventricles occurs along the specialized conducting system, resulting in a narrow QRS on the surface ECG and the absence of a pseudo–delta wave. In contrast, when the initial ventricular activation occurs in the epicardium, the intramyocardial delay of conduction produces a slurred initial part of the QRS complex.[14]

Several ECG intervals of ventricular activation can suggest an epicardial origin of the LV VT with RBBB pattern: (1) pseudo–delta wave (measured from the earliest ventricular activation to the earliest fast deflection in any precordial lead) of 34 milliseconds or more has a sensitivity of 83% and a specificity of 95%; (2) intrinsicoid deflection time in V_2 (measured from the earliest ventricular activation to the peak of the R wave in V_2) of more than 85 milliseconds has a sensitivity of 87% and a specificity of 90%; (3) shortest RS complex duration (measured from the earliest ventricular activation to the nadir of the first S wave in any precordial lead) of 121 milliseconds or more has a sensitivity of 76% and a specificity of 85%; and (4) QRS duration is more than 200 milliseconds (Fig. 18-7).[14]

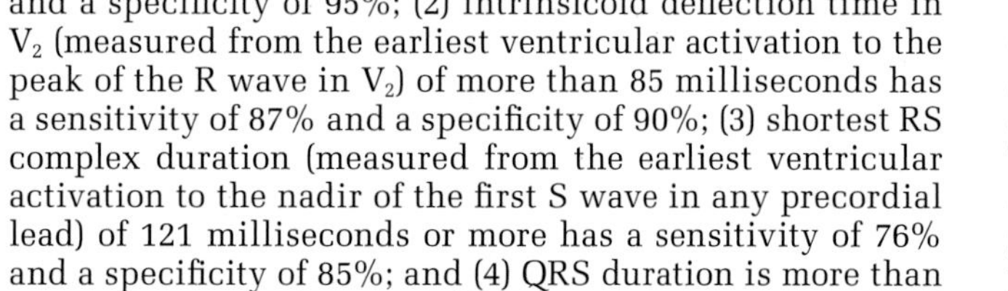

ELECTROPHYSIOLOGICAL TESTING

Induction of Tachycardia

Recommended Stimulation Protocols

The most commonly used stimulation protocol applies pacing output at twice the diastolic threshold current and a pulse width of 1 to 2 milliseconds. Single VESs during NSR and at pacing drive CLs of 600 and 400 milliseconds are delivered, first from the RV apex and then from the right ventricular outflow tract (RVOT). The prematurity of extrastimuli is increased until refractoriness or induction of sustained VT is achieved. Long-short cycle sequences may be tested. If that fails to induce VT, double and then triple VESs are used in the same manner. Because a VES with a very short coupling interval is more likely to induce VF as opposed to monomorphic VT, it may be reasonable to limit the prematurity of the VESs to a minimum of 180 milliseconds when studying patients for whom only inducible SMVT would be considered a positive endpoint. If VT still cannot be induced, rapid ventricular pacing is started at a CL of 400 milliseconds, gradually decreasing the pacing CL until 1:1 ventricular capture is lost or a pacing CL of 220 milliseconds is reached. Repeating the protocol at other pacing drive CLs, at other RV or LV stimulation sites, and/or after administration of isoproterenol or procainamide is then attempted.[1,2]

An alternative stimulation protocol uses a shorter pacing drive CL (350 milliseconds) and a reverse order of the pacing drive CL (i.e., starting the stimulation protocol at 350, then 400, and then 600 milliseconds). This *accelerated* protocol has been shown in one report to reduce the number of protocol steps and duration of time required to induce monomorphic VT by an average of more than 50% and improves the specificity of programmed electrical stimulation without impairing the yield of monomorphic VT.[14a]

Another proposed stimulation protocol exclusively uses four VESs; at no point are one, two, or three VESs used.[14b] At each basic drive train pacing CL, programmed electrical stimulation is initiated with coupling intervals of 290, 280, 270, and 260 milliseconds for the first through fourth VESs. The coupling intervals of the VESs are then shortened simultaneously in 10-millisecond steps until S_2 (the first VES) falls during the refractory period or a 200-millisecond coupling interval is reached. If S_2 is refractory at 290 milliseconds, all extrastimuli are lengthened by 30 milliseconds, and programmed electrical stimulation is then initiated. This *six-step* protocol was tested in a single report and was shown to improve the specificity and efficiency of programmed electrical stimulation without compromising the yield of monomorphic VT in patients with coronary artery disease.

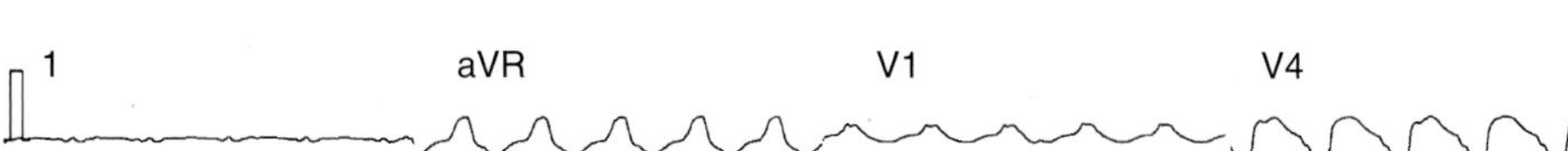

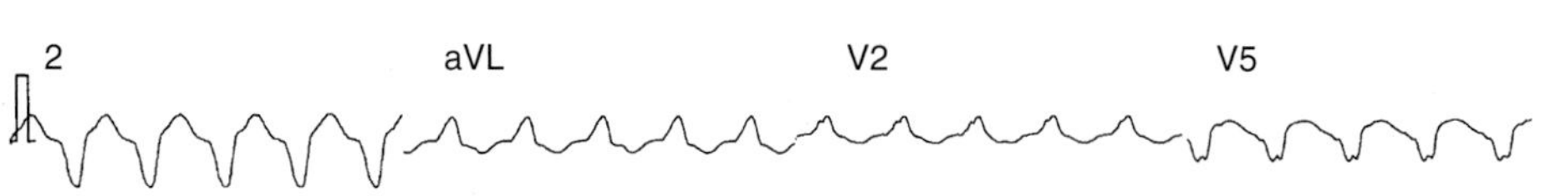

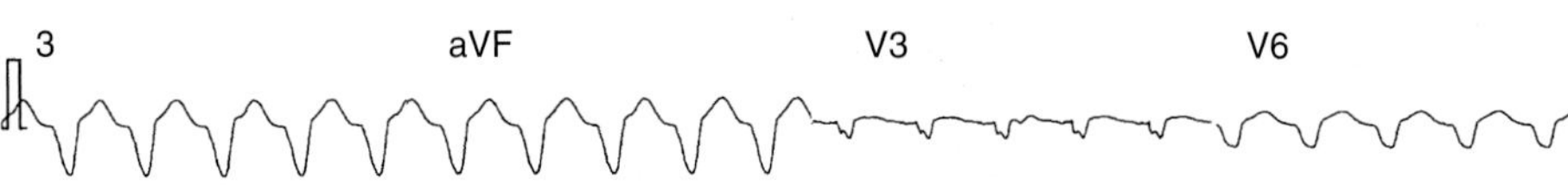

FIGURE 18–7 ECG of post–myocardial infarction ventricular tachycardia that required epicardial ablation. Note delayed QRS upstroke in V_2 and delayed S wave downstroke (pseudo–delta wave) and long RS interval in V_3 and V_4.

Number of Ventricular Extrastimuli. The sensitivity of programmed electrical stimulation to initiate SMVT increases with increasing the number of VESs used, but at the expense of decreasing specificity. The use of three VESs seems optimal because it offers the highest sensitivity associated with an acceptable specificity. More aggressive stimulation is likely to produce nonspecific responses, usually polymorphic VT or VF.

When SMVT is studied, the use of four VESs can be considered. However, when a patient resuscitated from cardiac arrest is studied, four VESs should not be used because the likelihood of inducing a nonspecific response (polymorphic VT/VF) is far higher than that of inducing SMVT (10:1). Triple VESs are required to induce SMVT in 20% to 40% of patients presenting with SMVT and in 40% to 60% of patients presenting with cardiac arrest.[1]

Atrial extrastimulation (AES) can initiate VT in approximately 5% of patients with SMVT. Usually, those VTs can also be initiated by VES, are usually slower, and are reproducibly initiated over a broad zone of VES coupling intervals. Initiation with AES is more common in patients without coronary artery disease.

Pacing Drive Cycle Length. The use of at least two pacing drive CLs (typically 600 and 400 milliseconds) is required to enhance the sensitivity of induction of SMVT in patients presenting with sustained VT of any morphology or those with cardiac arrest. VES at shorter or longer CLs or even in NSR may be necessary to initiate VT in some patients. Abrupt changes in CL can also facilitate VT induction. The CL used can also influence the number and prematurity of VESs required to initiate VT. Rapid ventricular pacing has a low yield in VT initiation.[1]

In 5% of patients with SMVT, and less in patients with cardiac arrest, VT can be initiated only with VES during NSR. On the other hand, most VTs that can be induced during NSR can also be induced during ventricular pacing or VESs delivered after a pacing drive.

Site of Ventricular Stimulation. In contrast to automatic or triggered activity VT, in which the stimulation site has no effect on initiating VT, reentrant VT can demonstrate absolute or relative site specificity for initiation. The direction of wavefront activation can be important in developing block and slow conduction necessary to initiate reentry. Therefore, the use of at least two sites of stimulation enhances the ability to induce VT.

If triple VESs are delivered only from the RV apex, 10% to 20% of patients will require the use of a second RV or LV pacing site for initiation of SMVT (less than 5% require an LV site). If double VESs are used, 20% to 30% will require a second pacing site (10% require an LV site). Because the number of VESs required for initiation can differ depending on the site of stimulation, which occurs in approximately 20% of patients with SMVT, the site that allows the use of the fewest number of VESs is preferred to avoid nonspecific responses. Thus, it is preferable to stimulate from both the RV apex and RVOT at each drive CL and number of VESs before proceeding to more aggressive stimulation.[1]

If stimulation from the RV apex and RVOT fails to initiate VT, stimulation from the LV may be used. However, the yield is low (2% to 5%) for patients with SMVT and somewhat higher in patients with cardiac arrest.

Pacing Current Output. Increasing the current (more than twice the diastolic threshold current or pulse width more than 2 milliseconds) produces only a small increase in sensitivity of initiating SMVT (more than 5%), but this is outweighed by a significant decrease in specificity and increase in the incidence of VF. The use of currents more than 5 mA is not recommended.[1]

Isoproterenol. Isoproterenol has a low yield in facilitating induction in patients with coronary artery disease and SMVT (more than 5%) and is more useful in initiation of exercise-related VTs or triggered activity outflow tract VTs.[1]

Reproducibility of Ventricular Tachycardia Initiation

More than 90% of patients with clinical SMVT will have their VT inducible, regardless of the underlying pathology, with the exception of exercise-induced VT. Patients with cardiac arrest or nonsustained VT have a lower incidence of inducibility; inducibility is higher in patients with coronary artery disease.

SMVT can be reproducibly initiated from day to day and year to year, especially in patients with coronary artery disease. However, the exact mode of initiation is not necessarily reproducible. The mere repetition of stimulation, either longitudinally (by repeating the entire protocol) or horizontally (by repeating each coupling interval), enhances the sensitivity and reproducibility of initiation. Once SMVT is initiated, it is easier to reinitiate.[1,15]

Relationship of Ventricular Extrastimulus Coupling Interval and Pacing Cycle Length to the Onset of Ventricular Tachycardia

Conduction delay is required for the initiation of reentrant rhythms; thus, an inverse relationship between the coupling interval of the VES initiating the VT or the pacing train CL and the interval from the VES to the first VT complex favors reentry. In contrast, a linear relationship of the pacing CL or VES coupling interval to the interval to the first VT complex and initial CL of the VT favors triggered activity. In reentrant VT, the initial CL would reflect conduction through the VT circuit, which in the absence of exit block should demonstrate the same or longer CL as the remaining VT cycles, depending on whether any conduction delay is produced in the circuit on initiation.[1]

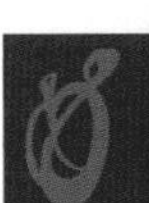

Endpoints of the Electrophysiology Stimulation Protocol

Induction of Sustained Monomorphic Ventricular Tachycardia. Induction of SMVT is very specific, especially with a VES coupling interval of more than 240 milliseconds, and only occurs in patients with spontaneous VT, cardiac arrest, or an arrhythmogenic substrate.

Induction of Polymorphic Ventricular Tachycardia or Ventricular Fibrillation. When EP testing is performed in patients presenting with SMVT, polymorphic VT and VF must be considered as nonspecific responses. Both sustained and nonsustained polymorphic VT and VF can be induced, even in normal subjects. In general, induction of VF requires multiple VESs delivered at shorter coupling intervals (usually less than 180 milliseconds) than induction of SMVT. Induction of polymorphic VT or VF in a patient who presents with cardiac arrest can have a different implication. Because cardiac arrest can be initiated by a polymorphic VT, the induction of polymorphic VT in this patient population can be significant. Therefore, although doubt will always exist, reproducible polymorphic VT induction is treated as a possible indicator of the clinical arrhythmia. Features that suggest that a polymorphic VT can be mechanistically meaningful are reproducible initiation of the same polymorphic VT template, especially from different stimulation sites, inducibility with relatively mild stimulation (single or double VESs), and transformation of the polymorphic VT to SMVT by procainamide. The induction of any arrhythmia (SMVT, polymorphic VT, or VF) in the setting of a recent MI (less than 1 month) may not have clinical significance.[1]

Induction of Multiple Sustained Monomorphic Ventricular Tachycardias. The endpoint of programmed electrical stimulation should be induction of the clinical arrhythmia or the assumed arrhythmia. However, patients with post-MI VT frequently (85%) have more than one VT morphology. Even in patients presenting with a single SMVT, multiple distinct uniform VTs may be induced in the EP laboratory, especially during antiarrhythmic therapy. Clinical VT is defined as an inducible SMVT that matches the morphology of the patient's documented, spontaneously occurring SMVT. Nonclinical VTs are defined as inducible SMVTs that were not previously known to have occurred spontaneously.

Multiple VT morphologies are defined as two or more inducible VTs having at least one of the following: (1) contralateral BBB patterns; (2) frontal plane axis of 30 degrees or more divergent; (3) marked differences in individual ECG leads recorded from the same electrode locations; (4) precordial transition zone in one or more leads or a different dominant deflection in more than one precordial lead; and/or (5) different tachycardia CL (more than 100 milliseconds for VTs with a similar morphology). A change in VT morphology need not reflect a change in a reentrant circuit or site of impulse formation but merely reflect the overall pattern of ventricular activation. In some cases, pacing can reverse the direction of wavefront propagation within the same reentrant loop. Approximately 85% of multiple morphologically distinct SMVTs arise from the same region of the heart (i.e., have closely located exit sites or shared components of an isthmus or diastolic pathway).[1]

Multiple uniform VTs inducible in the EP laboratory are of clinical significance because the distinction between clinical and nonclinical is often uncertain. Clinically, the ECG of spontaneous VTs terminated by an ICD or emergency medical technicians is often not available. The presence of

multiple VT morphologies might have been overlooked because of the lack of 12-lead ECGs obtained during multiple spontaneous episodes on a variety of different antiarrhythmic agents. The use of single-lead rhythm strips to record VT has been a major misleading factor suggesting that there is only one VT. Furthermore, inducible VTs never seen spontaneously in the preablation state can occur spontaneously following ablation of the clinical VT.

Tachycardia Features

His Bundle Activation

No Visible His Potential During Ventricular Tachycardia. The His potential cannot be observed during VT in many patients, likely because the retrograde His potential is masked by ventricular activation or because of suboptimal catheter position.[1] A proper His bundle (HB) catheter position can be verified by observation of the immediate appearance of the His potential on termination of the VT, the disappearance of the His potential on initiation of VT, or the sudden appearance of the His potential when spontaneous or induced supraventricular beats capture the HB (with or without ventricular capture) during VT. Additionally, when complete ventricular–His bundle (VH) block is present, dissociated His potentials will be observed.[1]

Visible His Potential During Ventricular Tachycardia. His potentials can be recorded during VT in approximately 80% of patients.[1] When the His potential is visible during VT, it is often difficult to determine whether the recorded His potential is anterograde or retrograde, and whether an apparent His potential is really a right bundle branch (RB) potential. Recording the RB or left bundle branch (LB) potentials to demonstrate that their activation precedes HB activation during VT, and HB pacing, producing a longer HV interval than the one noted during VT, usually help clarify the situation.[1]

In patients with coronary artery disease, the relative timing of the retrograde His potential in the QRS depends on how quickly the His-Purkinje system (HPS) is engaged and how slowly the impulse reaches the ventricle to produce the QRS. Thus, depending on the relative conduction time up the HPS and through the slowly conducting muscle to give rise to the QRS, the His potential can occur before, during, or after the QRS. The His potential can occasionally occur before ventricular activation (with a His bundle–ventricular [HV] interval during VT shorter than that during NSR; Fig. 18-8) and can also occur just after the onset of ventricular activation (with a short VH interval; Fig. 18-9). The occurrence of an HV interval (with the His potential before the QRS onset) shorter than that during NSR (in the absence of preexcitation) or a VH interval (with the His potential after the QRS onset) implies the presence of retrograde HB activation; it further implies that retrograde conduction from the exit of VT (defined by the onset of the QRS) to the HB is less than the anterograde conduction time over the HPS to activate the ventricle.[1] Some have suggested that the site of origin of such VTs is within the HPS (i.e., fascicular VTs), although proof that such VTs originate from the fascicles and differ from other forms of VT is often lacking. The retrograde His potential appears to reflect passive activation of the HPS, rather than involvement of the HPS in the reentrant circuit. This concept is supported by several

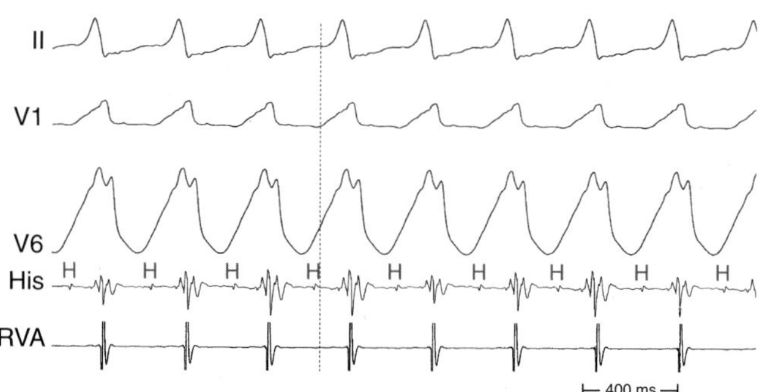

FIGURE 18–8 Ventricular tachycardia with short constant His bundle (HB)–ventricular (HV) interval, consistent with early retrograde activation of the HB.

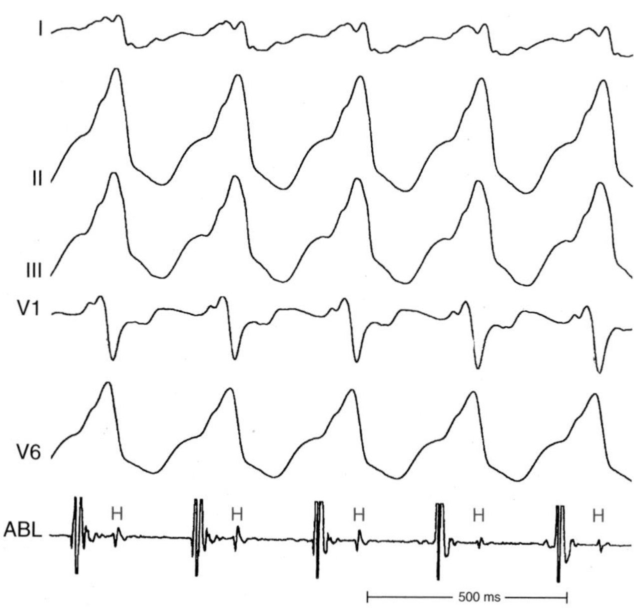

FIGURE 18–9 Ventricular tachycardia with long, constant ventricular–His bundle (VH) interval, consistent with retrograde activation of the His bundle (HB). HB activation is recorded by the ablation catheter positioned in the left ventricular outflow tract.

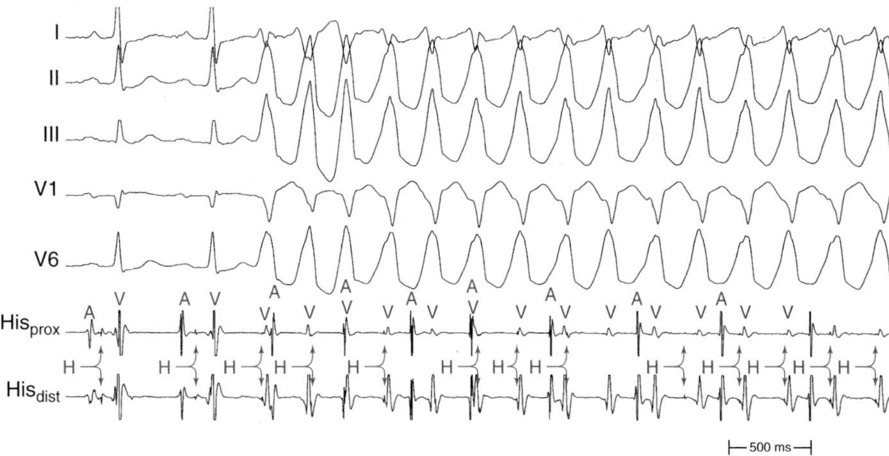

FIGURE 18–10 Ventricular tachycardia (VT) with variable relationship between ventricular and His bundle (HB) activation. HB catheter position is verified by observation of His potentials during normal sinus rhythm (NSR) at left. His potentials are observed intermittently during VT, with variable relationship to the QRS complexes, suggesting that the His-Purkinje system is not an essential part of the VT circuit.

observations. HB deflections can appear intermittently (typically in a 2 : 1 or 3 : 2 fashion, and occasionally in a Wenckebach periodicity), and changes in the VH interval can occur without changes in the tachycardia CL (Fig. 18-10). In fact, marked changes in the tachycardia CL can be present with no changes in the VH interval. Furthermore, AES or atrial pacing may result in anterograde capture of the HB in the presence or absence of ventricular capture or fusion beats. Such an event, linking atrial activation to the HB deflection, proves that HB deflections are caused by anterograde activation and are unrelated to the VT. These observations suggest that the HPS is passively activated in VTs associated with coronary artery disease and is not related to the reentrant circuit per se. Engagement of the HPS, when present, can allow for more rapid activation of the myocardium, which in turn results in a narrower QRS.[1]

The mere presence of a His potential before the QRS with a normal HV interval is not absolutely reliable evidence that the tachycardia is a supraventricular tachycardia (SVT).[1] The HV interval during VT is usually less than that during NSR; hence, if infranodal conduction delay is present during NSR, the VT can exist in the presence of an apparently normal HV interval (i.e., 35 to 55 milliseconds), but will be less than that during NSR. In post-MI VT, because ventricular activation is occurring in diastole (albeit slow enough not to be apparent on the surface ECG), the HPS could be activated during this time giving rise to a short or possibly normal HV interval during the VT. The time to conduct retrogradely to the HB can theoretically be less than the time required to exit from the VT circuit and produce the onset of the QRS, thereby producing an HV interval. Such VTs, which are rare, have a narrow QRS. BBR VT can also give rise to an HV interval that is longer than that during NSR.

For wide complex tachycardias (WCTs) with the His potential preceding the QRS, an $HV_{tachycardia} < HV_{NSR}$ suggests VT or preexcited SVT (see Fig. 14-3), whereas an $HV_{tachycardia} \geq HV_{NSR}$ suggests SVT with aberrancy (see Fig. 14-17), BBR VT (see Fig. 20-3), or, rarely, other VTs.[1] A changing AH interval and/or failure to observe anterograde His potential during VT with AV dissociation suggest that retrograde conduction is occurring and producing concealment in the AVN.

Right Ventricular Apical Local Activation Time

In the setting of apical MI, VT with an RBBB pattern and R/S ratio in V_1 more than 1 is common, but lateral versus septal surface ECG QRS morphologies significantly overlap, with variable early R wave progression and a similar frontal plane axis.[3] Assessing the activation time to a fixed reference endocardial recording at the RV apex can help regionalize a septal versus lateral origin for such VTs. For RBBB-type VT in the setting of an apical infarct, a QRS-RV apical activation time is consistently less than 100 milliseconds for an apical LV septal origin and more than 125 milliseconds for a lateral apical origin.[16] The same values for the QRS-RV apical activation time will also help identify a septal versus lateral wall origin in the setting of prior nonapical infarcts.

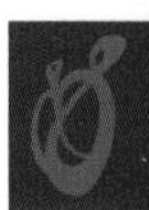

Diagnostic Maneuvers During Tachycardia

The response of VT to programmed stimulation can be studied only for SMVT. Nonsustained VT is too short and unpredictable in duration to allow reliable evaluation. Polymorphic VT is invariably associated with rapid hemodynamic collapse. Furthermore, SMVT must be well tolerated (tachycardia CL usually more than 280 milliseconds) and must have a stable CL to evaluate the response to stimulation. Fast, unstable SMVT usually can be slowed down by antiarrhythmic drugs (e.g., procainamide) to permit evaluation by programmed stimulation.

Ventricular Extrastimulation During Ventricular Tachycardia

Technique. Initially, a single VES is delivered at a coupling interval 10 to 20 milliseconds shorter than the tachycardia CL. The coupling interval is then gradually decreased by 5- to 10-millisecond decrements, until the local effective refractory period (ERP) is reached.[1] The RV apex is used as the initial site of stimulation. Stimulation from other sites (RVOT and LV) also can be used to gain information regarding site specificity of a given response. The return CL is analyzed to evaluate whether the VES has influenced the VT in terms of resetting, ability and pattern of termination, and site specificity for stimulation affecting the VT.

If resetting or termination of VT is not observed with single VESs, stimulation is repeated using double VESs.[1] The first VES is delivered at a coupling interval 20 milliseconds greater than the longest coupling interval at which a single VES resets the VT, or 20 milliseconds above the local ERP if a single VES fails to interact with the VT. The second VES is delivered at a coupling interval equal to the tachycardia CL, and then this coupling interval is progressively decreased in 5- to 10-millisecond decrements until the local ERP is reached. The use of double VESs allows comparable coupling intervals to reach the circuit at a greater relative degree of prematurity and ability to influence the VT than if the same coupling interval were used for a single VES. By this methodology, only a single VES interacts with the circuit; if the two VESs are delivered such that each VES interacts with the site of impulse formation, interpretation of the response would then be difficult. Thus, the first VES is delivered so that it would not interact with the circuit but would help the second VES to do so.

Ventricular Tachycardia Response to Ventricular Extrastimulation

Manifest Perpetuation. Manifest perpetuation is said to be present when the VES fails to influence the VT, resulting in a full compensatory pause surrounding the VES.[1] Factors influencing the ability of the VES to interact with the VT include tachycardia CL, local ventricular ERP at the stimulation site, and distance between the stimulation site and VT circuit. The tachycardia CL and duration of the excitable gap are the most important factors; the faster the VT (especially with CLs less than 300 milliseconds) and the shorter the duration of the reentrant circuit excitable gap, the more difficult it is for the VES to enter the VT circuit. Local ERP at the stimulation site and at the site of impulse formation also can limit the prematurity with which the VES can be introduced. Lastly, the farther the stimulation site from the VT circuit, the more difficult for the VES to reach the circuit with adequate prematurity.

Failure of a VES to affect the VT circuit helps demonstrate the extent of the ventricular myocardium that is not required for the VT. Thus, the ability to capture significant portions of the ventricle by the VES without affecting the VT suggests that those captured areas are not required for the VT circuit. Similarly, intermittent capture of the HPS during VT suggests that it also is not necessary to maintain the VT, regardless of where the His potential is located relative to the QRS during the VT. In an analogous fashion, sinus captures (occurring spontaneously or in response to atrial stimulation) may occur without influencing the VT. The demonstration that neither the proximal HPS nor the majority of the ventricles are required to sustain the VT suggests that the VT circuit must occupy a relatively small and electrocardiographically silent area of the heart.

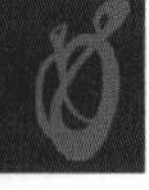

Concealed Perpetuation. Concealed perpetuation implies that the VES not only fails to influence the VT circuit, but also is followed by a pause that exceeds the tachycardia CL or that is occasionally interrupted by a sinus capture before the next VT beat. Such pauses are a form of functional exit block, because the VT impulse is unable to exit the circuit and depolarize the ventricles that have just been activated by the VES (Fig. 18-11).[1]

Resetting. Resetting is the advancement of VT by a timed VES with a pause that is less than fully compensatory before resumption of the VT (Fig. 18-12). The first return VT complexes should have the same morphology and CL as the VT before the VES, regardless of whether a single or multiple extrastimuli are used.[1]

The introduction of a single VES (S_2) during VT yields a return cycle (S_2-V_3) if the VT is not terminated. If S_2 does not affect the VT circuit, the coupling interval (V_1-S_2) plus the return cycle (S_2-V_3) will be equal to twice the VT cycle ($2 \times V_1V_1$)—that is, a fully compensatory pause will occur (see Fig. 1-12). Resetting of VT occurs when a less than fully compensatory pause occurs (by at least 20 milliseconds). In this situation, V_1-S_2 + S_2-V_3 will be less than $2 \times V_1V_1$, as measured from the surface ECG. Tachycardia CL oscillation should be taken into account when the return cycle is evaluated. To account for any tachycardia CL oscillation, at least a 20-millisecond shortening of the return cycle is required to demonstrate resetting.[1] When more than a single VES is used, the relative prematurity should be corrected by subtracting the coupling interval(s) from the spontaneous tachycardia cycles when the VESs are delivered.

To reset a reentrant VT, the stimulated wavefront must reach the reentrant circuit, encounter excitable tissue within the circuit (i.e., enter the excitable gap of the reentrant circuit), collide in the antidromic (retrograde) direction with the previous tachycardia beat, and continue in the orthodromic (anterograde) direction to exit at an earlier

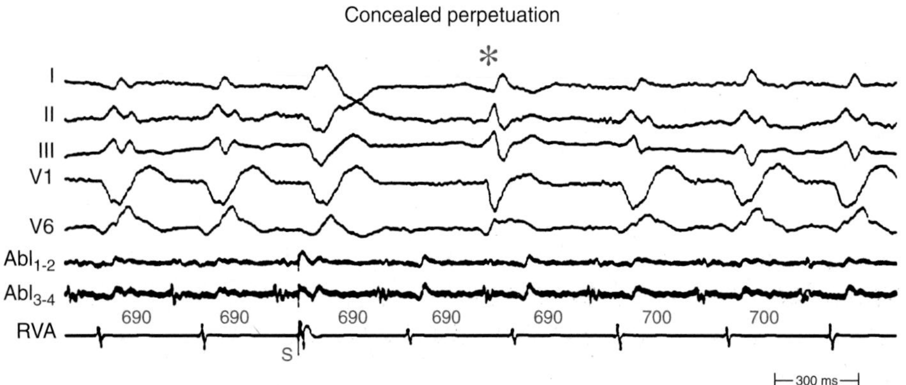

FIGURE 18–11 Concealed perpetuation in ventricular tachycardia (VT). Reentrant slow VT (cycle length = 690 msec); a single ventricular extrastimulus (VES) is introduced (S) that seems to terminate the VT; a conducted sinus complex (*) follows and then VT recurs. However, inspection of the distal ablation (Abl_{1-2}) electrogram shows that VT never actually terminated, because the mid-diastolic electrogram continues unperturbed by the VES.

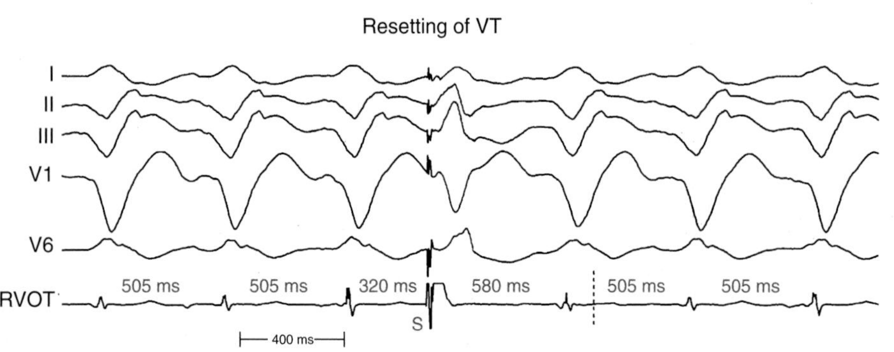

FIGURE 18–12 Resetting of ventricular tachycardia (VT). A single ventricular extrastimulus from the right ventricular outflow tract captures the ventricle during VT and causes the subsequent QRS to occur earlier than anticipated (dashed line), indicating resetting.

than expected time and perpetuate the tachycardia (see Fig. 1-13). If the VES encounters a fully excitable tissue, which commonly occurs in reentrant tachycardias with large excitable gaps, the tachycardia is advanced (made to occur earlier) by the extent that the stimulated wavefront arrives at the entrance site prematurely. If the tissue is partially excitable, which can occur in reentrant tachycardias with small or partially excitable gaps, or even in circuits with large excitable gaps when the VES is very premature, the stimulated wavefront will encounter some conduction delay in the orthodromic direction within the circuit. Consequently, the degree of advancement of the next tachycardia beat will depend on both the degree of prematurity of the VES and the degree of slowing of its conduction within the circuit. Therefore, the reset tachycardia beat can be early, on time, or later than expected.

EFFECT OF NUMBER OF VENTRICULAR EXTRASTIMULI. Approximately 60% of VTs can be reset with a single VES and 85% with double VESs using RV pacing. All VTs reset by a single VES can also be reset by double VESs.[1] Double VESs produce resetting over a longer range of coupling intervals and should therefore be used to characterize the excitable gap of the VT more fully. The resetting zone is approximately 70 milliseconds for most VTs, but is usually longer in those VTs reset by both single and double VESs than those requiring double VESs. Resetting zones in response to single VESs usually occupy 10% to 20% of the VT cycle. This is increased to approximately 25% in response to double VESs, but occasionally can exceed 30%, even in response to a single VES. VTs with LBBB morphology are less likely to require double VESs for resetting than VTs with RBBB morphology, regardless of the axis, because VTs with LBBB arise in or adjacent to the septum, closer to the RV stimulation site.

EFFECT OF SITE OF STIMULATION. Resetting does not require that the pacing site be located in the reentrant circuit. The closer the pacing site to the circuit, however, the less premature a single VES can be and reach the circuit without being extinguished by collision with the tachycardia wavefront emerging from the VT circuit. The longest coupling interval for a VES to be able to reset a reentrant tachycardia will depend on the tachycardia CL, the duration of the excitable gap of the tachycardia, local refractoriness at the pacing site, and conduction time from the stimulation site to the reentrant circuit.[1] Neither local ventricular ERP nor local activation time influences the number of VESs required for resetting. Approximately 10% to 20% of VTs demonstrate site specificity in response to VES. Using double VESs reduces this site specificity. Approximately 70% of VTs can be reset with a single VES delivered to the RV apex or RVOT. Resetting of VT by a single VES can always be achieved from some site in the LV, even when resetting cannot be achieved from RV sites.

RETURN CYCLE. The return cycle is the time interval from the resetting VES to the next excitation of the pacing site by the new orthodromic VT wavefront. This corresponds to the time required for the stimulated impulse to reach the circuit, conduct through the circuit, and exit. The noncompensatory pause following the VES and the return cycle are typically measured at the pacing site; however, they can also be measured to the onset of the surface ECG complex. When the return cycle is measured from the VES producing resetting to the onset of the first return tachycardia QRS on the surface ECG, conduction time into the tachycardia circuit is incorporated into that measurement. Conduction time between the pacing site and the VT circuit may or may not be equal to that from the VT circuit to the pacing site. Differences in the VT circuit entrance and exit can result in differences in conduction time to and from the pacing site. These differences depend on the site of stimulation and VT site of origin. In VTs reset by both single and double VESs, the shortest return cycle seen by both methods is usually the same.[1] If the return cycle is measured from the VES producing resetting to the onset of the QRS of the first return VT complex, the shortest return cycle will be less than the tachycardia CL in more than 40% to 45% of VTs. Because stimulation is usually performed from the RV, conduction time into the VT circuit is incorporated into that measurement. If one considers conduction time between the pacing site and the circuit to be equal to that from the circuit to the pacing site (i.e., local activation time) and subtracts this value from the return cycle as measured to the QRS, the resultant value for the return cycle is less than the tachycardia CL in 80% of VTs.

RESETTING RESPONSE CURVES. Flat or mixed (flat, and then increasing) response curves characterize reentrant VTs. A flat curve is noted in approximately two thirds of VTs, suggesting that a fully excitable gap is present. It also signifies anatomically separate entrance and exit sites of the circuit (see Fig. 1-14).[1] In approximately 40% of VTs, the types of resetting curves can vary, depending on the site of ventricular stimulation. VESs from different pacing sites likely engage different sites in the VT circuit that are in different states of excitability or refractoriness and, therefore, result in different conduction velocities and resetting patterns.

RESETTING WITH FUSION. The ability to reset a tachycardia after it has begun activating the myocardium (i.e., resetting with fusion) excludes automatic and triggered mechanisms and is diagnostic of reentry.[1] Resetting with ECG fusion requires wide separation (in time and/or distance) of entry and exit sites of the VT circuit, with the stimulus wavefront preferentially engaging the entrance. For resetting with fusion to occur, the premature paced wavefront has to reach the entrance of the reentrant circuit before it reaches the exit, and, at the same time, allow for the VT wavefront to exit the reentrant circuit, although the VT wavefront is unable to reach the entrance of the circuit before the paced wavefront (Fig. 18-13). Fusion of the stimulated impulse can be observed on the surface ECG and/or intracardiac recordings if the stimulated impulse is intermediate in morphology between a fully paced complex and the tachycardia complex. The ability to recognize surface ECG fusion requires a significant mass of myocardium to be depolarized by both the VES and VT. If presystolic activity in the reentrant circuit is present before delivery of the VES that resets the VT, this must be considered to represent local fusion. Thus, a VES delivered after the onset of the tachycardia QRS on the surface ECG and enters and resets the VT circuit will always demonstrate local fusion. Resetting with local fusion and a totally paced surface QRS complex suggests that the reentrant circuit is electrocardiographically small. The farther the stimulation site from the reentrant circuit, the less likely resetting with ECG fusion will occur; the VES should be delivered at a shorter coupling interval to enable the paced wavefront to reach the VT circuit with sufficient prematurity. Consequently, the stimulated impulse will reflect a purely paced QRS without ECG fusion.[1] Resetting with surface ECG fusion of the QRS during RV stimulation is observed in 60% of VTs, 40% of which are usually reset with a VES delivered after the onset of the VT QRS.[1] VTs reset with fusion have a higher incidence of flat resetting curves, longer resetting zones, and significantly shorter return cycle, measured from the stimulus to the onset of the VT QRS, than VTs not reset with fusion. The return cycle corrected to the tachycardia CL is shorter with VTs reset with fusion (0.89 versus 1.12). In 80% of VTs reset with fusion, the return cycle is shorter than the tachycardia CL measured at the onset of the QRS (versus only 4% of VTs reset without fusion). The return cycle minus local activa-

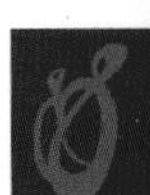

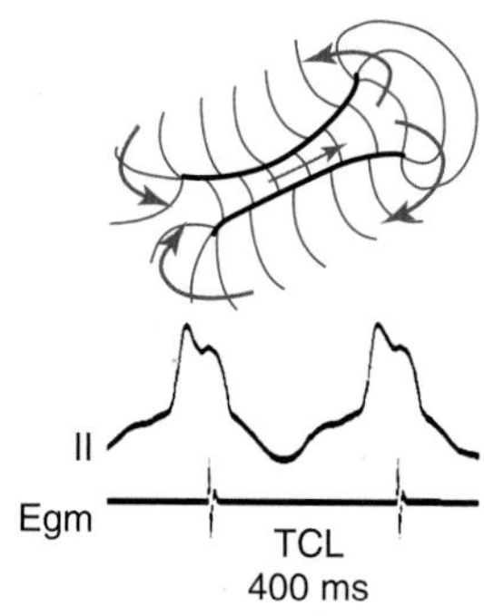

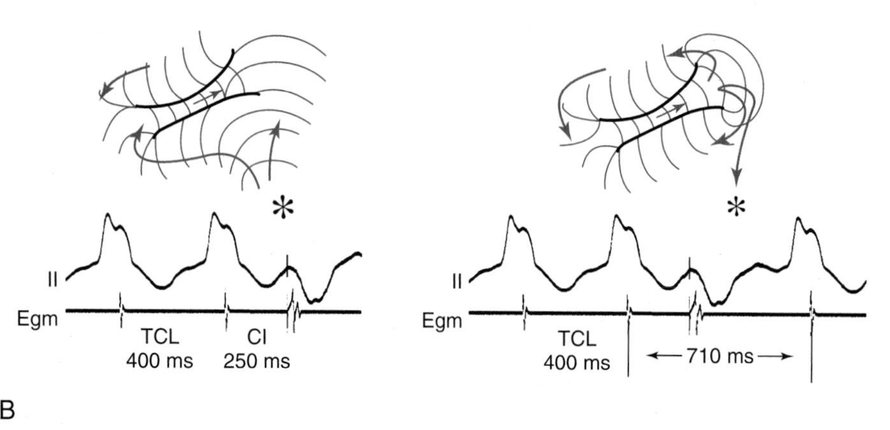

18

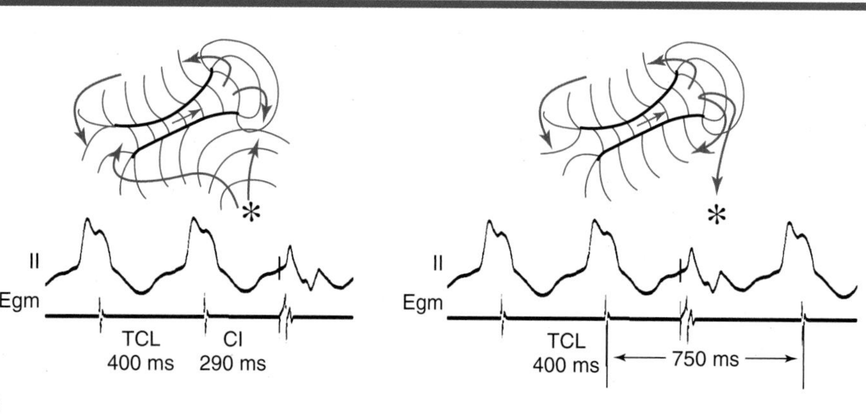

FIGURE 18–13 Schematic representation of the relationship of the return cycle during resetting of ventricular tachycardia (VT) to the absence or presence of surface ECG fusion. **A,** Stylized VT circuit, with direction of propagation as shown; electrogram is from a remote site. **B,** Single ventricular extrastimulus (VES) is introduced during VT at a coupling interval of 250 msec. **Left panel,** The VES occurs early enough that the circuit's exit site is captured; thus, there is no fusion. Meanwhile, the paced wavefront enters the entrance of the diastolic corridor before the approaching wavefront of the prior VT cycle (red arrow), allowing resetting. **Right panel,** Resetting is demonstrated in that the first VT cycle after the VES occurs at less than twice the tachycardia cycle length (TCL). **C,** A slightly later VES is introduced, with a paced wavefront approaching the diastolic pathway's exit after the VT wavefront has already left; this results in ECG fusion. Meanwhile, as before, the paced wave front arrives at the entrance site before the VT wavefront, allowing resetting. The right panel again shows resetting, this time with fusion. CI = coupling interval; Egm = intracardiac electrogram.

tion time is equal to the time for the wavefront to traverse the distance from the entrance to the exit of the circuit. This interval is less than the tachycardia CL in 100% of VTs reset with fusion. These findings are consistent with widely separate entrance and exit sites of the VT circuit.

Termination. Termination of VT by a VES occurs when the VES collides with the preceding tachycardia impulse antidromically and blocks in the reentrant circuit orthodromically (see Fig. 1-13). This occurs when the VES enters the reentrant circuit early enough in the relative refractory period, because it fails to propagate in the anterograde direction and encounters absolutely refractory tissue. In the retrograde direction, it meets increasingly recovered tissue and is able to propagate until it collides with the circulating wavefront and terminates the arrhythmia.[1]

Termination of VT by a single VES is uncommon, occurring in 10% to 46% of VTs. The closer the stimulation site to the circuit, the more prematurely a VES can engage the VT circuit, because the refractoriness and conduction delay in intervening myocardial tissue are avoided. The success of termination, however, is directly related to the number of VESs used.[1] Occasionally, when stimulation is performed at the critical isthmus of the VT circuit, termination can occur with a subthreshold VES that fails to depolarize the myocardium but is adequate to depolarize the isthmus and make it refractory to the incoming VT wavefront, resulting in termination of the VT (Fig. 18-14).

Ventricular Pacing During Ventricular Tachycardia

Technique. Rapid ventricular pacing is performed during VT at a pacing CL 10 to 20 milliseconds shorter than the tachycardia CL. The pacing CL is then decreased in 10-millisecond decrements in a stepwise fashion until the VT is terminated.[1] Pacing is stopped after each pacing CL and the response of VT to pacing is assessed. It is important to ensure that termination and reinitiation of the VT have not occurred during the pacing train, which would then affect the interpretation of the VT response.

It is critical to synchronize the initiation of pacing to the electrogram at the pacing site, because absence of synchronization will lead to a variable coupling interval of the first

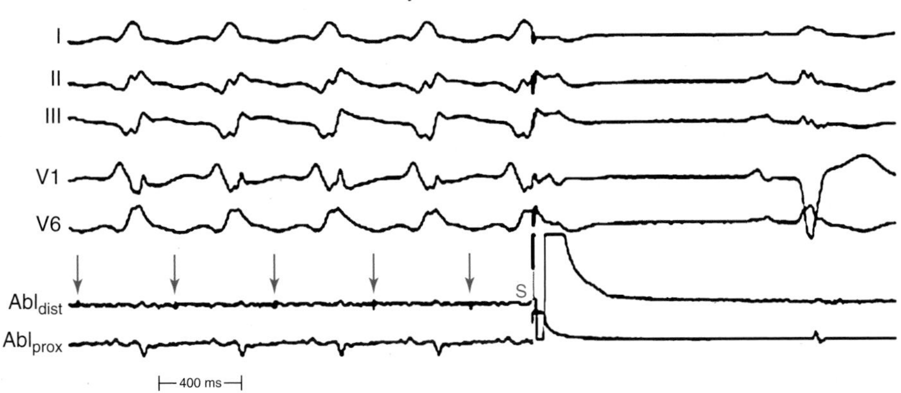

FIGURE 18–14 Ventricular tachycardia (VT) termination by a subthreshold ventricular extrastimulus (VES). VT is shown with the ablation electrode recording a small mid-diastolic potential (arrows). A single VES (S) is delivered during VT that does not appear to capture myocardium, yet terminates the tachycardia.

paced impulse to the VT. It is also important to perform overdrive ventricular pacing at each pacing CL for a long enough duration to allow the pacing drive to penetrate and affect the VT circuit. Pacing for a short period is a common mistake; it results in erroneous evaluation of the VT response. For VTs that are not stable enough to allow completion of an entire stimulation protocol, synchronized bursts of pacing at variable pacing CLs for a specified but variable number of beats, can usually be performed and can provide information about resetting or entrainment, overdrive suppression, and termination.

The response of VT to overdrive pacing is evaluated for overdrive suppression, acceleration, transformation into distinct uniform VT morphologies, entrainment, ability and pattern of termination, and site specificity for stimulation affecting the VT.

Ventricular Tachycardia Response to Ventricular Pacing

Overdrive Suppression. Overdrive suppression analogous to that seen with automatic rhythms has not been observed in post MI VTs, although prolonged return cycles can be seen at rapid pacing rates.

Acceleration. Acceleration by overdrive pacing refers to sustained shortening of the tachycardia CL following cessation of pacing. Acceleration occurs in 25% of VTs, and is more common with ventricular pacing than with VES (35% versus 5%). However, overdrive acceleration of VT analogous to that seen in triggered rhythms (i.e., linear relation of pacing CL to early acceleration of the tachycardia CL) is uncommon in post MI VT.[1] Since rapid ventricular pacing is usually required to terminate faster VTs, these VTs have a higher incidence of acceleration (40% of VTs with CL <300 ms with rapid ventricular pacing). Approximately 50% of the accelerated VTs can be terminated with even faster ventricular pacing; the other 50% (which can be polymorphic VT or ventricular flutter) require DC cardioversion.

Acceleration is classified according to the morphology of the accelerated VT: VT morphology identical to or different from the original VT, or polymorphic VT. An accelerated VT with a QRS morphology identical to the original VT suggests that the accelerated VT is using the same exit of the original VT circuit. The most likely mechanism underlying this form of VT acceleration is an area of block that determines the size of the reentrant circuit is determined to some extent by refractoriness. Rapid pacing can shorten the refractoriness in a proximal region of the arc of block, which would in turn shorten the length of the reentrant pathway. If the distal component of the arc of block remains unchanged, acceleration of the VT would occur with the same exit site and hence the same QRS morphology. Alternatively, rapid pacing can remove block in a shorter potential pathway, creating a smaller circuit.[1]

On the other hand, a VT morphology different from the original VT can be secondary to a change in the exit site from the same circuit, a reversal of the reentrant circuit, or the termination of the initial VT and reinitiation of a different VT elsewhere. Polymorphic VT with or without degeneration to VF can occur because of the inability of the myocardium to respond to the pacing CL with the development of changing activation wavefronts, leading to multiple reentrant wavelets that can degenerate into VF. There is no way to predict which type of acceleration will occur. However, in the presence of antiarrhythmic drugs, acceleration to different morphologically distinct VTs is common.

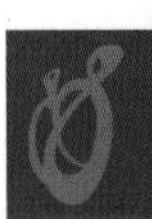

Transformation. Transformation of the index VT into multiple distinct uniform VT morphologies can occur in response to overdrive pacing. It is not infrequent for stimulation during one VT to induce another VT of different morphology and CL, only to be changed to a third or fourth one by continued stimulation.[1] The significance of all these multiple morphologically distinct VTs induced during overdrive pacing of the spontaneous VT is uncertain if they were never seen before spontaneously or induced by programmed stimulation. Usually, however, these VTs can also be induced by programmed electrical stimulation. Nevertheless, any VT (even if not seen before) that is uniform and has a CL more than 250 milliseconds is clinically important. Those VTs may not have been observed because the original VT dominates because it is more readily inducible. Induction of rapid unstable VTs (CL less than 250 milliseconds) in patients who presented with only stable VT does not have prognostic value.[1]

The ability to change from one VT to another with a different CL using single or double VESs is infrequent during triggered rhythms (other than those because of digitalis), and is another observation that is most compatible with a reentrant mechanism.

Entrainment. Overdrive ventricular pacing at long CLs (i.e., 10 to 30 milliseconds shorter than the tachycardia CL) can almost always entrain reentrant VTs. The slower the pacing rate and the farther the pacing site from the reentrant circuit, the longer the pacing drive required to penetrate and entrain the tachycardia.

Following the first beat of the pacing train that penetrates and resets the reentrant circuit, the subsequent stimuli will interact with the reset circuit, which has an abbreviated excitable gap. Depending on the degree that the excitable gap is preexcited by that first resetting stimulus, subsequent stimuli fall on fully or partially excitable tissue. Entrainment is said to be present when two consecutive extrastimuli conduct orthodromically through the circuit with the same conduction time while colliding antidromically with the preceding paced wavefront. During entrainment, the paced stimuli enter the reentrant circuit, block with the existing tachycardia wavefront in the antidromic direction, and conduct through the circuit in the orthodromic direction to produce the return cycle beat.

ENTRAINMENT CRITERIA. Classic criteria for recognition of entrainment are the following: (1) fixed fusion of the paced complexes at any single pacing CL; (2) progressive fusion as the pacing CL decreases (i.e., the surface ECG progressively looks more like the purely paced QRS complex than a pure tachycardia QRS complex); and (3) resumption of the same VT morphology following pacing with a nonfused tachycardia QRS complex at a return cycle equal to the pacing CL (see Figs. 3-15 and 3-16). The return cycle is measured from the surface QRS or RV electrograms. The return cycle is defined as the interval from the last paced beat to the first VT beat.

ENTRAINMENT WITH FUSION. As noted, fusion of the stimulated impulse can be observed on the surface ECG and/or intracardiac recordings. The stimulated impulse will have hybrid morphology between the fully paced QRS and the tachycardia QRS (see Figs. 3-15 and 3-16). The ability to demonstrate surface ECG fusion requires a significant mass of myocardium to be depolarized by both the extrastimulus and the tachycardia. The farther the stimulation site from the reentrant circuit, the less likely entrainment with ECG fusion will occur. Overdrive pacing of a tachycardia of any mechanism can result in a certain degree of fusion, especially when the pacing CL is only slightly

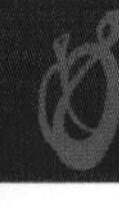

18

shorter than the tachycardia CL. Such fusion, however, is unstable during the same pacing drive at the same pacing CL, because pacing stimuli fall on a progressively earlier portion of the tachycardia cycle, producing progressively less fusion and more fully paced morphology. Such phenomena should be distinguished from entrainment, and sometimes this requires pacing for long intervals to demonstrate variable degrees of fusion. Focal tachycardias (automatic, triggered activity, or microreentrant) cannot manifest fixed or progressive fusion during overdrive pacing. Moreover, overdrive pacing frequently results in suppression (automatic) or acceleration (triggered activity) of focal VTs rather than resumption of the original tachycardia with an unchanged tachycardia CL.

ENTRAINMENT WITH MANIFEST FUSION. Entrainment of reentrant tachycardias commonly produces manifest fusion that is stable (fixed) during the pacing drive at a given pacing CL; repeated entrainment at pacing CLs progressively shorter than the tachycardia CL results in different degrees of QRS fusion, with the resultant QRS configuration looking more like fully paced configuration (see Figs. 3-15 and 3-16).[1]

ENTRAINMENT WITH INAPPARENT, LOCAL, OR INTRACARDIAC FUSION. Entrainment with inapparent fusion (also referred to as local or intracardiac fusion) is said to be present when a fully paced QRS morphology (with no ECG fusion) results, even when the tachycardia impulse exits the reentrant circuit (orthodromic activation of the presystolic electrogram is present). Fusion is limited to a small area and does not produce surface ECG fusion, and only intracardiac (local) fusion can be recognized (see Fig. 3-18). Local fusion can only occur when the presystolic electrogram is activated orthodromically. Collision with the last paced impulse must occur distal to the presystolic electrogram, either at the exit from the circuit or outside the circuit. In such cases, the return cycle measured at this local electrogram will equal the pacing CL.[1] Therefore, a stimulus delivered after the onset of the surface ECG QRS during entrainment will always demonstrate local fusion. This is to be distinguished from entrainment with antidromic capture. When pacing is performed at a CL significantly shorter than the tachycardia CL, the paced impulse can penetrate the circuit antidromically and retrogradely capture the presystolic electrogram so that no exit from the tachycardia circuit is possible. Consequently, the surface QRS appears fully paced. When pacing is stopped, the impulse that conducts antidromically also conducts orthodromically to reset the reentrant circuit with orthodromic activation of the presystolic electrogram. When antidromic (retrograde) capture of the local presystolic electrogram occurs, the return cycle, even when measured at the site of the presystolic electrogram, will exceed the pacing CL by the difference in time between when the electrogram is activated retrogradely (i.e., preexcited antidromically) and when it would have been activated orthodromically (see Fig. 3-15).

ENTRAINMENT WITH CONCEALED FUSION. Entrainment with concealed fusion (also called concealed entrainment) is defined as entrainment with orthodromic capture and a surface ECG complex identical to that of the tachycardia (Fig. 18-15). Entrainment with concealed fusion suggests that the pacing site is within a protected isthmus, either inside or outside but attached to the reentrant circuit (i.e., the pacing site can be in, attached to, or at the entrance to a protected isthmus that forms the diastolic pathway of the circuit). Entrainment with concealed fusion can occur by pacing from bystander pathways, such as a blind alley, alternate pathways, or inner loops, which are not critical for the maintenance of reentry. In this case, activation proceeds from the main circuit loop but is constrained by block lines having the shape of a cul-de-sac; ablation there does not terminate reentry.[1]

POST-PACING INTERVAL. The post-pacing interval (PPI) is the interval from the last pacing stimulus that entrained the tachycardia to the next recorded electrogram at the pacing site (see Fig. 18-15). The PPI should be measured to the near-field potential that indicates depolarization of tissue at the pacing site. The PPI remains relatively stable when entrainment of VT is performed at the same site, regardless of the length of the pacing drive. This is in contrast to overdrive suppression seen in automatic arrhythmias, which would be associated with progressive delay of the first tachycardia beat return cycle with progressively longer overdrive pacing drives.

Termination. The ability to terminate SMVT by rapid ventricular pacing and/or VES is influenced most importantly by the tachycardia CL (50% of VTs with CLs less than 300 milliseconds will require electrical cardioversion), but also by the local ERP at the pacing site, conduction time from the stimulation site to the site of origin of the VT, duration of the excitable gap, and presence of antiarrhythmic agents.

Failure of rapid ventricular pacing or VES to terminate VT has several potential explanations: the reentrant circuit is a protected focus; inability of VES to access the reentrant circuit because of local myocardial refractoriness; absence of an accessible excitable gap; termination of VT followed by reinitiation by a subsequent pacing impulse in the same pacing drive; and/or failure of conduction block to occur within the reentrant circuit, despite accelerating the VT to the faster pacing rate.

Factors influencing termination of VT can be modified. Refractoriness at the site of stimulation can be modified by the use of multiple VESs or a higher pacing current. The distance and/or conduction time from the site of stimulation to the VT site can be modified by changing the site of stimulation. The tachycardia CL can be increased by antiarrhythmic agents, but the response is unpredictable. However, two problems are frequently encountered in attempts to terminate VT—acceleration of the VT by overdrive pacing

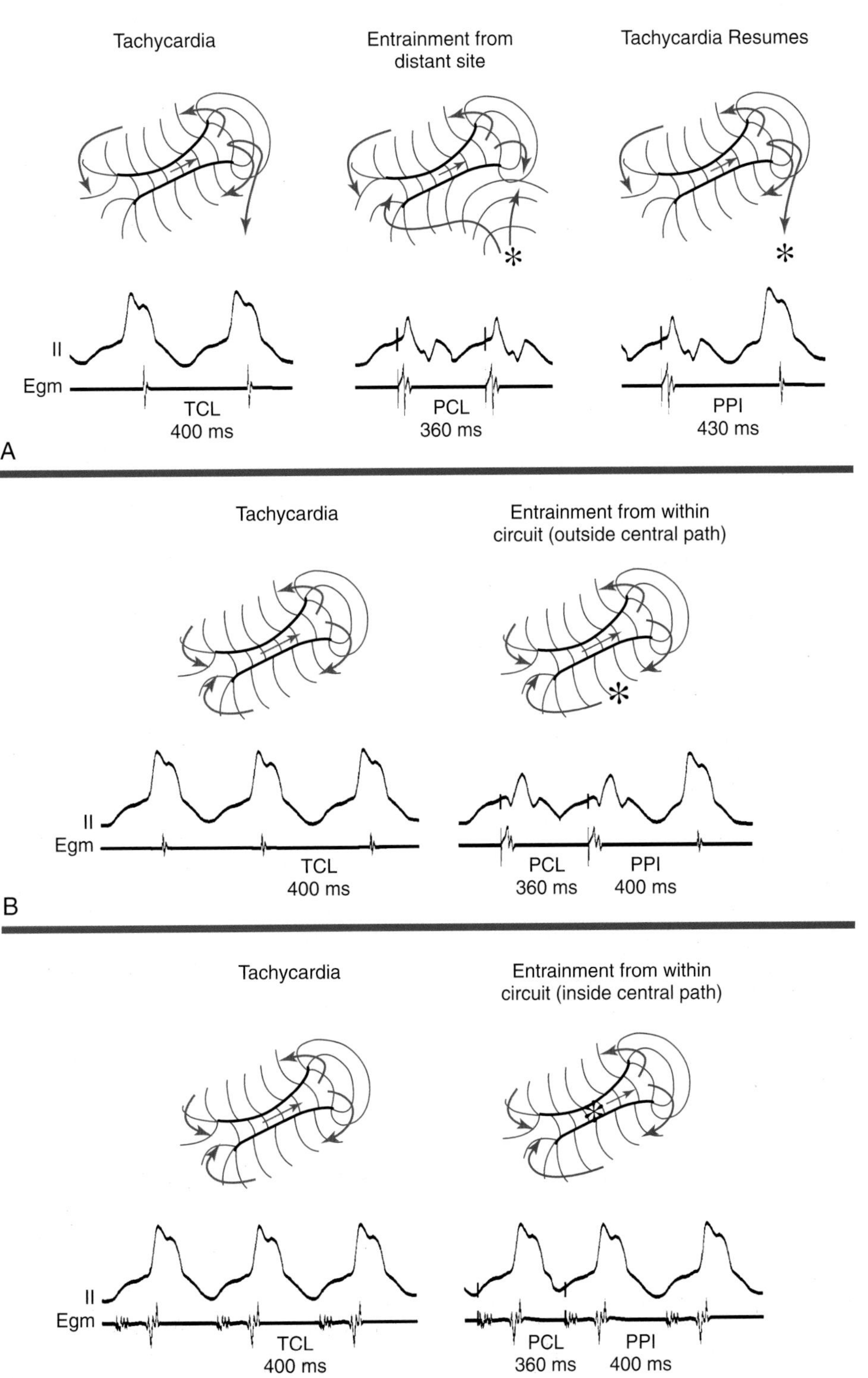

FIGURE 18–15 Entrainment mapping of ventricular tachycardia (VT). **A,** Entrainment of VT from distant site. Diagrammatic representation of a figure-of-8 VT circuit at left, with an electrogram recorded at a site remote from critical circuit elements. At center, during entrainment pacing, the paced wavefront from this remote site (*) interacts with the circuit by colliding with a VT wavefront that has exited the diastolic corridor while also entering the diastolic corridor at the opposite end. This results in fusion (part of the ventricle depolarized by VT wavefront, part by paced wavefront). For as long as pacing continues, this fusion of ventricular activation remains stable. With cessation of pacing (right figure), the last paced wavefront enters the diastolic corridor as on other cycles but there is no subsequent paced wavefront to collide with the wavefront that is exiting the corridor; thus the first return cycle complex is entrained, but not fused. The post- pacing interval (PPI) measured at the site of pacing reflects the time it takes to make one complete revolution around the circuit plus any time required to get from the pacing site to the circuit and back from the circuit to the pacing site. **B,** Entrainment of VT from a site within the circuit. The pacing site (*) is within the circuit but outside the diastolic corridor. As a result, the entrained QRS complex shows fusion and the PPI equals the VT cycle length (CL). **C,** Entrainment of VT from a site within the critical isthmus. The pacing site (*) is within the circuit and inside the diastolic corridor, recording the mid-diastolic electrogram. As a result, the entrained QRS complex shows no fusion and the PPI equals the VT CL. The S-QRS interval equals the electrogram-to-QRS interval during VT. This is the ideal ablation site. PCL = pacing cycle length; TCL = tachycardia cycle length.

and the appearance of multiple distinct uniform VT morphologies.[1]

Regardless of the mode of stimulation used, termination is usually abrupt, which distinguishes reentrant VTs from triggered VTs.[1] In reentrant VTs, termination must occur when an impulse penetrates the circuit and blocks in both directions. Rapid ventricular pacing is the most efficacious way of VT termination, regardless of the tachycardia CL. Approximately 80% of VTs terminated by a single VES had a tachycardia CL more than 400 milliseconds. All VTs terminated by single or double VESs could also be terminated by ventricular pacing. Termination is less likely to occur when the VT cannot be reset with very premature VES (i.e., the VES coupling interval is more than 75% of the tachycardia CL).[1]

A single VES delivered during entrainment of VT can facilitate termination of VT by allowing easier access to the excitable gap.[1] Even when a single VES or overdrive pacing alone fails to terminate the VT, the combination of both may be successful. Overdrive pacing ensures stable resetting of the VT circuit, allowing a single VES to interact with the circuit much more prematurely than it could in the absence of entrainment. Overdrive pacing also shortens the excitable gap of tissue in the reset circuit, making it possible for a single VES to terminate the VT. This technique avoids the need for multiple VESs, which can increase the heterogeneity of conduction and refractoriness in the intervening tissue and produce polymorphic VT, and the need for rapid pacing, which might induce acceleration of the VT. This method is especially helpful in VTs that were accelerated by rapid pacing and those resistant to standard pacing techniques in the presence of antiarrhythmic agents, especially in those VTs for which antiarrhythmic agents have made the VT more difficult to terminate.

Effects of Drugs on Ventricular Tachycardia

Class I agents are the most uniformly successful drugs for slowing the rate of or terminating SMVT.[1] These drugs can also facilitate the induction of SMVT in patients in whom SMVT cannot be induced by the standard programmed electrical stimulation protocol and in patients with coronary artery disease and nonsustained VT. These drugs can also occasionally produce incessant SMVT in patients who, before therapy, only had paroxysmal events. This phenomenon, almost always associated with a slower VT and prolongation of conduction by the agent, would not be expected if the mechanism were triggered activity. Adenosine, beta blockers, and calcium channel blockers are ineffective for termination of post-MI VT.

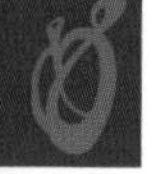

Exclusion of Other Arrhythmia Mechanisms

18

Exclusion of Triggered Activity Ventricular Tachycardia

Stimulation Site Specificity. The site of ventricular stimulation has no effect on the initiation of triggered activity VT as long as the impulse reaches the focus of the VT. Reentrant VT, on the other hand, can demonstrate absolute or relative site specificity for initiation.

Inducibility with Programmed Electrical Stimulation. Ventricular stimulation can initiate triggered activity VT in less than 65% of cases. Rapid ventricular pacing is usually more effective than VES, whereas it has a low yield in initiating reentrant VT. Multiple VESs during NSR or following a drive train of less than eight to ten beats usually fail to initiate triggered activity VT. Most episodes of triggered activity VT induced by ventricular stimulation are usually nonsustained. Induction of triggered activity VT with atrial pacing is not uncommon.

Reproducibility of Initiation. Reproducibility of triggered activity VT induction using all methods is less than 50%. Reproducibility of induction with single or double VESs is approximately 25%. Reproducibility is markedly affected by quiescence. Once a triggered rhythm is initiated, a period of quiescence is necessary to reinitiate the rhythm. Thus, the ability to initiate, terminate, and reinitiate sequence is uncommon, in contrast to reentrant VT.

Relationship of Pacing Cycle Length and Ventricular Extrastimulus Coupling Interval to Ventricular Tachycardia. Typically, both the initial cycle of the triggered activity VT (the return cycle) and the tachycardia CL following cessation of pacing bear a direct relationship to the pacing CL, and a direct relationship to the coupling interval of the VES, when used. Thus, the shorter the initiating ventricular pacing CL, or the shorter the initiating VES coupling interval, the shorter the interval to the first VT beat and the shorter the initial VT CL. Occasionally, with early VESs, a jump in the interval to the onset of the VT complex occurs, so that it is approximately twice the interval to the onset of the VT initiated by later coupled VESs. This is secondary to failure of the initial delayed afterdepolarization (DAD) to reach threshold while the second DAD reaches threshold. Thus, in triggered activity VTs caused by DADs, the coupling interval of the initial VT complex shortens or suddenly increases in response to progressively premature VES. It never demonstrates an inverse or gradually increasing relationship, in contrast to reentrant VT. Only with the addition of very early VESs or, occasionally, very rapid ventricular pacing (CL less than 300 milliseconds), a sudden jump in the interval to the first VT complex can be observed. Furthermore, ventricular pacing CLs longer or shorter than the critical CL window fail to induce triggered activity VT. This critical window may shift with changing autonomic tone.

Effects of Catecholamine. Inducibility of triggered activity VT is facilitated by catecholamines, whereas in reentrant VT, isoproterenol facilitates VT induction in only 5% of cases. However, induction of triggered activity VT can be inconsistent and is exquisitely sensitive to the immediate autonomic status of the patient. Therefore, noninducibility during a single EP study is not enough evidence to attribute the arrhythmia to a nontriggered activity mechanism.

Response to Antiarrhythmic Drugs. Triggered activity VTs respond favorably to calcium channel blockers and beta blockers. Conversely, those drugs fail to terminate more than 95% of VTs associated with coronary artery disease or cardiomyopathy.

Diastolic Electrical Activity. In reentrant VT, electrical activity occurs throughout the VT cycle. Thus, during diastole, conduction is extremely slow and in a small enough area that it is not recorded on the surface ECG. Demonstration that the VT initiation is dependent on a critical degree of slow conduction, manifested by fragmented electrograms spanning diastole, and that maintenance of the VT is associated with repetitive continuous activity, would be compatible with reentry.

Exclusion of Bundle Branch Reentrant Ventricular Tachycardia

His Bundle–Ventricular Interval. BBR should be suspected when the His potential precedes ventricular activation and the HV interval during VT is longer than that during NSR. In other VTs, the His potential is usually obscured within the local ventricular electrogram. Occasionally, the His potential can precede the onset of the QRS in post-MI VT; however, in contrast to BBR VT, the HV interval in those VTs is usually shorter than that during NSR.

Oscillation of Tachycardia Cycle Length. Spontaneous variation in the V-V intervals during BBR VT is dictated and preceded by similar changes in the H-H intervals. These changes can be demonstrated by ventricular stimulation during VT or can occur spontaneously following initiation. In other VTs, in contrast to BBR VT, the V-V interval variation usually dictates the subsequent H-H interval changes.

Activation Sequence. In the common type of BBR (LBBB pattern), the activation wavefront travels retrogradely up the LB to the HB and then anterogradely down the RB, with subsequent ventricular activation. This sequence is reversed in BBR with a RBBB pattern. Unfortunately, RB and/or LB potentials are not always recorded, so that the typical activation sequences (LB-HB-RB-V or RB-HB-LB-V) are not available for analysis. Even if either sequence is present, the HPS (usually the LB) could be activated passively in the retrograde fashion to produce an HB-RB-V sequence during a VT with an LBBB pattern without reentry requiring the LB. In these cases, other diagnostic criteria for BBR should be used.

Exclusion of Supraventricular Tachycardia

Supraventricular Tachycardia with Aberrancy. If VT exhibits 1:1 VA conduction, it can mimic SVT with aberrancy. Surface QRS morphology usually helps distinguish SVT with typical RBBB or LBBB from VT, as discussed in detail in Chapter 17. In VT, the atrium is not part of the tachycardia circuit and can be dissociated by atrial pacing. The HV interval in aberrantly conducted SVT is always equal to or longer than that during NSR, which is in contrast to intramyocardial VTs.

Preexcited Supraventricular Tachycardia. Differentiation between VT and preexcited SVT is particularly difficult on surface ECG, because ventricular activation begins outside the normal intraventricular conduction system in both tachycardias. As a result, many of the standard criteria cannot discriminate between preexcited SVT and VT. The HV interval is usually short or negative in both preexcited SVT and VT, and does not help in the differential diagnosis. However, in VT, the atrium is not part of the tachycardia circuit, and can be dissociated by atrial pacing.

MAPPING

The main goal of VT mapping is identification of the site of origin or critical isthmus of the VT. The site of origin of the tachycardia is the source of electrical activity producing the QRS. Although this is a discrete site of impulse formation in automatic and triggered rhythms, during reentrant VT it represents the exit site from the diastolic pathway (the critical isthmus) to the myocardium giving rise to the QRS. During VT, an isthmus is defined as a conductive myocardial tissue bounded by nonconductive tissue (conduction barriers). This nonconductive tissue can be a line of double potentials, a scar area, or an anatomical obstacle, such as the mitral annulus. The critical isthmus is an isthmus that the depolarization wavefront must cross to perpetuate the tachycardia. As a consequence, ablation of the critical isthmus should interrupt the tachycardia and prevent its reinducibility.

Mapping of post-MI VT has several prerequisites, including inducibility of VT at the time of EP testing, hemodynamic stability of the VT (which usually requires relatively slow VT rate), and stability of the VT reentry circuit (i.e., stable VT morphology and CL). If the tachycardia is not stable, mapping can still be performed by starting and stopping the VT after data acquisition at each site.[17] Additionally, poorly tolerated rapid VTs sometimes can be slowed by antiarrhythmic drugs to allow for mapping. Antiarrhythmic drugs do not alter the sequence of activation, despite slowing of the VT and widening of the QRS and, although the electrogram at the site of origin can widen, its relationship to the onset of the QRS remains unchanged.[1] Newer techniques such as basket catheter and noncontact mapping can also provide activation mapping data during nonsustained or unstable VT.

When multiple VTs are inducible, all mappable VTs should be completely mapped and targeted. However, some recommend targeting only the clinical VT, especially in very ill patients in whom the goal is decreasing the frequency of ICD shocks.

Mapping of VT circuits and identification of critical isthmuses are often challenging. The abnormal area of scarring, where the isthmus is located, is often large and contains false isthmuses (bystanders) that confuse mapping. Although in most cases a portion of the VT isthmus is located in the subendocardium, where it can be ablated, in rare cases the isthmuses or even the entire circuits are deep to the endocardium or even in the epicardium and cannot be identified or ablated from the endocardium. Additionally, multiple potential reentry circuits are frequently present, giving rise to multiple different monomorphic VTs in a single patient. Ablation in one area may abolish more than one VT or leave VT circuits in other locations intact.

Activation Mapping

Technical Considerations

Unipolar Recordings. The advantages of unfiltered unipolar recordings include providing a more precise measure of local activation (because the maximal negative dV/dt corresponds to the maximum sodium channel conductance), providing information about the direction of impulse propagation, allowing pacing and recording at the same location, and eliminating a possible anodal contribution to depolarization. On the other hand, unipolar recordings have a poor signal-to-noise ratio and distant activity can be difficult to separate from local activity. This is especially true when recording from areas of prior MI, where the QS potentials are ubiquitous and it is often impossible to select a rapid negative dV/dt when the entire QS potential is slowly inscribed (i.e., cavity potential). Another disadvantage is the inability to record an undisturbed electrogram during or immediately after pacing, in addition to sensing of far-field signals.

Bipolar Recordings. The advantages of bipolar recordings include providing an improved signal-to-noise ratio and observing high-frequency components more accurately. Although local activation is less precisely defined, the peak amplitude of a filtered (30 to 300 Hz or more) bipolar recording of a normal electrogram corresponds to the maximal negative dV/dt of the unipolar recording. However, bipolar recordings have several limitations. The electrogram amplitude can decrease when propagation is relatively perpendicular to the recording electrodes. One therefore cannot obtain directional information from an isolated bipolar electrogram. Moreover, bipolar recordings do not allow simultaneous pacing and recording from the same location. To simultaneously pace and record in bipolar fashion at endocardial sites as close together as possible, electrodes 1 and 3 of the mapping catheter are used for bipolar pacing and electrodes 2 and 4 are used for recording. Despite the limitations of bipolar recordings, they are preferred in scar-related VTs because noise is removed and high frequency components are more accurately seen.

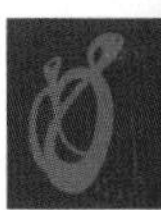

Typically, both bipolar and unipolar electrogram recordings are used during VT mapping.[1,7,18-20] The unipolar electrograms are open-filtered (0.05 to 300 Hz or more) when VT in a normal heart is studied and are filtered at comparable settings to those of bipolar electrograms (30 to 300 Hz or more) when scar-related VT is studied. The main goal of activation mapping of post-MI VT is to seek sites with continuous activity spanning diastole and/or isolated diastolic potentials.[21]

Endocardial activation time is the timing of the local electrogram measured relative to the earliest onset of the QRS complex in the 12-lead ECG. Using unipolar recordings, the earliest site should have a QS potential in the tip unipolar recording with a rapid negative intrinsic deflection earlier than that recorded from the proximal pole. However, unfiltered unipolar recordings are not helpful in scar-related VT to demonstrate that a presystolic site is earliest; the electrical signals in mid-diastolic electrograms are too small because they are generated by only a few fibers. Filtering gives reasonably clean signals; however, the signal is often of very low amplitude. Using bipolar recordings is preferred. Activation mapping is best taken from the onset of the high-frequency bipolar electrogram as it leaves the baseline. Using the peak deflection or the point of the most rapid deflection as it crosses the baseline is of less value in multicomponent fractionated electrograms. For the sake of simplicity, all signals whose maximal amplitude is less than 30 μV are considered as no local activity. The distal pole of the mapping catheter should be used for mapping of the earliest activation site, because it is the pole through which RF energy is delivered.

Contact is critical when standard quadripolar catheters are used. The degree of contact can be assessed by pacing threshold or impedance measurements at the recording electrode pair. Recording from multiple bipolar pairs from a multipolar electrode catheter in the LV is helpful in that if the proximal pair has a more attractive electrogram than the distal pair, the catheter can be withdrawn slightly to achieve the same position with the distal electrode. Using standard equipment, mapping a single SMVT requires recording and mapping performed at a number of sites, based on the ability of the investigator to recognize the mapping sites of interest from the morphology of the VT on the surface ECG.

Continuous Activity

Theoretically, if reentry were the mechanism of VT, electrical activity should occur throughout the VT cycle. Thus, during diastole, conduction should be extremely slow and in a small enough area such that it is not recorded on surface ECG. The QRS complex is caused by propagation of the wavefront from the exit of that isthmus to the surrounding myocardium.[1] Demonstration that VT initiation is dependent on a critical degree of slow conduction, manifested by fragmented electrograms spanning diastole, and that maintenance of the VT is associated with repetitive continuous activity, would be compatible with reentry.

Continuous activity, when observed, invariably occurs at sites that demonstrate markedly abnormal electrograms during NSR (Fig. 18-16).[1] However, continuous diastolic activity can be recorded in only 5% to 10% of post-MI VTs with detailed mapping using standard equipment. The ability to record continuous activity depends on the spatial and geometric arrangement of the involved tissue, the position of the catheter, and the interelectrode distance. Thus, continuous diastolic activity is likely to be recorded only if a bipolar pair records a small circuit. If a large circuit is recorded (i.e., VT circuit is larger than the recording area of the catheter and/or that the catheter is not covering the entire circuit), a nonholodiastolic activity will be recorded. In such VTs, when a nonholodiastolic activity is recorded at the site of origin, repositioning of the catheter to these other sites can allow visualization of the bridging of diastole (electrical activity in these adjacent sites spans diastole) (Fig. 18-17). Failure to record continuous activity is then not surprising, because catheter and intraoperative VT mapping suggest that most post-MI VTs incorporate a diastolic pathway 1 to 3 cm long and a few millimeters to 1 cm wide, with a circuit area probably larger than 4 cm^2.

All areas from which diastolic activity is recorded are not necessarily part of the reentrant circuit. Such sites may reflect late activation and may not be related to the VT site of origin. Analysis of the response of these electrograms to spontaneous or induced changes in tachycardia CL is critical in deciding their relationship to the VT circuit. Electrical signals that come and go throughout diastole should not be considered continuous. For continuous activity to be consistent with reentry, the following must be demonstrated: (1) VT initiation is dependent on continuous activity (i.e., broadening of electrograms that span diastole); (2) VT maintenance is dependent on continuous activity, so that termination of continuous activity, either spontaneously or following stimulation, without affecting the VT would exclude such continuous activity as requisite for sustaining the VT; (3) the recorded continuous diastolic activity is not just a broad electrogram whose duration equals the VT CL, which can be verified by analyzing the local electrogram during pacing at a CL comparable to VT CL—if pacing produces a continuous diastolic activity in the absence of VT, the continuous electrogram has no mechanistic significance; (4) motion artifact should be excluded (this is easiest because such electrograms are recorded only in infarcted ventricles and never from moving, contractile normal ventricles); (5) the continuous activity should be recorded from a circumscribed area; and (6) if possible, ablation of the area from which continuous activity is recorded will terminate the VT.

Mid-Diastolic Activity

An isolated mid-diastolic potential is defined as a low-amplitude, high-frequency diastolic potential separated from the preceding and subsequent ventricular electrograms by an isoelectric segment (Fig. 18-18).[22] It is likely that isolated mid-diastolic potentials that cannot be dissociated from the VT are generated in segments of the zone of slow conduction or common pathway (isthmus), which are integral components of the reentry circuit. The earliest presystolic electrogram closest to mid-diastole is the most commonly used definition for the site of origin of a VT circuit; however, continuous diastolic activity and/or bridging of diastole at adjacent sites or mapping a discrete diastolic pathway would be most consistent with a reentrant circuit (see Fig. 18-16).

In post-MI reentrant VT, the earliest presystolic electrogram is invariably abnormal and frequently fractionated and/or split, regardless of the QRS morphology of the VT or

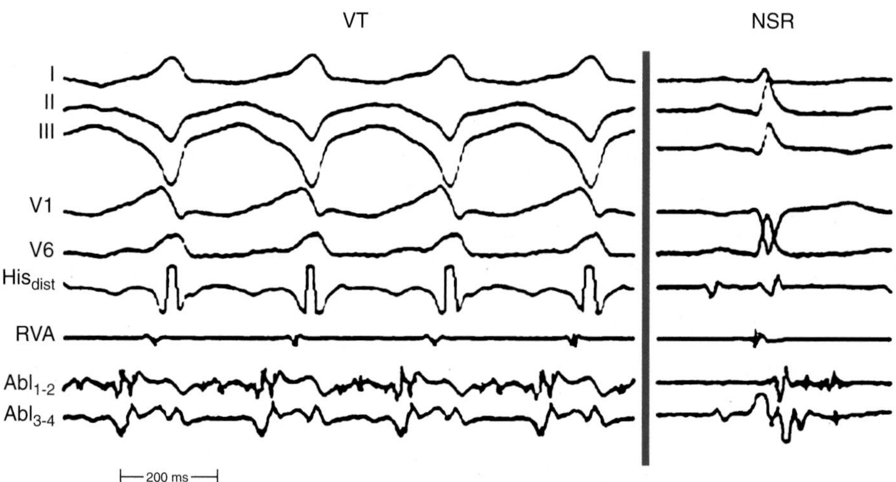

FIGURE 18–16 Continuous diastolic electrical activity during reentrant ventricular tachycardia (VT). VT is shown with almost continuous electrical activity in the distal ablation recording. During sinus rhythm (right), the electrogram is very fragmented and outlasts the surface QRS complex. NSR = normal sinus rhythm.

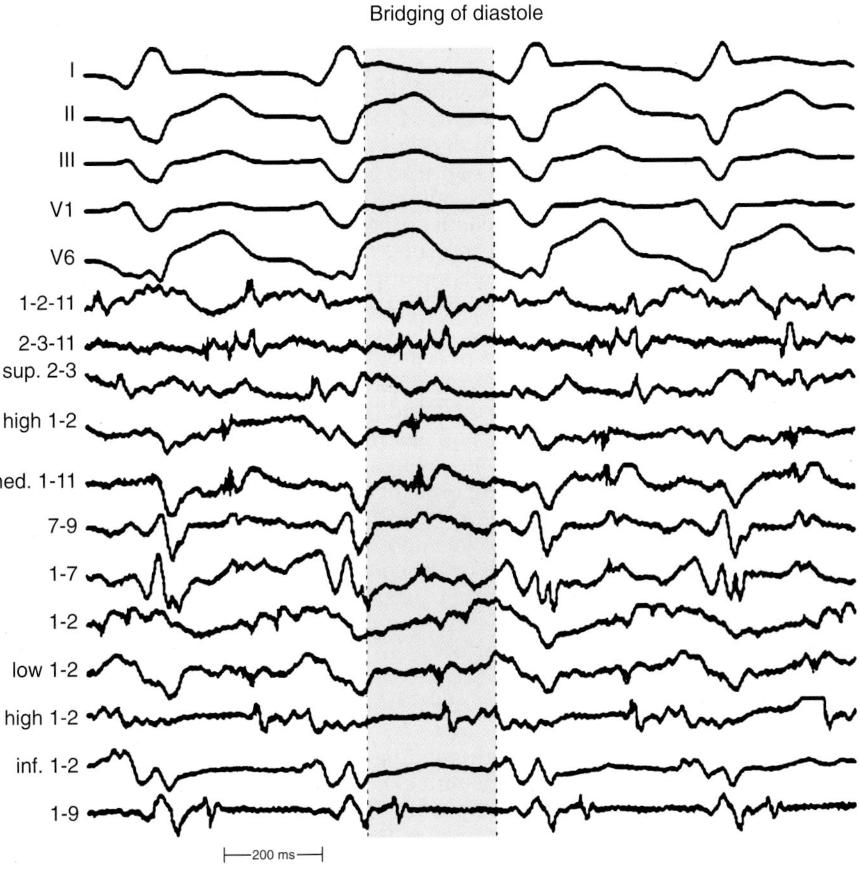

FIGURE 18–17 Bridging of diastole during reentrant ventricular tachycardia (VT). Shown is the compilation of numerous mapping sites around the left ventricular apical region during VT; diastole is shaded, showing progression of activation from early to mid to late diastole.

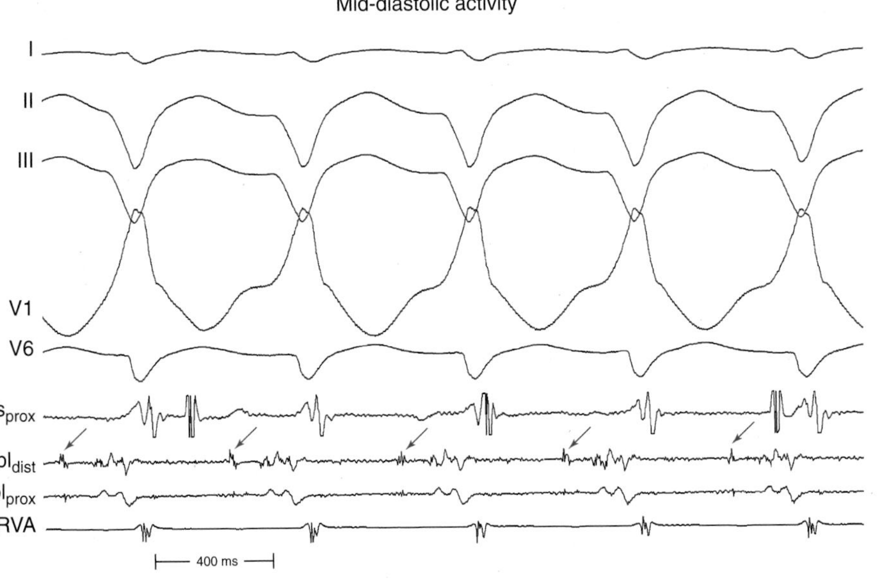

FIGURE 18–18 Mid-diastolic electrical activity during reentrant ventricular tachycardia (VT). VT is shown with a small mid-diastolic potential on the ablation recording.

the location of the site of origin. Thus, a normal presystolic bipolar electrogram (amplitude more than 3 mV, duration less than 70 milliseconds) should prompt further search for earlier activity. The early activity often appears focal, with spread from the early site to the remainder of the heart. The earliest electrogram in post-MI VT not infrequently has a diastolic and systolic component separated by an isoelectric component (see Fig. 18-18). Detailed mapping will usually reveal more than one site of presystolic activity. It is therefore essential to demonstrate that the presystolic site recorded is in fact the earliest site. This can be done by demonstrating that sites surrounding the assumed earliest site are activated later than that site, even though they may be presystolic in timing. If, after very detailed mapping, the earliest recorded site is not at least 50 milliseconds presystolic, this suggests that either the map is inadequate (most common) or that the VT arises deeper than the subendocardium, in the midmyocardium, or even incorporating the subepicardium.

It is important to recognize that mid-diastolic sites also can be part of a larger area of abnormal slow conduction unrelated to the VT circuit (i.e., a dead-end pathway), and can be recorded from a bystander site attached to the isthmus. Therefore, regardless of where in diastole the presystolic electrogram occurs (early, mid, or late), its appearance on initiation of VT and diastolic timing, although necessary, does not confirm its relevance to the VT mechanism. One must always confirm that the electrogram cannot be dissociated from the VT and is required for VT maintenance (see Fig. 3-12). Thus, during spontaneous changes in the tachycardia CL or those produced by programmed electrical stimulation, the electrogram, regardless of its position in diastole, should show a fixed relationship to the subsequent QRS and not the preceding QRS. Very early diastolic potentials, in the first half of diastole, can represent an area of slow conduction at the entrance of a protected isthmus. Such potentials will remain fixed to the prior QRS (exit site from the isthmus), and delay between it and the subsequent QRS would reflect delay entering or propagating through the protected diastolic pathway. This phenomenon is an uncommon response of presystolic electrograms occurring in the second half of diastole to pacing at rates slightly faster than the VT rate in post-MI VTs, but has been described in idiopathic and verapamil-sensitive VTs. Theoretically, such electrical activity may also arise from tissue between the site of impulse formation (the reentrant circuit) and the muscle mass that gives rise to the surface ECG. This response is also uncommon.

Limitations of Activation Mapping

Standard transcatheter endocardial mapping as performed in the EP laboratory is limited by the number, size, and type of electrodes that can be placed within the heart. Because these methods do not cover a vast area of the endocardial surface, time-consuming spot by spot maneuvering of the catheter is required to trace the origin of an arrhythmic event and its activation sequence in the neighboring areas.

The success of roving point mapping is predicated on the sequential beat by beat stability of the activation sequence being mapped and the ability of the patient to tolerate the sustained arrhythmia. Therefore, it can be difficult to perform activation mapping in the case of poorly inducible VT at the time of EP testing, hemodynamically unstable VT, and unstable VT morphology. Extensive mapping is not possible when the VT repeatedly changes, causing multiple different morphologies. However, as noted, mapping can still be facilitated by starting and stopping the tachycardia after data acquisition at each site, slowing the VT rate by antiarrhythmic agents, or the use of noncontact mapping.

Although activation mapping is adequate for defining the site of origin of focal tachycardias, it is deficient by itself in defining the critical isthmus of macroreentrant tachycardias. Adjunctive mapping modalities (e.g., entrainment mapping, pace mapping) are required in these cases.

Finally, using conventional activation mapping techniques, it is difficult to conceive the 3-D orientation of cardiac structures because these use a limited number of recording electrodes guided by fluoroscopy. Although catheters using multiple electrodes to acquire data points are available, the exact location of an acquired unit of EP data is difficult to ascertain because of inaccurate delineation of the location of anatomical structures. The inability to associate the intracardiac electrogram accurately with a specific endocardial site also limits the reliability with which the roving catheter tip can be placed at a site that was previously mapped. This results in limitations when the creation of long linear lesions is required to modify the substrate, and when multiple isthmuses, or channels, are present. This inability to identify, for example, the site of a previous ablation increases the risk of repeated ablation of areas already dealt with and the likelihood that new sites can be missed.

Entrainment Mapping

Focal ablation of all sites defined as in the reentrant circuit may not result in a cure of VT. Cure requires ablation of an isthmus bordered by barriers on either side, which is critical to the reentrant circuit. Because the circuit incorporates sites outside this critical isthmus, ablation of these external sites will not result in cure, although it may slightly alter the tachycardia CL or morphology. Stimulation at sites recording diastolic activity can provide evidence of its relationship to the VT circuit. Entrainment mapping is used to verify whether a diastolic electrogram (regardless of where in diastole it occurs, its position, and appearance on initiation of VT) is part of the VT circuit (see Fig. 18-15).[18,23,24] Entrainment mapping can be reliably carried out only if one can record and stimulate from the same area (e.g., for 2-5-2 mm spacing catheters, record from the second and fourth poles and stimulate from the first and third poles).

Pacing is usually started at a CL just shorter than the tachycardia CL. Pacing should be continued for a long enough duration to allow for entrainment; short pacing trains are usually not helpful. Pacing is then repeated at progressively shorter pacing CLs. After cessation of each pacing drive, the presence of entrainment should be verified by the presence of fixed fusion of the paced complexes at a given pacing CL, progressive fusion at faster pacing CLs, and resumption of the same tachycardia morphology following cessation of pacing with a nonfused complex at a return cycle that is equal to the pacing CL (see Figs. 3-15 and 3-16). The mere acceleration of the tachycardia to the pacing rate and then resumption of the original tachycardia after cessation of pacing does not establish the presence of entrainment, and evaluation of the PPI or other criteria are meaningless when the presence of true entrainment has not been verified. Moreover, it is important to verify the absence of termination and reinitiation of the tachycardia during the same pacing train. Once the presence of entrainment has been verified, several criteria can be used to indicate the relation of the pacing site to the reentrant circuit, as listed in Table 18-1 (also see Fig. 3-14).[18,23,24]

There are several limitations to the entrainment mapping technique. Entrainment requires the presence of sustained, hemodynamically well-tolerated tachycardia of stable morphology and CL. Furthermore, overdrive pacing can result in termination, acceleration, or transformation of the index tachycardia into a different one, making further mapping

TABLE 18–1 Entrainment Mapping Reentrant Ventricular Tachycardia (VT)

Pacing from Sites Outside VT Circuit
Manifest fusion on surface ECG and/or intracardiac recordings
PPI – tachycardia CL > 30 msec
S-QRS interval > local electrogram to QRS interval.
Pacing from Sites Inside VT Circuit but Outside Protected Isthmus
Manifest fusion on surface ECG and/or intracardiac recordings
PPI – tachycardia CL < 30 msec
S-QRS interval = local electrogram-to-QRS interval.
Pacing from Protected Isthmus Outside VT circuit
Concealed fusion
PPI – tachycardia CL > 30 msec
S-QRS interval > local electrogram to QRS interval
Pacing from Protected Isthmus Inside VT Circuit
Concealed fusion
PPI – tachycardia CL < 30 msec
S-QRS interval = local electrogram to QRS interval (±20 msec)

CL = cycle length; PPI = post-pacing interval.

challenging. Additionally, pacing and recording from the same area is required for entrainment mapping. This is usually satisfied by pacing from electrodes 1 and 3 and recording from electrodes 2 and 4 of the mapping catheter. However, this technique has its own limitations. Differences exist, albeit slight, of the area from which electrodes 2 and 4 record as compared with electrodes 1 and 3, as well as differences in the relationship of the site of stimulation from poles 1 and 3 to the recorded electrogram from poles 2 and 4 (i.e., proximal or distal to the recording site). Furthermore, the total area affected by the pacing stimulus can exceed the local area, especially when high currents (more than 10 mA) are required for stimulation, in addition to the fact that the pacing artifact can obscure the early part of the captured local electrogram. In such a case, a comparable component of the electrogram can be used to measure the PPI. The RV electrogram can also be used because it should have the same relationship to the paced site as it does from the electrogram during VT if the paced site is in the circuit. In both cases, these measurements provide indirect evidence of events in the circuit (i.e., the PPI will approximate the tachycardia CL if the stimulation site is in the circuit).

There are other criteria that suggest that the stimulation site is likely within the critical isthmus (see Fig. 3-14). A long stimulus-to-QRS (S-QRS) interval (the interval from the pacing stimulus to the onset of the earliest QRS on the 12-lead ECG) and an S-QRS interval–to–VT CL ratio of 0.7 or lower were found to predict successful ablation sites. In addition, alteration of the tachycardia CL or termination of VT by subthreshold or nonpropagated stimuli, repeated VT termination occurring with catheter manipulation or pacing at the site, and termination of VT by radiofrequency (RF) application without induction of premature ventricular complexes (PVCs) all are helpful predictors of the critical isthmus site. When RF application fails to terminate the VT at a site that appears to be in the circuit, the site may be a bystander. This technique is called RF current for thermal mapping. Similarly, termination by transient application of cryothermia would suggest an isthmus location.

Entrainment with Concealed Fusion

Entrainment with concealed fusion is defined by entrainment associated with an identical QRS to the VT QRS, and it suggests that the site is within, attached to, or at the entrance to a protected isthmus that forms the diastolic pathway of the circuit (Fig. 18-19; see Fig. 18-15). However, the positive predictive value of entrainment with concealed fusion in identifying effective ablation sites is only 50% to 60%, indicating that entrainment with concealed fusion can often occur at sites that are not critical to the maintenance of reentry (bystander pathway), such as a blind alley, alternate pathway, or inner loop. Even when such sites are believed to reside within the reentrant circuit isthmus, ablation can fail if lesions are too small to interrupt the circuit completely.

Other mapping criteria can be helpful in increasing the probability of identifying an effective site for ablation of VT in combination with entrainment with concealed fusion (Table 18-2). An isolated mid-diastolic potential that cannot be dissociated from VT increases the positive predictive value for identifying an effective ablation site to approximately 90%. Furthermore, if the electrogram-QRS interval is equal to the S-QRS interval at a site at which there is entrainment with concealed fusion, the positive predictive value increases to approximately 80%. Similarly, if the S-QRS interval–to–tachycardia CL ratio is lower than 0.7, the positive predictive value for successful ablation is approximately 70%.[18,23,24]

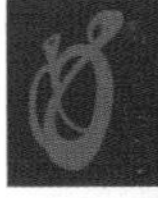

Post-Pacing Interval

Assessment of the PPI helps differentiate early presystolic electrical activity from late diastolic activity that can be unrelated to the tachycardia circuit (see Figs. 18-15 and 18-19). During entrainment from sites within the reentrant circuit, the orthodromic wavefront from the last stimulus propagates through the reentry circuit and returns to the pacing site following the same path as the circulating reentry wavefront. The conduction time required is the

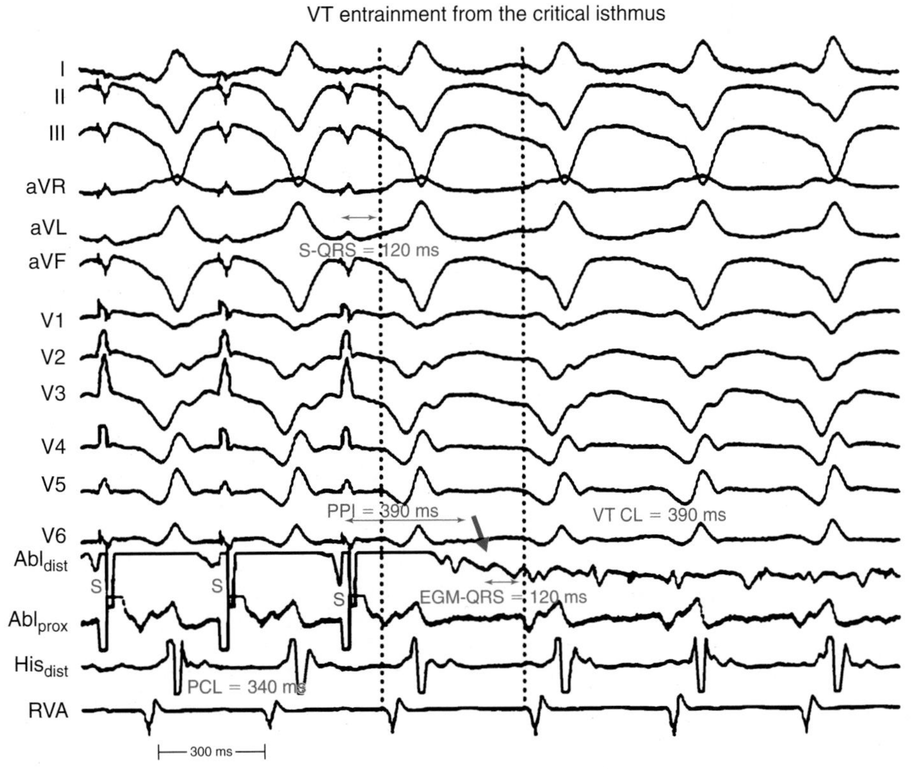

FIGURE 18–19 Entrainment during post–myocardial infarction ventricular tachycardia (VT) from the critical isthmus. The mid-diastolic potential (arrow) is present at the pacing site. Dashed lines denote QRS onset. Each stimulated complex is identical to that of VT at right (entrainment with concealed fusion). This, and findings that the S-QRS interval with pacing = electrogram–QRS interval in VT and post-pacing interval (PPI) = VT cycle length (CL) indicate that pacing is from with then protected diastolic corridor. Radiofrequency delivery at this site terminated VT in 4 seconds. PCL = pacing cycle length.

revolution time through the circuit. Thus, the PPI, measured from the pacing lead recording, should be equal (within 20 to 30 milliseconds) to the tachycardia CL. At sites distant from the circuit, stimulated wavefronts propagate to the circuit, then through the circuit, and finally back to the pacing site. Thus, the PPI should be equal to the tachycardia CL, plus the time required for the stimulus to propagate from the pacing site to the tachycardia circuit and back (see Fig. 3-14). The greater the difference between the PPI and the tachycardia CL, the longer the conduction time between the pacing site and the reentry circuit.[18]

The PPI should be measured to the near-field potential that indicates depolarization of tissue at the pacing site (see Figs. 18-15 and 18-19). In regions of scar, electrode catheters often record multiple potentials separated in time, some of which are far-field potentials that are caused by depolarization of adjacent myocardium. Far-field potentials are common during catheter mapping of infarct-related VT and can confound interpretation of the PPI. Assignment of an incorrect time of activation will render activation sequence maps misleading. The presence of far-field potentials also reduces the accuracy of entrainment mapping using the PPI. Measurement of the PPI to a far-field potential introduces an error, the magnitude of which is related to the conduction time between the pacing site and the source of the far-field potential (Fig. 18-20). When the PPI appears to be shorter than the tachycardia CL, the potential used for measurement is likely a far-field potential.[18] Analysis of the potentials recorded during entrainment often allows identification of the far-field potential so that it can be excluded from activation maps and the PPI measurement. These methods should improve the accuracy of mapping scar-related arrhythmias. The stimulus artifact obscures the potential produced in the tissue immediately at the stimulation site (i.e., near-field potentials). Thus, the local potential is not visible during pacing, but reappears after the last entrained QRS complex. On the other hand, far-field potentials usually fall sufficiently late after the pacing stimulus to be visible, and remain undisturbed during entrainment (see Fig. 18-20). These far-field potentials are accelerated to the pacing rate, but are not changed in morphology compared with those observed during tachycardia. The far-field potentials often precede the next stimulus by a short interval so that the tissue generating the far-field potential is probably refractory at the time of the next stimulus. Hence, the stimulus is not directly depolarizing the tissue generating the far-field potential. That these potentials are distant from the distal recording electrode is further supported by the lack of effect of RF ablation on the far-field potential.[18]

The validity of the difference between the PPI and VT CL [PPI – VT CL] is based on the assumption that the recorded electrogram represents depolarization at the pacing site. Ideally, electrograms are recorded from the mapping catheter electrodes used for stimulation, but this is sometimes difficult. Electrical noise introduced during pacing can obscure the electrograms at the stimulating electrodes, and many recording systems do not allow recording from the pacing site.[18] When the electrograms from the pacing site are not discernible because of stimulus artifact, relating the timing of the near-field potential to a consistent intracardiac electrogram or surface ECG wave can be used to determine the PPI. A reasonable alternative is calculating the PPI from electrograms recorded by electrodes adjacent to those used

TABLE 18–2 Sensitivity, Specificity, and Predictive Values of Analyzed Mapping Criteria in Association with Concealed Entrainment for Effective Ablation Sites

Mapping Criterion	Sensitivity (%)	Specificity (%)	Positive Predictive Value (%)	Negative Predictive Value (%)
Concealed entrainment	—	—	54	—
IMDP				
Overall	40	76	67	53
Not dissociable from VT	32	95	89	54
PPI = VT CL	58	19	45	29
S-QRS/VT CL < 0.7	96	52	71	92
S-QRS = EGM QRS				
Excluding IMDP	32	86	73	51
Including IMDP	56	86	82	62

From Bogun F, Bahu M, Knight BP, et al: Comparison of effective and ineffective target sites that demonstrate concealed entrainment in patients with coronary artery disease undergoing radiofrequency ablation of ventricular tachycardia. Circulation 1997;95:183.

CL = cycle length; EGM = electrogram; IMDP = isolated mid-diastolic potential; PPI = post-pacing interval; VT = ventricular tachycardia.

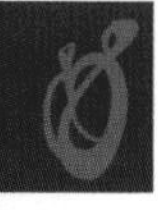

18

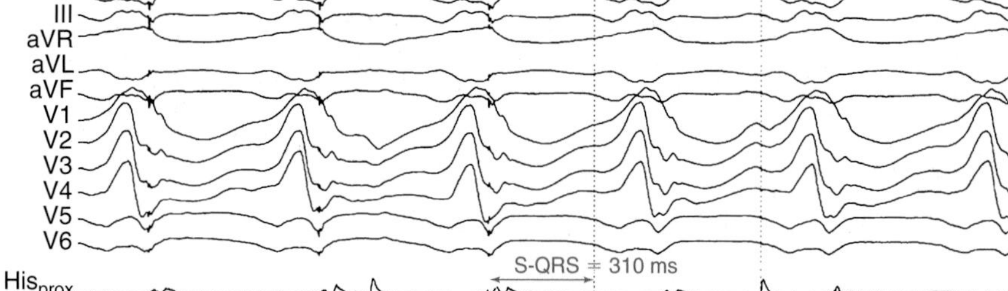

FIGURE 18–20 Entrainment during post-myocardial infarction ventricular tachycardia (VT) at site with both systolic and late diastolic (arrows) potentials. Stimulation (S) entrains VT with an identical QRS configuration (concealed fusion) and a very long S-QRS interval, suggesting pacing at the entrance of the protected isthmus. The sharp electrogram (arrows) at this site is present and accelerated to the pacing cycle length (PCL), suggesting that the tissue generating this potential is not directly depolarized by the pacing stimulus and is, therefore, a far-field potential. The post-pacing interval (PPI) measured from the last stimulus to this far-field potential is falsely short. The local potential (red arrow) is not discernible during pacing, consistent with direct capture, but reappears after the last stimulus. The true PPI is measured from the last stimulus to this local potential.

for pacing (i.e., from the proximal electrodes of the mapping catheter), provided such electrograms are also present in the distal electrode recordings. However, this does introduce potential error, particularly if low-amplitude local electrograms present at the pacing site are absent at the proximal recording site. A more accurate alternative is assessment of the [PPI – VT CL] value from the conduction time between the last pacing stimulus that entrains tachycardia and the second beat after the stimulus (the N + 1 beat) by comparing this interval with the electrogram timing at the pacing site in any following beat.[25] Additional errors can also be introduced by the decremental conduction properties of the zone of slow conduction that might cause a rate-dependent lengthening of the PPI.

Electrogram-QRS Interval Versus Stimulus-QR Interval

This criterion is helpful in differentiating a critical component of the zone of slow conduction from a blind alley or noncritical alternate (bystander) pathway, in a manner analogous to that of the [PPI – VT CL] method (see Fig. 3-14). An electrogram-QRS interval equal to the S-QRS interval (±20 milliseconds) indicates that the pacing site lies within the reentry circuit and excludes the possibility that the site is a dead-end bystander pathway attached to the circuit (see Figs. 18-19 and 18-20). This method requires that the stimulated orthodromic wavefronts exit from the circuit at the same site as the tachycardia wavefronts (i.e., presence of entrainment with concealed fusion). Any degree of QRS fusion indicates that the stimulated wavefronts could be exiting from another route, invalidating this analysis. However, QRS fusion is often difficult to detect when less than 22% of the QRS is fused, which poses a major limitation to the S-QRS method.

To avoid this limitation, a modification of the S-QRS method has been proposed whereby the S-QRS interval is measured to the second beat, which is unquestionably because of a wavefront that has emerged from the tachycardia circuit and is not fused.[25] The QRS complex and electrogram inscribed during or immediately after the pacing stimulus is defined as $QRS_{(N)}$ and $electrogram_{(N)}$, respectively; the following QRS and electrogram are defined as $QRS_{(N+1)}$ and $electrogram_{(N+1)}$, respectively. The $S\text{-}QRS_{(N+1)}$ interval and $electrogram_{(N+1)}$–$QRS_{(N+2)}$ interval are then determined; the difference between these two intervals is defined as the N + 1 difference. Because the $S\text{-}QRS_{(N+1)}$ interval is not influenced by QRS fusion during entrainment, an endocardial electrogram that is remote from the pacing site can potentially be used as the timing reference, instead of the QRS onset. Often, the endocardial recording is more precise and easily used for the fiducial point.[25]

The S-QRS criterion increases the positive predictive value of successful ablation outcome at sites demonstrating entrainment with concealed fusion to 80% (see Table 18-2). However, the electrogram-QRS interval may not be equal to the S-QRS interval at sites within the reentrant circuit. Several factors can explain this. Decremental conduction properties of the zone of slow conduction might result in lengthening of the S-QRS interval during pacing, and stimulus latency in an area of diseased tissue might also account for a delay in the S-QRS interval compared with the electrogram-QRS interval. In addition, failure of the recording electrodes to detect low-amplitude depolarizations at the pacing site can account for a mismatch of the S-QRS and electrogram-QRS intervals.

S-QRS Interval–to–Ventricular Tachycardia Cycle Length Ratio

Some investigators have proposed that critical areas of slow conduction within the reentrant circuit could be identified by overdrive pacing from LV sites associated with prolonged conduction times from the pacing site to the exit from the infarct scar, as reflected by the S-QRS interval. Although sites requisite for the reentrant circuit that exhibit slow conduction can behave in this manner, the mere presence of prolonged conduction from the S-QRS interval does not prove that the slow conduction is part of a reentrant circuit pathway. Multiple areas within the infarct zone can exhibit fractionated or abnormal electrograms and reduced excitability, which are associated with increased S-QRS intervals, yet may have nothing to do with the VT circuit itself.

Others have used a prolonged stimulus to local electrogram time during entrainment to identify pathways containing slow conduction. This again does not prove that the electrogram at the recording site has anything to do with the VT, because slow conduction involved in the orthodromic capture of this electrogram can occur inside or outside the circuit. In fact, whenever ECG fusion occurs, some electrograms outside the circuit (i.e., those activated after leaving the exit that is part of the VT wavefront) will be orthodromically activated and will fulfill the requirements for entrainment. For the same reason, termination with block before this orthodromically entrained electrogram does not mean that it was a critical component of the circuit.

On the other hand, during entrainment with concealed fusion, the S-QRS interval is an approximate indication of the location of the pacing site relative to the reentry circuit exit. A short S-QRS interval (less than 30% of the tachycardia CL) suggests a site near the exit. Long S-QRS intervals (more than 70% of the tachycardia CL) suggest bystander sites rather than critical isthmus. Therefore, at sites demonstrating entrainment with concealed fusion, an S-QRS interval–to–tachycardia CL ratio ≤0.7 suggests that the sites lie within the common pathway (isthmus) of the reentrant circuit, and sites at which the ratio ≥0.7 are considered to lie outside the common pathway (see Fig. 3-14). The S-QRS interval-to–VT CL ratio ≤0.7 criterion improves the positive predictive value of entrainment with concealed fusion to approximately 70%. Moreover, the negative predictive value of this criterion is 92%, indicating that ablation at sites with entrainment with concealed fusion at which the S-QRS interval–to–VT CL ratio is more than 0.7 is unlikely to be successful (see Table 18-2).

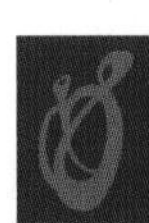

Pace Mapping

QRS Morphology During Pacing Versus Ventricular Tachycardia

When ventricular activation originates from a point-like source (e.g., during focal VT or during pacing from an electrode catheter), the QRS configuration recorded in the surface ECG is determined by the sequence of ventricular activation, which is largely determined by the initial site of ventricular depolarization. Analysis of specific QRS configurations in multiple leads allows estimation of the pacing site location to within several square centimeters (see Figs. 3-21 and 3-22). Therefore, comparing the paced QRS configuration with that of VT is particularly useful for locating a small arrhythmia focus in a structurally normal heart (e.g., idiopathic RVOT VT), whereas pace mapping has been less useful for guiding the ablation of post-MI VT.[26]

Reentry circuits in healed infarct scars often extend over several square centimeters and can have a variety of configurations. In many circuits, the excitation wavefront circulates through surviving myocytes within the scar, depolarization of which is not detectable on the standard surface ECG. The QRS complex is then inscribed after the reentry wavefront exits the scar and propagates across the ventricles. At sites at which the reentrant wavefront exits the scar, pace mapping is expected to produce a QRS configuration similar to that of VT (see Fig. 3-23). Pace mapping at sites more proximally located in the isthmus should also produce a similar QRS complex, but with a longer S-QRS interval. The S-QRS interval lengthens progressively as the pacing site is moved along the isthmus, consistent with pacing progressively farther from the exit (see Fig. 3-23).[22,27-32]

In infarct-related VT, however, a paced QRS configuration different from that during VT does not reliably indicate that the pacing site is distant from the reentry circuit. At many reentry circuit sites, pacing during NSR can produce a QRS configuration different from that during VT. In fact, it is uncommon to have similar or even almost identical morphology result from pacing from a known site of origin determined by mapping.[32] Several factors can explain this mismatch.[26] First, the pattern of ventricular activation and hence resultant QRS depends on how the wavefront propagates from the site of origin to the remainder of the heart, which can be totally different during VT than during pacing from the same site during NSR (see Fig. 3-23). In fact, such pacing would be expected to produce a different QRS than the VT because the paced wavefront spreads centrifugally to the heart while the VT wavefront spreads in one direction (i.e., orthodromically). This observation is one of the important limitations of the use of pace mapping to identify the site of origin of post-MI VT.[32] Propagation in the diseased myocardium is not homogeneous, and small differences in catheter location can cause grossly different propagation wavefronts and resulting QRS complexes. Even small differences in the angle of contact of catheter to the ventricular wall and site of initial ventricular activation can alter the precise QRS configuration. The relationship between conduction time, pacing site location in the isthmus, and conduction block determines whether pace mapping in an isthmus produces a QRS that resembles that of VT. When pace mapping in a defined isthmus is performed, the stimulated wavefront can only follow along its course, which occurs in at least two directions—orthodromic and antidromic (relative to the direction of VT propagation). The wavefront is only detected on the surface ECG when it leaves this protected channel. If the isthmus is long and the catheter is positioned in the distal part, near the exit, the orthodromic wavefront leaves the exit and rapidly depolarizes the region along the infarct, colliding with and preventing emergence of the antidromic wavefront from the infarct region. The resulting QRS complex is then similar to that of VT.[31] If the isthmus is short, or the catheter is positioned more proximally, the stimulated antidromic wavefront leaves the protected isthmus at the entrance, propagating to the surrounding myocardium and producing a different QRS morphology (see Fig. 3-23). If the orthodromic wavefront reaches the exit, a fusion QRS is produced that includes depolarization from both the antidromic and orthodromic wavefronts.

A second explanation is that the process whereby VT is generated in patients with structural heart disease usually involves the development of an area of functional block to conduction. Such functional block is not fixed, not anatomical, and variable in its extent. When formed, it combines with an area of fixed conduction block caused by, for example, the scar of MI, to create a protected channel for conduction that allows reentry to occur.[32] Regions of functional block, present during VT, can define propagation paths during tachycardia but not during pace mapping in NSR. Therefore, if block defining an isthmus is present only during VT and is absent during pace mapping in NSR, the stimulated wavefront produced by pacing at the isthmus site would propagate in all directions, resulting in a different QRS morphology. This is further exaggerated by the fact that pace mapping is usually performed at rates slower than the VT to avoid VT induction during the mapping process, which can reduce the likelihood of development of a line of functional block. Additionally, the area over which the current is delivered, especially where high current is required for relatively inexcitable tissue, can influence the pattern of subsequent ventricular activation, presumably by capturing more distant (i.e., far-field) tissue. When this occurs, it can indicate pacing in a region of a protected isthmus, where pacing at low output would capture only the isthmus, whereas pacing at a higher output can capture both the isthmus and far-field tissue, resulting in different QRS morphologies. Finally, some circuits can have more than one exit, with wavefronts emerging from the scar at multiple locations. Different exits can participate preferentially during VT but not during pace mapping, and vice versa.

On the other hand, pacing during NSR from sites attached to the reentrant circuit but not part of the circuit can occasionally produce QRS morphology identical to that of the VT, because the stimulated wavefront can be physiologically forced to follow the same route of activation as the VT as long as pacing is carried out between the entrance and exit of the protected isthmus. Although this strategy can result in the identification of irrelevant inner loop and adjacent bystander sites as well as the desired isthmus sites, it still can be helpful in gross identification of the region of the VT circuit.

Conduction away from the pacing site can potentially be influenced by the pacing output, rate, and antiarrhythmic drugs. To minimize the impact of rate-related changes in conduction, pacing is performed at a relatively slow rate. Pacing slower than the rate of the VT can further reduce the relationship of the paced QRS morphology to that of the VT target area.[32] During bipolar pacing, capture at the proximal electrode rather than the distal electrode can also modify the QRS morphology.[32] The sequence of ventricular activation can vary during pacing at different stimulus strengths. This phenomenon is more pronounced with bipolar than unipolar pacing, likely because of anodal capture at higher stimulus strengths. This potential problem can be avoided by using unipolar pacing and by limiting the current output to 10 mA and 2 milliseconds, which is within the range of routine programmed stimulation.[26,32]

S-QRS Interval During Pace Mapping

Parts of VT reentry circuit isthmuses can be traced during NSR by combining both the QRS morphology and the S-QRS delay during pace mapping in anatomical maps. Pacing in normal myocardium is associated with an S-QRS interval of less than 40 milliseconds. On the other hand, an S-QRS interval more than 40 milliseconds is consistent with slow conduction away from the pacing site, and is typically associated with abnormal fractionated electrograms recorded from that site. Thus, pace mapping can provide a measure of slow conduction, as indicated by the S-QRS interval, which can indicate a greater likelihood that the pacing site is in a reentry circuit. Creating a latency map using an electroanatomical mapping system to represent the regions of S-QRS latency graphically also can be a useful method for initially screening sites during NSR (see Fig. 3-23).[32] Data have suggested that sites with an S-QRS delay are always in the infarct region, as identified by electrogram voltage.[32] It is likely that pacing sites with long S-QRS delays are in a potential isthmus, adjacent to regions of conduction block. However, this isthmus can be part of the reentrant circuit (i.e., critical isthmus) or a bystander (see Fig. 3-14).

The reentry circuit exit, which is more likely to be at the border of the infarct and close to the normal myocardium, often has no delay during pace mapping during NSR, even though it is a desirable target for ablation. Sites with long S-QRS can be more proximal in the isthmuses; therefore, they are more likely to be associated with propagation of the paced wavefront in the antidromic direction away from the reentry circuit, producing a QRS different from that of the VT (see Fig. 3-23). Sites with prolonged S-QRS intervals during pace mapping are frequently associated with other markers of reentry circuit sites; however, this can be a somewhat limited mapping guide. Approximately 25% of likely reentry circuit sites have short S-QRS intervals during pace mapping, and more than 20% of sites with long S-QRS intervals do not appear to be in the reentry circuit.[1]

Value of Pace Mapping

At best, a pace map that matches the VT would only identify the exit site to the normal myocardium, and can be distant from the critical sites of the circuit required for ablation.[32] Thus, pace mapping remains only a corroborative method of localizing VT. It can be used to focus initial mapping to regions likely to contain the reentrant circuit exit or abnormal conduction but is not sufficiently specific or sensitive to be the sole guide for ablation. Pace mapping can also be used in conjunction with substrate mapping when other mapping techniques are not feasible, so that it can provide information on where ablation can be directed.

Technique of Pace Mapping

At isthmus sites, as identified by activation and entrainment mapping during VT, pace mapping in NSR is attempted after VT termination. Pace mapping is preferably performed with unipolar stimuli (10 mA, 2 milliseconds) from the distal electrode of the mapping catheter (cathode) and an electrode in the inferior vena cava (IVC; anode). The pacing CL is usually the same for each site in an individual patient (500 to 700 milliseconds), faster than the sinus rate and slower than the rate of the induced VTs.

The resulting 12-lead ECG morphology is compared with that of the VT. ECG recordings should be reviewed at the same gain and filter settings and at a paper-sweep speed of 100 mm/sec. It is often helpful to print regular 12-lead ECGs for side by side comparison on paper. The greater the degree of concordance between the morphology during pacing and tachycardia, the closer the catheter is to the site of origin of the tachycardia (see Fig. 3-22).

Evaluation of the S-QRS also is of value. The S-QRS interval is measured to the onset of the earliest QRS on the 12-lead ECG. Sites from which pace mapping produces the same QRS as that of the initial isthmus site with different S-QRS delays are identified in an attempt to trace the course of the VT isthmus (see Figs.3-14 and 3-23).

Sinus Rhythm (Substrate) Mapping

Post-MI VTs can be unstable or unsustainable and therefore not approachable by conventional entrainment maneuvers and point by point activation mapping. Therefore, mapping during NSR rather than during VT is of significant value during such unmappable VTs, and can help identify VT substrate.[30,31,33] Substrate mapping is also of value in ablation of stable VTs, because it can help focus activation-entrainment mapping efforts on a small region harboring the VT substrate, and therefore help minimize how long the patient is actually in VT.

Substrate mapping refers to delineation of the infarcted myocardium (VT substrate) based on the identification of abnormal local electrogram configuration during NSR (fractionated electrograms, multipotential electrograms, and/or electrograms with isolated delayed components),[27,29] and identification of abnormal local electrogram amplitude during NSR (voltage mapping; see later).[31,34,35]

Abnormal Electrograms During Normal Sinus Rhythm

The vast majority (approximately 85%) of post-MI VTs occur at sites that have abnormal and/or late electrograms during NSR (see Fig. 18-16).[1] Infarct regions are well delineated as areas of low-amplitude abnormal electrograms. Therefore, potential arrhythmogenic areas can be identified in the presence of abnormalities and/or late electrograms, which are associated with arrhythmogenic tissue.[29] However, abnormal sinus rhythm electrograms with multiple potentials are also frequently seen in bystander regions that are not integral parts of the reentrant circuit. Recording of simply abnormal low-voltage electrograms is highly nonspecific because the extensive areas in which they are located are not sufficiently specific to be the sole guide for ablation if the ablation approach seeks to target a small focal region. Resection of all areas of multiple potential electrograms abolishes VT, but probably includes bystander regions.[29] Therefore, additional electrogram characteristics have been proposed to improve the accuracy of sinus rhythm mapping.

Fractionated, Multipotential Electrograms. Reentry circuit isthmuses consist of a proximal part (entrance), a central part, and an exit from which the wavefront leaves the abnormal region and rapidly depolarizes the normal myocardium, resulting in the formation of the QRS complex. Conduction through the isthmus or at its entrance and/or exit is often slow because of decreased cell-to-cell coupling. During VT, multiple potentials and isolated potentials are often recorded from these regions. The presence of multiple discrete potentials suggests that conduction block is present between adjacent myocyte bundles. A typical local electrogram in the border of an infarct has a low voltage but is adjacent to more normal myocardium in the border, causing a multipotential electrogram that has markedly different amplitudes, with a large rounded potential (reflecting a far-field signal from activation of the large mass of surrounding tissue) and a small sharp potential (reflecting local depolarization of a small mass of fibers in the infarct). These electrograms are common in the infarct region and are not specific for the critical isthmus of the reentry circuit.[18,29]

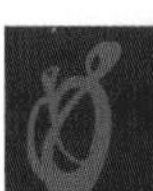

Wide Electrograms. Critical isthmus sites in the VT reentry circuit are likely to be located at sites with the latest activation during NSR. Most critical isthmus sites display electrograms that have a duration of more than 200 milliseconds and/or isolated diastolic potentials (see Fig. 18-16).[36] These findings are consistent with postinfarction remodeling, which results in progressive electrophysiological effects in the anatomical substrate for VT.[36] Moreover, there is a significant positive correlation between infarct age and the duration of the broadest endocardial electrograms (more than 200 milliseconds) during sinus rhythm mapping in the peri-infarct zone. The older the infarct, the broader the electrograms and the longer the delay between the electrogram and isolated potentials.[36] Sites with the broadest electrograms or isolated potentials detected during sinus rhythm mapping are typically identical to those at the critical isthmus of the reentrant circuit recorded during induced VT.[36]

Electrograms with Isolated Delayed Components. Electrograms with isolated delayed components are defined as electrograms with double or multiple components separated by more than a 50-millisecond very low-amplitude signal or an isoelectric interval. These electrograms can indicate greater separation of multiple fiber bundles, are relatively uncommon (15% of all multiple potentials), and have a relatively high specificity (99% during atrial pacing; 96% during RV pacing) for the critical isthmus region.[29,36] This type of electrogram, although unable to differentiate the central isthmus from a close bystander, can help reduce the area of interest, increasing the specificity. The areas demonstrating such electrograms are relatively small compared with scar areas; therefore, this method permits a focus on the diagnostic techniques and ablation in defined areas. Furthermore, recording of these electrograms before and during VT induction serves to relate them and VT within seconds, provided that the isolated diastolic component of the electrogram precedes the first VT beat and then becomes mid-diastolic. The ablation of all sites demonstrating electrograms with isolated diastolic component can overcome the lack of specificity of the selection of a single site as an ablation target when entrainment mapping criteria are not fulfilled. Ablation of these electrograms can also eliminate the substrate for different VTs otherwise not ablated by limited, conventional strategies.[22]

Changing Direction of Ventricular Activation Wavefront

Electrogram amplitude is in part a reflection of the depolarizing muscle mass as well as wavefront direction. Multipotential electrograms are sometimes detectable during NSR, but low-amplitude potentials can be obscured by the signal from the surrounding larger mass of myocardium. In regions of block, changing the direction of depolarization can produce greater separation between activation of adjacent bundles, altering the separation of multipotential electrograms.[22,37,38] Regions containing isthmuses and conduction block can be detected by analyzing electrograms recorded during two different ventricular activation sequences, such as atrial pacing (or NSR) and then RV pacing.[39]

Theoretically, a wavefront propagating parallel to the long axis of adjacent but separate fiber bundles would activate adjacent bundles simultaneously, reducing the time between potentials. Consequently, multiple potentials can become superimposed on each other, preventing their detection. On the other hand, a wavefront traveling perpendicular to a fiber long axis that encounters bundles would be expected to result in greater temporal separation of potentials in these regions. Conversely, multipotential electrograms that persist in both activation sequences are more likely to be associated with the reentry circuit isthmuses. Persistent multipotential electrograms may indicate greater separation from surrounding muscle, with fixed block and disordered conduction, regardless of the direction of activation.[22,37-39] Therefore, changing the direction of the activation wavefront can unmask some areas of block and slow conduction. Multipotential electrograms with more than two deflections, highly predictive of a reentrant circuit, are more frequently recorded during RV pacing. Theoretically, this can be related to the fact that during NSR several simultaneous activation wavefronts can coexist, making the probability of electrogram overlap higher than during RV pacing, when only one activation wavefront is present.[22]

Electroanatomical Mapping

Electroanatomical mapping can help in the precise description of VT reentrant circuits, sequence of ventricular activation during the VT and rapid visualization of the activation wavefront, and identification of slow-conducting pathways and appropriate sites for entrainment mapping. These systems also help in navigation of the ablation catheter, planning of ablation lines, and maintaining a log of sites of interest (e.g., sites with favorable entrainment or pace mapping findings), which can then be revisited with precision. Additionally, voltage (scar) mapping is a helpful feature of some of the electroanatomical mapping systems.[28,29,31,34,35,40]

The CARTO electroanatomical mapping system (Biosense Webster, Diamond Bar, Calif) has been extensively used in mapping and ablation of post-MI VT, and is described here as a model for 3-D mapping.[28,29,34,35,40] Other mapping systems, including the real-time position management system (RPM), have also been studied but to a lesser extent.

Activation Mapping

A 7 Fr, 4-mm-tip ablation catheter (Navistar, Biosense Webster) is typically used for electroanatomical mapping and temperature-guided RF ablation. Alternatively, a cool-tip ablation catheter (Navistar ThermoCool) or 8-mm tip ablation catheter (Navistar DS) may be used.

The electrical reference is chosen as a morphologically stable and regular electrogram obtained from an endocardial (e.g., RV apical electrogram) or surface lead (e.g., surface ECG lead with a QRS complex during VT demonstrating a sharp apex and a strong positive or negative deflection). The width of the window of interest varies from one VT map to another, inasmuch as it is correlated with the VT CL using the following formula: Window of interest width = tachycardia CL – 20 milliseconds. The middle of the window of interest is selected to coincide with the electrical reference. The local activation time for each endocardial position under the mapping catheter is calculated as the interval between the electrical reference and the peak deflection of the mapping bipolar electrogram. For double potentials, the earliest peak deflection of the doublet is used. Long-duration fractionated electrograms are marked to the highest peaklet.

Activation mapping is performed to define ventricular activation sequence during VT. A reasonable number of points have to be recorded. The LV is plotted during VT by dragging the mapping catheter over the endocardium. Stability is assessed by monitoring position on biplane fluoroscopy and on the electroanatomical mapping system and by continuous monitoring of electrogram morphology and timing. Points are added to the map only if stability criteria in space and local activation time are met. The local activation time at each site should have a beat to beat variability of less than 5 milliseconds. Infarct regions are sought first and more data points are acquired around these areas, as identified by low-amplitude potentials, with diastolic electrograms, or double potentials. The local activation time at each site is determined from the intracardiac bipolar electrogram and is measured in relation to the electrical reference. The mapping procedure is terminated when a density of points is achieved that is sufficient to allow an understanding of the VT circuit. The resulting reentrant circuit is considered to be the spatially shortest route of unidirectional activation encompassing a full range of mapped activation times (more than 90% of the tachycardia CL) and returning to the site of earliest activation.

The activation map can also be used to catalogue sites at which pacing maneuvers are performed during assessment of the VT. Silent areas are defined as a ventricular potential amplitude of less than 0.05 mV, which is the baseline noise in the Biosense system, and the absence of ventricular capture at 20 mA. Such areas are tagged as scar and therefore appear in gray on the 3-D maps.

Voltage (Scar) Mapping

Value. Voltage mapping is of value when activation mapping cannot be performed during VT because of hemodynamic instability. In these cases, voltage mapping can be used to delineate areas of low-voltage infarct scar that harbor the VT substrate to guide ablation. Even in well-tolerated VTs, the identification of these conducting channels by voltage mapping before induction of VT can facilitate subsequent mapping and/or ablation and minimize how long the patient is actually in VT.

Principles. More than 95% of electrograms recorded in normal ventricles have amplitudes exceeding 0.5 mV, and a bipolar electrogram amplitude less than 0.25 mV provides 84% specificity and 81% sensitivity for detection of electrical scars. Additionally, pacing provides complementary information to electrogram amplitude; only 2% of sites with amplitude more than 0.5 mV have a pacing threshold more than 10 mA, whereas a substantial number of very low-amplitude sites have high pacing thresholds, and many sites in reentry circuit isthmuses have very low amplitudes.[31,34,35]

The scar tissue is not homogeneous; there are areas of larger voltage shaped like a corridor of continuous electrograms, which connect with the tissue that surrounds the scar and serve as the diastolic pathway (isthmuses) of the VT reentrant circuit. Identification of these corridors is important for RF ablation procedures in patients with mappable or unmappable VT. Anatomical isthmuses are identified on the basis of voltage mapping as regions where the pacing threshold is less than 10 mA, located between two areas of electrically unexcitable scar or between electrically unexcitable scar and an anatomical obstacle, such as the mitral or aortic valve annulus.[31,34,35]

Recognition of conducting channels on voltage maps is a fast method for VT substrate identification. In one study, 86% of such channels were related to induced or clinical VT, which implies high arrhythmogenic potential. Conducting channels are relatively small compared with the scar areas; therefore, this method can permit focus on the diagnostic techniques and ablation to defined areas. This procedure can also allow the ablation of some nontolerated or noninducible VTs not approachable by conventional entrainment and activation mapping methods.[34]

The slow-conduction areas occur in narrow bundles of viable tissue that function as conducting channels bounded by scarred tissue. Because these conducting bundles should theoretically have a larger voltage amplitude than nonconducting scar, a careful step by step adjustment of voltage scar definition can identify these bundles. Nevertheless, for identification of conducting channels, the voltage limits of scar as a nonconducting tissue are not defined yet; the limit of 0.5 mV differentiates contractile and noncontractile areas but not bundles of viable myocardium. A single cutoff voltage amplitude may not be feasible in all cases, because voltage of the electrograms at sites at which RF ablation is effective has a wide range. Therefore, analysis of different voltage levels of scar definition may be required for the identification of conducting channels in each patient.[34]

Technique. The LV is mapped during NSR to construct a voltage map displaying peak to peak electrogram amplitude, with the color range set between 0.5 and 1.5 mV. Thus, purple areas represent normal-amplitude electrograms, and electrogram amplitude progressively diminishes as colors proceed to blue, green, yellow, and red. At low-amplitude (less than 0.5 mV) sites, pacing is performed with 10-mA, 2-millisecond pulse width stimuli. If pacing does not capture, the contact of the catheter is confirmed by observing the response to gentle manipulation. Sites with pacing threshold more than 10 mA are tagged as electrically unexcitable scar, marked as gray regions (see Fig. 3-35). A color-coded voltage map is then created and superimposed on the anatomical model to show the amplitudes of all selected points, with red as the lowest amplitude and orange, yellow, green, blue, and purple indicating progressively higher amplitudes (Fig. 18-21). As noted, careful step by step adjustment of voltage scar definition and analysis of different voltage levels of scar definition may be required for the identification of viable myocardium and conducting channels within the scar area. Points of interest (e.g., those with favorable pace maps) can also be marked or tagged as location only, enabling one to return precisely to the region of interest after several points have been investigated.

Limitations. Although an electrogram amplitude of 0.5 mV has been used to identify electrical scars, a minimum amplitude that distinguishes excitable tissue from unexcitable scar has not been established. The low-voltage infarct areas are relatively large (average area, 38.6 ± 34.6 cm^2; range, 6.4 to 205.4 cm^2), so that complete encirclement with RF ablation lesions is likely to be difficult. Additionally, although voltage mapping likely identifies large unexcitable

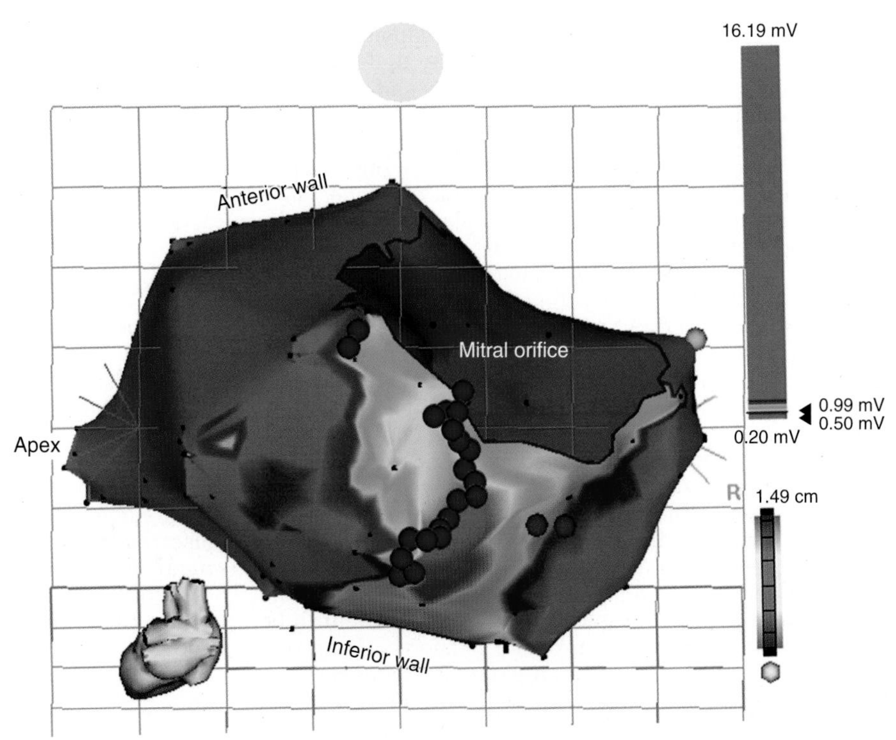

FIGURE 18–21 Electroanatomical voltage map of scar-based ventricular tachycardia (VT) in a patient with a prior inferior wall myocardial infarction (posterior view). The scale at right shows bipolar voltage; the red area denotes a very low-voltage (<0.5 mV) infarct zone with a small isthmus of higher voltage between this area and the mitral annulus. Red dots indicate a line of radiofrequency applications to transect this isthmus (additional red dots denote ablation at other sites that terminated VT).

areas of scar, small strands of fibrosis, which may still create important conduction block, may escape detection. Furthermore, it is likely that large sheets of surviving endocardial myocardium occur in some patients with circuits created by functional block during VT and no endocardial electrically unexcitable scar. When the boundaries of the isthmus are functional lines of block, they cannot be detected during NSR. The dispersion of voltage in some scar areas can appear only when activated at the VT rate. Even when conducting channels within the scar area can be identified by voltage mapping, their relationship to the VT circuit remains to be assessed by other mapping methods (e.g., entrainment mapping); plots of electrogram amplitude alone do not adequately identify VT circuit isthmuses. Finally, electrogram amplitude is influenced by precise recording methods, and these findings may differ with other electrode spacings and filter settings.

Noncontact Mapping

Value. When VT is short-lived, hemodynamically unstable, or cannot be reproducibly initiated, simultaneous multisite data acquisition using a noncontact mapping system (EnSite 3000, Endocardial Solutions, St. Paul, Minn) can help localize the VT site of origin. The system has been shown to reliably identify presystolic endocardial activation sites (potential exits) for reentrant VTs and thus starting points for conventional mapping. It may also help identify VT isthmuses and therefore suitable targets for ablation.[41-43]

The noncontact mapping system records electrical potentials from an electrode grid array surrounding a 7.5-mL balloon within the LV cavity.[41-43] Electrical potentials at the LV endocardial surface some distance away are calculated. Sites of early (presystolic) endocardial activity, which are likely adjacent to reentry circuit exits, are usually identifiable; in some cases, isthmuses can be identified.

Voltages are displayed as a colored isopotential map on the virtual endocardium. The color scale is adjusted to create a binary display, with negative unipolar potentials in white on a purple background, producing a unipolar activation map. Diastolic depolarization is defined as activity on the isopotential map that can be continuously tracked back in time from VT exit sites, defined on the map as synchronous with the QRS onset. Diastolic activity and exit sites are then marked on the virtual endocardium, and a mapping catheter is navigated to them by the locator.

Technique. The EnSite 3000 system requires a 9 Fr multielectrode array and a 7 Fr conventional (roving) deflectable mapping-ablation catheter. A standard, deflectable, mapping-ablation 4-mm-tip catheter is placed in the LV by a retrograde transaortic route. Using a separate arterial access site, the multielectrode catheter is advanced to the LV apex over a 0.032-inch J-tipped guidewire. The right anterior oblique (RAO) and left anterior oblique (LAO) views are used to assess the correct position of the balloon catheter, placed parallel to the long axis and with the pigtail end as close as possible to the LV apex. The guidewire is then withdrawn and the balloon inflated with a contrast-saline mixture. The balloon is positioned in the center of the LV and does not come in contact with the LV wall.[41,42]

Construction of the virtual endocardium model is preliminarily obtained during sinus rhythm by moving the ablation catheter along the LV endocardial surface to collect a series of geometric points. Unlike the CARTO mapping system, the noncontact system allows for the patient to be in NSR or VT during creation of the geometry. Using this geometric information, the computer creates a model of the LV. After the LV geometry is reconstructed, VT is induced by programmed stimulation and mapping of the arrhythmia can begin. A 15- to 20-second segment of any induced VT is recorded with the noncontact system and the VT may then be terminated by overdrive pacing or DC shock. The data acquisition process is performed automatically by the system, and all data for the entire LV are acquired simultaneously.

Once hemodynamic stability is regained during NSR, off-line analysis is performed. Starting from the beginning of the QRS, localization of the earliest endocardial activation, guided by the color-coded isopotential map, is assessed. Projection of the virtual endocardial electrograms over this area is performed at different high-pass filter settings (1, 2, 4, 8, 16, and 32 Hz) to avoid misinterpretation with repolarization waveforms. To identify the diastolic pathway and/or the exit point of the VT reentry circuit, a time cursor is moved backward in time until no endocardial activity can be observed on the isopotential map, even at the highest level of amplification and sensitivity. This process is repeated to reconfirm the identity of the diastolic pathway and/or exit point.

The locator technology is used to guide the ablation catheter to the proper location in the heart. The system allows the operator to create linear ablation lesions that transect critical regions and then return precisely to areas of interest, visualizing lines of ablation as they are being created and performing the ablation during NSR.

Limitations. Substrate mapping (based on scar or diseased tissue) is limited with this technology at present. Very low-amplitude signals may not be detected, particularly if the distance between the center of the balloon catheter and endocardial surface exceeds 40 mm, limiting the accurate identification of diastolic signals. This is the most important shortcoming.

The accurate identification of diastolic signals can be limited. Because the geometry of the cardiac chamber is contoured at the beginning of the study during NSR, changes of the chamber size and of the contraction pattern during tachycardia can adversely affect the accuracy of the location of the endocardial electrograms. Moreover, because isopotential maps are predominantly used, ventricular repolarization must be distinguished from atrial depolarization and diastolic activity. Early diastole can be challenging to map during VT.

Furthermore, the use of this system requires the maintenance of a greater degree of anticoagulation (activated clotting time [ACT] more than 350 sec) while the mapping balloon is in place than generally required for the point by point mapping techniques. Additionally, a second catheter is still required to be manipulated to the site identified for more precise localization of the target for ablation as well as RF energy delivery.

Basket Catheter Mapping

Value. Percutaneous endocardial mapping with multielectrode basket-shaped catheter has been shown to be feasible and safe in patients with post-MI VT. The multielectrode endocardial mapping system allows simultaneous recording of electrical activation from multiple sites and fast reconstruction of endocardial activation maps. This can limit the time endured in tachycardia compared with single-point mapping techniques without the insertion of multiple electrodes and facilitate endocardial mapping of hemodynamically unstable tachycardias.

Technique. The mapping catheter consists of an open-lumen catheter shaft with a collapsible, basket-shaped distal end (see Fig. 2-4). Currently, basket catheters consist of eight equidistant metallic arms, providing a total of 64 unipolar or 32 bipolar electrodes capable of simultaneously recording electrograms from a cardiac chamber. The catheters are constructed of a superelastic material to allow passive deployment of the array catheter and optimize endocardial contact. The size of the basket catheter used depends on the dimensions of the chamber to be mapped, requiring antecedent evaluation (usually by echocardiogram) to ensure proper size selection. The collapsed catheters are introduced percutaneously into the appropriate chamber where they are expanded.

Color-coded activation maps are reconstructed on-line. Fragmented early endocardial activation—suggesting a zone of slow conduction that can be a suitable ablation target—is frequently demonstrated. However, the relatively large interelectrode spacing in available catheters prevents high-resolution reconstruction of the reentrant circuit in most patients. More recently, a steerable sector basket catheter with improved spatial resolution (±1 cm) has been used to guide ablation procedures in patients with post-MI VT. This has enabled demonstration of early endocardial activation and localization of the area of slow conduction during VT.

Limitations. The spatial resolution (approximately 1 cm along the arms of the catheter and more than 1 cm between the arms) is generally not sufficient for a catheter-based ablation procedure given the small size and precise localization associated with RF lesions. Another limitation is that the electrode array does not expand to provide adequate contact with the entire ventricle. Good electrode contact at all sites on the endocardium is difficult to ensure because of irregularities in the ventricular surface, so areas crucial to reentry may not be recorded. Basket catheters also have limited torque capabilities, which hampers correct placement, and they may abrade the endocardium.

This mapping approach does not permit immediate correlation of activation times to precise anatomical sites. Additionally, a second catheter is still required to be manipulated to the site identified for more precise localization of the target for ablation as well as RF energy delivery. Furthermore, voltage, duration, or late potential maps are not provided by this mapping approach.

Mapping of Intramural and Epicardial Circuits

Mapping arrhythmia foci or circuits that are deep within the myocardium or in the epicardium is being attempted via the coronary sinus (CS) or pericardial space.[44-51] Small 2 Fr electrode catheters can be introduced into the CS and advanced out into the cardiac veins. The CS approach, however, has important limitations. Epicardial circuits may be identified only when the vessel cannulated happens to be in the region of the circuit. Additionally, catheter manipulation is limited by the anatomical distribution of these vessels. Furthermore, ablation through these small catheters is not feasible.

An alternative epicardial approach involves inserting an introducer sheath percutaneously into the pericardial space in the manner used for pericardiocentesis. The subxiphoid approach to the epicardial space is the only technique currently available that allows extensive and unrestricted mapping of the epicardial surface of both ventricles, and has been used most commonly for VT mapping and ablation. The epicardial approach may be used for VT ablation only after failure of a thorough endocardial mapping and ablation session, at a separate setting or the same setting after exhausting endocardial mapping efforts. Simultaneous endocardial and epicardial mapping can have several advantages, such as a better chance to map and ablate all inducible VTs and an opportunity to acquire more expertise with the technique. The epicardial approach can also be an option in patients with thrombus in the LV cavity or in patients with metallic prostheses in the aortic and mitral valves. Experimental studies have suggested that fat tissue attenuates epicardial lesion formation, which can limit the success of epicardial ablation. Irrigated-tip catheters may be more efficient to promote a more extensive and deep RF lesion. Closed irrigated systems to RF ablation are preferred. Open systems are not recommended because the fluid will need to be drained to prevent the development of tamponade physiology.[44,49-51]

The target for ablation is selected exactly like the endocardial target is selected. However, entrainment maneuvers are usually difficult to perform using bipolar pacing because of a very high epicardial stimulation threshold (more than 15 mA) in approximately 70% of cases, likely related to the presence of fat tissue. This procedure must be performed with the patient under general anesthesia because of the high-risk nature of the patients and also because RF pulses applied in the epicardial surface are painful. Additionally, the risk of damage to adjacent lung and epicardial vessels requires further evaluation.

Practical Approach to Ventricular Tachycardia Mapping

Evaluation Prior to Mapping

Evaluation of potential ischemia, which could contribute to instability during the ablation procedure, is necessary. Echocardiography, ventriculography, or nuclear, positron emission, and/or magnetic resonance (MR) imaging may be used to identify the size and location of the infarct, which potentially contains the arrhythmogenic scars (Fig. 18-22). These tests also help exclude the presence of LV thrombus, which can increase the risk of embolization during mapping. Organized thrombus can overly the area of interest for ablation and prevent effective energy delivery to target sites.

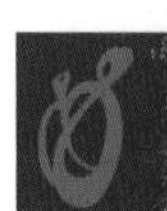

Mapping of Hemodynamically Stable Sustained Monomorphic Ventricular Tachycardia

Left Ventricular Access. The LV is approached through the retrograde approach, usually via a femoral arterial access. A transseptal approach may also be used, although accessing the entire LV is then more difficult. Both transseptal and retrograde approaches may be used concomitantly, so when a particular region of the LV cannot be mapped using one approach, it may be mapped using the other approach. Anticoagulation is started once the LV is accessed (with intravenous heparin) to maintain the ACT between 250 and 300 seconds.

A mapping catheter with a 4-mm ablation tip with 2-5-2 mm spacing for proximal electrodes is used. Poles 1-3 (distal) and 2-4 (proximal) of the ablation catheter are used for recording and poles 1-3 for stimulation. Catheter position is identified fluoroscopically in the RAO and LAO views. 3-D electroanatomical mapping can also aid catheter positioning.

First Step: Substrate Mapping During Normal Sinus Rhythm. Infarct regions are sought first and more data points are acquired around these areas. Refining the area under investigation relies on the usual clinical indicators, such as echocardiographic, ventriculographic, or MR imaging findings (e.g., regions of wall motion abnormalities, areas of scars), and 12-lead ECG recordings of spontaneous and induced VT are analyzed to regionalize the site of origin of the VT.

Activation mapping may be attempted initially during NSR (unless VT is incessant) to help reduce the area of interest and identify potential targets for further activation

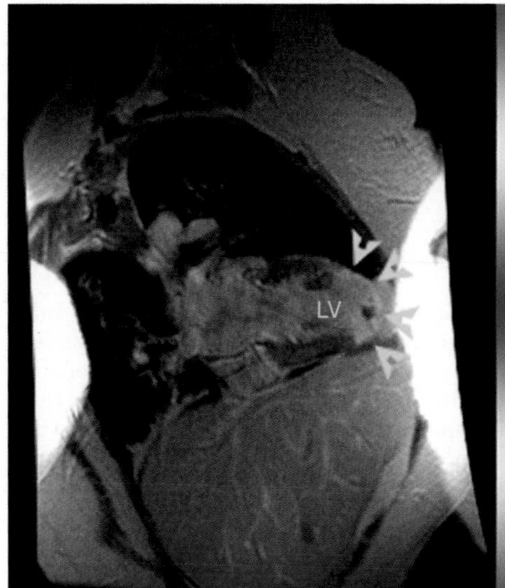

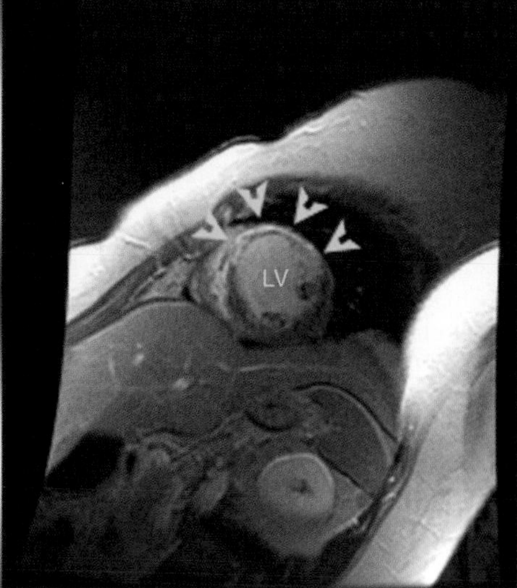

FIGURE 18–22 MR scans of the left ventricle (LV) in a patient with an old anterior myocardial infarction. Long axis (at left) and short axis (at right) views of the LV show a dense anteroapical scar (arrowheads), which can be visualized as a white thin area of the LV wall. (Courtesy of Dr. Nasar Nallamothu, Prairie Cardiovascular Consultants, Springfield, Ill.)

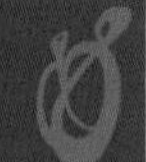

and entrainment mapping to be able to focus on the diagnostic techniques and ablation in defined areas. Goals of substrate mapping are the identification of abnormal local electrogram configuration during NSR and/or RV pacing and voltage mapping. Sites with fractionated electrograms, multipotential electrograms, and/or isolated diastolic electrograms are tagged and catalogued on the 3-D mapping system for future revisiting and guidance. Voltage mapping is performed using a 3-D mapping system to identify areas of abnormal low-amplitude local electrograms during NSR.

Second Step: Activation Mapping During Ventricular Tachycardia. Programmed stimulation is used to induce VT and to ascertain the ease of inducibility for subsequent testing, unless the VT is incessant. Activation mapping during VT is then carried out, initially focusing mapping to sites of VT substrate as identified during substrate mapping.

During activation mapping, particular sites of interest are sought, including the following: (1) sites with abnormal local bipolar electrogram (amplitude ≤.5 mV; duration ≥60 milliseconds); (2) sites at which the local electrogram precedes the QRS complex by ≥50 milliseconds (activation times are taken from the onset of the bipolar electrogram); and (3) sites with the earliest local activation closest to mid-diastole, isolated mid-diastolic potentials, or continuous activity. Filtered unipolar electrograms can help ensure that the tip electrode, which is the ablation electrode, is responsible for the early component of the bipolar electrograms. In addition, demonstration of a fixed relationship of the diastolic electrograms to the subsequent VT QRS, despite spontaneous or induced oscillations of the tachycardia CL, is important to exclude the possibility that those electrograms do not reflect late activation from unrelated dead-end pathways.

Third Step: Entrainment Mapping During Ventricular Tachycardia. Pacing is performed during VT at selected LV sites, as identified during activation mapping. Pacing trains at CLs 20 to 50 milliseconds shorter than the tachycardia CL are introduced using the least pacing output that captures the ventricle. Pacing should be continued long enough to ensure entrainment of the VT.

The presence of entrainment should be confirmed by the demonstration of fixed fusion of the paced QRS at any single pacing CL, progressive fusion as the pacing CL decreases (i.e., the surface ECG progressively looks more like the VT QRS than a purely paced QRS), and resumption of the VT following pacing with a nonfused VT QRS at a return cycle equal to the pacing CL. Once the presence of entrainment is confirmed, three parameters should be evaluated—the presence of manifest or concealed fusion, the PPI, and the local electrogram-to-QRS interval during VT versus the S-QRS interval during entrainment. The 12-lead ECGs during pacing and during VT are compared to evaluate whether manifest or concealed fusion is present. The PPI is measured from the stimulus artifact to the onset of the local electrogram of the first VT (unpaced) beat in the pacing lead recording. Finally, the local electrogram-to-QRS interval during VT and the S-QRS interval during entrainment are measured on the distal bipolar pair recording of the mapping catheter or with the use of the proximal bipolar pair when the presence of artifacts in the distal pole recording prevents reliable measurement.

The following three criteria are used to define the critical isthmus and predict the success of RF application in termination of the VT: (1) entrainment with concealed fusion; (2) PPI = tachycardia CL (±30 milliseconds); (3) and S-QRS interval = local electrogram to QRS interval (±20 ms). Other predictors of successful ablation sites include S-QRS interval–to–VT CL ratio ≤0.7, long S-QRS interval, alteration of the tachycardia CL and/or termination by subthreshold or nonpropagated stimuli, and repeated VT termination occurring with catheter manipulation or pacing at the site.

Fourth Step: Pace Mapping During Normal Sinus Rhythm. Pace mapping can be used to complement activation and entrainment mapping finding, although it may not be always necessary, especially when several criteria localizing the VT isthmus have been identified. At isthmus sites defined during VT, pace mapping during NSR is attempted after VT termination, with the mapping catheter being kept at the same location. Pace mapping is preferably performed with unipolar stimuli (10 mA, 2 milliseconds) from the distal electrode of the mapping catheter (cathode) and an electrode in the IVC (anode). The same pacing CL is usually used for each site in an individual patient (500 to 700 milliseconds), slightly faster than the sinus rate and slower than the rate of the induced VTs.

The resulting 12-lead ECG morphology is compared with that of the tachycardia. ECG recordings should be reviewed at the same gain and filter settings and at a paper-sweep speed of 100 mm/sec. It is often helpful to print regular 12-lead ECGs for side by side comparison on paper. The greater the degree of concordance between the morphology during pacing and tachycardia, the closer is the catheter to the site of origin of the tachycardia.

Evaluation of the S-QRS interval is of interest. The S-QRS interval is measured to the onset of the earliest QRS on the 12-lead ECG. Sites from which pace mapping produces the same QRS as that of the initial isthmus site with different S-QRS delays are identified in an attempt to trace the course of the VT isthmus.

Mapping of Hemodynamically Unstable or Unsustainable Monomorphic Ventricular Tachycardia

As noted, patients with post-MI VT often have multiple reentry circuits, with an average of three to four different inducible VTs. In addition, induced VTs are often unstable, preventing extensive mapping to localize all VT circuits. VT can be unstable for mapping because of hemodynamic collapse, frequent changes from one VT to another, or inability to induce the VT reproducibly.[17,22,27,29-31,33]

In patients in whom the induced VT is only marginally tolerated (hypotensive without syncope), several strategies can be used. Intravenous procainamide (infused with a maximum loading dose of 15 mg/kg at a rate of 50 mg/min, followed by a continuous infusion at a maximum rate of 0.11 mg/kg/min) can help slow and stabilize the VT rate. Additionally, circulatory support can be achieved with an intravenous infusion of dopamine, dobutamine (3- to 5-μg/kg/min infusion), or phenylephrine (small boluses of 50 μg or infusion of 1 to 5 μg/min), intraaortic balloon counterpulsation, partial or complete cardiopulmonary bypass, or LV assist device.

First Step: Substrate Mapping During Normal Sinus Rhythm. Infarct regions are sought first and more data points are acquired around these areas. Sites are identified to represent VT substrate based on their amplitude and configuration. Activation mapping is used to identify sites with abnormal local electrogram configuration (fractionated electrograms, multipotential electrograms, and isolated diastolic electrograms) during NSR and/or RV pacing. These sites are tagged and catalogued on the 3-D mapping system for future revisiting and guidance. Voltage mapping (using a 3-D mapping system) is used to identify areas of abnormal low-amplitude local electrograms during NSR. These sites are then used to guide designing linear ablation lesions targeting the VT exit sites or slow channels, or to guide other mapping maneuvers (activation and/or entrainment mapping) that then can be performed quickly during short periods of VT.

Second Step: Pace Mapping During Normal Sinus Rhythm. Pace mapping during NSR is performed at the border zone between scar and normal tissue to approximate the exit site of each inducible VT. Two measures are evaluated, paced QRS morphology matching that of the VT and long S-QRS interval. The resulting 12-lead ECG pace QRS morphology is compared with that of the VT. The greater the degree of concordance between the morphology during pacing and tachycardia, the closer is the catheter to the site of origin of the tachycardia. Sites with S-QRS latency are also sought, which may correlate with slow channels and isthmuses within the infarct area that may be in or close to the VT circuit.

Third Step: Limited Mapping During Ventricular Tachycardia. When hemodynamic compromise during the VT is the main limitation for conventional activation and entrainment mapping methods, brief inductions of VT (with the mapping catheter at the optimal site, as identified by substrate and pace mapping) can allow the assessment of the relationship of the abnormal electrograms to the VT circuit. This can also allow entrainment maneuvers to be performed at those sites to help distinguish sites critical to the VT circuit from bystander sites. VT is then quickly terminated before significant hemodynamic compromise ensues. This approach can be facilitated by hemodynamic support with the use of intravenous vasopressors and/or intraaortic balloon pump. This approach, however, requires being able to induce the same VT reproducibly.

Multisite Data Acquisition Mapping. This approach uses a system that simultaneously records electrograms throughout the ventricle during one or a few beats of the unstable VT, following which the VT can be terminated to allow ablation during stable sinus rhythm. Simultaneous multisite data acquisition using multielectrode basket catheters or a noncontact mapping system (EnSite 3000) may rapidly identify VT exit sites and thus starting points for conventional mapping. It can also help identify VT isthmuses and therefore suitable targets for ablation.

ABLATION

Target of Ablation

Hemodynamically Stable Ventricular Tachycardia

The critical isthmus of the VT circuit should be sought and targeted by ablation. These isthmuses are usually found at the border zone of the infarct and are defined as conductive myocardial tissue delineated by nonconductive tissue. This nonconductive tissue can be a line of double potentials or a scar area. It can also encompass an anatomical obstacle, such as the mitral annulus. As noted, focal ablation of all sites defined as in the reentrant circuit may not result in a cure of VT. Cure requires ablation of an isthmus bordered by barriers on either side. Because the circuit incorporates sites outside this critical isthmus, ablation of these external sites will not result in cure, although it may alter the VT CL or morphology slightly. The isthmuses are the preferred targets for VT ablation because they are usually narrow and critical parts of the VT reentry circuit.[52-55]

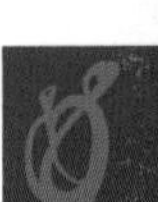

For stable VTs, reentry circuit isthmuses are defined by activation and entrainment mapping as sites with continuous activity or isolated mid-diastolic potentials, entrainment with concealed fusion, PPI equal to the VT CL, S-QRS interval < 70% of the VT CL, alteration of the tachycardia CL or termination of VT by subthreshold or nonpropagated stimuli, and repeated VT termination occurring with catheter manipulation or pacing at the site.

Results of ablation of infarct-related VTs have been improving over the last decade with our better understanding and selection of ablation sites. Initial attempts at ablation targeted early presystolic potentials. This was followed by the use of mid-diastolic potentials. Both approaches yielded unsatisfactory results. Presystolic potentials were found to be nonspecific, because they might be in an area at the scar tissue—for example, inner loop, bystander (inner sites attached to the central pathway), or not related to the VT circuit. Mid-diastolic potentials, which cannot be dissociated from the VT during entrainment, are uncommon (30% of patients) and can be at a bystander site. Demonstration of entrainment of VT with concealed fusion as a guide to VT ablation has increased ablation success rates over the last few years. However, entrainment with concealed fusion alone to guide VT ablation has only a 50% positive predictive value for terminating VT. The use of multiple criteria (e.g., S-QRS latency, mid-diastolic potentials) has been suggested, alone or in combination, to improve identification of the critical zone of the VT. These criteria have a different sensitivity and specificity with variable positive predictive values whenever they are used in different combinations. Recent data have shown that sites where the three entrainment criteria described are met have the highest ablation success rates, with a positive predictive value of 100% and negative predictive value of 96% (see Table 18-2).

The inability to find the appropriate target site can be caused by the presence of a large amount of scar tissue, intramyocardial or epicardial location of the VT isthmus, technical difficulty in catheter manipulation, and acceleration, termination, or changing of VT to a different arrhythmia during attempts at entrainment limiting mapping of the VT.

Multiple Inducible Ventricular Tachycardias

In patients referred for post-MI VT ablation, an average of three to four VTs is commonly inducible by programmed electrical stimulation. The presence of multiple morphologies of inducible or spontaneous VT has been associated with antiarrhythmic drug inefficacy and failure of surgical ablation. When multiple VTs are inducible during EP testing, several investigators have targeted the predominant morphology of VT.[28] Ablation that focused on the clinical VT but did not target other inducible VTs successfully abolished the clinical VT in 71% to 76% of cases. However, during follow-up, approximately one third of patients with acutely successful ablation of the clinical VT had arrhythmia recurrences, some of which occurred because of a VT different from that initially targeted for ablation. Furthermore, there are several difficulties with selecting a dominant, clinical VT for ablation. Often, it is not possible to determine which VT is the one that has occurred spontaneously. Only a limited recording of one or a few ECG leads may be available. In patients with ICD, VT is typically terminated by the device before an ECG is obtained. Even if one VT is identified as predominant, other VTs that are inducible can subsequently occur spontaneously.

An alternative approach is to attempt ablation of all inducible VTs that are sufficiently tolerated to allow mapping. The 3-year risk of recurrent VT after such approach is 33%. The goal(s) of ablation, however, should be individualized. In patients undergoing ablation because of frequent ICD shocks, elimination of problematic VT morphologies that result in frequent ICD discharges or tachycardia-induced cardiomyopathy is appropriate. Elimination of all inducible VTs should be considered, especially for patients who cannot undergo or decline ICD implantation.

Unmappable Ventricular Tachycardia

Over the past three decades, two effective surgical strategies have been developed. Subendocardial resection, guided by the presence of the endocardial scar and involving removal of the subendocardial layer containing the arrhythmogenic tissue, is associated with a 70% to 80% arrhythmia cure rate. Such surgical therapy is performed when uniform sustained VT cannot be initiated at the time of surgery. One technique is encircling endocardial ventriculotomy, whereby circumferential surgical lesions are placed through the border zone, presumably interrupting potential VT circuits.[56] This experience was critical in establishing the concepts on which substrate-based ablation is based; the arrhythmogenic substrate is predominantly located in the subendocardium and resides, at least partly, in the border zone between densely infarcted or fibrotic tissue and normal tissue. This substrate has distinguishing electrogram characteristics, and removal or interruption of this arrhythmogenic tissue can abolish the VT.

Ablation of post-MI VT during stable sinus rhythm, guided by delineation of the infarct region from sinus rhythm electrograms, maintains hemodynamic stability while ablation of unstable VTs and multiple VTs can potentially be achieved. However, how best to guide placement of ablation lesions is unclear. Single-point ablation guided by analysis of individual electrograms during NSR or pace mapping has proved insufficient to guide VT ablation. Eliminating all the border zone endocardium using current catheter-based ablative techniques would be impractical and possibly unsafe. Ablation over the entire infarct region or around the entire infarct border is difficult because of the large infarct size. Additionally, extensive lesions may not be desirable because the risk of complications, including damage to functioning myocardium, may increase.[17,27-29,35]

Currently, ablation strategies are guided by the identification of potential reentry circuit isthmuses and exit sites based on substrate, pace, and entrainment mapping.[27-31,33,35] Linear RF lesions are placed using one of several guiding principles:

1. Ablation lines extending across the borders of the endocardium that demonstrate abnormal bipolar electrogram voltage.
2. Ablation lines extending from the area of dense scar (i.e., areas demonstrating the lowest amplitude signals [less than 0.5 mV]) across the border zone and connecting out to normal myocardium (i.e., areas demonstrating a distinctly normal signal [more than 1.5 to 2.0 mV]) or to anatomical barriers (e.g., mitral annulus) (see Fig. 18-21).[29] This approach represents the closest approximation achieved by endocardial catheter ablation to subendocardial surgical resection of the VT substrate.
3. Ablation lines crossing through the border zones and intersecting sites where pace mapping approximates the QRS morphology of VT.[29]
4. Ablation lines extending perpendicular to all defined isthmuses within the scar areas or between islands of unexcitable segments within the infarct.[28,35]
5. Focal ablation lesions delivered at sites demonstrating electrograms with isolated diastolic components, provided that pace mapping at those sites reproduces target VT QRS morphology, with an S-QRS interval of more than 40 milliseconds, the electrogram at those sites becomes mid-diastolic during VT induction, and entrainment maneuvers during brief inductions of VT have confirmed relationship of those sites to the VT circuit.[28,35]

Ablation Technique

Once a target is selected, RF current is delivered generally during VT from a mapping catheter with a 4- or 8-mm tip. RF energy is delivered in a temperature-controlled mode for 60 to 120 seconds at each ablation site, with a maximal temperature target of 60° to 70°C and 50 W of maximum power delivered. Alternatively, RF energy is delivered at an initial power of 10 W and the power is titrated upward, as guided by temperature monitoring, to attain a temperature of 60°C. Once this endpoint is reached, the application of energy is continued for 20 seconds or longer. When VT fails to terminate, the energy application is discontinued and mapping is continued at other sites; if VT does terminate, the RF application is continued for a total of 60 seconds at the final power setting. Ablation can also be performed with a 4-mm-tip electrode with power titrated to a 5- to 10-Ω decrease in impedance or a maximum temperature of 60° to 65°C. Impedance is monitored during RF delivery. In case of an impedance rise, the ablation catheter is removed from the body and the distal electrode is wiped clean of the coagulum before continuing with the procedure.

Alternatively, cooled RF ablation may be performed using an external or internal irrigation system. The external irrigation system (ThermoCool, Biosense Webster) uses an 8 Fr catheter that has an electrode 3.5 mm in length with six holes in the tip through which saline flows at 30 mL/min during RF application.[31] In the internal irrigation system

(Chilli, Boston Scientific, Natick, Mass), saline flows at 36 mL/min through the electrode and returns through a second lumen to be discarded outside the patient.[57] For both cooled RF systems, RF application is initiated after saline irrigation decreases the measured electrode temperature to 28° to 32°C. Initial power is 20 to 30 W, and the power is gradually increased to achieve a fall in impedance of 5 to 10 Ω or a maximal measured electrode tip temperature of 40° to 45°C. Energy application is continued for a minimum of 30 to 120 seconds. RF current application is discontinued if measured impedance increases by more than 10 Ω, the catheter changes position, or VT fails to terminate after 30 to 60 seconds.

For the epicardial approach, the RF parameters used to ablate epicardial VT circuit are empirically chosen because there are no data about this issue. RF pulses are usually limited to 60°C during 10 seconds as a test and, if sufficient to stop VT, prolonged by approximately 30 seconds. A power of 5 W (and occasionally up to 30 W) is generally required to attain this temperature.

A second RF application is typically given at successful target sites if VT cannot immediately be reinitiated and the catheter has not moved. Successful ablation sites usually result in VT termination within 5 to 15 seconds of the RF application. Therefore, if there is no termination of VT by 30 seconds, it is suggested to discontinue RF energy application to decrease the likelihood of ablation of noninvolved myocardial tissue, with potential impairment of LV function.

For ablation of unstable VT, RF energy is delivered during NSR. A series of ablation lesions are made to transect the critical isthmus in the most convenient area, targeting the narrowest portion of the isthmus when allowed by catheter positioning and stability. To join the isthmus boundaries, RF lines are usually drawn perpendicular to the mitral annulus plane in perimitral circuits (see Fig. 18-21) and parallel to the mitral annulus plane in all other circuits. RF lesions are applied to the region until pacing with 10-mA, 2-millisecond strength stimuli fails to capture. After completion of each set of RF lesions, programmed electrical stimulation is repeated.

Application of RF energy at successful exit, central, or entry VT circuit sites usually results in termination of the VT within a mean time of 10 ± 11 seconds. When RF application at other sites terminates the VT, the average time to termination is 19 ± 16 seconds, which suggests that a larger region must be heated for interruption of reentry. Persistence of inducibility of VT after successful termination with a single RF application, despite further applications of RF energy at the same site, is probably secondary to inadequate lesion size because of a wide isthmus, epicardial location, and/or significant fibrosis, thrombus, or calcification.

When RF application fails to terminate the VT at a site that appears to be in the circuit, the site may be a bystander. Failure of ablation has been attributed to a number of factors, including inaccurate mapping because of failure to apply appropriate criteria for localizing a protected isthmus and/or inability to find such a site, and also to inadequate lesion size produced by the RF application. Occasionally, successful termination of VT is achieved with RF application at a site at which failure is predicted. This may occur if the site is not at the isthmus region but in the nearby vicinity, with good conduction of temperature.

Endpoints of Ablation

The complete protocol of programmed electrical stimulation is performed after ablation of target VT, and again repeated after a 30-minute waiting period. An effective target site is defined as a site at which RF energy terminates VT and prevents the reinduction of the targeted VT using the entire programmed electrical stimulation protocol. Ineffective target sites are defined as sites at which the application of RF energy does not terminate or prevent the reinduction of VT, despite an electrode-tissue interface temperature of more than 55°C.

Successful VT ablation is defined as noninducibility of any VT except polymorphic VT and/or VF. VT modification is defined as the absence of inducible clinical VT but with other monomorphic VTs remaining inducible. Modification of the reentry substrate is a common outcome of ablation. These VTs are usually faster and often not tolerated sufficiently to allow mapping. Modification is usually associated with a favorable outcome and a relatively low risk of arrhythmia recurrence. Following ablation of one or more reentry circuits, the remaining inducible VTs are often faster, suggesting that regions of slow conduction have been ablated; the remaining circuits that can form have shorter revolution time. Thus, the arrhythmia substrate appears to have been modified.

OUTCOME

Management after Ablation. After ablation, patients should be monitored on a cardiac step-down unit or intensive care unit. If amiodarone has been administered long term before the procedure, this medication is usually continued unless toxicity necessitates drug discontinuation. Other antiarrhythmic drugs are usually discontinued unless the ablation procedure is clearly unsuccessful.

Benefits of Post–Myocardial Infarction Ventricular Tachycardia Ablation. Catheter ablation results in improved arrhythmia control in two thirds of patients who have a mappable scar-related VT, can be life-saving for patients with incessant VT,[28] and can also decrease frequent episodes of VT triggering ICD therapies.[53,57]

Success and Recurrence. Generally, recurrent episodes of VT are abolished or diminished in frequency by RF ablation in 50% to 83% of patients.[24,52-55,57,58] Most reported series included patients who had at least one mappable VT. In a report of 72 patients who had a single clinical VT, RF ablation abolished the clinical VT in 74% of patients; 60% of all patients remained free of spontaneous VT recurrences during follow-up. In another report, RF ablation targeting multiple VTs was attempted in 108 patients with recurrent VT. An average of 3.6 to 4.7 different VTs was inducible per patient. All inducible SMVTs could be abolished in 33% of patients; in 22% of patients, ablation had no effect. In the remaining 45% of patients, the reentry substrate was modified; the VTs targeted for ablation were rendered noninducible, but other VTs remained. During mean follow-ups ranging from 12 to 18 months, 66% of patients remained free of recurrent VT and 24% suffered recurrences. The incidence of sudden death was 2.8%, but most patients had an ICD.

Following ablation, VT recurrence rate is approximately 25% to 40%.[24,52-55,57,58] Recurrence of the patient's initial spontaneous VT is usually presumed to occur if either the 12-lead ECG demonstrates the same VT morphology as the initial VT, or the VT CL as recorded from the ICD is within 20 milliseconds of the initial VT CL.

When the clinical VT recurs, it is invariably at a longer tachycardia CL. This occurs because of the following: (1) the RF lesion may produce slowing of conduction, and not block, in the critical isthmus, possibly because the width of the isthmus exceeds the size of the ablation lesion; (2) the RF lesion may increase the length of the central common pathway by increasing the barrier around which the impulse was circulated, without changing the circuit exit; and/or (3) the RF lesion might actually have been successful, but an inner loop, which was present and not part of the primary reentry circuit, becomes an active participant in a new longer circuit that has the same exit site as the original VT.

When a VT with different morphology occurs, it is usually one of the inducible VTs from the same region. This likely reflects different exit sites or different potential reentrant circuits in the same area of the infarct.

The variable success of post-MI VT ablation has been attributed to a number of factors, including inaccurate mapping because of failure to apply appropriate criteria for localizing a protected isthmus and/or inability to find such a site, and inadequate lesion size produced by RF.

Complications. Patients with post-MI VT typically have depressed LV function and concomitant illnesses. Ablation is often a late attempt in controlling refractory arrhythmias, sometimes after significant hemodynamic compromise has developed. Therefore, significant complications (e.g., stroke, transient ischemic attack, MI, cardiac perforation requiring treatment, or heart block) occur in approximately 5% to 8% of patients.[24,52-55,57,58] Procedure-related mortality is 1% in pooled data and 2.8% in a multicenter trial of cooled RF ablation.[57,58] During follow-up, the largest source of mortality is death from heart failure, with an incidence of approximately 10% over the following 12 to 18 months. Although this risk of death is not unexpected in this population, ablation injury to contracting myocardium outside the infarct or injury to the aortic or mitral valves during LV catheter manipulation are procedural complica-

tions that can potentially exacerbate heart failure. Therefore, it is prudent to restrict ablation lesions to areas of infarction, as identified from low-amplitude electrograms in regions observed to have little contractility on echocardiography or ventriculography.

Before considering ablation, possible aggravating factors should be addressed to reduce the risks of procedural complications. Although myocardial ischemia by itself does not generally cause recurrent monomorphic VT, it can be a trigger in patients with scar-related reentry circuits. Furthermore, severe ischemia during induced VT increases the risk of mapping and ablation procedures. An assessment of the potential for ischemia is generally warranted in these patients. Patients with LV dysfunction should also have an echocardiogram to assess the possible presence of LV thrombus that could be dislodged and embolize during catheter manipulation in the LV. Scar-related VTs are often associated with poor LV function and multiple inducible VTs; most patients will remain candidates for an ICD, with ablation used for control of symptoms caused by frequent arrhythmia recurrences.

REFERENCES

1. Josephson ME: Recurrent ventricular tachycardia. *In* Josephson ME (ed): Clinical Cardiac Electrophysiology, 3rd ed. Philadelphia, Lippincott, Williams & Wilkins, 2002, pp 425-610.
2. European Heart Rhythm Association; Heart Rhythm Society, Zipes DP, Camm AJ, Borggrefe M, et al; American College of Cardiology; American Heart Association Task Force; European Society of Cardiology Committee for Practice Guidelines: ACC/AHA/ESC 2006 guidelines for management of patients with ventricular arrhythmias and the prevention of sudden cardiac death: A report of the American College of Cardiology/American Heart Association Task Force and the European Society of Cardiology Committee for Practice Guidelines (Writing Committee to Develop Guidelines for Management of Patients With Ventricular Arrhythmias and the Prevention of Sudden Cardiac Death). J Am Coll Cardiol 2006;48:e247.
3. Miller JM, Marchlinski FE, Buxton AE, Josephson ME: Relationship between the 12-lead electrocardiogram during ventricular tachycardia and endocardial site of origin in patients with coronary artery disease. Circulation 1988;77:759.
4. Stevenson WG, Soejima K: Inside or out? Another option for incessant ventricular tachycardia. J Am Coll Cardiol 2003;41:2044.
5. Klein HU, Reek S. "The older the broader": Electrogram characteristics help identify the critical isthmus during catheter ablation of postinfarct ventricular tachycardia. J Am Coll Cardiol 2005 August 16;46(4):675-677.
6. de CC, Lacroix D, Klug D, et al: Isthmus characteristics of reentrant ventricular tachycardia after myocardial infarction. Circulation 2002;105:726.
7. Stevenson WG, Soejima K: Catheter ablation of ventricular tachycardia. *In* Zipes DP, Jalife J (eds): Cardiac Electrophysiology: From Cell to Bedside, 4th ed. Philadelphia, WB Saunders, 2004, pp 1087-1096.
8. Al-Khatib SM, Granger CB, Huang Y, et al: Sustained ventricular arrhythmias among patients with acute coronary syndromes with no ST-segment elevation: Incidence, predictors, and outcomes. Circulation 2002;106:309.
9. Volpi A, Cavalli A, Turato R, et al: Incidence and short-term prognosis of late sustained ventricular tachycardia after myocardial infarction: Results of the Gruppo Italiano per lo Studio della Sopravvivenza nell'Infarto Miocardico (GISSI-3) Data Base. Am Heart J 2001;142:87.
10. Domanski MJ, Sakseena S, Epstein AE, et al: Relative effectiveness of the implantable cardioverter-defibrillator and antiarrhythmic drugs in patients with varying degrees of left ventricular dysfunction who have survived malignant ventricular arrhythmias. AVID Investigators. Antiarrhythmics Versus Implantable Defibrillators. J Am Coll Cardiol 1999;34:1090.
11. Passman R, Kadish A: Sudden death prevention with implantable devices. Circulation 2007;116:561.
12. Josephson ME, Callans DJ: Using the twelve-lead electrocardiogram to localize the site of origin of ventricular tachycardia. Heart Rhythm 2005;2:443.
13. Segal OR, Chow AW, Wong T, et al: A novel algorithm for determining endocardial VT exit site from 12-lead surface ECG characteristics in human, infarct-related ventricular tachycardia. J Cardiovasc Electrophysiol 2007;18:161.
14. Berruezo A, Mont L, Nava S, et al: Electrocardiographic recognition of the epicardial origin of ventricular tachycardias. Circulation 2004;109:1842.

14a. Hummel JD, Strickberger SA, Daoud E, et al: Results and efficiency of programmed ventricular stimulation with four extrastimuli compared with one, two, and three extrastimuli. Circulation 1994;90:2827-2832.

14b. Morady F, Kadish A, De BM, et al: Prospective comparison of a conventional and an accelerated protocol for programmed ventricular stimulation in patients with coronary artery disease. Circulation 1991;83:764-773.

15. Miles WM, Prystowsky EN, Heger JJ, Zipes DP: The implantable transvenous cardioverter: Long-term efficacy and reproducible induction of ventricular tachycardia. Circulation 1986;74:518.
16. Patel VV, Rho RW, Gerstenfeld EP, et al: Right bundle-branch block ventricular tachycardias: Septal versus lateral ventricular origin based on activation time to the right ventricular apex. Circulation 2004;110:2582.
17. Ellison KE, Stevenson WG, Sweeney MO, et al: Catheter ablation for hemodynamically unstable monomorphic ventricular tachycardia. J Cardiovasc Electrophysiol 2000;11:41.
18. Tung S, Soejima K, Maisel WH, et al: Recognition of far-field electrograms during entrainment mapping of ventricular tachycardia. J Am Coll Cardiol 2003;42:110.
19. Delacretaz E, Soejima K, Gottipaty VK, et al: Single catheter determination of local electrogram prematurity using simultaneous unipolar and bipolar recordings to replace the surface ECG as a timing reference. Pacing Clin Electrophysiol 2001;24(Pt 1):441.
20. Stevenson WG, Soejima K: Recording techniques for clinical electrophysiology. J Cardiovasc Electrophysiol 2005;16:1017.
21. Bogun F, Hohnloser SH, Bender B, et al: Mechanism of ventricular tachycardia termination by pacing at left ventricular sites in patients with coronary artery disease. J Interv Card Electrophysiol 2002;6:35.
22. Arenal A, Glez-Torrecilla E, Ortiz M, et al: Ablation of electrograms with an isolated, delayed component as treatment of unmappable monomorphic ventricular tachycardias in patients with structural heart disease. J Am Coll Cardiol 2003;41:81.
23. Morton JB, Sanders P, Deen V, et al: Sensitivity and specificity of concealed entrainment for the identification of a critical isthmus in the atrium: Relationship to rate, anatomic location and antidromic penetration. J Am Coll Cardiol 2002;39:896.
24. Delacretaz E, Stevenson WG: Catheter ablation of ventricular tachycardia in patients with coronary heart disease. Part I: Mapping. Pacing Clin Electrophysiol 2001;24(Pt 1):1261.
25. Soejima K, Stevenson WG, Maisel WH, et al: The N + 1 difference: A new measure for entrainment mapping. J Am Coll Cardiol 2001;37:1386.
26. Brunckhorst CB, Delacretaz E, Soejima K, et al: Identification of the ventricular tachycardia isthmus after infarction by pace mapping. Circulation 2004;110:652.
27. Furniss S, nil-Kumar R, Bourke JP, et al: Radiofrequency ablation of haemodynamically unstable ventricular tachycardia after myocardial infarction. Heart 2000;84:648.
28. Soejima K, Suzuki M, Maisel WH, et al: Catheter ablation in patients with multiple and unstable ventricular tachycardias after myocardial infarction: short ablation lines guided by reentry circuit isthmuses and sinus rhythm mapping. Circulation 2001;104:664.
29. Marchlinski FE, Callans DJ, Gottlieb CD, Zado E: Linear ablation lesions for control of unmappable ventricular tachycardia in patients with ischemic and nonischemic cardiomyopathy. Circulation 2000;101:1288.
30. Kautzner J, Cihak R, Peichl P, et al: Catheter ablation of ventricular tachycardia following myocardial infarction using three-dimensional electroanatomical mapping. Pacing Clin Electrophysiol 2003;26(Pt 2):342.
31. Reddy VY, Neuzil P, Taborsky M, Ruskin JN: Short-term results of substrate mapping and radiofrequency ablation of ischemic ventricular tachycardia using a saline-irrigated catheter. J Am Coll Cardiol 2003;41:2228.

32. Brunckhorst CB, Stevenson WG, Soejima K, et al: Relationship of slow conduction detected by pace-mapping to ventricular tachycardia re-entry circuit sites after infarction. J Am Coll Cardiol 2003;41:802.
33. Kottkamp H, Wetzel U, Schirdewahn P, et al: Catheter ablation of ventricular tachycardia in remote myocardial infarction: substrate description guiding placement of individual linear lesions targeting noninducibility. J Cardiovasc Electrophysiol 2003;14:675.
34. Arenal A, del CS, Gonzalez-Torrecilla E, et al: Tachycardia-related channel in the scar tissue in patients with sustained monomorphic ventricular tachycardias: Influence of the voltage scar definition. Circulation 2004;110:2568.
35. Soejima K, Stevenson WG, Maisel WH, et al: Electrically unexcitable scar mapping based on pacing threshold for identification of the reentry circuit isthmus: Feasibility for guiding ventricular tachycardia ablation. Circulation 2002;106:1678.
36. Bogun F, Krishnan S, Siddiqui M, et al: Electrogram characteristics in postinfarction ventricular tachycardia: Effect of infarct age. J Am Coll Cardiol 2005;46:667.
37. Otomo K, Gonzalez MD, Beckman KJ, et al: Reversing the direction of paced ventricular and atrial wavefronts reveals an oblique course in accessory AV pathways and improves localization for catheter ablation. Circulation 2001;104:550.
38. Shah D, Haissaguerre M, Jais P, et al: Left atrial appendage activity masquerading as pulmonary vein potentials. Circulation 2002;105:2821.
39. Brunckhorst CB, Delacretaz E, Soejima K, et al: Ventricular mapping during atrial and right ventricular pacing: Relation of electrogram parameters to ventricular tachycardia reentry circuits after myocardial infarction. J Interv Card Electrophysiol 2004;11:183.
40. Reddy VY, Wrobleski D, Houghtaling C, et al: Combined epicardial and endocardial electroanatomic mapping in a porcine model of healed myocardial infarction. Circulation 2003;107:3236.
41. Strickberger SA, Knight BP, Michaud GF, et al: Mapping and ablation of ventricular tachycardia guided by virtual electrograms using a noncontact, computerized mapping system. J Am Coll Cardiol 2000;35:414.
42. Della BP, Pappalardo A, Riva S, et al: Non-contact mapping to guide catheter ablation of untolerated ventricular tachycardia. Eur Heart J 2002;23:742.
43. Ciaccio EJ, Chow AW, Davies DW, et al: Localization of the isthmus in reentrant circuits by analysis of electrograms derived from clinical noncontact mapping during sinus rhythm and ventricular tachycardia. J Cardiovasc Electrophysiol 2004;15:27.
44. Sosa E, Scanavacca M, D'avila A, et al: Nonsurgical transthoracic epicardial catheter ablation to treat recurrent ventricular tachycardia occurring late after myocardial infarction. J Am Coll Cardiol 2000;35:1442.
45. Soejima K, Stevenson WG, Sapp JL, et al: Endocardial and epicardial radiofrequency ablation of ventricular tachycardia associated with dilated cardiomyopathy: The importance of low-voltage scars. J Am Coll Cardiol 2004;43:1834.
46. Brugada J, Berruezo A, Cuesta A, et al: Nonsurgical transthoracic epicardial radiofrequency ablation: an alternative in incessant ventricular tachycardia. J Am Coll Cardiol 2003;41:2036.
47. Hsia HH, Marchlinski FE: Characterization of the electroanatomic substrate for monomorphic ventricular tachycardia in patients with nonischemic cardiomyopathy. Pacing Clin Electrophysiol 2002;25:1114.
48. Schweikert RA, Saliba WI, Tomassoni G, et al: Percutaneous pericardial instrumentation for endo-epicardial mapping of previously failed ablations. Circulation 2003;108:1329.
49. Sosa E, Scanavacca M: Epicardial mapping and ablation techniques to control ventricular tachycardia. J Cardiovasc Electrophysiol 2005;16:449.
50. Sosa E, Scanavacca M, D'avila A, et al: Nonsurgical transthoracic epicardial approach in patients with ventricular tachycardia and previous cardiac surgery. J Interv Card Electrophysiol 2004;10:281.
51. Sosa E, Scanavacca M, D'avila A: Transthoracic epicardial catheter ablation to treat recurrent ventricular tachycardia. Curr Cardiol Rep 2001;3:451.
52. O'Donnell D, Bourke JP, Anilkumar R, et al: Radiofrequency ablation for post infarction ventricular tachycardia. Report of a single centre experience of 112 cases. Eur Heart J 2002;23:1699.
53. Della BP, De PR, Uriarte JA, et al: Catheter ablation and antiarrhythmic drugs for haemodynamically tolerated post-infarction ventricular tachycardia; Long-term outcome in relation to acute electrophysiological findings. Eur Heart J 2002;23:414.
54. Stevenson WG, Delacretaz E: Radiofrequency catheter ablation of ventricular tachycardia. Heart 2000;84:553.
55. O'Callaghan PA, Poloniecki J, Sosa-Suarez G, et al: Long-term clinical outcome of patients with prior myocardial infarction after palliative radiofrequency catheter ablation for frequent ventricular tachycardia. Am J Cardiol 2001;87:975.
56. Miller JM, Rothman SA, Addonizio VP: Surgical techniques for ventricular tachycardia ablation. *In* Singer I (ed): Interventional Electrophysiology. Baltimore, Williams & Wilkins; 1997, pp 641-684.
57. Calkins H, Epstein A, Packer D, et al: Catheter ablation of ventricular tachycardia in patients with structural heart disease using cooled radiofrequency energy: Results of a prospective multicenter study. Cooled RF Multi Center Investigators Group. J Am Coll Cardiol 2000;35:1905.
58. Borger van der Burg AE, de Groot NM, van Erven L, et al: Long-term follow-up after radiofrequency catheter ablation of ventricular tachycardia: a successful approach? J Cardiovasc Electrophysiol 2002;13:417.

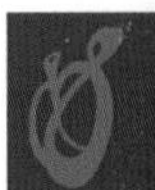

CHAPTER 19

Idiopathic Ventricular Tachycardia

CLASSIFICATION

Ventricular tachycardia (VT) is usually associated with structural heart disease, with coronary artery disease and cardiomyopathy being the most common causes. However, about 10% of patients who present with VT have no obvious structural heart disease (idiopathic VT).[1] Absence of structural heart disease is usually suggested if the ECG (except in Brugada syndrome and long-QT syndrome), echocardiogram, and coronary arteriogram collectively are normal.[2] Nevertheless, structural abnormalities can be identified by magnetic resonance (MR) imaging, even if all other test results are normal. In addition, focal dysautonomia in the form of localized sympathetic denervation has been reported in patients with VT and no other obvious structural heart disease.

Several distinct types of idiopathic VT have been recognized and classified with respect to the origin of VT (right ventricle [RV] VT versus left ventricle [LV] VT), VT morphology (left bundle branch block [LBBB] versus right bundle branch block [RBBB] pattern), response to exercise testing, response to pharmacological agents (adenosine-sensitive VT versus verapamil-sensitive VT versus propranolol-sensitive VT), and behavior of VT (repetitive salvos versus sustained).

ADENOSINE-SENSITIVE (OUTFLOW TRACT) VENTRICULAR TACHYCARDIA

Pathophysiology

Mechanism of Adenosine-Sensitive Ventricular Tachycardia

Most forms of outflow tract VTs are adenosine-sensitive, and are thought to be caused by catecholamine cyclic adenosine monophosphate (cAMP)–mediated delayed afterdepolarizations (DADs) and triggered activity, which is supported by several tachycardia features.[3,4] Heart rate acceleration facilitates VT initiation. This can be achieved by programmed stimulation, rapid pacing from either the ventricle or atrium, or infusion of a catecholamine alone or during concurrent rapid pacing. Additionally, termination of the VT is dependent on direct blockade of the dihydropyridine receptor by calcium channel blockers or by agents or maneuvers that lower cAMP levels (e.g., by activation of the M_2 muscarinic receptor with edrophonium or vagal maneuvers, inhibition of the beta-adrenergic receptor with beta blockers, or activation of the A_1 adenosine receptor with adenosine).[5] Furthermore, a direct relationship exists between the coupling interval of the initiating ventricular extrastimulus (VES) or ventricular pacing cycle length (CL) and the coupling interval of the first VT beat. Additionally, VT initiation is CL-dependent; pacing CLs longer or shorter than a critical CL window fail to induce VT. This critical window can shift with changing autonomic tone.[4,6,7]

Types of Adenosine-Sensitive Ventricular Tachycardia

Approximately 90% of idiopathic VTs are caused by one of two phenotypic forms of adenosine sensitive VT. Nonsustained, repetitive, monomorphic VT is characterized by frequent premature ventricular complexes (PVCs), couplets, and salvos of nonsustained VT, interrupted by brief periods of normal sinus rhythm (NSR) (Fig. 19-1). This form of VT usually occurs at rest or following a period of exercise, and typically decreases during exercise, but can be incessant. This is the most common form (60% to 90%).[4] On the other hand, paroxysmal exercise-induced VT is characterized by sustained episodes of VT precipitated by exercise or emotional stress, separated by long intervals of NSR with infrequent PVCs (Fig. 19-2).[4] Evidence has suggested that both types represent polar ends of the spectrum of idiopathic VT caused by cAMP-mediated triggered activity, and there is considerable overlap between the two types. Furthermore, this subtype classification, although useful, is not necessarily precise and depends on the means and duration of rhythm recordings. Patients are typically categorized based on their presenting or index arrhythmia. Prolonged telemetry and Holter recordings

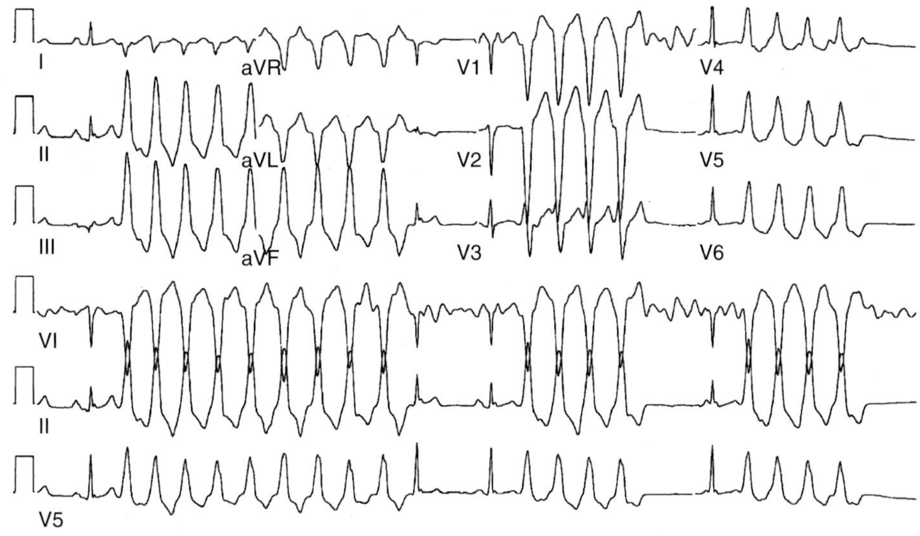

FIGURE 19–1 Surface ECG of repetitive monomorphic right ventricular outflow tract tachycardia. Repetitive bursts of ventricular tachycardia are present, with occasional sinus complexes.

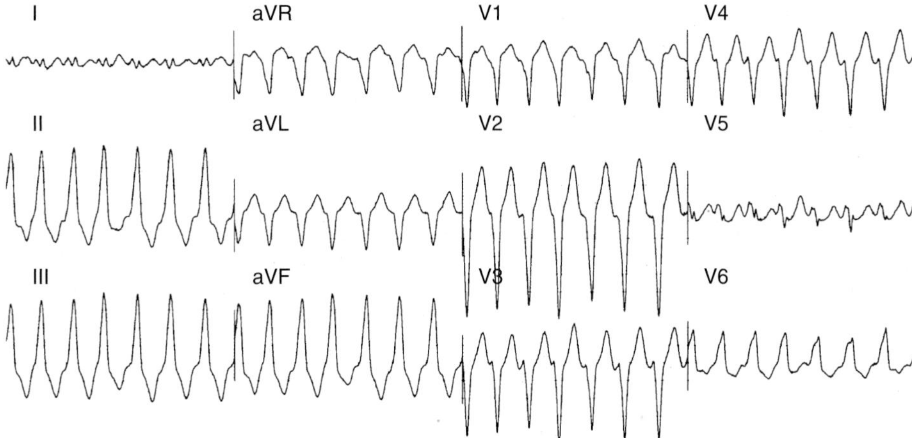

FIGURE 19–2 Surface ECG of sustained right ventricular outflow tract tachycardia.

have demonstrated that most patients with one subtype of outflow tract VT show evidence for at least one other subtype with an identical morphology. Almost all patients with nonsustained VT have high-density repetitive runs and frequent PVCs. In patients who present with repetitive PVCs, nonsustained VT can also be observed in approximately 70%; however, only 20% of these patients develop runs of more than five beats.[8]

Clinical Considerations

Epidemiology

Approximately 60% to 80% of idiopathic VTs arise from the RV (most commonly the right ventricular outflow tract [RVOT]). RVOT VT comprises 10% of all VTs referred to an electrophysiologist.[2] Age at presentation is usually 30 to 50 years (range, 6 to 80 years). Women are more commonly affected.[4,7]

Clinical Presentation

Most patients present with palpitations, 50% develop dizziness, and a minority (10%) present with syncope. Most commonly, symptoms are related to frequent PVCs or nonsustained VT. Less commonly, paroxysmal sustained VT is precipitated by exercise or emotional stress. The clinical course is benign and prognosis is excellent. Sudden cardiac death is rare. Spontaneous remission of the VT occurs in 5% to 20%.

Initial Evaluation

Diagnostic features include (1) structurally normal heart, (2) origin in the RVOT (although the VT can also originate from the RV inflow tract, RV apex, or LV), and (3) QRS with LBBB-like morphology and inferior axis. The diagnosis of idiopathic VT is one of exclusion; structural heart disease, coronary artery disease, catecholaminergic VT, and arrhythmogenic RV dysplasia-cardiomyopathy (ARVD) have to be excluded.

Exercise testing can help reproduce patients' clinical VT in 25% to 50% of the time, but is not clinically helpful in most cases. The echocardiogram is normal in most patients. Slight RV enlargement is observed rarely. The diagnosis of ARVD should be carefully considered. Signal-averaged ECG, MR imaging of the RV, RV biopsy, and RV angiography are all unremarkable in idiopathic RVOT VT and help exclude ARVD.

Principles of Management

Acute Management. Acute termination of outflow tract VT can be achieved by vagal maneuver or intravenous administration of adenosine (6 mg) which can be titrated up to 24 mg as needed. Intravenous verapamil (10 mg given over 1 minute) is an alternative, provided the patient has adequate blood pressure and has a previously established diagnosis of a verapamil-sensitive VT. Hemodynamic instability warrants emergent cardioversion.

Chronic Management. Long-term treatment options for outflow tract VT include medical therapy and catheter ablation. Medical therapy may be indicated in patients with mild to moderate symptoms. For patients with symptomatic, drug-refractory VT or those who are drug intolerant or who do not desire long-term drug therapy, catheter ablation is the treatment of choice. Medications, including beta blockers, verapamil, and diltiazem have a 25% to 50% rate of efficacy. Alternative therapy includes class IA, IC, and III agents, including amiodarone. Radiofrequency (RF) ablation now has cure rates of 90%, which makes it a preferable option, given the young age of most patients with outflow tract VT.

Electrocardiographic Features

ECG During Normal Sinus Rhythm. The surface ECG during NSR is usually normal. Up to 10% of patients can have complete or incomplete RBBB.

ECG Features of Ventricular Tachycardia. Repetitive monomorphic VT is characterized by frequent PVCs, couplets, and salvos of nonsustained VT, interrupted by brief periods of NSR (see Fig. 19-1). Paroxysmal exercise-induced VT is characterized by sustained episodes of VT precipitated by exercise or emotional stress (see Fig. 19-2). Both types characteristically have an LBBB pattern with a right inferior (more common) or left inferior axis. The tachycardia rate is frequently rapid (CL less than 300 milliseconds), but can be highly variable. A single morphology for the VT or PVC is characteristic.[3,4,6]

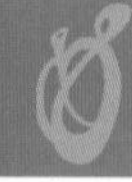

19

Differential Diagnosis of Ventricular Tachycardia with Left Bundle Branch Block Pattern. Idiopathic RVOT VT should be differentiated from other forms of VT with an LBBB pattern, including VT in ARVD, bundle branch reentrant (BBR) VT, reentrant VT following surgical repair of congenital heart disease, and post–myocardial infarction (MI) VT originating from the LV septum. In addition, antidromic atrioventricular reentrant tachycardia (AVRT) using an atriofascicular bypass tract (BT) also presents with wide complex tachycardia with an LBBB pattern. RVOT VT should, in particular, be distinguished from ARVD, a disorder with a more serious clinical outcome. The VT in ARVD also affects young adults, is commonly catecholamine-facilitated, and can originate from the RVOT. The VT in ARVD can have morphological features similar to RVOT VT (LBBB with inferior axis) but does not terminate with adenosine. In ARVD, the resting 12-lead ECG typically shows inverted T waves in the right precordial leads. When present, RV conduction delay with an epsilon wave, best seen in leads V_1 and V_2, is helpful in the diagnosis of ARVD. Furthermore, multiple spontaneous or inducible VT morphologies are typical for ARVD.[9]

Exercise ECG. Exercise testing reproduces VT in less than 25% to 50% of patients with clinical VT. The VT can manifest as nonsustained or, less commonly, sustained. There are two general positive response patterns, initiation of VT during the exercise test and initiation of VT during the recovery period.[3] Both scenarios likely represent examples of VT's dependence on a critical window of heart rates for induction. This window can be narrow and only transiently present during exercise, resulting in induction of VT only during recovery. In patients with repetitive monomorphic VT, the VT is often suppressed during exercise. Catecholaminergic VT, also exercise dependent, can be distinguished by the alternating QRS axis with 180-degree rotation on a beat to beat basis, so-called bidirectional VT, which can degenerate into polymorphic VT and ventricular fibrillation (VF).[10]

Ambulatory Monitoring. Several VT characteristics can be observed on ambulatory monitoring recordings. Ventricular ectopy typically occurs at a critical range of heart rates (CL dependence).[4,6] The coupling interval of the first PVC is relatively long (approximately 60% of the baseline sinus CL). A positive correlation exists between the sinus rate preceding the VT and the VT duration.[3,4] Additionally, the VT occurs in clusters, and is most prevalent on waking and during the morning and later afternoon hours. The VT is extremely sensitive to autonomic influences, resulting in poor day to day reproducibility.

ECG Localization of the Site of Origin of Outflow Tract Ventricular Tachycardia

The RVOT region is defined superiorly by the pulmonic valve and inferiorly by the superior margin of the RV inflow tract (tricuspid valve). The interventricular septum and RV free wall constitute the posteromedial and anterolateral aspects, respectively (Fig. 19-3).

RVOT VTs have LBBB morphology with precordial QRS transition (first precordial lead with R/S ratio >1) that begins no earlier than lead V_3 and more typically occurs in lead V_4. The frontal plane axis, precordial R/S transition, QRS width, and complexity of the QRS morphology in the inferior leads can pinpoint the origin of VT in RVOT. Most RVOT VTs originate from the anterosuperior aspect of the septum, just under the pulmonic valve. These tachycardias produce a characteristic 12-lead ECG appearance with large positive QRS complexes in leads II, III, and aVF and large negative complexes in leads aVR and aVL. The QRS morphology in lead I typically is multiphasic and has a net QRS vector of zero or only modestly positive (see Fig. 19-2).

However, not all VTs with a QRS morphology of LBBB and inferior or normal axis can be ablated successfully from the RVOT. Some VTs originate above the pulmonic valve, in the left ventricular outflow tract (LVOT, 10% to 15% of adenosine sensitive VTs), and occasionally in the aortic root. Idiopathic RV VTs with a superior QRS axis are generally located in the body of the RV on the anterior free wall, or in the mid and distal septum (Table 19-1).[1,11-18]

It is important to recognize that the prediction of the precise origin of outflow tract VT can still be challenging because of the close anatomical relationship of the different anatomical compartments of the outflow tract area. For example, an R/S transition zone in precordial lead V_3 is common in patients with idiopathic outflow tract VT, with a prevalence of up to 58%.[19] The prevalence of R/S transition in lead V_3 in RVOT VT is not statistically different from outflow tract tachycardia originating outside the RVOT; therefore, the predictive value for this ECG criterion is low. Approximately 50% of outflow tract tachycardia with R/S transition in V_3 could be successfully ablated from the RVOT; however, one study has shown that a relevant proportion of patients need different anatomical approaches for successful RF catheter ablation using up to six different anatomical accesses, including the LVOT, the aortic sinus of Valsalva, the coronary sinus (CS), the pulmonary artery, and the epicardium via percutaneous pericardial puncture.[19]

Right Ventricular Outflow Tract Versus Left Ventricular Outflow Tract. The absence of an R wave in lead V_1, or precordial transition zone in lead V_4, V_5, or V_6 predicts RVOT origin. On the other hand, the presence of an R wave in leads V_1 and V_2 and RS transition in leads V_1 or V_2 are characteristic of LVOT origin (Figs. 19-4 and 19-5). However,

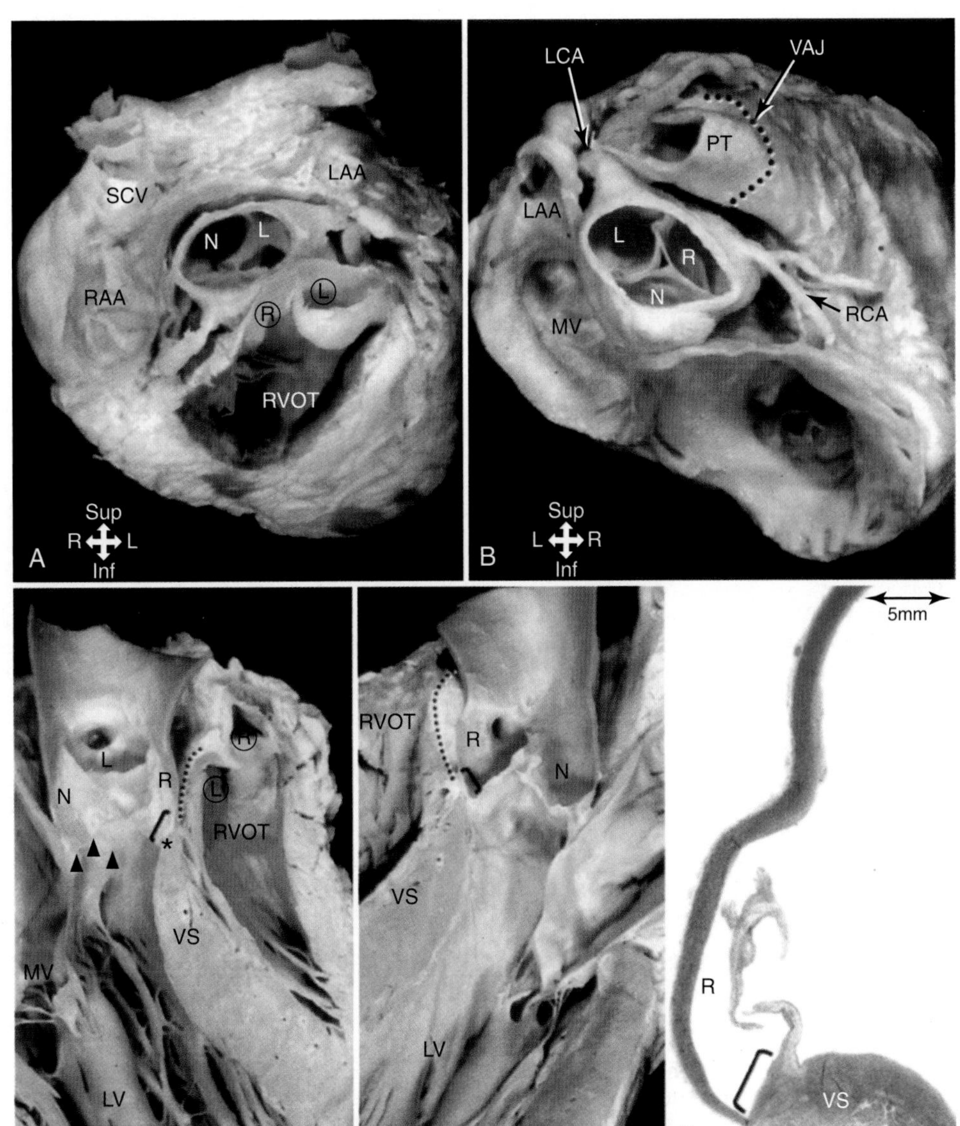

FIGURE 19–3 Anatomy of the outflow tracts and aortic sinuses. These heart specimens illustrate the anatomical arrangement between the right ventricular outflow tract (RVOT) and the aortic sinuses. **A,** Viewed anteriorly, the RVOT passes leftward and superior to the aortic valve. **B,** The posterior view shows the left (L) and right (R) coronary aortic sinuses adjacent to the pulmonary infundibulum. The noncoronary (N) aortic sinus is remote from the RVOT, but is related to the mitral valve (MV) and central fibrous body. The dotted line marks the ventriculoarterial junction (VAJ) between the wall of the pulmonary trunk (PT) and right ventricular muscle. Note the cleavage plane behind the pulmonary infundibulum and in front of the aortic root. **C and D,** These simulated parasternal long-axis sections show two halves of the same heart and display the left and right coronary orifices. The right- and left-facing pulmonary sinuses (R and L in circles, respectively) are situated superior to the aortic sinuses. The dotted line marks the epicardial aspect of the subpulmonary infundibulum in the so-called "septal" area (as illustrated in **E**). LAA = LA appendage; LCA = left coronary artery; RAA = RA appendage; RCA = right coronary artery; TV = tricuspid valve; VS = ventricular septum. *(From Ouyang F, Fotuhi P, Ho SY, et al: Repetitive monomorphic ventricular tachycardia originating from the aortic sinus cusp: Electrocardiographic characterization for guiding catheter ablation. J Am Coll Cardiol 2002;39:500.)*

TABLE 19–1 Estimation Indexes of RVOT VT Origins by 12-Lead ECG*

Anterior versus Posterior: QRS Duration, Leads II and III R Wave Pattern				
QRS duration	>140 msec	≤140 msec	Rr′ or rr′ in II and III	R in II and III
Free wall side	7	1	0	8
Septum	6	21	5	22
Left versus Right: Leads aVR and aVL QS Wave Amplitude, Lead I Polarity				
QS amplitude	aVR < aVL	aVR ≥ aVL	Lead I negative	Lead I positive
Left side	18	5	20	3
Right side	2	10	3	9
Superior versus Inferior: Leads V_1 and V_2 Initial r Wave Amplitude				
V_1 and V_2	High r*	†Low r		
Proximal side below pulmonic valve	14	8		
Distal side below pulmonic valve		4	9	
LVOT versus RVOT: Lead V_3 R/S Ratio				
V_3	R/S ≥ 1	R/S < 1		
LVOT side	4	1		
RVOT side	6	29		

*High r means initial r wave amplitude >0.2 mV in both leads.

†Low r means r wave amplitude <0.2 mV in one or both leads.

LV = left ventricle; LVOT = left ventricular outflow tract; RVOT = right ventricular outflow tract.

From Kottkamp H, Chen X, Hindricks G, et al: Idiopathic left ventricular tachycardia: New insights into electrophysiological characteristics and radiofrequency catheter ablation. Pacing Clin Electrophysiol 1995;18:1285.

R/S transition in lead V_3 is not specific. A QS complex in lead I is also consistent with LVOT origin.[11-13,19-22]

Septal Versus Free Wall Right Ventricular Outflow Tract. QRS duration less than 140 milliseconds, monophasic R wave without notching (i.e., no RR′ or Rr′) in leads II and III, and early precordial transition (by lead V_4) suggest a septal origin. On the other hand, the triphasic RR′ or Rr′ waves in VT of free wall origin probably reflect the longer QRS duration and the phased excitation from the RV free wall to the LV (see Fig. 19-4).[23]

Left (Anteromedial Attachment) Versus Right (Posterolateral Attachment) Side of the Right Ventricular Outflow Tract. In general, a QS complex in lead I is generated from sites at or near the anterior septum (the most leftward portion of the RVOT in the supine anteroposterior orientation). As the site of origin moves rightward, either on the septum or on the free wall, R waves appear in lead I and become progressively dominant and the QRS axis becomes more leftward. Similarly, a QS amplitude in aVL > aVR suggests an origin in the left side of the RVOT; a QS amplitude in aVR > aVL suggests an origin in the right side (see Fig. 19-4).[23]

Superior Versus Inferior Right Ventricular Outflow Tract. The R wave amplitude tends to be larger in leads V_1 and V_2 at superior and leftward sites; as the site of origin shifts to the right or inferiorly, there is a trend toward lower right precordial R wave amplitude and a shift in the precordial transition zone to the left. Furthermore, R wave amplitude in lead V_2 or "r" wave amplitude in leads V_1 and V_2 more than 0.2 mV suggests a superior origin. The closer the origin to the pulmonic valve, the more rightward and inferior the axis; the more posterior and inferior the origin, the more leftward the axis (see Fig. 19-4).

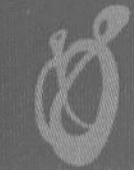

Ventricular Tachycardias Arising Above the Pulmonic Valve. VTs arising above the pulmonic valve are associated with an R/S ratio in lead V_2 and R wave amplitude in inferior leads that are significantly larger than those in RVOT VT. Furthermore, the Q wave amplitude in aVL is typically more than or equal to aVR, and a QS (or rS) wave is present in lead I.[18,24,25]

Ventricular Tachycardias Arising from the Tricuspid Annulus. VTs arising from the tricuspid annulus demonstrate LBBB QRS morphology and positive QRS polarity in leads I, V_5, and V_6. In contrast to VTs arising from the RVOT, no positive QRS polarities in any of the inferior leads characterize VTs arising from the tricuspid annulus. No negative component of the QRS complex is found in lead I, and the R wave magnitude in lead I is typically greater in the VTs arising from the tricuspid annulus than those arising from the RVOT.[26] Additionally, VTs arising from the tricuspid annulus have an rS or QS pattern in lead aVR, just as those arising from the RVOT; however, in lead aVL, a QS or rS pattern is rare (8%), and the QRS polarity in lead aVL is positive in almost all VTs arising from the annulus (89%), in contrast to those arising from the RVOT.[26,27]

Aortic Cusp Ventricular Tachycardias. VT originates from the right aortic (coronary) cusp more often than from the left aortic cusp, and rarely from the noncoronary cusp. The substrate of this VT likely originates from strands of ventricular myocardium present at the bases of the right and left aortic cusps. In contrast, the base of the noncoronary cusp is composed of fibrous tissue, which is in continuity with the mitral valve.

For LVOT VT, the absence of an S wave in leads V_5 or V_6 suggests a supravalvular location, whereas the presence of such waves indicates an infravalvular location (see Fig. 19-5). Origin from the aortic cusp is also strongly suggested by a longer duration and greater amplitude of the R wave in leads V_1 and V_2 (R/QRS duration more than 50% and R/S amplitude more than 30%) as compared with VT originating from the RVOT, because the aortic valve lies to the right and posterior to the RVOT.

Left aortic cusp VTs initially depolarize the LV and typically have a W pattern or notching in V_1 suggesting the transseptal activation (see Fig. 19-5).[13-15,17,28] The R wave is positive by lead V_2 or V_3 with VT from the right aortic cusp and by lead V_1 or V_2 from the left aortic cusp.[29] Additionally, left aortic cusp VTs tend to have a QS or rS complex in lead I, whereas right aortic cusp VTs have a greater R wave amplitude in lead I based on how posterior and rightward the right aortic cusp is positioned. In young patients with a vertical heart, the QRS complex in lead I can be negative in and around both the left and right aortic cusp regions. In patients with a horizontal heart, the area surrounding the aortic valve will be directed rightward relative to the LV apex–lateral wall, and a positive QRS complex in lead I can be seen.[29]

A recent report found that VTs originating from the aortic cusp often (25%) show preferential conduction to the RVOT, which can render pace mapping or some algorithms using

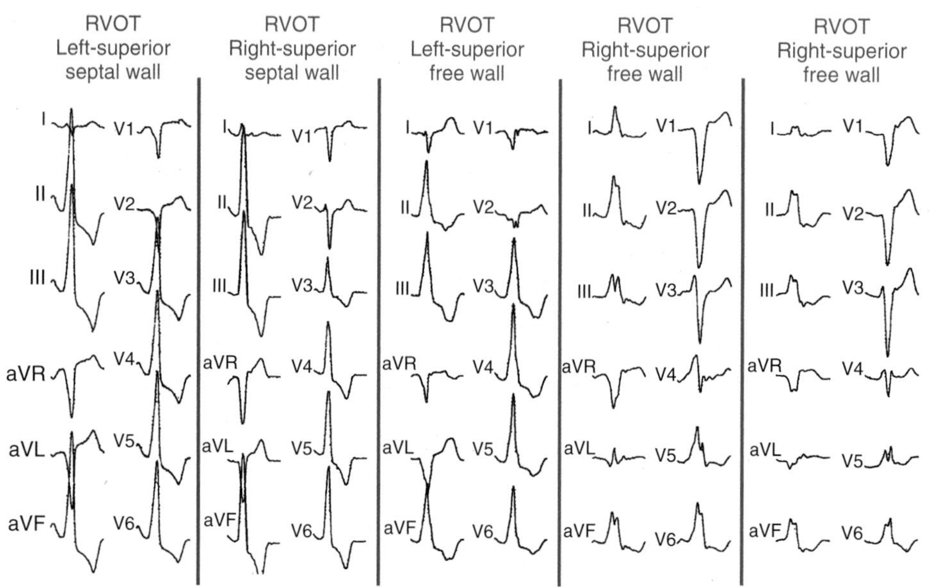

FIGURE 19–4 ECG of premature ventricular complexes from the right ventricular outflow tract (RVOT).

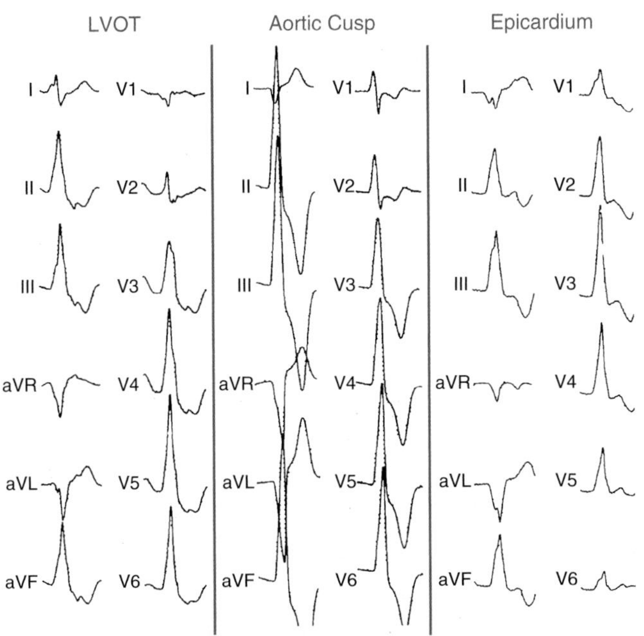

FIGURE 19–5 ECG of premature ventricular complexes (PVCs) from the left ventricular outflow tract (LVOT), aortic cusp, and epicardium.

the ECG characteristics less reliable. In fact, 20% of the VTs with an aortic cusp origin in that report showed a late QRS transition after V_3. In some of those cases, an insulated myocardial fiber across the ventricular outflow septum may exist.[30]

Epicardial Ventricular Tachycardia. Several QRS characteristics suggest an epicardial VT origin of LV VTs, including the presence of a very slurred upstroke (pseudo–delta wave ≥34 milliseconds), long intrinsicoid deflection time (≥85 milliseconds), and shortest precordial RS complex ≥121 milliseconds (see Fig. 19-5).[5] These criteria, however, do not seem to apply uniformly to all LV regions or to VTs originating from the RV. Other site-specific criteria have been suggested for identifying an epicardial origin for LV VTs: the presence of a Q wave in lead I for basal superior and apical superior VTs; the absence of a Q wave in any of the inferior leads for basal superior VTs; and the presence of a Q wave in the inferior leads for basal inferior and apical inferior VTs.[31] Epicardial VTs that appear to follow the anterior coronary vein often have a characteristic loss of R wave from leads V_1 and V_2 with broad R waves in leads V_3 through V_6.[16] For VTs originating from the RV, the presence of an initial Q wave in lead I and QS in lead V_2 for anterior sites in the RV strongly predicts an epicardial origin. Similarly, an initial Q wave in leads II, III, and aVF is observed with pace mapping from the inferior epicardial locations in the RV.[32]

Left Ventricular Sites of Origin of Adenosine-Sensitive Ventricular Tachycardias. VT can originate from multiple sites in the LVOT, the superior basal region of the left interventricular septum, aortomitral continuity, mitral annulus, aortic cusps, and epicardial sites in the region of the great cardiac and anterior interventricular veins. Most of these sites of origin are associated with an LBBB pattern and inferior axis. A basal LV septal origin is suggested by LBBB morphology associated with an early precordial transition in lead V_1 or V_2. An origin from the aortomitral continuity is associated with RBBB morphology and broad monophasic R waves across the precordial leads. As the origin moves laterally along the mitral annulus, the R wave in lead I and in the inferior leads decrease in amplitude. LVOT free wall VTs have early transition and persistent dominant R wave across the precordium, with a small or absent S wave out to the apex (see Fig. 19-5). The R wave in V_2 is broad and occupies a greater percentage of the QRS width than RVOT VTs. LVOT VT can rarely have an epicardial site of origin. This form is associated with an R wave in lead V_1, S wave in lead V_2, precordial transition in leads V_2 to V_4, deep QS in lead aVL, and tall R wave in the inferior leads.[4,33]

Electrophysiological Testing

Induction of Tachycardia

Frequently, VT foci can become inactive in the electrophysiology (EP) laboratory environment caused by sedative medications or deviation from daily activities (e.g., exercise or caffeine intake) that can affect VT activity. Thus, in preparation for a VT ablation procedure, antiarrhythmic drugs should be withheld for at least five half-lives before the EP study and minimal sedation should be used throughout the procedure. Additionally, it may be appropriate to monitor the patient in the EP laboratory initially without sedation. If no spontaneous tachycardia is observed, isoproterenol is administered. If no VT can be induced, a single quadripolar catheter is placed in the RV, and programmed electrical stimulation is performed. If VT focus remains quiescent, the procedure is aborted and retried at a future date. If VT is inducible at any step, the full EP catheter arrangement and EP study are undertaken.[6]

The programmed electrical stimulation protocol should include incremental ventricular burst pacing from the RV apex and RVOT (until 1:1 capture is lost or a pacing CL of 220 milliseconds is reached) and single, double, and triple VESs at multiple CLs (600 and 400 milliseconds) from the RV apex and RVOT. Additionally, VT inducibility can be facilitated by catecholamines.[4,6] Isoproterenol infusion (up to 4 μg/min, or 30% increase in heart rate) is frequently used. If VT is not induced with isoproterenol, rapid ventricular pacing and VES should be repeated. If VT is still noninducible, isoproterenol is discontinued because VT can develop during the washout phase, analogous to VT occurring during the recovery phase postexercise. If VT is still not inducible, isoproterenol is restarted and atropine (0.04 mg/kg) and aminophylline (2.8 mg/kg) are sequentially administered (with and without programmed electrical stimulation) to attenuate the potential antiarrhythmic effects of endogenous acetylcholine and adenosine, which inhibit cAMP.[6,23]

Ventricular stimulation can initiate the VT in less than 65% of patients and, in contrast to reentrant VT, rapid ventricular pacing is usually more effective than VES.[4,6] Induction of sustained VT is less common in patients with repetitive monomorphic VT. Moreover, multiple VESs during NSR or following a pacing drive train of less than 8 to 10 beats usually fail to initiate VT. Most episodes of triggered activity VT induced by ventricular stimulation are usually nonsustained. Reproducibility of VT induction using all methods is less than 50%, whereas reproducibility of induction with single or double VESs is approximately 25%. Induction with atrial pacing is not uncommon. Of note, VT initiation does not require associated ventricular conduction delay and/or block for initiation (in contrast to reentrant VT).

Typically, the initial cycle of the VT bears a direct relationship to the pacing CL (whether or not VESs are delivered following the pacing drive). Thus, the shorter the initiating ventricular pacing CL, the shorter the interval to the first VT beat and the shorter the initial VT CL. Similarly, the initial cycle of the VT bears a direct relationship to the

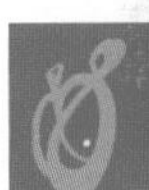

coupling interval of the VES initiating the VT.[4,6] Occasionally, with the addition of very early VESs or with very rapid ventricular pacing (CL less than 300 milliseconds), a sudden jump in the interval to the first VT complex can be observed, such that it is approximately twice the interval to the onset of the VT initiated by later coupled VESs. This can be caused by failure of the initial DAD to reach threshold, while the second DAD reaches threshold. Thus, in triggered activity VTs caused by DADs, the coupling interval of the initial VT complex either shortens or suddenly increases in response to progressively premature VES; it usually does not demonstrate an inverse or gradually increasing relationship (in contrast to reentrant VT).[6]

Ventricular pacing CLs longer or shorter than the critical CL window fail to induce VT. This critical window can shift with changing autonomic tone.[6] The site of ventricular stimulation has no effect on the initiation of triggered activity VT as long as the paced impulse reaches the focus of the VT (in contrast to reentrant VT).[6]

VT induction can be inconsistent. Induction is exquisitely sensitive to the immediate autonomic status of the patient. Therefore, noninducibility during a single EP study is not enough evidence to attribute the arrhythmia to a nontriggered activity mechanism.[4,6]

Tachycardia Features

As noted, the VT can be sustained or in the form of repetitive monomorphic VT (frequent PVCs, couplets, and salvos of nonsustained VT, interrupted by brief periods of NSR).[4,6] QRS morphology has an LBBB pattern with a right inferior or left inferior axis. The VT rate is frequently rapid (CL less than 300 milliseconds), but can be highly variable.

During VT, the His potential follows the onset of the QRS (i.e., negative His bundle–ventricular [HV] interval) and is usually buried inside the local ventricular electrogram. Ventriculoatrial (VA) conduction may or may not be present. The VT is very sensitive to adenosine, Valsalva maneuvers, carotid sinus massage, edrophonium, verapamil, and beta blockers.[3,4]

Diagnostic Maneuvers During Tachycardia

Response to Ventricular Extrastimulation. VES results in a decreasing resetting response curve characteristic of DAD-related triggered activity.[6]

Response to Overdrive Pacing. The VT cannot be entrained by ventricular pacing.[4,6] Rapid ventricular pacing during the VT can result in acceleration in the VT. There is a direct relationship between the overdrive pacing CL and the coupling interval and CL of the VT resuming after cessation of pacing.

Mapping

The RVOT is the tube-like portion of the RV cavity, above the supraventricular crest. The thickness of the RVOT wall is approximately 3 to 6 mm, and is thinnest at the level of the pulmonic valve. The RVOT region is defined superiorly by the pulmonic valve and inferiorly by the RV inflow tract and the top of the tricuspid valve. The lateral aspect of the RVOT region is the RV free wall, and the medial aspect is formed by the interventricular septum at the base of the RVOT and RV musculature opposite the root of the aorta at the region just inferior to the pulmonic valve (see Fig. 19-3).[23] From the coronal view above the pulmonic valve, the RVOT region is seen wrapping around the root of the aorta and extending leftward. The top of the RVOT can be convex or crescent-shaped, with the posteroseptal region directed rightward and the anteroseptal region directed leftward. The anteroseptal aspect of the RVOT actually is located in close proximity to the LV epicardium, adjacent to the anterior interventricular vein and in proximity to the left anterior descending coronary artery. The aortic valve cusps sit squarely within the crescent-shaped septal region of the RVOT and are inferior to the pulmonic valve (see Fig. 19-3). The posteroseptal aspect of the RVOT is adjacent to the region of the right coronary cusp, and the anterior septal surface is adjacent to the anterior margin of the right coronary cusp or the medial aspect of the left coronary cusp.[29]

VT origins in the RVOT are anatomically classified into 3-D directions: anterior and posterior, right and left, and superior and inferior. The anterior half of the RVOT by fluoroscopy in the 60-degree left anterior oblique (LAO) position is defined as the anterior side (or free wall side) and the posterior half is defined as the posterior side (or septal side; Fig. 19-6). When viewed by fluoroscopy in the 30-degree right anterior oblique (RAO) projection, the posterior half of the outflow is defined as the right side (or posterolateral attachment side), and the anterior half is defined as the left side (or anterolateral attachment side). The area within 1 cm of the pulmonic valve is defined as the superior side (the distal side just below the pulmonic valve), and the area over 1 cm away is defined as the inferior side (the proximal side). This means that the RVOT consists of eight subdivisions: free wall, right, and inferior side; free wall, right, and superior side; free wall, left, and inferior side; free wall, left, and superior side; septal, right, and inferior side; septal, right,

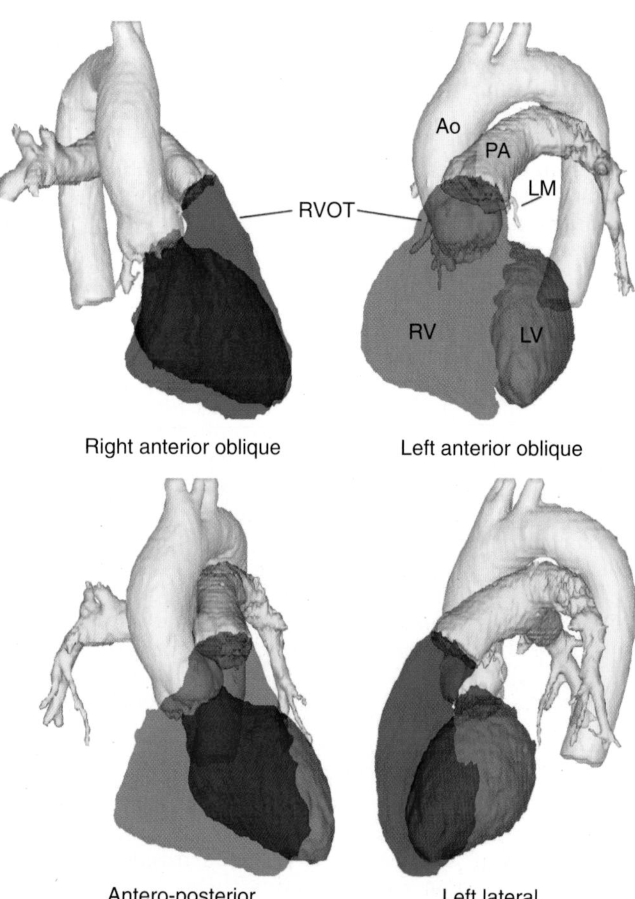

FIGURE 19–6 Anatomical relationships for ablation of outflow tract ventricular tachycardia (VT). Most RVOT VTs arise from just proximal to the pulmonic valve; note that the RVOT in this region is all free wall (not septal wall) and the leftward aspect of the RVOT is very near the LM, making it vulnerable to injury. Note also the close relationships between RVOT, aortic sinuses of Valsalva, and subaortic left ventricle (LV), explaining why VTs from this general region can have similar ECG morphologies. Ao = aorta; LM = left main coronary artery; PA = pulmonary artery; RVOT = RV outflow tract.

and superior side; septal, left, and inferior side; and septal, left, and superior side.

The prediction of the precise origin of outflow tract tachycardias can be challenging because of the close anatomical relationship of the different anatomical compartments of the outflow tract area. Therefore, a stepwise mapping procedure has been proposed, especially when the ECG does not provide clear criteria to guide localization of the VT site of origin, such as a precordial R/S transition in V_3.[19] Because most VTs originate from the RVOT, mapping is started there and, if that fails to identify the origin of the VT, mapping is extended to involve the pulmonary artery, although this site of origin is rare, but no additional anatomical access is required.[18,24,25] If activation mapping and pace mapping suggest a focus outside the RVOT and pulmonary artery, mapping of the CS can add useful information as to whether a left-sided epicardial origin is present. Successful RF catheter ablation through a CS access has been described in patients with ischemic VT and is possible in patients with idiopathic VT.[19] If a transvenous access is not successful, mapping the LVOT and aortic cusps via retrograde arterial access are usually the next steps.[13-15,17,28]

Finally, if all previous anatomical accesses are unsuccessful, epicardial mapping via a percutaneous pericardial access should be considered.[16] Mapping findings suggestive of epicardial origin include suboptimal pace maps generated from the ventricular endocardial surface, absence of sharp potentials more than 15 milliseconds prior to QRS onset, low-amplitude far-field potentials at the earliest endocardial sites, the occurrence of a very slurred upstroke and wide QS complex suggesting the possibility of an epicardial or intraseptal origin, and a large area of equally (and minimally) presystolic sites on CARTO or other activation map.

Activation Mapping

Initially, one should seek the general region of the origin of ectopy, as indicated by the surface ECG. All 12 leads should be inspected and the lead showing the earliest and most discernible onset of the QRS during VT or PVCs should be selected as the reference point for subsequent mapping. Subsequently, a single mapping catheter is moved under the guidance of fluoroscopy into the RVOT, and the bipolar signals are sampled from several endocardial sites.

Endocardial activation mapping is performed during VT to identify the site of earliest activation relative to the onset of the QRS. It is important to record examples of VT or PVCs prior to inserting catheters, because the catheters can cause ectopic complexes that resemble the target VT or PVCs (Fig. 19-7). The site of origin of the VT is defined as the site with the earliest bipolar recording in which the distal tip shows the earliest intrinsic deflection and QS unipolar electrogram configuration.

Activation times are generally measured from the onset or the first rapid deflection of the bipolar electrogram to the earliest onset of the QRS on the surface ECG during VT or PVCs. The distal pole of the mapping catheter should be used for searching for the earliest activation site, because it is the pole through which RF energy is delivered. Once an area of relatively early local activation is found, small movements of the catheter tip in that region are undertaken until the site is identified with the earliest possible local activation relative to the tachycardia beat.

Bipolar electrograms at the site of origin are modestly early (preceding the surface QRS by 10 to 45 milliseconds) and have high-amplitude and rapid slew rates. Fractionated complex electrograms and mid-diastolic potentials are rarely, if ever, seen and should raise the suspicion of underlying heart disease.[4,6] Once the site with the earliest bipolar signal is identified, the unipolar signal from the distal ablation electrode should be used to supplement conventional bipolar mapping (Fig. 19-8). The unfiltered (0.05 to ≥300 Hz) unipolar signal morphology should show a monophasic QS complex with a rapid negative deflection. Although this electrogram configuration is very sensitive for successful ablation sites, it is not specific (70% of unsuccessful ablation sites also manifest a QS complex). The size of the area with a QS complex can be larger than the focus, exceeding 1 cm

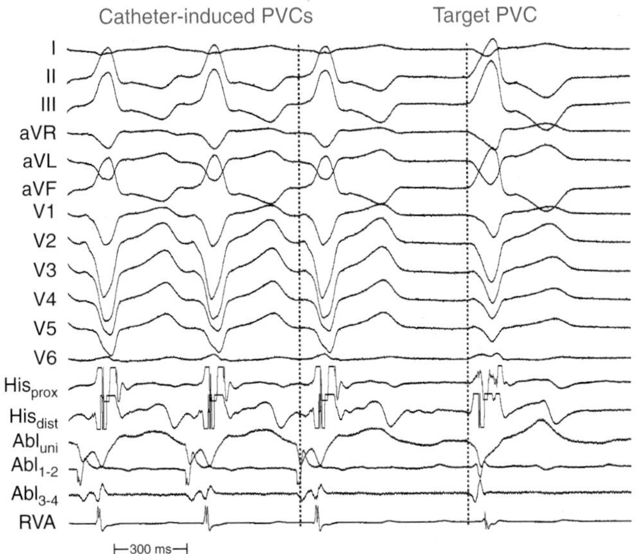

FIGURE 19-7 Catheter-induced premature ventricular complexes (PVCs) versus target spontaneous PVCs. Three complexes of catheter-induced PVCs are seen at left, during which both unipolar and bipolar signals are very early (as would be expected, because catheter tip irritation is causing these complexes). During the actual target PVC, however, this site is not early at all. This illustrates the need to be certain of the characteristics of the target PVC or ventricular tachycardia complex before beginning mapping.

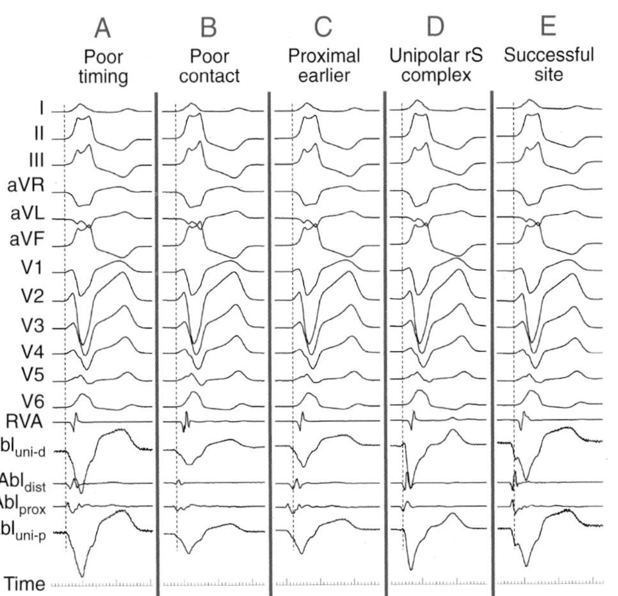

FIGURE 19-8 Activation mapping results from five sites are shown with 12 leads of a single ventricular tachycardia (VT) complex, as well as intracardiac recordings from the right ventricular apex, proximal and distal ablation electrode bipolar recordings, and unipolar recordings from the tip electrode (uni-d) and the second electrode (uni-p). A vertical line denotes QRS onset. Sites A to D are suboptimal ablation sites for reasons noted. Site E was where ablation terminated VT.

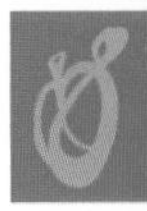

or more in diameter. Thus, a QS complex should not be the only mapping finding used to guide ablation (see Fig. 19-8). Successful ablation is unusual, however, at sites with an RS complex, because these are generally distant from the focus. Concordance of the timing of the onset of the bipolar electrogram with that of the filtered or unfiltered unipolar electrogram, with the rapid downslope of the S wave of the unipolar QS complex coinciding with the initial peak of the bipolar signal, helps ensure that the tip electrode, which is the ablation electrode, is responsible for the early component of the bipolar electrogram (see Fig. 19-8).[6] Additionally, the presence of ST elevation on the unipolar recording and the ability to capture the site with unipolar pacing are used to indicate good electrode contact.

Pace Mapping

Pace mapping is used to confirm the results of activation mapping and can be of great value, especially when the VT is scarcely inducible. Although there are some limitations to this technique, several studies have demonstrated efficacy using pace mapping to choose ablation target sites for idiopathic VT.[1,34]

Technique. Pace mapping during VT (at pacing CL 20 to 40 milliseconds shorter than the tachycardia CL) is preferable whenever possible, because it facilitates rapid comparison of VT and paced QRS at the end of pacing train in simultaneously displayed 12-lead ECGs. If sustained VT cannot be induced, mapping is performed during spontaneous nonsustained VT or PVCs. In this case, the pacing CL and coupling intervals of the VES should match those of spontaneous ectopy. Pace mapping is preferably performed with unipolar stimuli (10 mA, 2 milliseconds) from the distal electrode of the mapping catheter (cathode) and an electrode in the inferior vena cava (IVC) (anode) or from closely spaced bipolar pacing at twice the diastolic threshold to eliminate far-field stimulation effects.

Interpretation. Pace maps with identical or near-identical matches of VT morphology in all 12 surface ECG leads are indicative of the site of origin of VT (see Fig. 3-22). ECG recordings should be reviewed at the same gain and filter settings and at a paper-sweep speed of 100 mm/sec. It is often helpful to print regular 12-lead ECGs for side by side comparison on paper. Differences in the QRS morphology between pacing and spontaneous VT in a single lead can be critical. Pacing at a site 5 mm from the index pacing site can result in minor differences in QRS configuration (notching, new small component, change in amplitude of individual component, or overall change in QRS shape) in at least one lead in most patients. In contrast, if only major changes in QRS morphology are considered, pacing sites separated by as much as 15 mm can appear similar.

Although qualitative comparison of the 12-lead ECG morphology between a pace map and VT is frequently performed, there are few objective criteria for quantifying the similarity between two 12-lead ECG waveform morphologies. Such comparisons are frequently completely subjective or semiquantitative, such as a 10/12 lead match. Discrepancies in ablation results can result, in part, from subjective differences in the opinion of a pace map match to the clinical VT. Furthermore, the criteria for comparing the similarity in the 12-lead surface ECG waveforms from one laboratory to another or for describing such comparisons in the literature are lacking.[35] Two waveform comparison metrics, the correlation coefficient (CORR) and the mean absolute deviation (MAD) have been evaluated to quantify the similarity of the 12-lead ECG waveforms objectively during VT and pace mapping, and it has been suggested that an automated objective interpretation may have some advantage to human interpretation.[35] Although the CORR is the much more commonly used statistic, the MAD is much more sensitive to differences in waveform amplitude.

The most common human error when turning on RF energy is not appreciating subtle amplitude or precordial lead transition differences between two ECG patterns, and such subtle differences can be reflected in a single quantitative number.[35] The MAD score grades 12-lead ECG waveform similarity as a single number, ranging from 0% (identical) to 100% (completely different). A MAD score ≤12% was found to be 93% sensitive and 75% specific for a successful ablation site (Fig. 19-9). It is not surprising that the MAD

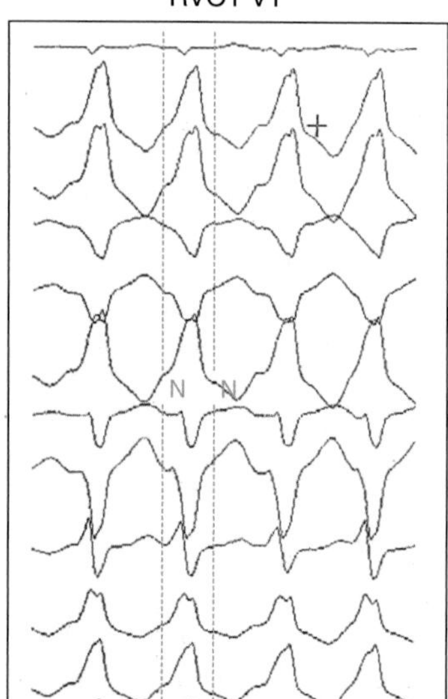

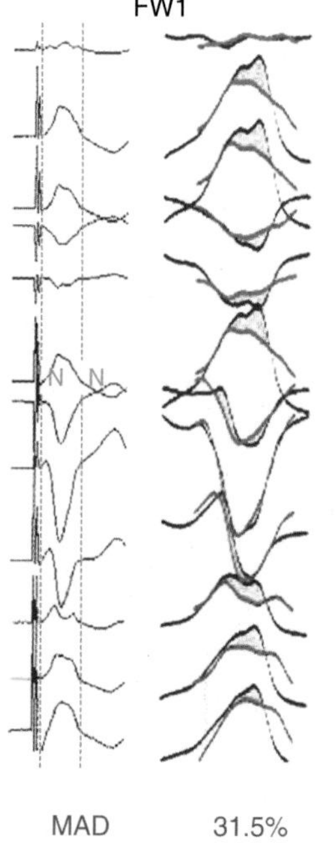

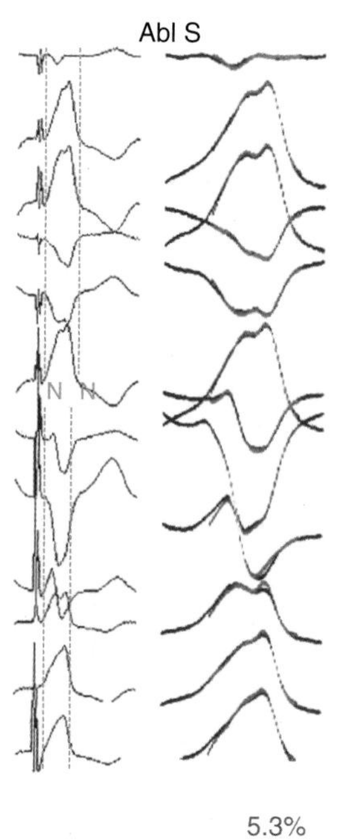

FIGURE 19-9 The mean absolute deviation (MAD) score. **Left panel,** Example of right ventricular outflow tract (RVOT) ventricular tachycardia (VT). The second VT complex has been identified as the target waveform by the annotation markers placed on either side of this complex. **Middle panel,** Pace map from a free wall site 1 (FW1) next to the superimposed VT and pace map waveforms after automatic computer alignment. There are substantial differences between these two waveforms (highlighted in gray), resulting in a MAD score of 31.5%. **Right panel,** Pace map from the successful ablation site (Abl S) near the posterior septum and the superimposed pace-map and VT waveform. Note in the Abl S panel that when these two waveforms are aligned they are nearly superimposable, and result in a very low MAD score of 5.3%. Correlation coefficients for these comparisons are also shown. *(From Gerstenfeld EP, Dixit S, Callans DJ, et al: Quantitative comparison of spontaneous and paced 12-lead electrocardiogram during right ventricular outflow tract ventricular tachycardia. J Am Coll Cardiol 2003;41:2046.)*

score is more sensitive than specific; characteristics other than a 12-lead ECG match are necessary for a successful ablation, including catheter-tissue contact, catheter orientation, and tissue heating.[35] A MAD score >12%, and certainly >15% (100% negative predictive value) suggests sufficient dissimilarity between pace map and clinical tachycardia to dissuade ablation at that site. A MAD score ≤12% should be considered an excellent match, and ablation at these sites is warranted if catheter contact and stability are adequate (see Fig. 19-9).[35] The MAD score is computationally simple and should be easy to incorporate into current EP recording systems, allowing feedback to the physician of pace map comparison before turning on the RF energy. The MAD score can also be used to standardize 12-lead ECG waveform morphology comparisons among different laboratories, and can be useful for guiding ablation of RVOT VT.[35]

A recent report using the CORR has found that the spatial resolution of a good pace map for targeting RVOT VT is 1.8 cm^2 in diameter and therefore is inferior to the spatial resolution of activation mapping.[35] In approximately 20% of patients, pace mapping is unreliable in identifying the site of origin.

Pitfalls. Current strengths up to 10 mA have little effect on unipolar paced ECG configuration. In contrast, bipolar pacing can introduce some variability in the paced ECG, which can be minimized by low pacing outputs and small interelectrode distance (≤5 mm). Additionally, the morphology of single paced QRS complexes can vary depending on coupling interval, and the QRS morphology during overdrive pacing is affected by the pacing CL. Therefore, the coupling interval or CL of the template arrhythmia should be matched during pace mapping; otherwise, rate-dependent changes in QRS morphology independent of the pacing site can confound mapping results. Similarly, spontaneous couplets from the same focus may have slight variations in QRS morphology that must be considered when seeking a pace match. Isoproterenol infusion has no significant effect on the QRS configuration.

Electroanatomical Mapping

Activation during RVOT VT is so rapid that minor differences between adjacent sites become difficult to detect, leading to a large number of sites with clinically indistinguishable activation times when examined on a site by site basis. However, when displayed simultaneously on a spatially precise electroanatomical reconstruction, the centers of the early activation area and the presumed site of VT origin become easy to identify (Fig. 19-10).[34] Electroanatomical mapping permits spatial discrimination between sites separated by less than 1 mm.

The CARTO (Biosense Webster, Diamond Bar, Calif) electromagnetic 3-D mapping system uses a single roving mapping catheter attached to a system that can precisely localize the catheter tip in 3-D space and store activation time on a 3-D anatomical reconstruction.[19,23,34] Initially, a stable reference electrogram is selected. This is the fiducial marker on which the entire mapping procedure is based. Preferably, a QRS on the surface ECG is selected as the reference signal. Alternatively, an intracardiac electrogram (e.g., RV apex) can be selected as the reference point, in which case care must be taken to avoid dislodging this catheter because, if it moves, timing of mapping catheter activations will not be comparable to previously mapped sites. Following selection of the reference electrogram, positioning of the anatomical reference, and determination of the window of interest, the mapping catheter is positioned in the RVOT under fluoroscopy guidance.

At the outset, the plane of the His bundle (HB) location and pulmonic valve are defined and tagged to outline the superior and inferior limits of the RVOT. The mapping catheter is advanced superiorly in the RVOT until no discrete bipolar electrograms are seen in the distal electrode pair. The catheter then is retracted until electrograms in the distal electrode pair reappear and pacing results in capture of the RVOT endocardium. This marks the level of pulmonic valve. At least three points are acquired and tagged to construct the pulmonic valve.[19,23] Next, a detailed electroanatomical activation map of the RVOT RV is constructed by acquiring multiple points during PVCs or VT. Points are color-coded (red for the earliest electrical activation areas; orange, yellow, green, blue, and purple for progressively delayed activation areas; see Fig. 19-10). The local activation time at each site is determined from the intracardiac bipolar electrogram and is measured in relation to the fixed reference electrogram (surface QRS or RV catheter). Display of activation times facilitate comparison of data from nearby sites, overcoming the imprecision of assigned activation times at single points, and permits rapid identification of a putative site of origin in the center of the early activation area. Points are added to the map only if stability criteria in space and local activation time are met. The end-diastolic location stability criterion is less than 2 mm and the local activation time stability criterion is less than 2 milliseconds.

The principles used for conventional activation mapping discussed above are also used here to define the site of

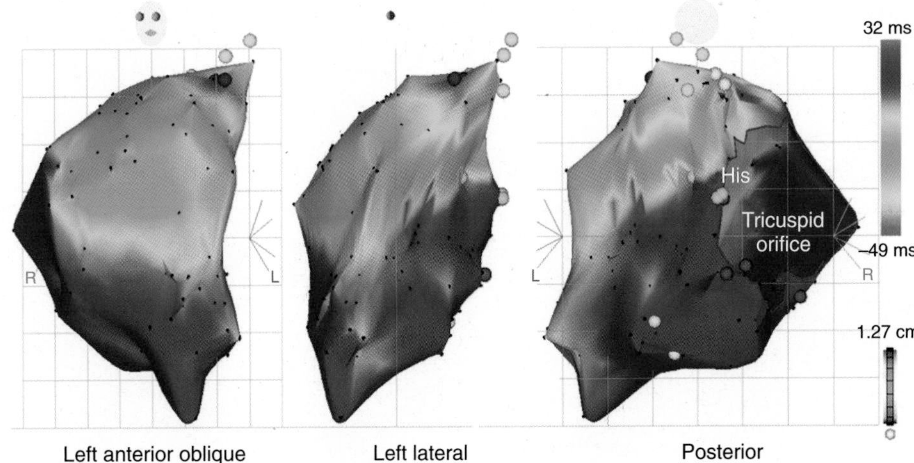

FIGURE 19–10 Electroanatomical (CARTO) maps of right ventricular activation during right ventricular outflow tract (RVOT) ventricular tachycardia. Yellow dots indicate approximate location of pulmonic valve annulus. His bundle location (orange dots) and tricuspid orifice are shown. The site of impulse origin during VT is in the basal superior leftward aspect of the RVOT (red area) at which ablation eliminated VT (red dots).

origin of VT. Although the traditional single-catheter mapping of the region of interest is still required, the ability to use the catheter localization system to steer precisely back to previously obtained sites of earliest activation greatly facilitates the ablation process. The activation map can also be used to catalogue sites at which pacing maneuvers are performed during assessment of the tachycardia (e.g., sites with good pace map).

Noncontact Mapping

When VT is scarcely inducible, simultaneous multisite data acquisition (basket catheter or noncontact mapping system) can help mapping the VT focus. More detailed mapping, however, is necessary to find the precise site to ablate.[19,36]

The EnSite 3000 noncontact mapping system (Endocardial Solutions, St. Paul, Minn) consists of a noncontact catheter (9 Fr) with a multielectrode array surrounding a 7.5-mL balloon mounted at the distal end. The system is able to reconstruct more than 3000 unipolar electrograms simultaneously and superimpose them onto the virtual endocardium, producing isopotential maps with a color range representing voltage amplitude (Fig. 19-11). Electrical potentials at the endocardial surface some distance away are calculated. Sites of early endocardial activity, which are likely adjacent to the VT focus, are usually identifiable.

To create a map, the balloon catheter is positioned over a 0.035-inch guidewire under fluoroscopy guidance in the RV. The balloon is then deployed; it can be filled with contrast dye, permitting it to be visualized fluoroscopically (see Fig. 19-11). Systemic anticoagulation is critical to prevent thromboembolic complications; intravenous heparin is usually administered to maintain the activated clotting time (ACT) at 250 to 300 seconds. A conventional (roving) deflectable mapping catheter is also positioned in the RVOT and used to collect geometry information. The tricuspid annulus, HB, and pulmonic valve are initially tagged and a detailed geometry of the RV and RVOT is reconstructed by moving the mapping catheter around the RV. Once the chamber geometry has been delineated, the tachycardia is induced, and mapping can begin. The data acquisition process is performed automatically by the system, and all data for the entire chamber are acquired simultaneously. Following this, the segment must be analyzed by the operator to find the site with early activation.

The system reconstructs over 3360 electrograms simultaneously over a computer-generated model of the RV ("virtual" endocardium) in an isochronal or isopotential mode. Color-coded isopotential maps are used to depict regions that are depolarized graphically, and wavefront propagation is displayed as a user-controlled 3-D movie

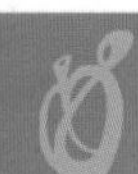

19

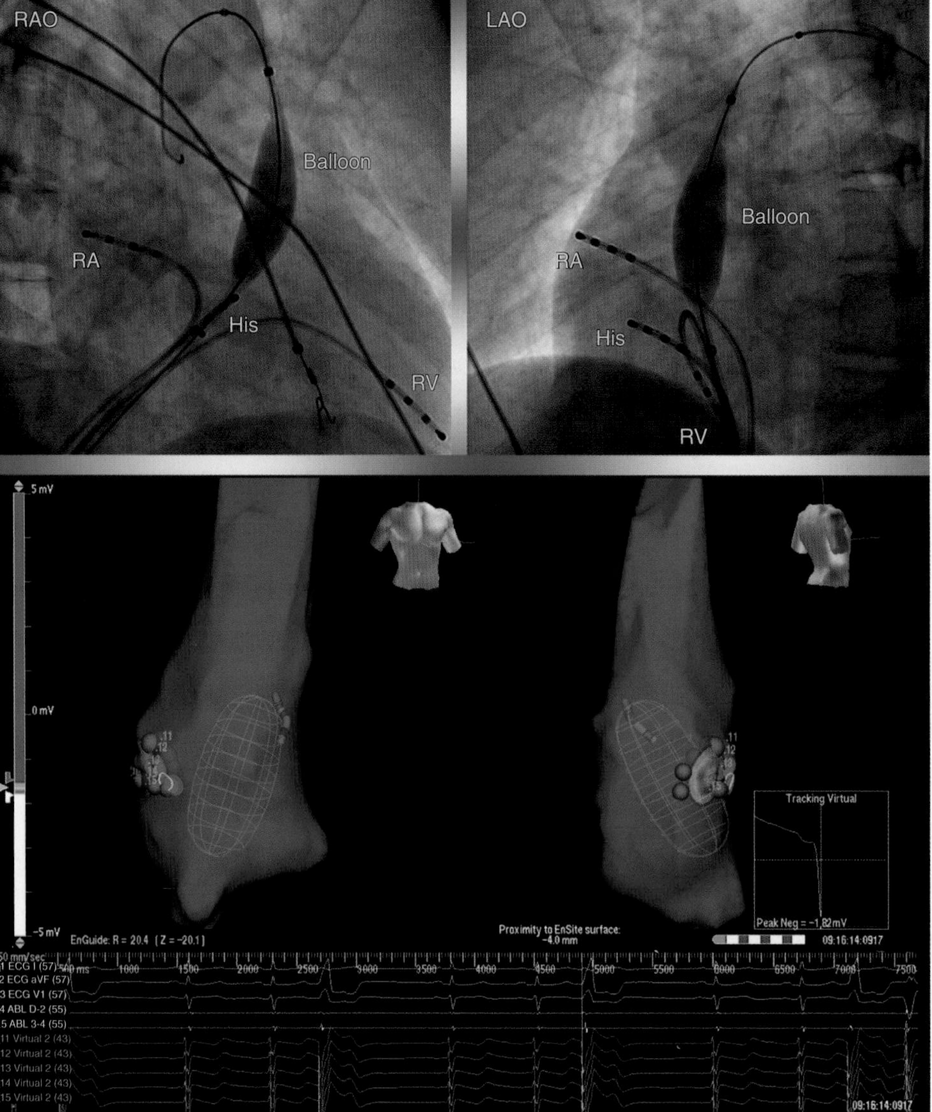

FIGURE 19–11 Noncontact mapping of idiopathic right ventricular outflow tract (RVOT) ventricular tachycardia. **Upper panel,** Fluoroscopic (right anterior oblique [RAO] and left anterior oblique [LAO]) views of the EnSite balloon catheter positioned in the RVOT. **Middle panel,** Color-coded isopotential map of RVOT activation during a single premature ventricular complex (PVC). The inset shows a virtual electrogram at the site of earliest activation (note QS pattern). Red dots indicate radiofrequency applications. Further detailed mapping using a standard mapping catheter localized the PVC focus to a site adjacent to the site, with the earliest local activation identified by the balloon catheter. **Lower panel,** Surface ECG and intracardiac contact (ABL) and virtual noncontact (green) electrograms are shown during mapping of PVCs. *(Courtesy of Dr. James Mullin, Prairie Cardiovascular Consultants, Springfield, Ill).*

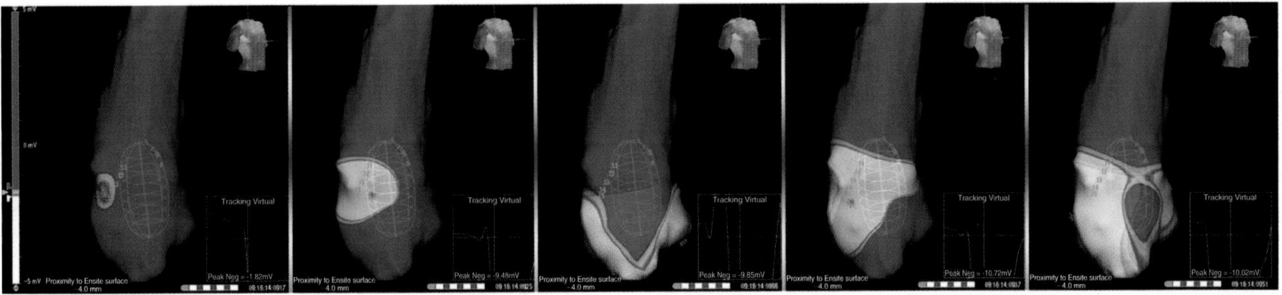

FIGURE 19–12 Noncontact color-coded propagation maps during a premature ventricular complex (PVC) originating from the right ventricular outflow tract. Wavefront propagation spreads radially from a small focus (from left to right). The inset shows a virtual electrogram with the bar indicating the timing of activation during the PVC.

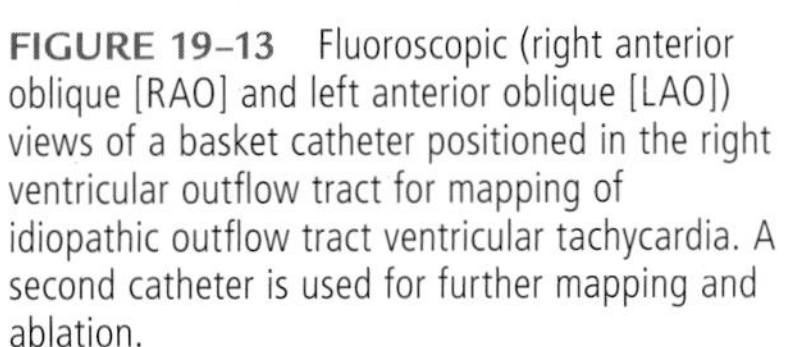
FIGURE 19–13 Fluoroscopic (right anterior oblique [RAO] and left anterior oblique [LAO]) views of a basket catheter positioned in the right ventricular outflow tract for mapping of idiopathic outflow tract ventricular tachycardia. A second catheter is used for further mapping and ablation.

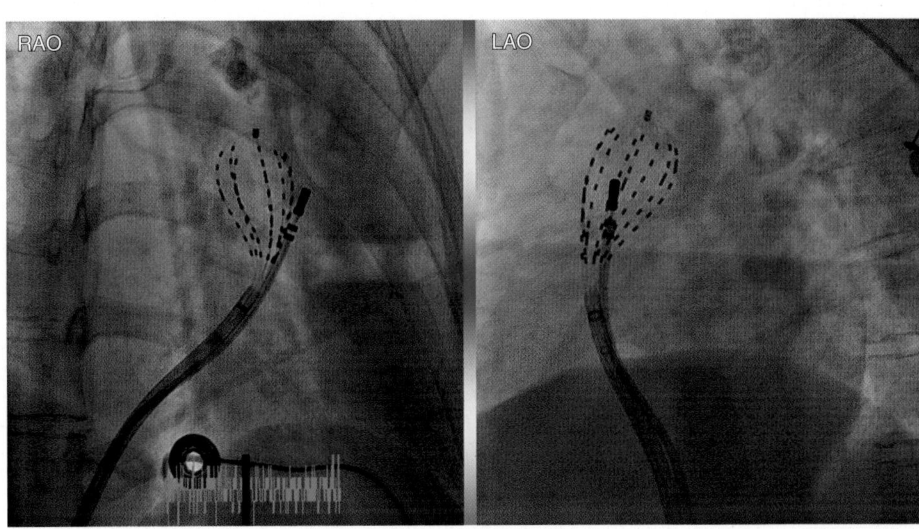

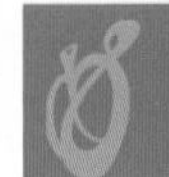

(Fig. 19-12). The color range represents voltage or timing of onset. The highest chamber voltage is at the site of origin of the electrical impulse. Additionally, the system can simultaneously display as many as 32 electrograms as waveforms. Unipolar or bipolar electrograms (virtual electrograms) can be selected at any given interval of the tachycardia cycle using the mouse from any part of the created geometry and displayed as waveforms as if from point, array, or plaque.

Although noncontact mapping can rapidly identify VT foci, a second catheter is still required for precise localization of the target site and delivery of RF energy. Thus, noncontact mapping helps identify starting points for conventional activation mappsing. Additionally, manipulation of the array into the RVOT can be difficult and contact of some portions of the area with myocardium may induce PVCs that appear similar to clinical PVCs or VT.

Basket Catheter Mapping

This mapping catheter consists of an open-lumen catheter shaft with a collapsible, basket-shaped distal end, which is composed of 64 electrodes mounted on eight flexible, self-expanding, equidistant metallic splines (each spline carrying eight ring electrodes; see Fig. 2-4). The electrodes are equally spaced 4 or 5 mm apart, depending on the size of the basket catheter used (with diameters of 48 or 60 mm, respectively). Each spline is identified by a letter (from A to H) and each electrode by a number (from 1 to 8), with electrode 1 having the distal position on the splines.[37]

The size of the RV is initially evaluated (usually with echocardiography) to help select the appropriate size of the basket catheter. The collapsed basket catheter is advanced under fluoroscopy guidance through an 11 Fr long sheath into the RV; the basket is then expanded. After basket catheter deployment, the conventional catheters are introduced and positioned in standard positions (Fig. 19-13). Several observations can help determine electrical-anatomical relations, including fluoroscopically identifiable markers (spline A has one marker and spline B has two markers located near the shaft of the basket catheter) and electrical signals recorded from certain electrodes (e.g., ventricular, atrial, or HB electrograms), which can help identify the location of those particular splines.

From the 64 electrodes, 64 unipolar signals and 32 to 56 bipolar signals can be recorded, by combining 1-2, 3-4, 5-6, 7-8, or 1-2, 2-3 until 7-8 electrodes are on each spline. The color-coded animation images simplify the analysis of multielectrode recordings and help in establishing the relation between activation patterns and anatomical structures. The degree of resolution is lower than that in 3-D mapping systems but appears satisfactory for clinical purposes.

The concepts of activation mapping discussed are then used to determine the site of origin of the tachycardia. The ablation catheter is placed in the region of earliest activity and is used for more detailed mapping of the site of origin of the VT. The Astronomer navigation system permits precise and reproducible guidance of the ablation catheter tip electrode to targets identified by the basket catheter. Without the use of this navigation system, it can be difficult to identify the alphabetical order of the splines by fluoroscopy guidance. The capacity of pacing from most basket electrodes allows the evaluation of activation patterns and pace mapping.

Basket catheter mapping has several limitations. Most basket catheters are difficult, if not impossible, to steer; thus, positioning in the RVOT can be challenging. In addition, firm contact with the tip of the basket and RVOT myocardium can induce ectopic complexes that mimic spontaneous VT or PVCs. A second catheter is still required to be manipulated to the site identified for more precise localization of the target for ablation as well as RF energy delivery.

Ablation

Target of Ablation

The ablation target site is defined as the site where the earliest endocardial activation time during VT or PVCs and exact or best pace map matches can be obtained.[22,38] Activation mapping and pace mapping are highly correlated techniques and both methods are typically used to select ablation sites—the more confirmatory information, the more likely the site of origin will fall within the range of the RF lesion produced (see Fig. 19-8).[34] There is little evidence to support the widely held notion that pace mapping provides superior spatial resolution for localizing idiopathic outflow tract VT.[34]

Ablation Technique

Ventricular Tachycardias Originating in the Right *Ventricular Outflow Tract.* The mapping-ablation catheter is initially positioned in the proximal pulmonary artery and slowly withdrawn into the RVOT until the first local endocardial electrogram is recorded. This site is just below the pulmonic valve, and is at the level where most RVOT VTs originate.[4,6] It is important to avoid trying to advance the catheter when its tip is perpendicular to the RVOT, because this can result in perforation and cardiac tamponade. Torque is applied to the catheter for circumferential mapping of the RVOT within 1 cm of the pulmonic valve, with a minimum of four sites (anterior and posterior septal, and anterior and posterior free wall, as determined by fluoroscopy). The plane of the septum in the LAO view is nearly perpendicular to the imaging plane. Delineating the boundaries within which mapping will be carried out is useful, rather than discovering after several minutes of mapping that more tissue lay in one direction or another from where efforts had previously been concentrated.

A catheter positioned at the proximal HB and/or midanterior septum helps in accurate localization, because septal sites are almost always within the same vertical plane or further rightward relative to these catheter positions in the LAO view. Based on the results of activation and pace mapping at these initial sites, and guided by surface QRS morphology, attention is then directed to sites of early activation and best pace map matches. If very thorough mapping in the RVOT fails to localize the VT site of origin, mapping is extended into the pulmonary artery.

Some physicians prefer to use a two-catheter leapfrog method. The catheter associated with the best pace map and activation time is left in place and a second catheter is used to explore the surrounding area. Once a site with better characteristics is located, the roving catheter is left in place and the initial catheter is used for the next step in mapping.

Ventricular Tachycardias Originating in the Left Ventricular Outflow Tract and Aortic Cusps. If very thorough mapping and ablation in the RVOT and pulmonary artery fail to localize or terminate the tachycardia, the femoral artery is cannulated and the ablation catheter is advanced into the aorta and prolapsed into the LV. The catheter is carefully manipulated in the LVOT and in the aortic root above the cusps of the aortic valve and in the region of the sinuses of Valsalva until an early ventricular electrogram is recorded and pace mapping shows a QRS identical to the clinical VT morphology. Pace mapping at these sites often requires high output pacing. Other parts of the LV can occasionally harbor the focus of the VT (Fig. 19-14).

In some VTs originating from the aortic cusps, a preferential conduction to the RVOT may render pace mapping less reliable. Therefore, when the local ventricular activation does not precede the QRS onset of the VT or PVCs adequately or RF ablation is not effective in the RVOT, despite obtaining a good pace map, mapping of the aortic cusp should be considered. On the other hand, in a recent report, 27% of patients with VTs with an aortic cusp origin had the local ventricular activation in the RVOT preceding the QRS onset of the VT or PVCs adequately.[30] Therefore, when a good pace map is not obtained or RF ablation is not effective in the RVOT, despite the fact that local ventricular activation adequately precedes the QRS onset of the VT or PVCs, mapping of the aortic cusp should be considered.[30,39]

When the earliest ventricular activation is identified in an aortic cusp, it is preferable to insert a 5 Fr pigtail catheter into the aortic root through the left femoral artery. The aortic root and the ostia of the right coronary artery and left main coronary artery are visualized by aortic root angiography.[12-15,17,19,28] If the origin of VT is in the left coronary cusp, it is preferable to cannulate the left main coronary artery with a 5 Fr left Judkin's catheter, which serves as a marker and for protection of the left main coronary artery in case of ablation catheter dislodgment during RF applica-

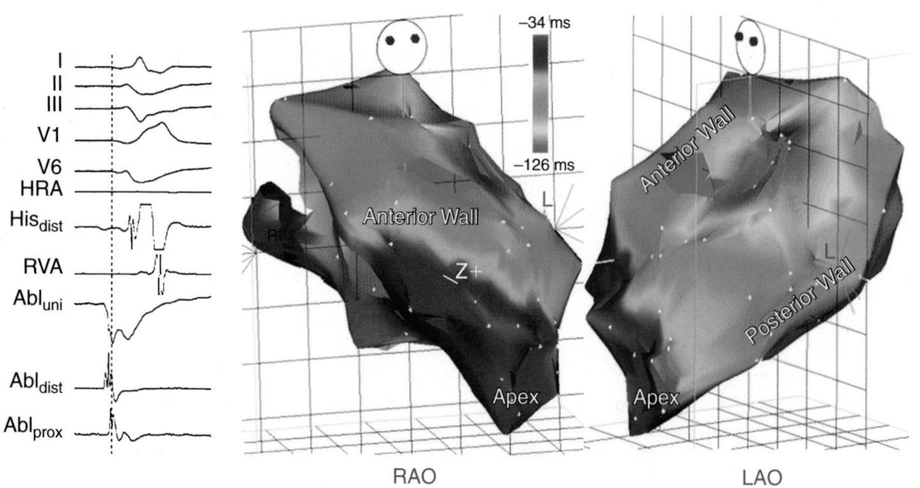

FIGURE 19–14 Focal left ventricle ventricular tachycardia (LV VT)—intracardiac recordings during VT and electroanatomical map of focal anterior wall LV VT. Note electrogram features of focality (QS on unipolar and slight presystolic timing of unipolar and bipolar electrograms during VT) as well as centrifugal spread of activation on the color map.

tion. Atrial electrograms often accompany ventricular potentials because the right and left coronary sinuses are in close proximity to the RA and LA appendages, respectively. Several other measures must be taken to avoid injuring the coronary arteries. RF energy delivery in the aorta should be started at a low power output (15 W), which can be increased to no more than 25 W to achieve a target temperature of approximately 55°C. Ablation should also be performed during continuous fluoroscopy to observe for catheter dislodgment, and energy delivery should be discontinued in case of even minimal dislodgment from the site showing the best mapping findings. RF application should also be stopped if the repetitive or sustained VT cannot be terminated after 10 seconds. Coronary angiography is often performed immediately after the ablative procedure to exclude coronary artery spasm, dissection, or thrombus.

Ablation of Epicardial Ventricular Tachycardias

Percutaneous Epicardial Mapping. Under a 15-degree LAO view, an 8.9-cm, 17-gauge epidural needle is gently advanced into the left subxyphoid region, with intermittent injection of a small amount of contrast material. Entry into the epicardial space is verified by injection of contrast showing characteristic layering in the epicardial space. A floppy guidewire is advanced through the needle and the position of the guidewire in the epicardial space is confirmed. An 8 Fr vascular sheath is advanced over the wire, through which a 7 Fr, 4-mm-tip deflectable catheter is placed in the epicardial space. Mapping of VT is carried out using a 3-D electroanatomical mapping system.[16,19]

Coronary Sinus Epicardial Mapping. Epicardial mapping via the coronary venous system can be achieved with small, flexible, multipolar electrode catheters introduced through a guiding catheter positioned at the coronary sinus ostium (CS os; Fig. 19-15). Before applying RF energy with a catheter in the pericardial space, CS venography and coronary arteriography should be performed to outline the spatial relationship between the target vein and the adjacent coronary artery. After ablation, coronary arteriography should be performed to rule out damage to coronary arteries.[19]

Radiofrequency Delivery. For VTs originating in the ROVT and LVOT, RF catheter ablation is performed during VT or NSR for 60 to 90 seconds with a preset temperature of 60° to 70°C and a power limit of 50 W.[18,19,34,38] For VTs originating in the aortic cusps, RF power setting should be limited to 15 to 25 W (see above).[13-15,17] Rarely, if ever, does one need more than 50 W or use of irrigated or large-tip electrodes to ablate outflow tract VTs successfully. RF delivery at successful ablation sites often can result in a rapid ventricular response (identical QRS morphology to that of VT), followed by gradual slowing and complete resolution (Fig. 19-16). This finding has a high specificity but low sensitivity for successful ablation sites.[4] When RF is delivered during VT, termination of VT at successful sites usually occurs within 10 seconds.

Typically, a few (range, two to eleven; mean, five) RF applications are required. Occasionally, following several RF applications, the first VT morphology is no longer seen

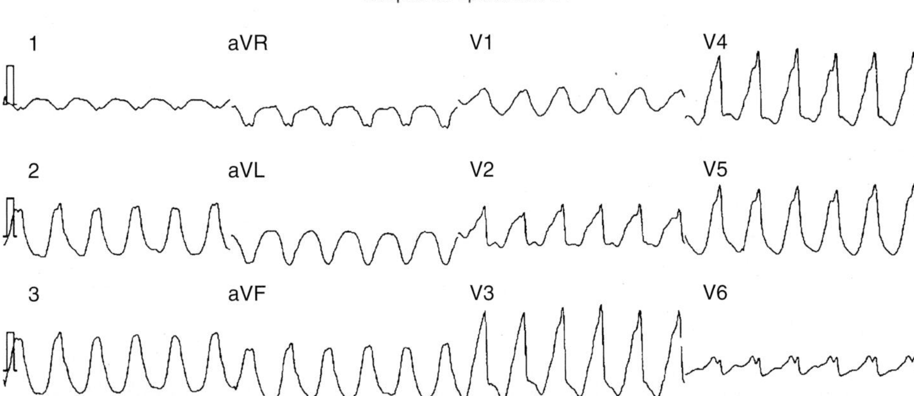

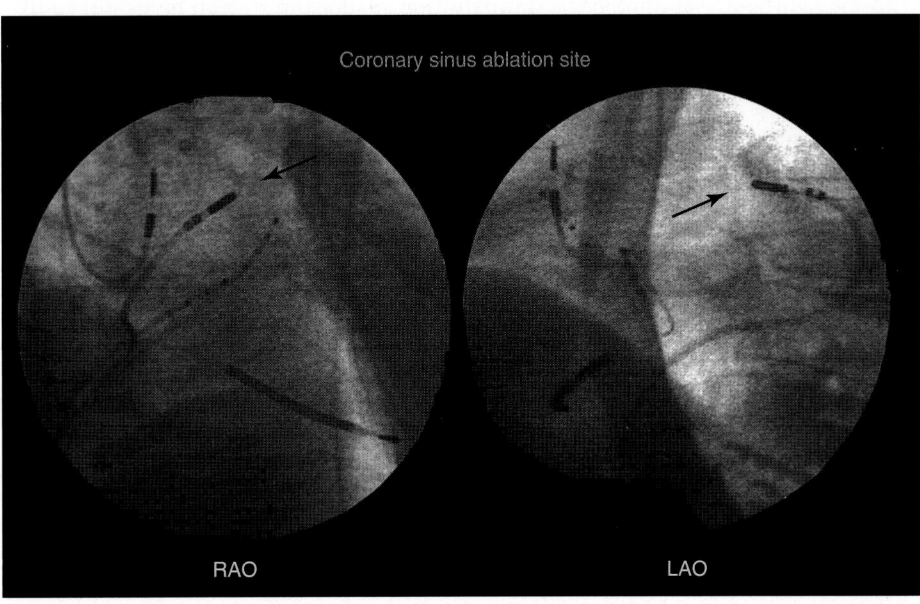

FIGURE 19–15 Idiopathic epicardial ventricular tachycardia (VT). **Top,** Surface ECG of a slow VT that was ablated from the coronary sinus (CS) after both endocardial and epicardial mapping failed to eliminate the VT. **Bottom,** Right anterior oblique (RAO) and left anterior oblique (LAO) fluoroscopic views of catheter location for VT ablation from the CS.

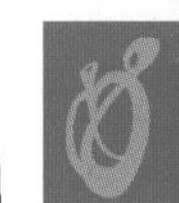

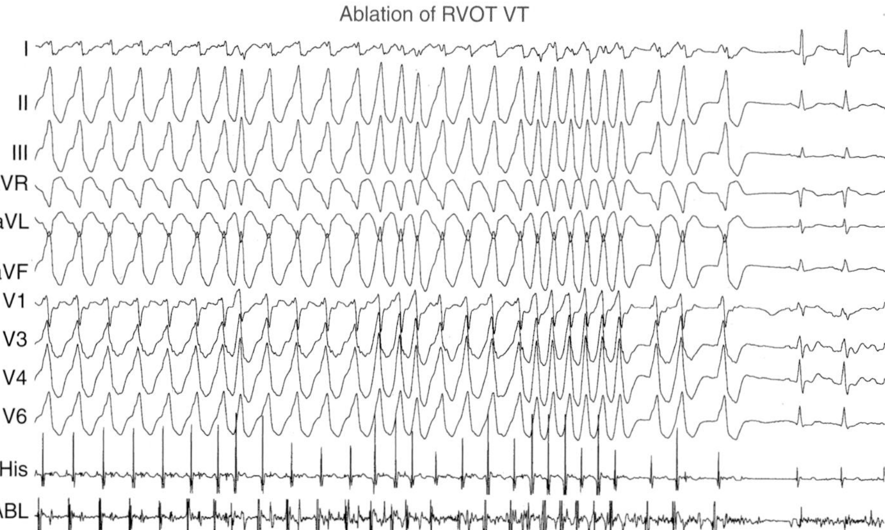

FIGURE 19–16 Ablation of right ventricular outflow tract (RVOT) ventricular tachycardia (VT). Radiofrequency (RF) energy delivery is started during sustained VT. Acceleration of the VT is observed within a few seconds, followed by slowing and termination of the VT.

but a second, similar one is now observed. This can be caused by an actual second focus near the first or modification of the exit site from the first focus. In this situation, ablation within 1 to 2 cm of the first site eliminates the second VT morphology.

Pitfalls of Ablation

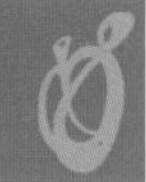

19

Catheter-induced PVCs frequently occur and can closely mimic target PVCs. The findings on the mapping catheter during these catheter-induced complexes are invariably excellent (e.g., substantial presystolic activation time, sharp QS on the unipolar recording). These complexes must be analyzed carefully to avoid delivery of RF energy at sites with no relevance to actual VT. Additionally, if an intracardiac reference ventricular electrogram is used (e.g., with a computerized mapping system), care must be taken to avoid dislodging this catheter, because if it moves, timing of mapping catheter activations will not be comparable to previously mapped sites.

Endpoints of Ablation

Successful ablation is defined as the noninducibility of VT, with and without isoproterenol administration (using the best method for induction documented before ablation), during at least 30 minutes after ablation.

Outcome

The acute success rate is more than 90%. The recurrence rate is approximately 7% to 10%. Of these, 40% recur during the first 24 to 48 hours after the ablation procedure. Recurrence of VT beyond the first year postablation is rare. Predictors of recurrences include poor pace map, late activation at target sites, reliance on pace mapping alone, and termination of VT inducibility with mechanical trauma by the mapping-ablation catheter before RF delivery.

Complications are rare. RBBB develops in 2% and cardiac tamponade is rare. Coronary artery injury and damage to the aortic valve may occur during ablation of LVOT or aortic cusp VTs.

Cryoablation

Initial experience suggests cryocatheter techniques to be a potent tool in treating monomorphic VT originating within the RVOT.[40] A major advantage of cryoablation is the virtual absence of pain, which makes the use of analgesia unnecessary. Moreover, reasonable fluoroscopy and procedure times can be achieved by an experienced investigator. Stability of the catheter during cryoablation can be advantageous because monitoring of catheter position by fluoroscopy is not necessary. Adhesion of the catheter, however, requires precise positioning before the start of cryoablation. Slight dislocations, as may easily occur with breathing, can delay ablation success. Furthermore, brushing of the catheter within a small defined area, as often observed with RF ablations, cannot occur; therefore, repositioning of the catheter to adjust for a dislocation is not possible during cryoablation. The cryocatheter differs substantially in size and rigidity from standard RF catheters and requires some experience in handling.

Complete disappearance of the arrhythmia is typically observed within 20 seconds of cryoablation. Therefore, cryoablation is stopped after 60 seconds if no positive effect is observed.

Given the high success rate and low risk of RF ablation of RVOT VT, it may be difficult to demonstrate a clinical advantage of cryoablation over RF ablation. Cryoablation can be useful in difficult or atypical sites when a maximal stability of the catheter is necessary—for example, to avoid dislodgment of the catheter into the coronary arteries during ablation of idiopathic VT originating from the aortic cusps. Also, the absence of pain during ablation may render the procedure more comfortable for the patient, especially when the use of sedative medications suppresses inducibility of the VT.

VERAPAMIL-SENSITIVE (FASCICULAR) VENTRICULAR TACHCYARDIA

Pathophysiology

Verapamil-sensitive LV VT is a reentrant tachycardia. The diagnosis of reentry as the mechanism of fascicular VT is supported by several observations. The VT can reproducibly be initiated and terminated by programmed electrical stimulation, entrainment and resetting with fusion can be demonstrated, and an inverse relationship between the coupling interval of the initiating VES or ventricular pacing CL and the first VT beat can be observed.

The exact nature of the reentry circuit in verapamil-sensitive LV VT has provoked considerable interest. Some investigators have suggested that it is a microreentry circuit in the territory of the left posterior fascicle (LPF). Others have suggested that the circuit is confined to the Purkinje system, which is insulated from the underlying ventricular myocardium. False tendons or fibromuscular bands that extend from the posteroinferior LV to the basal septum have also been implicated in the anatomical substrate of this tachycardia.

Currently, overwhelming evidence suggests that the VT is caused by a reentrant circuit confined to the posterior Purkinje system with an excitable gap and a slow conduction area.[4,28,41,42] The VT substrate can be a small macroreentrant circuit consisting of the LPF serving as one limb and abnormal Purkinje tissue with slow, decremental conduction serving as the other limb. The entrance site to the slow conduction zone is thought to be located closer to the base of the LV septum. The exit site (site of earliest ventricular activation) is located in the inferoposterior aspect of the LV septum (the region of the LPF) closer to the apex. The retrograde limb consists of Purkinje tissue from or contiguous to the LPF, which gives rise to the Purkinje potentials. The anterograde limb of the circuit appears to be composed of abnormal Purkinje tissue, which exhibits slow, decremental conduction, is verapamil-sensitive, gives rise to the late diastolic potentials along the midseptum, and appears to be insulated from the nearby ventricular myocardium (Fig. 19-17). The anterograde limb may be associated with longitudinal dissociation of the LPF or contiguous tissue that is directly coupled to the LPF (such as a false tendon) or, alternatively, has ventricular myocardium interposed. The zone of slow conduction appears to depend on the slow inward calcium current, because the degree of slowing of tachycardia CL in response to verapamil is entirely attributed to its negative dromotropic effects on the area of slow conduction.

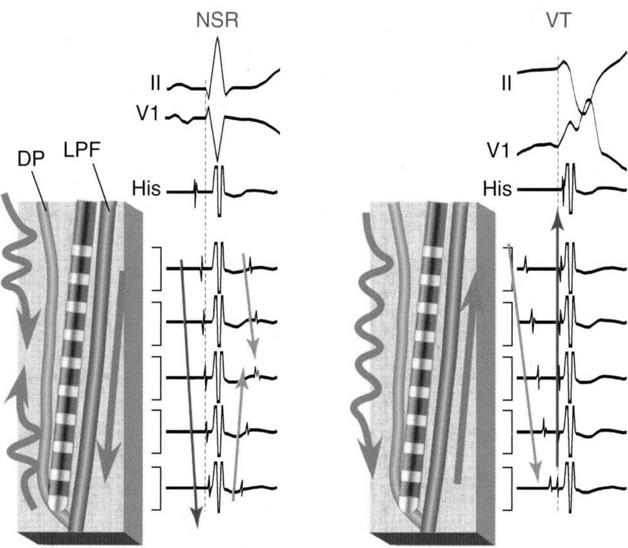

FIGURE 19–17 Schematic illustration of the reentrant circuit in verapamil-sensitive left ventricular tachycardia (LV VT). A block of the LV septum is depicted with the left posterior fascicle (LPF) and diastolic pathway (DP) running in parallel till they intersect at bottom. A 10-pole catheter is shown as recording between pathways; electrograms from each pair are shown along with surface ECG leads and His bundle recordings. **Left panel,** A sinus rhythm complex is shown; dashed line denotes QRS onset. Note the direction and speed of propagation over the LPF while the DP is activated after the QRS and in both directions (arrows). **Right panel,** During a VT complex, the DP is activated anterogradely and the LPF retrogradely (arrows). NSR = normal sinus rhythm. See text for discussion.

Clinical Considerations

Epidemiology

Age at presentation is typically 15 to 40 years (unusual after 55 years).[43] Males are more commonly affected (60% to 80%).[4,43] Fascicular VT is the most common form of idiopathic LV VT, and it accounts for 10% to 15% of idiopathic VTs.

Clinical Presentation

Most patients present with mild to moderate symptoms of palpitations and lightheadedness. Occasionally, symptoms are debilitating. The clinical course is benign and the prognosis is excellent. Sudden cardiac death is rare. Spontaneous remission of the VT may occur with time.

Initial Evaluation

Diagnostic features of fascicular VT include induction with atrial pacing, RBBB with left (or, less commonly, right) axis deviation, structurally normal heart, and verapamil sensitivity. Evaluation to exclude structural heart disease is necessary and typically includes echocardiographic examination, stress test, and/or cardiac catheterization, depending on patient age and risk factors.

Principles of Management

Acute Management. Intravenous verapamil is typically successful in terminating the VT. Termination with adenosine is rare, except for patients in whom isoproterenol is used for induction of the tachycardia in the EP laboratory.

Chronic Management. Long-term therapy with verapamil is useful in mild cases; however, it has little effect in patients with severe symptoms. RF ablation is highly effective (85% to 90%) and is recommended for patients with severe symptoms.

Electrocardiographic Features

ECG During Normal Sinus Rhythm. The resting ECG is usually normal. Symmetrical, inferolateral T wave inversion can be present after termination of the VT.

ECG During Ventricular Tachycardia. The QRS during VT has RBBB with left anterior fascicular (LAF) block or, less commonly (5% to 10%), LPF block pattern. The R/S ratio is less than 1 in leads V_1 and V_2 (Fig. 19-18).[41] VTs arising more toward the middle at the region of the posterior papillary muscle have a left superior axis and RS in leads V_5 and V_6, whereas those arising closer to the apex have a right superior axis with a tiny "r" and deep S (or even QS) in leads V_5 and V_6. QRS duration is 140 milliseconds, and

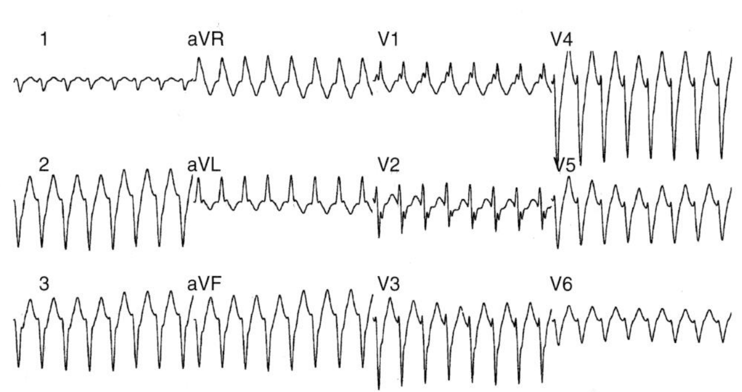

FIGURE 19–18 Surface ECGs of verapamil-sensitive left ventricular tachycardia. Note the right bundle branch block and left anterior fascicle block pattern characteristic of these VTs.

RS duration is 60 to 80 milliseconds; thus, the VT is frequently called fascicular VT. The VT rate is approximately 150 to 200 beats/min (range, 120 to 250 beats/min). Alternans in the CL is frequently noted during the VT; otherwise, the VT rate is stable.

The VT is paroxysmal, occurs with a precipitating factor, and can last for minutes to hours. Occasionally, the VT can be incessant, may be sustained for a long period (days), and does not revert spontaneously to NSR.[44]

Electrophysiological Testing

Induction of Tachycardia

The programmed electrical stimulation protocol used is similar to that used for adenosine-sensitive VT. VT can usually be initiated with atrial extrastimulation (AES), VES, atrial pacing, or ventricular pacing. Often, isoproterenol, alone or during concurrent programmed stimulation, facilitates induction. An inverse relationship is observed between the coupling interval of the initiating VES or ventricular pacing CL and the first VT beat.

Tachycardia Features

Site of Earliest Ventricular Activation. The site of earliest ventricular activation during VT is in the region of the LPF (inferoposterior LV septum) in 90% to 95% of LV VTs (explaining the RBBB–superior axis configuration of the QRS), and in the region of the LAF (anterosuperior LV septum) in 5% to 10% of LV VTs (explaining the RBBB–right axis configuration of the QRS). In most cases, ventricular electrograms are discrete during both NSR and VT. The HB is not a component of the reentrant circuit, because a retrograde His potential is often recorded 20 to 40 milliseconds after the earliest ventricular activation (Fig. 19-19).

Purkinje Potential. The Purkinje potential (PP) is a discrete, high-frequency potential that precedes the site of earliest ventricular activation by 15 to 42 milliseconds and is recorded in the posterior third of the LV septum during VT and NSR (Fig. 19-20; see also Fig. 19-19).[28,41,42] Because this potential also precedes ventricular activation during NSR, it is believed to originate from activation of a segment of the LPF, and to represent the exit site of the reentrant circuit.

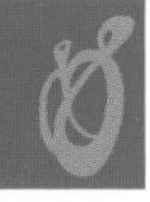

19

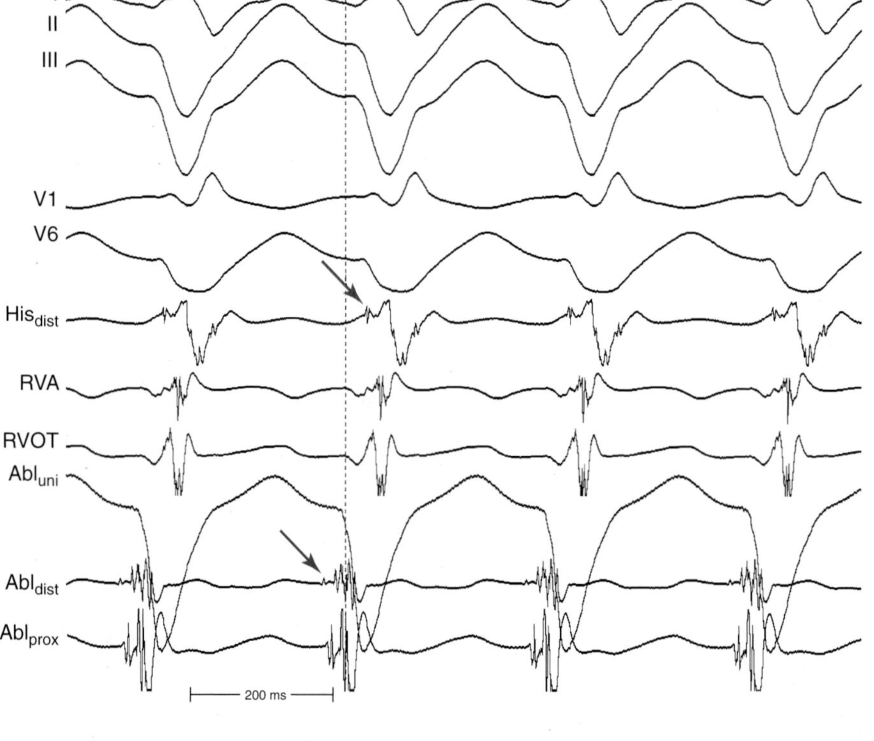

FIGURE 19–19 Idiopathic (fascicular) left ventricular tachycardia. The blue arrow shows late diastolic small potential, 45 msec prior to QRS onset. Distinct Purkinje-like potentials (*blue arrow*) are evident before the dotted line denoting QRS onset, as well as in the proximal ablation electrogram. The red arrow indicates retrograde His potential. Note the unipolar QS configuration just coinciding with QRS onset.

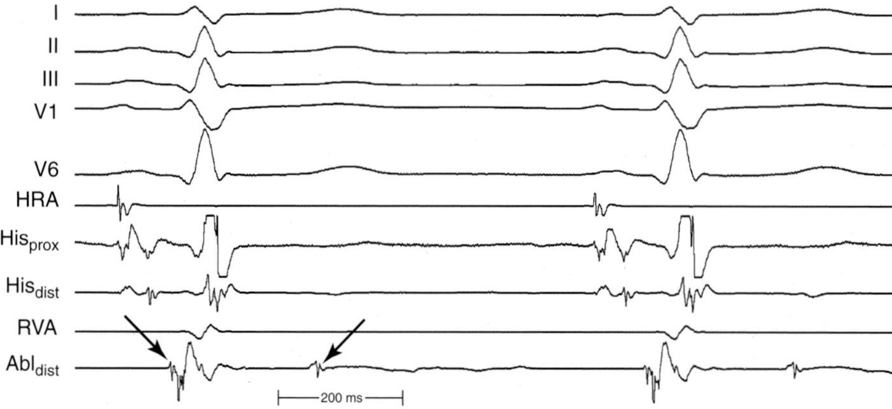

FIGURE 19–20 Sinus rhythm recordings at successful ablation site for idiopathic (fascicular) left ventricular tachycardia. The left arrow points to a Purkinje-like potential just prior to the local electrogram (also slightly preceding the onset of the QRS); the right arrow shows a sharp, delayed diastolic potential, purportedly from the slow-conducting limb of the circuit.

Late Diastolic Potential. The late diastolic potential (LDP) is a discrete potential that precedes the PP during VT, and is recorded at the basal, middle, or apical septum. The LDP is thought to originate from activation at the entrance to the abnormal Purkinje tissue that is thought to serve as the anterograde limb of the reentrant circuit.[28,41,42] The LDP differs in shape from the PP and has a relatively small amplitude and low-frequency component. The area with LDP recording is confined to a small region (0.5 to 1.0 cm^2) and is included in the larger area where the PP is recorded (2 to 3 cm^2). The LDP often is recorded simultaneously with the PP by the same electrode. The relative activation times of the LDP, PP, and local ventricular potential at the LDP recording site to the onset of QRS complex are −50.4 ± 18.9, −15.2 ± 9.6, and 3.0 ± 13.3 milliseconds, respectively (see Fig. 19-19). The earliest ventricular activation site (exit) during VT is identified at the posteroapical septum and is more apical in the septum than the region with LDP.[28]

Ventricular Activation Sequence. During NSR, conduction propagates anterogradely (proximal to distal or basal to apical) and rapidly down the LPF, generating an anterograde PP and followed by ventricular activation (see Fig. 19-17). In parallel, the impulse slowly conducts anterogradely over the abnormal Purkinje tissue, and such slow conduction and/or block in the proximal segment allows the wavefront traveling down the LPF to conduct retrogradely up the slow pathway, resulting in fusion of delayed (late) ascending and descending potentials that follow or are buried in local ventricular depolarization, which likely represent the LDPs recorded during VT (see Fig. 19-20). Those late potentials have been found only in patients with idiopathic LV VT and not in control, and have been recorded in the midinferior septum within or contiguous to the LPF.[28,41]

During ventricular pacing, the LPF is activated retrogradely generating a retrograde PP. In parallel, the impulse produces bidirectional activation of the abnormal Purkinje pathway in a manner similar to, but in reverse direction of that during NSR.[4]

During VT, activation propagates retrogradely (distal to proximal) over the LPF, generating a retrograde PP, and subsequently propagates anterogradely over the abnormal Purkinje tissue, producing an anterograde LDP. Thus, both limbs are activated in series (in contrast to NSR and ventricular pacing; see Fig. 19-17).[28,41] For a VES to initiate VT, retrograde block has to occur in the abnormal Purkinje tissue with retrograde conduction of the wavefront up the LPF (generating a retrograde PP) with some delay, and then down the abnormal Purkinje tissue (generating an anterograde LDP) to initiate reentry. Thus, during VT, the LDP precedes PP, which in turn precedes ventricular activation.

Response to Pharmacological and Physiological Maneuvers. Intravenous verapamil slows the rate of VT progressively and then terminates it. Diltiazem is equally effective. Nonsustained VT may continue to occur for a while after termination. VT is usually rendered noninducible after verapamil. Verapamil significantly prolongs the VT CL, LDP-PP interval, and PP-LDP interval during VT. However, the interval from PP to the onset of the QRS complex remains unchanged.[41,44]

Response of VT to lidocaine, procainamide, amiodarone, sotalol, and propranolol is less consistent, and these drugs are usually ineffective. Carotid sinus massage and Valsalva maneuvers have no effect on the VT. Fascicular VT is unresponsive to adenosine; however, when catecholamine stimulation (isoproterenol infusion) is required for the initiation of VT, the VT can become adenosine-sensitive.

Diagnostic Maneuvers During Tachycardia

Entrainment. Ventricular pacing can entrain the VT with antidromic or orthodromic capture.[28,41] Manifest entrainment is more frequently achieved when pacing is performed from the RVOT, because the RVOT is closer to the entrance site of the area of slow conduction in the reentrant circuit, located near the base of the LV septum. On the other hand, pacing from the RV apex is less likely to demonstrate entrainment and, when it does, it is unlikely to demonstrate manifest fusion because of the distance from the entrance site of the circuit and because of the narrow excitable gap of the reentrant circuit. During entrainment, the LDP (representing the entrance of the circuit) is orthodromically captured and, as the pacing rate is increased, the LDP-PP interval (representing an area of decremental Purkinje tissue) prolongs, whereas the stimulus-to-LDP and PP-V intervals typically remain constant. Entrainment can usually be demonstrated with ventricular pacing at a CL approximately 10 to 30 milliseconds shorter than the tachycardia CL.[4,28,41] Analysis of entrainment from different ventricular sites helps identify the relationship of those sites to the VT circuit (Table 19-2).

Resetting. VT can be reset with VES, with an increasing or mixed resetting response (characteristic of reentrant circuit with an excitable gap).[41]

Termination. VT can be reproducibly terminated with programmed electrical stimulation.[41]

Exclusion of Other Arrhythmia Mechanisms

The differential diagnosis of idiopathic LV VT should include interfascicular VT, which has several characteristic features: (1) bifascicular block QRS morphology during VT, which is identical to that during NSR; (2) reversal of activation sequence of HB and left bundle branch (LB) during VT; and (3) spontaneous oscillations in the VT CL caused by changes in the LB-LB interval that precede and drive the

TABLE 19–2 Entrainment Mapping of Verapamil-Sensitive Left Ventricle Ventricular Tachycardia

Pacing from Sites Outside VT Circuit (RV Apex or RVOT)
Manifest ventricular fusion on the surface ECG (fixed fusion at a single pacing CL and progressive fusion on progressively shorter pacing CLs) or fully paced QRS morphology
PPI – VT CL > 30 msec
Interval between stimulus artifact to onset of QRS on surface ECG > interval between local ventricular electrogram on pacing lead to onset of QRS on surface ECG
Pacing from Sites Inside VT Circuit (Posteroinferior LV Septum)
Manifest ventricular fusion on the surface ECG (fixed fusion at a single pacing CL and progressive fusion on progressively shorter pacing CLs).
PPI – VT CL < 30 msec
Interval between stimulus artifact to onset of QRS on surface ECG = interval between local ventricular electrogram on pacing lead to onset of QRS on surface ECG
Pacing from Protected Isthmus Inside VT circuit (Site Where Both PP and LDP are Recorded)
Concealed ventricular fusion (i.e., paced QRS is identical to the VT QRS)
PPI – VT CL < 30 msec
Interval between stimulus artifact to onset of QRS on surface ECG = interval between PP to onset of QRS on surface ECG
Stimulus-to-LDP interval is long and LDP is orthodromically captured from proximal to distal sites during activation

CL = cycle length; LDP = late diastolic potential; PP = Purkinje potential; PPI = post-pacing interval; RV = right ventricle; RVOT = right ventricular outflow tract; VT = ventricular tachycardia.

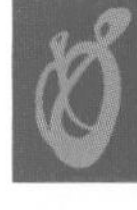

VT CL. Interfascicular VT terminates with VES or RF ablation that produces block in LAF or LPF.

When fascicular VT is associated with 1:1 VA conduction and, because of its responsiveness to verapamil and inducibility by atrial pacing, SVT with bifascicular block aberrancy can be misdiagnosed. The HV interval during SVT with aberrancy is equal to or slightly longer than that during NSR. In contrast, the HV interval during fascicular VT is negative or shorter than that during NSR. Furthermore, the HB is activated in an anterograde direction during SVT but in a retrograde direction during fascicular VT.

Ablation

Target of Ablation

Definition of the appropriate ablation target has evolved with better understanding of the anatomical substrate of the VT. Initially, the ablation target site was defined as the site where the best pace map and the earliest endocardial ventricular activation time could be obtained during VT.[1] Subsequently, in combination with pace mapping, the earliest PP, which likely represents LPF potential and VT circuit exit site, during VT was reported to be a marker for successful ablation, because the site of this potential is believed to be the exit site of the reentrant circuit. Successful ablation is achieved at sites where PP is recorded 30 to 40 milliseconds before QRS onset (Fig. 19-21). More recently, the LDP, which likely reflects the excitation within the critical slow conduction area participating in the reentry circuit, recorded during VT has been reported to be a useful marker in guiding successful ablation.[28,41,42]

Currently, ablation is targeted to a site over the middle or inferoapical portion of the LV septum where the earliest PP and LDP are recorded (Fig. 19-22). Verification of these sites can be achieved with entrainment mapping demonstrating concealed fusion and progressive prolongation of the LDP-PP interval with increasing pacing rate.[28] In addition, pressure applied to the catheter tip at the LDP region occasionally results in VT termination with conduction block between LDP and PP. Pace mapping can also be used as an adjunct to verify this site.

19

It is important to recognize that successful ablation is not necessarily predicted by targeting the earliest (most proximal) LDP. Success can actually be achieved by ablating an LDP distal to the earliest potential. This approach helps reduce the risk of damaging the trunk of the LB.[28] If such an LDP cannot be detected, the site with the earliest ventricular activation with a fused PP may then be targeted.[41]

Ablation Technique

It is helpful to initiate the VT reproducibly prior to entering the LV; if VT is not inducible, LV mapping may not be warranted. If VT can be readily initiated before but not after entering the LV, a portion of the circuit has probably been traumatized and one should wait several minutes and try to reinitiate before mapping any further.

Ablation is performed through the retrograde transaortic approach using a deflectable 4-mm-tip catheter. The catheter is advanced by prolapsing into the LV and directed to the LV septum. Mapping is initially concentrated at the inferoapical septum. If an ideal site is not found in this area, the ablation catheter is then moved upward to the midseptal area. It is important to move the catheter slowly and carefully to avoid mechanical trauma to the circuit. Endocardial activation mapping and entrainment mapping are performed to define the target site of ablation.

Once the target site is identified, a test RF current is applied for 20 seconds with an initial power of 20 to 35 W, targeting a temperature of 60°C.[41,45] If the VT is terminated or slowed within 15 seconds, additional current is applied for another 60 to 120 seconds and power is increased up to 40 W to reach the target temperature if necessary. If the test RF current is ineffective despite adequate catheter contact,

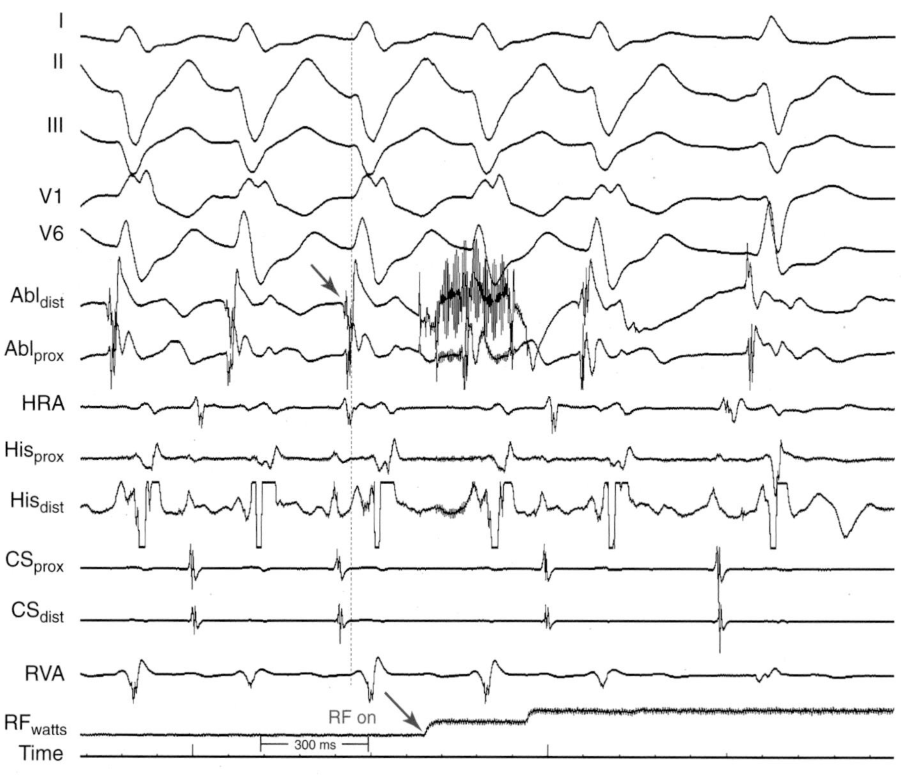

FIGURE 19–21 Ablation of idiopathic (fascicular) left ventricular tachycardia (LV VT). Radiofrequency (RF) delivery is begun (blue arrow) at the site of the diastolic Purkinje potential during idiopathic LV VT. Within less than 1 second, VT terminates. Red arrows indicate probable Purkinje potentials.

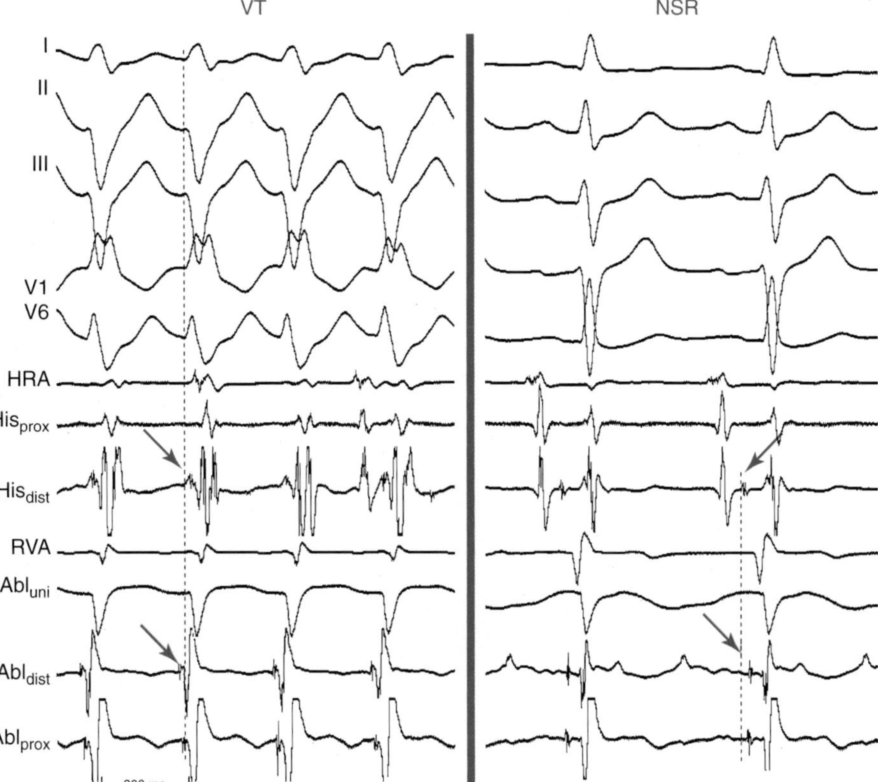

FIGURE 19–22 Ablation of idiopathic (fascicular) left ventricular tachycardia (LV VT). Shown are recordings during VT (left) and normal sinus rhythm (NSR; right) from a successful ablation site for idiopathic LV VT. Red arrows indicate probable Purkinje potentials, activated distal-to-proximal during VT and proximal-to-distal during sinus. Blue arrows show His potentials, occurring after QRS onset during VT.

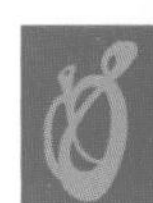

ablation should be directed to another site after additional mapping. This approach helps limit RF damage to the area of LPF and LB.

Successful ablation sites are often associated with progressive prolongation of the LDP-PP interval, with termination of VT coincident with conduction block between the two potentials.[41] Rarely, if ever, does one need more than 50 W or the use of irrigated or large-tip electrodes to ablate these VTs successfully.

Endpoints of Ablation

Successful ablation is defined as noninducibility of VT, with and without isoproterenol administration (using the best method for induction documented before ablation), during at least 30 minutes after ablation.

Outcome

The acute success rate is more than 90%, even when different mapping methods are used. The recurrence rate is approximately 7% to 10%, with most recurrences occurring in the first 24 to 48 hours after the ablation procedure. Complications are rare and include different degrees of fascicular block, LBBB, cardiac tamponade (rare), aortic regurgitation, and mitral regurgitation caused by torn chordae that may result from entrapment of the ablation catheter in a chordae of the mitral leaflet.[45]

Ablation of Noninducible Ventricular Tachycardia

Conventional activation mapping, guided by either the earliest PP or the LDP, although effective, depends on the inducibility and endurance of LV VT. However, the VT may not be inducible in the EP laboratory. Additionally, the critical substrate of LV VT is amenable to mechanical injury because of catheter manipulation, which will render the tachycardia noninducible. In these cases, substrate mapping and ablation during NSR have been suggested to eradicate LV VT.

Two approaches have been used for substrate mapping during sinus rhythm:

1. Ablation of the site where the earliest LDP is recorded during sinus rhythm (occurring 15 to 45 milliseconds after the PP). The PP-QRS interval at the successful ablation site with LDP is relatively short (mean, 13 ± 8 milliseconds).[41]
2. Anatomical linear ablation to transect the involved middle to distal LPF and destroy the substrate of LV VT.[41,46]

A recent study used the EnSite 3000 noncontact mapping system (Endocardial Solutions) to identify the sinus breakout point (i.e., the LV site with the earliest local activation during NSR) and used that point to guide linear ablation perpendicular to the conduction direction of LPF.[46,47] Particular attention is paid to the geometry detail in the areas of the HB, septum, and apex of the LV. Once the ventricular geometry had been generated, the system can then calculate electrograms from more than 3000 endocardial points simultaneously by reconstructing far-field signals to create the isopotential map of sinus rhythm using a single cardiac cycle. The HB, LB, fascicles, and sinus breakout point are tagged as special landmarks in the geometry. The sinus breakout point is located in the midposterior septum and the local virtual electrogram presents with QS morphology (Fig. 19-23). Virtual electrograms at points from the HB down to the sinus breakout point show a sharp, low-amplitude potential preceding the ventricular potential. The interval between these two potentials becomes progressively shorter as the activation propagates from the HB to the sinus breakout point, until the two potentials finally fuse together at the sinus breakout point. Virtual electrograms recorded from the points placed in the pattern of block above the sinus breakout point show the whole Purkinje network in the LPF area. An ablation line is created perpendicular to the activation direction of LPF and 1 cm

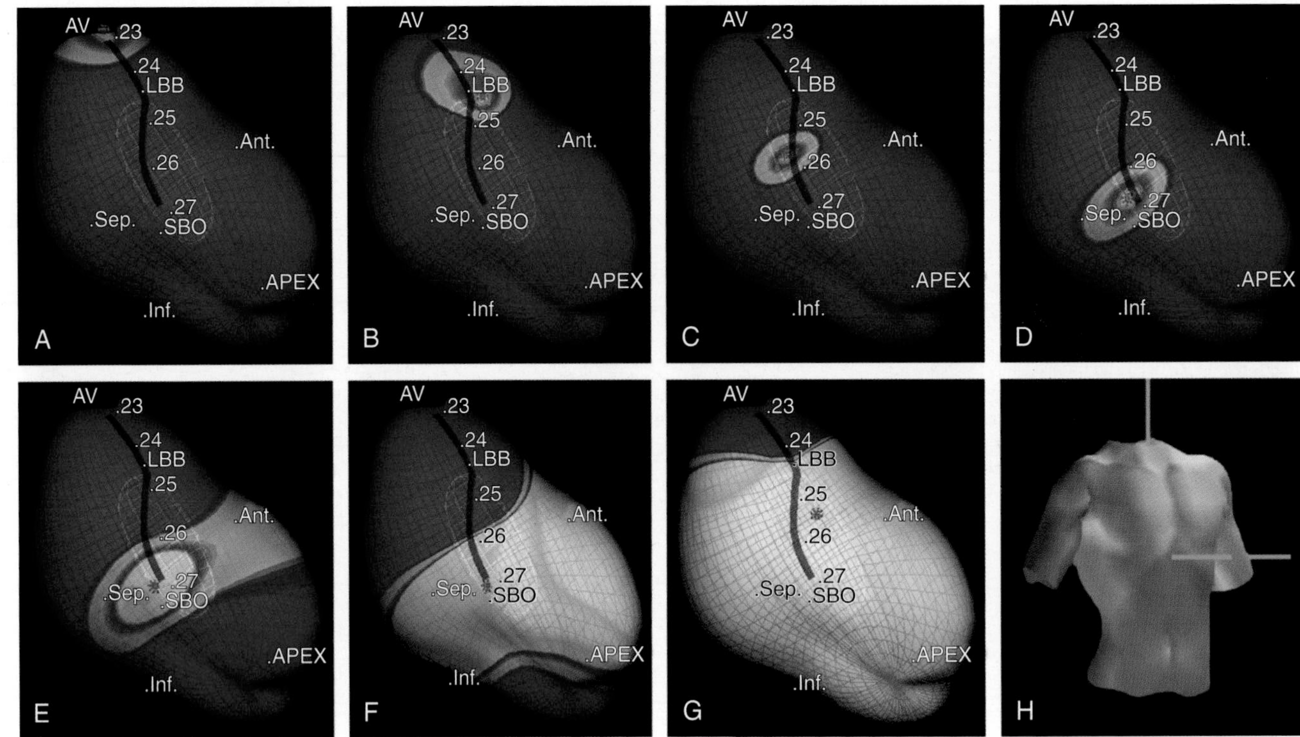

FIGURE 19–23 Noncontact mapping during normal sinus rhythm (NSR)—animated propagation map of the left ventricle (LV) from frames **A** to **G** in the right anterior oblique view during NSR. Note that the sinus activation propagates down from the His bundle (AV) to the left bundle branch (LBB), and then bifurcates into left anterior and left posterior fascicles before the entire LV is finally activated. The activation breakout point is at the midposterior septum and marked sinus breakout point (SBO) on the map. The thick black line indicates the propagation direction of the wavefronts from AV down to SBO. Ant = anterior; Inf = inferior; Sep = septal. *(From Chen M, Yang B, Zou J, et al: Non-contact mapping and linear ablation of the left posterior fascicle during sinus rhythm in the treatment of idiopathic left ventricular tachycardia. Europace 2005;7:138.)*

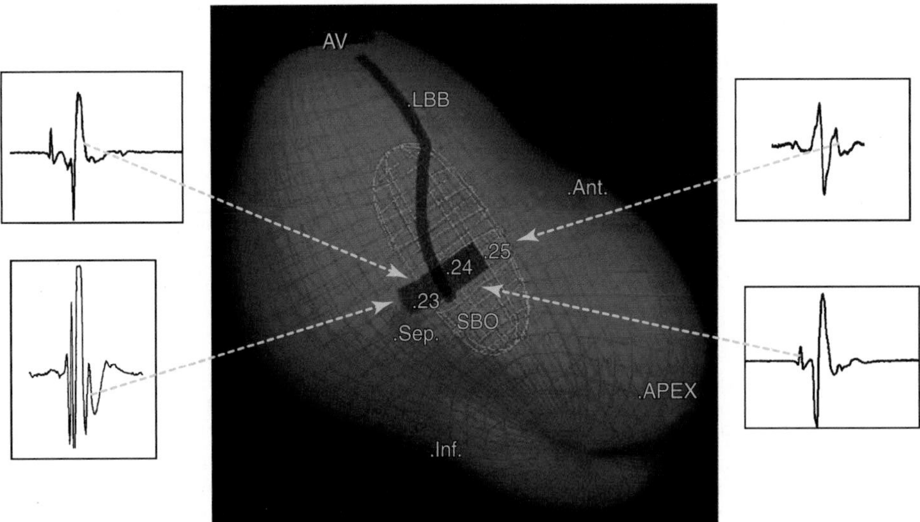

FIGURE 19–24 Noncontact mapping during normal sinus rhythm (NSR). A linear ablation lesion was created perpendicular to the wavefront propagation direction and 1 cm above the sinus breakout point (SBO). Both the starting and ending lesion points have a small Purkinje potential preceding the ventricular activation. Ant = anterior; AV = His recording area; Inf = inferior; LBB = left bundle branch; Sep = septal. *(From Chen M, Yang B, Zou J, et al: Non-contact mapping and linear ablation of the left posterior fascicle during sinus rhythm in the treatment of idiopathic left ventricular tachycardia. Europace 2005;7:138.)*

above the sinus breakout point (Fig. 19-24). There was a small Purkinje potential preceding the ventricular activation at its starting and ending points (see Fig. 19-24). The mean length of the deployed line was 2.0 ± 0. 4 cm, requiring a mean of 5.5 ± 1.6 RF applications. A significant rightward shift of the QRS axis in the surface limb leads was observed in all patients after the ablation procedure.

REFERENCES

1. Klein LS, Shih HT, Hackett FK, et al: Radiofrequency catheter ablation of ventricular tachycardia in patients without structural heart disease. Circulation 1992;85:1666.
2. Miles WM: Idiopathic ventricular outflow tract tachycardia: Where does it originate? J Cardiovasc Electrophysiol 2001;12:536.
3. Lerman BB, Stein KM, Markowitz SM, et al: Ventricular arrhythmias in normal hearts. Cardiol Clin 2000;18:265.

4. Lerman BB, Stein KM, Markowitz SM, et al: Ventricular tachycardia in patients with structurally normal hearts. *In* Zipes DP, Jalife J (eds): Cardiac Electrophysiology: From Cell to Bedside, 4th ed. Philadelphia, WB Saunders, 2004, pp 668-682.
5. Berruezo A, Mont L, Nava S, et al: Electrocardiographic recognition of the epicardial origin of ventricular tachycardias. Circulation 2004;109:1842.
6. Josephson ME. Recurrent ventricular tachycardia. *In* Josephson ME (ed): Clinical Cardiac Electrophysiology, 3rd. ed. Philadelphia, Lippincott, Williams & Wilkins, 2004, pp 425-610.
7. Iwai S, Cantillon DJ, Kim RJ, et al: Right and left ventricular outflow tract tachycardias: evidence for a common electrophysiologic mechanism. J Cardiovasc Electrophysiol 2006;17:1052.
8. Kim RJ, Iwai S, Markowitz SM, et al: Clinical and electrophysiological spectrum of idiopathic ventricular outflow tract arrhythmias. J Am Coll Cardiol 2007;49: 2035.
9. Gaita F, Giustetto C, Di DP, et al: Long-term follow-up of right ventricular monomorphic extrasystoles. J Am Coll Cardiol 2001;38:364.
10. Francis J, Sankar V, Nair VK, Priori SG: Catecholaminergic polymorphic ventricular tachycardia. Heart Rhythm 2005;2:550.
11. Dixit S, Marchlinski FE: Clinical characteristics and catheter ablation of left ventricular outflow tract tachycardia. Curr Cardiol Rep 2001;3:305.
12. Hachiya H, Aonuma K, Yamauchi Y, et al: Electrocardiographic characteristics of left ventricular outflow tract tachycardia. Pacing Clin Electrophysiol 2000;23(Pt 2):1930.
13. Hachiya H, Aonuma K, Yamauchi Y, et al: How to diagnose, locate, and ablate coronary cusp ventricular tachycardia. J Cardiovasc Electrophysiol 2002;13:551.
14. Kanagaratnam L, Tomassoni G, Schweikert R, et al: Ventricular tachycardias arising from the aortic sinus of Valsalva: An under-recognized variant of left outflow tract ventricular tachycardia. J Am Coll Cardiol 2001;37:1408.
15. Ouyang F, Fotuhi P, Ho SY, et al: Repetitive monomorphic ventricular tachycardia originating from the aortic sinus cusp: Electrocardiographic characterization for guiding catheter ablation. J Am Coll Cardiol 2002;39:500.
16. Schweikert RA, Saliba WI, Tomassoni G: Percutaneous pericardial instrumentation for endo-epicardial mapping of previously failed ablations. Circulation 2003;108: 1329.
17. Tada H, Nogami A, Naito S, et al: Left ventricular epicardial outflow tract tachycardia: A new distinct subgroup of outflow tract tachycardia. Jpn Circ J 2001;65:723.
18. Timmermans C, Rodriguez LM, Crijns HJ, et al: Idiopathic left bundle-branch block-shaped ventricular tachycardia may originate above the pulmonary valve. Circulation 2003;108:1960.
19. Tanner H, Hindricks G, Schirdewahn P, et al: Outflow tract tachycardia with R/S transition in lead V_3: Six different anatomical approaches for successful ablation. J Am Coll Cardiol 2005;45:418.
20. Kautzner J, Cihak R, Vancura V: ECG signature of idiopathic monomorphic ventricular tachycardia from the outflow tract. Eur Heart J 2000;21;332.
21. Krebs ME, Krause PC, Engelstein ED, et al: Ventricular tachycardias mimicking those arising from the right ventricular outflow tract. J Cardiovasc Electrophysiol 2000;11:45.
22. Lee SH, Tai CT, Chiang CE, et al: Determinants of successful ablation of idiopathic ventricular tachycardias with left bundle branch block morphology from the right ventricular outflow tract. Pacing Clin Electrophysiol 2002;25:1346.
23. Dixit S, Gerstenfeld EP, Callans DJ, Marchlinski FE: Electrocardiographic patterns of superior right ventricular outflow tract tachycardias: Distinguishing septal and free wall sites of origin. J Cardiovasc Electrophysiol 2003;14:1.
24. Sekiguchi Y, Aonuma K, Takahashi A, et al: Electrocardiographic and electrophysiologic characteristics of ventricular tachycardia originating within the pulmonary artery. J Am Coll Cardiol 2005;45:887.
25. Timmermans C, Rodriguez LM, Medeiros A, et al: Radiofrequency catheter ablation of idiopathic ventricular tachycardia originating in the main stem of the pulmonary artery. J Cardiovasc Electrophysiol 2002;13:281.
26. Tada H, Tadokoro K, Ito S, et al: Idiopathic ventricular arrhythmias originating from the tricuspid annulus: Prevalence, electrocardiographic characteristics, and results of radiofrequency catheter ablation. Heart Rhythm 2007;4:7.
27. Tada H, Ito S, Naito S, et al: Prevalence and electrocardiographic characteristics of idiopathic ventricular arrhythmia originating in the free wall of the right ventricular outflow tract. Circ J 2004;68:909.
28. Ouyang F, Cappato R, Ernst S, et al: Electroanatomical substrate of idiopathic left ventricular tachycardia: Unidirectional block and macroreentry within the Purkinje network. Circulation 2002;105:462.
29. Bala R, Marchlinski FE: Electrocardiographic recognition and ablation of outflow tract ventricular tachycardia. Heart Rhythm 2007;4:366.
30. Yamada T, Murakami Y, Yoshida N, et al: Preferential conduction across the ventricular outflow septum in ventricular arrhythmias originating from the aortic sinus cusp. J Am Coll Cardiol 2007;50:884.
31. Bazan V, Gerstenfeld EP, Garcia FC, et al: Site-specific twelve-lead ECG features to identify an epicardial origin for left ventricular tachycardia in the absence of myocardial infarction. Heart Rhythm 2007;4:1403.
32. Bazan V, Bala R, Garcia FC, et al: Twelve-lead ECG features to identify ventricular tachycardia arising from the epicardial right ventricle. Heart Rhythm 2006;3: 1132.
33. Tada H, Ito S, Naito S, et al: Idiopathic ventricular arrhythmia arising from the mitral annulus: a distinct subgroup of idiopathic ventricular arrhythmias. J Am Coll Cardiol 2005;45:877.
34. Azegami K, Wilber DJ, Arruda M, et al: Spatial resolution of pacemapping and activation mapping in patients with idiopathic right ventricular outflow tract tachycardia. J Cardiovasc Electrophysiol 2005;16:823.
35. Gerstenfeld EP, Dixit S, Callans DJ, et al: Quantitative comparison of spontaneous and paced 12-lead electrocardiogram during right ventricular outflow tract ventricular tachycardia. J Am Coll Cardiol 2003;41:2046.
36. Friedman PA, Beinborn DA, Shultz J, Hammill SC: Ablation of noninducible idiopathic left ventricular tachycardia using a non-contact map acquired from a premature complex with tachycardia morphology. Pacing Clin Electrophysiol 2000;23: 1311.
37. Aiba T, Shimizu W, Taguchi A, et al: Clinical usefulness of a multielectrode basket catheter for idiopathic ventricular tachycardia originating from right ventricular outflow tract. J Cardiovasc Electrophysiol 2001;12:511.
38. Takemoto M, Yoshimura H, Ohba Y, et al: Radiofrequency catheter ablation of premature ventricular complexes from right ventricular outflow tract improves left ventricular dilation and clinical status in patients without structural heart disease. J Am Coll Cardiol 2005;45:1259.
39. Storey J, Iwasa A, Feld GK: Left ventricular outflow tract tachycardia originating from the right coronary cusp: Identification of location of origin by endocardial noncontact activation mapping from the right ventricular outflow tract. J Cardiovasc Electrophysiol 2002;13:1050.
40. Kurzidim K, Schneider HJ, Kuniss M, et al: Cryocatheter ablation of right ventricular outflow tract tachycardia. J Cardiovasc Electrophysiol 2005;16:366.
41. Nogami A, Naito S, Tada H, et al: Demonstration of diastolic and presystolic Purkinje potentials as critical potentials in a macroreentry circuit of verapamil-sensitive idiopathic left ventricular tachycardia. J Am Coll Cardiol 2000;36:811.
42. Tsuchiya T, Okumura K, Honda T, et al: Effects of verapamil and lidocaine on two components of the re-entry circuit of verapamil-senstitive idiopathic left ventricular tachycardia. J Am Coll Cardiol 2001;37:1415.
43. Iwai S, Lerman BB: Management of ventricular tachycardia in patients with clinically normal hearts. Curr Cardiol Rep 2000;2:515.
44. Wu D, Wen MS, Yeh SJ: Ablation of idiopathic left ventricular tachycardia. *In* Huang SKS, Wilber DJ (eds): Radiofrequency Catheter Ablation of Cardiac Arrhythmias: Basic Concepts and Clinical Applications, 2nd ed. Armonk, NY, Futura, 2000, pp 601-620.
45. Li D, Guo J, Xu Y, Li X: The surface electrocardiographic changes after radiofrequency catheter ablation in patients with idiopathic left ventricular tachycardia. Int J Clin Pract 2004;58:11.
46. Chen M, Yang B, Zou J, et al: Non-contact mapping and linear ablation of the left posterior fascicle during sinus rhythm in the treatment of idiopathic left ventricular tachycardia. Europace 2005;7:138.
47. Friedman PA, Asirvatham SJ, Grie S: Noncontact mapping to guide ablation of right ventricular outflow tract tachycardia. J Am Coll Cardiol 2002;39:1808.

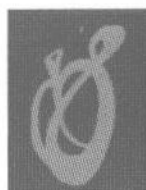

CHAPTER 20

Bundle Branch Reentrant Ventricular Tachycardia

PATHOPHYSIOLOGY

Bundle branch reentrant (BBR) VT is the only reentrant ventricular tachycardia (VT) with a well-defined reentry circuit, incorporating the right bundle branch (RB) and left bundle branch (LB) as obligatory limbs of the circuit, connected proximally by the His bundle (HB) and distally by the ventricular septal myocardium (Fig. 20-1).[1]

Single BBR beats can be induced in up to 50% of patients with normal intraventricular conduction undergoing electrophysiological (EP) study. The QRS during BBR can display either left bundle branch block (LBBB) or right bundle branch block (RBBB) when anterograde ventricular activation occurs over the RB or LB, respectively. The vast majority have LBBB configuration. BBR with a bundle branch block (BBB) pattern can also occur occasionally during right ventricular (RV) pacing. This requires that the effective refractory period of the LB be longer than that of the RB, or that retrograde conduction over the RB is resumed after an initial bilateral block in the His-Purkinje system (HPS) (i.e., gap phenomenon). Left ventricular (LV) pacing does not seem to increase the yield of induction of BBR with RBBB morphology.[1,2]

In patients with normal intraventricular conduction, BBR is a self-limited phenomenon. The rapid conduction and long refractory period of the HPS prevent sustained BBR in normal hearts. Spontaneous termination of BBR most commonly occurs in the retrograde limb between the ventricular muscle and the HB.[2] Sometimes, anterograde block can also occur, making refractoriness in the RB-Purkinje system the limiting factor. Continuation of BBR as a tachycardia is critically dependent on the interplay between conduction velocity and recovery of the tissue ahead of the reentrant wavefront; the presence of conduction abnormalities in the HPS sets the stage for sustained BBR to develop by slowing conduction in the reentrant pathway.

Rarely, self-terminating BBR can occur with a narrow QRS during ventricular extrastimulation (VES) in the setting of normal intraventricular conduction. After retrograde conduction via the left anterior fascicle (LAF) or left posterior fascicle (LPF), anterograde propagation occurs over the RB and the remaining LB fascicle, resulting in a narrow QRS with either LAF or LPF block.

Two changes from normal physiology must occur for BBR to become sustained: (1) anatomically longer reentrant pathway caused by a dilated heart, providing sufficiently longer conduction time around the HPS; and (2) slow conduction in the HPS caused by HPS disease.[2] These two factors are responsible for sufficient prolongation of conduction time to permit expiration of the refractory period of the HPS.

CLINICAL CONSIDERATIONS

Epidemiology

Sustained BBR is a monomorphic VT that usually occurs in patients with structural heart disease, especially dilated cardiomyopathy.[3] Idiopathic dilated cardiomyopathy is the anatomical substrate for BBR VT in 45% of cases, and BBR VT accounts for up to 41% of all inducible sustained VTs in this population. BBR VT can also be associated with cardiomyopathy secondary to valvular or ischemic heart disease, and has been reported with Ebstein's anomaly, hypertrophic cardiomyopathy, and even in patients without structural heart disease other than intraventricular conduction abnormalities.[3-6]

In patients with spontaneous sustained monomorphic VT, the incidence of inducible BBR VT ranges from 4.5% to 6% in patients with ischemic heart disease to 16.7% to 41% in patients with nonischemic cardiomyopathy.[3] BBR VT accounts for up to 6% of all forms of induced sustained monomorphic VT.[3] In patients with BBR VT, additional myocardial VTs occur in 25%.

Clinical Presentation

Sustained BBR VT is typically unstable secondary to very rapid ventricular rates (often 200 to 300 beats/min) and poor underlying ventricular function; 75% of patients present with syncope or cardiac arrest.

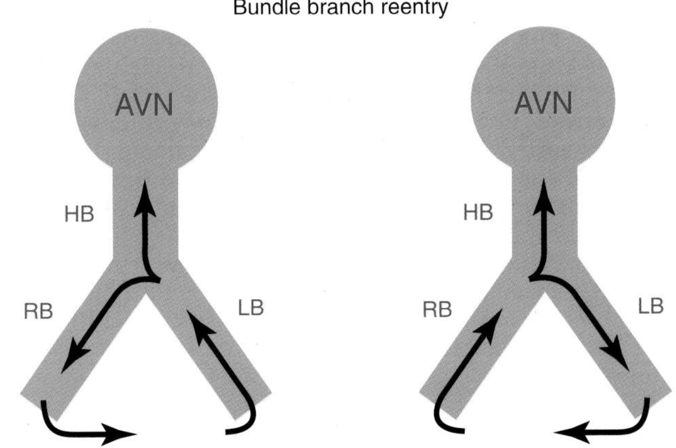

FIGURE 20–1 Schematic illustration of the two types of bundle branch reentry (BBR) circuits. At left is the most commonly seen type of BBR ventricular tachycardia (VT). Retrograde conduction occurs via the left bundle branch (LB) and anterograde conduction occurs via the right bundle branch (RB). This yields a VT in which the QRS has a left bundle branch block (LBBB) pattern. At right is the uncommon type of BBR VT. Retrograde conduction occurs via the RB and anterograde conduction occurs via the LB, which yields a VT in which the QRS has a RBBB pattern. AVN = atrioventricular node; HB = His bundle.

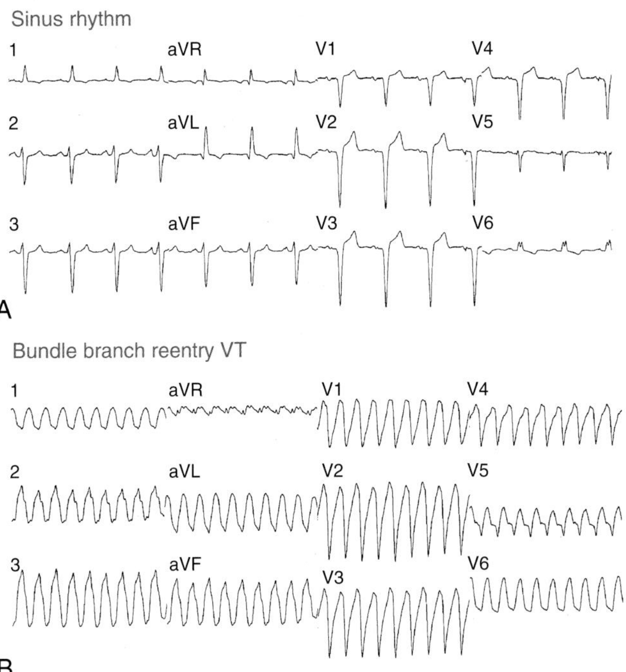

FIGURE 20–2 ECG of bundle branch reentrant (BBR) ventricular tachycardia (VT). **A,** Normal sinus rhythm baseline with intraventricular conduction delay resembling left bundle branch block. **B,** BBR VT. Note typical-appearing complete LBBB in this rapid VT.

Initial Evaluation

BBR VT should be suspected in the presence of typical ECG QRS morphology during NSR and VT (see later), especially in a patient with dilated cardiomyopathy. Echocardiographic examination and coronary arteriography are required in most patients to evaluate for structural heart disease.

Principles of Management

Pharmacological antiarrhythmic therapy is usually ineffective. Radiofrequency (RF) catheter ablation of a bundle branch (typically the RB) can cure BBR VT and is currently regarded as first-line therapy.

Associated myocardial VT occurs in approximately 25% of patients postablation, and these patients continue to be at a high risk of sudden cardiac death. Therefore, implantable cardioverter-defibrillator (ICD) implantation is indicated for secondary prevention, and additional antiarrhythmic therapy is required for some patients. ICD implantation will also provide back-up pacing, which is frequently required postablation secondary to the development of atrioventricular (AV) block or an excessively prolonged His bundle–ventricular (HV) interval. Implantation of a dual-chamber or biventricular ICD should be considered in these patients.

Because BBR VT has a limited response to antiarrhythmic drugs and can be an important cause of repetitive ICD therapies, catheter ablation of the arrhythmia should always be considered as an important adjunct to the device therapy.

ELECTROCARDIOGRAPHIC FEATURES

Baseline ECG. The baseline rhythm is usually normal sinus rhythm (NSR) or atrial fibrillation (AF). Almost all patients with BBR VT demonstrate intraventricular conduction abnormalities. The most common ECG abnormality is nonspecific intraventricular conduction delay (IVCD) of an LBBB pattern and PR interval prolongation (Fig. 20-2).[3] Complete RBBB is rare but does not preclude BBR as the mechanism of VT. Although total interruption of conduction in one of the bundle branches would theoretically prevent occurrence of BBR, an ECG pattern of complete BBB may not be an accurate marker of *complete* conduction block.

ECG During Ventricular Tachycardia. Twelve-lead ECG documentation of BBR VT is usually unavailable because the VT is rapid and hemodynamically unstable. The VT rate is usually 180 to 300 beats/min.[3] QRS morphology during VT is a typical BBB pattern and can be identical to that in NSR. BBR VT with LBBB pattern is the most common VT morphology, and it usually has normal or left axis deviation (see Fig. 20-2).[3] In contrast to VT of myocardial origin, BBR with an LBBB pattern characteristically shows rapid intrinsicoid deflection in the right precordial leads, suggesting that initial ventricular activation occurs through the HPS and not ventricular muscle. BBR VT with an RBBB pattern usually has a leftward axis, but it can have a normal or rightward axis, depending on which fascicle is used for anterograde propagation.

ELECTROPHYSIOLOGICAL TESTING

Baseline Observations During Normal Sinus Rhythm

Conduction abnormalities in the HPS are almost invariably present and are a critical prerequisite for the development of sustained BBR, regardless of the underlying anatomical substrate (Fig. 20-3).[3,7] The average HV interval is about 80 milliseconds (range, 60 to 110 milliseconds).[3,7] Although some patients can have the HV interval in NSR within normal limits, functional HPS impairment in these patients manifests as HV interval prolongation or split HB potentials, commonly becoming evident during atrial programmed stimulation or burst pacing.[8] Nonspecific IVCD of an LBBB pattern and PR interval prolongation are the most common abnormalities.[3]

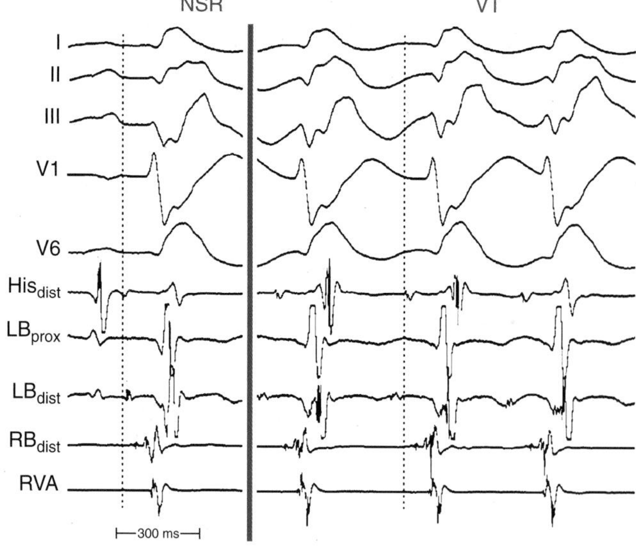

FIGURE 20–3 Bundle branch reentrant (BBR) ventricular tachycardia (VT) versus normal sinus rhythm (NSR). Sinus and BBR VT with His, left bundle branch (LB) and right bundle branch (RB) recordings in a patient with a prior septal myocardial infarction. Dashed lines mark onset of His deflection. During NSR, the His potential is followed first by the LB potential; RB activation is further delayed. The fact that left bundle branch block (LBBB) is present on the ECG suggests that, although the LB is activated prior to the RB, delay is encountered more distally in the LV His-Purkinje system such that LBBB is evident on ECG. During BBR VT, activation propagates in a LB-His-RB sequence. Retrograde LB activation is very delayed, most likely because of the same factors responsible for the ECG in NSR.

Induction of Tachycardia

VES from the RV apex is the usual method used to induce BBR with an LBBB pattern. Induction is consistently dependent on the achievement of a critical conduction delay in the HPS (i.e., critical ventricular–His bundle [VH] interval) following the VES.

During RV pacing at a constant cycle length (CL) and during introduction of VES at relatively long coupling intervals, retrograde conduction to the HB occurs via the RB. At shorter coupling intervals, retrograde delay and block occur in the RB when its relative and effective refractory periods are encountered, respectively. When retrograde block occurs in the RB, the impulse propagates across the septum and retrogradely up the LB to the HB, producing a long V_2-H_2 interval. The LB would still be capable of retrograde conduction because of its shorter refractoriness and because of the delay associated with transseptal propagation. Further shortening of the coupling intervals is associated with increasing delay in LB conduction (i.e., increasing V_2-H_2 interval). Within a certain range of coupling intervals, increasing retrograde LB delay allows for recovery of anterograde conduction via the RB, and another ventricular activation ensues, displaying a wide QRS with an LBBB pattern. This beat is called a BBR beat or V_3 phenomenon.[1,7,9]

An inverse relationship exists between retrograde conduction delay in the LB (V_2-H_2 interval) and the time of anterograde conduction in the RB (H_2-V_3 interval). This is because the faster the impulse propagates transseptally and up the LB, the more likely it will reach the RB while it is still refractory from the previous activation (concealment) by the VES, resulting in slower anterograde conduction down the RB.

BBR is more likely to occur when the VES is delivered following pacing drives incorporating short to long CL changes as compared with constant CL drives, because of CL dependency of the HPS refractoriness. An abrupt change in CL (i.e., long to short) can result in a more distal site of retrograde block, and less concealment, along the myocardium-Purkinje-RB axis, which can allow sufficient recovery of excitability in the anterograde limb of the circuit (i.e., the RB -Purkinje- myocardium axis) for reentry to develop. In addition, earlier recovery of excitability along this axis, because of the more distal site of block and less concealment, is associated with a shorter H_2-V_3 interval in this reentrant beat.[1,7]

Procainamide, which increases conduction time within the HPS, especially in the diseased HPS and, potentially, isoproterenol can facilitate induction of sustained BBR.[3] In some patients, the arrhythmia can be inducible only with atrial pacing.[7]

Tachycardia Features

BBR VT can only be diagnosed using intracardiac recording. AV dissociation is typically present, but 1 : 1 ventriculoatrial (VA) conduction can occur. EP criteria for the diagnosis of BBR VT include the following: (1) the His potential precedes the QRS; and (2) the HV interval during BBR with an LBBB pattern is usually similar to or longer than that during baseline rhythm (the HV interval is usually 55 to 160 milliseconds; see Fig. 20-3). However, in rare cases, the HV interval during BBR VT can be slightly shorter (by less than 15 milliseconds) than the HV interval in NSR, because during BBR the HB is activated in the retrograde direction simultaneously (in parallel) with the proximal part of the bundle branch serving as the anterograde limb of the reentry circuit, whereas during NSR, activation of the HB and bundle branch occur in sequence.[2,10,11]

The relative duration of the HV interval recorded during VT as compared with NSR would depend on two factors: the balance between anterograde and retrograde conduction times from the upper turnaround point of the reentry circuit, and the site of HB recording relative to the upper turnaround point (i.e., the HB catheter electrode positioned at the proximal versus distal HB).[10] Conduction delay in the bundle branch used as the anterograde limb of the circuit would tend to prolong the HV interval during VT, whereas retrograde conduction delay to the HB recording site, as well as the use of a relatively proximal HB recording site (far from the turnaround point), would tend to shorten it. The RB-V interval during VT with LBBB morphology must always be longer than that recorded in sinus rhythm, emphasizing the importance of recording the RB potential during VT.[2] The HV interval during BBR with an RBBB pattern can be significantly different from that during NSR (HV interval = 65 to 250 milliseconds). During NSR, the HV interval is usually determined by conduction over whichever bundle branch conducts most rapidly, whereas during BBR it is determined by conduction over the typically diseased LB.

In the common type of BBR VT (LBBB pattern), the activation wavefront propagates retrogradely up the LB to the HB and then anterogradely down the RB, with subsequent ventricular activation. This sequence is reversed in BBR with an RBBB pattern. The HV and RB-V (during VT with LBBB morphology) or LB-V (during VT with RBBB morphology) intervals are relatively stable. Spontaneous variations in the V-V intervals are preceded and dictated by similar changes in the H-H (RB-RB or LB-LB) intervals. These changes can occur spontaneously, most common immediately after induction of the VT, or be demonstrated by ventricular stimulation during VT. In other words, the VT CL is affected by variation in the V-H (V-RB or V-LB) intervals. However, oscillations in the V-V intervals can occasionally precede those of the H-H intervals during BBR VT because of conduction variations in the anterograde, rather than the retrograde, conducting bundle branch.

Recording from both sides of the septum can help in the identification of BBR mechanism. Documentation of a typical H-RB-V-LB (during VT with LBBB morphology), or H-LB-V-RB (during VT with RBBB morphology), activation sequence would further support BBR diagnosis (see Fig. 20-3).[9,12] Unfortunately, RB and/or LB potentials are not always recorded, so that the typical activation sequences (LB-H-RB-V or RB-H-LB-V) are not available for analysis.[2] Even if either activation sequence is present, the HPS (usually the LB) could be activated passively in a retrograde fashion to produce an H-RB-V sequence during a VT with an LBBB pattern without reentry requiring the LB. In these cases, other diagnostic criteria for BBR should be used. In addition, during VT with LBBB morphology, RV activation must precede the LV activation. The opposite is true for the VT with RBBB morphology.

BBR can be terminated by block in the HPS—spontaneous, pacing-induced, secondary to catheter trauma, or caused by ablation.

Diagnostic Maneuvers During Tachycardia

Pacing maneuvers, if feasible, can be extremely helpful to establish the diagnosis of BBR; however, application of the pacing maneuvers during BBR is often not feasible because of the hemodynamic compromise commonly associated with these VTs.

Entrainment. BBR VT can be entrained by ventricular pacing. Entrainment with manifest QRS fusion during ventricular pacing is classic for BBR VT.[13] Entrainment with concealed fusion can be demonstrated by pacing at the LB or RB (i.e., within the reentrant circuit). During entrainment from the RV apex, a post-paving interval (PPI) – VT CL > 30 milliseconds excludes a BBR mechanism, provided that the RV apex catheter is correctly positioned. The greater this value, the more reliable the certainty of exclusion. Conversely, a PPI – VT CL < 30 milliseconds is consistent with but not diagnostic of a BBR mechanism.

Entrainment of BBR VT with concealed QRS fusion can also occur during atrial pacing. This approach, however, demands that the patient is not in AF and usually requires the infusion of atropine, isoproterenol, or both to avoid AV block during rapid atrial pacing. However, observation of manifest fusion during entrainment by atrial pacing does not exclude BBR when it has an RBBB morphology. The combination of entrainment with concealed QRS fusion during atrial pacing and entrainment with manifest QRS fusion during ventricular pacing has been recently proposed as a useful diagnostic criterion for BBR VT with LBBB QRS morphology.[13]

Resetting. VES can reset the VT by advancing the HB or bundle branch potential. In addition, VES can reverse the direction of impulse propagation during BBR. Theoretically this requires double VESs, with the first VES producing block and the second initiating the reentry in the opposite direction.

Other Pacing Maneuvers. The ability to dissociate the HB or, particularly, bundle branch (RB or LB) potential would strongly argue against a BBR mechanism. An atrial extrastimulus (AES) that blocks below the HB deflection should terminate BBR. Additionally, simultaneous LV and RV pacing should prevent BBR.[2]

Exclusion of Other Arrhythmia Mechanisms

Myocardial Ventricular Tachycardias

Myocardial VTs are rarely associated with classic LBBB (or RBBB) QRS morphology, as is expected with BBR VT. Additionally, in myocardial VTs, the His potential is often obscured within the local ventricular electrogram. Occasionally, the His potential can precede the onset of the QRS, thus resembling BBR VT; however, the HV interval in myocardial VTs is usually shorter than that during NSR. In contrast to BBR VT, spontaneous or induced V-V cycle length variations during myocardial VTs usually precede and dictate H-H interval changes.

Entrainment with concealed QRS fusion during atrial pacing excludes myocardial VT and should be expected in BBR VT. When entrainment with concealed fusion can be demonstrated by pacing at the LB or RB, BBR VT is very likely. In addition, a PPI – VT CL < 30 milliseconds after entrainment of the VT from the RV apex is suggestive of BBR VT; in contrast, in myocardial VTs, the PPI – VT CL is > 30 milliseconds, unless the VT originates in the apex.

Idiopathic (Fascicular) Left Ventricular Tachycardia

The QRS and HV interval are normal during NSR in idiopathic VT. In contrast, BBR VT is rare in the absence of baseline HPS conduction abnormalities. Additionally, the His potential falls within or before the QRS in idiopathic LV VT, producing a negative or short HV interval, and HB activation follows activation of the left fascicles, which is inconsistent with RBBB-type BBR VT.

Supraventricular Tachycardia with Aberrancy

BBR VT typically exhibits AV dissociation, which excludes atrial tachycardia (AT) and atrioventricular reentrant tachycardia (AVRT). Occasionally, BBR VT can be associated with 1:1 VA conduction, and it can then mimic supraventricular tachycardia (SVT) with aberrancy.

Multiple HB recordings, using a hexapolar or octapolar catheter, may help demonstrate the direction of HB depolarization—anterograde during SVT and retrograde during BBR VT. In addition, recording of LB and RB potentials in addition to HB potential can be helpful; activation of the HB occurs anterogradely via the atrioventricular node (AVN) during SVT and precedes the RB potential by an interval equal to or longer that that during NSR.

The atrium is not part of the circuit in the BBR VT and can be dissociated by atrial pacing, which excludes AT and AVRT as the mechanism of wide complex tachycardia. Moreover, during entrainment from the RV apex, a PPI – tachycardia CL > 30 milliseconds excludes a BBR mechanism. Conversely, a PPI – tachycardia CL < 30 milliseconds excludes atrioventricular nodal reentrant tachycardia (AVNRT). Additionally, entrainment with manifest fusion during ventricular pacing excludes AVNRT and AT and should be expected in BBR tachycardia. The ability to terminate or reset the tachycardia with VES introduced when HB is refractory excludes AT and AVNRT.

Antidromic Atrioventricular Reentrant Tachycardia Using an Atriofascicular Bypass Tract

During antidromic AVRT, the impulse propagates retrogradely over the RB to the HB, a sequence inconsistent with BBR with an LBBB pattern. The AV relationship is always 1:1 during AVRT and rarely so during BBR VT. Because the atrium is not part of the circuit in the BBR VT, it can be dissociated by atrial pacing, which excludes AVRT. Moreover, resetting the tachycardia with an AES from the right atrial (RA) free wall, timed when the AV junctional atrium is refractory, excludes VT. Similarly, the ability of an AES to terminate the tachycardia without conduction to the ventricle or to retard ventricular activation excludes VT (see Figs. 14-20 and 15-4).

Target of Ablation

The ablation target is either the RB or LB; however, RB ablation is easier and usually is the method of choice.[3,14] In most patients with BBR VT, although diffuse conduction system disease is present, the conduction abnormality in the LB is more severe than that in the RB. However, in most patients, the LB can still maintain 1:1 AV conduction during NSR. For these occasional patients in whom anterograde conduction down the LB is known to be inadequate for maintaining AV conduction, ablation of the RB will commit the patient to a permanent pacemaker. Therefore, ablation of the LB in these patients is preferable because it can prevent BBR and still preserve anterograde conduction.[14]

The mere presence of LBBB on ECG does not mean complete block in the LB. Signs that can indicate that conduction down the LB may be inadequate in maintaining 1:1 AV conduction and favor ablation of the LB over the RB include (1) development of high-grade AV block below the HB on transient RBBB that can occur secondary to RV catheter manipulation, and (2) observation of an LB potential following the ventricular electrogram either intermittently or during every sinus beat.

Ablation Technique

Ablation of the Right Bundle Branch

The RB is a long, thin, and discrete structure that courses down the right side of the interventricular septum near the endocardium in its upper third, deeper in the muscular portion of the septum in the middle third, and then again near the endocardium in its lower third. The RB does not divide throughout most of its course, and begins to ramify as it approaches the base of the right anterior papillary muscle, with fascicles going to the septal and free walls of the RV.

A quadripolar catheter is positioned at the HB region and maintained as a reference. The ablation catheter is initially positioned in the HB region and the area of the septum at which the largest His potential is recorded. The catheter is then advanced gradually (in the right anterior oblique [RAO] view) superiorly and to the patient's left side, with clockwise torque to ensure adequate catheter tip contact with the septum and RB and continuous adjustment of the catheter's curvature until the RB potential is recorded.[14] Attempts should be made to obtain the distal RB recording to ensure that the catheter tip is away from the HB and LB.

The RB potential can be distinguished from the HB potential by the absence of or minimal atrial electrogram on the recording and presence of a sharp deflection inscribed at least 15 to 20 milliseconds later than the His potential (Fig. 20-4). An RB-V interval value of <30 milliseconds may not be a reliable marker of the RB potential in these patients because disease of the HPS can cause prolongation of the RB-V conduction time.[14]

When there is RB conduction delay at baseline, the RB potential can become hidden within the ventricular electrogram, and it may be impossible to map in NSR, especially when the surface ECG shows complete or incomplete RBBB. However, the RB potential should be readily observed during BBR beats induced by RV stimulation or during BBR VT. In this case, anatomically guided lesions or a linear ablation perpendicular to the axis of the RB distal to the HB recording may be effective.[14]

A 4-mm-tip ablation catheter is typically used for RB ablation. RF delivery is usually started at low levels (5 W) and gradually increased every 10 seconds, targeting a temperature of 60°C. In general, RBBB develops at 15 to 20 W.[14] Successful ablation will result in clear development of RBBB in V_1 (Fig. 20-5; see Fig. 20-4). Occasionally, an accelerated rhythm from the RB is observed during ablation (analogous to accelerated junctional rhythm with HB ablation; see Fig. 20-5).

Ablation of the Left Bundle Branch

Whereas the RB is anatomically a continuation of the HB, the LB arises as a broad band of fibers from the HB in a perpendicular direction toward the inferior septum. The main LB penetrates the membranous portion of the interventricular septum under the aortic ring and then divides into several fairly discrete branches. The LPF arises more proximally than the LAF, appears as an extension of the main LB, and is large in its initial course. It then fans out extensively posteriorly toward the papillary muscle and inferoposteriorly to the free wall of the LV. The LAF crosses the LV outflow tract and terminates in the Purkinje system of the anterolateral wall of the LV. In the RAO view, the LPF extends from the HB region toward the inferior diaphragmatic wall and the LAF extends toward the apex of the heart. However, considerable variability exists.

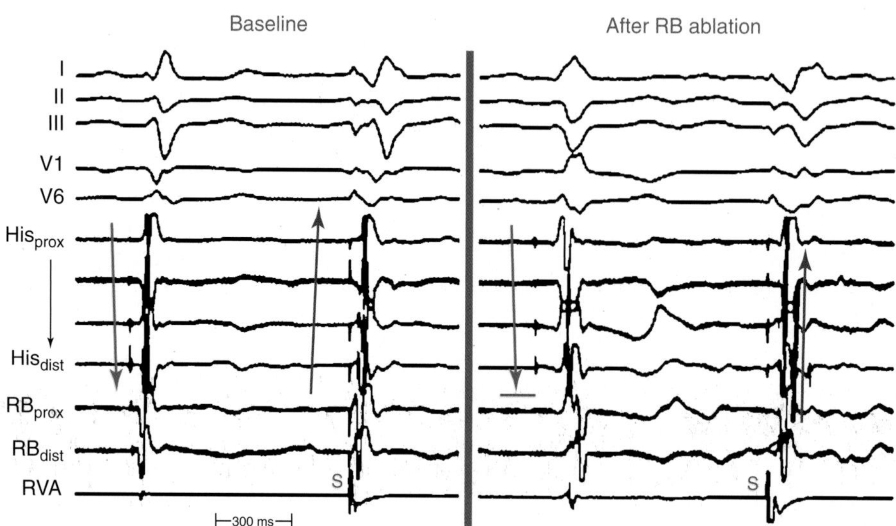

FIGURE 20–4 Ablation of bundle branch reentry (BBR). Sinus and right ventricular apical paced complexes from before (left) and after (right) catheter ablation of the right bundle branch (RB) in a patient with BBR VT. Four bipolar recordings from a catheter at the His position and RB are shown. Prior to RB ablation, propagation along the His-RB axis is linear, anterograde during sinus rhythm (green arrow) and retrograde during RV pacing (purple arrow). After RB ablation, anterograde propagation is interrupted (green arrow, red line) and retrograde activation of the His electrograms occurs after the local ventricular electrogram (purple arrow) indicating block in the RB with transseptal propagation, then up the left bundle.

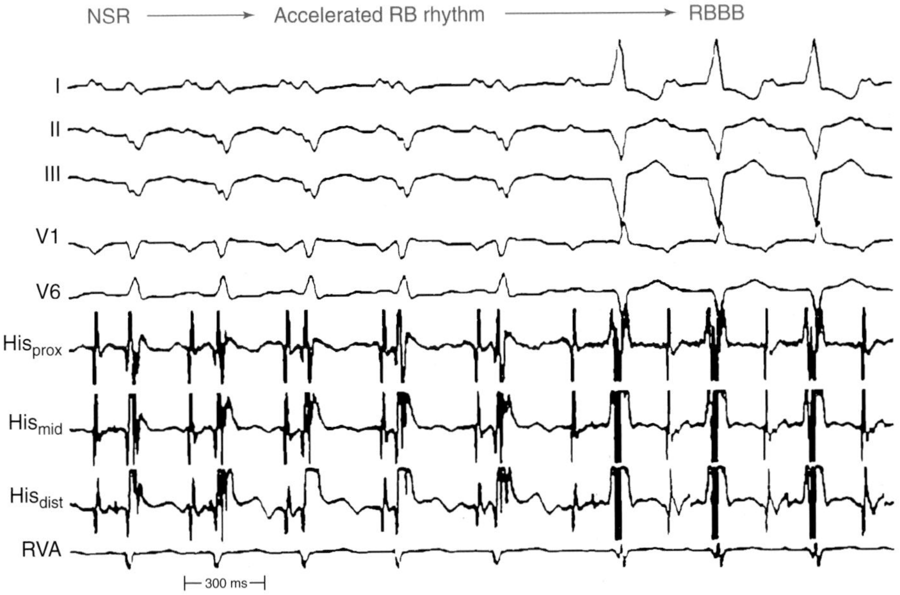

FIGURE 20–5 Right bundle branch (RB) ablation. During RB ablation, delivery of radiofrequency current causes accelerated rhythm from RB until complete block occurs (note lead V_1). The His bundle–ventricular interval after ablation is 145 msec (baseline, 80 msec). NSR = normal sinus rhythm; RBBB = right bundle branch block.

The mapping catheter is placed via a transaortic approach into the LV. The inferoapical septum is a starting point. The catheter is then gradually withdrawn toward the HB until a discrete LB potential is recorded. The LB-V interval should be ≤20 milliseconds, and the A:V electrogram amplitude ratio should be ≤1 : 10. At this position, the tip of the catheter typically is 1 to 1.5 cm inferior to the optimal HB recording site near the distal portion of the common LB.[14]

Because the LB is a broad band of fibers (typically 1 to 3 cm long and 1 cm wide), it can be difficult to ablate with a single RF application. Furthermore, the fascicles can diverge proximally; thus, ablation of the LB can be difficult without harming the HB. In these situations, it may be necessary to deliver several lesions along the left side of the septum in an arc distal to the HB, extending from the anterior superior septum (a point near the RB in the RAO view) to the inferior basal septum to transect both fascicles.

It is more difficult to monitor the progress of LB ablation during RF delivery. Most patients will already have some IVCD localized to the LB system. As opposed to the usually clear development of RBBB in V_1 during RB ablation, LB ablation can produce relatively subtle ECG changes, primarily manifesting as widening of the QRS and changes in the QRS axis. One can also monitor the presence of retrograde conduction during VES after each RF application. Elimination of the retrograde V_2-H_2 conduction that was present before ablation is a good indication that sufficient ablation of the LB has been achieved to eliminate BBR.

Endpoints of Ablation

Endpoints of RB ablation include the development of an RBBB pattern (see Fig. 20-5), noninducibility of BBR, and reversal of the direction of HB and RB activation during RV pacing. Prior to ablation, HB electrodes are depolarized during RV pacing from distal to proximal (RB-HB); after RB ablation, HB activation is delayed and reversed (HB-RB; see Fig. 20-4).

Endpoints of LB ablation include elimination of retrograde conduction of VESs over the LB and noninducibility of BBR.

After ablation, aggressive ventricular stimulation should be performed to evaluate the inducibility of VT. Also, decremental atrial pacing should be performed to evaluate the conduction properties of the HPS and the propensity for infra-Hisian AV block.

Outcome

Recurrence after successful ablation is extremely rare. The reported incidence of clinically significant conduction system impairment requiring implantation of a permanent pacemaker varies from 10% to 30%.[3,7,8]

Pacemaker implantation is indicated when infra-Hisian AV block is demonstrated with atrial pacing, or when the postablation HV interval is ≥100 milliseconds. As noted, associated myocardial VT is seen in approximately 25% of patients postablation, and these patients continue to be at a high risk of sudden cardiac death. Therefore, ICD implantation is indicated for secondary prevention, and additional antiarrhythmic therapy is required for some patients.

INTERFASCICULAR REENTRANT VENTRICULAR TACHYCARDIA

VT secondary to interfascicular reentry is extremely rare; when it does occur, it is most commonly seen in patients with coronary artery disease, specifically those with anterior myocardial infarction (MI) with LAF or LPF block. In these patients, RBBB is complete and bidirectional, so true BBR cannot occur. Additionally, there is slow conduction in the apparently blocked fascicle.[2,3,7]

Interfascicular reentry incorporates the LAF and LPF as obligatory limbs of the circuit, connected proximally by the main trunk of the LB and distally by the ventricular myocardium (Fig. 20-6). The tachycardia usually has RBBB morphology. The orientation of the frontal plane axis is variable and may depend on the direction of propagation in the reentrant circuit. Anterograde activation over the LAF and retrograde through the LPF would be associated with right axis deviation, wherea the reversed activation sequence shows left axis deviation (see Fig. 20-6).[7,12]

In contrast to BBR VT, the HV interval during interfascicular VT is usually shorter by less than 40 milliseconds than that recorded in NSR.[12] This is because the upper turnaround point of the circuit, the distal end of LB bifurcation

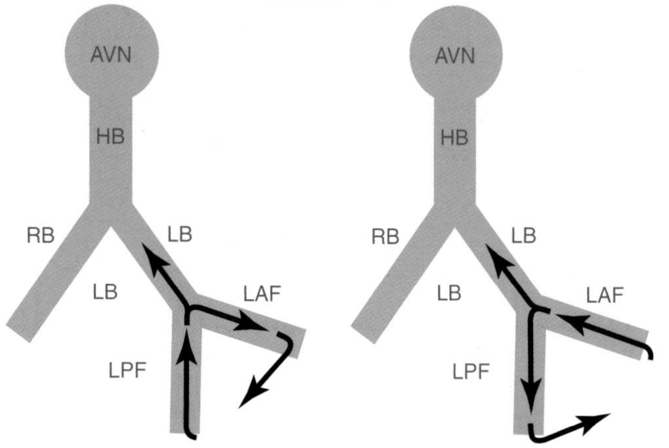

FIGURE 20–6 Schematic illustration of the two types of interfascicular ventricular tachycardia (VT) circuits. **Left,** The interfascicular reentrant VT uses the left posterior fascicle (LPF) as the retrograde limb of the reentrant circuit and the left anterior fascicle (LAF) as the anterograde limb. At right, the interfascicular reentrant VT utilizes the LAF as the retrograde limb of the reentrant circuit and the LPF as the anterograde limb. In both types, because the ventricle is activated via the left bundle branch (LB), the QRS has right bundle branch block morphology. The QRS axis will depend on which fascicle serves as the anterograde route of ventricular activation. The right bundle branch (RB) is activated in a bystander fashion and is not necessary for sustaining the tachycardia. AVN = atrioventricular node; HB = His bundle.

point, is relatively far from the retrogradely activated HB. During interfascicular VT, the LB potential should be inscribed before the His potential.[12] In contrast, during BBR VT with RBBB morphology, the His potential usually precedes the LB potential, although the reverse is theoretically possible if the retrograde conduction time to the HB recording point is significantly prolonged. Interfascicular reentry also demonstrates variations in the V-V interval preceded by similar changes in the H-H interval.

Atrial pacing, AES, VES, and ventricular pacing can initiate interfascicular reentry by producing transient anterograde block in the slowly conducting fascicle (LAF or LPF), with subsequent impulse anterograde conduction over the healthy fascicle, giving rise to a QRS morphology identical to that during NSR, and then retrogradely in the initially blocked fascicle to initiate reentry.

When interfascicular reentry occurs in the setting of an anterior MI, complete cure by ablation is usually not possible because other myocardial VTs are always present, and the LV ejection fraction is usually poor, thereby mandating ICD implantation for improved survival. When interfascicular reentry occurs without coronary artery disease, in association with degenerative disease of the conduction system, LV systolic function is usually normal and cure of the VT is possible by ablation of the diseased fascicle, although a pacemaker would likely be required.

Ablation of interfascicular tachycardia is guided by fascicular potentials. Successful ablation of the arrhythmia can be performed by targeting the LAF or LPF.[7]

REFERENCES

1. Akhtar M, Damato AN, Batsford WP, et al: Demonstration of re-entry within the His-Purkinje system in man. Circulation 1974;50:1150.
2. Josephson ME: Recurrent ventricular tachycardia. *In* Josephson M (ed): Clinical Cardiac Electrophysiology, 3rd ed. Philadelphia, Lippincott, Williams & Wilkins, 2002, pp 425-610.
3. Blanck Z, Dhala A, Deshpande S, et al: Bundle branch reentrant ventricular tachycardia: Cumulative experience in 48 patients. J Cardiovasc Electrophysiol 1993;4:253.
4. Lloyd EA, Zipes DP, Heger JJ, Prystowsky EN: Sustained ventricular tachycardia due to bundle branch reentry. Am Heart J 1982;104(Pt 1):1095.
5. Chalvidan T, Cellarier G, Deharo JC, et al: His-Purkinje system reentry as a proarrhythmic effect of flecainide. Pacing Clin Electrophysiol 2000;23(Pt 1):530.
6. Mazur A, Iakobishvili Z, Kusniec J, Strasberg B: Bundle branch reentrant ventricular tachycardia in a patient with the Brugada electrocardiographic pattern. Ann Noninvasive Electrocardiol 2003;8:352.
7. Lopera G, Stevenson WG, Soejima K, et al: Identification and ablation of three types of ventricular tachycardia involving the His-Purkinje system in patients with heart disease. J Cardiovasc Electrophysiol 2004;15:52.
8. Li YG, Gronefeld G, Israel C, et al: Bundle branch reentrant tachycardia in patients with apparent normal His-Purkinje conduction: The role of functional conduction impairment. J Cardiovasc Electrophysiol 2002;13:1233.
9. Glassman RD, Zipes DP: Site of antegrade and retrograde functional right bundle branch block in the intact canine heart. Circulation 1981;64:1277.
10. Fisher JD: Bundle branch reentry tachycardia: Why is the HV interval often longer than in sinus rhythm? The critical role of anisotropic conduction. J Interv Card Electrophysiol 2001;5:173.
11. Daoud EG: Bundle branch reentry. *In* Zipes D, Jalife J (eds): Cardiac Electrophysiology: From Cell to Bedside, 4th ed. Philadelphia, WB Saunders, 2004, pp 683-688.
12. Josephson ME: Recurrent ventricular tachycardia. *In* Josephson ME (ed): Clinical Cardiac Electrophysiology: Technique and Interpretation, 3rd ed. Philadelphia, Lippincott, Williams & Wilkins, 2002, pp 425-610.
13. Merino JL, Peinado R, Fernandez-Lozano I, et al: Bundle-branch reentry and the postpacing interval after entrainment by right ventricular apex stimulation: A new approach to elucidate the mechanism of wide-QRS-complex tachycardia with atrioventricular dissociation. Circulation 2001;103:1102.
14. Mehdirad AA, Tchou P: Catheter ablation of bundle branch reentrant ventricular tachycardia. *In* Huang D, Wilber DJ (eds): Radiofrequency Catheter Ablation of Cardiac Arrhythmias: Basic Concepts and Clinical Applications, 2nd ed. Armonk, NY, Futura, 2000, pp 653-658.

CHAPTER 21

Ventricular Tachycardia in Arrhythmogenic Right Ventricular Dysplasia

PATHOPHYSIOLOGY

The diagnosis of arrhythmogenic right ventricular dysplasia-cardiomyopathy (ARVD) has been used to describe the right ventricular (RV) myopathy associated with multiple left bundle branch block (LBBB)-type ventricular tachycardias (VTs). ARVD is a progressive disease in which normal myocardium is replaced by fibrofatty tissue. This disorder usually involves the RV, but the left ventricle (LV) and septum also can be affected. Fibrofatty replacement of myocardium produces "islands" of scar region that can lead to reentrant VTs, and these patients have an increased risk of sudden cardiac death, mostly secondary to VT.[1,2]

The exact cause of ARVD is not fully understood. Several theories for the pathogenesis of ARVD have been proposed, some of which reflect acquired rather than familial disease: dysontogenic, degenerative, inflammatory, and apoptotic. Progressive myocyte replacement can be secondary to a metabolic disorder affecting the RV. This process would be analogous to the situation involving skeletal muscle in patients with muscular dystrophy, in whom progressive degeneration of muscle occurs with time. The loss of myocardial tissue also can reflect increased apoptosis (programmed cell death) of myocardial cells. A possible infectious or immunological cause resulting in postinflammatory RV fibrofatty cardiomyopathy has also been suggested—up to 80% of hearts at autopsy documenting inflammatory infiltrates.[2]

ARVD can also represent a congenital abnormality of development, resulting in a progressive increase in RV size because of atrophy and weakness of the wall muscle. RV dilation then predisposes to the development of ventricular arrhythmias. Evidence has suggested that typical ARVD is a disease of the cardiac desmosome. Desmosomes are specialized cadherin-based cell–cell adhesion structures abundant in cardiac muscle and skin epidermis. Mutations in one or more desmosomal proteins, including desmoglein-2, desmoplakin, desmocollin-2, junctional plakoglobin, and plakophilin-2 have been identified in patients with ARVD. Mechanisms by which the affected desmosomes cause myocytes apoptosis, fibrogenesis, and adipogenesis, thus leading to impaired RV function and increased arrhythmogenicity, have been shown in vitro and in animal models. The effect of age and exercise on disease progression at the desmosomal level has also been shown in a mouse model.[3-16]

Two patterns of inheritance have been described in ARVD: autosomal dominant disease and Naxos disease. ARVD has been associated with an autosomal dominant inheritance pattern, with 30% to 50% of family members of index patients having manifestations of the disease. Disease loci for the autosomal dominant disorder have been mapped to chromosomes 14q23-q24 (ARVD1), 1q42-q43 (ARVD2), 14q12-q22 (ARVD3), 2q32 (ARVD4), 3p23 (ARVD5), 10p12-p14 (ARVD6), 10q22, 6p24 (ARVD8), and 12p11 (ARVD9). Some of the genes responsible have been identified. The gene at locus 1q42-q43 (ARVD2) encodes the cardiac ryanodine receptor RyR2. Affected patients have exercise-induced polymorphic VT. Mutations in RyR2 have also been associated with familial polymorphic VT without ARVD. RyR2 mediates the release of calcium from the sarcoplasmic reticulum that is required for myocardial contraction. The FK506 binding protein (FKBP12.6) stabilizes RyR2, preventing aberrant activation. The mutations in RyR2 interfere with the interaction with FKBP12.6, increasing channel activity under conditions that simulate exercise. The mutations in ARVD appear to act differently from those in familial polymorphic VT without ARVD. The gene at locus 6p24 (ARVD 8) encodes desmoplakin. Desmoplakin is a key component of desmosomes and adherens junctions that is important for maintaining the tight adhesion of many cell types, including those in the heart and skin; when junctions are disrupted, cell death and fibrofatty replacement occur.[13,17-23]

A variant form of ARVD with autosomal recessive inheritance is familial palmoplantar keratosis, also called Naxos disease and mal de Meleda disease. This disorder is characterized by typical features of ARVD accompanied by nonepidermolytic palmoplantar keratosis, a disorder of the epidermis causing hyperkeratosis of the palms and soles and woolly hair. All patients who are homozygotes for Naxos disease have diagnostic cardiac abnormalities, which are 100% penetrant by adolescence. These include ECG abnormalities (92%), RV structural alterations (100%), and LV involvement (27%). A minority of heterozygotes has minor ECG and echo changes, but clinically significant disease is not seen.[3,10,12,24]

Regardless of the mechanism, the patchy replacement of the RV myocardium by fatty and fibrous tissue provides a substrate for reentrant ventricular arrhythmias. The most striking morphological feature of the disease is the diffuse or segmental loss of RV myocytes, with replacement by fibrofatty tissue and thinning of the RV wall. Fibrofatty replacement usually begins in the subepicardium or midmural layers and progresses to the subendocardium. Only the endocardium and myocardium of the trabeculae may be spared. Anatomical malformations of the RV consist of mild to severe global RV dilation, RV aneurysms (Fig. 21-1), and segmental RV hypokinesia. The sites of involvement are found in the so-called triangle of dysplasia—namely, the RV outflow tract, apex, and inferolateral wall near the tricuspid valve. However, the fibrofatty pattern of ARVD is limited not only to the RV; the disease also can migrate to the interventricular septum and the LV free wall, with a predilection for the posteroseptal and posterolateral areas. LV involvement may even be the first manifestation of the disease.[25]

CLINICAL CONSIDERATIONS

Epidemiology

ARVD occurs in young adults (80% are younger than 40 years) and is more common in men. The mean age at diagnosis of familial ARVD is approximately 31 years. The disease is almost never diagnosed in infancy and rarely before the age of 10.[19]

The true incidence and prevalence of the disease are unknown because the diagnosis may be missed in a substantial number of patients. The prevalence of the disease

in the general population is estimated at 0.02% to 0.1% but is dependent on geographic circumstances. In certain regions of Italy (Padua, Venice) and Greece (island of Naxos), an increased prevalence of 0.4% to 0.8% for ARVD has been reported.[1,2]

Clinical Presentation

The clinical presentation varies widely because ARVD includes a spectrum of different conditions rather than a single identity. Different pathological processes can manifest a diversity of symptoms, such as fatigue, atypical chest pain, syncope, or acute coronary syndrome. ARVD can have a temporal progression and can present differently according to the time of presentation. Overall, judging the accurate position of the patient on the time scale of the spectrum is difficult, and some patients may remain stable for several decades.[2]

Approximately 50% of patients with ARVD present with symptomatic ventricular arrhythmias, most commonly sustained and nonsustained VT with LBBB configuration, although right bundle branch block (RBBB) configuration also can be observed, manifested by palpitations, dizziness, and/or syncope. The frequency of ventricular arrhythmias in ARVD varies with the severity of the disease, ranging from 23% in patients with mild disease to almost 100% in patients with severe disease. Ventricular arrhythmias characteristically occur during exercise; up to 50% to 60% of patients with ARVD show monomorphic VT during exercise testing.

Sudden cardiac death occurs in patients with ARVD and can be the first presentation of the disease. ARVD is an important cause of sudden cardiac death in young adults in northern Italy, accounting for approximately 11% of cases overall and 22% in athletes. In contrast, ARVD is rarely diagnosed in the United States. This probably reflects a difference in genetic predisposition.[1,19,25,26] The occurrence of arrhythmic cardiac arrest due to ARVD is significantly increased in athletes. The risk of exercise can be caused in part by increased stress on the RV.

Patients with ARVD at increased risk for sudden death include the following: (1) younger patients; (2) patients who present with or have recurrent syncope, (3) patients with a previous history of cardiac arrest or a history of VT with hemodynamic compromise; (4) patients with LV involvement; (5) patients with ARVD2, who can develop polymorphic VT and juvenile sudden death associated with sympathetic stimulation; (6) patients with an increase in QRS dispersion (maximum measured QRS duration minus minimum measured QRS duration $\geq$ 40 milliseconds); (7) patients with S wave upstroke $\geq$0 milliseconds on the 12-lead ECG; and (8) patients with Naxos disease.[12,17,27-29]

Supraventricular tachycardias (SVTs) are present in approximately 25% of patients with ARVD referred for treatment of ventricular arrhythmias; less often, they are

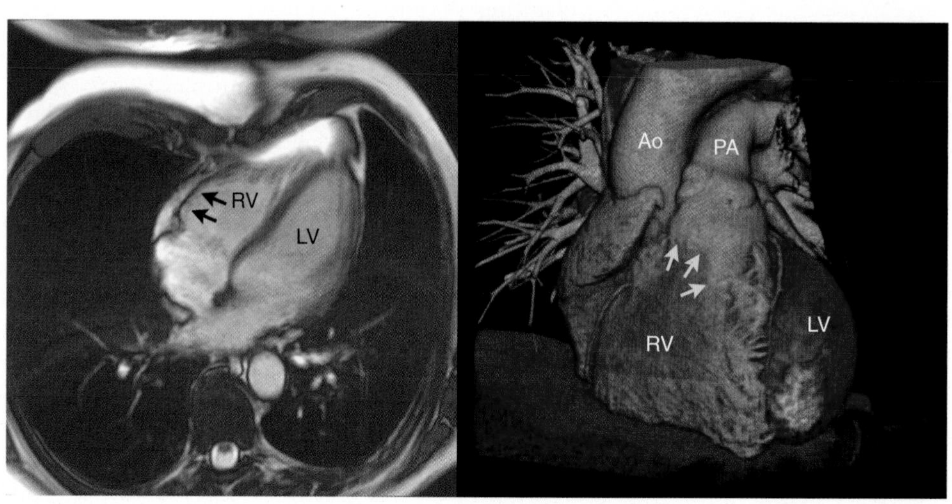

FIGURE 21–1 Right ventricular (RV) aneurysm. This cardiac CT angiogram shows thinning and aneurysmal dilation of the RV anterior wall and outflow tract (arrows) in a patient with arrhythmogenic right ventricular dysplasia-cardiomyopathy and ventricular tachycardia. Ao = aorta; LV = left ventricle; PA = pulmonary artery. *(Courtesy of Dr. Nasar Nallamothu, Prairie Cardiovascular Consultants, Springfield, Ill.)*

TABLE 21–1 Task Force Diagnostic Criteria for Arrhythmogenic Right Ventricular Dysplasia-Cardiomyopathy (ARVD)

Parameter	Major Criteria	Minor Criteria
I. Global and/or regional dysfunction and structural alterations	· Severe dilation and reduction of RV ejection fraction with no (or only mild) LV impairment · Localized RV aneurysms (akinetic or dyskinetic areas with diastolic bulging) · Severe segmental dilation of the RV	· Mild global RV dilation and/or ejection fraction reduction, with normal LV · Mild segmental dilation of the RV · Regional RV hypokinesia
II. Tissue characterization of walls	· Fibrofatty replacement of myocardium on endomyocardial biopsy	
III. Repolarization abnormalities		· Inverted T waves on right precordial leads (V_2 and V_3) (age > 12 yr, in absence of RBBB)
IV. Depolarization, conduction abnormalities	· Epsilon waves or localized prolongation (>110 msec) of the QRS complex in right precordial leads (V_1– V_3)	· Late potentials (signal-averaged ECG)
V. Arrhythmias		· LBBB-type VT, sustained and nonsustained (ECG, Holter, exercise testing) · Frequent PVCs, >1000/24 hr (Holter)
VI. Family history	· Familial disease confirmed at necropsy or surgery	· Familial history of premature sudden death (<35 yr) caused by suspected ARVD · Familial history (clinical diagnosis based on present criteria)

Adapted from McKenna WJ, Thiene G, Nava A, et al: Diagnosis of arrhythmogenic right ventricular dysplasia/cardiomyopathy. Task Force of the Working Group Myocardial and Pericardial Disease of the European Society of Cardiology and of the Scientific Council on Cardiomyopathies of the International Society and Federation of Cardiology. Br Heart J 1994;71:215.

To fulfill the appropriate criteria for ARVD, patients must meet two major criteria, one major plus two minor criteria, or four minor criteria.

LBBB = left bundle branch block; LV = left ventricle; PVC = premature ventricular complex; RBBB = right bundle branch block; RV = right ventricle.

the only arrhythmia present. In decreasing order of frequency, SVTs in these patients include atrial (AF), atrial tachycardia (AT), and atrial flutter (AFL).

Some patients are asymptomatic and ARVD is only suspected by the finding of ventricular ectopy and other abnormalities on routine ECG or other testing because of a positive family history. In a review of 37 families, only 17 of 168 patients with ARVD (10%) were healthy carriers. In one report, 9.6% of those initially unaffected subjects developed structural signs of disease on echocardiography during a mean follow-up of 8.5 years; almost 50% had symptomatic ventricular arrhythmias. Progression from mild to moderate disease occurred in 5% of patients, and progression from moderate to severe disease occurred in 8%.[19]

Unless sudden cardiac death occurs, progressive impairment of cardiac function can result in right or biventricular heart failure late in the evolution of ARVD, usually within 4 to 8 years after typical development of complete RBBB. In most patients, the mechanism of sudden death in ARVD is acceleration of VT, with ultimate degeneration into ventricular fibrillation (VF). Generally, RV failure and LV dysfunction are independently associated with cardiovascular mortality.

Initial Evaluation

Definitive diagnosis of ARVD requires histological confirmation of transmural fibrofatty replacement of the RV myocardium at postmortem or surgery; however, this criterion is not practical in the clinical setting. Furthermore, myocardial biopsy lacks sufficient sensitivity (67% in one report) because, for safety reasons, the biopsy is performed mostly in the interventricular septum, whereas the typical pathological changes of ARVD are more pronounced in the RV free wall.[2]

A study group has proposed diagnostic criteria based on family history as well as structural, functional, and ECG abnormalities (Table 21-1).[30] The diagnosis of ARVD is based on the presence of two major criteria, one major plus two minor criteria, or four minor criteria. These criteria are highly specific but lack sensitivity. Furthermore, this diagnostic approach does not specify the preferred order of imaging techniques to examine and score RV morphology and function. This diagnostic framework is being prospectively evaluated, but it is likely that less severe forms of the disease may not be encompassed by these criteria. When available, genetic diagnosis will improve diagnostic accuracy. A stepwise diagnostic approach has been suggested in patients with suspected ARVD (Table 21-2).[31]

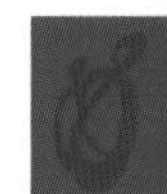

Principles of Management

Pharmacological Therapy

Therapy with beta blockers, sotalol, or amiodarone can be effective in suppressing ventricular arrhythmias and possibly in preventing sudden cardiac death. Among asymptomatic patients and those with mild disease, beta blockers are a reasonable recommendation to reduce the possibility of adrenergically induced arrhythmia.

Patients with well tolerated and non–life-threatening ventricular arrhythmias are at relatively low risk for sudden death and can be treated with antiarrhythmic drugs, guided either noninvasively with ambulatory monitoring or with EP testing.[1,31,32] The usefulness of antiarrhythmic drugs for primary prevention is considered less well established. Sotalol is more effective than beta blockers and amiodarone in patients with inducible VT and in those with noninducible VT. Among patients who have VT, those who are treated with antiarrhythmic drugs generally have a low risk of arrhythmic death, with an overall mortality rate of 0.08% per year.[19] The prognosis of ARVD is thus considerably better than the outcome with sustained VT of LV origin seen in patients with structural heart disease. The lower mortality in ARVD probably reflects a better hemodynamic tolerance of VT because of maintained LV function, and a lesser likelihood of degeneration to VF.

Thus, initial therapy with sotalol is a reasonable option for many patients for primary prevention. For those that do not respond to sotalol, response to other drugs is unlikely, and consideration should be given to nonpharmacological therapy. Sotalol can also be given to reduce the frequency of implantable cardioverter-defibrillator (ICD) discharges.

When the disease has progressed to right or biventricular failure, treatment consists of the current therapy for heart failure, including diuretics, beta blockers, angiotensin-converting enzyme inhibitors, and anticoagulants (if appropriate). For intractable RV failure, cardiac transplantation can be the only remaining alternative.[2,32]

Because of the association between exercise and the induction of ventricular tachyarrhythmias, a diagnosis of ARVD is considered incompatible with competitive sports and/or moderate- to high-intensity level recreational activities. Furthermore, any activity, competitive or not, that causes symptoms of palpitations, presyncope, or syncope should be avoided.[2,19,32]

Cardioverter-Defibrillator Implantation

Patients who are considered to be at high risk for sudden cardiac death should receive an ICD. This includes patients who have been resuscitated from cardiac arrest, with history of syncope, or who have life-threatening arrhythmias that are not completely suppressed by antiarrhythmic drug therapy (secondary prevention), and those with the disease who have a family history of cardiac arrest in first-degree relatives (primary prevention).

There are risks with this approach. Areas of the RV myocardium in patients with ARVD are thin and noncontractile and can be penetrated during placement of the RV leads, with subsequent cardiac tamponade. Also, the fibrofatty nature of the RV can lead to difficulty in attaining a location with acceptable R wave amplitude and pacing threshold. Marginal parameters may prevent adequate sensing of arrhythmias, resulting in improper ICD function or failure. Therefore, ICD implantation is reserved for patients who do not tolerate or respond to drug therapy or who have had unstable VT or sudden death. In all other patient categories, it may be preferable to start with sotalol as the primary drug of choice.[1,2,27,31-38]

Catheter Ablation

Catheter ablation of VT may be indicated for some ARVD patients, either as a primary therapy or as an adjunct to ICD implantation in patients with numerous VT episodes or those who are intolerant of antiarrhythmic drugs, to reduce the number of ICD therapies and improve quality of life.[39-41] However, given the high long-term recurrence rate, this technique is far from curative.

TABLE 21–2 Stepwise Approach to the Diagnosis of Arrhythmogenic Right Ventricular Dysplasia-Cardiomyopathy (ARVD)

Step	Test	Indication
I.	· Clinical history (family history of sudden death or ARVD; personal history of syncope · ECG (12-lead, 24-hour Holter monitoring, exercise testing, signal-averaged ECG) · Echocardiography	· Baseline clinical evaluation of patients with suspected ARVD
II.	· Contrast ventricular angiography · Cardiac MRI · Radionuclide ventricular angiography	· Patients with borderline findings at previous clinical evaluation
III.	· Electrophysiology testing	· Assessment of ventricular electrical stability and guide for antiarrhythmic therapy
IV.	· Endomyocardial biopsy	· Histological validation of diagnosis in select patients
V.	· Molecular genetic testing	· Genetic diagnosis

From Corrado D, Basso C, Nava A, Thiene G: Arrhythmogenic right ventricular cardiomyopathy: Current diagnostic and management strategies. Cardiol Rev 2001;9:259.

ELECTROCARDIOGRAPHIC FEATURES

Approximately 40% to 50% of patients with ARVD have a normal ECG at presentation. However, by 6 years, almost all patients with ARVD have one or more of several findings on ECG during normal sinus rhythm (NSR), including epsilon wave, T wave inversion, QRS duration ≥ 110 milliseconds in leads V_1 through V_3, and RBBB. Significant differences exist in most ECG features among ARVD patients according to the degree of RV involvement, and they are more prevalent in diffuse ARVD than in the localized form of the disease.[19]

The hallmark feature of ARVD, the epsilon wave, is a marker of delayed activation of the RV and is considered a major diagnostic criterion for ARVD (Fig. 21-2). This is a highly specific but insensitive criterion and is observed in 25% to 33% of ARVD patients when evaluated by standard ECG. The epsilon wave has the appearance of a distinct wave just beyond the QRS, particularly in lead V_1, and represents low-amplitude potentials caused by delayed activation of some portion of the RV.

Other markers of delayed activation of the RV include prolongation of the QRS duration ≥10 milliseconds in leads V_1 through V_3, and the ratio of the sum of the QRS duration in leads $(V_1 + V_2 + V_3) / (V_4 + V_5 + V_6) \geq 2$. In fact, a QRS duration > 110 milliseconds in lead V_1 has a sensitivity of 55% and a specificity of 100% in patients suspected of having

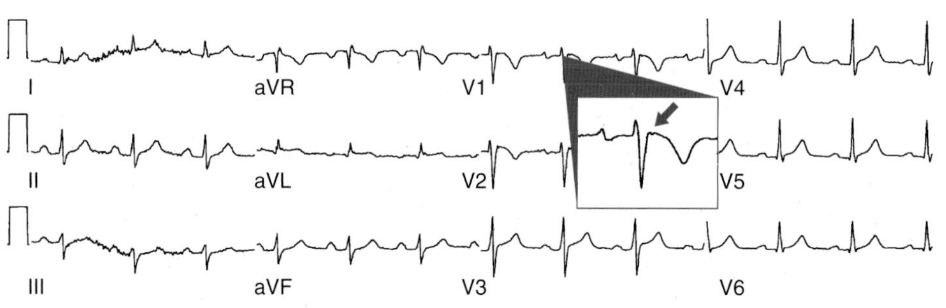

FIGURE 21–2 Surface ECG of sinus rhythm in a patient with arrhythmogenic right ventricular dysplasia-cardiomyopathy. **Inset,** Magnified view of a single complex in V_1 showing epsilon waves (arrow).

ARVD based on historical features. Additionally, incomplete (18%) or complete (15%) RBBB can be present. Epicardial mapping suggests that these patterns are usually caused by parietal block, rather than by disease of the bundle branch. In the presence of an RBBB pattern, selective prolongation of the QRS duration in leads V_1 to V_3 compared with lead V_6 (>25 milliseconds, parietal block) is an important hallmark of ARVD. Furthermore, T wave inversion in leads V_1 through V_3 in the absence of RBBB is considered a minor diagnostic criterion for ARVD and its prevalence in ARVD has been reported as 55% to 94% in different series. The extent of right precordial T wave inversion relates to the degree of RV involvement. Increased QT dispersion (i. e., interlead variability of the QT interval) has been observed in ARVD.[2,32]

Prolongation of the upstroke of the S wave (≥55 milliseconds) in leads V_1 through V_3 in the absence of RBBB is a new ECG criterion that was found to be present in all cases with diffuse ARVD and was also highly prevalent (90%) in the localized form of the disease.[42] This measurement has the highest diagnostic usefulness for differentiating the localized form of ARVD from right ventricular outflow tract (RVOT) VT, correlates with the degree of RV involvement, and is an independent predictor of VT induction. It is recognized that a prolonged S wave upstroke directly relates to QRS width in the right precordial leads; nonetheless, it is superior to localized QRS prolongation in distinguishing the mild form of ARVD from RVOT VT.[42]

Ventricular ectopy in ARVD usually arises from the RV and therefore has an LBBB pattern similar to that seen in idiopathic RVOT VT. The ECG morphology of the VT is predominantly LBBB, but RBBB can be observed and does not exclude an RV origin (Fig. 21-3). The QRS axis during VT is typically between −90 and +11 degrees; an extreme rightward direction of the QRS axis is uncommon.[43] No correlation has been observed between any specific ECG morphology and a particular activation pattern, although all RBBB morphology VTs exhibit a peritricuspid circuit.

ELECTROPHYSIOLOGICAL FEATURES

As noted, in ARVD, the normal myocardium is replaced by fatty and then fibrous tissue, causing thinning and scarring, predominantly in the RV. Studies have found that regions of abnormal voltage suggestive of scar were observed in all patients.[41,44] The endocardial bipolar voltage abnormalities tend to be perivalvular and, although affecting predominantly the RV free wall, involve some aspect of the septum in most patients (76%). This pattern is consistent with path-

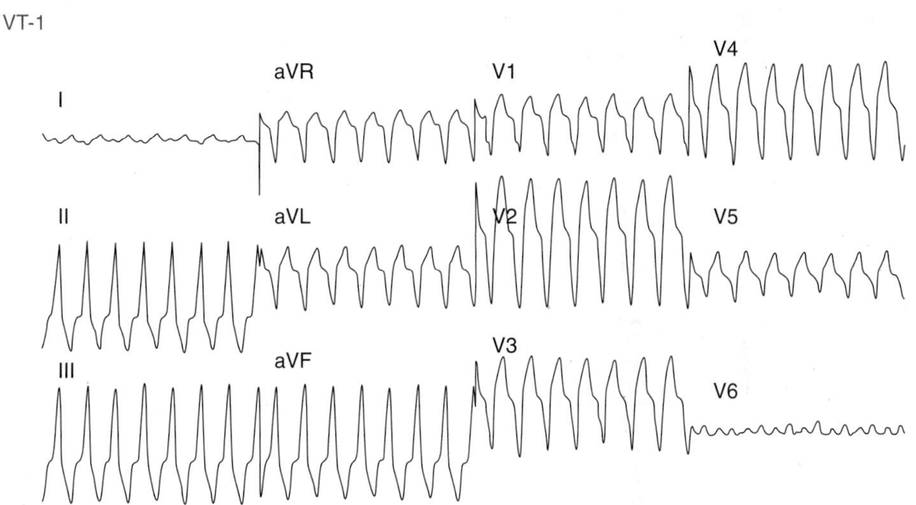

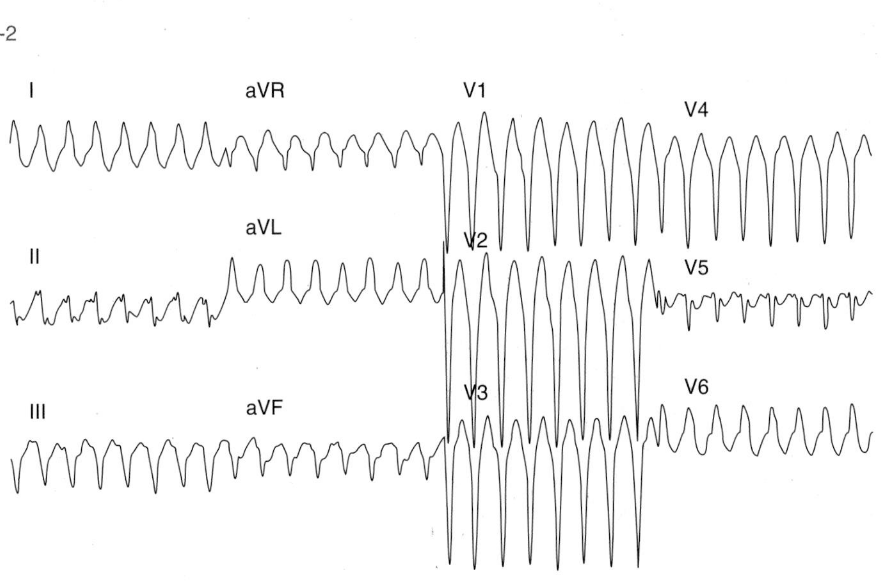

FIGURE 21–3 Surface lead ECGs of ventricular tachycardia (VT) in a patient with arrhythmogenic right ventricular dysplasia-cardiomyopathy. Both have left bundle branch block–type morphology but with very different frontal axes.

ological studies demonstrating a predilection for scar to occur in these particular areas in ARVD. It is unclear why these specific regions develop scar, although local apoptosis or inflammation may play a role.

In ARVD, the regions of abnormal myocardium do not always follow the pattern of dense scar surrounded by a ring of abnormal myocardium, often referred to as the scar border zone. Sometimes, abnormal voltages are found alone, without dense scar defining the regions. This is because ARVD is a different process from scarring caused by myocardial infarction (MI). Infarction causes dense scar surrounded by a border zone because of the ischemic penumbra that surrounds the infarcted territory. In ARVD, however, the process is patchy and can cause inhomogeneous scarring in anatomically disparate areas. Nevertheless, previous data have shown that it is still possible to identify well-demarcated borders around these abnormal regions.

A monomorphic VT in the setting of ARVD is associated with a predominantly perivalvular distribution of endocardial electrogram abnormalities and arrhythmia origin. Perivalvular LV endocardial involvement is also common, both in pathological studies and in voltage mapping studies, and can be associated with the origin of additional VTs from that chamber.[44]

The disease in ARVD has been reported to begin epicardially and progress to the endocardium.[30,39,45] Therefore, endocardial fibrosis, as reflected by the voltage map findings, can be a manifestation of more extensive disease involvement and can be anticipated to be the more common substrate for uniform sustained VT. Whether an extensive perivalvular fibrotic process is fairly specific for patients who present with sustained monomorphic VT in the setting of RV cardiomyopathy is yet to be determined.

Reentry in areas of abnormal myocardium is the most likely mechanism of VT in ARVD, as demonstrated by entrainment mapping. The repetitive initiation of these VTs by ventricular programmed stimulation also suggests a reentrant mechanism. Most reentrant circuits cluster around the tricuspid annulus and the RVOT. The critical isthmus of each reentrant circuit typically is bounded by an area of low scar (as identified by voltage mapping) on one side and an anatomical barrier (tricuspid annulus) on the other side, or by two parallel lines of double potentials. VTs in patients with ARVD exhibiting a focal activation pattern have also been described; however, an epicardial reentrant circuit with a defined endocardial exit may explain the focal activation pattern of the RV endocardium.[43]

Multiple morphologies of inducible VT are common. A variety of different reentry circuit sites can be identified with entrainment mapping. A single region can give rise to multiple VT morphologies.

The association with exercise and stress and the frequent induction of arrhythmia by isoproterenol infusion suggests a role for catecholamines. The sensitivity to catecholamines, which may be acquired, can result from abnormalities in cardiac sympathetic function.[46]

It is important to distinguish idiopathic RVOT VT from VT caused by ARVD, both of which generally have LBBB morphology. Idiopathic RVOT VT has a much more benign prognosis than ARVD and can be successfully treated with radiofrequency (RF) ablation. The resting ECG in NSR is typically normal in patients with idiopathic VT. The surface ECG is also normal in 40% to 50% of patients with ARVD at presentation, but in almost no patient after 6 years. Patients with idiopathic VT have a normal signal-averaged ECG when in NSR and normal imaging studies of RV size and function. Other clues suggesting the presence of an RV cardiomyopathy include the presence of RV dilation, multiple VT morphologies, and a well-defined anatomical substrate. VTs in ARVD patients generally have lower QRS amplitude and more fragmentation, but these are qualitative differences not always present.

The response during electrophysiological (EP) testing is also helpful in distinguishing idiopathic RVOT VT from ARVD. In one report, programmed electrical stimulation induced VT in all but 1 of 15 patients with ARVD compared with only 2 patients with idiopathic RVOT VT (93% versus 3%). Additionally, fractionated diastolic electrograms recorded during VT or NSR at the VT site of origin or other RV sites were present in all but one patient with ARVD, but were not seen in any patient with idiopathic RVOT VT. Furthermore, the induction of VTs with different QRS morphologies was seen only in ARVD (73% versus 0%). Although isoproterenol infusion can induce VT in patients with idiopathic RVOT VT, it has a similar effect in ARVD and therefore does not help distinguish between these disorders. Reentry was the mechanism of tachycardia in 80% of the ARVD group, whereas 97% of RVOT VT had features of triggered activity.[47]

MAPPING

Activation Mapping

Endocardial activation mapping during VT can detect abnormal fragmented electrograms with diastolic potentials (Fig. 21-4). The site of origin for mappable VT demonstrates presystolic activity and entrainment with concealed fusion and a post-pacing interval (PPI) within 30 milliseconds of tachycardia CL.[44]

Entrainment Mapping

Entrainment mapping is used to characterize reentry circuits in ARVD, identify critical isthmuses, and guide ablation. VT circuits in ARVD share many features observed in post-MI VTs. First, the circuits are comprised of zones of abnormal conduction, characterized by low-amplitude abnormal electrograms, with identifiable exit regions to the surrounding myocardium. Second, outer loops, which can be broad portions of the reentry circuit in communication with the surrounding myocardium, have also been observed. Third, the same types of targets for ablation previously identified in post-MI VT (critical isthmus) can also be useful for targeting VT in ARVD.

In ARVD, reentrant circuit sites, as determined by entrainment mapping, tend to cluster around the RVOT and the inferolateral tricuspid annulus, which are typical areas of fibrous and fatty infiltration in ARVD. Interestingly, VTs from these locations appear to be more susceptible to ablation than VTs originating from the body of the RV.[44]

Pace Mapping

Pace mapping helps confirm ablation target sites. For VT that is not mappable, the circuit's exit site is approximated by the site of pace mapping that generates QRS complexes similar to those of VT. When detailed activation mapping and entrainment mapping cannot be performed, limited activation and entrainment information can be used to corroborate pace map information when available.[44]

Electroanatomical Substrate Mapping

Electroanatomical mapping provides a helpful tool in reconstructing the VT circuit in patients with ARVD and hemodynamically stable VTs.[43] Additionally, in a subset of ARVD patients, conventional mapping during VT can be limited by changing multiple morphologies, nonsustain-

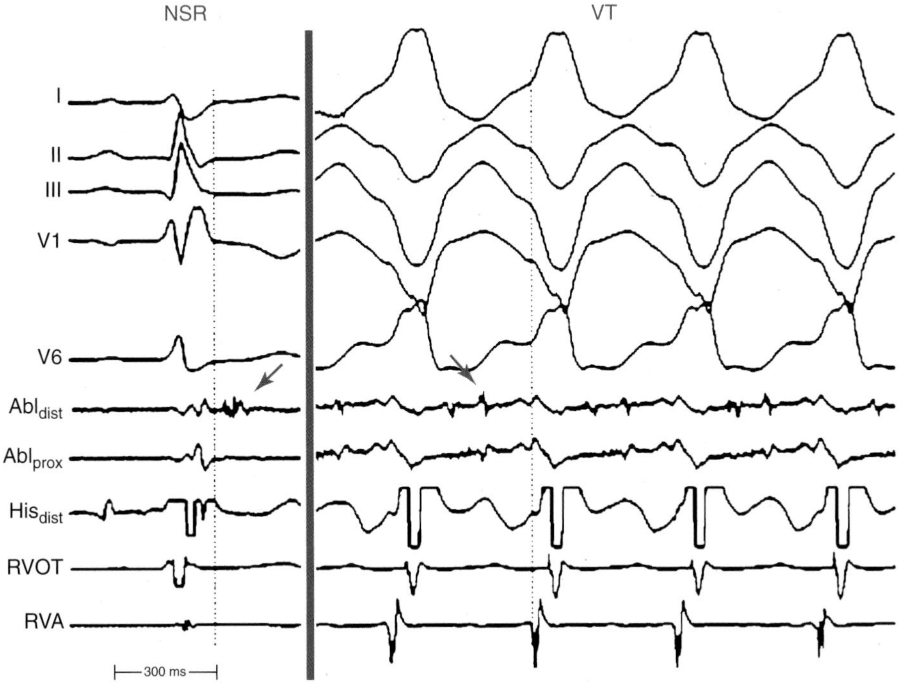

FIGURE 21–4 ECG and intracardiac recordings during normal sinus rhythm (NSR; left) and ventricular tachycardia (VT; right) in a patient with arrhythmogenic right ventricular dysplasia-cardiomyopathy. During NSR, a late potential is present (arrow); the same potential occurs during mid-diastole during VT.

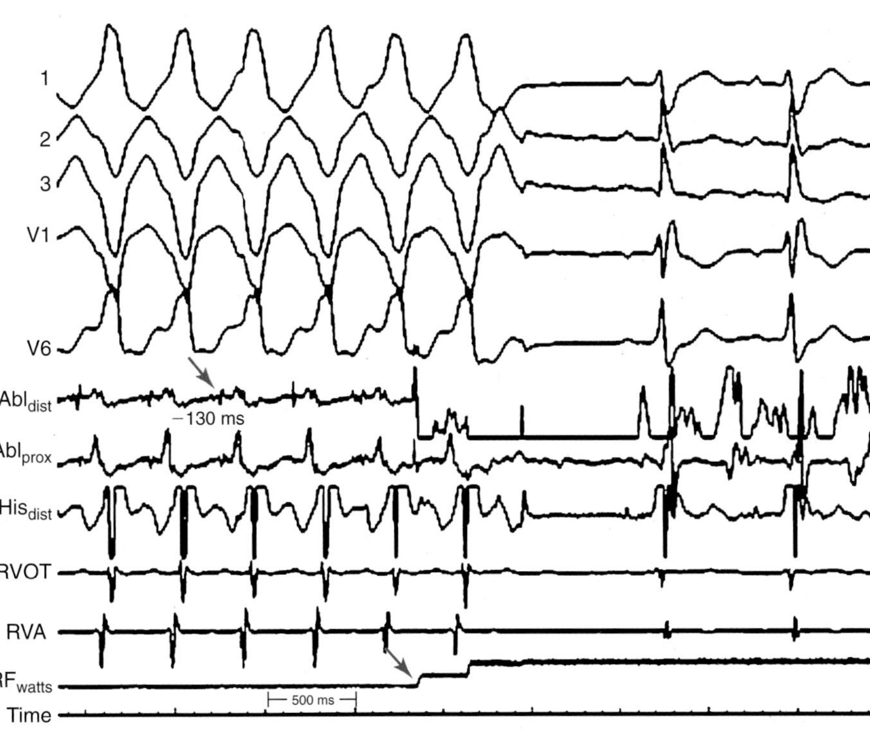

FIGURE 21–5 Ablation of arrhythmogenic right ventricular dysplasia-cardiomyopathy (ARVD) ventricular tachycardia. Shown is radiofrequency (RF) energy delivery in the basal lateral right ventricle in a patient with ARVD. Note the mid-diastolic potential (red arrow) 130 msec prior to QRS onset and almost immediate cessation of ventricular tachycardia on RF delivery. Blue arrow marks initiation of RF energy delivery.

ability, or hemodynamic instability. Substrate-based voltage mapping during sinus rhythm can be used in these cases to identify regions of scar and abnormal myocardium and guide, in conjunction with pace mapping, ablation of linear lesions to connect or encircle the abnormal regions.[41]

The dysplastic regions can be identified, quantified, and differentiated from healthy myocardium by the presence of electrograms with low amplitudes and longer durations, reflecting replaced myocardial tissue. Voltage mapping is performed during sinus rhythm, atrial pacing, or ventricular pacing. The peak to peak signal amplitude of the bipolar electrogram is measured automatically.[44] Endocardial regions with a bipolar electrogram amplitude > 1.5 mV are defined as normal, and dense scar areas are defined as those with an amplitude < 0.5 mV. Abnormal myocardium is defined as an area of contiguous recordings with a bipolar electrogram amplitude between 0.5 and 1.5 mV.[41,43,44] These abnormal regions are mostly located around the lateral tricuspid annulus, proximal RVOT, anterior-anteroapical wall, and inferior-inferoapical wall.

ABLATION

For stable VT, RF ablation targets the critical isthmus of the reentrant circuit, as defined by activation, entrainment, and pace mapping. Most VTs can be entrained and critical isthmuses can be identified and ablated to terminate the tachycardia successfully (Fig. 21-5).[43]

For unmappable VT, RF ablation can be performed as linear lesions targeting potential exit sites and isthmuses of VT circuits based on the location of the best pace map, location of valvular anatomical boundaries, and the substrate defined by the voltage mapping. Typically, linear lesions are created over target regions by sequential point lesions designed to accomplish the following: (1) connect scar or abnormal myocardium to a valve continuity; (2) connect scar or abnormal myocardium to another scar; (3) extend from the most abnormal endocardium (<0.5 mV) to normal myocardium (>1.5 mV); or (4) encircle the scar or abnormal region, depending on the scar location and size.[41,44,48]

Ablation of VT in ARVD still remains a clinical challenge and should be viewed as a potential palliative procedure in selected patients, although more cases are being reported in the literature. Although VT ablation is feasible in ARVD patients with relatively high short-term success, up to 88% in one series, long-term success is low and VT recurs in up to 85% of patients, even following extensive or repeated ablation attempts.[38,41,43,49]

One reason for the poor long-term outcome is that ARVD is a progressive disease, with new regions of scar developing over time and creating new circuits or changes in current ones. Furthermore, multiple morphologies, hemodynamic instability, or noninducibility can limit the success of VT ablation.[30] Additionally, ARVD can create a large number of potential circuits; an empirical approach may not eliminate all the possible pathways. Achieving adequate energy delivery can also be a problem, particularly in regions difficult to access by catheter—in particular, abnormal regions along the tricuspid annulus, which can require the use of 8-mm-tip or irrigation-tip ablation to achieve effective lesions underneath the tricuspid valve. It must be emphasized that caution must be taken when using irrigation-tip ablation in patients with very thin ventricular walls. The risk of creating deeper lesions in thin walls of the RV body or apex potentially increases the risk of perforation, although the magnitude of this risk is not well known.[41]

REFERENCES

1. Corrado D, Fontaine G, Marcus FI, et al: Arrhythmogenic right ventricular dysplasia/cardiomyopathy: Need for an international registry. Study Group on Arrhythmogenic Right Ventricular Dysplasia/Cardiomyopathy of the Working Groups on Myocardial and Pericardial Disease and Arrhythmias of the European Society of Cardiology and of the Scientific Council on Cardiomyopathies of the World Heart Federation. Circulation 2000;101:E101.
2. Gemayel C, Pelliccia A, Thompson PD: Arrhythmogenic right ventricular cardiomyopathy. J Am Coll Cardiol 2001;38:1773.
3. Alcalai R, Metzger S, Rosenheck S, et al: A recessive mutation in desmoplakin causes arrhythmogenic right ventricular dysplasia, skin disorder, and woolly hair. J Am Coll Cardiol 2003;42:319.
4. Awad MM, Dalal D, Cho E, et al: DSG2 mutations contribute to arrhythmogenic right ventricular dysplasia/cardiomyopathy. Am J Hum Genet 2006;79:136.
5. Bauce B, Basso C, Rampazzo A, et al: Clinical profile of four families with arrhythmogenic right ventricular cardiomyopathy caused by dominant desmoplakin mutations. Eur Heart J 2005;26:1666.
6. Dalal D, Molin LH, Piccini J, et al: Clinical features of arrhythmogenic right ventricular dysplasia/cardiomyopathy associated with mutations in plakophilin-2. Circulation 2006;113:1641.
7. Garcia-Gras E, Lombardi R, Giocondo MJ, et al: Suppression of canonical Wnt/beta-catenin signaling by nuclear plakoglobin recapitulates phenotype of arrhythmogenic right ventricular cardiomyopathy. J Clin Invest 2006;116:2012.
8. Gerull B, Heuser A, Wichter T, et al: Mutations in the desmosomal protein plakophilin-2 are common in arrhythmogenic right ventricular cardiomyopathy. Nat Genet 2004;36:1162.
9. Kirchhof P, Fabritz L, Zwiener M, et al: Age- and training-dependent development of arrhythmogenic right ventricular cardiomyopathy in heterozygous plakoglobin-deficient mice. Circulation 2006;114:1799.
10. McKoy G, Protonotarios N, Crosby A, et al: Identification of a deletion in plakoglobin in arrhythmogenic right ventricular cardiomyopathy with palmoplantar keratoderma and woolly hair (Naxos disease). Lancet 2000;355:2119.
11. Pilichou K, Nava A, Basso C, et al: Mutations in desmoglein-2 gene are associated with arrhythmogenic right ventricular cardiomyopathy. Circulation 2006;113:1171.
12. Protonotarios N, Tsatsopoulou A, Anastasakis A: Genotype-phenotype assessment in autosomal recessive arrhythmogenic right ventricular cardiomyopathy (Naxos disease) caused by a deletion in plakoglobin. J Am Coll Cardiol 2001;38:1477.
13. Rampazzo A, Nava A, Malacrida S, et al: Mutation in human desmoplakin domain binding to plakoglobin causes a dominant form of arrhythmogenic right ventricular cardiomyopathy. Am J Hum Genet 2002;71:1200.
14. Syrris P, Ward D, Asimaki A, et al: Clinical expression of plakophilin-2 mutations in familial arrhythmogenic right ventricular cardiomyopathy. Circulation 2006;113:356.
15. Syrris P, Ward D, Evans A, et al: Arrhythmogenic right ventricular dysplasia/cardiomyopathy associated with mutations in the desmosomal gene desmocollin-2. Am J Hum Genet 2006;79:978.
16. van Tintelen JP, Entius MM, Bhuiyan ZA, et al: Plakophilin-2 mutations are the major determinant of familial arrhythmogenic right ventricular dysplasia/cardiomyopathy. Circulation 2006;113:1650.
17. Bauce B, Nava A, Rampazzo A, et al: Familial effort polymorphic ventricular arrhythmias in arrhythmogenic right ventricular cardiomyopathy map to chromosome 1q42-43. Am J Cardiol 2000;85:573.
18. Li D, Ahmad F, Gardner MJ, et al: The locus of a novel gene responsible for arrhythmogenic right-ventricular dysplasia characterized by early onset and high penetrance maps to chromosome 10p12-p14. Am J Hum Genet 2000;66:148.
19. Nava A, Bauce B, Basso C, et al: Clinical profile and long-term follow-up of 37 families with arrhythmogenic right ventricular cardiomyopathy. J Am Coll Cardiol 2000;36:2226.
20. Priori SG, Napolitano C, Memmi M, et al: Clinical and molecular characterization of patients with catecholaminergic polymorphic ventricular tachycardia. Circulation 2002;106:69.
21. Tiso N, Stephan DA, Nava A, et al: Identification of mutations in the cardiac ryanodine receptor gene in families affected with arrhythmogenic right ventricular cardiomyopathy type 2 (ARVD2). Hum Mol Genet 2001;10:189.
22. Tiso N, Salamon M, Bagattin A, et al: The binding of the RyR2 calcium channel to its gating protein FKBP12.6 is oppositely affected by ARVD2 and VTSIP mutations. Biochem Biophys Res Commun 2002;299:594.
23. Wehrens XH, Lehnart SE, Huang F, et al: FKBP12.6 deficiency and defective calcium release channel (ryanodine receptor) function linked to exercise-induced sudden cardiac death. Cell 2003;113:829.
24. Norgett EE, Hatsell SJ, Carvajal-Huerta L, et al: Recessive mutation in desmoplakin disrupts desmoplakin-intermediate filament interactions and causes dilated cardiomyopathy, woolly hair and keratoderma. Hum Mol Genet 2000;9:2761.
25. Tabib A, Loire R, Chalabreysse L, et al: Circumstances of death and gross and microscopic observations in a series of 200 cases of sudden death associated with arrhythmogenic right ventricular cardiomyopathy and/or dysplasia. Circulation 2003;108:3000.
26. Maron BJ, Carney KP, Lever HM, et al: Relationship of race to sudden cardiac death in competitive athletes with hypertrophic cardiomyopathy. J Am Coll Cardiol 2003;41:974.
27. Corrado D, Leoni L, Link MS, et al: Implantable cardioverter-defibrillator therapy for prevention of sudden death in patients with arrhythmogenic right ventricular cardiomyopathy/dysplasia. Circulation 2003;108:3084.
28. Le GD, Gauthier H, Porcher R, et al: Prognostic value of radionuclide angiography in patients with right ventricular arrhythmias. Circulation 2001;103:1972.
29. Turrini P, Corrado D, Basso C, et al: Dispersion of ventricular depolarization-repolarization: A noninvasive marker for risk stratification in arrhythmogenic right ventricular cardiomyopathy. Circulation 2001;103:3075.
30. McKenna WJ, Thiene G, Nava A, et al: Diagnosis of arrhythmogenic right ventricular dysplasia/cardiomyopathy. Task Force of the Working Group Myocardial and Pericardial Disease of the European Society of Cardiology and of the Scientific Council on Cardiomyopathies of the International Society and Federation of Cardiology. Br Heart J 1994;71:215.
31. Corrado D, Basso C, Nava A, Thiene G: Arrhythmogenic right ventricular cardiomyopathy: Current diagnostic and management strategies. Cardiol Rev 2001;9:259.
32. Kies P, Bootsma M, Bax J, et al: Arrhythmogenic right ventricular dysplasia/cardiomyopathy: screening, diagnosis, and treatment. Heart Rhythm 2006;3:225.
33. Gatzoulis K, Protonotarios N, Anastasakis A, et al: Implantable defibrillator therapy in Naxos disease. Pacing Clin Electrophysiol 2000;23:1176.
34. Priori SG, Aliot E, Blomstrom-Lundqvist C, et al: Task Force on Sudden Cardiac Death of the European Society of Cardiology. Eur Heart J 2001;22:1374.
35. Tavernier R, Gevaert S, De SJ, et al: Long term results of cardioverter-defibrillator implantation in patients with right ventricular dysplasia and malignant ventricular tachyarrhythmias. Heart 2001;85:53.
36. Basso C, Wichter T, Danieli GA, et al: Arrhythmogenic right ventricular cardiomyopathy: Clinical registry and database, evaluation of therapies, pathology registry, DNA banking. Eur Heart J 2004;25:531.
37. D'Amati G, di Gioia CR, Giordano C, Gallo P: Myocyte transdifferentiation: A possible pathogenetic mechanism for arrhythmogenic right ventricular cardiomyopathy. Arch Pathol Lab Med 2000;124:287.
38. Thiene G, Basso C: Arrhythmogenic right ventricular cardiomyopathy: An update. Cardiovasc Pathol 2001;10:109.
39. Basso C, Fox PR, Meurs KM, et al: Arrhythmogenic right ventricular cardiomyopathy causing sudden cardiac death in boxer dogs: A new animal model of human disease. Circulation 2004;109:1180.
40. Danieli GA, Rampazzo A: Genetics of arrhythmogenic right ventricular cardiomyopathy. Curr Opin Cardiol 2002;17:218.
41. Verma A, Kilicaslan F, Schweikert RA, et al: Short- and long-term success of substrate-based mapping and ablation of ventricular tachycardia in arrhythmogenic right ventricular dysplasia. Circulation 2005;111:3209.

42. Nasir K, Bomma C, Tandri H, et al: Electrocardiographic features of arrhythmogenic right ventricular dysplasia/cardiomyopathy according to disease severity: A need to broaden diagnostic criteria. Circulation 2004;110:1527.
43. Miljoen H, State S, de Chillou C, et al: Electroanatomic mapping characteristics of ventricular tachycardia in patients with arrhythmogenic right ventricular cardiomyopathy/dysplasia. Europace 2005;7:516.
44. Marchlinski FE, Zado E, Dixit S, et al: Electroanatomic substrate and outcome of catheter ablative therapy for ventricular tachycardia in setting of right ventricular cardiomyopathy. Circulation 2004;110:2293.
45. Peters S, Brattstrom A, Gotting B, Trummel M: Value of intracardiac ultrasound in the diagnosis of arrhythmogenic right ventricular dysplasia-cardiomyopathy. Int J Cardiol 2002;83:111.
46. Wichter T, Schafers M, Rhodes CG, et al: Abnormalities of cardiac sympathetic innervation in arrhythmogenic right ventricular cardiomyopathy: Quantitative assessment of presynaptic norepinephrine reuptake and postsynaptic beta-adrenergic receptor density with positron emission tomography. Circulation 2000;101:1552.
47. Niroomand F, Carbucicchio C, Tondo C, et al: Electrophysiological characteristics and outcome in patients with idiopathic right ventricular arrhythmia compared with arrhythmogenic right ventricular dysplasia. Heart 2002;87:41.
48. Marchlinski FE, Callans DJ, Gottlieb CD, Zado E: Linear ablation lesions for control of unmappable ventricular tachycardia in patients with ischemic and nonischemic cardiomyopathy. Circulation 2000;101:1288.
49. Dalal D, Jain R, Tandri H, et al: Long-term efficacy of catheter ablation of ventricular tachycardia in patients with arrhythmogenic right ventricular dysplasia/cardiomyopathy. J Am Coll Cardiol 2007;50:432.

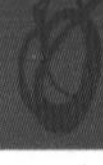

CHAPTER 22

Other Ventricular Tachycardias

VENTRICULAR TACHYCARDIA LATE AFTER REPAIR OF CONGENITAL HEART DEFECTS

General Considerations

The most information concerning patients with ventricular tachycardia (VT) and congenital heart disease pertains to tetralogy of Fallot, as compared with other forms of congenital heart disease. Tetralogy of Fallot is the most common cyanotic malformation. The core lesion is an underdeveloped subpulmonary infundibulum, which is superiorly and anteriorly displaced, resulting in the well-known tetrad—pulmonary stenosis, ventricular septal defect, aortic override, and right ventricular (RV) hypertrophy.[1] Correction of the defect involves patch closure of the ventricular septal defect and relief of right ventricular outflow tract (RVOT) obstruction, which typically requires resection of a large amount of RV muscle. When the procedure was first performed, it was not done through the tricuspid valve but required a ventriculotomy. The pulmonary annulus is usually small, and repair with a transannular patch leads to chronic pulmonic insufficiency, which can be severe if associated with downstream obstruction caused by significant pulmonary arterial stenosis. It has been hypothesized that ventricular arrhythmias in these patients are of the result of years of chronic cyanosis, followed by the placement of a ventriculotomy, increased RV pressures caused by inadequate relief of obstruction, and severe pulmonic regurgitation with RV dysfunction. Such factors can lead to myocardial fibrosis and result in the substrate for reentrant ventricular arrhythmias.[1,2]

Ventricular arrhythmias late after repair of congenital heart disease are a common finding, predominantly in those with tetralogy of Fallot, and potentially contribute to sudden death in this population. The incidence of late sudden death has been debated but ranges from 1% to 5% during a follow-up period of 7 to 20 years after surgery. Patients with surgical correction of ventricular septal defect or pulmonary stenosis also have a higher than normal risk of serious ventricular arrhythmias and sudden death.[2] In a multicenter study of 359 surgically treated patients with tetralogy of Fallot, sustained VT was noted in 33 patients (9.2%).[2]

Although controversy still exits, considerable progress has been made toward identifying noninvasive risk factors for VT and sudden cardiac death in corrected tetralogy of Fallot. Independent predictors of clinical VT include QRS duration ≥180 milliseconds, late and rapid increase in QRS duration after surgery, dispersion of QRS duration on the surface ECG, increased QT interval dispersion, high-grade ventricular ectopy on Holter monitoring, complete heart block, older age at surgery (especially older than 10 years), presence of a transannular RVOT patch, increased RV systolic pressures, RVOT aneurysm, and pulmonic and tricuspid regurgitation.[2,3]

QRS widening after tetralogy of Fallot repair is probably the result of a combined effect of the surgical injury on the myocardium and on the right bundle, and of the RV enlargement. Therefore, a prolonged QRS duration cannot be considered the specific expression of delayed intraventricular conduction from an arrhythmogenic substrate, but a nonspecific marker of electrical instability.[4]

Electrophysiological Features

Despite advances in noninvasive risk stratification, identification of high-risk subgroups has not been sufficiently accurate to guide management decisions reliably. More recently, inducible sustained VT by programmed ventricular stimulation was found to be a significant independent predictor of events in patients with and without antiarrhythmic agents, VT ablation, and defibrillators.[5] In this patient population, the rate of inducible sustained VT is approximately 35%, which is similar to that reported in post–myocardial infarction (MI) patients with left ventricular (LV) ejection fractions <40% and nonsustained VT.[5] Additionally, the diagnostic value of electrophysiological (EP) testing (sensitivity, 77.4%; specificity, 79.5%; diagnostic accuracy, 79.0%) and prognostic significance (relative ratio, 4.7 for subsequent clinical VT or sudden cardiac death) compares favorably with programmed ventricular stimulation after MI.[5] However, patient selection for screening with EP testing and the timing and frequency of testing remain to be elucidated.

Using intraoperative mapping, VT after surgical correction of tetralogy of Fallot has been classified into two types: VT originating from the RVOT, which is considered to be related to prior right ventriculotomy or reconstruction of the RVOT (Fig. 22-1); and VT originating from the RV inflow tract septum, which is thought to be related to closure of the ventricular septal defect. The VT is most commonly monomorphic and macroreentrant, rotating clockwise or counterclockwise around myotomy scars or surgical patches. QRS morphology during VT is dictated by the pattern of ventricular activation around the scar. Most commonly, a left bundle branch block (LBBB) or right bundle branch block (RBBB) and right inferior axis morphology is seen during clockwise rotation around the scar. Less commonly, an LBBB and left axis morphology is observed (Fig. 22-2).[6]

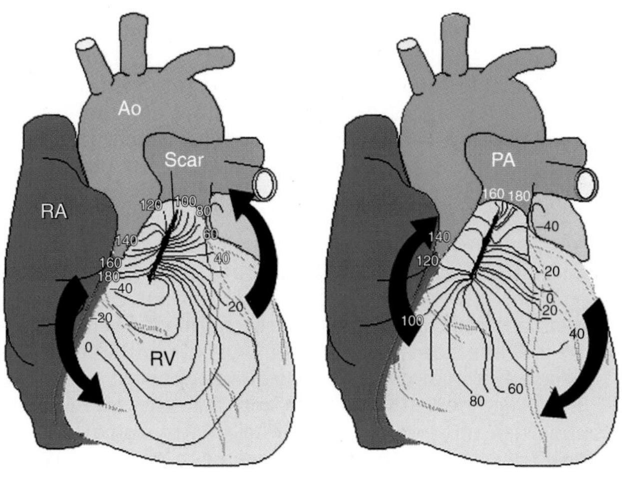

FIGURE 22–1 Ventricular tachycardia (VT) postsurgical repair of tetralogy of Fallot. Illustrated is scar-based reentry in surgically repaired tetralogy of Fallot with a right ventriculotomy. The incision heals as a nonconductive scar, leaving a small rim of muscle between the pulmonic valve annulus and scar. This is the diastolic corridor for rotation in either direction as shown, giving rise to VT with left bundle branch block–like QRS morphology and left superior axis or; in the opposite direction of rotation, right bundle branch block–like QRS morphology and right inferior axis. Ao = aorta; PA = pulmonary artery; RA = right atrium; RV = right ventricle.

The arrhythmic substrate in tetralogy of Fallot has been likened to post-MI scar-related VT. The sites of the presystolic activation and delayed conduction along the reentrant circuit have been shown to have significant abnormalities such as fibrosis, adiposis, and degeneration of the myocardium. The scattered myocyte islets in the extensive adiposis and/or fibrosis can form an electrical maze around the surgical suture area.

Mapping

Detailed knowledge of the congenital and surgical anatomy is essential before ablation. Transthoracic and transesophageal echocardiography, right and left ventricular catheterization, computed tomography (CT), and/or magnetic resonance (MR) imaging should be considered to clarify the anatomic landmarks for mapping.

The mechanism of VT is macroreentry involving the RVOT, either at the site of anterior right ventriculotomy or at the site of a ventricular septal defect patch. The mapping procedure to detect an adequate site for ablation includes pace mapping during sinus rhythm, endocardial activation mapping, and entrainment mapping during VT. Activation mapping during VT is used to identify sites with presystolic and mid-diastolic activity. Entrainment mapping is performed in a manner analogous to that used for post-MI VT, and can be used to characterize ventricular sites' relationship to the reentrant circuit and to verify that a diastolic electrogram, regardless of where in diastole it occurs and its position and appearance on initiation of VT, is part of the VT circuit. Entrainment with concealed fusion and prolonged stimulus-to-QRS interval helps identify the critical isthmus of the reentrant circuit targeted by catheter ablation. Pace mapping during sinus rhythm is used to identify exit sites of the reentrant circuit and confirm potential ablation target sites identified by activation and/or entrainment mapping, as indicated by a paced QRS morphology matching that of the VT morphology. Electroanatomical mapping can be of value because the presence of multiple circuits and the complexity of anatomical alteration, particularly in the vicinity of surgical scar, can pose significant challenges to mapping and ablation procedures. Additionally, voltage mapping of the area of interest can help identify the area of scar and border zone and guide conventional mapping techniques. Additionally, most reentrant circuit isthmuses are located within anatomically defined isthmuses bordered by unexcitable tissue. These boundaries can be identified by 3-D mapping during normal sinus rhythm (NSR). Radiofrequency (RF) ablation of the anatomic isthmus during

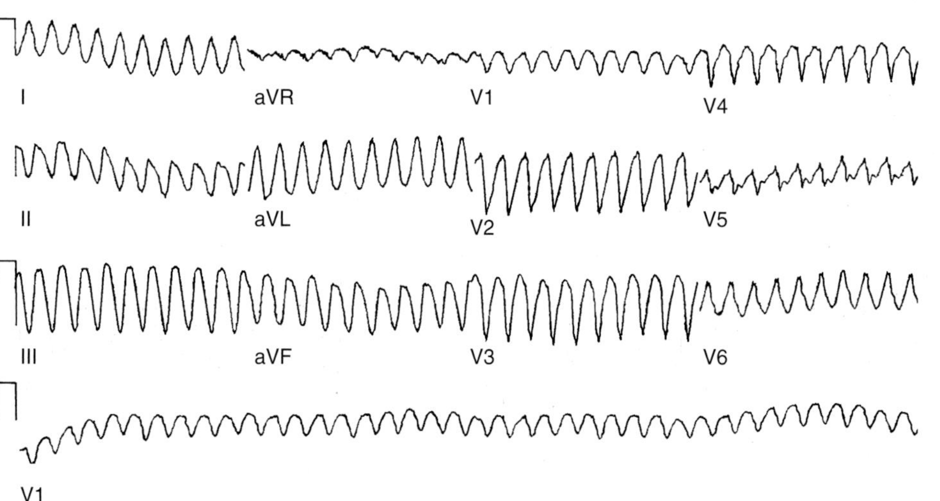

FIGURE 22–2 Surface ECG of ventricular tachycardia postsurgical repair of tetralogy of Fallot. Note the left bundle branch block pattern and left superior axis morphology characteristic of clockwise macroreentry around the right ventriculotomy scar.

NSR can potentially eliminate the tachycardia, even when conventional mapping is not feasible. An isthmus between unexcitable tissue in the RVOT free wall and either the tricuspid annulus or the pulmonic valve is the most common cause of VT.[2,4,7,8]

Ablation

The critical isthmus of the VT circuit is the usual target of ablation. A good pace map and entrainment with concealed QRS fusion and a prolonged stimulus-to-QRS interval indicate more precisely an adequate site for ablation. Linear ablation lesions can also be performed using data obtained from substrate mapping to target anatomical isthmuses between surgical and structural lines of block.[7] Most VT circuits use the anatomic isthmus between the RVOT free wall scar or patch and the tricuspid annulus or pulmonic valve, and/or the septal scar or patch and either the tricuspid annulus or the pulmonic valve. Ablation lines transecting these anatomical isthmuses eliminate the VT in most patients.[8]

The experience with catheter ablation of VT in congenital heart disease is limited.[2] Several reports have described single-center experiences spanning several eras of technological advances. In a report of 20 patients with VT and congenital heart disease, 50% of patients were unable to undergo ablation because of VT noninducibility, hemodynamic instability, access or anatomical problems, or proximity of the ablation target to the His bundle (HB). The acute success rate for mappable VTs was 83%, with a long-term recurrence rate of 40%.[9] In another report, immediate noninducibility of sustained or nonsustained VT was achieved in 15 of 16 patients (94%) after the ablation procedure. Repeat ventricular stimulation 5 to 7 days later revealed noninducibility in 14 patients (88%). At successful ablation sites, a good pace map during sinus rhythm could be found in 15 of the 16 patients (94%). However, an area of slow conduction, defined as mid-diastolic low-amplitude endocardial potential, could be found in only 3 patients (19%). The mean activation time of the endocardial electrogram preceding the QRS complex on the surface ECG at the ablation site was −69 ± 16 milliseconds. In 9 of 11 patients with inducible sustained VT (82%), entrainment with concealed fusion and a prolonged stimulus-QRS interval (10 to 120 milliseconds) could be demonstrated. A recent report of 11 patients with VT after repair of congenital heart disease used electroanatomical substrate mapping during NSR in addition to conventional mapping, when feasible. RF ablation eliminated VT in all patients, with 91% remaining free of VT at 30 ± 29 months' follow-up.[8]

VENTRICULAR TACHYCARDIA IN NONISCHEMIC DILATED CARDIOMYOPATHY

Electrophysiological Substrate

The diagnosis of nonischemic cardiomyopathy is established by the absence of significant (>75% stenosis) coronary artery disease, prior MI, or primary valvular abnormalities. In contrast to ischemic heart disease, the EP substrate for sustained monomorphic ventricular tachycardia (SMVT) in patients with nonischemic cardiomyopathy is not clearly defined. Premature ventricular complexes (PVCs) and nonsustained VTs induced by programmed electrical stimulation or occurring spontaneously in patients with end-stage idiopathic dilated cardiomyopathy initiate primarily in the subendocardium by a focal mechanism without evidence of macroreentry. The nature of the focal mechanism remains unknown; triggered activity arising from early or delayed afterdepolarizations seems to be more likely than microreentry. On the other hand, reentry within the myocardium is the most common mechanism underlying SMVT in patients with nonischemic cardiomyopathy, although bundle branch reentrant and focal VTs also occur.[10-15] Bundle branch reentrant VT is discussed separately in Chapter 20.

Myocardial fibrosis is an important factor in the substrate causing VT in patients with dilated cardiomyopathy. Sustained VT is associated with more extensive myocardial fibrosis and nonuniform anisotropy, involving both the endocardium and epicardium, compared with those without sustained reentry.[10-15] The reentry circuits are typically associated with regions of low-voltage electrograms, consistent with scar.[12-15] Catheter mapping studies of patients with nonischemic cardiomyopathy point to reentry around scar deep in the myocardium, near the ventricular base and in the perivalvular region, as the underlying mechanism for VT. Studies of explanted hearts have found unexcitable fibrosis creating regions of conduction block and surviving myocardium creating potential reentry circuit paths in dilated nonischemic cardiomyopathy. Slow conduction through muscle bundles separated by interstitial fibrosis can cause a zigzag path, producing slow conduction that promotes reentry. Patients with nonischemic cardiomyopathy and predominance of scar distribution involving 26% to 75% of wall thickness (as quantified by MR imaging) are more likely to have inducible VT.[16] In most patients, it appears that the VT site of origin is consistent with the location of the abnormal anatomical substrate demonstrating low endocardial voltage. The cause of fibrosis in cardiomyopathy is not well defined. Scattered regions of replacement fibrosis are commonly seen at autopsy, but confluent regions of scar are not common. The unique propensity for abnormal basal endocardial voltage and VT site of origin in patients with nonischemic cardiomyopathy remains unexplained. Low-voltage areas have also been observed during electroanatomical mapping in patients with focal VT and bundle branch reentry, although the scar areas appeared to be smaller.[15]

Several similarities of the arrhythmia substrate exist in myocardial reentry VT in patients with dilated nonischemic cardiomyopathy to that in patients with previous MI.[15] Low-voltage areas are observed in all patients, and the regions of scar are frequently adjacent to a valve annulus, as is often the case in VT after inferior wall MI. The annulus often seems to form a border for an isthmus in the reentry path, which suggests the formation of a long channel, or isthmus, along an annulus contributes to the formation of reentry circuits that can support VT.

The diagnosis of sarcoidosis or Chagas' cardiomyopathy should be considered in patients with dilated cardiomyopathy of unknown cause, particularly in those with marked regional wall motion abnormalities. Epicardial reentrant circuits can be more prevalent in these cardiomyopathies, especially in those with VT related to chronic Chagas' disease, in whom approximately 70% of VTs are epicardial in origin.[17]

Mapping

QRS morphology during VT can be used to regionalize the site of origin of the VT. Endocardial activation mapping is performed in the RV and/or LV in patients with stable VTs. Most VTs are localized to the area around the mitral annulus. Entrainment and pace mapping are used to define the relationship of different endocardial sites to the circuit of the

VT. Furthermore, the relationship of reentry circuits to regions of scar supports the feasibility of a substrate mapping approach, targeting the abnormal area based on voltage mapping during sinus rhythm, to guide ablation of unstable VT, similar to that described for patients with post-MI VT.[15]

Electroanatomical Voltage Mapping

In patients with nonischemic cardiomyopathy, the predominant distribution of abnormal low-voltage endocardial electrogram recordings is typically located near the ventricular base, frequently surrounding the mitral annulus. Voltage mapping typically demonstrates a modest-sized basal area of endocardial electrogram abnormalities (ranging from 6% to 48% of the LV endocardial surface, but uncommonly involving more than 25% of the total endocardial surface area). The amount of dense scar (<0.5 mV) accounts for approximately 27% ± 20% (range, 0% to 64%) of the overall abnormal low-voltage endocardial substrate. The VT site of origin corresponds to these basal electrogram abnormalities. Therefore, voltage mapping during sinus rhythm can be used to guide further mapping techniques (entrainment and pace mapping) and also guide ablation lesions (especially in patients with unmappable VTs).

Activation Mapping

After construction of an endocardial voltage map during sinus rhythm (or ventricular pacing), VT is induced by programmed ventricular stimulation. The average number of induced VT morphologies is 3 ± 1 per patient, with a range of one to six VTs. Because surface ECG documentation of the presenting arrhythmia is often not available, clinical versus nonclinical VT is difficult to define with certainty. Mapping is therefore directed at all SMVTs induced by programmed stimulation. For hemodynamically tolerated SMVT, activation mapping is performed to identify sites with early presystolic or mid-diastolic activity (Fig. 22-3).

Entrainment Mapping

Entrainment can be demonstrated in most patients with SMVT. The site of origin for hemodynamically tolerated VT is defined as the site of entrainment with concealed fusion and the return cycle length (CL) equaled to the VT CL (see Fig. 22-3). For unstable VT, limited entrainment mapping can be feasible with brief induction and termination of the tachycardia.

Pace Mapping

Pace mapping has been shown to be an effective corroborative method to regionalize the site of origin of VT and define potential exit sites along the border of any low-voltage region. Pace mapping with the paced QRS morphology mimicking that of VT on the 12-lead ECG can help identify the site of origin of the VT. Additionally, pace mapping can identify regions of slow conduction with a stimulus-QRS interval (S-QRS) >40 milliseconds and a pace map match consistent with the exit region from an isthmus. For the unmappable VT (because of hemodynamic intolerance, inconsistent induction, altering QRS morphology, and/or nonsustained duration), pace mapping is the predominant mapping technique and is directed to the scar border zone as defined by voltage mapping.

Epicardial Mapping

When endocardial mapping and ablation fail, the epicardial (transvenous or percutaneous) approach should be consid-

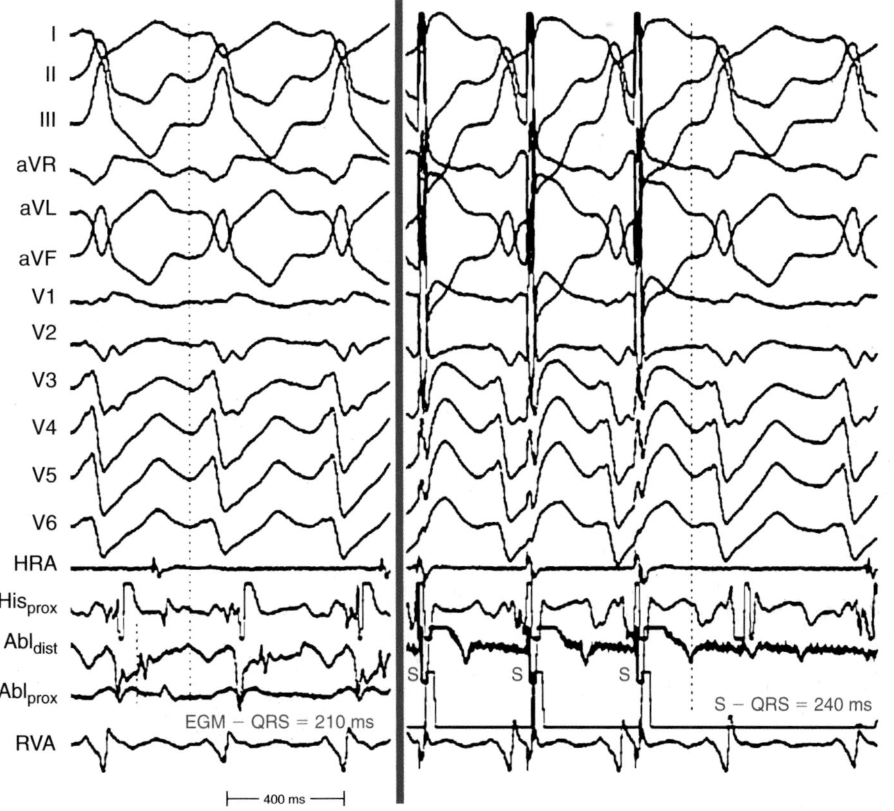

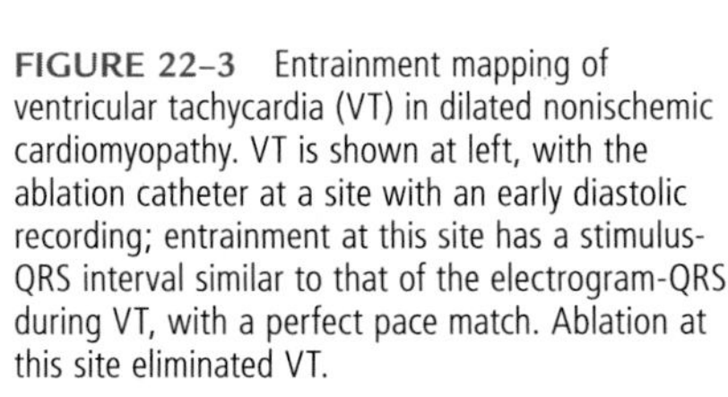
FIGURE 22–3 Entrainment mapping of ventricular tachycardia (VT) in dilated nonischemic cardiomyopathy. VT is shown at left, with the ablation catheter at a site with an early diastolic recording; entrainment at this site has a stimulus-QRS interval similar to that of the electrogram-QRS during VT, with a perfect pace match. Ablation at this site eliminated VT.

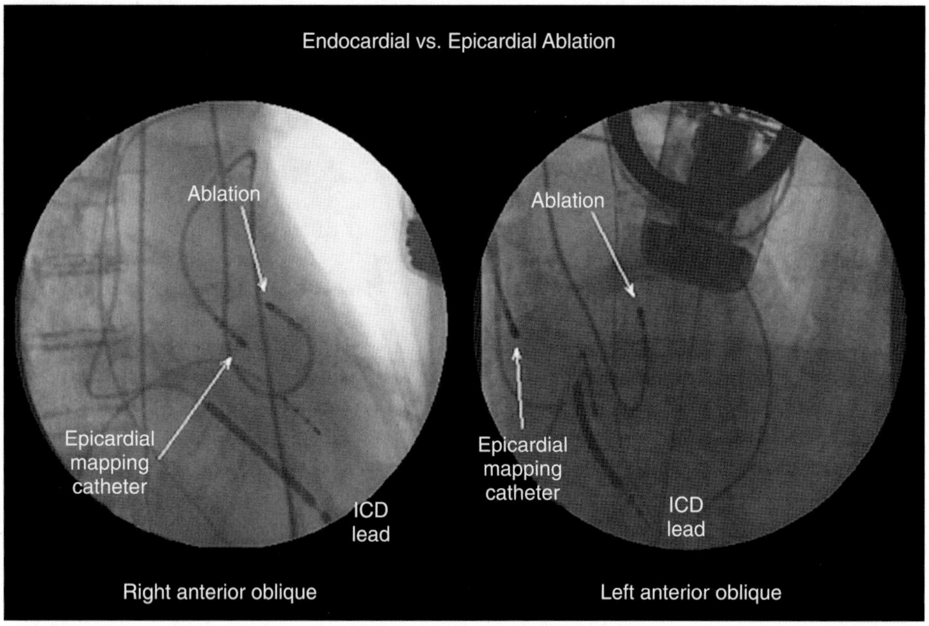

FIGURE 22–4 Combined endocardial and epicardial mapping of ventricular tachycardia (VT) in dilated nonischemic cardiomyopathy. Shown are fluoroscopic views of endocardial and epicardial ablation catheter positions. VT was eventually eliminated with endocardial ablation at the site shown (basal left ventricle). ICD = implantable cardioverter-defibrillator.

ered. The importance of epicardial reentry circuits in cardiomyopathy has been demonstrated for patients with Chagas' disease and, more recently, for patients with dilated cardiomyopathy unrelated to Chagas' disease (Fig. 22-4).[13,15] Percutaneous epicardial ablation of VT can be guided by activation, entrainment, and pace mapping. Limited epicardial mapping can be performed via the coronary venous system.[13]

Ablation

For patients with mappable VTs, focal ablation targets the critical isthmus of the reentrant circuit as defined by activation, entrainment, and pace mapping techniques. For unmappable VTs, linear ablation lesions are guided by QRS morphology on the 12-lead surface ECG during VT and pace mapping in the scar border zone. Linear lesions are created in regions that cross the border zone and intersect the best pace map site, which approximates the exit site of the VT circuit, similar to strategies described for unmappable post-MI VT.[14]

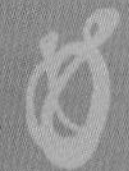

22 The success of endocardial ablation is lower than that observed for post-MI VT. Reentry circuits deep to the endocardium and in the epicardium appear to be a likely explanation. Combined endocardial and epicardial mapping approaches are likely to improve the success of ablation.[15]

In one report, 39 of 57 VTs were targeted with RF ablation based on mapping information.[13] RF energy delivery resulted in noninducibility in 30 targeted VTs using focal and/or linear ablation strategies. Additional VTs became noninducible after ablating different arrhythmia morphologies. Of the 19 patients, 14 had no VT inducible at the end of procedure. After a follow-up of 22 ± 12 months, 5 patients were alive without VT recurrence and 8 patients were alive with only rare VT recurrences (less than one event every 6 months).

Limited data exist on the catheter ablation of VTs associated with Chagas' cardiomyopathy. Success rates are limited when only endocardial mapping and ablation techniques are used. Epicardial ablation has been shown to improve outcome and should be considered in these cases.[17]

POLYMORPHIC VENTRICULAR TACHYCARDIA AND VENTRICULAR FIBRILLATION

Mechanism

The mechanisms underlying the initiation and maintenance of polymorphic VT and VF are poorly understood. Emerging evidence has suggested that the underlying mechanisms of cardiac fibrillation may be similar, regardless of the chamber it affects. An initiating trigger interacts with factors that perpetuate and maintain the arrhythmia (the substrate) and that results in sustained fibrillation. In the atria, this results in atrial fibrillation (AF), whereas in the ventricle it results in ventricular fibrillation (VF).[18-23] Analogous to our understanding of the mechanisms of AF, the mechanisms of VF can be broadly classified into initiation by triggers and maintenance by substrate.

Different mechanisms of VF initiation have been observed. VF can be triggered by ectopy occurring during the vulnerable period of the ventricle, the so-called R on T phenomenon. These can represent delayed afterdepolarizations and triggered activity. The importance of this vulnerable period is apparent with the induction of VF during defibrillation threshold testing.[22] Alternatively, VF can be initiated by spontaneous reentry caused by the interaction of a single wave, with a fixed anatomical obstacle causing the wave to break and give rise to multiple wavelets that are self-sustained and result in high-frequency electrical activity. Automaticity or reentry involving different structures that constitute the ventricle—namely, the myocardium and Purkinje network—is a third potential mechanism. Based on the multiple reentrant wavelet hypothesis, it has now been accepted that the maintenance of VF is similarly caused by different forms of reentry or rotors. Experimental studies have suggested the possibility that these arrhythmias may be maintained by migrating scroll waves, intramural reentry, and Purkinje network reentry. However, it is possible that VF is the endpoint of a heterogeneous group of electrical disturbances and it may not be possible to identify a single mechanism that adequately accounts for all cases.[22]

Studies in patients with polymorphic VT and/or VF in a variety of clinical scenarios have implicated an important role for triggers originating from the distal Purkinje arborization and RVOT in the initiation of these malignant arrhythmias.[18-25] Triggers from the Purkinje arborization or the RVOT have a crucial role in initiating idiopathic VF and VF associated with the ischemic heart disease and long QT and Brugada syndromes. Ambulatory monitoring and stored electrograms of the defibrillator in these patients have revealed that up to 67% of spontaneous episodes of VF are preceded by isolated PVCs identical to the triggering PVC (Fig. 22-5).[26] The finding that such PVCs were consistently preceded by low-amplitude, high-frequency Purkinje-like potentials supports the hypothesis that triggered activity from Purkinje fibers is responsible for the PVCs that initiate polymorphic VT and/or VF. Closely coupled extrasystoles, and even VF-like disorganized rhythms, can experimentally result from reentry involving both antidromic (muscle to Purkinje) and orthodromic activation or scroll waves at the Purkinje-muscle junctions.

The mechanism of focal PVC triggers of polymorphic VT and/or VF is under investigation. In vitro studies have extensively shown that the Purkinje system can generate or maintain arrhythmias by automaticity, reentry, or triggered activity during a number of conditions, such as electrolyte imbalance, catecholaminergic stimulation, other drug exposure, and myocardial ischemia. Triggered activity in the distal Purkinje arborizations seems to be the most likely mechanism. At least the first tachycardia beats appear to be triggered by local potentials, whereas later, local fibers can be bystanders or passively activated. In some patients with electrical storm complicating MI, overdrive pacing at a rate of 120 beats/min was able to suppress PVCs and VF, but only for the time of pacing. When the pacing rate was reduced, PVCs recurred immediately. These findings favor triggered activity as the underlying mechanism of the PVCs. Furthermore, in animal models, triggered activity from surviving distal Purkinje arborizations in the scar border is required for the development of VF. Purkinje fibers are more resistant to ischemia than myocardial cells, and endocardial Purkinje fibers may be nourished from cavity blood. This may be sufficient to keep them structurally intact, even though function can be impaired, giving rise to afterdepolarization and triggered activity. Microreentry in small parts of the Purkinje network as the underlying mechanism of the PVCs has also been suggested. The combination of coexisting scar and viable myocardium create the substrate required for reentry.

Although the mechanisms of polymorphic VT associated with a normal or long QT interval are probably different, the morphological characteristics of the VT are surprisingly similar. Intracardiac recordings during polymorphic VT associated with normal QT interval demonstrate that chaotic electrical activity usually follows a period of rapid VT, and either spreads from one area through the entire heart or appears simultaneously in several parts of the heart. Moreover, similar polymorphic VT can be associated with discrete electrograms that are asynchronous. These observations suggest that regardless of the exact mechanism of the primary arrhythmia, multiple simultaneous wavefronts on the heart are necessary for the surface QRS to look polymorphic. Therefore, ECG characteristics alone should not be used to imply a specific mechanism for the arrhythmia. As such, one must continue to think that polymorphic VT and/or VF associated with normal QT interval, congenital long-QT syndrome, and acquired long QT syndrome are distinct disorders, each having a specific mechanism whose ultimate ECG expression is polymorphic VT.

A novel mapping-ablation treatment strategy has been described that targets the triggers for recurrent polymorphic VT and/or VF associated with repolarization abnormalities (long QT and Brugada syndromes), ischemic heart disease, or no apparent structural heart disease (idiopathic VF).[18-23] It is now recognized that the triggering events for recurrent polymorphic VT and/or VF that occurs in the periinfarction period appear to be a PVC with a reproducible QRS morphology. The reproducible QRS morphology suggests a specific triggering site of origin. Indeed, these triggers have been identified and, in the setting of infarction, appear most commonly to originate from the Purkinje network adjacent to the infarcted myocardium. Because the same triggers may be observed without the initiation of the polymorphic arrhythmia, they can be localized and targeted for ablation.

Electrophysiological Testing

Polymorphic Ventricular Tachycardia in the Presence of Normal QT Interval

The most common cause of polymorphic VT with normal QT interval is ischemic heart disease, followed by other types of structural heart disease. In patients with coronary artery disease and a normal QT interval who have polymorphic VT and/or VF, a similar tachycardia can be induced by programmed ventricular stimulation using the standard protocol 75% to 85% of the time. Polymorphic VT and VF can be a nonspecific response to aggressive stimulation, and occur in approximately 28% of patients with a normal heart and normal QT interval with programmed stimulation using triple ventricular extrastimuli (VESs). Most nonspecific responses are associated with very short VES coupling intervals (<180 milliseconds). The reproducible initiation of polymorphic VT with the same template of changing QRSs, despite changes in pacing site or CL, suggests some structural basis (functional or anatomical) for the induced arrhythmia. Rarely, polymorphic VT and/or VF are induced with single or double VESs during NSR. This is extremely rare in the absence of a clinical history of syncope or cardiac arrest. Induction of polymorphic VT and VF can be site-dependent. VF can also arise by spontaneous degeneration from VT or by stimulation during VT. Patients with coronary artery disease, prior MI, LV dysfunction, and nonsustained VT who have VF or polymorphic VT induced during programmed ventricular stimulation have similar rates of

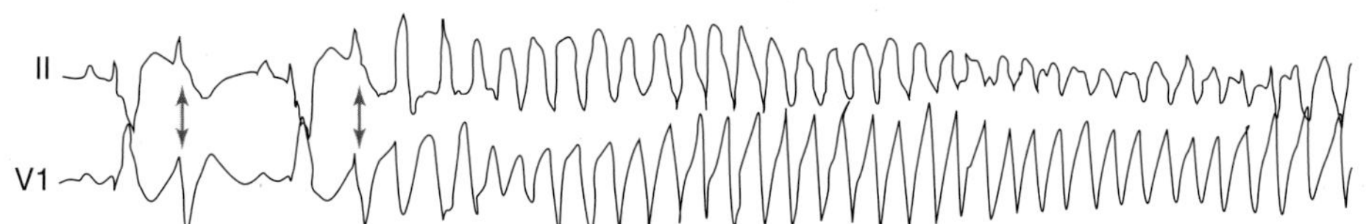

FIGURE 22–5 Polymorphic ventricular tachycardia (VT) triggered by premature ventricular complexes (PVCs). The telemetry rhythm strips show normal sinus rhythm with PVCs that trigger an episode of polymorphic VT. Note that the morphology of the triggering PVCs is similar to that of the isolated PVC (arrows).

subsequent clinical ventricular tachyarrhythmias as patients with inducible monomorphic VT.[27]

Why some patients have self-terminating polymorphic VT and some go on to VF is not well understood. In those who develop VF, an accelerated phase of VT occurs. Progressive conduction delay in local electrograms is observed until total fractionation and irregular activity are noted in all electrograms throughout the heart. Whether polymorphic VT will develop into VF is determined by whether such abnormal and chaotic activity persists in all regions in the heart. Spontaneous reversion of polymorphic VT to NSR occurs when localized chaotic activity is confined to small areas of the heart and gradually becomes regular. Occasionally, what appears to be polymorphic VT or VF is not associated with chaotic activity in the RV but is associated with discordant (asynchronous) discrete electrograms at multiple ventricular rates. Termination of polymorphic VT is always associated with regularization and synchronization of electrograms. Sometimes, polymorphic VT goes through periods of uniform VT. Thus, polymorphic VT persists if all areas recorded have regular activity but are asynchronously activated, or if several (but not all) sites in the ventricles exhibit chaotic fibrillatory activity, but the remainder of the ventricles exhibit regular activity.

Many polymorphic VTs (and occasionally VF) can be changed by class IA antiarrhythmic agents to a typical SMVT, which has identical characteristics as reentrant SMVT. Usually, these are patients who have presented with syncope or cardiac arrest and are subsequently treated with antiarrhythmic agents. The response to these agents is different from that in drug-induced long QT syndrome, in which polymorphic VT is produced by the drug. Such a response is seen mainly in patients with structural heart disease and history of arrhythmia, especially patients with coronary artery disease and prior MI. Generally, rapid pacing and isoproterenol do not facilitate induction of polymorphic VT in patients with a normal QT interval.

Polymorphic Ventricular Tachycardia in the Presence of Long QT Interval

Polymorphic VT and/or VF associated with congenital or acquired long QT syndromes cannot be reproducibly initiated with programmed electrical stimulation. Although in 25% to 50% of these patients polymorphic VTs can be initiated with vigorous stimulation protocols, this is not significantly different from the response to comparable stimulation with patients with no history of ventricular arrhythmias. These polymorphic VTs can be sustained or nonsustained, and most likely represent nonspecific responses. Failure to initiate specific polymorphic VTs in patients with long QT syndrome is consistent with an automatic mechanism or an initiating mechanism caused by triggered activity secondary to early afterdepolarizations. On the other hand, isoproterenol can initiate polymorphic VT in patients with congenital long QT syndrome. Also, it has been suggested that the short-long-short sequence that characterizes torsades de pointes (i.e., bradycardia-dependent arrhythmias) can facilitate the induction of polymorphic VT that otherwise would not be induced with typical stimulation protocols.

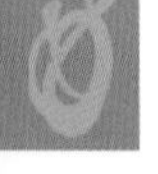

Mapping

Localization of arrhythmogenic triggers (PVCs) requires an adequate frequency of ectopy to allow mapping. It is helpful to perform the ablation procedure while the patient clinically presents with frequent polymorphic VT or VF (e.g., electrical storm) and frequent spontaneous PVCs. The 12-lead surface ECG documentation of PVC morphologies during a period of arrhythmia storm, even if months earlier, may allow localization in sinus rhythm based on initial pace mapping, followed by RF delivery at sites exhibiting local Purkinje potential.

Activation Mapping

In patients with frequent PVCs resembling the PVC morphology that initiated their polymorphic VT and/or VF, activation mapping is used to localize the source of PVCs, which is indicated by the earliest electrogram relative to the onset of the ectopic QRS complex (Fig. 22-6).

Careful attention should be made to identify any low-amplitude, high-frequency, Purkinje-like potentials preceding the PVCs at the earliest activation sites of the PVC.[18-25] An initial local sharp (<10 milliseconds in duration), high-frequency, low-amplitude potential preceding (by <15 milliseconds) the larger and slower ventricular electrogram during NSR represents a peripheral Purkinje component, whereas longer intervals indicate proximal Purkinje fascicle activation. The presence of a Purkinje potential preceding ventricular activation during PVCs suggests that the latter originated from the Purkinje system, whereas its absence at the site of earliest activation suggests an origin from ventricular muscle.

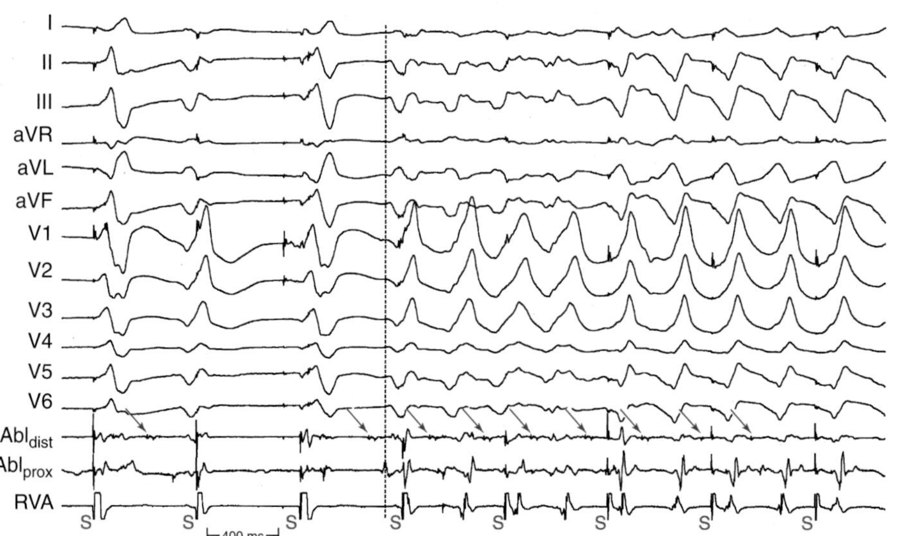

FIGURE 22–6 Premature ventricular complexes (PVCs) triggering polymorphic ventricular tachycardia (VT). Shown are 12 surface ECG leads and intracardiac recordings in a patient with recurrent episodes of polymorphic VT–ventricular fibrillation (VF) resulting in up to 70 implantable cardioverter-defibrillator shocks in 1 day. Ventricular pacing to prevent pauses is ongoing throughout the tracing. Arrows point to fragmented diastolic potentials preceding the PVCs that often initiated episodes of polymorphic VT-VF. Ablation at this site caused cessation of all episodes of VT-VF.

The site of origin of triggering PVCs can be localized in either the RV or LV. Triggering PVCs can be elicited from the Purkinje system, notably in long QT syndrome and idiopathic VF, or from the RVOT, notably in Brugada syndrome. In ischemic heart disease, triggering PVCs originate from the distal Purkinje network arborization located in the infarct border zone, regardless of the duration after the initial MI.[18,21,23]

In a report of post-MI patients, Purkinje potentials preceded each PVC by a mean of 68 ± 20 milliseconds.[18,21,23] Activation times varied among different PVCs, but Purkinje potentials were always found in a defined region close to the anatomic border of the infarction. At the same location, a Purkinje potential was observed during sinus rhythm, preceding the QRS complex by 23 to 26 milliseconds. In contrast, activation time between Purkinje fibers and ventricular muscle has been reported to be much shorter in patients without structural heart disease during NSR (11 ± 5 milliseconds) and PVCs (38 ± 28 milliseconds). This can be related to a conduction delay between Purkinje fibers and myocardial tissue and can also account for the changes in morphology and width of the PVCs, which were wider than expected for PVCs originating from Purkinje fibers in normal hearts.[19,20]

Pace Mapping

Pace mapping can be used to confirm the results of activation mapping, and can be of great value, especially when the tachycardia is scarcely inducible. Concordance of QRS morphology occurring in 12 of 12 leads on the surface ECG is suggestive of the site of origin of the PVC.[18,21,23]

Electroanatomical Mapping

Electroanatomical mapping is often used to help activation mapping of the triggering PVCs. In patients with ischemic heart disease, simultaneous voltage mapping is of value to identify infarct-related scar, define the scar border zone, and facilitate both trigger mapping (mapping along the border zone to identify Purkinje-like potentials) and sinus rhythm substrate mapping in patients in whom PVCs cannot be detected in sufficient quantity to permit trigger mapping.[21-23]

Noncontact Mapping

Noncontact mapping (EnSite 3000, Endocardial Solutions, St. Paul, Minn) can offer a potential advantage for patients with infrequent PVCs.[28,29]

Ablation

Target of Ablation

Analogous to AF, elimination of the triggers and modification of the substrate, individually or in combination, can theoretically be targeted for the ablation of polymorphic VT and VF. Reports thus far have only targeted the triggers. This perhaps reflects our limited understanding of the substrate maintaining VF and the large mass of ventricular myocardium involved.

Therefore, the focus of the triggering PVCs is the target of ablation. Such focus is identified by the earliest endocardial activation during PVCs and by pace mapping with an exact match of QRS morphology.[18-23]

Whether eliminating all potential triggers along the border zone in post-MI patients is superior to targeting a single PVC focus is unclear and warrants further study. In patients with ischemic heart disease in whom PVCs cannot be detected in sufficient quantity to permit PVC mapping, sinus rhythm substrate mapping can be performed using electroanatomical mapping systems. Ablation is performed along the scar border zone in locations at which the Purkinje-like potentials are identified.[21]

Technique

A 4-mm standard or irrigated-tip ablation catheter may be used. A typical RF setting targets a temperature of 55° to 60°C and a maximum power of 50 W for a duration of 60 to 120 seconds. When the maximum power delivered is limited to less than 30 W, an external irrigated-tip catheter (17 mL/min; maximum 50 W) can be used to allow higher power delivery.

Ablation of ectopy elicited from the Purkinje system can produce temporary exacerbation of arrhythmia (increased number of PVCs and polymorphic VT) during the first minute of local RF application, followed by disappearance of the PVCs.

Endpoints

In patients with spontaneous or inducible PVCs, complete elimination of ectopy is the endpoint of the ablation procedure. Electrograms after ablation typically show the abolition of the local Purkinje potential, but the QRS complex during sinus rhythm remains unchanged. For post-MI patients without inducible PVCs, the endpoint is the application of scar border zone ablation lesions until all Purkinje-like potentials are abolished.

Outcome

Approximately 20% of patients with defibrillators have frequent episodes of VF. Provided the triggers of these arrhythmias can be localized, whatever their origin in Purkinje or muscle tissue, focal ablation of the sources of those triggers can offer significant palliative control of VF storm and prevent the recurrence of drug-refractory, sustained ventricular arrhythmias, which can reduce defibrillation requirements and defibrillator generator replacement and improve the patient's quality of life.[18-26] Studies in small series of patients have demonstrated success of this approach in patients with incessant ventricular tachyarrhythmias or electrical storm after MI, long QT and Brugada syndromes, and idiopathic VF. Therefore, catheter ablation of the triggering PVCs may be used as a bailout therapy in these patients, with reported success rates of 88% to 100%.

REFERENCES

1. Van Hare GF: Ventricular tachycardia in patients following surgery for congenital heart disease. *In* Zipes DP, Jalife J (eds): Cardiac Electrophysiology: From Cell to Bedside, 4th ed. Philadelphia, WB Saunders, 2004, pp 618-624.
2. Walsh EP: Interventional electrophysiology in patients with congenital heart disease. Circulation 2007;115:3224.
3. Gatzoulis MA, Balaji S, Webber SA, et al: Risk factors for arrhythmia and sudden cardiac death late after repair of tetralogy of Fallot: A multicentre study. Lancet 2000;356:975.
4. Folino AF, Daliento L: Arrhythmias after tetralogy of Fallot repair. Indian Pacing Electrophysiol 2005;5:312.
5. Khairy P, Landzberg MJ, Gatzoulis MA, et al: Value of programmed ventricular stimulation after tetralogy of Fallot repair: a multicenter study. Circulation 2004;109:1994.
6. Josephson ME: Catheter and surgical ablation in the therapy of arrhythmias. *In* Josephson ME (ed): Clinical Cardiac Electrophysiology, 3rd ed. Philadelphia, Lippincott, Williams & Wilkins, 2002, pp 710-836.
7. Rostock T, Willems S, Ventura R, et al: Radiofrequency catheter ablation of a macroreentrant ventricular tachycardia late after surgical repair of tetralogy of Fallot using the electroanatomic mapping (CARTO). Pacing Clin Electrophysiol 2004;27(Pt 1):801.
8. Zeppenfeld K, Schalij MJ, Bartelings MM, et al: Catheter ablation of ventricular tachycardia after repair of congenital heart disease: Electroanatomic identification of the critical right ventricular isthmus. Circulation 2007;116:2241.
9. Morwood JG, Triedman JK, Berul CI, et al: Radiofrequency catheter ablation of ventricular tachycardia in children and young adults with congenital heart disease. Heart Rhythm 2004;1:301.
10. Delacretaz E, Stevenson WG, Ellison KE, et al: Mapping and radiofrequency catheter ablation of the three types of sustained monomorphic ventricular tachycardia in nonischemic heart disease. J Cardiovasc Electrophysiol 2000;11:11.

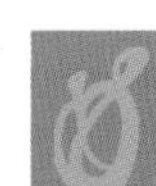

11. Hsia HH, Marchlinski FE: Electrophysiology studies in patients with dilated cardiomyopathies. Card Electrophysiol Rev 2002;6:472.
12. Hsia HH, Marchlinski FE: Characterization of the electroanatomic substrate for monomorphic ventricular tachycardia in patients with nonischemic cardiomyopathy. Pacing Clin Electrophysiol 2002;25:1114.
13. Hsia HH, Callans DJ, Marchlinski FE: Characterization of endocardial electrophysiological substrate in patients with nonischemic cardiomyopathy and monomorphic ventricular tachycardia. Circulation 2003;108:704.
14. Marchlinski FE, Callans DJ, Gottlieb CD, Zado E: Linear ablation lesions for control of unmappable ventricular tachycardia in patients with ischemic and nonischemic cardiomyopathy. Circulation 2000;101:1288.
15. Soejima K, Stevenson WG, Sapp JL, et al: Endocardial and epicardial radiofrequency ablation of ventricular tachycardia associated with dilated cardiomyopathy: The importance of low-voltage scars. J Am Coll Cardiol 2004;43:1834.
16. Nazarian S, Bluemke DA, Lardo AC, et al: Magnetic resonance assessment of the substrate for inducible ventricular tachycardia in nonischemic cardiomyopathy. Circulation 2005;112:2821.
17. Sosa E, Scanavacca M, D'Avila A, et al: Nonsurgical transthoracic epicardial approach in patients with ventricular tachycardia and previous cardiac surgery. J Interv Card Electrophysiol 2004;10:281.
18. Bansch D, Oyang F, Antz M, et al: Successful catheter ablation of electrical storm after myocardial infarction. Circulation 2003;108:3011.
19. Haissaguerre M, Shoda M, Jais P, et al: Mapping and ablation of idiopathic ventricular fibrillation. Circulation 2002;106:962.
20. Haissaguerre M, Extramiana F, Hocini M, et al: Mapping and ablation of ventricular fibrillation associated with long-QT and Brugada syndromes. Circulation 2003;108:925.
21. Marrouche NF, Verma A, Wazni O, et al: Mode of initiation and ablation of ventricular fibrillation storms in patients with ischemic cardiomyopathy. J Am Coll Cardiol 2004;43:1715.
22. Saunders P, Hsu LF, Hocini M, et al: Mapping and ablation of ventricular fibrillation. Minerva Cardioangiol 2004;52:171-181.
23. Szumowski L, Sanders P, Walczak F, et al: Mapping and ablation of polymorphic ventricular tachycardia after myocardial infarction. J Am Coll Cardiol 2004; 44:1700.
24. Haissaguerre M, Shah DC, Jais P, et al: Role of Purkinje conducting system in triggering of idiopathic ventricular fibrillation. Lancet 2002;359:677.
25. Weerasooriya R, Hsu LF, Scavee C, et al: Catheter ablation of ventricular fibrillation in structurally normal hearts targeting the RVOT and Purkinje ectopy. Herz 2003;28:598.
26. Kakishita M, Kurita T, Matsuo K, et al: Mode of onset of ventricular fibrillation in patients with Brugada syndrome detected by implantable cardioverter defibrillator therapy. J Am Coll Cardiol 2000;36:1646.
27. Greenberg SL, Mauricio SJ, Cooper JA, et al: Sustained polymorphic arrhythmias induced by programmed ventricular stimulation have prognostic value in patients receiving defibrillators. Pacing Clin Electrophysiol 2007;30:1067.
28. Betts TR, Yue A, Roberts PR, Morgan JM: Radiofrequency ablation of idiopathic ventricular fibrillation guided by noncontact mapping. J Cardiovasc Electrophysiol 2004;15:957.
29. Darmon JP, Bettouche S, Deswardt P, et al: Radiofrequency ablation of ventricular fibrillation and multiple right and left atrial tachycardia in a patient with Brugada syndrome. J Interv Card Electrophysiol 2004;11:205.

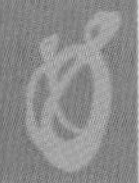

Index

Page numbers followed by f or t indicate figures or tables, respectively.

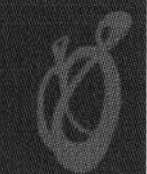